D0184788

2013

the calorie carb and fat bible 2013

Juliette Kellow BSc RD, Lyndel Costain BSc RD & Laurence Beeken

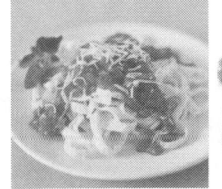 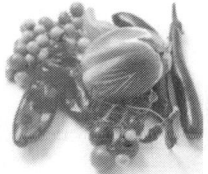 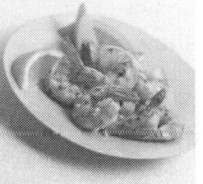 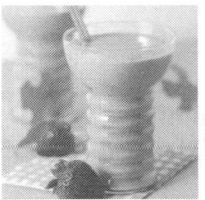 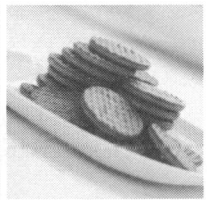 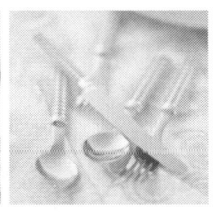

The UK's Most Comprehensive Calorie Counter

The Calorie, Carb & Fat Bible 2013

© Weight Loss Resources 2013
Lyndel Costain's contributions © Lyndel Costain 2007

Published by:
Weight Loss Resources Ltd
29 Metro Centre
Woodston,
Peterborough
PE2 7UH.

Tel: 01733 345592
www.weightlossresources.co.uk

Companies and other organisations wishing to make bulk purchases of the Calorie, Carb and Fat Bible should contact their local bookstore or Weight Loss Resources direct.

Except as otherwise permitted under the Copyright Designs and Patents Act 1988 this publication may only be reproduced, stored or transmitted in any form or by any means, with the prior permission of the publisher, in the case of reprographic reproduction, in accordance with the terms of a licence issued by The Copyright Licensing Agency. Enquiries concerning reproduction outside those terms should be sent to the address above.

Whilst every effort has been made to ensure accuracy, the publishers cannot be held responsible for any errors or omissions.

ISBN 978-1-904512-11-0

Authors: Lyndel Costain BSc RD
Juliette Kellow BSc RD
Laurence Beeken, Weight Loss Resources

Database Editor: Laurence Beeken

Design and Layout: Joanne Readshaw

Printed and bound by:
CPI Group (UK) Ltd, Croydon, CR0 4YY

Contents

Losing weight – the easy way

Juliette Kellow BSc RD

CHINESE TAKEAWAYS, curries, chocolate, chips and a glass of wine! Imagine being told the best diet to help you lose weight includes all these foods and more. It sounds too good to be true, doesn't it? But the truth is, these are exactly the types of foods you can still enjoy if you opt to lose weight by counting calories.

But you'd be forgiven for not knowing you can still eat all your favourite foods *and* lose weight. In recent years, endless trendy diets that cut carbs, boost protein intake or skip entire groups of foods, have helped to make dieting a complicated business. Added to this, an increasing number of celebrities and so-called nutrition experts have helped mislead us into thinking that dieting is all about restriction and denial. Is it any wonder then that most of us have been left feeling downright confused and miserable about what we should and shouldn't be eating to shift those pounds?

Dieting doesn't have to be complicated or an unhappy experience. In fact, there's really only one word you need to remember if you want to shift those pounds healthily and still eat all your favourite foods. And that's CALORIE!

It's calories that count

When it comes to losing weight, there's no getting away from the fact that it's calories that count. Ask any qualified nutrition expert or dietitian for advice on how to fight the flab and you'll receive the same reply: quite simply you need to create a calorie deficit or shortfall. In other words, you need to take in fewer calories than you use up so that your body has to draw on its fat stores to provide it with the energy it needs to function properly. The result: you start losing fat and the pounds start to drop off!

Fortunately, it couldn't be easier to create this calorie deficit. Regardless of your age, weight, sex, genetic make up, lifestyle or eating habits, losing weight is as simple as reducing your daily calorie intake slightly by modifying your diet and using up a few more calories by being slightly more active each day.

Better still, it's a complete myth that you need to change your eating and exercise habits dramatically. You'll notice I've said you need to reduce your calorie intake 'slightly' and be 'slightly' more active. It really is just LITTLE differences between the amount of calories we take in and the amount we use up that make BIG differences to our waistline over time. For example, you only need to consume one can of cola more than you need each day to gain a stone in a year. It's no wonder then that people say excess weight tends to 'creep up on them'.

10 simple food swaps you can make every day (and won't even notice!)

Make these simple swaps every day and in just 4 weeks you'll lose 7lb!

SWAP THIS...	FOR THIS...	SAVE...
300ml full-fat milk (195 calories)	300ml skimmed milk (100 calories)	95 calories
1tsp butter (35 calories)	1tsp low-fat spread (20 calories)	15 calories
1tbsp vegetable oil (100 calories)	10 sprays of a spray oil (10 calories)	90 calories
1tsp sugar (16 calories)	Artificial sweetener (2 calories)	14 calories
1tbsp mayonnaise (105 calories)	1tbsp fat-free dressing (10 calories)	95 calories
Regular sandwich (600 calories)	Low-fat sandwich (350 calories)	250 calories
Can of cola (135 calories)	Can of diet cola (1 calorie)	134 calories
Large (50g) packet of crisps (250 calories)	Small (25g) packet of crisps (125 calories)	125 calories
1 chocolate digestive (85 calories)	1 small chocolate chip cookie (55 calories)	30 calories
1 slice thick-cut wholemeal bread (95 calories)	1 slice medium-cut wholemeal bread (75 calories)	20 calories
	TOTAL CALORIE SAVING:	868 calories

The good news is the reverse is also true. You only need to swap that daily can of cola for the diet version or a glass of sparking water and you'll lose a stone in a year – it really is as easy as that!

Of course, most people don't want to wait a year to shift a stone. But there's more good news. To lose 1lb of fat each week you need to create a calorie deficit of just 500 calories a day. That might sound like a lot, but you can achieve this by simply swapping a croissant for a wholemeal fruit scone, a regular sandwich for a low-fat variety, a glass of dry white wine for a gin and slimline tonic and using low-fat spread on two slices of toast instead of butter. It is also important to become more active and increase your level of exercise. Losing 1lb a week, amounts to a stone in 14 weeks, or just under 4 stone in a year!

Taking control of calories

By now you've seen it really is calories that count when it comes to shifting those pounds. So it should be no surprise that a calorie-controlled diet is the only guaranteed way to help you shift those pounds – and that's a scientific fact! But better still, a calorie-controlled diet is one of the few that allows you to include anything, whether it's pizza, wine or chocolate. A healthy diet means including a wide range of foods (see 'Healthy Eating Made Easy' page 32).

And that's where this book can really help. Gone are the days when it was virtually impossible to obtain information about the calorie contents of foods. This book provides calorie information for more than 22,000 different branded and unbranded foods so that counting calories has never been easier.

The benefits of counting calories
• *It's guaranteed to help you lose weight providing you stick to your daily calorie allowance*
• *You can include favourite foods*
• *No foods are banned*
• *It's a great way to lose weight slowly and steadily*
• *Nutrition experts agree that it's a proven way to lose weight*

Calorie counting made easy

Forget weird and wacky science, complicated diet rules and endless lists of foods to fill up on or avoid every day! Counting calories to lose weight couldn't be easier. Quite simply, you set yourself a daily calorie allowance to help you lose between ½-2lb (¼-1kg) a week and then add up the calories of everything you eat and drink each day, making sure you don't go over your limit.

To prevent hunger from kicking in, it's best to spread your daily calorie allowance evenly throughout the day, allowing a certain amount of calories for breakfast, lunch, dinner and one or two snacks. For example, if you are allowed 1,500 calories a day, you could have 300 calories for breakfast, 400 calories for lunch, 500 calories for dinner and two snacks or treats of 150 calories each. You'll find more detailed information on p26-31 (Your step-by-step guide to using this book and shifting those pounds).

QUESTION
What affects the calorie content of a food?

ANSWER:
Fat, protein, carbohydrate and alcohol all provide the body with calories, but in varying amounts:

- *1g fat provides 9 calories*

- *1g alcohol provides 7 calories*

- *1g protein provides 4 calories*

- *1g carbohydrate provides 3.75 calories*

The calorie content of a food depends on the amount of fat, protein and carbohydrate it contains. Because fat provides more than twice as many calories as an equal quantity of protein or carbohydrate, in general, foods that are high in fat tend to contain more calories. This explains why 100g of chips (189 calories) contains more than twice as many calories as 100g of boiled potato (72 calories).

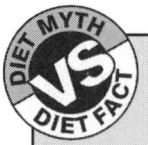

DIET MYTH:
Food eaten late at night stops you losing weight

DIET FACT:
It's not eating in the evening that stops you losing weight. It's consuming too many calories throughout the day that will be your dieting downfall! Providing you stick to your daily calorie allowance you'll lose weight, regardless of when you consume those calories. Nevertheless, it's a good idea to spread your calorie allowance throughout the day to prevent hunger from kicking in, which leaves you reaching for high-calorie snack foods.

Eat for good health

While calories might be the buzz word when it comes to shifting those pounds, it's nevertheless important to make sure your diet is healthy, balanced and contains all the nutrients you need for good health. Yes, you can still lose weight by eating nothing but, for example, chocolate, crisps and biscuits providing you stick to your calorie allowance. But you'll never find a nutrition expert or dietitian recommending this. And there are plenty of good reasons why.

To start with, an unbalanced diet is likely to be lacking in essential nutrients such as protein, vitamins, minerals and fibre, in the long term putting you at risk of nutritional deficiencies. Secondly, research proves that filling up on foods that are high in fat and/or salt and sugar can lead to many different health problems. But most importantly, when it comes to losing weight, it's almost impossible to stick to a daily calorie allowance if you're only eating high-calorie foods.

Filling up on lower-calorie foods also means you'll be able to eat far more with the result that you're not constantly left feeling unsatisfied. For example, six chocolates from a selection box contain around 300 calories, a lot of fat and sugar, few nutrients – and are eaten in just six mouthfuls! For 300 calories, you could have a grilled skinless chicken breast (packed with protein and zinc), a large salad with fat-free dressing (a great source of fibre, vitamins and minerals), a slice of wholemeal bread with low-fat spread (rich in fibre and B vitamins) and a satsuma (an excellent source of vitamin C). That's a lot more food that will take you a lot more time to eat! Not convinced? Then put six chocolates on one plate, and the chicken, salad, bread and fruit on another!

Bottom line: while slightly reducing your calorie intake is the key to losing weight, you'll be healthier and far more likely to keep those pounds off if you do it by eating a healthy diet *(see 'Healthy Eating Made Easy' page 32).*

Eight steps to a healthy diet

1 *Base your meals on starchy foods.*

2 *Eat lots of fruit and vegetables.*

3 *Eat more fish.*

4 *Cut down on saturated fat and sugar.*

5 *Try to eat less salt - no more than 6g a day.*

6 *Get active and try to be a healthy weight.*

7 *Drink plenty of water.*

8 *Don't skip breakfast.*

SOURCE: www.nhs.uk/Livewell/Goodfood/Pages/eatwell-plate.aspx

Fat facts

Generally speaking, opting for foods that are low in fat can help slash your calorie intake considerably, for example, swapping full-fat milk for skimmed, switching from butter to a low-fat spread, not frying food in oil and chopping the fat off meat and poultry. But don't be fooled into believing that all foods described as 'low-fat' or 'fat-free' are automatically low in calories or calorie-free. In fact, some low-fat products may actually be higher in calories than standard products, thanks to them containing extra sugars and thickeners to boost the flavour and texture. The solution: always check the calorie content of low-fat foods, especially for things like cakes, biscuits, crisps, ice creams and ready meals. You might be surprised to find there's little difference in the calorie content when compared to the standard product.

Uncovering fat claims on food labels

Many products may lure you into believing they're a great choice if you're trying to cut fat, but you need to read between the lines on the labels if you want to be sure you're making the best choice. Here's the lowdown on what to look for:

LOW FAT	by law the food must contain less than 3g of fat per 100g for solids. These foods are generally a good choice if you're trying to lose weight.
REDUCED FAT	by law the food must contain 25 percent less fat than a similar standard product. This doesn't mean the product is low-fat (or low-calorie) though! For example, reduced-fat cheese may still contain 14g fat per 100g.
FAT FREE	the food must contain no more than 0.5g of fat per 100g or 100ml. Foods labelled as Virtually Fat Free must contain less than 0.3g fat per 100g. These foods are generally a good choice if you're trying to lose weight.
LESS THAN 8% FAT	this means the product contains less than 8g fat per 100g. It's only foods labelled 'less than 3% fat' that are a true low-fat choice.
X% FAT FREE	claims expressed as X% Fat Free shall be prohibited.
LIGHT OR LITE	claims stating a product is 'light' or 'lite' follows the same conditions as those set for the term 'reduced'.

10 easy ways to slash fat (and calories)

1 Eat fewer fried foods – grill, boil, bake, poach, steam, roast without added fat or microwave instead.

2 Don't add butter, lard, margarine or oil to food during preparation or cooking.

3 Use spreads sparingly. Butter and margarine contain the same amount of calories and fat – only low fat spreads contain less.

4 Choose boiled or jacket potatoes instead of chips or roast potatoes.

5 Cut off all visible fat from meat and remove the skin from chicken before cooking.

6 Don't eat too many fatty meat products such as sausages, burgers, pies and pastry products.

7 Use semi-skimmed or skimmed milk instead of full-fat milk.

8 Try low-fat or reduced-fat varieties of cheese such as reduced-fat Cheddar, low-fat soft cheese or cottage cheese.

9 Eat fewer high-fat foods such as crisps, chocolates, cakes, pastries and biscuits.

10 Don't add cream to puddings, sauces or coffee.

Getting Ready for Weight Loss Success

Lyndel Costain BSc RD

THIS BOOK not only provides tools to help you understand more about what you eat and how active you are, but guidance on how to use this information to develop a weight loss plan to suit your needs. Getting in the right frame of mind will also be a key part of your weight control journey, especially if you've lost weight before, only to watch the pounds pile back on.

The fact is that most people who want to lose weight know what to do. But often there is something that keeps stopping them from keeping up healthier habits. The same may be true for you. So what's going on? For many it's a lack of readiness. When the next diet comes along with its tempting promises it's so easy to just jump on board. But if you have struggled with your weight for a while, will that diet actually help you to recognise and change the thoughts and actions that have stopped you shifting the pounds for good?

Check out your attitude to weight loss programmes

Before starting any new weight loss programme, including the Weight Loss Resources approach, ask yourself:

Am I starting out thinking that I like myself as a person right now?	(YES or NO)
OR I feel I can only like myself once I lose weight?	(YES or NO)
Do I want to stop overeating, but at the same time find myself justifying it – in other words I want to be able to eat what I want, but with no consequences?	(YES or NO)
Do I believe that I need to take long-term responsibility for my weight?	(YES or NO)
OR Am I relying on 'it' (the diet) to do it for me?	(YES or NO)

Keep these questions, and your replies, in mind as you read through this chapter.

Next Steps

You may have already assessed the healthiness of your weight using the BMI guide on page 37. If not, why not do it now, remembering that the tools are a guide only. The important thing is to consider a weight at which you are healthy and comfortable – and which is realistic for the life you lead *(see opposite - What is a healthy weight?)*.

The next step is to have a long hard think about why you want to lose weight. Consider all the possible benefits, not just those related to how you look. Psychologists have found that if we focus only on appearance we are less likely to succeed in the long-term. This is because it so often reflects low self-esteem or self-worth – which can sabotage success – as it saps confidence and keeps us stuck in destructive thought patterns. Identifying key motivations other than simply how you look - such as health and other aspects of physical and emotional well being - is like saying that you're an OK person right now, and worth making changes for. Making healthy lifestyle choices also has the knock on effect of boosting self-esteem further.

Write down your reasons for wanting to lose weight in your Personal Plan *(see page 42)* – so you can refer back to them. This can be especially helpful when the going gets tough. It may help to think of it in terms of what your weight is stopping you from doing now. Here's some examples: to feel more confident; so I can play more comfortably with my kids; my healthier diet will give me more energy; to improve my fertility.

GETTING READY FOR WEIGHT LOSS SUCCESS

What is a Healthy Weight?

With all the 'thin is beautiful' messages in the media it can be easy to get a distorted view about whether your weight is healthy or not. However, as the BMI charts suggest, there is no single 'ideal' weight for anybody. Research also shows that modest amounts of weight loss can be very beneficial to health and are easier to keep off. Therefore, health professionals now encourage us to aim for a weight loss of 5-10%. The ideal rate of weight loss is no more than 1-2 pounds (0.5-1kg) per week – so averaging a pound a week is great, and realistic progress.

The health benefits of modest weight loss include:

- *Reduced risk of developing heart disease, stroke and certain cancers*

- *Reduced risk of developing diabetes and helping to manage diabetes*

- *Improvements in blood pressure*

- *Improvements in mobility, back pain and joint pain*

- *Improvements with fertility problems and polycystic ovarian syndrome*

- *Less breathlessness and sleep/snoring problems*

- *Increased self esteem and control over eating*

- *Feeling fitter and have more energy*

Are You Really Ready to Lose Weight?

When you think of losing weight, it's easy just to think of what weight you'd like to get to. But weight loss only happens as a result of making changes to your usual eating and activity patterns – which allow you to consume fewer calories than you burn *(see 'It's calories that count' page 5)*.

So here comes the next big question. Are you really ready to do it? Have you thought about the implications of your decision? If you have lost weight in the past, and put it all back on - have you thought about why that was? And how confident do you feel about being successful this time?

CALORIE, CARB AND FAT BIBLE 2013　　15

To help you answer these questions, try these short exercises.

Where would you place yourself on the following scales?

Importance

How important is it to you, to make the changes that will allow you to lose weight?

0 1 2 3 4 5 6 7 8 9 10

Not at all important   *Extremely important*

If you ranked yourself over half way along the scale then move on to the next question. If you were half way or less along the scale, you may not be mentally ready to make the required changes to lose weight. To further explore this, go to *'The Pros and Cons of Weight Loss' (page 17).*

Confidence

How confident are you in your ability to make the changes that will allow you to lose weight?

0 1 2 3 4 5 6 7 8 9 10

Not at all confident   *Extremely confident*

Now ask yourself (regarding your confidence ratings):

1. Why did I place myself here?

2. What is stopping me moving further up the scale (if anything)?

3. What things, information, support would help me move further up the scale? (if not near 10)

If you aren't sure about answers to question 3, then keep reading for some pointers.

The Pros and Cons of Weight Loss

Making lifestyle changes to lose weight is simpler if there are lots of clear benefits or pros, for example, clothes fit again, more energy, helps back pain - but there will also be associated downsides or cons. For example, some may feel it interferes with their social life, or don't have the time to plan meals or check food labels. Or overeating can help, if only temporarily, as a way of coping with unwanted feelings. Being overweight allows some people to feel strong and assertive, or to control their partner's jealousy. So in these cases there are downsides to losing weight, even if the person says they are desperate to do it.

If you are aware of the possible downsides, as well as the pros, you will be better prepared to deal with potential conflicts. Understanding what could be (or were with past weight loss efforts) barriers to success gives you the chance to address them. This boosts confidence in your ability to succeed this time, which in turn maintains your motivation.

Have a go at weighing up the pros and cons using the charts below and on page 18. Some examples are included. If you decide that the pros outweigh the cons, then great. You can also use the cons as potential barriers to plan strategies for *(see page 42)*. If you find it's the other way around, this may not be the best time to actively lose weight. Try the exercise again in a month or so.

Making Lifestyle Changes to Lose Weight Now

CONS *e.g. Must limit eating out, take aways*	PROS *e.g. Feel more energetic, slimmer*

Not Making Changes Now – how would I feel in 6 months time?

PROS *e.g. Haven't had to worry about failing; Still able to eat take aways a lot*	CONS *e.g. Probably gained more weight; Back pain may be worse*

To change your weight, first change your mind

To lose weight you may already have a list of things to change, such as eating more fruit and veg, calculating your daily calorie intake, going for a walk each morning or buying low fat options. Others could also give you tips to try. But knowing what to do isn't the same as feeling motivated or able to do it. To be effective, you have to believe the changes are relevant, do-able and worth it.

What you think, affects how you feel, and in turn the actions you take.

Self-efficacy

In fact, research is telling us that one of the most important factors that influences weight loss success are your feelings of 'self-efficacy'. Self-efficacy is a term used in psychology to describe a person's belief that any action they take will have an effect on the outcome. It reflects our inner expectation that what we do will lead to the results we want. Not surprisingly, high levels of self-efficacy can enhance motivation, and allow us to deal better with uncertainty and conflict, and recovery from setbacks. But low levels, can reduce our motivation. We fear that whatever we do will not bring about our desired goal. This can lead self-defeating thoughts or 'self-talk', which make it hard to deal with set-backs, meaning we are more likely to give up. Here's some examples.

Examples: Low self-efficacy

' No matter how carefully I diet, I don't lose weight . . . '

*' I have eaten that chocolate and as usual blown my diet,
so I may as well give up now. '*

*' I had a rich dessert – I have no willpower to say no.
I can't stand not being able to eat what I want. '*

If you have a strong sense of self-efficacy, your mindset and 'self-talk' will be more like:

Examples: High self-efficacy

*' I know from previous weight loss programmes, that if I stay
focussed on what I am doing I do lose weight. I have always
expected to lose too much too quickly which frustrates me. I
know that I will lose weight if I keep making the right changes,
and this time it is important to me. '*

*' The chocolate bar won't ruin my diet, but if I think it has and
keep on eating, then my negative self-talk will. So I will get
back on track. '*

*' I don't like having to eat differently from others, but losing
weight is very important to me, so I **can** stand it. After all,
the world won't stop if I say no to dessert, and I will feel great
afterwards. If I think about it, I am not hungry so would just
feel bloated and guilty if I ate it. '*

Willpower is a Skill

Many people feel that they just need plenty of willpower or a good telling off to lose weight. But willpower isn't something you have or you don't have. Willpower is a skill. Like the dessert example on page 19, it's a sign that you've made a conscious choice to do something, because you believe the benefits outweigh any downsides. In reality everything we do is preceded by a thought. This includes everything we eat. It just may not seem like it because our actions often feel automatic *(see 'Look out for trigger eating' page 21)*.

When it comes to weight loss, developing a range of skills – including choosing a lower calorie diet, coping with negative self-talk and managing things that don't go to plan - will boost your sense of self-efficacy to make the changes you want. This is especially important because we live in such a weight-promoting environment.

Our weight-promoting environment

We are constantly surrounded by tempting food, stresses that can trigger comfort eating and labour-saving devices that make it easy not to be physically active. In other words, the environment we live in makes it easy to gain weight, unless we stop and think about the food choices we make and how much exercise we do. In fact, to stay a healthy weight/maintain our weight, just about all of us need to make conscious lifestyle choices everyday. This isn't 'dieting' but just part of taking care of ourselves in the environment we live in.

It is also true that some people find it more of a challenge than others to manage their weight, thanks to genetic differences in factors such as appetite control, spontaneous activity level and emotional responses to food – rather than metabolic rate, as is often believed. The good news is that with a healthy diet and active lifestyle a healthier weight can still be achieved. But do talk to your doctor if you feel you need additional support.

Coping with Common Slimming Saboteurs

Lyndel Costain BSc RD

Look out for 'trigger' eating

Much of the overeating we do or cravings we have are actually down to unconscious, habitual, responses to a variety of triggers. These triggers can be external, such as the sight or smell of food, or internal and emotion-led, such as a response to stress, anger, boredom or emptiness. Your food diary (see page 43) helps you to recognise 'trigger' or 'non-hungry' eating which gives you the chance to think twice before you eat (see below).

Get some support

A big part of your success will be having someone to support you. It could be a friend, partner, health professional, health club or website. Let them know how they can help you most.

Make lapses your ally

Don't let a lapse throw you off course. You can't be, nor need to be perfect all the time. Doing well 80-90% of the time is great progress. Lapses are a normal part of change. Rather than feel you have failed and give up, look at what you can learn from a difficult day or week and use it to find helpful solutions for the future.

Understand why you eat

When I ask people what prompts them to eat, hunger usually comes down near the bottom of their list of reasons. Some people struggle to remember or appreciate what true hunger feels like. We are lucky that we have plenty of food to eat in our society. But its constant presence makes it harder to control what we eat, especially if it brings us comfort or joy.

If you ever find yourself in the fridge even though you've recently eaten, then you know hunger isn't the reason but some other trigger. The urge to eat can be so automatic that you feel you lack willpower or are out of control. But it is in fact a learned or conditioned response. A bit like Pavlov's dogs. He rang a bell every time he fed them, and from then on, whenever they heard the bell ring they were 'conditioned' to salivate in anticipation of food.

Because this 'non-hungry' eating is learned, you can reprogramme your response to the situations or feelings that trigger it. The first step is to identify when these urges strike. When you find yourself eating when you aren't hungry ask yourself 'why do I want to eat, what am I feeling?' If you aren't sure think back to what was happening before you ate. Then ask yourself if there is another way you can feel better without food. Or you could chat to your urge to eat in a friendly way, telling it that you don't want to give into it, you have a planned meal coming soon, and it's merely a learned response. Whatever strategy you choose, the more often you break into your urges to eat, the weaker their hold becomes.

Practise positive self-talk

Self-talk may be positive and constructive (like your guardian angel) or negative and irrational (like having a destructive devil on your shoulder).

If you've had on-off battles with your weight over the years, it's highly likely that the 'devil' is there more often. 'All or nothing' self-talk for example, 'I ate a "bad food" so have broken my diet', can make you feel like a failure which, can then trigger you into the action of overeating and/or totally giving up *(see 'Diet-binge cycle' page 23)*. One of the most powerful things about it is that the last thoughts we have are what stays in our mind. So if we think 'I still look fat' or 'I will never be slim', these feelings stay with us.

To change your self-talk for the better, the trick is to first recognise it's happening (keeping a diary really helps, *see Keep a Food Diary, page 29*). Then turn it around into a positive version of the same events *(see Self-efficacy, page 18)* where the resulting action was to feel good and stay on track. Reshaping negative self-talk helps you to boost your self-esteem and feelings of self-efficacy, and with it change your self-definition - from someone who can't 'lose weight' or 'do this or that', to someone 'who can'. And when you believe you can…

The Diet – Binge Cycle

If this cycle looks familiar, use positive self-talk, and a more flexible dietary approach, to help you break free.

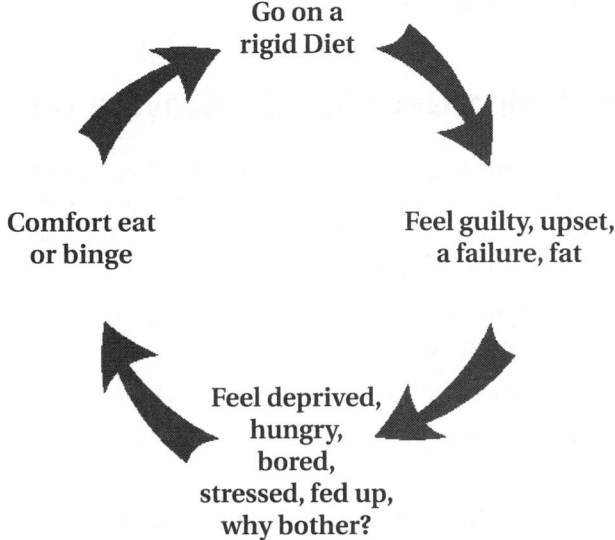

Go on a rigid Diet

Feel guilty, upset, a failure, fat

Feel deprived, hungry, bored, stressed, fed up, why bother?

Comfort eat or binge

Really choose what you want to eat

This skill is like your personal brake. It also helps you to manage 'trigger/ non-hungry' eating and weaken its hold. It legalises food and stops you feeling deprived. It helps you to regularly remind yourself why you are making changes to your eating habits, which keeps motivation high. But it doesn't just happen. Like all skills it requires practise. Sometimes it will work well for you, other times it won't – but overall it will help. Basically, ask yourself if you really want to eat that food in front of you. This becomes the prompt for you to make a conscious choice, weighing up the pros and cons or consequences of making that choice, and feeling free to have it, reject it or just eat some. Remembering all the while that you can eat this food another time if you want to.

Action Planning

Successful people don't just wait for things to happen. They believe in themselves, plan ahead, take action and then refine their plan until it gets, and keeps on getting the results they want. Successful slimmers use a very similar approach. They don't rely on quick-fixes or magic formulas, but glean information from reliable sources to develop a plan or approach that suits their needs, tastes and lifestyle. Thinking of weight management as a lifelong project, which has a weight loss phase and a weight maintenance phase, is also a route to success.

When the Going Gets Tough - Staying on Track

If things start to go off track, don't panic. Learning new habits takes time. And life is never straightforward so there will be times when it all seems too much, or negative 'self- talk' creeps in to try and drag you back into old ways. So if the going gets tough:

- Value what you've achieved so far, rather than only focus on what you plan to do.

- Look back at your reasons to lose weight and refer to the list often.

- Don't expect to change too much, too quickly. Take things a step at a time.

- Accept difficulties as part of the learning and skill building process.

- Enjoy a non-food reward for achieving your goals (including maintaining your weight).

- Use recipes and meal ideas to keep things interesting.

- Talk to your supporters and get plenty of encouragement. This is really vital!

Strategies of Successful Slimmers

Thanks to research conducted by large studies such as the US National Weight Control Registry and the German Lean Habits Study, we now know more about what works best for people who have lost weight and successfully kept it off. So be inspired!

The key elements of success are to:

- Believe that you can control your weight and the changes involved are really worth it.
- Stay realistic and value what you have achieved rather than dwell on a weight you 'dream' of being.
- Be more active – plan ways to fit activity into your daily life – aim for 1 hour of walking daily.
- Plan ahead for regular meals and snacks, starting with breakfast.
- Choose a balanced, low-fat diet with plenty of fruit and vegetables *(see Healthy Eating Made Easy, page 32)*.
- Watch portion size and limit fast food.
- Sit down to eat and take time over meals, paying attention to what you are eating.
- Have a flexible approach – plan in and enjoy some favourite foods without guilt.
- Recognise and address 'all or nothing' thinking and other negative 'self-talk'.
- Keep making conscious choices.
- Learn to confront problems rather than eat, drink, sleep or wish they would go away.
- Enlist ongoing help and support from family, friends, professionals or websites.
- Regularly (at least once a week but not more than once daily) check your weight.
- Take action before your weight increases by more than 4-5lb (2kg).
- Accept that your weight management skills need to be kept up long-term.
- Take heart from successful slimmers, who say that it gets easier over time.

Your step-by-step guide to using this book and shifting those pounds

Juliette Kellow BSc RD and Rebecca Walton

1. Find your healthy weight

Use the weight charts, body mass index table and information on pages 36-43 to determine the right weight for you. Then set yourself a weight to aim for. Research shows it really helps if you make losing 10% of your weight your first overall target. It also brings important health benefits too *(see 'What is a Healthy Weight?' page 15)*. You can break this down into smaller manageable steps, for example, 3kg/6.5lbs at a time. If 10% is too much, then go for a 5% loss – this has important health benefits too. In fact, just keeping your weight stable is a great achievement these days, because of our weight-promoting environment *(see page 20)*.

Waist Management

In addition to BMI, another important way to assess your weight is by measuring your waist just above belly button level. It is especially useful for men as they tend to carry more excess weight around their bellies, but women should test it out too. Having excess weight around your middle (known as being 'apple-shaped') increases your risk of heart disease and type 2 diabetes. A simple way to stay aware of your waist is according to how well, or otherwise, skirts and trousers fit. Talk to your doctor about any weight and health concerns.

WAIST MEASUREMENT

	Increased Health Risk	High Risk to Health
Women	32-35in (81-88cm)	more than 35in (88cm)
Men	37-40in (94-102cm)	more than 40in (102cm)

2. Set a realistic time scale

With today's hectic lifestyles, everything tends to happen at breakneck speed, so it's no wonder that when it comes to losing weight, most of us want to shift those pounds in an instant. But it's probably taken years to accumulate that extra weight, with the result that it's unrealistic to expect to lose the excess in just a few weeks! Instead, prepare yourself to lose weight slowly and steadily. It's far healthier to lose weight like this. But better still, research shows you'll be far more likely to maintain your new, lower weight.

If you only have a small amount of weight to lose, aim for a weight loss of around 1lb (½kg) a week. But if you have more than 2 stone (28kg) to lose, you may prefer to aim for 2lb (1kg) each week. Remember though, it's better to keep going at 1lb (½kg) a week than to give up because trying to lose 2lb (1kg) a week is making you miserable! The following words may help you to keep your goal in perspective:

'Never give up on a goal because of the time it will take to achieve it – the time will pass anyway.'

Weight Fluctuations

Weight typically fluctuates on a day to day basis. You know that shock/horror feeling when you weigh yourself in the morning then later in the day, or after a meal out, and it looks like youve gained pounds in hours! But this is due to fluid not fat changes. Real changes in body fat can only happen more gradually (remember, to gain 1lb you need to eat 3500 calories more than you usually do). Don't be confused either by seemingly very rapid weight loss in the first week or so.

When calorie intake is initially cut back, the body's carbohydrate stores in the liver and muscles (known as glycogen) are used up. Glycogen is stored with three times its weight in water, meaning that rapid losses of 4.5- 6.6lb (2 -3 kg) are possible. These stores can be just as rapidly refilled if normal eating is resumed. True weight loss happens more gradually and this book helps you to lose weight at the steady and healthy rate of no more than 1-2 lbs per week.

---

3. Calculate your calorie allowance

Use the calorie tables on pages 39-40 to find out how many calories you need each day to maintain your current weight. Then use the table below to discover the amount of calories you need to subtract from this amount every day to lose weight at your chosen rate. For example, a 35 year-old woman who is moderately active and weighs 12 stone (76kg) needs 2,188 calories a day to keep her weight steady. If she wants to lose ½lb (¼kg) a week, she needs 250 calories less each day, giving her a daily calorie allowance of 1,938 calories. If she wants to lose 1lb (½kg) a week, she needs 500 calories less each day, giving her a daily calorie allowance of 1,688 calories, and so on.

TO LOSE...	Cut your daily calorie intake by	In three months you could lose...	In six months you could lose...	In one year you could lose...
½lb a week	250	6.5lb	13lb	1st 12lb
1lb a week	500	13lb	1st 12lb	3st 10lb
1½lb a week	750	1st 5.5lb	2st 11lb	5st 8lb
2lb a week	1,000	1st 12lb	3st 10lb	7st 6lb

TO LOSE...	Cut your daily calorie intake by	In three months you could lose...	In six months you could lose...	In one year you could lose...
¼kg a week	250	3.25kg	6.5kg	13kg
½kg a week	500	6.5kg	13kg	26kg
¾kg a week	750	9.75kg	19.5kg	39kg
1kg a week	1,000	13kg	26kg	52kg

4. Keep a food diary

Writing down what you eat and drink and any thoughts linked to that eating helps you become more aware of your eating habits. Recognising what is going on helps you feel in control and is a powerful way to start planning change. Keeping a food diary before you start to change your eating habits will also help you identify opportunities for cutting calories by substituting one food for another, cutting portion sizes of high-calorie foods or eating certain foods less often. Simply write down every single item you eat or drink during the day and use this book to calculate the calories of each item. Then after a few days of eating normally, introduce some changes to your diet to achieve your daily calorie allowance. Remember to spread your daily calorie allowance fairly evenly throughout the day to prevent hunger. You'll find a template for a daily food and exercise diary on page 43. Try to use it as carefully as you can as research shows that people who do, do best.

Top Tip

If you only fill in your main food diary once a day, keep a pen and notepad with you to write down all those little extras you eat or drink during the day – that chocolate you ate in the office, the sliver of cheese you had while cooking dinner and the few chips you pinched from your husband's plate, for example! It's easy to forget the little things if they're not written down, but they can make the difference between success and failure.

QUESTION: Why are heavier people allowed more calories than those who have smaller amounts of weight to lose?

ANSWER: This confuses a lot of people but is easily explained. Someone who is 3 stone overweight, for example, is carrying the equivalent of 42 small packets of butter with them everywhere they go – up and down the stairs, to the local shops, into the kitchen. Obviously, it takes a lot more energy simply to move around when you're carrying that extra weight. As a consequence, the heavier you are, the more calories you need just to keep your weight steady. In turn, this means you'll lose weight on a higher calorie allowance. However, as you lose weight, you'll need to lower your calorie allowance slightly as you have less weight to carry around.

5. Control your portions

As well as making some smart food swaps to cut calories, it's likely you'll also need to reduce your serving sizes for some foods to help shift those pounds. Even 'healthy' foods such as brown rice, wholemeal bread, chicken, fish and low-fat dairy products contain calories so you may need to limit the amount you eat. When you first start out, weigh portions of foods like rice, pasta, cereal, cheese, butter, oil, meat, fish, and chicken rather than completing your food diary with a 'guesstimated' weight! That way you can calculate the calorie content accurately. Don't forget that drinks contain calories too, alcohol, milk, juices and sugary drinks all count.

6. Measure your success

Research has found that regular weight checks do help. Weighing yourself helps you assess how your eating and exercise habits affect your body weight. The important thing is to use the information in a positive way – to assess your progress - rather than as a stick to beat yourself up with. Remember that weight can fluctuate by a kilogram in a day, for example, due to fluid changes, premenstrually, after a big meal out, so weigh yourself at the same time of day and look at the trend over a week or two.

People who successfully lose weight and keep it off, also tend to continue weighing themselves at least once a week, and often daily (but not in an obsessive way), because they say it helps them stay 'on track'. Probably because they use it as an early warning system. People who weigh themselves regularly (or regularly try on a tight fitting item of clothing) will notice quickly if they have gained a couple of kilograms and can take action to stop gaining more. Checking your weight less often can mean that you might discover one day that you gained 6kg. That can be pretty discouraging, and it might trigger you to just give up.

Top Tip

Don't just focus on what the bathroom scales say either – keep a record of your vital statistics, too. Many people find it doubly encouraging to see the inches dropping off, as well as the pounds!

7. Stay motivated

Each time you lose half a stone, or reach your own small goal – celebrate! Treat yourself to a little luxury – something new to wear, a little pampering or some other (non-food) treat. It also helps replace the comfort you once got from food and allows you to take care of yourself in other ways. Trying on an item of clothing that used to be tight can also help to keep you feeling motivated. Make sure you keep in touch with your supporters, and if the going gets tough take another look at the *'Coping with Common Slimming Saboteurs' section on page 21*. Once you've reviewed how well you've done, use this book to set yourself a new daily calorie allowance based on your new weight to help you lose the next half stone *(see point 3 - page 28 - Calculate your calorie allowance)*.

8. Keep it off

What you do to stay slim is just as important as what you did to get slim. Quite simply, if you return to your old ways, you are likely to return to your old weight. The great thing about calorie counting is that you will learn so much about what you eat, and make so many important changes to your eating and drinking habits, that you'll probably find it difficult to go back to your old ways – and won't want to anyway. It's still a good idea to weigh yourself at least once a week to keep a check on your weight. The key is to deal with any extra pounds immediately, rather than waiting until you have a stone to lose *(see page 30)*. Simply go back to counting calories for as long as it takes to shift those pounds and enjoy the new slim you. Page 25 has more information about how successful slimmers keep it off.

QUESTION: Do I need to stick to exactly the same number of calories each day or is it OK to have a lower calorie intake during the week and slightly more at the weekend?

ANSWER: The key to losing weight is to take in fewer calories than you need for as long as it takes to reach your target, aiming for a loss of no more than 2lb (1kg) a week. In general, most nutrition experts recommend a daily calorie allowance. However, it's just as valid to use other periods of time such as weeks. If you prefer, simply multiply your daily allowance by seven to work out a weekly calorie allowance and then allocate more calories to some days than others. For example, a daily allowance of 1,500 calories is equivalent to 10,500 calories a week. This means you could have 1,300 calories a day during the week and 2,000 calories a day on Saturday and Sunday.

Healthy Eating Made Easy

Juliette Kellow BSc RD

GONE ARE THE DAYS when a healthy diet meant surviving on bird seed, rabbit food and carrot juice! The new approach to eating healthily means we're positively encouraged to eat a wide range of foods, including some of our favourites – it's just a question of making sure we don't eat high fat, high sugar or highly processed foods too often.

Eating a healthy diet, together with taking regular exercise and not smoking, has huge benefits to our health, both in the short and long term. As well as helping us to lose or maintain our weight, a healthy diet can boost energy levels, keep our immune system strong and give us healthy skin, nails and hair. Meanwhile, eating well throughout life also means we're far less likely to suffer from health problems such as constipation, anaemia and tooth decay or set ourselves up for serious conditions in later life such as obesity, heart disease, stroke, diabetes, cancer or osteoporosis.

Fortunately, it couldn't be easier to eat a balanced diet. To start with, no single food provides all the calories and nutrients we need to stay healthy, so it's important to eat a variety of foods. Meanwhile, most nutrition experts also agree that mealtimes should be a pleasure rather than a penance. This means it's fine to eat small amounts of our favourite treats from time to time.

To help people eat healthily, the Food Standards Agency recommends eating plenty of different foods from four main groups of foods and limiting the amount we eat from a smaller fifth group. Ultimately, we should eat more fruit, vegetables, starchy, fibre-rich foods and fresh products, and fewer fatty, sugary, salty and processed foods.

The following guidelines are all based on the healthy eating guidelines recommended by the Food Standards Agency.

Bread, other cereals and potatoes

Eat these foods at each meal. They also make good snacks.

Foods in this group include bread, breakfast cereals, potatoes, rice, pasta, noodles, yams, oats and grains. Go for high-fibre varieties where available, such as wholegrain cereals, wholemeal bread and brown rice. These foods should fill roughly a third of your plate at mealtimes.

TYPICAL SERVING SIZES

* *2 slices bread in a sandwich or with a meal*

* *a tennis ball sized serving of pasta, potato, rice, noodles or couscous*

* *a bowl of porridge*

* *around 40g of breakfast cereal*

Fruit and vegetables

Eat at least five portions every day.

Foods in this group include all fruits and vegetables, including fresh, frozen, canned and dried products, and unsweetened fruit juice. Choose canned fruit in juice rather than syrup and go for veg canned in water without added salt or sugar.

TYPICAL PORTION SIZES

* *a piece of fruit eg: apple, banana, pear*

* *2 small fruits eg: satsumas, plums, apricots*

* *a bowl of fruit salad, canned or stewed fruit*

* *a small glass of unsweetened fruit juice*

* *a cereal bowl of salad*

* *3tbsp vegetables*

Milk and dairy foods

Eat two or three servings a day.

Foods in this group include milk, cheese, yoghurt and fromage frais. Choose low-fat varieties where available such as skimmed milk, reduced-fat cheese and fat-free yoghurt.

TYPICAL SERVING SIZES

* *200ml milk*

* *a small pot of yoghurt or fromage frais*

* *a small matchbox-sized piece of cheese*

Meat, fish and alternatives

Eat two servings a day

Foods in this group include meat, poultry, fish, eggs, beans, nuts and seeds. Choose low-fat varieties where available such as extra-lean minced beef and skinless chicken and don't add extra fat or salt.

TYPICAL SERVING SIZES

* *a piece of meat, chicken or fish the size of a deck of cards*

* *1-2 eggs*

* *3 heaped tablespoons of beans*

* *a small handful of nuts or seeds*

Healthy Eating on a plate

A simple way to serve up both balance and healthy proportions is to fill one half of your plate with salad or vegetables and divide the other half between protein-rich meat, chicken, fish, eggs or beans, and healthy carbs (potatoes, rice, pasta, pulses, bread or noodles).

Fatty and sugary foods

Eat only small amounts of these foods

Foods in this group include oils, spreading fats, cream, mayonnaise, oily salad dressings, cakes, biscuits, puddings, crisps, savoury snacks, sugar, preserves, confectionery and sugary soft drinks.

TYPICAL SERVING SIZES:

• *a small packet of sweets or a small bar of chocolate*

• *a small slice of cake*

• *a couple of small biscuits*

• *1 level tbsp mayo, salad dressing or olive oil*

• *a small packet of crisps*

Useful Tools

Body Mass Index

The Body Mass Index (BMI) is the internationally accepted way of assessing how healthy our weight is. It is calculated using an individual's height and weight. Use the Body Mass Index Chart to look up your BMI, and use the table below to see what range you fall into.

BMI Under 18.5	Underweight
BMI 18.5-25	Healthy
BMI 25-30	Overweight
BMI 30-40	Obese
BMI Over 40	Severely Obese

This is what different BMI ranges mean.

- **Underweight:** you probably need to gain weight for your health's sake. Talk to your doctor if you have any concerns, or if you feel frightened about gaining weight.

- **Healthy weight:** you are a healthy weight, so aim to stay in this range (note that most people in this range tend to have a BMI between 20-25).

- **Overweight:** aim to lose some weight for your health's sake, or at least prevent further weight gain.

- **Obese:** your health is at risk and losing weight will benefit your health.

- **Severely obese:** your health is definitely at risk. You should visit your doctor for a health check. Losing weight will improve your health.

Please note that BMI is not as accurate for athletes or very muscular people (muscle weighs more than fat), as it can push them into a higher BMI category despite having a healthy level of body fat. It is also not accurate for women who are pregnant or breastfeeding, or people who are frail.

Body Mass Index Table

	HEIGHT IN FEET / INCHES														
	4'6	4'8	4'10	5'0	5'2	5'4	5'6	5'8	5'10	6'0	6'2	6'4	6'6	6'8	6'10
6st 7	22.0	20.5	19.1	17.8	16.7	15.7	14.7	13.9	13.1	12.4	11.7	11.1	10.6	10.0	9.5
7st 0	23.7	22.1	20.6	19.2	18.0	16.9	15.9	15.0	14.1	13.3	12.6	12.0	11.4	10.8	10.3
7st 7	25.4	23.6	22.0	20.6	19.3	18.1	17.0	16.0	15.1	14.3	13.5	12.8	12.2	11.6	11.0
8st 0	27.1	25.2	23.5	22.0	20.6	19.3	18.1	17.1	16.1	15.2	14.4	13.7	13.0	12.3	11.8
8st 7	28.8	26.8	25.0	23.3	21.8	20.5	19.3	18.2	17.1	16.2	15.3	14.5	13.8	13.1	12.5
9st 0	30.5	28.4	26.4	24.7	23.1	21.7	20.4	19.2	18.1	17.2	16.2	15.4	14.6	13.9	13.2
9st 7	32.2	29.9	27.9	26.1	24.4	22.9	21.5	20.3	19.2	18.1	17.1	16.2	15.4	14.7	14.0
10st 0	33.9	31.5	29.4	27.4	25.7	24.1	22.7	21.4	20.2	19.1	18.0	17.1	16.2	15.4	14.7
10st 7	35.6	33.1	30.8	28.8	27.0	25.3	23.8	22.4	21.2	20.0	18.9	18.0	17.0	16.2	15.4
11st 0	37.3	34.7	32.3	30.2	28.3	26.5	24.9	23.5	22.2	21.0	19.8	18.8	17.9	17.0	16.2
11st 7	39.0	36.2	33.8	31.6	29.6	27.7	26.1	24.6	23.2	21.9	20.7	19.7	18.7	17.8	16.9
12st 0	40.7	37.8	35.2	32.9	30.8	28.9	27.2	25.6	24.2	22.9	21.6	20.5	19.5	18.5	17.6
12st 7	42.3	39.4	36.7	34.3	32.1	30.1	28.3	26.7	25.2	23.8	22.5	21.4	20.3	19.3	18.4
13st 0	44.0	41.0	38.2	35.7	33.4	31.4	29.5	27.8	26.2	24.8	23.5	22.2	21.1	20.1	19.1
13st 7	45.7	42.5	39.6	37.0	34.7	32.6	30.6	28.8	27.2	25.7	24.4	23.1	21.9	20.8	19.8
14st 0	47.4	44.1	41.1	38.4	36.0	33.8	31.7	29.9	28.2	26.7	25.3	23.9	22.7	21.6	20.6
14st 7	49.1	45.7	42.6	39.8	37.3	35.0	32.9	31.0	29.2	27.6	26.2	24.8	23.5	22.4	21.3
15st 0	50.8	47.3	44.0	41.2	38.5	36.2	34.0	32.0	30.2	28.6	27.1	25.7	24.4	23.2	22.0
15st 7	52.5	48.8	45.5	42.5	39.8	37.4	35.2	33.1	31.2	29.5	28.0	26.5	25.2	23.9	22.8
16st 0	54.2	50.4	47.0	43.9	41.1	38.6	36.3	34.2	32.3	30.5	28.9	27.4	26.0	24.7	23.5
16st 7	55.9	52.0	48.5	45.3	42.4	39.8	37.4	35.2	33.3	31.4	29.8	28.2	26.8	25.5	24.2
17st 0	57.6	53.6	49.9	46.6	43.7	41.0	38.6	36.3	34.3	32.4	30.7	29.1	27.6	26.2	25.0
17st 7	59.3	55.1	51.4	48.0	45.0	42.2	39.7	37.4	35.3	33.3	31.6	29.9	28.4	27.0	25.7
18st 0	61.0	56.7	52.9	49.4	46.3	43.4	40.8	38.5	36.3	34.3	32.5	30.8	29.2	27.8	26.4
18st 7	62.7	58.3	54.3	50.8	47.5	44.6	42.0	39.5	37.3	35.3	33.4	31.6	30.0	28.6	27.2
19st 0	64.4	59.9	55.8	52.1	48.8	45.8	43.1	40.6	38.3	36.2	34.3	32.5	30.8	29.3	27.9
19st 7	66.1	61.4	57.3	53.5	50.1	47.0	44.2	41.7	39.3	37.2	35.2	33.3	31.7	30.1	28.6
20st 0	67.8	63.0	58.7	54.9	51.4	48.2	45.4	42.7	40.3	38.1	36.1	34.2	32.5	30.9	29.4
20st 7	69.4	64.6	60.2	56.3	52.7	49.4	46.5	43.8	41.3	39.1	37.0	35.1	33.3	31.6	30.1
21st 0	71.1	66.2	61.7	57.6	54.0	50.6	47.6	44.9	42.3	40.0	37.9	35.9	34.1	32.4	30.9
21st 7	72.8	67.7	63.1	59.0	55.3	51.9	48.8	45.9	43.3	41.0	38.8	36.8	34.9	33.2	31.6
22st 0	74.5	69.3	64.6	60.4	56.5	53.1	49.9	47.0	44.4	41.9	39.7	37.6	35.7	34.0	32.3
22st 7	76.2	70.9	66.1	61.7	57.8	54.3	51.0	48.1	45.4	42.9	40.6	38.5	36.5	34.7	33.1
23st 0	77.9	72.5	67.5	63.1	59.1	55.5	52.2	49.1	46.4	43.8	41.5	39.3	37.3	35.5	33.8
23st 7	79.6	74.0	69.0	64.5	60.4	56.7	53.3	50.2	47.4	44.8	42.4	40.2	38.2	36.3	34.5
24st 0	81.3	75.6	70.5	65.9	61.7	57.9	54.4	51.3	48.4	45.7	43.3	41.0	39.0	37.0	35.3
24st 7	83.0	77.2	71.9	67.2	63.0	59.1	55.6	52.3	49.4	46.7	44.2	41.9	39.8	37.8	36.0
25st 0	84.7	78.8	73.4	68.6	64.2	60.3	56.7	53.4	50.4	47.6	45.1	42.8	40.6	38.6	36.7
25st 7	86.4	80.3	74.9	70.0	65.5	61.5	57.8	54.5	51.4	48.6	46.0	43.6	41.4	39.4	37.5
26st 0	88.1	81.9	76.3	71.3	66.8	62.7	59.0	55.5	52.4	49.5	46.9	44.5	42.2	40.1	38.2
26st 7	89.8	83.5	77.8	72.7	68.1	63.9	60.1	56.6	53.4	50.5	47.8	45.3	43.0	40.9	38.9
27st 0	91.5	85.1	79.3	74.1	69.4	65.1	61.2	57.7	54.4	51.5	48.7	46.2	43.8	41.7	39.7
27st 7	93.2	86.6	80.8	75.5	70.7	66.3	62.4	58.7	55.4	52.4	49.6	47.0	44.7	42.4	40.4
28st 0	94.9	88.2	82.2	76.8	72.0	67.5	63.5	59.8	56.4	53.4	50.5	47.9	45.5	43.2	41.1
28st 7	96.5	89.8	83.7	78.2	73.2	68.7	64.6	60.9	57.5	54.3	51.4	48.7	46.3	44.0	41.9
29st 0	98.2	91.4	85.2	79.6	74.5	69.9	65.0	62.0	58.5	55.3	52.3	49.6	47.1	44.8	42.6
29st 7	99.9	92.9	86.6	80.9	75.8	71.1	66.9	63.0	59.5	56.2	53.2	50.5	47.9	45.5	43.3

WEIGHT IN STONES / LBS

Weight Chart

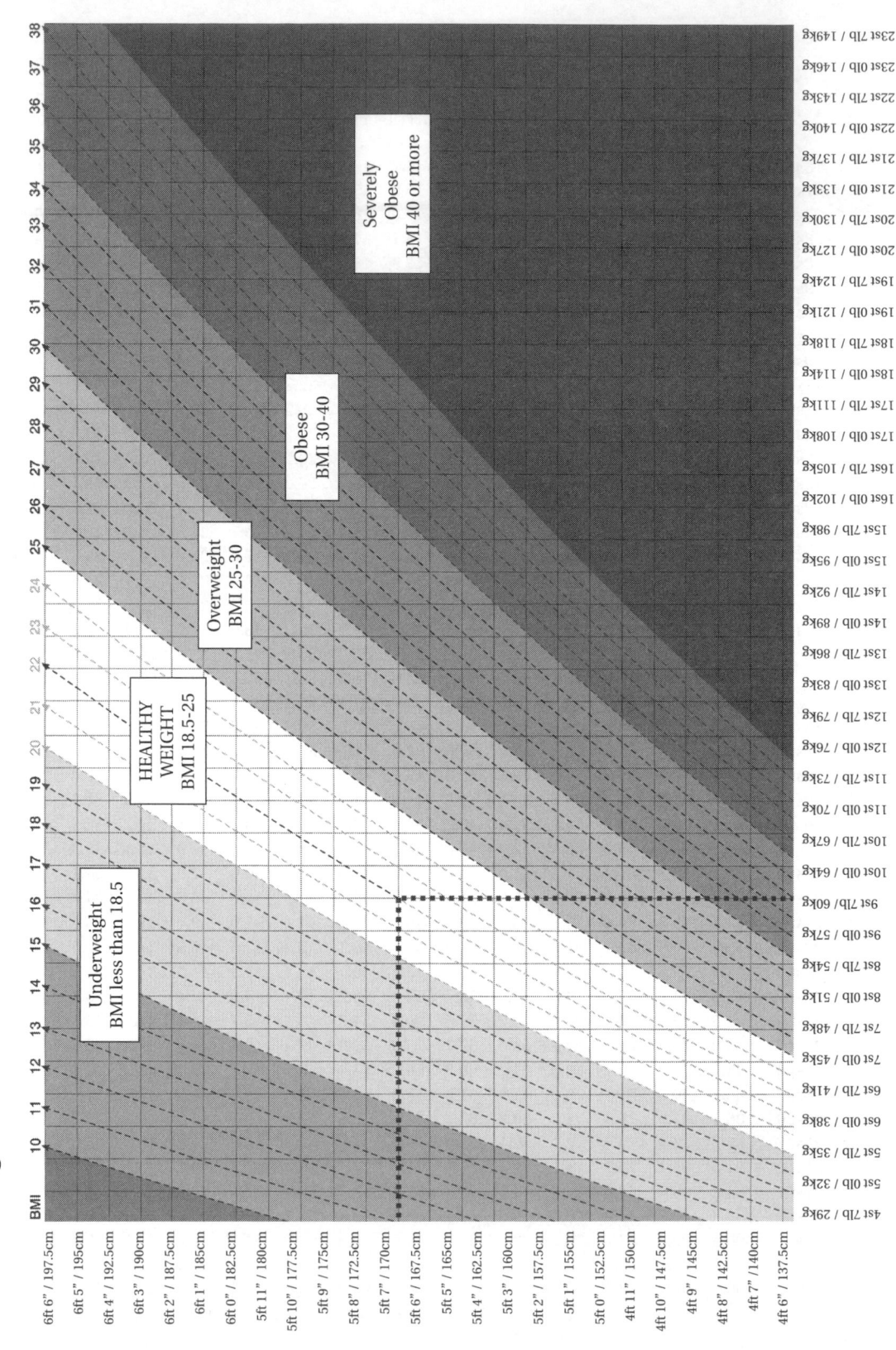

Calories Required to Maintain Weight
Adult Females

ACTIVITY LEVEL / AGE

WEIGHT IN STONES / LBS	VERY SEDENTARY			MODERATELY SEDENTARY			MODERATELY ACTIVE			VERY ACTIVE		
	<30	30-60	60+	<30	30-60	60+	<30	30-60	60+	<30	30-60	60+
7st 7	1425	1473	1304	1544	1596	1412	1781	1841	1630	2138	2210	1956
8st 0	1481	1504	1338	1605	1629	1450	1852	1880	1673	2222	2256	2008
8st 7	1537	1535	1373	1666	1663	1487	1922	1919	1716	2306	2302	2059
9st 0	1594	1566	1407	1726	1696	1524	1992	1957	1759	2391	2349	2111
9st 7	1650	1596	1442	1787	1729	1562	2062	1996	1802	2475	2395	2163
10st 0	1706	1627	1476	1848	1763	1599	2133	2034	1845	2559	2441	2214
10st 7	1762	1658	1511	1909	1796	1637	2203	2073	1888	2644	2487	2266
11st 0	1819	1689	1545	1970	1830	1674	2273	2111	1931	2728	2534	2318
11st 7	1875	1720	1580	2031	1863	1711	2344	2150	1975	2813	2580	2370
12st 0	1931	1751	1614	2092	1897	1749	2414	2188	2018	2897	2626	2421
12st 7	1987	1781	1648	2153	1930	1786	2484	2227	2061	2981	2672	2473
13st 0	2044	1812	1683	2214	1963	1823	2555	2266	2104	3066	2719	2525
13st 7	2100	1843	1717	2275	1997	1861	2625	2304	2147	3150	2765	2576
14st 0	2156	1874	1752	2336	2030	1898	2695	2343	2190	3234	2811	2628
14st 7	2212	1905	1786	2397	2064	1935	2766	2381	2233	3319	2858	2680
15st 0	2269	1936	1821	2458	2097	1973	2836	2420	2276	3403	2904	2732
15st 7	2325	1967	1855	2519	2130	2010	2906	2458	2319	3488	2950	2783
16st 0	2381	1997	1890	2580	2164	2047	2976	2497	2362	3572	2996	2835
16st 7	2437	2028	1924	2640	2197	2085	3047	2535	2405	3656	3043	2887
17st 0	2494	2059	1959	2701	2231	2122	3117	2574	2449	3741	3089	2938
17st 7	2550	2090	1993	2762	2264	2159	3187	2613	2492	3825	3135	2990
18st 0	2606	2121	2028	2823	2298	2197	3258	2651	2535	3909	3181	3042
18st 7	2662	2152	2062	2884	2331	2234	3328	2690	2578	3994	3228	3093
19st 0	2719	2182	2097	2945	2364	2271	3398	2728	2621	4078	3274	3145
19st 7	2775	2213	2131	3006	2398	2309	3469	2767	2664	4162	3320	3197
20st 0	2831	2244	2166	3067	2431	2346	3539	2805	2707	4247	3366	3249
20st 7	2887	2275	2200	3128	2465	2383	3609	2844	2750	4331	3413	3300
21st 0	2944	2306	2235	3189	2498	2421	3680	2882	2793	4416	3459	3352
21st 7	3000	2337	2269	3250	2531	2458	3750	2921	2836	4500	3505	3404
22st 0	3056	2368	2303	3311	2565	2495	3820	2960	2879	4584	3552	3455
22st 7	3112	2398	2338	3372	2598	2533	3890	2998	2923	4669	3598	3507
23st 0	3169	2429	2372	3433	2632	2570	3961	3037	2966	4753	3644	3559
23st 7	3225	2460	2407	3494	2665	2608	4031	3075	3009	4837	3690	3611
24st 0	3281	2491	2441	3554	2699	2645	4101	3114	3052	4922	3737	3662
24st 7	3337	2522	2476	3615	2732	2682	4172	3152	3095	5006	3783	3714
25st 0	3394	2553	2510	3676	2765	2720	4242	3191	3138	5091	3829	3766
25st 7	3450	2583	2545	3737	2799	2757	4312	3229	3181	5175	3875	3817
26st 0	3506	2614	2579	3798	2832	2794	4383	3268	3224	5259	3922	3869
26st 7	3562	2645	2614	3859	2866	2832	4453	3307	3267	5344	3968	3921
27st 0	3618	2676	2648	3920	2899	2869	4523	3345	3310	5428	4014	3973
27st 7	3675	2707	2683	3981	2932	2906	4594	3384	3353	5512	4060	4024
28st 0	3731	2738	2717	4042	2966	2944	4664	3422	3397	5597	4107	4076
28st 7	3787	2768	2752	4103	2999	2981	4734	3461	3440	5681	4153	4128

Calories Required to Maintain Weight
Adult Males

ACTIVITY LEVEL / AGE

WEIGHT IN STONES / LBS	VERY SEDENTARY			MODERATELY SEDENTARY			MODERATELY ACTIVE			VERY ACTIVE		
	<30	30-60	60+	<30	30-60	60+	<30	30-60	60+	<30	30-60	60+
9st 0	1856	1827	1502	2010	1979	1627	2320	2284	1878	2784	2741	2254
9st 7	1913	1871	1547	2072	2026	1676	2391	2338	1933	2870	2806	2320
10st 0	1970	1914	1591	2134	2074	1724	2463	2393	1989	2955	2871	2387
10st 7	2027	1958	1636	2196	2121	1772	2534	2447	2045	3041	2937	2454
11st 0	2084	2001	1680	2258	2168	1820	2605	2502	2100	3127	3002	2520
11st 7	2141	2045	1724	2320	2215	1868	2677	2556	2156	3212	3067	2587
12st 0	2199	2088	1769	2382	2262	1916	2748	2611	2211	3298	3133	2654
12st 7	2256	2132	1813	2444	2310	1965	2820	2665	2267	3384	3198	2720
13st 0	2313	2175	1858	2506	2357	2013	2891	2719	2322	3470	3263	2787
13st 7	2370	2219	1902	2568	2404	2061	2963	2774	2378	3555	3329	2854
14st 0	2427	2262	1947	2630	2451	2109	3034	2828	2434	3641	3394	2920
14st 7	2484	2306	1991	2691	2498	2157	3106	2883	2489	3727	3459	2987
15st 0	2542	2350	2036	2753	2545	2205	3177	2937	2545	3813	3525	3054
15st 7	2599	2393	2080	2815	2593	2253	3248	2992	2600	3898	3590	3120
16st 0	2656	2437	2125	2877	2640	2302	3320	3046	2656	3984	3655	3187
16st 7	2713	2480	2169	2939	2687	2350	3391	3100	2711	4070	3721	3254
17st 0	2770	2524	2213	3001	2734	2398	3463	3155	2767	4155	3786	3320
17st 7	2827	2567	2258	3063	2781	2446	3534	3209	2823	4241	3851	3387
18st 0	2884	2611	2302	3125	2828	2494	3606	3264	2878	4327	3917	3454
18st 7	2942	2654	2347	3187	2876	2542	3677	3318	2934	4413	3982	3520
19st 0	2999	2698	2391	3249	2923	2591	3749	3373	2989	4498	4047	3587
19st 7	3056	2741	2436	3311	2970	2639	3820	3427	3045	4584	4112	3654
20st 0	3113	2785	2480	3373	3017	2687	3891	3481	3100	4670	4178	3721
20st 7	3170	2829	2525	3434	3064	2735	3963	3536	3156	4756	4243	3787
21st 0	3227	2872	2569	3496	3112	2783	4034	3590	3211	4841	4308	3854
21st 7	3285	2916	2614	3558	3159	2831	4106	3645	3267	4927	4374	3921
22st 0	3342	2959	2658	3620	3206	2880	4177	3699	3323	5013	4439	3987
22st 7	3399	3003	2702	3682	3253	2928	4249	3754	3378	5098	4504	4054
23st 0	3456	3046	2747	3744	3300	2976	4320	3808	3434	5184	4570	4121
23st 7	3513	3090	2791	3806	3347	3024	4392	3862	3489	5270	4635	4187
24st 0	3570	3133	2836	3868	3395	3072	4463	3917	3545	5356	4700	4254
24st 7	3627	3177	2880	3930	3442	3120	4534	3971	3600	5441	4766	4321
25st 0	3685	3220	2925	3992	3489	3168	4606	4026	3656	5527	4831	4387
25st 7	3742	3264	2969	4054	3536	3217	4677	4080	3712	5613	4896	4454
26st 0	3799	3308	3014	4116	3583	3265	4749	4135	3767	5699	4962	4521
26st 7	3856	3351	3058	4177	3630	3313	4820	4189	3823	5784	5027	4587
27st 0	3913	3395	3103	4239	3678	3361	4892	4243	3878	5870	5092	4654
27st 7	3970	3438	3147	4301	3725	3409	4963	4298	3934	5956	5158	4721
28st 0	4028	3482	3191	4363	3772	3457	5035	4352	3989	6042	5223	4787
28st 7	4085	3525	3236	4425	3819	3506	5106	4407	4045	6127	5288	4854
29st 0	4142	3569	3280	4487	3866	3554	5177	4461	4101	6213	5354	4921
29st 7	4199	3612	3325	4549	3913	3602	5249	4516	4156	6299	5419	4987
30st 0	4256	3656	3369	4611	3961	3650	5320	4570	4212	6384	5484	5054

Calories Burned in Exercise

This table shows the approximate number of extra* calories that would be burned in a five minute period of exercise activity.

ACTIVITY	CALORIES BURNED IN 5 MINUTES	ACTIVITY	CALORIES BURNED IN 5 MINUTES
Aerobics, Low Impact	25	Situps, Continuous	17
Badminton, Recreational	17	Skiing, Moderate	30
Cross Trainer	30	Skipping, Moderate	30
Cycling, Recreational, 5mph	17	Squash Playing	39
Dancing, Modern, Moderate	13	Tennis Playing, Recreational	26
Fencing	24	Toning Exercises	17
Gardening, Weeding	19	Trampolining	17
Hill Walking, Up and Down, Recreational	22	Volleyball, Recreational	10
Jogging	30	Walking, Uphill, 15% Gradient, Moderate	43
Kick Boxing	30	Walking Up and Down Stairs, Moderate	34
Netball Playing	23	Walking, 4mph	24
Rebounding	18	Weight Training, Moderate	12
Roller Skating	30	Yoga	13
Rowing Machine, Moderate	30		
Running, 7.5mph	48		

*Extra calories are those in addition to your normal daily calorie needs.

My Personal Plan

Date:

Body Mass Index:

Weight:

Waist Measurement:

Height:

Body Fat % (if known)

10% Weight Loss Goal:

Current weight	16stone (224lb)	100kg
- 10% weight	1stone 8½lb (22½lb)	10kg
= 10% loss goal	14stone 5½lb (201½lb)	90kg

My smaller weight targets on the way to achieving my 10% goal will be:

Reasons why I want to lose weight:

Changes I will make to help me lose weight:
Diet:

Activity:

Potential saboteurs or barriers will be:

Ways I will overcome these:

My supporters will be:

I will monitor my progress by:

I will reward my progress with:
In the short term:

In the long term:

© LYNDEL COSTAIN. THIS PAGE MAY BE PHOTOCOPIED FOR PERSONAL USE

Food and Exercise Diary

Date:

/ /

Daily Calorie Allowance: **A**

Food/Drink Consumed	Serving Size	Calories
_____	_____	_____
_____	_____	_____
_____	_____	_____
_____	_____	_____
_____	_____	_____
_____	_____	_____
_____	_____	_____
_____	_____	_____
_____	_____	_____
_____	_____	_____
_____	_____	_____
_____	_____	_____
_____	_____	_____
_____	_____	_____
_____	_____	_____

You are aiming for your Calorie Balance (Box D) to be as close to zero as possible - ie. you consume the number of calories you need.

Your Daily Calorie Allowance (Box A) should be set to lose ½-2lb (¼-1kg) a week, or maintain weight, depending on your goals.

Total calories consumed **B**

Exercise/Activity	No. mins	Calories
_____	_____	_____
_____	_____	_____
_____	_____	_____

Daily Calorie Allowance (A) *plus* Extra Calories used in Exercise (C) *minus* Total Calories Consumed (B) *equals* Calorie Balance (D)

$A + C - B = D$

Calories used in exercise **C**

Calorie balance **D**

You can also write down any comments or thoughts related to your eating if you want to.

FOOD DIARY PADS AVAILABLE FROM www.dietandfitnessresources.co.uk
© WEIGHT LOSS RESOURCES. THIS PAGE MAY BE PHOTOCOPIED FOR PERSONAL USE

Food Information

Nutritional Information

CALORIE AND FAT values are given per serving, plus calorie and nutrition values per 100g of product. This makes it easy to compare the proportions of fat, protein, carbohydrate and fibre in each food.

The values given are for uncooked, unprepared foods unless otherwise stated. Values are also for only the edible portion of the food unless otherwise stated. ie - weighed with bone.

Finding Foods

The Calorie, Carb & Fat Bible has an Eating Out section which is arranged alphabetically by brand. In the General Foods and Drinks A-Z most foods are grouped together by type, and then put in to alphabetical order. This makes it easy to compare different brands, and will help you to find lower calorie and/or fat alternatives where they are available.

This format also makes it easier to locate foods. Foods are categorised by their main characteristics so, for example, if it is bread, ciabatta or white sliced, you'll find it under "Bread".

Basic ingredients are highlighted to make them easier to find at a glance. You'll find all unbranded foods in bold - making the index easier to use, whether it's just an apple or all the components of a home cooked stew.

There are, however, some foods which are not so easy to categorise, especially combination foods like ready meals. The following pointers will help you to find your way around the book until you get to know it a little better.

FILLED ROLLS AND SANDWICHES - Bagels, baguettes, etc which are filled are listed as "Bagels (filled)" etc. Sandwiches are under "Sandwiches".

CURRIES - Popular types of curry, like Balti or Jalfrezi, are listed under their individual types. Unspecified or lesser known types are listed under their main ingredient.

BURGERS - All burgers, including chicken-type sandwiches from fast-food outlets, are listed under "Burgers". CHIPS & FRIES - Are listed separately, depending on the name of the particular brand. All other types of potato are listed under "Potatoes".

SWEETS & CHOCOLATES - Well-known brands, eg. Aero, Mars Bar, are listed under their brand names. Others are listed under "Chocolate" (for bars) and "Chocolates" (for individual sweets).

READY MEALS - Popular types of dishes are listed under their type, eg. "Chow Mein", "Casserole", "Hot Pot", etc. Others are listed by their main ingredient, eg. "Chicken With", "Chicken In", etc.

EATING OUT & FAST FOODS - By popular demand this edition has the major eating out and fast food brands listed separately, at the back of the book. They are alphabetised first by brand, then follow using the same format as the rest of the book.

Serving Sizes

Many ready-meal type foods are given with calories for the full pack size, so that an individual serving can be worked out by estimating the proportion of the pack that has been consumed. For example, if you have eaten a quarter of a packaged pasta dish, divide the calorie value given for the whole pack by 4 to determine the number of calories you have consumed. Where serving sizes are not appropriate, or unknown, values are given per 1oz/28g. Serving sizes vary greatly from person to person and, if you are trying to lose weight, it's very important to be accurate – especially with foods that are very high in calories such as those that contain a fair amount of fat, sugar, cream, cheese, alcohol etc.

Food Data

Nutrition information for basic average foods has been compiled by the Weight Loss Resources food data team using many sources of information to calculate the most accurate values possible. Some nutrition information for non-branded food records is from The Composition of Foods 6th Edition (2002). Reproduced under licence from The Controller of Her Majesty's Stationary Office. Where basic data is present for ordinary foodstuffs such as 'raw carrots'; branded records are not included.

Nutrition information for branded goods is from details supplied by retailers and manufacturers, and researched by Weight Loss Resources staff. The Calorie Carb & Fat Bible contains data for over 1400 UK brands, including major supermarkets and fast food outlets.

The publishers gratefully acknowledge all the manufacturers and retailers who have provided information on their products. All product names, trademarks or registered trademarks belong to their respective owners and are used only for the purpose of identifying products.

Calorie & nutrition data for all food and drink items are typical values.

Caution
The information in The Calorie, Carb and Fat Bible is intended as an aid to weight loss and weight maintenance, and is not medical advice. If you suffer from, or think you may suffer from a medical condition you should consult your doctor before starting a weight loss and/or exercise regime. If you start exercising after a period of relative inactivity, you should start slowly and consult your doctor if you experience pain, distress or other symptoms.

Weights, Measures & Abbreviations

ABBREVIATIONS

kcal	kilocalories / calories
prot	protein
carb	carbohydrate
sm	small
med	medium
av	average
reg	regular
lge	large
tsp	teaspoon
tbsp	tablespoon
dtsp	dessertspoon

BRAND ABBREVIATIONS USED

ASDA

Good for You	GFY

MARKS & SPENCER — M & S

Count on Us	COU

MORRISONS

Better For You	BFY

SAINSBURY'S

Be Good to Yourself	BGTY
Way to Five	WTF
Taste the Difference	TTD

TESCO

Healthy Living	HL

WAITROSE

Perfectly Balanced	PB

Weights, Measures
& Abbreviations

	Measure INFO/WEIGHT	per Measure KCAL	per Measure FAT	Nutrition Values per 100g / 100ml KCAL	PROT	CARB	FAT	FIBRE
ABALONE								
Cooked, Fried, Weighed without Shells	1 Serving/85g	161	5.8	189	19.6	11.0	6.8	0.0
Raw, Weighed without Shells	1 Serving/85g	89	0.6	105	17.1	6.0	0.8	0.0
ABSINTHE								
Average	*1 Shot/35ml*	*127*	*0.0*	*363*	*0.0*	*38.8*	*0.0*	*0.0*
ACKEE								
Canned, Drained, Average	*1oz/28g*	*43*	*4.3*	*151*	*2.9*	*0.8*	*15.2*	*0.0*
ADVOCAAT								
Average	*1 Shot/35ml*	*91*	*2.2*	*260*	*4.7*	*28.4*	*6.3*	*0.0*
AERO								
Creamy White Centre, Nestle*	1 Bar/46g	244	13.8	530	7.6	57.4	30.0	0.0
Milk, Medium, Bar, Nestle*	1 Bar/43g	232	13.3	539	6.6	57.7	30.9	2.2
Milk, Snacksize, Bar, Nestle*	1 Bar/21g	110	6.5	537	6.6	55.9	31.9	2.2
Milk, Standard, Bar, Nestle*	1 Bar/31g	165	9.6	531	6.3	56.9	30.9	0.8
Minis, Nestle*	1 Bar/11g	57	3.2	518	6.8	58.1	28.7	0.8
Mint, Bubbles, Aero, Nestle*	1 Bubble/3g	16	0.9	538	5.4	60.5	30.1	1.4
Mint, Nestle*	1 Bar/46g	245	13.7	533	4.9	61.2	29.8	0.4
Mint, Snack Size, Nestle*	1 Bar/21g	112	6.7	548	7.7	55.3	32.8	0.9
Mint, Standard, Aero, Nestle*	1 Bar/43g	233	13.2	542	5.2	60.5	30.8	0.9
Orange, Bubbles, Aero, Nestle*	1 Bubble/3g	16	0.9	538	5.4	60.5	30.0	1.4
Orange, Nestle*	6 Squares/22g	119	6.8	542	5.1	60.7	30.7	0.9
ALFALFA SPROUTS								
Raw, Average	1 Serving/33g	8	0.3	24	3.0	3.0	0.9	3.0
ALLSPICE								
Ground, Schwartz*	1 Tsp/3g	11	0.1	358	6.1	74.3	4.0	0.0
ALMONDS								
Blanched, Average	*1 Serving/100g*	*617*	*54.3*	*617*	*25.1*	*6.9*	*54.3*	*8.1*
Candied, Sugared	1 Serving/100g	458	16.3	458	8.4	69.2	16.3	2.2
Flaked, Average	*1oz/28g*	*172*	*15.2*	*613*	*24.9*	*6.5*	*54.3*	*7.6*
Flaked, Toasted, Average	*1oz/28g*	*176*	*15.8*	*629*	*24.6*	*5.8*	*56.4*	*7.5*
Ground, Average	*1 Serving/10g*	*62*	*5.6*	*625*	*24.0*	*6.6*	*55.8*	*7.4*
Marcona, Average	*1 Serving/100g*	*608*	*53.7*	*608*	*22.1*	*13.0*	*53.7*	*9.7*
Sugared, Co-Op*	1 Almond/6g	25	0.8	455	7.0	74.0	14.0	2.0
Toasted, Average	*1oz/28g*	*178*	*15.8*	*634*	*24.9*	*6.6*	*56.4*	*6.6*
Whole, Average	*1 Serving/20g*	*122*	*11.0*	*612*	*23.4*	*21.2*	*54.8*	*8.4*
ALOO TIKKI								
Average	1 Serving/25g	48	2.0	191	4.5	25.2	8.0	3.5
AMARANTH								
Grain, Cooked	1 Serving/100g	102	2.0	102	4.0	19.0	2.0	2.0
ANCHOVIES								
Fillets, Flat, John West*	1 Can/50g	113	7.0	226	25.0	0.1	14.0	0.0
Fillets, Tesco*	1 Serving/15g	34	2.1	226	25.0	0.0	14.0	0.0
in Oil, Canned, Drained	1 Anchovy/4g	8	0.5	195	23.4	0.0	11.3	0.0
Marinated, Sainsbury's*	¼ Pot/44g	78	4.0	177	22.0	2.0	9.0	0.1
Provencale, Finest, Tesco*	1 Anchovy/10g	20	1.3	201	22.0	0.0	12.6	0.0
Salted, Finest, Tesco*	1 Serving/10g	9	0.2	93	18.2	0.0	2.2	0.0
ANGEL DELIGHT								
Banana Flavour, Kraft*	1 Sachet/59g	280	12.3	474	2.3	69.3	20.9	0.3
Banana Toffee Flavour, No Added Sugar, Kraft*	1 Sachet/59g	292	15.6	495	4.8	58.5	26.5	0.0
Butterscotch Flavour, No Added Sugar, Kraft*	1 Sachet/47g	226	11.3	480	4.5	61.0	24.0	0.0
Chocolate Flavour, Kraft*	1 Sachet/67g	305	12.1	455	3.7	69.5	18.0	0.4
Raspberry Flavour, No Added Sugar, Kraft*	1 Sachet/59g	292	15.3	495	4.8	59.5	26.0	0.0
Strawberry Flavour, No Added Sugar, Kraft*	1 Sachet/47g	230	12.5	490	4.8	59.0	26.5	0.0
Toffee Flavour, Kraft*	1 Sachet/59g	283	12.4	480	2.0	70.0	21.0	0.0

	Measure INFO/WEIGHT	per Measure		Nutrition Values per 100g / 100ml				
		KCAL	FAT	KCAL	PROT	CARB	FAT	FIBRE
ANGEL DELIGHT								
Vanilla Ice Cream Flavour, Kraft*	1 Sachet/59g	289	12.7	490	2.5	71.5	21.5	0.0
Vanilla Ice Cream Flavour, No Added Sugar, Kraft*	1 Sachet/59g	295	15.9	500	4.8	59.5	27.0	0.0
ANGEL HAIR								
Pasta, Dry	1 Serving/50g	181	1.1	362	12.4	73.6	2.2	4.4
ANTIPASTO								
Artichoke, Sainsbury's*	1 Serving/50g	67	6.2	135	2.0	3.6	12.5	2.3
Mixed Pepper, Sainsbury's*	½ Jar/140g	48	1.8	34	1.3	4.2	1.3	3.5
Parma Ham, from Selection Platter, TTD, Sainsbury's*	1 Serving/100g	236	12.9	236	29.9	0.1	12.9	0.0
Roasted Pepper, Drained, Tesco*	1 Jar/170g	127	9.3	75	0.9	5.5	5.5	4.1
Seafood, Drained, Sainsbury's*	½ Jar/84g	150	9.7	178	14.3	4.1	11.6	1.4
Sun Dried Tomato, Sainsbury's*	¼ Jar/70g	275	25.0	393	4.5	13.4	35.7	6.2
APPLES								
Bites, Average	1 Pack/118g	58	0.1	49	0.3	11.6	0.1	2.2
Braeburn, Average	*1 Apple/123g*	*58*	*0.1*	*47*	*0.3*	*11.4*	*0.1*	*2.0*
Cooking, Baked with Sugar, Flesh Only, Average	*1 Serving/140g*	*104*	*0.1*	*74*	*0.5*	*19.2*	*0.1*	*1.7*
Cooking, Raw, Peeled, Average	*1oz/28g*	*10*	*0.0*	*35*	*0.3*	*8.9*	*0.1*	*1.6*
Cooking, Stewed with Sugar, Average	*1 Serving/140g*	*104*	*0.1*	*74*	*0.3*	*19.1*	*0.1*	*1.2*
Cooking, Stewed without Sugar, Average	*1 Serving/140g*	*46*	*0.1*	*33*	*0.3*	*8.1*	*0.1*	*1.5*
Cox, English, Average	*1 Apple/108g*	*52*	*0.1*	*48*	*0.4*	*11.3*	*0.1*	*2.0*
Discovery, Average	*1 Apple/182g*	*82*	*0.9*	*45*	*0.3*	*10.5*	*0.5*	*0.9*
Dried, Average	*1 Pack/250g*	*537*	*0.7*	*215*	*0.8*	*52.8*	*0.3*	*5.9*
Empire, Average	*1 Apple/120g*	*58*	*0.1*	*48*	*0.4*	*11.8*	*0.1*	*2.0*
Fuji, Average	1 Apple/132g	64	0.1	48	0.4	11.8	0.1	1.8
Gala, Average	*1 Apple/152g*	*73*	*0.2*	*48*	*0.4*	*11.6*	*0.1*	*1.6*
Golden Delicious, Average	*1 Med/102g*	*48*	*0.2*	*47*	*0.3*	*11.2*	*0.1*	*1.7*
Granny Smith, Average	*1 Sm/125g*	*62*	*0.1*	*50*	*0.4*	*11.9*	*0.1*	*2.0*
Green, Raw, Average	*1 Med/182g*	*86*	*0.2*	*47*	*0.3*	*11.3*	*0.1*	*1.7*
Mackintosh, Red, Average	*1 Apple/165g*	*81*	*0.5*	*49*	*0.2*	*12.8*	*0.3*	*1.8*
Pink Lady, Average	*1 Apple/125g*	*62*	*0.1*	*50*	*0.4*	*11.7*	*0.1*	*2.1*
Sliced, Average	*1oz/28g*	*14*	*0.0*	*49*	*0.4*	*11.6*	*0.1*	*1.8*
APPLETISER*								
Juice Drink, Sparkling, Appletiser, Coca-Cola*	1 Glass/200ml	94	0.0	47	0.0	11.0	0.0	0.4
APRICOTS								
Canned, in Syrup, Average	*1oz/28g*	*18*	*0.0*	*63*	*0.4*	*16.1*	*0.1*	*0.9*
Dried, Average	*1 Apricot/10g*	*17*	*0.1*	*171*	*3.6*	*37.4*	*0.5*	*6.3*
Dried, Soft, Average	*1 Serving/50g*	*104*	*0.2*	*208*	*2.4*	*48.5*	*0.4*	*5.2*
Halves, in Fruit Juice, Average	*1 Can/221g*	*87*	*0.1*	*40*	*0.5*	*9.2*	*0.1*	*1.0*
Raw, Flesh Only, Average	*1 Apricot/37g*	*19*	*0.2*	*52*	*1.5*	*12.0*	*0.4*	*2.1*
Raw, Weighed with Stone, Average	*1 Apricot/40g*	*19*	*0.2*	*48*	*1.4*	*11.1*	*0.4*	*2.0*
ARCHERS*								
Aqua, Peach, Archers*	1 Bottle/275ml	206	0.0	75	0.3	5.1	0.0	0.0
Peach (Calculated Estimate), Archers*	1 Shot/35ml	91	0.0	260	0.0	0.0	0.0	0.0
ARTICHOKE								
Chargrilled, in Olive Oil, Cooks Ingredients, Waitrose*	1 Serving/40g	52	4.9	129	1.7	2.7	12.3	2.7
Fresh, Raw, Average	*1oz/28g*	*13*	*0.0*	*47*	*3.3*	*10.5*	*0.1*	*5.4*
Hearts, Canned, Drained, Average	*½ Can/117g*	*35*	*0.1*	*30*	*1.9*	*5.4*	*0.0*	*2.1*
Hearts, Sliced with Extra Virgin Olive Oil, Waitrose*	1 Serving/40g	24	1.6	59	1.3	4.4	4.0	7.0
Marinated in Oil with Parsley & Garlic, Drained, M & S*	1 Serving/100g	115	11.9	115	1.5	0.5	11.9	4.7
ASAFOETIDA								
Powder, Schwartz*	1 Tbsp/0.7g	2	0.0	271	6.5	56.2	2.2	0.0
ASPARAGUS								
Boiled, in Salted Water, Average	*5 Spears/125g*	*32*	*1.0*	*26*	*3.4*	*1.4*	*0.8*	*1.4*
Canned, Average	*1 Can/250g*	*47*	*0.5*	*19*	*2.3*	*2.0*	*0.2*	*1.6*

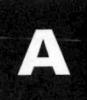

	Measure INFO/WEIGHT	per Measure		Nutrition Values per 100g / 100ml				
		KCAL	FAT	KCAL	PROT	CARB	FAT	FIBRE
ASPARAGUS								
Spears, Frozen, Asda*	1 Serving/80g	23	0.6	29	3.4	1.4	0.8	1.4
Trimmed, Raw, Average	*1 Serving/80g*	*20*	*0.4*	*24*	*2.9*	*1.9*	*0.5*	*1.7*
ASPIRE								
Cranberry Flavoured Soft Drink, Aspire*	1 Can/250ml	12	0.0	5	0.0	1.1	0.0	0.0
AUBERGINE								
Fried, Average	*1oz/28g*	*85*	*8.9*	*302*	*1.2*	*2.8*	*31.9*	*2.3*
Marinated & Grilled, Waitrose*	½ Pack/100g	106	10.0	106	1.0	3.0	10.0	2.0
Raw, Fresh, Average	*1 Sm/250g*	*37*	*1.0*	*15*	*0.9*	*2.2*	*0.4*	*2.0*
AVOCADO								
Flesh Only, Average	*1 Med/145g*	*275*	*28.3*	*190*	*1.9*	*1.9*	*19.5*	*3.4*

	Measure INFO/WEIGHT	per Measure		Nutrition Values per 100g / 100ml				
		KCAL	FAT	KCAL	PROT	CARB	FAT	FIBRE
BACARDI*								
& Diet Cola, Bacardi*	1 Bottle/275ml	85	0.0	31	0.0	1.0	0.0	0.0
*37.5% Volume, Bacardi**	*1 Shot/35ml*	*72*	*0.0*	*207*	*0.0*	*0.0*	*0.0*	*0.0*
*40% Volume, Bacardi**	*1 Shot/35ml*	*78*	*0.0*	*222*	*0.0*	*0.0*	*0.0*	*0.0*
Breezer, Apple, Half Sugar, Crisp, Bacardi*	1 Bottle/275ml	121	0.0	44	0.0	3.7	0.0	0.0
Breezer, Cranberry, Bacardi*	1 Bottle/275ml	154	0.0	56	0.0	7.1	0.0	0.0
Breezer, Half Sugar, Bacardi*	1 Bottle/275ml	122	0.0	44	0.0	0.0	0.0	0.0
Breezer, Lemon, Diet, Bacardi*	1 Bottle/275ml	96	0.0	35	0.0	1.2	0.0	0.0
Breezer, Lime, Bacardi*	1 Bottle/275ml	181	0.0	66	0.0	9.1	0.0	0.0
Breezer, Orange, Bacardi*	1 Bottle/275ml	179	0.0	65	0.0	8.2	0.0	0.0
Breezer, Orange, Diet, Bacardi*	1 Bottle/275ml	80	0.0	29	0.0	0.0	0.0	0.0
Breezer, Pineapple, Bacardi*	1 Bottle/275ml	102	0.0	37	0.0	3.1	0.0	0.0
Breezer, Raspberry, Half Sugar, Refreshing, Bacardi*	1 Bottle/275ml	99	0.0	36	0.0	3.3	0.0	0.0
Breezer, Watermelon, Bacardi*	1 Bottle/275ml	100	0.0	36	0.0	3.2	0.0	0.0
BACON								
Back, Dry Cured, Average	*1 Rasher/31g*	*77*	*4.7*	*250*	*28.1*	*0.3*	*15.1*	*0.3*
Back, Dry Fried or Grilled, Average	*1 Rasher/25g*	*72*	*5.4*	*287*	*23.2*	*0.0*	*21.6*	*0.0*
Back, Lean, Average	*1 Rasher/33g*	*57*	*4.0*	*173*	*16.3*	*0.1*	*12.0*	*0.5*
Back, Smoked, Average	*1 Rasher/25g*	*66*	*5.0*	*265*	*20.9*	*0.0*	*19.9*	*0.0*
Back, Smoked, Lean, Average	*1 Rasher/25g*	*41*	*1.2*	*163*	*28.2*	*1.1*	*5.0*	*0.2*
Back, Smoked, Rindless, Average	*1 Rasher/25g*	*60*	*4.3*	*241*	*21.0*	*0.1*	*17.4*	*0.0*
Back, Tendersweet, Average	*1 Rasher/25g*	*63*	*3.6*	*250*	*29.8*	*0.4*	*14.3*	*0.0*
Back, Unsmoked, Average	*1 Rasher/32g*	*78*	*5.5*	*243*	*21.3*	*0.4*	*17.3*	*0.0*
Back, Unsmoked, Rindless, Average	*1 Rasher/23g*	*56*	*3.9*	*241*	*22.5*	*0.0*	*16.9*	*0.0*
Chops, Average	*1oz/28g*	*62*	*4.2*	*222*	*22.3*	*0.0*	*14.8*	*0.0*
Collar Joint, Lean & Fat, Boiled	*1oz/28g*	*91*	*7.6*	*325*	*20.4*	*0.0*	*27.0*	*0.0*
Collar Joint, Lean & Fat, Raw	*1oz/28g*	*89*	*8.1*	*319*	*14.6*	*0.0*	*28.9*	*0.0*
Collar Joint, Lean Only, Boiled	*1oz/28g*	*53*	*2.7*	*191*	*26.0*	*0.0*	*9.7*	*0.0*
Fat Only, Cooked, Average	*1oz/28g*	*194*	*20.4*	*692*	*9.3*	*0.0*	*72.8*	*0.0*
Fat Only, Raw, Average	*1oz/28g*	*209*	*22.7*	*747*	*4.8*	*0.0*	*80.9*	*0.0*
Lean, Average	*1 Rasher/33g*	*47*	*2.2*	*142*	*19.6*	*0.9*	*6.7*	*0.2*
Lean Only, Fried, Average	*1 Rasher/25g*	*83*	*5.6*	*332*	*32.8*	*0.0*	*22.3*	*0.0*
Lean Only, Grilled, Average	*1 Rasher/25g*	*73*	*4.7*	*292*	*30.5*	*0.0*	*18.9*	*0.0*
Loin Steaks, Grilled, Average	*1 Serving/120g*	*229*	*11.6*	*191*	*25.9*	*0.0*	*9.7*	*0.0*
Medallions, Average	*1 Rasher/18g*	*27*	*0.6*	*151*	*29.3*	*0.9*	*3.3*	*0.1*
Middle, Fried	*1 Rasher/40g*	*140*	*11.4*	*350*	*23.4*	*0.0*	*28.5*	*0.0*
Middle, Grilled	*1 Rasher/40g*	*123*	*9.2*	*307*	*24.8*	*0.0*	*23.1*	*0.0*
Middle, Raw	*1 Rasher/43g*	*104*	*8.6*	*241*	*15.2*	*0.0*	*20.0*	*0.0*
Rashers, Lean Only, Trimmed, Average	1 Rasher/20g	24	0.8	119	20.6	0.0	4.0	0.0
Rindless, Average	*1 Rasher/20g*	*30*	*1.7*	*150*	*18.5*	*0.0*	*8.5*	*0.0*
Smoked, Average	*1 Rasher/28g*	*46*	*2.1*	*166*	*24.7*	*0.2*	*7.3*	*0.0*
Smoked, Crispy, Cooked, Average	*1 Serving/10g*	*46*	*2.7*	*460*	*53.0*	*2.1*	*26.9*	*0.0*
Smoked, Rindless, Average	*1 Rasher/20g*	*21*	*0.6*	*106*	*19.8*	*0.0*	*3.0*	*0.0*
Streaky, Average	*1oz/28g*	*76*	*5.9*	*270*	*20.0*	*0.0*	*21.0*	*0.0*
Streaky, Cooked, Average	*1 Rasher/20g*	*68*	*5.6*	*342*	*22.4*	*0.3*	*27.8*	*0.0*
Vegetarian, Rashers	*1 Rasher/16g*	*33*	*1.7*	*206*	*19.5*	*8.6*	*10.4*	*2.8*
BACON BITS								
Average	*1oz/28g*	*75*	*5.9*	*268*	*18.6*	*0.7*	*21.2*	*0.1*
BACON VEGETARIAN								
Rashers, Cheatin', The Redwood Co*	1 Rasher/16g	32	1.2	196	25.9	7.3	7.3	0.5
Rashers, Tesco*	1 Rasher/20g	41	2.2	203	22.5	3.3	11.1	3.9
Realeat*	1 Rasher/19g	49	1.1	260	27.0	25.0	5.8	1.6
Streaky Style Rashers, Tesco*	1 Rasher/8g	17	0.8	215	23.7	5.0	10.6	2.2
Strips, Morningstar Farms*	1 Strip/8g	30	2.3	375	12.5	12.5	28.1	6.2

	Measure INFO/WEIGHT	per Measure KCAL	FAT	Nutrition Values per 100g / 100ml KCAL	PROT	CARB	FAT	FIBRE
BAGEL								
Bacon, & Soft Cheese, Boots*	1 Serving/148g	481	25.2	325	12.0	31.0	17.0	2.2
Cream Cheese, & Salmon, Smoked, M & S*	1 Bagel/23g	64	2.8	280	10.9	31.7	12.2	2.9
Cream Cheese, M & S*	1 Bagel/23g	79	4.9	352	7.8	31.0	21.8	1.8
Ham, & Pesto, COU, M & S*	1 Pack/173g	259	2.4	150	11.1	23.5	1.4	1.7
Soft Cheese, & Salmon, Smoked, Finest, Tesco*	1 Pack/173g	396	10.0	229	13.1	31.2	5.8	1.7
Tuna, & Salad, BGTY, Sainsbury's*	1 Bagel/170g	325	7.1	191	10.4	26.0	4.2	1.0
Turkey, & Cranberry, Bagelmania*	1 Pack/198g	325	7.3	164	9.0	24.5	3.7	1.1
Turkey, Pastrami & American Mustard, Shapers, Boots*	1 Bagel/146g	296	5.0	203	11.0	32.0	3.4	1.4
BAGUETTE								
All Day Breakfast, Darwins Deli*	1 Serving/184g	498	21.5	271	13.4	31.9	11.7	0.0
Beef & Horseradish, Freshly Prepared, M & S*	1 Baguette/274g	795	31.0	290	12.1	37.2	11.3	2.0
Brie, Tomato & Rocket, Freshly Prepared, M & S*	1 Baguette/219g	570	21.7	260	10.3	33.2	9.9	1.9
Cheese, & Tomato, Tesco*	1 Baguette/108g	243	8.3	225	9.7	29.3	7.7	1.8
Cheese, Tomato, & Basil, Asda*	¼ Baguette/42g	138	5.9	329	10.0	40.8	14.0	1.3
Cheese & Ham, Average	1 Baguette/203g	593	20.8	292	13.9	35.9	10.3	1.3
Chicken, & Mayonnaise, Asda*	1 Pack/190g	407	16.5	214	9.7	30.5	8.7	1.3
Chicken, & Salad, Asda*	1 Serving/158g	326	9.5	206	9.0	29.0	6.0	2.1
Chicken, & Salad, Shapers, Boots*	1 Baguette/132g	222	2.6	168	11.0	27.0	2.0	1.5
Chicken, Honey & Mustard, BGTY, Sainsbury's*	1 Pack/187g	340	3.7	182	11.0	30.0	2.0	0.0
Chicken, Oakham, Fresh, M & S*	1 Baguette/225g	450	10.8	200	12.4	26.7	4.8	1.5
Chicken, Tikka, Asda*	1 Pack/190g	439	17.9	231	10.4	32.8	9.4	1.3
Chicken, Tikka, Hot, Sainsbury's*	1 Pack/190g	386	11.6	203	8.5	28.4	6.1	0.0
Egg, Bacon & Tomato, Freshly Prepared, M & S*	1 Baguette/182g	455	17.3	250	12.9	28.0	9.5	1.7
Egg Mayonnaise, & Cress, Cafe, Sainsbury's*	1 Pack/100g	480	20.4	480	13.8	60.2	20.4	0.0
Ham, & Cheese, Freshly Prepared, M & S*	1 Baguette/231g	555	11.3	240	13.4	35.9	4.9	2.4
Ham, & Salad with Mustard Mayonnaise, Sainsbury's*	1 Baguette/100g	412	15.9	412	17.6	49.6	15.9	0.1
Ham, & Turkey, Asda*	1 Baguette/360g	774	18.4	215	11.6	30.7	5.1	1.3
Prawn, French, Shell*	1 Baguette/63g	171	7.2	272	9.7	32.4	11.5	0.0
Prawn Mayonnaise, Asda*	1 Pack/190g	399	9.3	210	9.1	32.5	4.9	1.3
Smoked Salmon & Egg, Freshly Prepared	1 Baguette/178g	455	17.3	255	13.7	28.4	9.7	1.6
Steak, & Onion, Snack 'n' Go, Sainsbury's*	1 Baguette/177g	398	8.8	225	14.3	30.6	5.0	2.2
Tuna, Crunch, Shapers, Boots*	1 Pack/138g	315	4.8	228	14.0	35.0	3.5	3.1
Tuna, Melt, Sainsbury's*	1 Serving/204g	373	8.0	183	11.3	25.8	3.9	0.0
BAILEYS*								
Glide, Baileys*	1 Serving/200ml	212	2.4	106	0.0	18.0	1.2	0.0
Irish Cream, Original, Baileys*	1 Serving/50ml	163	6.5	327	3.0	25.0	13.0	0.0
BAKE								
Aubergine & Mozzarella, Finest, Tesco*	1 Pack/400g	288	13.6	72	3.6	6.7	3.4	2.6
Aubergine & Mozzarella Cheese, BGTY, Sainsbury's*	1 Pack/360g	194	7.2	54	3.0	6.0	2.0	1.3
Beef, Minced, & Root Vegetable, COU, M & S*	1 Pack/400g	320	11.6	80	6.6	6.0	2.9	3.0
Bolognese, Mini Classics, Co-Op*	1 Pack/300g	345	13.2	115	5.8	12.5	4.4	2.1
Broccoli & Cheese, Asda*	1 Bake/132g	269	15.4	204	5.3	19.3	11.7	2.5
Broccoli & Cheese, M & S*	1 Pack/400g	380	22.8	95	4.8	5.6	5.7	1.1
Cheese & Spinach, Tesco*	1 Bake/140g	269	10.9	192	4.5	26.0	7.8	1.4
Cheesy Broccoli, Asda*	1 Pack/400g	400	17.6	100	4.5	10.6	4.4	1.4
Chicken, & Mushroom, COU, M & S*	1 Serving/360g	324	8.3	90	7.3	10.3	2.3	1.1
Chicken Arrabiatta, M & S*	1 Pack/450g	540	13.5	120	7.6	16.0	3.0	2.0
Chicken Spiralli, M & S*	1 Serving/400g	400	15.2	100	7.9	9.1	3.8	1.1
Cod, & Prawn, 327, Oakhouse Foods Ltd*	1 Meal/340g	466	23.5	137	8.6	10.3	6.9	0.3
Cod, & Prawn, COU, M & S*	1 Pack/400g	320	8.0	80	6.5	8.8	2.0	1.0
Courgette, & Tomato, Cauldron Foods*	1 Pack/285g	593	37.0	208	10.0	17.0	13.0	6.4
Fish, & Vegetable, Youngs*	1 Serving/375g	446	23.6	119	5.6	10.0	6.3	1.3
Fish, Haddock, Average	1 Serving/400g	312	9.2	78	6.4	8.0	2.3	0.9

	Measure INFO/WEIGHT	per Measure KCAL	FAT	Nutrition Values per 100g / 100ml KCAL	PROT	CARB	FAT	FIBRE
BAKE								
Fish, Haddock, Smoked, Light & Easy, Youngs*	1 Pack/310g	242	7.1	78	6.4	8.0	2.3	0.9
Fish, with Carrots & Peas, Light & Easy, Youngs*	1 Pack/240g	168	4.1	70	8.3	5.4	1.7	1.4
Haddock, Smoked, Light & Easy, Youngs*	1 Pack/300g	234	6.9	78	6.4	8.0	2.3	0.9
Haddock, Smoked, Luxury, Light & Easy, Youngs*	1 Pack/355g	390	17.0	110	7.5	9.2	4.8	0.6
Lentil, Spiced, Vegetarian, TTD, Sainsbury's*	1 Bake/132g	245	8.4	186	4.8	27.3	6.4	4.2
Mediterranean Vegetable Bistro, Frozen, Cauldron Foods*	1 Bake/100g	190	10.0	190	4.0	21.0	10.0	3.0
Mushroom, Cauldron Foods*	1 Serving/100g	164	12.0	164	6.0	15.0	12.0	6.0
Mushroom, Leek & Spinach, Cumberland, Sainsbury's*	1 Pack/450g	518	24.3	115	3.6	12.9	5.4	1.2
Penne Bolognese, BGTY, Sainsbury's*	1 Pack/400g	492	10.8	123	7.0	17.7	2.7	1.3
Peppercorn, Vegetarian, Creamy, Tesco*	1 Serving/140g	322	16.8	230	3.6	27.0	12.0	1.2
Potato, Cheese, & Bacon, Homepride*	1 Serving/210g	277	26.2	132	1.6	3.2	12.5	0.0
Potato, Cheese, & Onion, Tesco*	1 Pack/400g	376	19.6	94	2.4	10.0	4.9	1.0
Potato, Mushroom & Leek, M & S*	1 Serving/225g	225	13.3	100	3.5	10.0	5.9	2.0
Potato & Vegetable, Co-Op*	1 Bake/340g	425	27.2	125	4.0	11.0	8.0	1.0
Roast Onion & Potato, COU, M & S*	1 Pack/450g	337	5.8	75	1.9	13.6	1.3	1.5
Salmon, & Broccoli, Youngs*	1 Bake/375g	409	19.1	109	6.3	9.6	5.1	1.3
Salmon, & Broccoli 329, Oakhouse Foods Ltd*	1 Meal/400g	624	44.4	156	5.0	9.1	11.1	0.6
Salmon, & Prawn, M & S*	1 Bake/329g	460	31.2	140	7.4	6.6	9.5	0.7
Smoked Haddock, & Prawn, BGTY, Sainsbury's*	1 Pack/350g	318	2.4	91	7.5	13.6	0.7	1.1
Vegetable, Multigrain, Grassington's Food Co*	1 Bake/106g	148	3.6	140	4.9	22.4	3.4	5.0
BAKING POWDER								
Average	*1 Tsp/2g*	*3*	*0.0*	*163*	*5.2*	*37.8*	*0.0*	*0.0*
BAKLAVA								
Average	2 Pieces/50g	239	14.2	478	8.0	47.4	28.3	2.8
BALTI								
Chick Pea, & Spinach, Cauldron Foods*	1 Pack/400g	356	8.0	89	2.3	15.5	2.0	1.0
Chicken, & Mushroom, Tesco*	1 Serving/350g	325	10.5	93	12.3	4.2	3.0	0.7
Chicken, & Rice, M & S*	1 Pack/400g	380	6.0	95	6.9	14.1	1.5	1.2
Chicken, Asda*	1 Pack/450g	324	9.9	72	8.0	5.0	2.2	0.0
Chicken, Indian Takeaway, Iceland*	1 Pack/402g	362	19.3	90	7.8	4.0	4.8	0.7
Chicken, Morrisons*	1 Pack/350g	441	26.6	126	12.1	2.3	7.6	1.5
Chicken, Takeaway, Sainsbury's*	1 Pack/400g	404	18.0	101	10.4	4.8	4.5	1.4
Chicken, with Garlic & Coriander Naan, Frozen, Patak's*	1 Pack/375g	431	18.7	115	6.3	11.1	5.0	1.1
Chicken, with Naan Bread, Perfectly Balanced, Waitrose*	1 Pack/375g	450	13.5	120	12.1	9.7	3.6	2.8
Chicken, with Naan Bread, Sharwood's*	1 Pack/375g	529	23.2	141	7.3	14.1	6.2	2.2
Chicken, with Pilau Rice, Asda*	1 Pack/504g	625	24.7	124	5.0	15.0	4.9	1.2
Chicken, with Pilau Rice, Weight Watchers*	1 Pack/329g	306	4.3	93	6.9	13.4	1.3	1.2
Chicken, with Pilau Rice & Naan Bread, Tesco*	1 Meal/550g	660	19.8	120	6.1	15.5	3.6	1.4
Chicken, with Potato Wedges, HL, Tesco*	1 Pack/450g	387	9.4	86	6.0	10.8	2.1	1.1
Chicken, with Rice, Curry Break, Patak's*	1 Pack/220g	198	6.2	90	4.7	11.6	2.8	0.0
Chicken, with Rice, Patak's*	1 Pack/370g	440	12.9	119	6.1	16.7	3.5	1.7
Chicken Ceylon, Finest, Tesco*	1 Pack/400g	588	38.0	147	14.4	0.9	9.5	5.0
Chicken Tikka, & Wedges, HL, Tesco*	1 Pack/450g	391	9.9	87	6.0	10.7	2.2	1.3
Lamb, Bhuna, Tesco*	1 Pack/400g	360	14.8	90	9.2	4.8	3.7	1.1
Prawn, Budgens*	1 Pack/350g	374	24.8	107	5.6	5.2	7.1	1.3
Vegetable, & Rice, Tesco*	1 Pack/450g	378	7.2	84	2.0	15.6	1.6	1.3
Vegetable, Average	1 Serving/200g	182	8.3	91	1.9	11.3	4.1	1.7
Vegetable, Chosen By You, Asda*	1 Pack/200g	190	11.6	95	2.0	7.7	5.8	2.0
Vegetable, GFY, Asda*	1 Pack/450g	324	4.0	72	1.9	14.0	0.9	1.5
BAMBOO SHOOTS								
Canned, Average	*1 Can/120g*	*11*	*0.2*	*9*	*1.1*	*0.9*	*0.1*	*0.9*
BANANA								
Raw, Flesh Only, Average	*1 Sm/95g*	*90*	*0.3*	*95*	*1.2*	*20.9*	*0.3*	*4.2*

B

	Measure INFO/WEIGHT	per Measure KCAL	FAT	Nutrition Values per 100g / 100ml KCAL	PROT	CARB	FAT	FIBRE
BANANA								
Raw, Weighed with Skin, Average	*1 Lge/185g*	*176*	*0.6*	*95*	*1.2*	*20.9*	*0.3*	*4.2*
Slices, Dried, Love Life, Waitrose*	1 Serving/25g	74	0.1	295	4.8	66.5	0.6	5.2
BANANA CHIPS								
Average	*1oz/28g*	*143*	*8.8*	*511*	*1.0*	*59.9*	*31.4*	*1.7*
BANGERS & MASH								
& Beans, Blue Parrot Cafe, Sainsbury's*	1 Pack/300g	354	12.6	118	5.3	14.8	4.2	2.1
Asda*	1 Pack/400g	636	28.0	159	9.0	15.0	7.0	1.6
Co-Op*	1 Pack/300g	375	18.0	125	4.0	13.0	6.0	0.8
Morrisons*	1 Pack/300g	306	14.7	102	3.0	12.3	4.9	0.8
BARS								
All Bran, Apple, Kellogg's*	1 Bar/40g	158	7.6	395	8.0	48.0	19.0	5.0
All Bran, Honey & Oat, Kellogg's*	1 Bar/27g	99	2.2	366	6.0	67.0	8.0	12.0
All Fruit, Frusli, Strawberry, Jordans*	1 Bar/30g	94	0.1	313	2.3	81.3	0.3	5.0
Almond & Cranberry, Day Break, Atkins*	1 Bar/37g	137	5.9	371	37.0	23.0	16.0	15.0
Am, Breakfast Muffin, Apple & Sultana, McVitie's*	1 Bar/45g	168	7.5	373	4.4	54.9	16.7	1.6
Am, Cereal, Apricot, McVitie's*	1 Bar/30g	146	6.1	486	6.5	68.8	20.5	0.5
Am, Cereal, Berry, McVitie's*	1 Bar/30g	146	6.1	486	6.5	68.8	20.5	0.5
Am, Cereal, Fruit & Nut, McVitie's*	1 Bar/35g	167	7.5	477	6.6	64.9	21.4	3.4
Am, Cereal, Raisin & Nut, McVitie's*	1 Bar/35g	148	5.8	422	6.4	62.1	16.4	2.4
Am, Granola, Almond, Raisin & Cranberry, McVitie's*	1 Bar/35g	133	4.0	380	7.1	62.9	11.4	4.0
Am, Muesli Fingers, McVitie's*	1 Bar/35g	154	6.9	440	6.0	59.8	19.6	3.1
Apple, & Cinnamon, Breakfast Snack, Tesco*	1 Bar/38g	137	4.7	365	4.3	58.8	12.5	2.0
Apple, & Cinnamon, Chewy, GFY, Asda*	1 Bar/27g	95	0.7	351	6.0	76.0	2.6	3.5
Apple, & Raisin, Snack, Geobar, Traidcraft*	1 Bar/35g	127	1.7	362	3.3	76.4	4.8	2.3
Apple, Geobar, Traidcraft*	1 Bar/35g	132	3.1	376	5.3	69.0	8.8	3.5
Apple, Granola, McVitie's*	1 Bar/35g	128	3.4	366	6.6	63.1	9.7	4.3
Apricot, & Almond, Eat Natural*	1 Bar/50g	202	8.1	403	11.2	53.3	16.1	0.0
Apricot, & Almond, Truly Juicy, Raw Health*	1 Bar/45g	182	10.3	405	17.0	49.0	23.0	9.0
Apricot, & Orange, Diet Chef Ltd*	1 Bar/25g	97	1.7	388	4.3	75.2	7.0	2.4
Apricot, & Peach, Multigrain, BGTY, Sainsbury's*	1 Bar/25g	70	0.6	282	6.6	58.2	2.5	23.1
Apricot, Fruity Grain, Tesco*	1 Bar/37g	135	2.6	366	6.5	65.0	7.0	2.5
Banoffee, Weight Watchers*	1 Bar/18g	68	0.9	379	6.3	77.0	5.1	3.0
Berry Delight, Gluten Free, Nak'd*	1 Bar/35g	135	5.2	385	9.0	52.0	15.0	6.0
Berry Snack, Diet Chef Ltd*	1 Bar/27g	96	2.2	356	7.2	64.0	8.2	5.5
Biscuit, Chocolate, Penguin, McVitie's*	1 Bar/25g	130	6.9	520	5.2	62.4	27.7	2.4
Biscuit, Medley, Raisin & Chocolate Hob Nob, McVitie's*	1 Bar/31g	131	4.1	422	5.5	69.4	13.3	3.6
Black Forest, Weight Watchers*	1 Bar/23g	94	2.0	408	3.9	78.4	8.8	1.4
Blue Riband, 99 Calories, Nestle*	1 Bar/19g	99	4.9	513	4.8	66.4	25.3	0.0
Blue Riband, Double Choc, Nestle*	1 Bar/22g	113	5.6	513	4.8	66.4	25.3	1.1
Blueberry, Fruit & Grain, Asda*	1 Bar/37g	124	2.6	335	4.1	64.0	7.0	3.9
Blueberry, Weight Watchers*	1 Bar/25g	91	1.8	365	4.5	74.9	7.4	2.2
Boohbah, Milk & White Chocolate, M & S*	1 Bar/75g	405	24.2	540	7.9	54.7	32.3	1.2
Breakfast, Apple Crisp, Morning Start, Atkins*	1 Bar/37g	145	7.9	392	29.2	25.4	21.3	13.8
Breakfast, Chocolate Chip Crisp, Morning Start, Atkins*	1 Bar/37g	137	7.0	370	31.8	22.5	18.8	15.0
Breakfast, Vitality, Fruit & Fibre, Asda*	1 Bar/29g	113	2.9	390	6.0	69.0	10.0	4.1
Breakfast, Vitality, Tropical Fruit, Asda*	1 Bar/28g	101	1.1	361	6.0	75.0	4.1	4.4
Brunch, Hazelnut, Cadbury*	1 Bar/35g	160	7.4	460	7.0	60.5	21.4	2.2
Brunch, Snack, Raisin, Cadbury*	1 Bar/35g	150	5.4	430	5.6	66.4	15.5	1.8
Caramel, Double, Chocolate, Crunch, Atkins*	1 Bar/44g	160	9.0	364	22.7	50.0	20.4	25.0
Caramel, Nut Chew, Endulge, Atkins*	1 Bar/34g	130	2.7	382	5.0	17.0	8.0	6.0
Cereal, 3 Berries & Cherries, Dorset Cereals*	1 Bar/35g	127	1.7	363	5.7	73.9	4.9	5.2
Cereal, 3 Fruit, Nuts & Seeds, Dorset Cereals*	1 Bar/35g	136	3.6	389	7.4	66.6	10.3	6.2
Cereal, Apple & Blackberry with Yoghurt, Alpen*	1 Bar/29g	117	3.1	404	5.4	71.8	10.6	5.0

BARS

	Measure INFO/WEIGHT	per Measure KCAL	FAT	Nutrition Values per 100g / 100ml KCAL	PROT	CARB	FAT	FIBRE
Cereal, Apple & Cinnamon, Fruit 'n' Grain, Asda*	1 Bar/37g	131	2.6	353	4.5	68.0	7.0	2.9
Cereal, Apple & Cinnamon, Tesco*	1 Bar/38g	137	4.7	365	4.3	58.9	12.5	2.1
Cereal, Apple & Raisin, Harvest, Quaker Oats*	1 Bar/22g	87	2.5	396	5.0	70.0	11.5	4.0
Cereal, Apple & Raspberry, Waitrose*	1 Bar/25g	90	0.8	359	5.0	77.1	3.4	4.6
Cereal, Apple & Sultana, Light, Alpen*	1 Bar/20g	63	0.7	330	4.1	59.4	3.6	21.7
Cereal, Apricot & Yoghurt, Shapers, Boots*	1 Bar/27g	99	1.5	366	3.7	75.0	5.7	3.3
Cereal, Balance with Fruit, Sainsbury's*	1 Bar/25g	100	2.1	401	5.8	75.2	8.6	1.9
Cereal, Banoffee, COU, M & S*	1 Bar/20g	75	0.4	375	4.5	82.5	2.0	2.5
Cereal, Banoffee, Vitality, Asda*	1 Bar/22g	73	0.6	331	6.5	69.6	2.9	13.5
Cereal, Berry & Cream, COU, M & S*	1 Bar/20g	72	0.5	360	5.3	79.7	2.3	3.1
Cereal, Blackcurrant & Apple, GFY, Asda*	1 Bar/25g	72	0.6	287	7.0	59.0	2.6	22.0
Cereal, Bran, Apple & Pomegranate, Morrisons*	1 Bar/25g	89	1.1	357	7.0	72.5	4.3	7.5
Cereal, Brownie, COU, M & S*	1 Bar/21g	75	0.5	365	5.5	79.7	2.6	4.6
Cereal, Chewy, BGTY, Sainsbury's*	1 Bar/25g	85	0.5	342	4.9	75.8	2.1	1.9
Cereal, Chewy & Crisp with Choc Chips, Tesco*	1 Bar/27g	125	6.3	463	9.2	54.0	23.4	3.8
Cereal, Chewy Pomegranate, Vitality, Asda*	1 Bar/22g	76	0.6	346	4.1	69.3	2.8	13.4
Cereal, Chocolate, Geobar, Traidcraft*	1 Bar/32g	130	2.7	407	4.3	78.5	8.4	0.0
Cereal, Chocolate & Fudge, Light, Alpen*	1 Bar/21g	63	1.4	301	4.8	55.4	6.7	22.0
Cereal, Chocolate & Orange, Officially Low Fat, Fox's*	1 Bar/19g	54	0.4	286	5.0	61.6	2.3	17.5
Cereal, Chocolate & Pear, Fitnesse, Nestle*	1 Bar/24g	88	1.3	374	4.7	76.3	5.5	3.2
Cereal, Cinnamon Grahams, Nestle*	1 Bar/25g	106	3.7	426	7.2	66.2	14.7	1.9
Cereal, Citrus Fruits, Light, Alpen*	1 Bar/21g	59	0.9	283	5.6	55.9	4.1	22.4
Cereal, Cranberry, Raisin & Nut, Shapers, Boots*	1 Bar/35g	140	4.4	400	7.1	65.7	12.6	3.7
Cereal, Cranberry & Blackcurrant, HL, Tesco*	1 Bar/25g	121	7.0	485	7.2	50.3	27.9	3.8
Cereal, Cranberry & Orange, Weight Watchers*	1 Bar/28g	102	1.1	365	4.5	77.6	4.1	2.3
Cereal, Double Milk Chocolate, Special K, Kellogg's*	1 Bar/20g	79	1.8	396	9.0	66.0	9.0	10.0
Cereal, Fig & Prune, Eurodiet*	1 Bar/50g	162	5.8	324	30.0	31.5	11.6	7.5
Cereal, Fruit & Fibre, You Count, Love Life, Waitrose*	1 Bar/25g	88	0.2	351	6.0	76.5	0.9	6.3
Cereal, Fruit & Nut, Ainsley Harriott*	1 Bar/35g	151	6.1	431	5.4	63.2	17.4	3.8
Cereal, Fruit & Nut, Alpen*	1 Bar/28g	109	2.3	390	5.8	73.0	8.3	2.9
Cereal, Fruit & Nut with Milk Chocolate, Alpen*	1 Bar/29g	123	3.8	425	6.4	70.5	13.0	2.2
Cereal, Frusli, Blueberry Burst, Jordans*	1 Bar/30g	118	2.9	392	5.8	70.1	9.8	5.1
Cereal, Frusli, Cranberry & Apple, Jordans*	1 Bar/30g	118	3.0	393	5.7	70.0	10.0	5.3
Cereal, Frusli, Red Berries, Jordans*	1 Bar/30g	113	2.4	378	5.1	71.7	7.9	4.5
Cereal, Ginger, Essential, Waitrose*	1 Bar/23g	81	0.6	353	4.9	77.7	2.5	3.2
Cereal, Ginger, Perfectly Balanced, Waitrose*	1 Bar/26g	90	0.5	352	4.0	79.2	2.1	3.0
Cereal, Granola, Alpen*	1 Bar/29g	119	3.1	410	5.9	72.4	10.7	0.0
Cereal, Hazelnut & Sultana, Organic, Seeds of Change*	1 Bar/29g	116	3.7	399	5.9	65.5	12.6	5.1
Cereal, Marmite*	1 Bar/25g	93	2.0	372	18.5	56.2	8.1	6.0
Cereal, Milk Chocolate, Weetos, Weetabix*	1 Bar/20g	88	2.9	440	5.9	70.9	14.7	1.6
Cereal, Mint Chocolate, Kellogg's*	1 Bar/22g	88	2.2	401	4.5	74.0	10.0	3.5
Cereal, Multigrain, Peach & Apricot, BGTY, Sainsbury's*	1 Bar/28g	77	0.6	274	6.4	57.0	2.3	24.2
Cereal, Multigrain Balance, Maple, BGTY, Sainsbury's*	1 Bar/27g	75	0.8	276	6.4	56.2	2.8	25.5
Cereal, Oat & Raisin, Basics, Sainsbury's*	1 Bar/25g	98	2.2	391	5.1	72.8	8.8	3.8
Cereal, Oats & More, Chocolate, Nestle*	1 Bar/30g	118	3.1	395	6.8	68.3	10.5	3.4
Cereal, Oaty, Milk Chocolate, Weetabix*	1 Bar/23g	80	1.5	342	6.9	51.7	6.5	24.3
Cereal, Oaty, Strawberry, Weetabix*	1 Bar/23g	69	1.4	299	6.2	54.7	6.1	24.5
Cereal, Peach Melba, Tesco*	1 Bar/25g	103	3.2	413	4.4	63.7	13.0	2.5
Cereal, Pomegranate with Prebiotic, GFY, Asda*	1 Bar/22g	76	0.6	345	6.2	69.3	2.8	13.4
Cereal, Raisin & Chocolate Chip, Fairtrade, Co-Op*	1 Bar/49g	185	4.6	378	5.3	69.2	9.4	3.7
Cereal, Raisin & Coconut, Value, Tesco*	1 Bar/21g	84	2.4	400	5.5	67.2	11.6	5.0
Cereal, Roast Hazelnut, Organic, Jordans*	1 Bar/33g	150	7.2	455	8.0	56.7	21.8	7.8
Cereal, Special Flake with Cranberries, Tesco*	1 Bar/23g	90	1.4	390	4.9	78.9	5.9	1.8

BARS

INFO/WEIGHT	Measure	per Measure KCAL	per Measure FAT	Nutrition per 100g KCAL	PROT	CARB	FAT	FIBRE
Cereal, Strawberry, BGTY, Sainsbury's*	1 Bar/26g	100	1.2	385	3.8	82.0	4.6	5.2
Cereal, Strawberry, Fruit 'n' Grain, Asda*	1 Bar/37g	126	2.6	340	4.2	65.0	7.0	4.5
Cereal, Sultana & Apple, Sainsbury's*	1 Bar/27g	101	1.4	374	6.7	75.3	5.1	4.3
Cereal, Sultana & Honey, Jordans*	1 Bar/36g	130	3.0	361	6.0	65.9	8.2	9.2
Cereal, Super High Fibre, Dorset Cereals*	1 Bar/35g	149	5.6	425	9.6	60.8	16.0	7.1
Cereal, Tropical Fruit & Nut, Organic, Dove's Farm*	1 Bar/40g	196	4.6	490	6.5	63.3	11.5	5.3
Cereal, Tropical Fruit & Nut Bar, Delicious, Boots*	1 Bar/40g	201	12.0	502	7.5	52.5	30.0	2.2
Cereal, White Chocolate & Strawberry, Value, Tesco*	1 Bar/21g	85	1.7	405	6.2	76.2	8.1	2.4
Cherries, & Almonds, & a Yoghurt Coating, Eat Natural*	1 Bar/45g	200	9.5	444	6.6	58.8	21.1	3.6
Choc Crunch, Meal Replacement, The Biggest Loser*	1 Bar/55g	204	8.1	371	33.5	25.1	14.7	14.2
Choc Nut, Snack, The Biggest Loser*	1 Bar/30g	132	6.9	440	29.3	30.3	23.0	8.0
Chocolate, Milk, Crispy, Endulge, Atkins*	1 Bar/30g	141	9.6	469	13.0	48.0	32.0	2.0
Chocolate, Milkshake, Crisp, Weight Watchers*	1 Bar/21g	82	2.1	391	4.4	59.6	10.0	13.4
Chocolate, Slim Fast*	1 Bar/39g	107	3.5	274	20.6	35.3	9.0	5.5
Chocolate, Soya, Dairy Free, Free From, Sainsbury's*	1 Bar/50g	274	17.5	548	10.8	47.5	35.0	4.3
Chocolate & Crispy Rice, Organic, Dove's Farm*	1 Bar/35g	147	5.3	421	4.4	66.9	15.1	3.0
Chocolate & Orange, Nutrition, Exante*	1 Bar/59g	209	5.7	354	30.4	41.8	9.7	8.4
Chocolate & Orange, Shapers, Boots*	1 Bar/26g	98	3.4	378	4.2	73.0	13.0	1.5
Chocolate & Raisin, Shapers, Boots*	1 Bar/30g	99	2.0	331	5.4	55.0	6.8	5.0
Chocolate & Raspberry, COU, M & S*	1 Bar/25g	90	0.7	360	5.4	78.2	2.7	3.2
Chocolate Banana, Recovery, Mule Refuel*	1 Bar/65g	253	5.8	390	21.0	56.0	9.0	2.0
Chocolate Brownie	1 Bar/68g	240	4.0	353	14.7	60.3	5.9	8.8
Chocolate Brownie, Big Softies, to Go, Fox's*	1 Bar/25g	87	0.7	348	5.5	74.9	2.9	0.0
Chocolate Caramel, Wacko, Belmont, Aldi*	1 Bar/21g	100	4.7	478	4.9	63.8	22.6	1.4
Chocolate Caramel, Weight Watchers*	1 Bar/20g	80	2.5	400	5.0	70.0	12.5	0.0
Chocolate Caramel Whip, Weight Watchers*	1 Bar/25g	88	2.7	353	2.7	72.4	10.8	1.0
Chocolate Chip, Snack, Slim Fast*	1 Bar/26g	99	3.0	382	4.9	70.4	11.4	1.8
Chocolate Chip & Hazelnut, Snack, Benecol*	1 Bar/25g	99	3.3	395	4.7	64.5	13.1	2.5
Chocolate Creme, Endulge, Atkins*	1 Bar/14g	70	4.8	504	12.5	38.6	34.3	2.5
Chocolate Crisp, Weight Watchers*	1 Bar/25g	92	2.5	369	5.4	75.1	10.2	0.8
Chocolate Crispy, Free From, Tesco*	1 Bar/30g	132	4.6	440	4.1	71.2	15.4	0.5
Chocolate Decadence, Atkins*	1 Bar/60g	227	12.2	378	27.1	30.7	20.4	11.6
Chocolate Double, Dark, Zone Perfect*	1 Bar/45g	190	5.5	422	24.5	44.9	12.2	2.0
Chocolate Fruit & Nut, M & S*	1 Bar/50g	235	12.0	470	6.5	57.1	24.1	2.5
Chocolate Toffee Pecan, M & S*	1 Bar/36g	179	9.8	498	4.9	58.3	27.3	0.7
Club, Fruit, Jacob's*	1 Biscuit/25g	124	6.2	496	5.6	62.2	25.0	2.3
Club, Milk Chocolate, Jacob's*	1 Biscuit/24g	123	6.3	511	5.8	62.6	26.4	2.0
Club, Mint, Jacob's*	1 Biscuit/24g	124	6.5	517	5.6	62.5	27.2	1.7
Club, Orange, Jacob's*	1 Biscuit/23g	117	6.1	509	5.7	61.8	26.5	2.3
Cocoa Brownie, Trek, The Natural Health Company*	1 Bar/68g	223	4.1	328	17.0	53.0	6.0	8.0
Cocoa Loco, Wildly Different, Nak'd*	1 Bar/30g	100	3.0	332	8.0	65.0	10.0	7.0
Cocoa Mint, Gluten Free, Raw, Wholefood, Nak'd*	1 Bar/35g	135	5.2	386	9.0	49.0	15.0	7.0
Cocoa Orange, Gluten Free, Nak'd*	1 Bar/35g	145	7.0	415	11.0	45.0	20.0	6.0
Coconut Cream Pie, Larabar*	1 Bar/48g	200	10.0	417	6.2	56.2	20.8	10.4
Coconut Whip, Weight Watchers*	1 Bar/20g	81	2.8	404	2.4	70.6	14.1	1.5
Cookie, Apple Crumble, COU, M & S*	1 Bar/27g	90	0.7	335	5.8	72.6	2.6	2.3
Cookie, Oreo, Nabisco*	1 Bar/35g	180	10.1	514	2.0	66.0	29.0	0.0
Corn Flakes, & Chocolate Milk, Kellogg's*	1 Bar/40g	176	6.4	440	9.0	66.0	16.0	2.0
Cranberry, & Raisin, Geobar, Traidcraft*	1 Bar/35g	131	2.8	374	3.7	72.6	8.0	2.3
Cranberry, Crunch, Cambridge Weight Plan*	1 Bar/50g	152	5.3	305	23.7	28.7	10.6	17.9
Crazy Caramel, Tesco*	1 Bar/40g	192	9.2	480	3.9	64.0	23.0	1.0
Crunchy Crispy Treat, Kids, Tesco*	1 Bar/24g	100	5.0	453	3.6	62.5	20.9	1.5
Crunchy Nut, Chocolate Peanut Crisp, Kellogg's*	1 Bar/35g	169	8.7	483	12.0	53.0	25.0	3.5

BARS	Measure INFO/WEIGHT	per Measure KCAL	FAT	Nutrition Values per 100g / 100ml KCAL	PROT	CARB	FAT	FIBRE
Crunchy Nut, Kellogg's*	1 Bar/30g	119	1.5	397	6.0	82.0	5.0	2.5
Crunchy Nut, Nuts About Nuts, Kellogg's*	1 Bar/40g	212	14.0	530	15.0	40.0	35.0	5.0
Date & Fig, Lyme Regis Foods*	1 Bar/42g	143	4.9	341	7.0	52.0	11.7	9.3
Date & Walnut, Eat Natural*	1 Bar/50g	220	10.0	441	8.0	57.1	20.1	3.3
Digestive, Milk Chocolate, McVitie's*	1 Bar/23g	118	5.8	511	6.6	64.6	25.1	1.9
Digestive, Milk Chocolate, Tesco*	1 Bar/19g	96	4.9	506	6.8	61.6	25.8	2.4
Digestive, Milk Chocolate, Value, Tesco*	1 Bar/19g	96	4.9	505	6.6	61.8	25.8	3.0
Echo, Fox's*	1 Bar/25g	126	6.6	513	7.1	60.7	26.7	2.3
Energize, Banana Punch, Power Bar*	1 Bar/55g	203	2.2	369	10.5	71.7	4.0	2.0
Energize, Berry Blast, Power Bar*	1 Bar/55g	199	2.0	362	10.9	70.8	3.7	2.0
Energize, Cherry, Cranberry Twister, Power Bar*	1 Bar/55g	199	1.9	363	10.8	71.1	3.5	2.0
Energy, Cocoa Brownie, Natural Balance Foods*	1 Bar/68g	216	4.1	318	17.0	51.0	6.0	0.0
Energy, Cool Mint, Chocolate, Clif*	1 Bar/68g	256	5.0	377	14.7	63.2	7.3	7.3
Energy, Strawberry & Cranberry, Power Bar*	1 Bar/40g	153	3.0	384	7.9	68.7	7.5	4.8
Fair Break, Traidcraft*	1 Bar/22g	116	6.2	528	6.0	63.0	28.0	0.0
Fig & Mango, The Food Doctor*	1 Bar/35g	103	0.9	293	8.6	58.6	2.7	10.3
Four Fruits, Organic, Trophy, The Village Bakery*	1 Bar/43g	150	2.5	353	3.8	71.2	5.9	4.2
Four Seeds, Organic, Trophy, The Village Bakery*	1 Bar/43g	164	3.7	385	8.1	68.7	8.7	2.5
Frosties, & Milk, Kellogg's*	1 Bar/25g	102	2.7	408	7.0	71.0	11.0	1.0
Frosties, Chocolate, Kellogg's*	1 Bar/25g	103	3.0	412	6.0	72.0	12.0	1.6
Fruit, Nut & Seed Bars, The Village Bakery*	1 Bar/25g	93	1.5	373	5.7	73.7	6.2	0.1
Fruit, Strawberry, Fruitina*	1 Bar/15g	43	0.2	289	1.9	61.9	1.1	12.2
Fruit & Fibre, Whole Grain, Sainsbury's*	1 Bar/27g	109	3.0	405	6.2	70.1	11.1	3.8
Fruit & Grain, Apple, Aldi*	1 Bar/37g	129	3.0	349	4.2	65.0	8.0	4.5
Fruit & Nut, Eat Natural*	1 Bar/50g	223	11.1	446	11.6	49.8	22.3	5.3
Fruit & Nut, Ginger Snap, Larabar*	1 Bar/51g	220	14.0	431	9.8	47.1	27.4	9.8
Fruit & Nut, Organic, Eat Natural*	1 Bar/50g	244	15.3	488	10.2	42.9	30.6	0.0
Fruit 'n' Fibre, Bakes with Sultanas, Kellogg's*	1 Bar/40g	146	5.2	365	4.5	58.0	13.0	9.0
Fruit 'n' Fibre, Kellogg's*	1 Bar/25g	95	2.2	380	5.0	71.0	9.0	5.0
Fruit to Go, Apple Wildberry, Evernat*	1 Bar/14g	49	0.0	350	1.4	85.7	0.0	5.7
Fruits of the Forest, Advantage, Atkins*	1 Bar/60g	224	10.4	374	31.0	32.9	17.4	7.7
Fruity, Oat, Low Fat, Organic, Dove's Farm*	1 Bar/40g	142	1.1	354	5.0	71.5	2.7	2.4
Fruity Cereal Bar, Free From, Sainsbury's*	1 Bar/25g	100	2.6	399	4.4	72.3	10.2	2.6
Fudge Mallow Delight, Whipple Scrumptious, Wonka*	1 Bar/38g	205	12.0	537	4.6	59.2	31.3	0.6
Ginger, Solo Slim, Rosemary Conley*	1 Bar/35g	117	1.3	335	27.2	48.1	3.8	8.5
Ginger Bread, Nak'd*	1 Bar/35g	157	10.8	450	10.0	35.0	31.0	9.0
Granola, Crunchy, Roasted Almond, Nature Valley*	1 Bar/42g	193	7.6	459	8.1	65.6	18.2	3.7
Granola, Peanut Butter, Advantage, Atkins*	1 Bar/48g	210	11.0	437	29.2	39.6	22.9	10.4
Granola, with Peanut Butter, Natco*	1 Bar/29g	129	4.1	445	10.0	69.0	14.1	5.5
Groove, Lemon, Alpen*	1 Bar/32g	124	1.9	389	5.6	78.4	5.9	1.9
Groove, Sassy Strawberry, Alpen*	1 Bar/32g	124	1.7	386	5.6	78.8	5.4	1.9
Harvest Cheweee, Choc Chip, Quaker Oats*	1 Bar/22g	95	3.5	430	5.5	68.0	16.0	3.5
Harvest Cheweee, Toffee, Quaker Oats*	1 Bar/22g	94	3.3	427	5.0	68.0	15.0	3.0
Harvest Cheweee, White Chocolate Chip, Quaker Oats*	1 Bar/22g	93	3.4	425	6.0	67.0	15.5	3.5
Hazelnut Sandwich, Finn Crisp*	1 Bar/25g	134	8.5	535	7.0	50.0	34.0	0.0
Healthy Meal, Herbalife*	1 Bar/56g	207	6.0	369	23.7	37.1	10.7	14.7
Honey, Natural, Trail Mix, Kallo*	1 Bar/40g	196	13.3	490	15.7	40.9	33.2	5.7
Honey Nut, Special K, Special K, Kellogg's*	1 Bar/22g	90	2.0	409	9.1	72.7	9.1	13.6
Luna, Chocolate Pecan Pie, Luna*	1 Bar/48g	180	4.5	375	20.8	50.0	9.4	2.1
Luna, Nutz Over Chocolate, Luna*	1 Bar/48g	180	4.5	375	20.8	50.0	9.4	2.1
Luxury, Absolute Nut, Jordans*	1 Bar/45g	251	18.6	557	12.7	33.3	41.4	7.0
Luxury, Cranberry & Almond, Jordans*	1 Bar/50g	217	9.6	434	8.6	56.6	19.2	5.8
Luxury, Exotic Fruit & Nut, Jordans*	1 Bar/50g	196	2.7	393	5.0	69.1	5.4	4.8

BARS

INFO/WEIGHT	Measure	per Measure KCAL	per Measure FAT	Nutrition Values per 100g / 100ml KCAL	PROT	CARB	FAT	FIBRE
Macadamia, & Fruit, Eat Natural*	1 Bar/50g	242	15.4	485	7.3	44.6	30.8	0.0
Macaroon, Lees*	1 Bar/70g	276	4.7	395	1.2	82.5	6.7	0.0
Mango, & Brazil, Tropical Whole Foods*	1 Bar/40g	172	7.6	429	4.7	61.4	19.1	4.2
Marshmallow, Chewy, Rice Krispies Squares, Kellogg's*	1 Bar/28g	119	3.4	424	3.0	76.0	12.0	0.9
Marshmallow Mudslide, Advantage, Atkins*	1 Bar/48g	210	10.0	437	31.2	39.6	20.8	10.4
Milk Chocolate, Crispy Wafer, Tasty Little Numbers*	1 Bar/20g	100	5.0	499	6.1	61.4	25.1	3.0
Milk Chocolate Whirls, Asda*	1 Bar/26g	116	4.2	447	3.7	72.0	16.0	0.8
Mint, Double Take, Sainsbury's*	1 Bar/20g	107	6.2	534	7.2	56.9	30.8	1.3
Mint Chocolate Whip, Weight Watchers*	1 Bar/20g	80	2.0	402	3.6	74.0	9.9	0.7
Mixed Berry, Trek, Natural Balance Foods*	1 Bar/68g	204	1.5	300	15.6	56.5	2.2	6.0
Mixed Nut Feast, Eat Natural*	1 Bar/50g	278	20.5	556	18.8	28.0	41.0	0.0
Muesli, Apricot & Almond, Carmen's*	1 Bar/45g	190	8.2	423	10.4	50.6	18.2	7.4
Muesli, Cherry & Milk, Sirius*	1 Bar/25g	104	2.8	417	7.2	71.3	11.4	3.9
Muesli, Cookie Coach*	1 Bar/75g	289	8.3	385	6.8	65.1	11.1	0.0
Muffin, Cadbury*	1 Bar/68g	274	17.3	403	5.6	38.0	25.4	0.0
Multigrain, Apple & Sultana, Jordans*	1 Bar/40g	141	2.5	353	4.4	70.0	6.2	4.8
Multigrain, Cranberry & Raspberry, Jordans*	1 Bar/37g	135	2.4	364	4.8	71.3	6.6	4.8
Multigrain, Fruit & Nut, Jordans*	1 Bar/40g	164	6.5	410	7.0	59.1	16.2	5.7
Munch, Apricot Flavour, Tony Ferguson*	1 Bar/60g	211	4.1	351	25.1	43.1	6.8	8.9
Natural Energy, Cacao Crunch, Power Bar*	1 Bar/40g	156	3.8	391	8.3	65.5	9.4	5.7
Nine Bar, Mixed Seed with Hemp, Original, Wholebake*	1 Bar/40g	222	16.2	555	18.3	29.2	40.5	5.2
Nine Bar, Nutty, Wholebake*	1 Bar/50g	277	20.3	555	18.3	29.9	40.6	5.2
Noisettes & Amandes, Special K, Kellogg's*	1 Bar/21g	83	2.1	397	8.0	66.0	10.0	7.0
Nougat, Cool Mint, & Dark Chocolate, Shapers, Boots*	1 Bar/23g	83	3.2	362	2.6	70.0	14.0	1.1
Nougat, Summer Strawberry, Shapers, Boots*	1 Bar/23g	83	3.0	361	2.7	73.0	13.0	0.6
Nut, Dark Chocolate & Apricot, Natural, Nice & Natural*	1 Bar/35g	163	10.2	465	15.2	35.2	29.1	5.4
Nutri-Grain, Apple, Kellogg's*	1 Bar/37g	131	3.3	355	4.0	67.0	9.0	4.0
Nutri-Grain, Blackberry & Apple, Kellogg's*	1 Bar/37g	131	3.3	355	4.0	67.0	9.0	4.0
Nutri-Grain, Blueberry, Kellogg's*	1 Bar/37g	133	3.0	359	3.5	69.0	8.0	3.5
Nutri-Grain, Cherry, Kellogg's*	1 Bar/37g	129	3.0	348	4.0	67.0	8.0	4.0
Nutri-Grain, Chocolate, Kellogg's*	1 Bar/37g	136	3.7	367	4.5	66.0	10.0	4.0
Nutri-Grain, Chocolate Chip, Chewy, Kellogg's*	1 Bar/25g	103	3.0	413	4.5	73.0	12.0	2.5
Nutri-Grain, Elevenses, Choc Chip, Kellogg's*	1 Bar/45g	179	5.8	397	4.0	66.0	13.0	2.0
Nutri-Grain, Elevenses, Ginger, Kellogg's*	1 Bar/45g	168	4.0	373	5.0	68.0	9.0	3.0
Nutri-Grain, Elevenses, Raisin, Kellogg's*	1 Bar/45g	164	4.0	364	5.0	66.0	9.0	3.5
Nutri-Grain, Honey Oat & Raisin, Chewy, Kellogg's*	1 Bar/25g	98	2.0	393	3.5	78.0	8.0	2.5
Nutri-Grain, Oat Bakes, Cherry, Kellogg's*	1 Bar/50g	204	7.0	408	4.5	66.0	14.0	2.5
Nutri-Grain, Oat Bakes, Totally Oaty, Kellogg's*	1 Bar/50g	205	7.5	411	5.0	64.0	15.0	3.0
Nutri-Grain, Raspberry, Kellogg's*	1 Bar/37g	131	3.3	355	4.0	67.0	9.0	4.0
Nutri-Grain, Strawberry, Kellogg's*	1 Bar/37g	133	3.0	359	3.5	69.0	8.0	3.5
Nuts & Berry, Weight Watchers*	1 Bar/24g	92	2.9	383	5.9	52.1	11.9	12.7
Nutty Crunch Surprise, Wonka*	1 Bar/37g	202	11.9	543	4.9	58.7	32.1	0.9
Nutty Nougat Caramel, Tesco*	1 Bar/20g	99	5.4	493	8.5	54.0	27.0	2.4
Oat, Mixed Berry, Quaker Oats*	1 Bar/38g	137	3.3	360	6.8	64.5	8.8	8.0
Oat, Original with Golden Syrup, Quaker Oats*	1 Bar/38g	139	3.6	366	7.1	64.5	9.5	7.9
Oat, Quaker Oats*	1 Bar/38g	137	3.4	360	6.8	64.5	8.8	8.0
Oats, Raisins, Honey & Apricots, Geobar, Traidcraft*	1 Bar/35g	132	3.1	376	5.3	69.0	8.8	3.5
Oaty, Strawberry Crusher, Weetabix*	1 Bar/23g	79	1.4	345	6.1	55.2	6.1	22.2
Oaty with Cranberry & Blueberry, Tesco*	1 Bar/38g	141	2.8	370	5.5	69.0	7.5	6.2
Optivita, Berry Oat, Kellogg's*	1 Bar/28g	101	2.0	360	7.0	68.0	7.0	9.0
Orango Crunch, Go Ahead, McVitie's*	1 Bar/23g	99	2.9	430	4.1	78.0	12.8	0.8
Orange Truffle, M & S*	1 Bar/33g	177	10.5	535	6.6	55.6	31.9	1.4
Orchard Fruits & Yoghurt, Fruit & Fibre, Sainsbury's*	1 Bar/27g	102	1.6	379	5.9	75.3	6.0	4.1

BARS

	Measure INFO/WEIGHT	per Measure KCAL	FAT	Nutrition Values per 100g / 100ml KCAL	PROT	CARB	FAT	FIBRE
Original, Crunchy, Honey & Almond, Jordans*	1 Bar/30g	139	6.8	463	8.3	56.7	22.7	6.7
Original, Nut Free, Get Buzzing*	1 Bar/62g	248	12.0	400	6.8	51.6	19.3	3.7
Original Muesli, Diet Chef Ltd*	1 Bar/50g	199	6.9	398	6.1	59.0	13.8	6.4
Peach, Apricot & Almond, Altu*	1 Bar/40g	158	4.6	395	7.9	65.2	11.4	4.3
Peanut, Cashew & Thai Sweet Chilli, Altu*	1 Bar/40g	172	8.1	430	14.7	47.0	20.3	3.1
Peanut, Mr Toms*	1 Bar/40g	210	13.0	525	20.0	42.5	32.5	2.5
Peanut, Protein Blast, Natural Energy Ball, Bounce*	1 Ball/49g	210	8.0	429	28.6	38.8	16.3	4.1
Peanut, Raisin & Chocolate, Weight Watchers*	1 Bar/25g	97	2.8	388	7.6	60.0	11.2	12.8
Peanut & Caramel Whip, Weight Watchers*	1 Bar/20g	76	2.7	381	4.4	73.7	13.7	1.2
Peanut & Oat, Trek, Nak'd*	1 Bar/68g	239	7.5	352	16.0	49.0	11.0	7.0
Peanut Butter, Chewy, Granola, Slim Fast*	1 Bar/56g	123	3.4	220	8.0	35.0	6.0	0.0
Peanut Fudge Granola, Advantage, Atkins*	1 Bar/48g	210	10.0	437	33.3	35.4	20.8	18.7
Pear & Ginger, Fruit Break, Lyme Regis Foods*	1 Bar/42g	160	8.8	381	2.7	45.4	20.9	9.9
Pecan Apricot & Peach, M & S*	1 Bar/50g	255	17.7	510	9.3	38.2	35.5	4.9
Pecan Pie, Gluten Free, Nak'd*	1 Bar/35g	156	10.8	447	8.0	36.0	31.0	9.0
Pecan Pie, Larabar*	1 Bar/45g	200	14.0	444	6.7	48.9	31.1	8.9
Penguin, Chukka, McVitie's*	1 Bar/28g	135	6.1	481	6.1	65.1	21.8	0.0
Penguin Bigstix, McVitie's*	1 Biscuit/13g	63	3.2	508	6.4	62.8	25.7	2.6
Protein, Chocolate Chewy Crisp, Pro-Bar Xs*	1 Bar/70g	239	4.5	341	44.0	6.0	6.5	12.0
Protein, Flapjack, Oat Crunch, Natural Balance Foods*	1 Bar/56g	249	12.9	444	18.0	43.0	23.0	3.0
Protein, Low Carb, Pro-Lite 25, Peak Body*	1 Bar/50g	177	3.4	354	50.0	7.8	6.8	0.0
Protein, Peanut Chewy Crisp, Chemical Protein Pro-Xs*	1 Bar/70g	243	5.2	347	42.9	5.5	7.5	12.5
Protein, Vanilla, Low Carb, Protein Plus, Power Bar*	1 Bar/35g	131	7.3	373	16.0	21.5	21.0	26.5
Protein Pack, X-Treme with White Chocolate, Inkospor*	1 Bar/35g	136	3.5	388	32.0	43.0	10.0	0.3
Raisin, Munch, Tesco*	1 Bar/30g	126	4.4	420	5.4	66.3	14.8	3.8
Raisin & Apricot, Geobar, Traidcraft*	1 Bar/35g	132	3.1	376	5.3	69.0	8.8	3.5
Raisin & Hazelnut, Weight Watchers*	1 Bar/24g	95	2.4	396	5.0	71.2	10.0	2.9
Raisin & Oatmeal, Breakfast Snack, Tesco*	1 Bar/38g	133	4.4	355	5.6	56.8	11.7	2.8
Raspberry, Baked, Asda*	1 Bar/27g	104	2.1	385	3.4	74.2	7.6	1.8
Raspberry, Fruit Bake, Go Ahead, McVitie's*	1 Bar/35g	124	2.5	354	2.7	73.8	7.2	1.2
Raspberry, Yoghurt Breaks, Go Ahead, McVitie's*	1 Pack/35g	143	3.6	408	5.4	73.6	10.2	2.3
Raspberry & White Chocolate Crispie, Shapers, Boots*	1 Bar/24g	93	2.0	387	3.8	68.0	8.5	11.0
Rice Crisp, Cranberry & Orange, Go Ahead, McVitie's*	1 Bar/22g	92	2.3	417	3.9	77.0	10.4	1.0
Rice Krispies, Snack, Kellogg's*	1 Bar/20g	83	2.0	415	7.0	70.0	10.0	0.5
Rice Krispies & Milk, Kellogg's*	1 Bar/20g	83	2.4	416	7.0	71.0	12.0	0.3
Rocky Road, Rice Krispies Squares, Kellogg's*	1 Square/34g	143	3.7	420	4.0	76.0	11.0	1.5
Sandwich, Chocolate, Rik & Rok*	1 Bar/22g	105	4.2	477	6.5	70.0	19.0	0.0
Sandwich, Chocolate Viennese, Fox's*	1 Biscuit/14g	76	4.4	542	6.9	57.4	31.6	1.6
Sandwich, Milk Chocolate, Smart Price, Asda*	1 Bar/25g	132	7.0	528	6.0	63.0	28.0	0.0
Sandwich, Milk Chocolate, Value, Tesco*	1 Bar/26g	130	6.4	504	5.4	64.5	24.9	2.4
Sandwich, Milk Chocolate Orange, Tesco*	1 Biscuit/25g	136	7.4	536	6.2	62.2	29.1	1.8
School, Apple, Fruit Bowl*	1 Bar/20g	67	0.6	337	0.7	75.0	3.0	6.0
School, Apricot, Fruit Bowl*	1 Bar/20g	67	0.6	337	0.7	75.0	3.0	6.0
School, Blackcurrant, Fruit Bowl*	1 Bar/20g	67	0.6	337	0.7	75.0	3.0	2.0
School, Cherry, Fruit Bowl*	1 Bar/20g	67	0.6	337	0.7	75.0	3.0	6.0
Sesame Snaps, Anglo-Dal*	1 Pack/30g	163	9.4	542	2.8	61.8	31.5	0.0
Sesame Snaps in Chocolate, Anglo-Dal*	1 Pack/40g	211	11.9	527	9.3	55.6	29.7	0.0
Sesame Snaps with Coconut, Anglo-Dal*	1 Pack/30g	155	8.8	517	9.7	52.9	29.5	0.0
Slow Fig & Macadamia, Southern Alps, Slow Puck*	1 Bar/45g	200	7.4	444	4.0	70.2	16.4	4.4
Snack, Ginger, Diet Chef Ltd*	1 Bar/27g	94	1.9	348	5.5	65.6	7.1	4.4
Special Fruit Muesli, Jordans*	1 Bar/40g	140	2.4	349	5.0	68.8	6.0	5.0
Special K, Apple & Pear, Kellogg's*	1 Bar/23g	92	1.8	400	8.0	73.0	8.0	2.0
Special K, Cereal with Chocolate Chip, Kellogg's*	1 Bar/21g	83	1.3	396	9.0	77.0	6.0	1.5

	Measure INFO/WEIGHT	per Measure		Nutrition Values per 100g / 100ml				
		KCAL	FAT	KCAL	PROT	CARB	FAT	FIBRE
BARS								
Special K, Chocolate Chip, Kellogg's*	1 Bar/22g	90	1.6	401	9.0	76.0	7.0	1.5
Special K, Fruits of the Forest, Kellogg's*	1 Bar/22g	87	1.8	397	8.0	74.0	8.0	2.5
Special K, Mint Chocolate, Bliss, Special K, Kellogg's*	1 Bar/22g	88	2.2	401	4.5	74.0	10.0	3.5
Special K, Peach & Apricot, Kellogg's*	1 Bar/21g	80	1.3	383	8.0	75.0	6.0	2.5
Special K, Red Berry, Kellogg's*	1 Bar/23g	90	1.2	383	8.0	77.0	5.0	2.0
Special Muesli, Jordans*	1 Bar/40g	152	4.8	379	6.0	61.6	12.1	5.8
Strawberry, Breakfast, Carb Control, Tesco*	1 Bar/37g	144	8.6	389	7.0	40.5	23.2	4.0
Strawberry, Fruit Bakes, Go Ahead, McVitie's*	1 Bar/35g	131	3.0	375	3.5	72.0	8.5	4.0
Strawberry, Morning Shine, Atkins*	1 Bar/37g	145	8.0	392	28.9	24.9	21.6	14.1
Strawberry, Shapers, Boots*	1 Bar/22g	75	2.4	343	2.5	77.0	11.0	0.9
Sultana, Apple & Yoghurt, Balance, Sainsbury's*	1 Bar/27g	104	1.6	387	6.1	77.4	5.9	2.3
Three Musketeer, Candy, Mars*	1 Bar/60g	260	8.0	430	3.3	76.2	13.2	1.7
Toffee, Nut & Raisin, Exante*	1 Bar/59g	215	6.6	364	31.7	38.9	11.2	8.8
Toffee, Slim Fast*	1 Bar/39g	122	3.3	314	19.7	47.1	8.5	5.6
Toffee & Banana, Weight Watchers*	1 Bar/18g	67	0.7	372	6.1	77.2	3.9	1.7
Toffee Crunch, Simply Lite, Perfect Days*	1 Bar/51g	200	9.0	392	23.5	49.0	17.6	9.8
Totally Chocolatey, Rice Krispies Squares, Kellogg's*	1 Bar/36g	156	4.7	432	4.5	74.0	13.0	1.5
Tracker, Breakfast, Banana, Mars*	1 Bar/37g	176	8.4	476	4.7	63.3	22.6	9.4
Tracker, Breakfast, Lemon, Mars*	1 Bar/26g	124	5.8	477	4.6	64.3	22.4	0.0
Tracker, Chocolate Chip, Mars*	1 Bar/37g	178	8.7	480	6.8	58.0	23.6	3.8
Tracker, Forest Fruits, Mars*	1 Bar/26g	123	5.8	474	4.6	64.1	22.2	0.0
Tracker, Roasted Nut, Mars*	1 Bar/26g	127	6.6	489	8.1	55.0	25.3	4.9
Tracker, Strawberry, Mars*	1 Bar/26g	118	4.8	452	4.2	63.2	18.4	2.9
Tracker, Yoghurt, Mars*	1 Bar/27g	133	6.3	491	6.3	64.2	23.2	0.0
Triple Dazzle, Wonka*	1 Bar/39g	195	10.0	504	5.9	61.9	25.9	0.0
Ultimate Oat, Organic, Honeyrose Bakery*	1 Bar/75g	309	9.0	412	7.0	44.2	12.0	4.5
Vanilla Caramel, Eurodiet*	1 Bar/45g	162	5.5	360	31.7	24.5	12.3	11.1
Very Berry, Cookie, Big Softies, Fox's*	1 Bar/26g	85	0.7	325	5.7	69.7	2.5	2.5
Vyomax Lite, Vyomax*	1 Bar/45g	170	6.0	378	33.3	32.4	13.3	7.6
Wafer, Chocolate Flavour Crisp, Carbolite*	1 Bar/25g	120	8.7	482	8.5	52.3	34.8	2.0
Wafer Biscuit, Milk Chocolate Coated, Value, Tesco*	1 Bar/24g	126	6.7	526	6.9	61.4	28.1	1.7
White Chocolate, Crispy Wafer, Tasty Little Numbers*	1 Bar/20g	100	5.2	498	7.0	59.0	26.0	3.0
White Chocolate & Hazelnuts, Porridge Oat, Stoats*	1 Bar/85g	398	26.8	468	10.1	64.8	31.5	8.0
Zippy Fruit, Mini Chefs, Natco*	1 Bar/20g	60	0.0	300	1.0	70.0	0.0	5.0
BASA								
Tempura, Fillets, Northern Catch*	1 Fillet/160g	248	11.0	155	17.5	7.9	6.9	1.9
BASIL								
Dried, Ground	*1 Tsp/1g*	*4*	*0.1*	*251*	*14.4*	*43.2*	*4.0*	*0.0*
Fresh, Average	*1 Tbsp/5g*	*2*	*0.0*	*40*	*3.1*	*5.1*	*0.8*	*0.0*
BASKETS								
Brandy Snap, Askeys*	1 Basket/20g	98	4.3	490	1.9	72.7	21.3	0.0
BATTER MIX								
for Yorkshire Puddings, Baked, Aunt Bessie's*	1 Pudding/13g	48	1.1	356	9.8	34.0	8.1	2.3
for Yorkshire Puddings & Pancakes, Morrisons*	1 Pudding/30g	43	0.8	143	6.4	23.1	2.8	4.1
for Yorkshire Puddings & Pancakes, Tesco*	1 Serving/17g	34	0.3	200	2.3	43.3	1.5	2.5
Green's*	1 Bag/125g	296	9.0	237	8.7	34.3	7.2	0.0
Pancake, Sainsbury's*	1 Pancake/63g	96	1.1	152	6.5	27.4	1.8	3.1
Smart Price, Asda*	1 Pack/128g	268	5.8	209	8.0	34.0	4.5	2.7
Tesco*	1 Pack/130g	467	1.8	359	12.3	74.4	1.4	7.7
BAY LEAVES								
Dried, Average	*1 Tsp/0.6g*	*2*	*0.1*	*313*	*7.6*	*48.6*	*8.4*	*0.0*
BEAN MIX								
Great Fire Dragon, Graze*	1 Pack/25g	123	7.0	491	15.0	48.1	20.1	2.5

	Measure INFO/WEIGHT	per Measure		Nutrition Values per 100g / 100ml				
		KCAL	FAT	KCAL	PROT	CARB	FAT	FIBRE
BEAN MIX								
Mexican Style, Tinned, Asda*	1 Serving/81g	71	0.6	88	8.7	11.8	0.7	10.4
Wasabi, Whitworths*	1 Serving/25g	107	3.4	430	30.9	40.1	13.7	10.7
BEAN SPROUTS								
Mung, Canned, Drained, Average	*1 Serving/90g*	*9*	*0.1*	*10*	*1.6*	*0.8*	*0.1*	*0.7*
Mung, Raw, Average	*1oz/28g*	*9*	*0.1*	*31*	*2.9*	*4.0*	*0.5*	*1.5*
Mung, Stir-Fried in Blended Oil, Average	*1 Serving/90g*	*65*	*5.5*	*72*	*1.9*	*2.5*	*6.1*	*0.9*
Raw, Average	*1 Serving/150g*	*55*	*2.6*	*37*	*2.2*	*3.2*	*1.8*	*1.2*
Sainsbury's*	½ Pack/200g	122	11.4	61	1.8	0.7	5.7	1.0
BEANFEAST								
Bolognese Style, Dry, Batchelors*	1 Pack/120g	362	6.7	302	23.9	39.0	5.6	13.5
Mexican Chilli, Batchelors*	1 Serving/65g	203	3.2	312	24.3	42.7	4.9	13.6
BEANS								
Aduki, Cooked in Unsalted Water, Average	*1 Tbsp/30g*	*37*	*0.1*	*123*	*9.3*	*22.5*	*0.2*	*5.5*
Aduki, Dried, Raw	*1 Tbsp/30g*	*82*	*0.1*	*272*	*19.9*	*50.1*	*0.5*	*11.1*
Adzuki, Dry, Love Life, Waitrose*	1 Serving/100g	340	0.5	340	19.9	62.9	0.5	12.7
Adzuki in Water, Canned, Drained, Tesco*	½ Can/118g	117	0.5	100	6.5	13.6	0.4	6.5
Baked, & Jumbo Sausages, Asda*	1 Serving/210g	317	14.7	151	7.0	15.0	7.0	2.6
Baked, & Pork Sausages, Sainsbury's*	1 Serving/210g	248	9.2	118	5.7	13.9	4.4	3.4
Baked, & Pork Sausages, Tesco*	½ Can/210g	231	5.7	110	5.5	15.6	2.7	3.0
Baked, & Sausage, Asda*	½ Can/203g	211	4.0	104	6.7	13.0	2.0	3.5
Baked, & Sausage, GFY, Asda*	1 Serving/217g	178	5.6	82	4.7	10.0	2.6	1.8
Baked, & Sausages, Basics, Sainsbury's*	1 Serving/175g	149	2.6	85	4.8	13.1	1.5	2.6
Baked, & Sausages, Meatfree, Sainsbury's*	1 Can/420g	500	16.8	119	8.0	12.6	4.0	2.7
Baked, & Sausages, Value, Tesco*	½ Can/202g	232	7.1	115	5.6	15.0	3.5	2.8
Baked, Barbecue, Smokey, Beanz, Heinz*	1 Can/420g	332	0.8	79	4.9	14.3	0.2	3.8
Baked, Basics, Sainsbury's*	1 Can/420g	206	1.3	49	4.2	7.4	0.3	4.4
Baked, Cheezy, Heinz*	1oz/28g	53	1.4	189	11.6	24.5	4.9	6.2
Baked, Curried, Average	*½ Can/210g*	*203*	*1.9*	*96*	*4.8*	*17.2*	*0.9*	*3.6*
Baked, Curry, Beanz, Heinz*	1 Can/200g	218	3.2	109	4.8	17.0	1.6	4.0
Baked, Eat Smart, Morrisons*	1 Can/420g	294	1.7	70	5.3	11.4	0.4	5.6
Baked, HL, Tesco*	1 Can/420g	315	2.1	75	4.3	12.1	0.5	3.8
Baked, in Barbeque Sauce, Tesco*	1 Can/220g	198	1.3	90	5.0	13.6	0.6	5.2
Baked, in Tomato Sauce, Average	*1 Can/400g*	*318*	*1.6*	*80*	*4.6*	*13.9*	*0.4*	*3.7*
Baked, in Tomato Sauce, Beanz, Heinz*	½ Can/208g	164	0.4	79	4.7	12.9	0.2	3.7
Baked, in Tomato Sauce, Corale, Aldi*	½ Can/220g	200	0.9	91	5.2	14.4	0.4	4.3
Baked, in Tomato Sauce, Everyday Value, Tesco*	½ Can/210g	185	1.0	90	3.7	14.6	0.5	4.4
Baked, in Tomato Sauce, Light Choices, Tesco*	½ Can/210g	150	1.1	70	4.3	12.1	0.5	3.8
Baked, in Tomato Sauce, Organic, Beanz, Heinz*	1 Can/415g	336	0.8	81	4.8	12.9	0.2	3.8
Baked, in Tomato Sauce, Reduced Sugar & Salt	*½ Can/210g*	*159*	*0.7*	*75*	*4.5*	*13.6*	*0.3*	*3.8*
Baked, in Tomato Sauce, Reduced Sugar & Salt, Asda*	½ Tin/211g	158	1.1	75	4.6	13.0	0.5	4.5
Baked, in Tomato Sauce, Smart Price, Asda*	1 Can/410g	403	1.7	96	5.0	16.4	0.4	3.5
Baked, in Tomato Sauce, Snap Pot, Beanz, Heinz*	1 Pot/200g	159	0.4	79	4.7	12.9	0.2	3.7
Baked, in Tomato Sauce, Tesco*	1 Can/220g	198	1.1	90	4.3	14.1	0.5	4.1
Baked, Jalfrezi, Mean, Beanz, Heinz*	1 Serving/195g	135	2.5	69	4.5	9.8	1.3	3.6
Baked, Mexican, Mean, Beanz, Heinz*	½ Can/208g	158	1.0	76	5.0	12.9	0.5	4.0
Baked, Reduced Sugar & Salt, Sainsbury's*	½ Can/210g	168	1.0	80	5.2	16.1	0.5	5.0
Baked, Sweet Chilli, Mean, Beanz, Heinz*	½ Can/195g	142	0.6	73	4.5	13.0	0.3	3.6
Baked, Tikka, Mean, Beanz, Heinz*	1 Serving/195g	172	5.9	88	4.8	10.6	3.0	3.5
Baked, Virtually Fat Free, Heinz*	½ Can/207g	164	0.4	79	4.7	12.9	0.2	3.7
Baked, with Chicken Nuggets, Beanz, Heinz*	1 Can/200g	210	6.3	105	6.7	12.4	3.1	3.2
Baked, with Hidden Veg, Beanz, Heinz*	½ Can/208g	156	0.6	75	4.7	13.5	0.3	4.1
Baked, with HP Sauce, Beanz, Heinz*	½ Can/208g	158	0.6	76	4.8	13.7	0.3	3.9
Baked, with Lea & Perrins Sauce, Beanz, Heinz*	1 Can/415g	303	0.8	73	4.8	13.1	0.2	3.8

BEANS

	Measure INFO/WEIGHT	per Measure KCAL	FAT	Nutrition Values per 100g / 100ml KCAL	PROT	CARB	FAT	FIBRE
Baked, with Sausages, Branston, Crosse & Blackwell*	½ Can/202g	233	6.5	115	6.9	12.2	3.2	5.0
Baked, with Spicy Meatballs, Beanz, Heinz*	1 Can/400g	372	9.6	93	5.8	12.0	2.4	2.9
Baked, with Steak Chunks, Beanz, Heinz*	1 Can/415g	340	2.9	82	6.9	12.1	0.7	3.5
Black, Cooked, Average	*1 Cup/172g*	*227*	*0.9*	*132*	*8.8*	*23.7*	*0.5*	*8.7*
Black, Dried, Average	*1 Serving/100g*	*341*	*1.4*	*341*	*21.6*	*62.4*	*1.4*	*15.2*
Black Turtle, Dried, Love Life, Waitrose*	1 Serving/100g	351	0.9	351	21.3	63.3	0.9	24.9
Blackeye, Canned, Average	*1 Can/172g*	*206*	*1.3*	*119*	*8.4*	*19.7*	*0.7*	*3.3*
Blackeye, Dried, Raw	*1oz/28g*	*87*	*0.4*	*311*	*23.5*	*54.1*	*1.6*	*8.2*
Borlotti, Canned, Asda*	½ Can/87g	96	0.4	110	8.0	18.4	0.5	7.0
Borlotti, Canned, Average	*1oz/28g*	*29*	*0.1*	*103*	*7.6*	*16.9*	*0.5*	*4.7*
Borlotti, Dried, Love Life, Waitrose*	1 Serving/100g	348	1.2	348	23.0	60.1	1.2	24.7
Borlotti, Dried, Raw, Average	*1 Serving/100g*	*335*	*1.2*	*335*	*23.0*	*60.0*	*1.2*	*24.7*
Broad, Canned, Drained, Average	*1 Can/195g*	*136*	*1.1*	*70*	*6.9*	*9.2*	*0.6*	*6.8*
Broad, Crispy, Wasabi Flavoured, Khao Shong*	1 Serving/30g	116	3.0	386	17.0	57.0	10.0	7.0
Broad, Dried, Raw, Average	*1oz/28g*	*69*	*0.6*	*245*	*26.1*	*32.5*	*2.1*	*27.6*
Broad, Frozen, Sainsbury's*	1 Serving/80g	64	0.5	80	7.9	10.7	0.6	6.5
Broad, in Water, Drained, Asda*	1 Serving/98g	73	0.5	75	7.4	10.1	0.5	7.1
Broad, Weighed with Pod, Raw, Average	*1oz/28g*	*17*	*0.3*	*59*	*5.7*	*7.2*	*1.0*	*6.1*
Butter, Canned, Drained, Average	*1oz/28g*	*24*	*0.1*	*86*	*6.3*	*13.5*	*0.5*	*4.6*
Butter, Canned, Drained, Wholefoods, Tesco*	½ Can/125g	100	0.6	80	5.9	13.0	0.5	4.6
Butter, Drained Weight, M & S*	1 Serving/119g	125	0.6	105	7.2	15.3	0.5	5.6
Butter, Dried, Boiled, Average	*1oz/28g*	*30*	*0.2*	*106*	*7.2*	*18.6*	*0.6*	*5.2*
Butter, Dried, Raw, Average	*1oz/28g*	*81*	*0.5*	*290*	*19.1*	*52.9*	*1.7*	*16.0*
Cannellini, Canned, Asda*	½ Can/87g	76	0.3	87	7.0	14.0	0.3	6.0
Cannellini, Canned, Average	*1 Can/400g*	*375*	*2.1*	*94*	*7.2*	*15.0*	*0.5*	*5.7*
Cannellini, Dried, Tesco*	1 Serving/32g	83	0.3	260	24.8	37.4	0.8	20.9
Chilli, Canned, Average	*1 Can/420g*	*381*	*3.1*	*91*	*5.2*	*15.8*	*0.7*	*4.3*
Curried, Mixed, Morrisons*	1 Can/420g	420	16.4	100	4.2	12.1	3.9	5.6
Dwarf, Sainsbury's*	1oz/28g	7	0.1	24	1.9	3.1	0.5	2.2
Edamame, Sainsbury's*	1 Serving/150g	211	9.6	141	12.3	6.8	6.4	4.2
Flageolet, Canned, Average	*1 Can/265g*	*235*	*1.6*	*89*	*6.7*	*14.0*	*0.6*	*3.5*
Flageolet, Dried, Love Life, Waitrose*	1 Serving/50g	125	3.1	250	30.4	19.8	6.2	40.4
French, Boiled, Average	*1 Serving/150g*	*37*	*0.0*	*25*	*2.3*	*3.8*	*0.0*	*3.7*
French, Canned, Average	*1oz/28g*	*6*	*0.1*	*22*	*1.6*	*3.5*	*0.3*	*2.5*
French, Raw	*1oz/28g*	*7*	*0.1*	*24*	*1.9*	*3.2*	*0.5*	*2.2*
Green, Cut, Average	*1oz/28g*	*7*	*0.1*	*24*	*1.7*	*3.6*	*0.2*	*2.7*
Green, Extra Fine, in Salted Water, Lidl*	1 Serving/220g	37	0.4	17	1.3	2.5	0.2	3.5
Green, Fine, Average	*1 Serving/75g*	*18*	*0.3*	*23*	*1.8*	*3.1*	*0.4*	*2.9*
Green, Fresh, Value, Tesco*	1 Pack/100g	27	0.1	27	1.9	3.2	0.1	4.1
Green, Sliced, Average	*1oz/28g*	*6*	*0.1*	*23*	*1.9*	*3.5*	*0.2*	*2.1*
Green, Sliced, Frozen, Average	*1 Serving/50g*	*13*	*0.0*	*26*	*1.8*	*4.4*	*0.1*	*4.1*
Green, Very Fine, Field Fresh, Birds Eye*	1 Serving/80g	20	0.4	25	1.8	2.9	0.5	2.4
Green, Whole, Average	*1oz/28g*	*6*	*0.1*	*22*	*1.6*	*3.0*	*0.4*	*1.7*
Green, Whole, Frozen, Boiled, Chosen By You, Asda*	1 Portion/80g	28	0.1	35	1.7	4.7	0.1	4.1
Haricot, Canned, Average	1 Can/400g	77	0.5	77	6.2	10.7	0.5	5.9
Haricot, Dried, Boiled in Unsalted Water	*1oz/28g*	*27*	*0.1*	*95*	*6.6*	*17.2*	*0.5*	*6.1*
Haricot, Dried, Raw	*1oz/28g*	*80*	*0.4*	*286*	*21.4*	*49.7*	*1.6*	*17.0*
Haricot, in Water, Canned, Drained, Tesco*	½ Can/118g	76	0.6	65	5.7	9.0	0.5	7.8
Kidney, Curried, Rajmah, Sohna *	½ Can/225g	217	1.1	97	3.7	17.6	0.5	1.4
Kidney, Red, Canned, Drained, Average	*½ Can/90g*	*88*	*0.5*	*98*	*7.6*	*21.2*	*0.6*	*5.7*
Kidney, Red, Drained, Savers, Morrisons*	½ Can/120g	125	0.8	104	7.7	12.9	0.7	7.8
Kidney, Red, Dried, Boiled in Unsalted Water	*1oz/28g*	*29*	*0.1*	*103*	*8.4*	*17.4*	*0.5*	*6.7*
Kidney, Red, Dried, Raw	*1oz/28g*	*74*	*0.4*	*266*	*22.1*	*44.1*	*1.4*	*15.7*

B

BEANS	Measure INFO/WEIGHT	per Measure KCAL	FAT	Nutrition Values per 100g / 100ml KCAL	PROT	CARB	FAT	FIBRE
Kidney, Red, in Chilli Sauce, Sainsbury's*	1 Can/420g	365	1.7	87	5.3	15.6	0.4	4.5
Kidney, Red, in Chilli Sauce, Waitrose*	½ Can/201g	175	0.8	87	5.5	15.3	0.4	3.2
Kidney, Red, Value, Tesco*	1 Serving/65g	60	0.4	93	6.9	15.0	0.6	6.2
Kidney, White, Dry, Raw, Unico*	½ Cup/80g	270	0.9	337	22.5	61.2	1.1	21.2
Mixed, Canned, Average	*1 Can/300g*	*300*	*3.5*	*100*	*6.7*	*15.6*	*1.2*	*4.1*
Mixed, in Mild Chilli Sauce, Sainsbury's*	1 Can/420g	328	1.3	78	4.9	13.8	0.3	3.7
Mixed, Spicy, Average	*1 Serving/140g*	*108*	*0.7*	*77*	*4.8*	*13.4*	*0.5*	*3.9*
Mixed, with Lentils, Waitrose*	1 Pack/300g	399	21.9	133	5.1	11.6	7.3	3.1
Mixed, with Passata, Tesco*	1 Can/300g	237	2.1	79	6.0	12.1	0.7	3.9
Mung, Whole, Dried, Boiled in Unsalted Water	*1oz/28g*	*25*	*0.1*	*91*	*7.6*	*15.3*	*0.4*	*3.0*
Mung, Whole, Dried, Raw	*1oz/28g*	*78*	*0.3*	*279*	*23.9*	*46.3*	*1.1*	*10.0*
Pinto, Dried, Boiled in Unsalted Water	*1oz/28g*	*38*	*0.2*	*137*	*8.9*	*23.9*	*0.7*	*0.0*
Pinto, Dried, Love Life, Waitrose*	1 Serving/80g	288	1.0	360	21.4	62.6	1.2	15.5
Pinto, Dried, Raw	*1oz/28g*	*92*	*0.4*	*327*	*21.1*	*57.1*	*1.6*	*14.0*
Refried, Average	*1 Serving/215g*	*162*	*1.5*	*75*	*4.6*	*12.7*	*0.7*	*1.7*
Runner, Average	*1 Serving/80g*	*16*	*0.3*	*20*	*1.4*	*2.8*	*0.4*	*2.2*
Soya, Dried, Average	*1oz/28g*	*104*	*5.1*	*370*	*34.2*	*15.4*	*18.3*	*19.6*
Soya, Dried, Boiled in Unsalted Water	*1oz/28g*	*39*	*2.0*	*141*	*14.0*	*5.1*	*7.3*	*6.1*
Soya, Frozen, Birds Eye*	1 Serving/80g	98	5.1	123	12.4	4.0	6.4	4.2
Soya, in Water, Salt Added, Sainsbury's*	1 Serving/100g	102	7.3	102	4.0	5.1	7.3	6.1
Soya, Shelled, Frozen, Raw, Average	*1 Serving/80g*	*99*	*4.3*	*124*	*12.2*	*6.9*	*5.3*	*4.4*
Soya, Tesco*	1 Pack/200g	240	11.6	120	10.2	6.7	5.8	2.0
White, Campo Largo*	½ Jar/200g	180	1.0	90	7.1	11.2	0.5	0.0
Wholesome, 10 Mix, Dried, Love Life, Waitrose*	1 Pack/500g	1850	17.0	370	13.3	71.5	3.4	10.0
BEEF								
Brisket, Boiled, Lean	1 Serving/100g	225	11.0	225	31.4	0.0	11.0	0.0
Brisket, Boiled, Lean & Fat	1 Serving/100g	268	17.4	268	27.8	0.0	17.4	0.0
Brisket, Braised, Lean	1 Serving/100g	280	17.4	280	29.0	0.0	17.4	0.0
Brisket, Raw, Lean	*1oz/28g*	*39*	*1.7*	*139*	*21.1*	*0.0*	*6.1*	*0.0*
Brisket, Raw, Lean & Fat	*1oz/28g*	*61*	*4.5*	*218*	*18.4*	*0.0*	*16.0*	*0.0*
Cooked, Sliced, From Supermarket, Average	*1 Slice/35g*	*47*	*1.2*	*135*	*23.6*	*2.0*	*3.5*	*0.5*
Escalope, Healthy Range, Average	*1 Serving/170g*	*233*	*6.7*	*137*	*24.2*	*1.2*	*4.0*	*0.4*
Flank, Pot-Roasted, Lean	*1oz/28g*	*71*	*3.9*	*253*	*31.8*	*0.0*	*14.0*	*0.0*
Flank, Pot-Roasted, Lean & Fat	*1oz/28g*	*87*	*6.2*	*309*	*27.1*	*0.0*	*22.3*	*0.0*
Flank, Raw, Lean	*1oz/28g*	*49*	*2.6*	*175*	*22.7*	*0.0*	*9.3*	*0.0*
Flank, Raw, Lean & Fat	*1oz/28g*	*74*	*5.8*	*266*	*19.7*	*0.0*	*20.8*	*0.0*
for Casserole, Lean, Diced, Average	*1oz/28g*	*35*	*1.1*	*126*	*23.0*	*0.0*	*3.8*	*0.0*
Fore Rib, Lean & Fat, Average	*1oz/28g*	*40*	*1.7*	*143*	*21.7*	*0.0*	*6.2*	*0.2*
Fore Rib, Raw, Lean	*1oz/28g*	*41*	*1.8*	*145*	*21.5*	*0.0*	*6.5*	*0.0*
Fore Rib, Roasted, Lean	*1oz/28g*	*66*	*3.2*	*236*	*33.3*	*0.0*	*11.4*	*0.0*
Fore Rib, Roasted, Lean & Fat	*1oz/28g*	*84*	*5.7*	*300*	*29.1*	*0.0*	*20.4*	*0.0*
Grill Steak, Average	*1 Steak/170g*	*501*	*39.5*	*295*	*19.3*	*2.1*	*23.2*	*0.1*
Grill Steak, Peppered, Average	*1 Serving/172g*	*419*	*24.4*	*243*	*23.6*	*5.2*	*14.2*	*0.3*
Joint, for Roasting, Average	*1oz/28g*	*38*	*1.0*	*134*	*24.5*	*1.4*	*3.4*	*0.2*
Joint, Sirloin, Roasted, Lean	*1oz/28g*	*53*	*1.8*	*188*	*32.4*	*0.0*	*6.5*	*0.0*
Joint, Sirloin, Roasted, Lean & Fat	*1oz/28g*	*65*	*3.5*	*233*	*29.8*	*0.0*	*12.6*	*0.0*
Mince, Cooked, Average	*1 Serving/75g*	*214*	*15.3*	*286*	*23.9*	*0.0*	*20.3*	*0.0*
Mince, Extra Lean, Raw, Average	*1 Serving/100g*	*124*	*5.0*	*124*	*21.2*	*0.1*	*5.0*	*0.0*
Mince, Extra Lean, Stewed	*1oz/28g*	*50*	*2.4*	*177*	*24.7*	*0.0*	*8.7*	*0.0*
Mince, Lean, Raw, Average	*1oz/28g*	*48*	*2.8*	*172*	*20.8*	*0.0*	*10.0*	*0.1*
Mince, Raw, Average	*1oz/28g*	*68*	*5.1*	*242*	*19.6*	*0.2*	*18.1*	*0.0*
Mince, Raw, Frozen, Average	*1 Serving/100g*	*176*	*10.0*	*176*	*20.4*	*0.0*	*10.0*	*0.0*
Mince, Steak, Extra Lean, Average	*1oz/28g*	*37*	*1.6*	*131*	*20.5*	*0.4*	*5.6*	*0.0*

	Measure INFO/WEIGHT	per Measure KCAL	FAT	Nutrition Values per 100g / 100ml KCAL	PROT	CARB	FAT	FIBRE
BEEF								
Mince, Steak, Raw, Average	1 Serving/125g	317	25.0	254	17.2	0.0	20.0	0.0
Mince, Stewed	1oz/28g	59	3.8	209	21.8	0.0	13.5	0.0
Peppered, Sliced, Average	1 Slice/20g	26	1.1	129	18.2	1.3	5.6	1.0
Roast, Sliced, Average	1 Slice/35g	48	1.3	136	26.1	0.4	3.6	0.2
Salt, Average	1 Serving/70g	80	1.7	114	21.7	1.0	2.5	0.1
Salted, Dried, Raw	1oz/28g	70	0.4	250	55.4	0.0	1.5	0.0
Silverside, Pot-Roasted, Lean	1oz/28g	54	1.8	193	34.0	0.0	6.3	0.0
Silverside, Pot-Roasted, Lean & Fat	1oz/28g	69	3.8	247	31.0	0.0	13.7	0.0
Silverside, Raw, Lean	1oz/28g	38	1.2	134	23.8	0.0	4.3	0.0
Silverside, Raw, Lean & Fat	1oz/28g	60	4.1	215	20.4	0.0	14.8	0.0
Silverside, Salted, Boiled, Lean	1oz/28g	52	1.9	184	30.4	0.0	6.9	0.0
Silverside, Salted, Boiled, Lean & Fat	1oz/28g	63	3.5	224	27.9	0.0	12.5	0.0
Silverside, Salted, Raw, Lean	1oz/28g	39	2.0	140	19.2	0.0	7.0	0.0
Silverside, Salted, Raw, Lean & Fat	1oz/28g	64	5.0	227	16.3	0.0	18.0	0.0
Steak, Braising, Braised, Lean	1oz/28g	63	2.7	225	34.4	0.0	9.7	0.0
Steak, Braising, Braised, Lean & Fat	1oz/28g	69	3.6	246	32.9	0.0	12.7	0.0
Steak, Braising, Lean, Raw, Average	1oz/28g	40	1.4	144	24.8	0.0	5.0	0.0
Steak, Braising, Raw, Lean & Fat	1oz/28g	45	2.4	160	20.7	0.0	8.6	0.0
Steak, Economy, Average	1oz/28g	53	2.4	190	26.9	1.2	8.7	0.4
Steak, Fillet, Cooked, Average	1oz/28g	54	2.4	191	28.6	0.0	8.5	0.0
Steak, Fillet, Lean, Average	1oz/28g	42	2.0	150	21.0	0.0	7.3	0.0
Steak, Fillet, Lean, Cooked, Average	1oz/28g	52	2.2	186	28.6	0.0	7.9	0.0
Steak, Frying, Average	1 Steak/110g	128	2.7	116	23.7	0.0	2.5	0.0
Steak, Rump, Cooked, Average	1oz/28g	69	4.0	245	29.1	0.5	14.1	0.0
Steak, Rump, Grilled, Rare, Lean	1 Steak/227g	381	15.6	168	26.5	0.0	6.9	0.0
Steak, Rump, Lean, Cooked, Average	1oz/28g	50	1.7	179	31.0	0.0	6.1	0.0
Steak, Rump, Raw, Lean	1oz/28g	35	1.1	125	22.0	0.0	4.1	0.0
Steak, Rump, Raw, Lean & Fat	1oz/28g	49	2.8	174	20.7	0.0	10.1	0.0
Steak, Sirloin, Fried, Rare, Lean	1oz/28g	53	2.3	189	28.8	0.0	8.2	0.0
Steak, Sirloin, Fried, Rare, Lean & Fat	1oz/28g	65	3.9	233	26.8	0.0	14.0	0.0
Steak, Sirloin, Grilled, Medium-Rare, Lean	1oz/28g	49	2.2	176	26.6	0.0	7.7	0.0
Steak, Sirloin, Grilled, Medium-Rare, Lean & Fat	1oz/28g	60	3.5	213	24.8	0.0	12.6	0.0
Steak, Sirloin, Grilled, Rare, Lean	1oz/28g	46	1.9	166	26.4	0.0	6.7	0.0
Steak, Sirloin, Grilled, Rare, Lean & Fat	1oz/28g	60	3.6	216	25.1	0.0	12.8	0.0
Steak, Sirloin, Grilled, Well-Done, Lean	1oz/28g	63	2.8	225	33.9	0.0	9.9	0.0
Steak, Sirloin, Grilled, Well-Done, Lean & Fat	1oz/28g	72	4.0	257	31.8	0.0	14.4	0.0
Steak, Sirloin, Raw, Lean	1oz/28g	38	1.3	135	23.5	0.0	4.5	0.0
Steak, Sirloin, Raw, Lean & Fat	1oz/28g	56	3.6	201	21.6	0.0	12.7	0.0
Stewed Steak, Average	1 Serving/220g	258	10.1	117	15.8	3.3	4.6	0.0
Stewing Steak, Lean & Fat, Raw, Average	1 Serving/100g	135	4.3	135	24.2	0.1	4.3	0.1
Stewing Steak, Raw, Lean	1oz/28g	34	1.0	122	22.6	0.0	3.5	0.0
Stewing Steak, Stewed, Lean	1oz/28g	52	1.8	185	32.0	0.0	6.3	0.0
Stewing Steak, Stewed, Lean & Fat	1oz/28g	57	2.7	203	29.2	0.0	9.6	0.0
Stir Fry Strips, Raw, Average	1 Serving/125g	149	3.7	119	23.0	0.0	3.0	0.2
Topside, Lean & Fat, Average	1oz/28g	61	3.4	219	27.5	0.0	12.2	0.0
Topside, Raw, Lean	1oz/28g	32	0.8	116	23.0	0.0	2.7	0.0
BEEF &								
Beer, Princes*	½ Can/205g	215	6.1	105	14.0	5.5	3.0	0.0
Black Bean, Sizzling, Oriental Express*	1 Pack/400g	420	8.4	105	7.2	14.0	2.1	2.1
Black Bean, with Rice, Weight Watchers*	1 Pack/320g	288	4.2	90	5.0	14.6	1.3	0.1
Onions, Minced, Asda*	½ Can/196g	314	19.6	160	13.0	4.6	10.0	0.1
Potatoes, Minced, Light Choices, Tesco*	1 Pack/450g	400	9.5	80	4.3	10.3	1.9	2.3
Yorkshire Pudding, Minced, Sainsbury's*	1 Pack/350g	374	11.9	107	8.4	10.7	3.4	1.1

	Measure INFO/WEIGHT	per Measure KCAL	FAT	Nutrition Values per 100g / 100ml KCAL	PROT	CARB	FAT	FIBRE
BEEF BORDELAISE								
Sainsbury's*	1 Pack/401g	525	25.7	131	8.7	9.7	6.4	1.0
BEEF BOURGUIGNON								
Extra Special, Asda*	1 Serving/300g	279	11.0	93	9.3	5.7	3.7	0.7
Finest, Tesco*	½ Pack/300g	247	7.8	82	9.9	4.8	2.6	0.5
BEEF BRAISED								
Steak, & Cabbage, COU, M & S*	1 Pack/380g	323	9.9	85	8.3	6.7	2.6	1.9
Steak, & Carrots, Mini Favourites, M & S*	1 Serving/200g	140	5.0	70	8.0	4.2	2.5	1.3
Steak, & Mash, GFY, Asda*	1 Pack/400g	260	3.2	65	3.4	11.0	0.8	0.7
Steak, & Mash, HL, Tesco*	1 Pack/450g	418	12.1	93	7.0	10.2	2.7	0.7
Steak, & Mash, M Kitchen, Morrisons*	1 Meal/250g	209	6.0	87	6.4	9.1	2.5	1.1
Steak, & Red Wine, Veg Mash, HL, Tesco*	1 Pack/500g	360	13.5	72	5.1	6.9	2.7	1.2
Steak, with Colcannon Mash, Tesco*	1 Pack/450g	477	15.7	106	9.5	9.0	3.5	0.9
Tender, Pub Specials, Birds Eye*	1 Pack/450g	243	3.6	54	5.5	6.1	0.8	1.8
BEEF CANTONESE								
Sainsbury's*	½ Pack/175g	199	2.3	114	5.5	20.1	1.3	0.5
BEEF CHASSEUR								
& Potato Mash, BGTY, Sainsbury's*	1 Pack/450g	387	10.8	86	7.8	8.4	2.4	1.3
BEEF DINNER								
British Cuisine, Tesco*	1 Pack/433g	390	10.0	90	6.3	10.0	2.3	2.3
Roast, Iceland*	1 Serving/340g	354	12.6	104	8.5	9.1	3.7	1.6
Roast, Sainsbury's*	1 Pack/400g	356	6.8	89	6.5	12.0	1.7	1.9
Roast with Trimmings	1 Dinner/840g	1310	63.0	156	6.1	17.7	7.5	2.3
Tesco*	1 Pack/400g	380	11.2	95	6.1	10.1	2.8	1.7
BEEF HOT & SOUR								
Chef's Selection, M & S*	1 Pack/329g	395	17.4	120	9.2	8.4	5.3	1.3
with Garlic Rice, BGTY, Sainsbury's*	1 Pack/400g	428	6.8	107	5.9	17.0	1.7	0.6
with Vegetable Rice, COU, M & S*	1 Pack/400g	360	5.6	90	5.5	14.4	1.4	0.6
BEEF IN								
Ale Gravy, Chunky, Birds Eye*	1 Pack/340g	272	6.8	80	7.4	8.3	2.0	1.5
Ale with Mushrooms, BGTY, Sainsbury's*	1 Pack/251g	193	3.8	77	10.2	5.6	1.5	0.4
Black Bean, with Egg Noodles, M & S*	1 Pack/400g	460	6.0	115	8.6	16.7	1.5	1.8
Black Bean Sauce, Chinese, Tesco*	1 Pack/400g	396	12.4	99	9.1	8.7	3.1	0.5
Black Bean Sauce, M & S*	1 Pack/350g	402	22.4	115	8.9	5.7	6.4	1.1
Black Pepper Sauce, & Egg Fried Rice, Tesco*	1 Pack/451g	622	24.8	138	7.0	15.2	5.5	1.2
Black Velvet Porter, Diet Chef Ltd*	1 Meal/300g	201	3.6	67	8.2	6.0	1.2	2.1
Burgundy Red Wine, GFY, Asda*	1 Pack/405g	348	8.1	86	8.0	9.0	2.0	1.1
Creamy Peppercorn Sauce, Steak, Tesco*	1 Steak/150g	189	8.2	126	16.5	2.6	5.5	0.1
Gravy, Roast, Birds Eye*	1 Pack/227g	177	3.9	78	13.4	2.2	1.7	0.0
Gravy, Sliced, Iceland*	1 Pack/200g	172	3.2	86	12.1	5.9	1.6	0.3
Gravy, Sliced, Sainsbury's*	1 Serving/125g	100	2.2	80	13.5	2.6	1.8	0.2
Gravy, Sliced, Tesco*	1 Serving/200g	152	4.2	76	11.3	3.1	2.1	0.2
Madeira & Mushroom Gravy, Sliced, Finest, Tesco*	1 Pack/400g	536	24.8	134	15.2	4.3	6.2	1.0
Oriental Sauce, Lean Cuisine, Findus*	1 Pack/350g	420	8.7	120	4.5	20.0	2.5	1.5
Oyster Sauce, Asda*	1 Serving/100g	82	4.0	82	7.0	4.4	4.0	1.7
Red Wine, 117, Oakhouse Foods Ltd*	1 Meal/380g	403	17.1	106	7.7	8.1	4.5	1.5
Red Wine Sauce, Milson's Kitchen, Aldi*	1 Pack/400g	256	6.0	64	5.6	9.6	1.5	2.1
Red Wine Sauce, Simply Bistro, Aldi*	1 Pack/400g	316	6.0	79	5.6	9.2	1.5	2.1
Strips, Chilli Sauce, Tesco*	1 Pack/166g	290	7.8	175	23.2	9.6	4.7	0.0
Velvet Porter, with Potatoes, Look What We Found*	1 Pack/300g	201	3.6	67	8.2	6.0	1.2	2.1
BEEF SZECHUAN								
Sizzling Hot Spicy, Oriental Express*	1 Pack/400g	380	7.6	95	6.4	13.2	1.9	2.0
BEEF TERIYAKI								
Incredibly Tender, Charlie Bigham's*	½ Pack/300g	477	26.7	159	5.0	10.9	8.9	0.9

	Measure INFO/WEIGHT	per Measure KCAL	FAT	Nutrition Values per 100g / 100ml KCAL	PROT	CARB	FAT	FIBRE
BEEF TERIYAKI								
with Noodles, BGTY, Sainsbury's*	1 Pack/400g	320	4.0	80	7.7	10.1	1.0	1.0
BEEF WELLINGTON								
Average	1 Serving/200g	530	33.3	265	12.3	16.9	16.6	1.0
BEEF WITH								
Black Bean Sauce, Chilli, Sainsbury's*	1 Pack/300g	336	14.4	112	8.7	8.6	4.8	1.0
Black Bean Sauce, Rice Bowl, Uncle Ben's*	1 Pack/350g	367	4.9	105	5.6	17.4	1.4	0.0
Diane Sauce, Rump Steak, Tesco*	1 Steak/165g	181	8.1	110	15.1	1.1	4.9	0.3
Horseradish Dressing, Slow Cooked, HL, Tesco*	1 Pack/356g	285	10.3	80	5.4	7.5	2.9	1.4
Onion & Gravy, Minced, Princes*	1 Serving/200g	342	24.4	171	9.9	5.5	12.2	0.0
Onions & Gravy, Minced, Tesco*	1 Can/198g	224	10.1	113	14.0	2.8	5.1	0.8
Oyster Sauce, Ooodles of Noodles, Oriental Express*	1 Pack/425g	378	5.5	89	4.9	14.2	1.3	1.5
Peppercorn Sauce, Rib Eye Joint, Sainsbury's*	1 Serving/181g	299	12.7	165	22.2	3.4	7.0	0.1
Peppercorn Sauce, Steak, Just Cook, Sainsbury's*	½ Pack/128g	174	7.3	136	17.7	3.4	5.7	1.2
Red Wine Sauce, Rump Steak, Tesco*	1 Serving/150g	180	8.5	120	17.2	0.1	5.7	3.3
Red Wine Sauce, Steaks, Just Cook, Sainsbury's*	½ Pack/70g	83	2.3	118	20.0	2.0	3.3	0.2
Shiraz Wine Sauce, Pot Roast, Finest, Tesco*	1 Pack/350g	350	9.1	100	14.1	5.1	2.6	0.9
Vegetables, Tesco*	1 Pot/300g	102	3.0	34	2.9	3.3	1.0	1.1
Vegetables & Gravy, Minced, Birds Eye*	1 Pack/178g	155	6.1	87	9.1	5.1	3.4	0.6
BEER								
Ale, Bottled, Old Speckled Hen*	1 Bottle/330ml	124	0.3	37	0.2	1.8	0.1	0.2
Ale, Freeminer, Organic, Fairtrade, Co-Op*	1 Bottle/480ml	240	0.5	50	0.2	2.7	0.1	0.0
Ale, Hopping Hare, Hall & Woodhouse Ltd*	1 Bottle/500ml	188	0.0	38	0.4	3.0	0.0	0.0
Ale, Pale, IPA, Greene King*	1 Pint/570ml	158	0.1	28	0.3	1.6	0.0	0.3
Ale, Pale, Sierra Nevada*	1 Bottle/350g	175	0.0	50	0.4	4.0	0.0	0.0
Ale, Scarecrow, Wychwood, Marstons PLC*	1 Bottle/500ml	214	0.0	43	0.3	4.3	0.0	0.0
Bitter, Canned, Average	*1 Can/440ml*	*141*	*0.0*	*32*	*0.3*	*2.3*	*0.0*	*0.0*
Bitter, Cask, Draught, London Pride, Fullers*	1 Pint/568ml	201	0.0	35	0.0	0.0	0.0	0.0
Bitter, Draught, Average	*1 Pint/568ml*	*182*	*0.0*	*32*	*0.3*	*2.3*	*0.0*	*0.0*
Bitter, Keg, Average	*1 Pint/568ml*	*176*	*0.0*	*31*	*0.3*	*2.3*	*0.0*	*0.0*
Bitter, Low Alcohol, Average	*1 Pint/568ml*	*74*	*0.0*	*13*	*0.2*	*2.1*	*0.0*	*0.0*
Bitter, Original, Tetley's*	1 Can/440ml	140	0.0	32	0.2	4.5	0.0	0.0
Especial, Modelo*	1 Bottle/355ml	145	0.0	41	0.0	1.1	0.0	0.0
Guinness, Draught*	*1 Can/440ml*	*158*	*0.2*	*36*	*0.3*	*3.0*	*0.0*	*0.0*
Guinness, Stout*	*1 Pint/568ml*	*170*	*0.0*	*30*	*0.4*	*3.0*	*0.0*	*0.0*
Guinness Extra Stout, Bottled*	*1 Bottle/500ml*	*215*	*0.0*	*43*	*4.0*	*0.0*	*0.0*	*0.0*
Honey Dew, Fullers*	1 Bottle/500ml	232	0.0	46	0.0	4.6	0.0	0.0
Kilkenny, Diageo*	1 Pint/568ml	210	0.0	37	0.3	3.0	0.0	0.0
Low Calorie, Low Carb, Cobra*	1 Bottle/330ml	96	0.0	29	0.1	1.3	0.0	0.0
Mackeson, Stout	*1 Pint/568ml*	*205*	*0.0*	*36*	*0.4*	*4.6*	*0.0*	*0.0*
Mild, Draught, Average	*1 Pint/568ml*	*136*	*0.0*	*24*	*0.2*	*1.6*	*0.0*	*0.0*
Non Alcoholic, Cobra*	1 Bottle/330ml	79	0.0	24	0.8	2.0	0.0	0.0
Oak Aged, Innis & Gunn*	1 Bottle/330ml	120	0.0	36	0.0	3.6	0.0	0.0
Resolution, Low Carb, Marstons PLC*	1 Glass/250ml	77	0.2	31	0.3	0.6	0.1	0.0
Ultra, Michelob*	1 Bottle/275ml	88	0.0	32	0.0	0.9	0.0	0.0
Weissbier, Alcohol Free, Erdinger*	1 Bottle/500ml	125	0.0	25	0.4	5.3	0.0	0.0
Wheat, Tesco*	1 Bottle/500ml	155	0.0	31	0.5	0.4	0.0	0.0
BEETROOT								
Cooked, Boiled, Drained, Average	*1 Serving/100g*	*44*	*0.2*	*44*	*1.7*	*10.0*	*0.2*	*2.0*
Crinkle Cut, Drained, Baxters*	1 Slice/10g	3	0.0	26	1.2	5.1	0.1	1.2
Pickled, in Sweet Vinegar, Average	*1oz/28g*	*16*	*0.0*	*57*	*1.2*	*12.8*	*0.1*	*1.5*
Pickled, in Vinegar, Average	*1 Serving/50g*	*19*	*0.0*	*37*	*1.6*	*7.5*	*0.1*	*1.2*
Raw, Average	*1oz/28g*	*9*	*0.0*	*32*	*1.5*	*6.0*	*0.1*	*1.8*

	Measure INFO/WEIGHT	per Measure KCAL	FAT	Nutrition Values per 100g / 100ml KCAL	PROT	CARB	FAT	FIBRE
BHAJI								
Aubergine & Potato, Fried in Vegetable Oil, Average	1oz/28g	36	2.5	130	2.0	12.0	8.8	1.7
Cabbage & Pea, Fried in Vegetable Oil, Average	1oz/28g	50	4.1	178	3.3	9.2	14.7	3.4
Cauliflower, Fried in Vegetable Oil, Average	1oz/28g	60	5.7	214	4.0	4.0	20.5	2.0
Mushroom, Fried in Vegetable Oil, Average	1oz/28g	46	4.5	166	1.7	4.4	16.1	1.3
Okra, Bangladeshi, Fried in Butter Ghee, Average	1oz/28g	27	1.8	95	2.5	7.6	6.4	3.2
Onion, Asda*	1 Bhaji/49g	96	4.9	196	6.0	20.0	10.0	2.0
Onion, Sainsbury's*	1 Bhaji/38g	93	5.1	245	6.5	24.7	13.4	6.4
Onion, Tesco*	1 Bhaji/47g	85	4.9	181	5.7	16.2	10.4	4.3
Onion with Tomato & Chilli Dip, M & S*	1 Bhaji/54g	111	6.3	205	4.1	21.1	11.7	3.6
Potato, Onion & Mushroom, Fried, Average	1oz/28g	58	4.9	208	2.0	12.0	17.5	1.5
Potato, Spinach & Cauliflower, Fried, Average	1oz/28g	47	4.2	169	2.2	7.1	15.1	1.4
Potato & Onion, Fried in Vegetable Oil, Average	1oz/28g	45	2.8	160	2.1	16.6	10.1	1.6
Spinach, Fried in Vegetable Oil, Average	1oz/28g	23	1.9	83	3.3	2.6	6.8	2.4
Spinach & Potato, Fried in Vegetable Oil, Average	1oz/28g	53	3.9	191	3.7	13.4	14.1	2.3
Turnip & Onion, Fried in Vegetable Oil, Average	1oz/28g	36	3.1	128	1.3	7.1	10.9	2.2
Vegetable, Fried in Vegetable Oil, Average	1oz/28g	59	5.2	212	2.1	10.1	18.5	2.4
BHUNA								
Chicken, & Rice, Sainsbury's*	1 Pack/501g	696	31.5	139	7.3	13.3	6.3	1.5
Chicken, Curry, Tesco*	1 Serving/300g	396	22.8	132	11.4	4.5	7.6	0.5
Chicken, Hyderabadi, Sainsbury's*	1 Pack/400g	472	20.8	118	12.6	5.2	5.2	1.3
Chicken, Indian Takeaway, Tesco*	1 Pack/350g	437	27.6	125	8.3	4.6	7.9	2.2
Chicken, with Naan Bread, Sharwood's*	1 Pack/375g	465	19.1	124	6.8	12.8	5.1	2.8
Chicken Tikka, Tesco*	1 Pack/350g	437	23.4	125	11.3	5.0	6.7	0.9
King Prawn, Chosen By You, Asda*	1 Pack/375g	296	17.2	79	4.4	4.3	4.6	1.4
King Prawn, M & S*	1 Pack/350g	262	13.3	75	6.7	3.3	3.8	1.5
King Prawn, Morrisons*	1 Pack/350g	301	20.6	86	6.5	1.8	5.9	0.5
Lamb, & Rice, Sainsbury's*	1 Pack/500g	619	26.5	124	7.4	11.6	5.3	2.0
Prawn, Co-Op*	1 Pack/400g	300	16.0	75	3.0	6.0	4.0	1.0
Prawn, Tandoori, Indian, Sainsbury's*	½ Pack/200g	152	8.0	76	5.5	4.5	4.0	1.7
BIERWURST								
Average	*1 Slice/10g*	*25*	*2.1*	*252*	*14.4*	*0.9*	*21.2*	*0.0*
BILBERRIES								
Fresh, Raw	*1oz/28g*	*8*	*0.1*	*30*	*0.6*	*6.9*	*0.2*	*1.8*
BILTONG								
Average	*1 Serving/25g*	*64*	*1.0*	*256*	*50.0*	*0.0*	*4.0*	*0.0*
BIRYANI								
Chicken, COU, M & S*	1 Pack/400g	360	8.4	90	6.9	10.8	2.1	1.9
Chicken, Easy Steam, HL, Tesco*	1 Pack/400g	424	7.2	106	7.0	15.5	1.8	0.6
Chicken, Indian, Asda*	1 Pack/450g	778	22.5	173	9.0	23.0	5.0	0.7
Chicken, Light Choices, Tesco*	1 Serving/450g	495	10.3	110	7.0	15.0	2.3	3.4
Chicken, Ready Meal, Average	1 Pack/400g	521	17.1	130	7.5	15.2	4.3	1.6
Chicken, Ready Meal, Healthy Range, Average	1 Pack/400g	369	5.5	92	7.4	12.6	1.4	0.9
Chicken, Tikka, Ready Meal, Average	1 Pack/400g	460	11.5	115	7.3	14.8	2.9	1.5
Chicken, Weight Watchers*	1 Pack/330g	308	3.7	93	6.2	14.6	1.1	0.6
Chicken Tikka, BGTY, Sainsbury's*	1 Pack/400g	316	3.8	84	6.8	10.7	1.0	2.9
Chicken Tikka, Northern Indian, Sainsbury's*	1 Pack/450g	697	25.6	155	9.4	16.5	5.7	1.2
Lamb, Average	1 Serving/200g	390	19.4	195	7.3	20.9	9.7	0.0
Lamb, HL, Tesco*	1 Pack/400g	560	17.6	140	5.1	19.0	4.4	3.1
Lamb, Ready Meal, Average	1 Pack/400g	535	18.9	134	6.0	16.6	4.7	2.2
Seafood, M & S*	1 Pack/450g	619	25.7	138	7.1	14.4	5.7	1.7
Vegetable, & Rice, Sainsbury's*	½ Pack/125g	229	5.0	183	4.4	32.4	4.0	0.7
Vegetable, HL, Tesco*	1 Pack/450g	454	9.4	101	2.7	17.9	2.1	1.6
Vegetable, Sainsbury's*	1 Serving/225g	328	17.8	146	2.4	16.3	7.9	1.1

	Measure INFO/WEIGHT	per Measure KCAL	FAT	Nutrition Values per 100g / 100ml KCAL	PROT	CARB	FAT	FIBRE
BIRYANI								
Vegetable, Tikka, Vegelicious, Tesco*	1 Pack/340g	340	10.5	100	4.6	11.4	3.1	3.0
Vegetable, Waitrose*	1 Pack/450g	521	19.8	116	2.4	14.9	4.4	3.6
Vegetable with Rice, Patak's*	½ Pack/125g	194	1.9	155	3.6	32.9	1.5	1.2
BISCOTTI								
Almond, Pan Ducale*	1 Serving/30g	130	5.0	433	10.0	60.0	16.7	3.3
Chocolate, Heinz*	1 Biscuit/20g	80	1.7	398	8.5	72.0	8.7	5.8
Chocolate Chip, Kate's Cakes Ltd*	1 Biscotti/36g	134	4.6	372	6.5	57.9	12.7	2.7
BISCUITS								
Abbey Crunch, McVitie's*	1 Biscuit/9g	43	1.6	477	6.0	72.8	17.9	2.5
Abernethy, Simmers*	1 Biscuit/12g	61	2.7	490	5.7	69.2	21.9	0.0
Aero, Nestle*	1 Bar/19g	99	5.5	534	6.4	59.4	29.4	2.1
Aero, Orange, Aero, Nestle*	1 Biscuit/19g	101	5.6	534	6.0	60.6	29.3	1.7
After Eight, Nestle*	1 Biscuit/5g	26	1.4	525	6.5	62.6	27.7	1.5
All Butter, Tesco*	1 Biscuit/9g	44	2.1	486	6.3	63.5	23.0	1.9
Almond, Artisan Bakery, Extra Special, Asda*	1 Biscuit/19g	103	6.1	548	7.9	54.3	32.3	4.2
Almond & Chocolate, Biscotti, TTD, Sainsbury's*	1 Biscuit/30g	132	4.8	440	8.4	65.6	16.0	3.1
Almond Butter Thins, Extra Special, Asda*	1 Biscuit/4g	15	0.5	375	5.0	60.0	12.5	2.5
Almond Fingers, Tesco*	1 Finger/46g	180	6.8	391	6.2	58.4	14.7	1.0
Almond Thins, Continental, Tesco*	1 Biscuit/3g	15	0.5	450	6.7	72.8	14.7	3.1
Almond Thins, TTD, Sainsbury's*	1 Biscuit/4g	16	0.5	450	6.7	72.8	14.7	3.1
Amaretti, Doria*	1 Biscuit/4g	17	0.3	433	6.0	84.8	7.8	0.0
Amaretti, M & S*	1 Biscuit/6g	30	1.1	480	9.6	71.3	17.2	3.8
Amaretti, Sainsbury's*	1 Biscuit/6g	27	0.7	450	6.5	80.5	11.3	1.1
Animals, Milk Chocolate, Cadbury*	1 Biscuit/19g	94	4.0	493	6.6	69.8	20.9	0.0
Apple & Raspberry, Minis, Officially Low Fat, Fox's*	1 Bag/40g	140	1.1	350	3.9	76.9	2.7	3.8
Apple & Sultana, Go Ahead, McVitie's*	1 Biscuit/15g	56	1.1	386	6.0	72.7	7.9	3.3
Apple Crumble, Officially Low Fat, Fox's*	1 Biscuit/23g	85	0.6	365	5.4	80.4	2.4	2.5
Apricot, Low Fat, M & S*	1 Biscuit/23g	79	1.0	343	6.1	69.6	4.4	7.8
Arrowroot, Thin, Crawfords*	1 Biscuit/7g	35	1.2	450	6.9	71.4	15.2	2.8
Belgian Chocolate, Selection, Finest, Tesco*	1 Biscuit/10g	51	2.7	515	6.0	62.0	27.0	3.0
Belgian Milk Chocolate, M & S*	1 Biscuit/12g	60	2.5	490	6.2	70.1	20.3	2.5
Berry GI, Diet Chef Ltd*	1 Biscuit/20g	87	3.2	435	7.0	65.2	16.1	7.2
Biscbits, Honeycomb Crunch, Cadbury*	7 Pieces/25g	120	5.2	480	6.0	67.3	20.9	1.4
Blackcurrant with Wheat Bran, Bisca*	1 Biscuit/8g	31	0.9	420	6.0	72.0	12.0	5.5
Blueberry, Biscuit Moments, Special K, Kellogg's*	2 Biscuits/25g	99	2.3	394	4.5	73.0	9.0	1.5
Blueberry & Vanilla, Oaty, Weight Watchers*	1 Biscuit/22g	101	4.1	460	7.1	65.6	18.8	4.2
Bn, Chocolate Flavour, McVitie's*	1 Biscuit/18g	83	3.0	460	6.6	71.0	16.7	2.6
Bn, Strawberry Flavour, McVitie's*	1 Biscuit/18g	71	1.2	395	5.6	78.0	6.8	0.0
Bn, Vanilla Flavour, McVitie's*	1 Biscuit/18g	85	3.0	470	5.9	74.0	16.6	1.2
Bourbon, Average	1 Biscuit/13g	63	2.8	488	5.7	68.2	21.3	2.1
Bourbon, Gluten & Wheat Free, Lovemore*	1 Biscuit/15g	70	2.9	469	4.1	67.9	19.1	4.7
Bourbon, Trufree*	1 Biscuit/13g	61	2.8	486	7.5	62.6	22.6	1.1
Brandy Snaps, Average	1 Biscuit/15g	69	2.2	460	2.7	79.7	14.4	0.5
Breakfast, Forest Fruits, Belvita, Nabisco*	1 Biscuit/13g	60	2.1	460	8.5	67.0	16.0	5.3
Breakfast, Honey & Nuts, Belvita, Nabisco*	1 Biscuit/13g	58	2.1	464	8.0	68.0	17.0	3.5
Breakfast, Muesli, Belvita, Nabisco*	1 Biscuit/13g	59	2.1	455	8.2	67.0	16.0	4.1
Breakfast, Original, All Bran, Kellogg's*	1 Pack/40g	176	8.0	440	8.0	49.0	20.0	16.0
Breakfast, Yogurt Crunch, Belvita, Nabisco*	2 Biscuits/50g	230	8.6	455	7.6	66.0	17.0	4.0
Butter, Crinkle Crunch, Fox's*	1 Biscuit/11g	50	1.9	460	5.8	69.8	17.5	2.4
Cafe Noir, McVitie's*	1 Biscuit/9g	39	0.5	420	4.5	87.0	5.5	1.1
Cantuccini, with Almonds, Average	1 Biscotti/30g	130	5.0	433	10.0	60.0	16.7	3.3
Caramel & Honeycomb Cream, Velverty, Fox's*	1 Biscuit/19g	104	6.3	546	6.7	55.0	32.9	1.4
Caramel Crunch, Go Ahead, McVitie's*	1 Bar/24g	106	3.3	440	4.7	76.6	13.8	0.8

B

	Measure INFO/WEIGHT	per Measure KCAL	FAT	Nutrition Values per 100g / 100ml KCAL	PROT	CARB	FAT	FIBRE
BISCUITS								
Caramelised, Lotus*	1 Biscuit/9g	43	1.7	483	4.9	72.7	18.9	1.3
Caramels, Milk Chocolate, McVitie's*	1 Serving/17g	81	3.6	478	5.6	65.8	21.4	1.8
Cheddars, Real Cheddar Cheese, Jacob's*	1 Biscuit/4g	20	1.2	526	11.0	48.6	32.1	3.0
Cheese, & Chutney, Delicious, Boots*	1 Pack/134g	290	14.7	217	9.0	19.0	11.0	2.3
Cheese Melts, Carr's*	1 Biscuit/4g	20	0.9	483	11.2	57.0	22.5	3.9
Cheese Sandwich, Ritz*	1 Biscuit/9g	50	2.8	530	9.5	55.0	30.2	2.0
Choc Chip, Paterson's*	1 Biscuit/17g	79	3.6	474	5.6	64.0	21.6	3.1
Chocahoops, Cadbury*	1 Biscuit/13g	65	3.4	510	5.8	62.7	26.4	0.0
Choco Leibniz, Dark Chocolate, Bahlsen*	1 Biscuit/14g	69	3.6	493	6.8	59.0	26.0	5.1
Choco Leibniz, Milk, Bahlsen*	1 Biscuit/10g	51	2.5	515	7.9	63.4	25.5	0.0
Choco Leibniz, Orange Flavour, Bahlsen*	1 Biscuit/14g	70	3.7	504	7.9	58.5	26.4	0.0
Chocolate, Belgian Chocolate, Weight Watchers*	1 Biscuit/18g	87	4.1	481	7.1	61.8	22.8	4.5
Chocolate, Fingers, Average	1 Biscuit/6g	31	1.6	514	6.7	61.4	26.8	1.5
Chocolate, Golden Crunch, Free From Milk, Tesco*	1 Biscuit/17g	85	4.9	510	4.2	57.2	29.4	4.6
Chocolate, Quirks, Mcvitie's*	1 Biscuit/13g	66	3.6	509	5.0	58.7	27.7	2.5
Chocolate & Coconut, Duchy Originals*	1 Biscuit/13g	68	4.3	543	6.3	52.1	34.4	2.6
Chocolate & Hazelnut, Quirks, Mcvitie's*	1 Biscuit/13g	66	3.6	511	5.0	58.4	28.0	2.6
Chocolate Break, Plain Chocolate, Tesco*	1 Biscuit/21g	112	6.1	535	6.7	61.2	29.2	3.8
Chocolate Chip & Peanut, Trufree*	1 Biscuit/11g	55	2.6	496	4.0	66.0	24.0	2.0
Chocolate Chip Gl, Diet Chef Ltd*	1 Pack/20g	90	3.6	450	7.4	64.4	17.9	6.4
Chocolate Fingers, Caramel, Cadbury*	1 Finger/8g	39	1.9	490	5.8	63.2	23.8	0.0
Chocolate Fingers, Milk, Cadbury*	1 Biscuit/6g	31	1.6	515	6.8	60.8	27.1	1.7
Chocolate Fingers, Milk, Extra Crunchy, Cadbury*	1 Biscuit/5g	25	1.2	505	6.6	66.2	23.6	0.0
Chocolate Fingers, Plain, Cadbury*	1 Biscuit/6g	30	1.6	508	6.2	60.6	26.8	0.0
Chocolate Florentine, M & S*	1 Serving/39g	195	9.7	500	7.4	64.5	24.9	1.7
Chocolate Ginger, Organic, Duchy Originals*	1 Biscuit/12g	64	3.6	518	4.6	59.7	29.0	2.1
Chocolate Ginger, Thorntons*	1 Biscuit/19g	96	5.3	512	5.9	58.2	28.4	0.0
Chocolate Kimberley, Jacob's*	1 Biscuit/20g	86	3.4	428	3.9	64.4	17.2	1.1
Chocolate Mini Shorties, Mcvities*	1 Pack/25g	131	7.1	524	6.0	61.2	28.3	2.0
Chocolate Viennese, Fox's*	1 Biscuit/16g	85	4.9	530	6.7	56.6	30.7	1.7
Chocolinis, Milk Chocolate, Go Ahead, McVitie's*	1 Biscuit/12g	56	1.7	466	7.7	77.2	14.0	2.0
Christmas Shapes, Assorted, Sainsbury's*	1 Biscuit/15g	77	4.3	525	5.2	59.0	29.8	1.7
Classic, Creams, Fox's*	1 Biscuit/14g	72	3.6	516	4.4	65.2	25.8	1.7
Classic, Milk Chocolate, Fox's*	1 Biscuit/13g	67	3.1	517	6.1	64.9	24.0	1.6
Coconut Crinkle, Sainsbury's*	1 Biscuit/11g	54	2.8	500	6.4	59.6	26.2	3.7
Coconut Crinkles, Fox's*	1 Biscuit/11g	53	2.5	487	5.2	63.8	22.6	3.7
Coconut Ring, Asda*	1 Biscuit/8g	37	1.7	486	6.0	66.0	22.0	2.6
Crispy Slices, Raspberry, Go Ahead, McVitie's*	1 Slice/14g	54	1.0	389	5.9	75.9	6.9	3.0
Crispy Slices, Red Cherry, Go Ahead, McVitie's*	3 Slice/39g	147	2.7	380	5.5	73.9	7.0	2.9
Crunchers, Salted, Savoury, Crackers, Sainsbury's*	1 Cracker/5g	22	1.0	448	6.1	59.4	20.4	1.4
Crunchy Caramel, Tesco*	1 Bar/21g	98	5.2	467	4.6	56.0	25.0	1.4
Crunchy Oats, Breakfast, Belvita, Nabisco*	1 Biscuit/13g	59	2.1	455	8.0	67.0	16.0	5.5
Custard Creams, 25% Less Fat, Asda*	1 Biscuit/10g	47	1.8	474	6.0	72.0	18.0	1.2
Custard Creams, 25% Less Fat, Sainsbury's*	1 Biscuit/13g	59	2.2	469	5.8	72.7	17.3	1.3
Custard Creams, BGTY, Sainsbury's*	1 Biscuit/12g	56	2.1	473	5.8	72.2	17.9	1.2
Custard Creams, Crawfords*	1 Biscuit/11g	57	2.7	517	5.9	69.2	24.1	1.5
Custard Creams, Jacob's*	1 Biscuit/16g	77	3.3	481	5.3	68.0	20.9	1.6
Custard Creams, Trufree*	1 Biscuit/12g	60	2.8	504	8.7	65.0	23.0	1.0
Dark Chocolate All Butter, M & S*	1 Biscuit/15g	72	4.1	480	6.9	52.4	27.2	11.4
Dark Chocolate Ginger, M & S*	1 Biscuit/21g	105	5.7	505	5.0	58.8	27.6	4.2
Dark Chocolate Gingers, Border*	1 Biscuit/17g	74	3.4	445	4.4	61.4	20.1	2.9
Digestive, 25% Less Fat, Asda*	1 Biscuit/16g	73	2.6	455	7.3	69.8	16.3	2.6
Digestive, 25% Less Fat, Tesco*	1 Biscuit/14g	65	2.3	462	7.3	71.0	16.5	3.8

BISCUITS

	Measure INFO/WEIGHT	per Measure KCAL	FAT	Nutrition Values per 100g / 100ml KCAL	PROT	CARB	FAT	FIBRE
Digestive, Caramels, Milk Chocolate, McVitie's*	1 Biscuit/17g	81	3.7	478	5.6	65.1	21.7	2.3
Digestive, Caramels, Plain Chocolate, McVitie's*	1 Biscuit/17g	82	3.8	481	5.7	65.5	22.1	2.1
Digestive, Chocolate	1 Biscuit/17g	84	4.1	493	6.8	66.5	24.1	2.2
Digestive, Chocolate, Cadbury*	1 Biscuit/17g	85	4.2	495	6.8	62.3	24.4	0.0
Digestive, Cracker Selection, Tesco*	1 Biscuit/12g	56	2.3	464	7.1	65.2	19.4	4.3
Digestive, Crawfords*	1 Biscuit/12g	58	2.4	484	7.1	68.8	20.0	3.4
Digestive, Creams, McVitie's*	1 Biscuit/12g	60	2.8	502	5.6	68.2	23.0	2.1
Digestive, Dark Chocolate, McVitie's*	1 Biscuit/17g	82	4.0	487	6.0	61.6	24.0	4.0
Digestive, Everyday Value, Tesco*	1 Biscuit/16g	80	3.4	490	6.7	66.5	21.0	3.0
Digestive, GFY, Asda*	1 Biscuit/14g	65	2.4	461	6.0	71.0	17.0	3.6
Digestive, Gluten & Wheat Free, Lovemore*	1 Biscuit/15g	55	2.7	378	3.4	49.3	18.5	18.4
Digestive, Gluten Free, Barkat*	1 Biscuit/15g	56	2.7	378	3.4	49.3	18.5	18.4
Digestive, Happy Shopper*	1 Biscuit/13g	64	2.9	498	6.8	66.3	22.8	3.3
Digestive, Hovis*	1 Biscuit/6g	27	1.1	447	10.2	60.0	18.5	4.4
Digestive, Jacob's*	1 Biscuit/14g	67	3.0	479	6.6	65.7	21.1	3.4
Digestive, Lemon & Ginger, McVitie's*	1 Biscuit/15g	72	3.1	480	6.7	66.7	20.7	2.7
Digestive, Light, McVitie's*	1 Biscuit/15g	65	2.1	437	7.3	69.5	14.4	3.6
Digestive, McVitie's*	1 Biscuit/15g	70	3.2	470	7.2	62.7	21.5	3.6
Digestive, Milk Chocolate, 25% Less Fat, Tesco*	1 Biscuit/17g	79	3.0	466	7.4	69.0	17.8	2.6
Digestive, Milk Chocolate, Basics, Sainsbury's*	1 Biscuit/14g	71	3.4	496	6.5	62.9	23.7	2.9
Digestive, Milk Chocolate, GFY, Asda*	1 Biscuit/17g	78	2.9	457	7.0	69.0	17.0	3.2
Digestive, Milk Chocolate, Homewheat, McVitie's*	1 Biscuit/17g	83	4.1	486	6.0	61.5	24.0	4.0
Digestive, Milk Chocolate, McVitie's*	1 Biscuit/17g	84	4.0	488	6.7	62.7	23.4	2.9
Digestive, Milk Chocolate, Trufree*	1 Biscuit/12g	63	3.0	521	4.0	70.0	25.0	2.0
Digestive, Milk Chocolate Mint, McVitie's*	1 Biscuit/17g	81	3.9	487	6.7	62.6	23.4	2.9
Digestive, Munch Bites, McVitie's*	1 Pack/40g	205	10.2	512	6.5	64.5	25.5	2.0
Digestive, Oat, Weight Watchers*	1 Biscuit/11g	50	2.1	457	6.0	66.3	18.6	6.9
Digestive, Organic, Sainsbury's*	1 Biscuit/12g	60	2.9	483	6.6	60.9	23.7	5.8
Digestive, Plain, Average	1 Biscuit/14g	67	2.9	480	7.1	65.6	20.5	3.5
Digestive, Reduced Fat, M & S*	1 Biscuit/16g	75	2.7	480	7.2	73.3	17.5	3.4
Digestive, Reduced Fat, McVitie's*	1 Biscuit/15g	70	2.4	467	7.1	72.8	16.3	3.4
Digestive, Reduced Fat, Tesco*	1 Biscuit/16g	70	2.6	453	7.0	69.1	16.6	3.4
Digestive, Sweetmeal, Asda*	1 Biscuit/14g	68	3.1	499	7.0	66.0	23.0	3.5
Digestive, Sweetmeal, Sainsbury's*	1 Biscuit/14g	72	3.3	498	6.0	66.4	23.1	3.3
Digestive, Whole Wheat, Organic, Dove's Farm*	1 Biscuit/13g	56	2.4	446	5.9	61.6	19.5	7.8
Digestive with Wheatgerm, Hovis*	1 Biscuit/12g	37	2.2	306	6.2	66.8	18.5	5.8
Double Choc Chip, Trufree*	1 Biscuit/11g	58	3.0	523	3.0	67.0	27.0	1.8
Double Chocolate, Quirks, Mcvitie's*	1 Biscuit/13g	66	3.6	505	5.0	57.2	27.8	3.2
First Class, Bahlsen*	1 Serving/125g	711	45.2	569	7.5	53.4	36.2	0.0
Florentines, Sainsbury's*	1 Florentine/8g	40	2.5	506	10.0	47.2	30.8	7.0
Fruit, All Butter, Sainsbury's*	1 Biscuit/9g	45	2.0	477	5.6	66.0	21.2	1.9
Fruit, Oat, GI, Diet Chef Ltd*	1 Biscuit/20g	85	2.9	425	7.8	65.3	14.7	7.6
Fruit Bake, Organic, Tesco*	1 Biscuit/12g	53	2.1	453	7.5	65.1	18.1	5.6
Fruit Shortcake, McVitie's*	1 Biscuit/8g	37	1.6	464	5.7	65.1	20.1	2.7
Fruit Shrewsbury, Mini Pack, Paterson's*	1 Biscuit/17g	81	3.8	483	4.9	64.9	22.7	1.9
Fruity Iced, Blue Parrot Cafe, Sainsbury's*	1 Pack/20g	83	1.4	415	6.0	82.0	7.0	1.1
Fruity Oat, Organic, Dove's Farm*	1 Biscuit/12g	53	2.1	453	7.5	65.1	18.1	5.6
Fudge Flavour Choc Chip, Go Eat*	1 Biscuit/15g	76	4.1	510	6.5	59.2	27.4	1.7
Garibaldi, Asda*	1 Biscuit/10g	39	0.9	375	4.7	68.5	9.1	2.2
Garibaldi, Sainsbury's*	1 Biscuit/9g	35	1.0	389	5.7	67.1	10.9	3.3
Ginger, Belgian Dark Chocolate, Thins, Waltrose*	1 Biscuit/10g	48	2.2	481	6.2	61.2	22.5	4.6
Ginger, Traditional, Fox's*	1 Biscuit/8g	33	1.0	404	4.4	70.1	11.7	1.4
Ginger Crinkle, Sainsbury's*	1 Biscuit/11g	53	2.5	486	6.2	63.8	22.9	2.9

BISCUITS

INFO/WEIGHT	Measure	per Measure KCAL	FAT	Nutrition Values per 100g / 100ml KCAL	PROT	CARB	FAT	FIBRE
Ginger Crinkle Crunch, Fox's*	1 Biscuit/12g	50	1.4	435	4.7	75.3	12.5	1.6
Ginger Crunches, Organic, Against the Grain*	1 Biscuit/15g	71	3.4	474	2.8	65.6	23.0	1.2
Ginger GI, Diet Chef Ltd*	1 Biscuit/20g	87	3.0	435	8.8	65.6	15.2	6.1
Ginger Nuts, Asda*	1 Biscuit/10g	45	1.5	447	5.0	73.0	15.0	0.0
Ginger Nuts, Value, Tesco*	1 Biscuit/12g	55	1.9	460	5.2	74.2	15.8	1.6
Ginger Snap, BGTY, Sainsbury's*	1 Biscuit/12g	51	1.2	427	6.5	78.2	9.8	1.8
Ginger Snap, Fox's*	1 Biscuit/8g	35	1.0	443	4.6	77.1	12.8	1.5
Ginger Snap, Less Than 10% Fat, Sainsbury's*	1 Biscuit/12g	51	1.1	424	6.5	78.9	9.1	1.9
Gingerbread Man, Gluten & Wheat Free, Lovemore*	1 Biscuit/37g	179	7.6	485	4.7	70.1	20.5	1.7
Gingernut	1 Biscuit/11g	50	1.7	456	5.6	79.1	15.2	1.4
Golden Crunch, Bronte*	1 Biscuit/15g	69	3.3	474	5.1	62.5	22.6	0.0
Golden Crunch, Go Ahead, McVitie's*	1 Biscuit/9g	38	0.9	419	7.7	75.2	9.7	2.1
Golden Crunch Creams, Fox's*	1 Biscuit/15g	75	3.8	515	4.7	64.8	26.3	1.2
Golden Shortie, Jacob's*	1 Biscuit/11g	54	2.6	492	6.0	64.9	23.2	0.0
Gruyere & Spinach Twists, Savoury, Ardens*	1 Twist/7g	33	1.4	466	13.0	56.0	20.0	5.0
Happy Faces, Jacob's*	1 Biscuit/16g	78	3.6	485	4.8	66.1	22.3	1.6
Hob Nobs, Chocolate Creams, McVitie's*	1 Biscuit/12g	60	3.1	503	6.7	60.3	26.1	4.0
Hob Nobs, McVitie's*	1 Biscuit/14g	67	3.1	466	7.1	60.8	21.7	5.5
Hob Nobs, Milk Chocolate, McVitie's*	1 Biscuit/19g	92	4.5	479	6.8	60.7	23.3	4.5
Hob Nobs, Milk Chocolate, Mini, McVitie's*	1 Pack/25g	121	5.9	483	6.6	61.3	23.5	4.4
Hob Nobs, Munch Bites, McVitie's*	1 Pack/40g	203	10.1	508	6.8	63.4	25.2	2.8
Hob Nobs, Vanilla Creams, McVitie's*	1 Biscuit/12g	60	3.0	501	6.1	62.3	25.2	3.6
Iced Gems, Jacob's*	1 Serving/30g	118	0.9	393	5.0	86.3	3.1	2.0
Jaffa Cakes, Asda*	1 Cake/12g	43	1.0	368	4.7	67.5	8.8	1.9
Jaffa Cakes, Blackcurrant, McVitie's*	1 Cake/12g	45	1.0	371	4.8	69.7	8.1	2.3
Jaffa Cakes, Free From, Asda*	1 Cake/12g	42	0.9	340	5.8	62.6	7.4	8.0
Jaffa Cakes, Lemon & Lime, McVitie's*	1 Cake/12g	45	1.0	370	4.7	69.5	8.1	2.1
Jaffa Cakes, Lunch Box, McVitie's*	1 Cake/7g	26	0.6	395	4.2	74.3	9.0	1.4
Jaffa Cakes, McVitie's*	1 Cake/12g	45	1.0	374	4.8	70.6	8.0	2.1
Jaffa Cakes, Mini, Orange Pods, McVitie's*	1 Cake/40g	150	3.4	380	4.3	71.2	8.7	3.5
Jaffa Cakes, Mini Roll, McVitie's*	1 Cake/30g	115	3.3	382	3.5	67.2	11.0	1.3
Jaffa Cakes, Plain Chocolate, Sainsbury's*	1 Cake/13g	50	1.1	384	4.4	73.3	8.1	1.3
Jaffa Cakes, Sainsbury's*	1 Cake/11g	41	1.0	373	4.3	69.3	8.8	2.0
Jam Rings, Crawfords*	1 Biscuit/12g	56	2.1	470	5.5	73.0	17.2	1.9
Jam Sandwich Creams, M & S*	1 Biscuit/17g	80	3.7	485	5.7	64.5	22.6	1.8
Jam Sandwich Creams, Sainsbury's*	1 Biscuit/16g	77	3.4	486	5.0	67.0	21.8	1.6
Jammie Dodgers, Minis, Lunchbox, Burton's*	1 Pack/20g	90	2.9	452	5.5	72.7	14.7	2.5
Jammie Dodgers, Original, Burton's*	1 Biscuit/19g	83	3.0	437	5.1	69.5	15.9	1.9
Lebkuchen, Sainsbury's*	1 Biscuit/10g	39	0.8	400	5.7	76.1	8.0	1.3
Lemon, All Butter, Half Coated, Finest, Tesco*	1 Biscuit/17g	84	4.5	505	5.6	60.4	26.9	3.6
Lemon Butter, Thins, Sainsbury's*	1 Biscuit/13g	65	3.5	515	5.3	60.7	27.9	2.2
Lemon Curd Sandwich, Fox's*	1 Biscuit/14g	69	3.3	494	4.7	66.2	23.4	1.3
Lemon Puff, Jacob's*	1 Biscuit/13g	69	4.1	533	4.3	58.8	31.2	2.8
Lincoln, McVitie's*	1 Biscuit/8g	41	1.9	514	6.3	69.0	23.6	2.0
Malted Milk, Average	1 Biscuit/9g	42	1.9	490	7.0	65.5	22.1	1.8
Malted Milk, Chocolate, Tesco*	1 Biscuit/10g	52	2.5	500	6.7	64.4	24.0	1.9
Malted Milk, Milk Chocolate, Asda*	1 Biscuit/11g	56	2.7	509	7.0	64.0	25.0	1.7
Marie, Crawfords*	1 Biscuit/7g	33	1.1	475	7.5	76.3	15.5	2.3
Melts, Carr's*	1 Biscuit/4g	20	0.9	468	11.0	58.3	21.2	4.9
Melts, Sesame with Chive, Carr's*	1 Biscuit/5g	23	1.2	498	8.2	57.4	26.2	3.5
Milk Chocolate, All Butter, M & S*	1 Biscuit/14g	70	3.6	490	7.9	57.4	25.5	1.4
Mini Assortment, M & S*	1 Biscuit/3g	12	0.6	480	6.1	63.9	22.5	2.8
Mini Clotted Cream, Fosters Traditional Foods*	1 Biscuit/13g	66	3.6	507	5.4	59.5	27.4	0.0

BISCUITS

	Measure INFO/WEIGHT	per Measure KCAL	per Measure FAT	Nutrition Values per 100g / 100ml KCAL	PROT	CARB	FAT	FIBRE
Mint, Plain Chocolate, Tesco*	1 Biscuit/25g	136	7.5	538	5.1	63.0	29.5	1.7
Mint, Viscount*	1 Biscuit/13g	73	3.8	552	5.1	60.6	28.8	1.3
Mixed Seed & Honey, Oaty, Weight Watchers*	1 Biscuit/22g	106	5.1	482	9.2	59.0	23.2	4.9
Nice, Average	1 Biscuit/8g	36	1.6	484	6.3	67.3	21.0	2.5
Nice, Cream, Tesco*	1 Serving/10g	50	2.4	503	5.3	66.2	24.1	1.9
Nice, Fox's*	1 Biscuit/9g	39	1.7	450	6.3	62.4	19.4	5.0
Nice, Jacob's*	1 Biscuit/7g	33	1.3	471	6.1	68.5	19.2	1.8
Oat, Fruit & Spice, Nairn's*	1 Biscuit/10g	43	1.5	425	7.8	65.3	14.7	7.6
Oat, Santiveri*	1 Biscuit/5g	23	0.9	428	10.0	58.8	17.0	7.0
Oat, Stem Ginger, Nairn's*	1 Biscuit/10g	43	1.5	434	8.8	65.6	15.2	6.1
Oat & Chocolate Chip, Cadbury*	1 Biscuit/17g	80	3.9	485	6.9	60.2	23.9	4.2
Oat & Wholemeal, Crawfords*	1 Biscuit/14g	67	3.0	482	7.7	64.2	21.6	4.8
Oat Crunch, Weight Watchers*	1 Biscuit/12g	52	2.1	448	7.4	65.2	17.8	6.1
Oat Digestives, Nairn's*	1 Biscuit/11g	50	2.0	437	12.0	57.8	17.5	7.8
Oaten, Organic, Duchy Originals*	1 Biscuit/16g	71	2.7	441	9.8	62.3	16.9	5.3
Oatmeal, Asda*	1 Biscuit/12g	54	2.5	470	6.0	62.0	22.0	6.0
Oatmeal Crunch, Jacob's*	1 Biscuit/8g	37	1.5	458	6.8	65.9	18.6	3.6
Oaty Thins, Rude Health*	1 Thin/6g	23	0.3	380	11.5	68.5	4.7	8.7
Orange Munchy Bites, Blue Riband, Nestle*	1 Box/125g	652	34.9	522	5.2	61.4	27.9	2.0
Orange Sultana, Go Ahead, McVitie's*	1 Biscuit/15g	58	1.2	400	5.1	75.7	8.1	3.0
Parmesan Cheese, Sainsbury's*	1 Biscuit/3g	18	1.0	553	14.7	56.4	29.9	1.8
Peanut Butter, American Style, Sainsbury's*	1 Biscuit/13g	63	2.9	504	5.2	68.7	23.1	2.2
Petit Beurre, Stella Artois*	1 Biscuit/6g	26	0.9	440	9.0	73.0	15.0	0.0
Pink Wafers, Crawfords*	1 Measure/7g	36	1.9	521	2.5	68.6	26.5	1.1
Raspberry & Cream Viennese, Melts, Fox's*	1 Biscuit/16g	84	4.5	521	4.0	62.1	28.1	1.7
Rich Shorties, Asda*	1 Biscuit/10g	50	2.3	486	6.0	66.0	22.0	2.0
Rich Tea, 25% Less Fat, Tesco*	1 Biscuit/10g	43	1.1	435	7.1	77.0	11.0	1.3
Rich Tea, Average	1 Biscuit/10g	45	1.5	451	6.8	72.8	14.5	2.5
Rich Tea, BGTY, Sainsbury's*	1 Biscuit/10g	43	1.1	430	7.8	75.9	10.6	2.4
Rich Tea, Creams, Fox's*	1 Biscuit/11g	52	2.3	456	5.3	62.7	20.4	1.4
Rich Tea, Finger, Essential, Waitrose*	1 Biscuit/5g	22	0.7	450	7.2	72.5	14.3	3.0
Rich Tea, Light, McVitie's*	1 Biscuit/8g	36	0.9	431	7.5	75.0	11.3	3.1
Rich Tea, Low Fat, M & S*	1 Biscuit/9g	40	1.0	435	8.3	76.7	10.5	2.4
Rich Tea, Milk Chocolate Covered, Cadbury*	1 Biscuit/12g	60	2.6	490	6.6	67.6	21.4	0.0
Rich Tea, Plain Chocolate, Sainsbury's*	1 Biscuit/13g	65	3.0	497	6.6	66.0	23.0	2.6
Riva Milk, McVitie's*	1 Biscuit/25g	136	7.9	540	6.4	57.7	31.5	1.6
Rolo, Nestle*	1 Biscuit/22g	110	5.6	498	5.4	62.0	25.4	0.6
Rosemary & Thyme, Savoury, Weight Watchers*	1 Biscuit/8g	33	1.5	419	8.1	55.0	18.7	13.1
Savoury, Gluten, Wheat & Dairy Free, Sainsbury's*	1 Biscuit/17g	77	2.9	467	11.7	65.1	17.7	2.4
Savoury, Organic, M & S*	1 Biscuit/7g	28	1.0	395	7.0	58.4	14.6	8.7
Savoury Oat, with Thyme, Rick Stein*	1 Biscuit/10g	46	2.1	460	9.8	66.9	21.4	10.4
Scotch Finger, Arnotts Australia*	1 Biscuit/18g	88	3.9	489	6.6	65.8	21.5	0.0
Scottish Sweet Oatie, Organic, Daylesford Organic*	1 Biscuit/23g	119	7.1	516	6.1	53.9	30.7	4.7
Shortcake, Average	1 Biscuit/11g	55	3.0	501	6.3	66.1	27.1	2.1
Shortcake, Caramel, Average	1 Biscuit/37g	183	10.5	494	4.8	54.7	28.3	0.8
Shortcake, Caramel, Squares, M & S*	1 Square/40g	190	9.6	475	5.5	59.7	23.9	1.0
Shortcake, Caramel, Squares, Tesco*	1 Square/54g	274	16.4	507	4.6	54.1	30.4	0.4
Shortcake, Crawfords*	1 Biscuit/10g	52	2.4	504	6.2	63.5	24.4	2.6
Shortcake, Fruit, Crawfords*	1 Biscuit/8g	34	1.5	419	5.4	55.9	19.3	2.4
Shortcake, Jacob's*	1 Biscuit/10g	48	2.2	485	6.7	65.6	21.8	2.0
Shortcake, Mini Pack, Paterson's*	1 Biscuit/17g	82	4.2	490	5.5	60.8	25.0	3.2
Shortcake, Organic, Waitrose*	1 Biscuit/13g	64	3.2	495	5.8	63.0	24.4	1.8
Shortcake, Rounds, Value, Tesco*	1 Biscuit/22g	120	7.0	540	5.5	58.8	31.4	2.1

	Measure INFO/WEIGHT	per Measure KCAL	FAT	Nutrition Values per 100g / 100ml KCAL	PROT	CARB	FAT	FIBRE
BISCUITS								
Shortcake, Snack, Cadbury*	1 Biscuit/7g	35	1.8	515	7.2	61.0	26.7	1.8
Shortcake with Real Milk Chocolate, Cadbury*	1 Biscuit/15g	75	3.5	500	6.3	65.8	23.5	0.0
Shorties, Cadbury*	1 Biscuit/15g	77	3.6	511	6.5	67.3	24.0	0.0
Shorties, Fruit, Value, Tesco*	1 Serving/10g	46	1.7	457	5.7	69.3	17.4	3.0
Shorties, Rich Highland, Tesco*	1 Biscuit/10g	48	2.2	485	6.1	65.3	21.7	2.6
Shorties, Sainsbury's*	1 Biscuit/10g	50	2.2	500	6.4	69.8	21.8	2.0
Sports, Fox's*	1 Biscuit/9g	41	1.7	483	6.7	67.0	20.0	2.0
Stem Ginger, Brakes*	1 Biscuit/13g	62	3.1	495	5.6	62.6	24.7	0.0
Sugar Wafers, Vanilla, Flavoured, Triunfo*	1 Biscuit/10g	53	2.5	511	4.1	70.1	24.3	0.6
Sultana & Cinnamon, Weight Watchers*	1 Biscuit/12g	51	1.7	441	4.3	72.3	15.0	3.0
Taxi, McVitie's*	1 Biscuit/27g	134	6.9	504	4.2	63.3	26.0	0.7
Teddy Bear, Mini, M & S*	1 Biscuit/17g	80	3.8	475	5.4	62.6	22.7	3.2
Toffee Apple Crumbles, Border Biscuits Ltd*	1 Biscuit/18g	77	3.7	427	5.0	56.7	20.4	2.3
Toffee Dodgers, Burtons*	1 Biscuit/18g	84	3.1	468	5.7	71.4	17.5	1.1
Treacle Crunch Creams, Fox's*	1 Biscuit/13g	65	3.2	502	4.5	65.3	24.8	1.4
Triple Chocolate, Fox's*	1 Biscuit/21g	100	5.2	478	5.7	57.3	25.1	2.5
Turkish Delight, Cadbury*	1 Biscuit/16g	70	3.1	445	5.5	62.0	20.0	0.9
Viennese, Bronte*	1 Biscuit/25g	106	6.2	424	4.4	45.6	24.8	0.0
Viennese, Chocolate, Melts, Fox's*	1 Biscuit/12g	64	3.4	526	6.1	60.5	28.3	2.4
Viennese, Jaffa, M & S*	1 Biscuit/17g	80	3.7	465	5.9	61.1	21.7	0.9
Viennese, Mini Pack, Paterson's*	1 Biscuit/20g	106	6.2	527	5.4	67.1	30.8	1.6
Viennese Creams, Raspberry, M & S*	1 Biscuit/17g	90	4.9	520	4.6	60.4	28.6	1.3
Viennese Creams, Strawberry, M & S*	1 Biscuit/17g	80	3.7	485	6.4	63.0	22.2	1.7
Viennese Finger, Mr Kipling*	1 Finger/32g	167	10.2	523	4.3	54.9	31.8	0.0
Viennese Whirl, Chocolate, Border*	1 Biscuit/19g	96	4.3	512	6.5	61.9	23.2	0.0
Water, Average	1 Biscuit/6g	24	0.7	440	10.8	75.8	12.5	3.1
Water, High Bake, Jacob's*	1 Biscuit/5g	22	0.4	414	10.5	76.4	7.4	3.0
Water, Table, Large, Carr's*	1 Biscuit/8g	30	0.6	400	9.9	73.1	7.5	4.1
Water, Table, Small, Carr's*	1 Biscuit/3g	14	0.3	406	10.1	80.0	7.6	4.2
Wholemeal Brans, Fox's*	1 Biscuit/20g	90	4.0	451	8.5	58.8	20.2	7.5
Yorkie, Nestle*	1 Biscuit/25g	127	6.7	510	6.7	60.4	26.8	1.3
Yumbles, Oat Nibbles, Organic, McVitie's*	1 Biscuit/11g	50	2.5	449	7.9	53.2	22.7	6.6
BISON								
Raw	***1oz/28g***	***31***	***0.5***	***109***	***21.6***	***0.0***	***1.8***	***0.0***
BITES								
All Butter, Chocolate, M & S*	1 Biscuit/10g	55	3.1	530	7.9	57.0	30.1	3.5
Apple & Cinnamon, All Butter, M & S*	1 Biscuit/10g	50	2.5	510	5.5	64.6	25.2	2.1
Cake, Triple Choc Crisp, Cadbury*	1 Cake/14g	63	3.3	450	4.3	54.7	23.4	1.3
Cheese & Garlic, M & S*	1 Bite/11g	40	3.1	350	8.3	17.2	27.3	5.8
Chicken, Southern Fried, Fridge Raiders*	1 Bag/65g	120	6.5	184	20.1	3.3	10.0	1.5
Ciabatta, Fried Onion, Occasions, Sainsbury's*	1 Bite/12g	44	2.3	368	10.9	37.6	19.3	1.0
Ciabatta, Garlic & Herb, Occasions, Sainsbury's*	1 Bite/12g	48	2.6	398	8.9	42.2	21.5	3.2
Coconut, Sainsbury's*	1 Bite/80g	339	16.9	424	5.3	53.0	21.2	4.2
Corn Flake, Chocolate, Mini, Tesco*	1 Bite/14g	62	2.5	446	7.1	64.1	17.9	5.9
Crispy, Cheese & Pickle, Go Ahead, McVitie's*	1 Bag/27g	112	1.8	415	6.4	82.6	6.6	1.2
Crispy, Chicken & Herb, Go Ahead, McVitie's*	1 Bag/27g	109	1.6	404	6.7	81.1	5.9	1.2
Crispy Potato, Salt & Vinegar, BGTY, Sainsbury's*	1 Bag/20g	71	0.5	356	5.9	77.4	2.5	4.4
Egg & Bacon, Mini, Savoury, Tesco*	1 Bite/18g	55	3.8	305	8.8	20.2	21.0	2.7
Milk Chocolate, Mini, Luxury, Holly Lane*	1 Mini Bite/15g	72	3.9	479	5.1	55.5	26.3	2.5
BITTER LEMON								
Fever-Tree*	1 Glass/200ml	77	0.0	38	0.0	9.2	0.0	0.0
Low Calorie, Tesco*	1 Glass/200ml	6	0.2	3	0.1	0.3	0.1	0.1
Sainsbury's*	1 Glass/250ml	45	0.2	18	0.1	4.4	0.1	0.1

B

	Measure INFO/WEIGHT	per Measure		Nutrition Values per 100g / 100ml				
		KCAL	FAT	KCAL	PROT	CARB	FAT	FIBRE
BITTER LEMON								
Schweppes*	1 Glass/250ml	85	0.0	34	0.0	8.2	0.0	0.0
BLACK GRAM								
Urad Gram, Dried, Raw	*1oz/28g*	*77*	*0.4*	*275*	*24.9*	*40.8*	*1.4*	*0.0*
BLACK PUDDING								
Average, Uncooked	*1 Serving/40g*	*101*	*6.0*	*252*	*10.2*	*19.0*	*14.9*	*0.6*
VLH Kitchens	1 Serving/40g	105	39.0	262	11.0	20.3	15.6	0.4
BLACKBERRIES								
Fresh, Raw, Average	*1oz/28g*	*7*	*0.1*	*25*	*0.9*	*5.1*	*0.2*	*3.1*
Frozen, Average	1 Serving/80g	37	0.1	46	0.9	9.6	0.2	2.9
in Fruit Juice, Average	*½ Can/145g*	*52*	*0.3*	*36*	*0.6*	*7.9*	*0.2*	*1.3*
BLACKCURRANTS								
Fresh, Raw	*1oz/28g*	*8*	*0.0*	*28*	*0.9*	*6.6*	*0.0*	*3.6*
in Fruit Juice, Average	*1 Serving/30g*	*11*	*0.0*	*37*	*0.6*	*8.6*	*0.1*	*2.4*
Stewed with Sugar	*1oz/28g*	*16*	*0.0*	*58*	*0.7*	*15.0*	*0.0*	*2.8*
Stewed without Sugar	*1oz/28g*	*7*	*0.0*	*24*	*0.8*	*5.6*	*0.0*	*3.1*
BLINIS								
Cocktail, M & S*	½ Pack/81g	154	1.9	190	6.3	35.9	2.3	2.0
Sausage, Cocktail, Waitrose*	1 Blini/16g	30	0.4	190	6.3	35.9	2.3	2.0
Smoked Salmon, M & S*	1oz/28g	67	3.6	240	11.9	18.9	13.0	1.8
BLUEBERRIES								
Chocolate Covered, Waitrose*	1 Serving/25g	120	5.6	481	4.0	65.6	22.4	3.0
Dried, Love Life, Waitrose*	1 Serving/30g	107	0.2	358	1.1	80.1	0.8	3.6
Dried, Whitworths*	1 Pack/75g	226	0.1	301	0.9	74.2	0.1	11.4
Dried, Wholefoods, Tesco*	1 Serving/20g	66	0.2	329	2.0	77.9	1.0	3.2
Dried & Sweetened, Sainsbury's*	1oz/28g	77	0.2	275	1.7	65.7	0.6	11.7
Frozen, Average	1 Serving/80g	41	0.2	51	0.6	13.8	0.2	4.4
Shearway*	1 Serving/80g	41	0.5	51	0.4	12.2	0.6	0.0
BOAR								
Wild, Raw, Average	*1 Serving/200g*	*244*	*6.7*	*122*	*21.5*	*0.0*	*3.3*	*0.0*
BOILED SWEETS								
Average	1 Sweet/7g	21	0.0	327	0.0	87.1	0.0	0.0
Blackcurrant & Liquorice, Co-Op*	1 Sweet/8g	32	0.4	405	0.9	91.0	5.0	0.0
Cherry Drops, Bassett's*	1 Sweet/5g	18	0.0	390	0.0	98.1	0.0	0.0
Clear Fruits, Sainsbury's*	1 Sweet/7g	26	0.0	372	0.1	92.9	0.0	0.0
Cough Sweets, Fundays, Bassett's*	1oz/28g	107	0.0	383	0.0	94.9	0.0	0.0
Fruit Drops, Co-Op*	1 Sweet/6g	24	0.0	395	0.2	98.0	0.0	0.0
Fruit Rocks, Assorted, M & S*	1oz/28g	107	0.0	381	0.0	95.2	0.0	0.0
Fruit Sherbets, Assorted, M & S*	1 Sweet/8g	34	0.6	425	0.0	89.7	7.3	0.0
Lockets, Mars*	1 Pack/43g	165	0.0	383	0.0	95.8	0.0	0.0
Mentho-Lyptus, Extra Strong, Hall's*	1 Lozenge/4g	14	0.0	389	0.0	96.9	0.0	0.0
Pear Drops, Bassett's*	1 Sweet/4g	16	0.0	390	0.0	96.4	0.0	0.0
Soothers, Cherry, Hall's*	1 Pack/45g	165	0.0	365	0.0	91.3	0.0	0.0
Soothers, Strawberry Flavour, Hall's*	1 Sweet/5g	19	0.0	385	0.0	96.0	0.0	0.0
BOMBAY MIX								
Average	1oz/28g	141	9.2	503	18.8	35.1	32.9	6.2
Suma*	½ Pack/125g	595	35.6	476	13.6	41.2	28.5	10.1
BON BONS								
Apple, Lemon & Strawberry, Co-Op*	¼ Bag/50g	202	2.5	405	1.0	88.0	5.0	0.0
Bassett's*	1 Sweet/7g	28	0.5	417	1.1	85.4	7.5	0.0
Fruit, Bassett's*	1 Serving/7g	25	0.0	380	0.1	94.2	0.0	0.0
Lemon, Bassett's*	1 Sweet/7g	30	0.7	425	0.0	83.7	9.8	0.0
BOOST								
Standard Bar, Cadbury*	1 Bar/61g	305	17.0	510	5.8	57.0	28.5	0.9

	Measure INFO/WEIGHT	per Measure KCAL	FAT	Nutrition Values per 100g / 100ml KCAL	PROT	CARB	FAT	FIBRE
BOOST								
Treat Size, Cadbury*	1 Bar/24g	130	7.4	535	5.3	59.6	30.5	0.0
with Glucose, Cadbury*	1 Bar/61g	315	17.8	521	5.6	58.0	29.4	4.0
with Glucose & Guarana, Cadbury*	1 Bar/61g	314	18.0	515	5.5	56.7	29.5	0.0
BOUILLON								
Beef, Benedicta*	1 fl oz/30ml	22	0.1	73	7.5	9.5	0.5	0.0
Chicken, Benedicta*	1 fl oz/30ml	22	0.9	75	4.0	8.0	3.0	5.6
Miso, Powder, Marigold*	1 Tsp/5g	12	0.5	248	7.0	34.0	9.3	1.4
Vegetable, Benedicta*	1 fl oz/30ml	30	0.1	101	7.5	17.0	0.3	0.0
Vegetable, Powder, Swiss, Marigold*	1 Tsp/5g	12	0.4	243	10.5	29.4	8.1	0.7
BOUNTY								
Calapuno, Mars*	1 Pack/175g	919	54.9	525	6.3	54.3	31.4	0.0
Dark, Mars*	1 Funsize/29g	142	8.0	488	3.7	55.7	27.6	0.0
Milk, Mars*	1 Funsize/29g	137	7.4	471	3.7	56.4	25.6	0.0
BOURNVITA								
Powder, Made Up with Semi-Skimmed Milk	1 Mug/227ml	132	3.6	58	3.5	7.8	1.6	0.0
Powder, Made Up with Whole Milk	1 Mug/227ml	173	8.6	76	3.4	7.6	3.8	0.0
BOVRIL								
Beef Extract, Drink, Made Up with Water, Bovril*	1 Serving/12g	22	0.1	184	38.9	4.6	1.2	0.0
Chicken Savoury Drink, Bovril*	1 Serving/13g	16	0.2	129	9.7	19.4	1.4	2.1
BRANDY								
37.5% Volume, Average	*1 Shot/35ml*	*72*	*0.0*	*207*	*0.0*	*0.0*	*0.0*	*0.0*
40% Volume, Average	*1 Shot/35ml*	*78*	*0.0*	*222*	*0.0*	*0.0*	*0.0*	*0.0*
Cherry, Average	*1 Shot/35ml*	*89*	*0.0*	*255*	*0.0*	*32.6*	*0.0*	*0.0*
BRAZIL NUTS								
Average	*6 Whole/20g*	*136*	*13.7*	*681*	*15.3*	*2.8*	*68.3*	*5.4*
Milk Chocolate, Tesco*	1 Nut/8g	47	3.5	585	9.9	38.0	43.7	1.9
BREAD								
50/50, Wholemeal & White, Medium Sliced, Kingsmill*	1 Slice/40g	90	0.9	225	9.9	41.2	2.3	4.9
Arabic, El Amar Bakery*	1 Serving/110g	318	1.3	289	11.6	57.9	1.2	0.0
Bagel, 4 Everything, Finest, Tesco*	1 Bagel/100g	268	1.8	268	11.1	51.9	1.8	2.5
Bagel, Baked with Marmite, Marmite*	1 Bagel/85g	240	2.6	282	12.9	49.3	3.1	2.8
Bagel, Blueberry, Sara Lee*	1 Bagel/104g	290	1.5	279	9.6	58.6	1.4	1.9
Bagel, Caramelised Onion & Poppy Seed, Tesco*	1 Bagel/85g	221	2.1	260	10.9	47.6	2.5	3.8
Bagel, Caramelised Onion & Poppyseed, Waitrose*	1 Bagel/86g	222	2.1	258	9.7	49.2	2.5	2.4
Bagel, Cinnamon & Raisin, Morrisons*	1 Bagel/85g	215	1.7	253	7.7	51.1	2.0	4.5
Bagel, Cinnamon & Raisin, New York Bagel Co*	1 Bagel/90g	231	1.0	257	10.1	49.9	1.1	3.6
Bagel, Cinnamon & Raisin, Tesco*	1 Bagel/85g	223	1.6	262	10.3	51.0	1.9	2.1
Bagel, Fruit & Spice, Sainsbury's*	1 Bagel/85g	234	1.8	275	9.7	54.3	2.1	3.8
Bagel, Granary, Bagel Factory*	1 Bagel/100g	288	2.1	288	11.9	57.4	2.1	4.5
Bagel, High Bran & Seed, The Food Doctor*	1 Bagel/85g	239	6.6	281	10.7	41.3	7.8	6.3
Bagel, Mini, Sainsbury's*	1 Bagel/25g	67	0.4	268	11.2	52.4	1.6	2.8
Bagel, Multi Seed, New York Bagel Co*	1 Bagel/90g	244	4.3	271	12.4	41.6	4.8	5.8
Bagel, Multigrain, Sainsbury's*	1 Bagel/113g	293	3.5	259	10.0	49.6	3.1	2.0
Bagel, Onion, New York Bagel Co*	1 Bagel/85g	222	1.6	261	10.6	50.3	1.9	3.1
Bagel, Onion, Tesco*	1 Bagel/85g	233	2.0	274	10.5	52.4	2.4	1.9
Bagel, Onion & Poppy Seed, Average	1 Bagel/85g	225	2.8	264	9.0	50.5	3.3	3.2
Bagel, Original, Organic, New York Bagel Co*	1 Bagel/85g	220	1.2	259	9.3	52.2	1.4	4.1
Bagel, Plain, Average	*1 Bagel/78g*	*202*	*1.5*	*259*	*10.1*	*50.4*	*1.9*	*3.1*
Bagel, Plain, Bagel Factory*	1 Bagel/150g	318	1.3	212	9.4	41.6	0.9	2.1
Bagel, Plain, Free From, Tesco*	1 Bagel/80g	215	5.5	270	3.4	47.7	6.9	4.7
Bagel, Plain, GFY, Asda*	1 Bagel/84g	218	1.8	259	10.0	50.0	2.1	1.8
Bagel, Plain, New York Bagel Co*	1 Bagel/85g	216	1.6	255	9.1	50.4	1.9	2.9
Bagel, Plain, Organic, Tesco*	1 Bagel/85g	216	2.3	254	9.0	48.4	2.7	3.6

B

BREAD

	Measure INFO/WEIGHT	per Measure		Nutrition Values per 100g / 100ml				
		KCAL	FAT	KCAL	PROT	CARB	FAT	FIBRE
Bagel, Plain, So Organic, Sainsbury's*	1 Bagel/85g	216	2.3	254	9.0	48.4	2.7	3.6
Bagel, Poppy Seed, New York Bagel Co*	1 Bagel/85g	233	2.4	274	11.4	50.8	2.8	3.2
Bagel, Rye, Bagel Factory*	1 Bagel/85g	279	1.3	329	14.5	64.3	1.5	6.2
Bagel, Sesame, M & S*	1 Bagel/87g	240	2.8	275	10.2	51.2	3.2	2.1
Bagel, Sesame, New York Bagel Co*	1 Bagel/85g	226	2.6	266	10.3	49.2	3.1	4.0
Bagel, Sesame Seed, Essential, Waitrose*	1 Bagel/85g	243	2.7	286	9.6	54.6	3.2	3.6
Bagel, Sesame Seed, GFY, Asda*	1 Bagel/84g	227	2.1	271	11.0	51.0	2.5	2.6
Bagel, Soda, Round, Genesis Crafty*	1 Bagel/135g	307	5.3	227	6.9	41.3	3.9	2.9
Bagel, Wee Soda, Genesis Crafty*	1 Bagel/65g	148	2.5	227	6.9	41.3	3.9	2.9
Bagel, White, Asda*	1 Bagel/86g	227	2.7	264	10.0	49.0	3.1	0.0
Bagel, White, Original, Weight Watchers*	1 Bagel/67g	158	0.5	236	9.5	42.4	0.8	10.7
Bagel, Wholemeal, Average	1 Bagel/90g	235	2.7	261	12.7	44.6	3.0	7.7
Bagel, Wholemeal, New York Bagel Co*	1 Bagel/90g	223	2.1	248	11.4	41.5	2.3	7.5
Baguette, French, Tesco*	1 Serving/60g	144	0.7	240	7.8	49.5	1.2	3.4
Baguette, Gluten Free, Glutafin*	1 Serving/100g	401	4.4	401	5.6	79.3	4.4	11.0
Baguette, Granary, Average	1 Serving/100g	250	2.7	250	20.0	46.0	2.7	6.0
Baguette, Homebake, Half, Tesco*	1 Serving/60g	141	0.5	235	7.8	49.1	0.8	1.2
Baguette, Mediterranean Herb, Sainsbury's*	1 Serving/60g	203	9.4	339	8.5	40.8	15.7	2.3
Baguette, White, Ready to Bake, Asda*	1 Serving/60g	168	1.1	280	10.0	56.0	1.8	2.6
Baguette, White, Sainsbury's*	1 Serving/50g	131	0.7	263	9.3	53.1	1.5	2.7
Baps, Brown, Large, Asda*	1 Bap/58g	140	0.9	242	10.0	47.0	1.6	0.0
Baps, Brown, Malted Grain, Large, Tesco*	1 Bap/93g	228	3.1	245	9.9	42.7	3.3	5.3
Baps, Cheese Top, Sainsbury's*	1 Bap/75g	218	6.4	291	12.1	41.6	8.5	2.0
Baps, Cheese Topped, Baker's Soft, Tesco*	1 Bap/65g	180	3.7	275	10.2	45.8	5.6	2.2
Baps, Cheese Topped, White, Tesco*	1 Bap/65g	179	3.6	275	10.2	45.8	5.6	0.7
Baps, Floured, M & S*	1 Bap/60g	168	3.7	280	11.5	46.8	6.2	2.0
Baps, Giant Malted, Sainsbury's*	1 Bap/109g	282	5.2	260	8.6	45.7	4.8	5.7
Baps, Malted, Large, Co-Op*	1 Bap/85g	208	2.6	245	10.2	44.3	3.1	5.0
Baps, Multigrain, Tesco*	1 Bap/98g	238	3.1	244	8.7	45.1	3.2	1.9
Baps, White, Average	1 Bap/65g	167	2.3	257	9.5	46.9	3.5	1.9
Baps, White, Warburton's*	1 Bap/57g	144	2.5	252	9.8	43.4	4.3	2.7
Baps, White Sandwich, Kingsmill*	1 Bap/80g	209	3.2	261	10.1	46.2	4.0	2.2
Baps, Wholemeal, Brace's*	1 Bap/59g	137	2.6	234	10.5	42.5	4.4	4.3
Baps, Wholemeal, Country Oven*	1 Bap/40g	92	1.3	231	9.5	41.0	3.3	4.1
Baps, Wholemeal, Giant, Rathbones*	1 Bap/110g	230	2.1	209	9.4	39.0	1.9	8.0
Baps, Wholemeal, Giant, Sainsbury's*	1 Bap/86g	230	3.5	268	9.7	48.1	4.1	7.7
Baps, Wholemeal, Large, Tesco*	1 Bap/95g	223	3.9	235	10.5	39.1	4.1	7.6
Baps, Wholemeal, Tesco*	1 Bap/46g	104	2.4	227	9.6	41.4	5.3	5.6
Baps, Wholemeal, Village Green*	1 Bap/65g	151	2.3	232	10.0	40.0	3.5	3.8
Baps, Wholemeal, Waitrose*	1 Bap/67g	156	3.2	234	10.6	37.2	4.8	6.7
Best of Both, Farmhouse, Hovis*	1 Slice/44g	99	1.4	226	9.5	40.0	3.1	4.9
Best of Both, Medium, Hovis*	1 Slice/40g	91	0.9	227	9.0	40.4	2.2	4.7
Best of Both, Thick Sliced, Hovis*	1 Slice/50g	113	0.9	224	9.0	40.4	1.8	5.0
Bloomer, COU, M & S*	1 Slice/33g	78	0.5	235	9.5	45.5	1.5	3.6
Bloomer, Multiseed, Average	1 Slice/50g	120	2.4	240	11.8	37.2	4.9	7.7
Bloomer, Soft Grain, M & S*	1 Slice/34g	80	0.5	235	9.5	45.5	1.5	3.6
Bloomer, White, Sliced, Waitrose*	1 Slice/50g	129	0.9	259	8.5	52.1	1.8	2.6
Bloomer, Wholemeal, Organic, M & S*	1 Slice/50g	110	2.1	220	10.2	35.5	4.2	6.4
Brace's*	1 Slice/25g	60	0.7	238	10.4	43.2	2.6	4.7
Brown, Danish, Sliced, Weight Watchers*	1 Slice/20g	48	0.4	233	9.9	40.7	1.8	7.6
Brown, Danish, Weight Watchers*	1 Slice/20g	47	0.4	235	9.8	40.7	2.0	7.3
Brown, Farmhouse, Linwoods*	1 Slice/25g	56	0.4	225	7.3	44.4	1.7	5.8
Brown, Gluten & Wheat Free, Sliced	1 Slice/25g	56	1.3	224	3.4	41.0	5.2	9.4

BREAD

	Measure INFO/WEIGHT	per Measure		Nutrition Values per 100g / 100ml				
		KCAL	FAT	KCAL	PROT	CARB	FAT	FIBRE
Brown, Gluten Free, Genius*	1 Slice/35g	97	4.7	277	6.7	42.2	13.3	9.5
Brown, Good Health, Warburton's*	1 Slice/35g	79	1.0	226	10.3	39.6	2.9	7.2
Brown, Granary Malted, Thick Sliced, Waitrose*	1 Slice/40g	95	0.9	238	9.4	44.8	2.3	5.1
Brown, High Fibre, Ormo*	1 Slice/24g	57	0.6	239	9.2	42.9	2.6	7.5
Brown, Irwin's Bakery*	1 Slice/64g	137	0.4	214	10.4	41.8	0.6	6.1
Brown, Kingsmill Gold, Seeds & Oats, Kingsmill*	1 Slice/45g	126	4.4	280	12.2	35.6	9.8	4.9
Brown, Malted, Average	1 Slice/25g	60	0.6	242	9.4	45.5	2.4	4.2
Brown, Malted, Farmhouse Gold, Morrisons*	1 Slice/38g	94	0.5	248	8.2	49.6	1.4	3.0
Brown, Medium Sliced	*1 Slice/34g*	*74*	*0.7*	*218*	*8.5*	*44.3*	*2.0*	*3.5*
Brown, Medium Sliced, Premium, Warburton's*	1 Slice/24g	59	0.9	249	10.5	43.2	3.7	4.3
Brown, Mixed Grain, Original, Vogel*	1 Slice/45g	102	0.6	227	9.8	47.1	1.2	6.4
Brown, Multi Grain, Wheat Free, Gluten Free	1 Slice/33g	76	1.7	229	5.1	40.8	5.1	5.6
Brown, Sainsbury's*	1 Slice/34g	81	0.7	239	8.4	46.8	2.1	4.2
Brown, Seeded Batch, Large Loaf, 800g, Warburton's*	1 Slice/46g	132	4.1	288	12.3	39.7	8.9	6.0
Brown, Sliced, By Brennans, Weight Watchers*	1 Slice/20g	51	0.4	257	9.5	45.4	2.1	6.8
Brown, Sliced, Free From, Tesco*	1 Slice/45g	121	3.7	268	5.4	43.2	8.2	3.6
Brown, Soda, M & S*	1 Slice/40g	92	1.4	229	9.2	43.6	3.6	4.9
Brown, Sunflower & Barley, Vogel*	1 Slice/42g	100	1.9	239	9.4	40.3	4.5	6.7
Brown, Thick, Warburton's*	1 Slice/38g	80	0.7	211	9.4	39.2	1.8	6.2
Brown, Thin Sliced, Sainsbury's*	1 Slice/29g	65	0.5	225	8.2	43.8	1.9	3.9
Brown, Toasted, Average	*1 Slice/24g*	*65*	*0.5*	*272*	*10.4*	*56.5*	*2.1*	*4.5*
Brown, Toastie, Thick Sliced, Kingsmill*	1 Slice/44g	101	1.4	230	9.5	40.5	3.3	4.7
Brown, Very Dark, Albert Heijn*	1 Slice/35g	84	1.4	240	12.0	35.0	4.0	7.4
Brown, Wholemeal, Healthy Choice, Warburton's*	1 Slice/24g	58	0.6	244	10.4	40.7	2.5	6.5
Buns, Burger, American Style, Sainsbury's*	1 Bun/50g	131	2.1	261	10.5	45.6	4.1	3.6
Buns, Burger, Giant, Sainsbury's*	1 Bun/95g	249	4.9	262	8.7	45.2	5.2	2.9
Buns, Burger, Sainsbury's*	1 Bun/56g	154	2.9	275	9.2	47.8	5.2	4.1
Buns, Burger, Sesame, American Style, Sainsbury's*	1 Bun/60g	162	3.8	270	7.3	46.2	6.3	2.2
Buns, Burger, Sesame, Sliced, Tesco*	1 Bun/60g	168	4.0	280	7.9	47.3	6.6	2.1
Buns, White, Stay Fresh, Tesco*	1 Bun/56g	152	3.7	271	7.5	45.5	6.6	0.0
Carrot & Raisin, Sprouted, Sunnyvale*	1 Loaf/400g	800	2.2	200	9.5	48.1	0.5	7.9
Challah, Average	*1 Slice/50g*	*143*	*3.6*	*286*	*8.9*	*53.6*	*7.1*	*3.6*
Cheese, Bites, Planet Lunch*	1 Bag/20g	83	2.7	415	8.5	65.0	13.5	4.5
Cheese, Morrisons*	1 Serving/96g	297	13.6	311	9.9	35.9	14.2	3.0
Cheese, Onion & Garlic, Tear & Share, Waitrose*	¼ Bread/112g	326	14.6	290	9.4	33.9	13.0	2.1
Cheese, Onion Mustard Seed, Cluster, Sainsbury's*	1 Cluster/100g	276	8.1	276	10.0	40.6	8.1	3.1
Cheese, Tear & Share, Tesco*	¼ Loaf/73g	225	7.8	310	8.8	44.0	10.7	0.8
Cheese & Garlic, Pizza Style, Sainsbury's*	¼ Bread/63g	199	8.1	318	10.7	39.7	13.0	2.2
Cheese & Garlic, Stonebaked, Morrisons*	¼ Bread/69g	228	9.9	331	10.9	39.5	14.4	1.9
Cheese & Onion, Tear & Share, Sainsbury's*	¼ Bread/71g	202	6.6	285	9.8	40.6	9.3	1.9
Cheese & Onion, Toastie, Warburton's*	1 Slice/42g	120	5.8	286	7.5	33.1	13.7	0.0
Cheese & Tomato, Tear & Share, Sainsbury's*	¼ Bread/72g	211	9.5	293	8.0	35.7	13.2	1.5
Cholla, Average	*1/10 Loaf/154g*	*421*	*14.3*	*274*	*6.9*	*40.8*	*9.3*	*1.0*
Ciabatta, Black Olive, Part Baked, Sainsbury's*	¼ Ciabatta/67g	172	2.5	257	8.8	46.8	3.8	2.4
Ciabatta, Gluten & Wheat Free, Average	1 Slice/55g	136	1.6	248	2.0	52.4	2.9	4.2
Ciabatta, Green Olive, Tesco*	¼ Ciabatta/70g	155	3.1	222	7.4	38.2	4.4	1.9
Ciabatta, Half, Organic, Sainsbury's*	½ Ciabatta/63g	152	0.6	241	9.1	48.7	1.0	2.3
Ciabatta, Half, Part Baked, TTD, Sainsbury's*	¼ Pack/67g	173	3.3	257	8.6	44.6	4.9	3.5
Ciabatta, Italian Style, Waitrose*	1 Ciabatta/89g	231	1.2	260	10.7	51.2	1.3	2.2
Ciabatta, Olive & Rosemary, Mini, Tesco*	1 Pack/75g	319	8.2	425	17.8	63.0	10.9	3.6
Ciabatta, Plain, Tesco*	¼ Ciabatta/73g	174	2.8	240	9.8	41.5	3.9	2.4
Ciabatta, Ready to Bake, M & S*	1 Serving/150g	393	6.1	262	10.3	48.1	4.1	2.1
Ciabatta, Ready to Bake, Sainsbury's*	½ Ciabatta/66g	172	2.4	260	8.9	47.7	3.7	2.2

BREAD

	Measure INFO/WEIGHT	per Measure KCAL	FAT	Nutrition Values per 100g / 100ml KCAL	PROT	CARB	FAT	FIBRE
Ciabatta, Spicy Topped, Finest, Tesco*	1 Serving/73g	163	4.0	223	9.2	34.0	5.5	1.7
Ciabatta, Sun Dried Tomato & Basil, Tesco*	¼ Ciabatta/75g	193	4.3	257	8.9	42.4	5.7	2.4
Ciabatta, Tomato & Basil, GFY, Asda*	1 Serving/55g	143	1.2	260	9.0	51.0	2.2	0.0
Ciabatta, TTD, Sainsbury's*	¼ Pack/68g	185	4.0	274	10.4	44.8	5.9	2.7
Ciabatta Stick, Organic, M & S*	1 Stick/140g	315	2.0	225	8.9	48.5	1.4	4.2
Cinnamon & Fruit Swirl, Genesis Crafty*	1 Slice/40g	133	4.1	332	6.7	53.7	10.2	0.0
Cinnamon Swirl, Asda*	1 Serving/25g	87	3.2	349	6.0	52.0	13.0	1.6
Cottage Loaf, Stonebaked, Asda*	1 Serving/67g	155	0.9	232	10.0	45.0	1.3	3.2
Danish, Lighter, White, Warburton's*	1 Slice/26g	62	0.3	238	10.5	45.8	1.2	2.6
Danish, White, Medium Sliced, Tesco*	1 Slice/20g	47	0.3	234	9.4	45.4	1.7	3.3
Danish, White, Thick Sliced, Tesco*	1 Slice/24g	60	0.6	250	9.7	47.4	2.3	2.9
Dinkel, Coop Naturaplan*	1 Slice/27g	57	0.4	211	8.0	38.0	1.5	5.0
Farmhouse, Batch, Multiseed, Love Life, Waitrose*	1 Slice/50g	130	3.5	259	9.9	39.2	7.0	7.2
Farmhouse, Poppy Seed, Crusty, Loaf, M & S*	1 Slice/40g	104	1.3	260	9.4	47.6	3.3	2.3
Farmhouse, Wholemeal, Average	1 Slice/43g	94	1.4	219	10.7	36.2	3.3	7.3
Farmhouse Soft Grained, Sliced, Warburton's*	1 Slice/42g	109	1.7	258	10.2	44.6	4.0	5.0
Farmhouse with Oatmeal, Batch, Finest, Tesco*	1 Slice/44g	110	1.4	240	9.8	43.2	3.1	5.2
Fig & Almond, Bröderna Cartwright*	4 Slices/100g	267	7.5	267	9.2	39.7	7.5	0.0
Focaccia, Onion & Herb, Tesco*	½ Pack/190g	547	23.7	288	8.7	35.2	12.5	3.7
Focaccia, Roast Cherry Tomato & Olive, GFY, Asda*	½ Pack/148g	350	6.0	237	9.0	41.0	4.1	2.8
Focaccia, Roasted Onion & Cheese, M & S*	1 Serving/89g	240	4.1	270	10.4	45.7	4.6	2.8
Fougasse, Caramelised Onion & Cheese, Tesco*	1oz/28g	80	1.8	284	11.1	43.1	6.3	3.5
French	1.5" Slice/45g	110	0.0	244	8.9	53.3	0.0	2.2
French Stick, Average	*1 Serving/60g*	*147*	*0.2*	*245*	*8.7*	*52.2*	*0.4*	*2.1*
Fruit, Continental, Schneider Brot*	1 Slice/65g	198	3.5	305	5.4	57.0	5.4	0.0
Fruit, Loaf, Banana, Lunchbox, Soreen*	1 Bar/30g	100	1.3	332	8.2	63.3	4.4	2.9
Fruit, Loaf, Toasted, Cafe Instore, Asda*	1 Slice/33g	89	1.2	269	8.0	51.0	3.7	2.9
Fruit, Raisin Swirl, Sun-Maid*	1 Slice/33g	95	1.9	287	8.3	50.4	5.8	2.6
Fruit & Cinnamon Loaf, Finest, Tesco*	1 Slice/37g	134	4.9	363	6.4	54.6	13.2	1.5
Fruit Loaf, Apple, M & S*	1 Slice/39g	100	0.6	255	8.5	51.9	1.5	3.3
Fruit Loaf, Apple & Cinnamon, Soreen*	1 Serving/10g	31	0.4	307	6.9	60.5	4.2	0.0
Fruit Loaf, Banana, Soreen*	1 Slice/25g	78	1.2	313	6.8	60.9	4.7	0.0
Fruit Loaf, Cinnamon & Raisin, Soreen*	1/8 Loaf/25g	77	1.0	308	7.7	54.1	4.0	4.1
Fruit Loaf, Fresh, Free From, Sainsbury's*	1 Slice/33g	93	2.5	279	3.2	45.5	7.5	8.1
Fruit Loaf, Fruity Five, Snack Pack, Soreen*	1 Pack/61g	200	5.5	329	7.1	54.9	9.0	2.7
Fruit Loaf, Luxury, Christmas, Soreen*	1 Serving/28g	85	0.6	303	4.5	66.6	2.1	0.0
Fruit Loaf, Mixed Berry, Weight Watchers*	1 Slice/34g	79	0.9	231	7.6	44.3	2.6	7.7
Fruit Loaf, Mother's Pride*	1 Slice/36g	92	1.0	256	8.2	49.3	2.9	2.6
Fruit Loaf, Plum, Lincolnshire, Soreen*	1 Slice/25g	65	0.8	261	8.4	49.3	3.4	2.1
Fruit Loaf, Sliced, Asda*	1 Serving/33g	89	1.2	269	8.0	51.0	3.7	2.9
Fruit Loaf, Sliced, Sainsbury's*	1 Slice/40g	104	1.4	260	8.9	47.9	3.6	2.4
Fruit Loaf, Sliced, Tesco*	1 Slice/36g	100	1.8	278	6.9	51.2	5.1	3.7
Fruit Loaf, Sultana & Cherry, Sainsbury's*	1 Slice/50g	178	6.1	357	2.7	59.0	12.2	1.7
Garlic, & Cheese, Tesco*	1 Serving/143g	490	24.0	343	9.4	38.5	16.8	2.0
Garlic, & Herb, Giant Feast, Sainsbury's*	1 Serving/50g	158	6.4	317	8.0	42.1	12.9	2.6
Garlic, & Herb, Tear & Share, Tesco*	1 Serving/73g	217	9.2	300	6.3	40.0	12.7	1.7
Garlic, & Tomato, Pizza, Italiano, Tesco*	½ Bread/140g	405	15.1	289	7.5	40.5	10.8	2.5
Garlic, 30% Less Fat, Morrisons*	1 Serving/80g	231	7.4	289	7.9	43.8	9.2	2.7
Garlic, Average	1 Serving/100g	327	13.8	327	8.1	43.7	13.8	1.4
Garlic, Baguette, 25% Less Fat, Tesco*	1 Serving/100g	292	11.3	292	7.0	40.7	11.3	1.8
Garlic, Baguette, Average	1 Slice/20g	66	2.8	330	7.8	43.1	14.2	1.8
Garlic, Baguette, with Cheese, HL, Tesco*	1 Serving/50g	114	1.1	229	9.4	43.0	2.2	2.1
Garlic, Ciabatta, Finest, Tesco*	1 Serving/65g	205	8.9	316	8.1	40.1	13.7	2.4

BREAD

INFO/WEIGHT	Measure	per Measure KCAL	FAT	Nutrition Values per 100g / 100ml KCAL	PROT	CARB	FAT	FIBRE
Garlic, Ciabatta, Hand Stretched, Sainsbury's*	¼ Pack/75g	244	10.6	325	8.4	41.0	14.1	2.9
Garlic, Ciabatta, HL, Tesco*	¼ Ciabatta/60g	151	2.5	251	8.6	44.6	4.2	2.6
Garlic, Ciabatta, Italian, Sainsbury's*	1 Serving/145g	454	17.1	313	10.0	41.6	11.8	2.9
Garlic, Ciabatta, Italiano, Tesco*	1 Ciabatta/65g	211	9.4	324	7.7	40.9	14.4	2.2
Garlic, Ciabatta, Mini, Italiano, Tesco*	½ Ciabatta/47g	150	6.9	320	8.2	38.5	14.6	2.8
Garlic, Ciabatta, TTD, Sainsbury's*	1 Serving/67g	199	8.1	298	8.3	38.7	12.2	3.1
Garlic, Ciabatta with Herbs, Weight Watchers*	1 Pack/88g	216	3.5	245	9.2	43.0	4.0	2.9
Garlic, Finest, Tesco*	¼ Loaf/60g	187	7.9	311	7.7	40.3	13.2	1.8
Garlic, Flatbread, BGTY, Sainsbury's*	¼ Bread/56g	177	5.7	316	9.6	46.6	10.1	2.7
Garlic, Flatbread, Tesco*	1 Serving/83g	249	8.6	302	6.7	45.3	10.4	3.0
Garlic, Foccacia, & Rosemary, Tesco*	¼ Loaf/73g	193	4.9	266	9.0	42.1	6.8	3.7
Garlic, Homebake, Tesco*	1 Serving/60g	209	12.3	348	7.1	33.7	20.5	1.5
Garlic, Italian Style Stone Baked, Morrisons*	½ Pack/115g	420	22.0	365	7.9	40.4	19.1	1.9
Garlic, Pizza Bread, Co-Op*	1 Pizza/240g	756	31.2	315	8.0	41.0	13.0	2.0
Garlic, Slices, Asda*	1 Slice/27g	88	3.3	328	8.0	46.2	12.4	2.8
Garlic, Slices, BGTY, Sainsbury's*	1 Slice/27g	82	2.2	305	9.4	48.9	8.0	2.9
Garlic, Slices, Chilled, Sainsbury's*	1 Pack/368g	1369	60.0	372	9.1	47.3	16.3	3.2
Garlic, Slices, GFY, Asda*	1 Slice/31g	80	1.0	259	8.9	48.1	3.3	3.0
Garlic, Slices, HL, Tesco*	1 Slice/52g	131	2.2	251	8.6	44.6	4.2	2.6
Garlic, Slices, Italian, Chilled, Tesco*	1 Slice/27g	110	6.0	415	6.2	46.8	22.4	2.7
Garlic, Slices, Light Choices, Tesco*	1 Slice/30g	75	1.7	250	7.3	42.3	5.7	2.9
Garlic, Slices, Morrisons*	1 Slice/30g	82	2.7	272	7.3	40.2	9.1	2.6
Garlic, Stonebaked, M & S*	1 Loaf/85g	263	10.1	310	9.3	41.4	11.9	3.1
Garlic, to Share, M & S*	¼ Loaf/82g	230	10.7	280	6.5	33.2	13.0	1.3
Garlic, with Cheese, Asda*	1 Slice/34g	130	6.1	382	11.0	44.0	18.0	0.0
Garlic & Cheese, Slices, Tesco*	1 Slice/31g	118	5.2	380	11.7	43.9	16.8	2.0
Garlic & Gruyere, Fougasse, TTD, Sainsbury's*	¼ Bread/76g	219	6.8	288	9.5	42.6	8.9	2.9
Garlic & Herb, Ciabatta, GFY, Asda*	¼ Ciabatta/60g	137	1.4	230	8.8	43.2	2.4	1.0
Garlic & Herb, Flatbread, Tear & Share, Sainsbury's*	¼ Bread/68g	201	6.3	297	10.9	42.5	9.3	3.7
Garlic & Herb, Tear & Share, Chosen By You, Asda*	¼ Portion/63g	185	6.7	295	9.2	39.0	10.7	2.7
Granary, Average	**1 Slice/35g**	**85**	**1.0**	**242**	**9.8**	**43.9**	**2.8**	**4.8**
Granary, Country, Multiseeded, Hovis*	1 Slice/44g	96	1.3	218	11.1	37.0	2.9	6.5
Granary, Malted, Medium Brown, Asda*	1 Slice/35g	81	0.9	231	9.0	43.0	2.6	3.3
Granary, Oatmeal, Hovis*	1 Slice/44g	104	0.9	236	9.2	45.3	2.1	3.1
Granary, Original, All Sizes, Hovis*	1 Slice/33g	85	0.8	256	10.6	46.4	2.4	3.7
Granary, Original, Thick Sliced, Hovis*	1 Slice/44g	112	1.0	256	10.3	46.4	2.4	3.7
Granary, Seeded, Sunflower, Hovis*	1 Slice/44g	119	2.5	271	10.1	44.9	5.7	2.9
Granary, White, Seeded, Medium Sliced, Hovis*	1 Slice/44g	109	1.8	248	10.9	41.7	4.2	3.8
Granary, Wholemeal, Average	1 Slice/35g	80	0.9	227	10.8	38.4	2.6	6.6
Granary, Wholemeal, Hovis*	1 Slice/44g	104	1.1	237	10.6	39.8	2.4	6.8
Granary, Wholemeal, Seeded, Medium Sliced, Hovis*	1 Slice/44g	104	1.1	237	10.6	39.8	2.4	6.8
Half Wheat Rye, The Polish Bakery, Tesco*	1 Slice/44g	140	0.7	319	8.0	38.3	1.7	0.0
Heyford Sliced Bloomer, Waitrose*	1 Slice/50g	104	1.5	208	10.1	35.0	3.1	6.6
Hi Bran, M & S*	1 Slice/26g	55	0.8	210	12.6	32.5	3.0	6.3
Hi Fibre, Seed, Lifefibre*	1 Slice/35g	109	3.5	313	12.5	43.6	10.1	2.7
High Bran, M & S*	1 Slice/26g	60	0.8	230	13.4	34.2	3.0	7.4
Irish Barm Brack, Tesco*	1 Serving/75g	232	5.2	310	16.0	47.6	6.9	3.0
Irish Brown, Ormo*	1 Serving/100g	229	3.6	229	9.2	43.6	3.6	4.9
Irish Brown, Soda, Sainsbury's*	1 Serving/100g	208	3.0	208	8.8	36.4	3.0	5.3
Irish Brown Soda, Tesco*	1 Serving/50g	109	1.9	219	9.2	36.2	3.8	6.4
Irish Cottage Wheaten, Tesco*	1 Serving/40g	79	0.8	198	9.1	35.4	1.9	6.1
Irish Sliced Fruit Soda, Irwin's Bakery*	2 Slices/80g	218	4.2	273	2.4	53.8	5.3	2.5
Juvela*	1 Slice/25g	60	0.7	240	3.3	50.0	3.0	1.7

BREAD

	Measure INFO/WEIGHT	per Measure KCAL	FAT	Nutrition Values per 100g / 100ml KCAL	PROT	CARB	FAT	FIBRE
Lavash, Flax, Oat Bran, Whole Flour, Wrap, Joseph's*	1 Serving/32g	50	2.0	156	15.6	21.9	6.2	9.4
Loaf, Tasty Grains & Seeds, Warburton's*	1 Slice/38g	100	1.6	264	10.6	45.6	4.3	5.2
Low GI, Multiseed, Percy Ingle*	1 Slice/35g	99	3.1	283	0.0	0.0	8.9	6.0
Malt Loaf, Family, Asda*	1 Serving/20g	54	0.3	270	8.0	56.0	1.5	5.0
Malt Loaf, Fruity, Sliced, Soreen*	1 Slice/33g	101	0.7	303	7.6	62.1	2.2	3.8
Malt Loaf, Organic, Tesco*	1 Slice/28g	82	0.6	292	7.2	61.2	2.0	2.3
Malt Loaf, Sticky, M & S*	1 Slice/16g	47	0.4	295	6.9	64.9	2.3	3.1
Malt Loaf, Tesco*	1 Slice/50g	145	1.3	291	8.6	58.0	2.7	4.8
Malt Loaf, Value, Tesco*	1 Slice/25g	72	0.3	289	8.9	60.2	1.4	3.3
Malt Loaf, Weight Watchers*	1 Slice/23g	68	0.4	294	8.9	60.2	1.9	3.6
Malted, & Seeded, Batch, Organic, Waitrose*	1 Slice/50g	118	1.9	236	10.9	39.5	3.9	6.2
Malted, Crusty, Sainsbury's*	1 Slice/42g	109	1.4	259	8.6	48.6	3.3	4.4
Malted, Danish, Sliced, Weight Watchers*	1 Slice/20g	51	0.3	249	11.8	45.1	1.5	4.2
Malted, Sunblest*	1 Serving/45g	115	1.0	256	9.9	49.1	2.2	3.8
Malted, Wheat Loaf, Crusty, Finest, Tesco*	1 Slice/50g	115	0.7	230	9.8	44.2	1.5	4.4
Malted Brown, Slice, BGTY, Sainsbury's*	1 Slice/22g	53	0.6	239	12.1	41.4	2.8	5.8
Malted Brown, Thick Sliced, Organic, Tesco*	1 Slice/44g	111	0.9	249	8.9	48.8	2.0	3.5
Malted Danish, Weight Watchers*	1 Slice/20g	49	0.3	241	12.3	44.5	1.7	4.3
Malted Grain, Co-Op*	1 Slice/43g	99	0.9	230	8.0	46.0	2.0	3.0
Malted Grain, Good As Gold, Kingsmill*	1 Slice/47g	114	1.2	243	9.5	45.4	2.6	4.2
Malted Oat, Duchy Originals*	1 Serving/80g	195	3.0	244	8.8	43.6	3.8	3.7
Malted Wheatgrain, Roberts Bakery*	1 Slice/30g	79	1.0	265	11.0	48.0	3.3	3.6
Malted Wholegrain, Nimble*	1 Slice/22g	49	0.3	222	10.4	41.9	1.4	6.7
Mediterranean Olive, Waitrose*	1 Slice/30g	82	2.8	273	7.4	40.1	9.2	4.9
Mediterranean Style, M & S*	1/6 Loaf/48g	150	5.3	315	10.9	42.5	11.1	1.2
Milk Roll, Warburton's*	1 Slice/18g	46	0.5	253	11.0	45.1	2.7	2.7
Mixed Seed, Organic, Duchy Originals*	1 Slice/43g	114	3.4	269	10.9	39.1	8.1	5.3
Multi Seeded Loaf, Gluten & Wheat Free, Lovemore*	1 Serving/35g	102	4.3	291	0.0	3.0	12.3	0.0
Multigrain, Batch, Finest, Tesco*	1 Slice/50g	117	1.4	235	10.8	40.4	2.9	5.5
Multigrain, Brennans*	1 Slice/40g	110	1.3	275	8.8	48.0	3.3	6.3
Multigrain, Brown, Farmhouse Baker's, M & S*	1 Slice/51g	115	2.8	225	13.0	31.2	5.4	5.1
Multigrain, Crusty, Finest, Tesco*	1 Slice/40g	98	1.4	245	9.0	44.7	3.4	5.0
Multigrain, Gluten Free, Sainsbury's*	1 Slice/17g	39	0.8	229	5.1	40.8	5.0	5.6
Multigrain, Sliced, Fresh And Easy*	1 Slice/40g	110	1.0	275	10.0	52.5	2.5	5.0
Multigrain, Soft Batch, Sainsbury's*	1 Slice/44g	106	2.9	242	11.3	34.5	6.5	5.6
Multigrain, Sub Rolls, Asda*	1 Sub/150g	357	6.3	238	0.0	0.0	4.2	0.0
Multigrain, Sunblest*	1 Slice/30g	76	0.7	254	9.0	47.0	2.5	4.5
Multigrain, Tesco*	1 Slice/31g	66	1.0	214	11.1	36.8	3.2	8.9
Multigrain, Thick Sliced, Tesco*	1 Slice/50g	112	1.2	225	8.4	42.2	2.5	3.9
Multiseed, Farmhouse, Finest, Tesco*	1 Slice/50g	135	3.8	270	12.5	37.0	7.7	5.8
Multiseed Farmhouse Batch, Finest, Tesco*	1 Slice/44g	108	1.9	245	9.9	40.4	4.4	7.5
Naan, Average	**1 Naan/130g**	**344**	**5.6**	**264**	**8.3**	**48.5**	**4.3**	**2.0**
Naan, Chilli & Mango, Finest, Tesco*	½ Naan/90g	229	5.1	255	8.4	41.9	5.7	3.2
Naan, Garlic & Coriander, Free From, Tesco*	1 Naan/90g	215	6.0	240	5.1	38.7	6.7	4.9
Naan, Garlic & Coriander, Large, TTD, Sainsbury's*	¼ Pack/70g	194	3.8	277	9.4	47.7	5.4	2.2
Naan, Garlic & Coriander, M & S*	1 Naan/150g	375	2.1	250	9.8	50.1	1.4	2.0
Naan, Garlic & Coriander, Mild, Patak's*	1 Naan/140g	452	15.1	323	9.0	47.5	10.8	0.0
Naan, Garlic & Coriander, Mini, Asda*	1 Naan/110g	320	12.5	291	6.9	40.2	11.4	2.5
Naan, Garlic & Coriander, Mini, Finest, Tesco*	1 Naan/50g	160	6.7	320	6.7	42.4	13.5	0.8
Naan, Garlic & Coriander, Mini, Sainsbury's*	1 Naan/50g	140	2.0	280	8.2	51.2	4.1	2.6
Naan, Garlic & Coriander, Mini, Sharwood's*	1 Naan/59g	144	2.0	244	7.1	46.2	3.4	2.0
Naan, Garlic & Coriander, Mini, Tesco*	1 Naan/65g	185	5.0	285	7.6	45.6	7.7	2.6
Naan, Garlic & Coriander, Mini, Weight Watchers*	1 Naan/40g	100	1.0	250	9.3	47.6	2.5	4.2

BREAD

INFO/WEIGHT	Measure	per Measure KCAL	FAT	Nutrition Values per 100g / 100ml KCAL	PROT	CARB	FAT	FIBRE
Naan, Garlic & Coriander, Weight Watchers*	1 Naan/60g	155	2.6	259	8.9	46.0	4.3	3.4
Naan, Light Choices, Tesco*	1 Naan/71g	181	1.6	255	7.5	50.7	2.2	2.3
Naan, Mini, Light Choices, Tesco*	1 Naan/65g	149	1.8	230	8.1	42.5	2.8	2.9
Naan, Onion & Mint, M & S*	½ Naan/135g	351	11.7	260	8.9	35.8	8.7	2.5
Naan, Onion Bhaji, M & S*	1 Naan/140g	400	17.0	285	9.5	34.2	12.1	2.0
Naan, Onion Bhaji, Sharwood's*	1 Pack/130g	378	9.9	291	7.3	48.4	7.6	2.2
Naan, Peshwari, Apple & Coconut, Mini, Sharwood's*	1 Naan/40g	112	2.7	281	6.9	46.6	6.7	3.1
Naan, Peshwari, Finest, Tesco*	1 Naan/130g	338	7.3	260	8.6	43.7	5.6	4.9
Naan, Peshwari, M & S*	1 Serving/127g	394	12.8	310	9.2	45.8	10.1	1.9
Naan, Peshwari, Mega, Asda*	1 Naan/220g	680	26.4	309	7.1	43.1	12.0	2.7
Naan, Peshwari, Sainsbury's*	1 Naan/166g	511	18.3	308	7.1	45.1	11.0	4.7
Naan, Peshwari, Sharwood's*	1 Naan/130g	334	6.9	257	7.2	45.1	5.3	2.5
Naan, Peshwari, Tesco*	1 Naan/215g	684	26.7	318	7.5	48.9	12.4	4.8
Naan, Peshwari, TTD, Sainsbury's*	1 Serving/80g	247	10.1	309	6.3	42.5	12.6	4.4
Naan, Plain, Average	1 Naan/160g	437	10.5	273	8.0	45.7	6.5	2.1
Naan, Plain, GFY, Asda*	1 Naan/130g	307	2.7	236	8.4	45.9	2.1	2.4
Naan, Plain, Mini, BGTY, Sainsbury's*	1 Naan/50g	113	1.1	226	8.2	43.2	2.2	3.3
Naan, Plain, Mini, Weight Watchers*	1 Naan/44g	108	1.1	245	9.1	46.5	2.5	4.9
Naan, Plain, Sharwood's*	1 Naan/120g	326	8.9	272	8.5	42.9	7.4	2.4
Naan, Tandoori, Sharwood's*	1 Naan/130g	330	6.5	254	7.3	45.0	5.0	2.0
Naan, Tandoori Baked, Waitrose*	1 Naan/140g	372	4.3	266	9.8	49.6	3.1	2.9
Oatmeal, Farmhouse, Extra Special, Asda*	1 Slice/44g	102	1.1	231	11.0	41.0	2.6	6.0
Oatmeal, Farmhouse, Soft, M & S*	1 Slice/45g	110	2.0	245	11.1	39.5	4.4	5.2
Oatmeal, Farmhouse, Waitrose*	1 Slice/40g	110	2.1	276	9.4	47.9	5.2	4.6
Oatmeal, Sliced Loaf, Tesco*	1 Slice/50g	111	1.7	222	7.4	40.5	3.4	2.8
Olive, Waitrose*	1 Slice/28g	86	3.0	306	9.0	43.6	10.6	2.0
Olive Oval, la Brea Bakery*	1 Serving/100g	249	3.8	249	7.0	46.4	3.8	2.7
Pain Au Raisin, M & S*	1 Pain/74g	215	9.5	290	5.3	38.7	12.8	1.2
Pave, Walnut, Sainsbury's*	1 Serving/50g	140	4.7	280	9.0	40.0	9.5	3.5
Pea, Artisan*	1 Slice/50g	102	1.2	204	9.5	31.8	2.4	9.4
Pitta, Garlic, Pride Valley*	1 Pitta/63g	157	1.1	249	9.7	51.1	1.8	2.7
Pitta, Garlic, Sainsbury's*	1 Pitta/60g	153	0.6	255	9.5	52.0	1.0	2.5
Pitta, Garlic & Coriander, Asda*	1 Pitta/55g	116	0.5	212	7.0	44.0	0.9	1.8
Pitta, Garlic & Herb, Tesco*	1 Pitta/60g	134	1.2	223	9.6	44.6	2.0	3.0
Pitta, Mexican, Santa Maria*	1 Pitta/66g	165	0.7	250	7.5	52.0	1.0	0.0
Pitta, Multi Seed & Cereal, The Food Doctor*	1 Pitta/70g	157	1.9	224	10.1	39.9	2.7	10.2
Pitta, Organic, Tesco*	1 Pitta/60g	124	0.8	206	8.3	40.2	1.4	5.7
Pitta, Pockets, Pride Valley*	1 Pitta/63g	151	0.6	239	9.3	48.4	0.9	3.2
Pitta, Pockets, Sainsbury's*	1 Pitta/75g	187	0.7	250	8.5	52.0	1.0	3.5
Pitta, Sd Tomato, Olive & Oregano, Extra Special, Asda*	1 Pitta/75g	194	0.8	259	7.1	55.2	1.1	1.6
Pitta, Seeded, HL, Tesco*	1 Pitta/60g	153	3.6	255	10.8	39.4	6.0	12.8
Pitta, Sesame, Sainsbury's*	1 Pitta/59g	156	1.4	264	9.8	50.8	2.4	3.1
Pitta, Tex Mex Style, Mini, Morrisons*	1 Pitta/18g	43	0.2	240	9.2	48.7	0.9	3.3
Pitta, White, Average	**1 Pitta/75g**	**191**	**1.1**	**255**	**9.2**	**50.8**	**1.5**	**2.7**
Pitta, White, Free From, Tesco*	1 Pitta/55g	140	1.2	255	6.5	52.6	2.1	5.5
Pitta, White, Greek Style, Asda*	1 Pitta/50g	126	0.9	253	8.0	51.0	1.9	0.0
Pitta, White, Organic, Sainsbury's*	1 Pitta/59g	150	0.6	254	10.3	50.7	1.1	2.5
Pitta, White, Soft, Sandwich, Warburton's*	½ Pitta/36g	81	0.9	228	9.8	41.4	2.6	1.8
Pitta, White, Speciality Breads, Waitrose*	1 Pitta/60g	149	0.7	249	10.3	49.3	1.2	3.5
Pitta, White, Weight Watchers*	1 Pitta/45g	106	0.3	238	8.7	45.9	0.7	6.7
Pitta, White Picnic, Waitrose*	1 Pitta/30g	75	0.4	249	10.3	49.3	1.2	3.5
Pitta, Wholemeal, Acropolis, Lidl*	1 Pitta/57g	136	0.9	238	12.0	44.0	1.6	6.0
Pitta, Wholemeal, Average	**1 Pitta/64g**	**154**	**1.1**	**241**	**11.0**	**45.8**	**1.7**	**6.4**

B

BREAD

	Measure INFO/WEIGHT	per Measure KCAL	per Measure FAT	Nutrition Values per 100g / 100ml KCAL	PROT	CARB	FAT	FIBRE
Pitta, Wholemeal, Healthy Eating, Co-Op*	1 Pitta/63g	135	1.3	215	12.0	37.0	2.0	9.0
Pitta, Wholemeal, Hollyland Bakery*	1 Pitta/20g	48	0.3	242	13.1	43.7	1.6	6.0
Pitta, Wholemeal, Lemon & Black Pepper, Finest, Tesco*	1 Pitta/80g	215	4.8	270	10.8	42.4	6.0	6.0
Pitta, Wholemeal, Mini, Organic, Newbury Phillips*	1 Pitta/100g	144	1.7	144	10.3	50.8	1.7	6.4
Pitta, Wholemeal, Round, SuperValu*	1 Pitta/48g	57	0.4	118	4.9	20.7	0.8	2.9
Pitta, Wholemeal, So Organic, Sainsbury's*	1 Pitta/60g	140	1.0	233	9.8	44.8	1.6	8.1
Pitta, Wholemeal, Weight Watchers*	1 Pitta/46g	106	0.6	229	8.7	44.5	1.2	7.6
Pitta, Wholemeal with Extra Virgin Olive Oil, Tesco*	1 Pitta/60g	135	1.6	225	8.3	41.5	2.6	5.5
Potato & Rosemary, M & S*	1 Serving/40g	108	2.7	270	9.4	42.2	6.8	2.3
Potato Farls, Irish, Rankin Selection, Irwin's Bakery*	1 Farl/60g	110	2.2	184	2.3	34.4	3.6	2.5
Potato Farls, M & S*	1 Farl/55g	79	0.2	144	4.2	33.8	0.4	4.7
Potato Farls, Sunblest*	1 Farl/100g	156	0.9	156	3.8	33.2	0.9	1.9
Pumpernickel, Organic, Bavarian Pumpernickel*	1 Slice/50g	90	0.5	180	6.0	38.0	1.0	10.0
Pumpernickel Rye, Kelderman*	1 Slice/50g	92	0.5	185	6.0	38.0	1.0	0.0
Pumpkin Seed, Raisin & Sunflower Seed, Sainsbury's*	1 Slice/30g	76	0.8	255	11.6	45.9	2.8	3.4
Raisin & Pumpkin Seed, Organic, Tesco*	1 Slice/30g	76	1.7	253	9.7	40.6	5.8	3.8
Raisin Loaf with Cinnamon, Warburton's*	1 Slice/36g	96	1.3	267	7.2	51.1	3.7	3.2
Roasted Onion, M & S*	1 Slice/50g	125	1.6	250	9.0	46.7	3.3	2.1
Rolls, 3 Seeded, Sandwich, Warburton's*	1 Roll/77g	242	6.7	314	13.3	41.2	8.7	6.0
Rolls, American Style Deli, Tesco*	1 Roll/65g	162	2.2	249	7.8	46.8	3.4	1.6
Rolls, Batched Sandwich, Warburton's*	1 Roll/60g	148	2.5	246	9.6	42.7	4.1	0.0
Rolls, Best of Both, Hovis*	1 Roll/62g	148	2.9	239	9.8	39.7	4.6	5.0
Rolls, Brioche	1 Roll/53g	191	7.5	361	8.8	50.1	14.1	1.5
Rolls, Brioche, Average	1 Roll/49g	177	6.9	361	8.8	50.1	14.1	1.5
Rolls, Brioche, Brialys*	1 Roll/35g	121	3.9	347	8.8	52.8	11.2	1.5
Rolls, Brioche, Butter, Tesco*	1 Serving/35g	126	4.5	360	8.8	51.3	12.8	2.0
Rolls, Brioche, Continental Classics*	1 Roll/35g	122	3.3	349	8.2	58.3	9.3	0.0
Rolls, Brioche, Finest, Tesco*	1 Roll/52g	207	11.6	398	10.8	38.3	22.4	2.0
Rolls, Brioche, Milk Chocolate Chip, Chosen By You, Asda*	1 Roll/25g	91	3.6	363	8.0	50.0	14.5	1.8
Rolls, Brioche, Plain Chocolate Chip, Sainsbury's*	1 Roll/35g	131	5.6	374	8.5	49.0	16.0	5.9
Rolls, Brioche, Sainsbury's*	1 Roll/32g	116	3.7	362	8.5	56.0	11.5	3.6
Rolls, Brioche, Tesco*	1 Roll/26g	92	2.9	349	8.5	54.0	11.0	0.0
Rolls, Brown, Carb Control, Tesco*	1 Roll/45g	98	2.7	218	20.5	20.7	5.9	10.7
Rolls, Brown, Crusty	*1 Roll/50g*	*127*	*1.4*	*255*	*10.3*	*50.4*	*2.8*	*3.5*
Rolls, Brown, Free From, Tesco*	1 Roll/65g	174	5.3	268	5.4	43.2	8.2	3.6
Rolls, Brown, Large, Asda*	1 Roll/57g	138	0.9	242	10.0	47.0	1.6	0.0
Rolls, Brown, M & S*	1 Roll/105g	241	6.4	230	9.2	37.3	6.1	4.4
Rolls, Brown, Malted Grain, Tesco*	1 Roll/58g	144	1.9	248	8.7	46.2	3.2	1.9
Rolls, Brown, Mini, M & S*	1 Roll/33g	80	2.5	245	9.8	35.5	7.6	3.8
Rolls, Brown, Morning, Farmfoods*	1 Roll/50g	134	1.8	269	12.0	47.0	3.7	4.2
Rolls, Brown, Old Fashioned, Waitrose*	1 Roll/63g	152	2.6	241	9.6	41.3	4.1	4.7
Rolls, Brown, Seeded, Organic, Sainsbury's*	1 Roll/70g	166	3.2	237	9.9	39.1	4.6	6.5
Rolls, Brown, Snack, Allinson*	1 Roll/44g	119	2.9	270	10.8	41.6	6.7	5.6
Rolls, Brown, Soft, Average	*1 Roll/50g*	*134*	*1.9*	*268*	*10.0*	*51.8*	*3.8*	*3.5*
Rolls, Brown, Soft, Organic, Sainsbury's*	1 Roll/70g	166	3.2	237	9.9	39.1	4.6	6.6
Rolls, Brown, Square, M & S*	1 Roll/105g	241	6.4	230	9.2	37.3	6.1	4.4
Rolls, Cheese & Tomato, Seeded, White, M & S*	1 Pack/160g	480	25.0	300	13.7	26.1	15.6	2.1
Rolls, Cheese Topped, Sandwich Rolls, Warburton's*	1 Roll/62g	168	4.0	270	12.1	40.7	6.5	2.6
Rolls, Cheese Topped, Village Green*	1 Roll/56g	159	4.1	284	13.1	41.2	7.4	4.8
Rolls, Ciabatta, Cheese Topped, Mini, Finest, Tesco*	1 Roll/30g	85	2.4	282	11.5	40.9	8.1	3.8
Rolls, Ciabatta, Garlic, Asda*	1 Roll/93g	333	16.7	358	9.0	40.0	18.0	2.3
Rolls, Ciabatta, M & S*	1 Roll/80g	210	3.3	262	10.3	48.1	4.1	2.1
Rolls, Ciabatta, Mini, Finest, Tesco*	1 Roll/30g	89	2.0	297	9.9	49.1	6.8	4.1

BREAD

	Measure INFO/WEIGHT	per Measure KCAL	FAT	Nutrition Values per 100g / 100ml KCAL	PROT	CARB	FAT	FIBRE
Rolls, Ciabatta, Sun Dried Tomato, Mini, Finest, Tesco*	1 Roll/30g	79	1.9	262	8.7	42.3	6.4	2.6
Rolls, Ciabatta, Tesco*	1 Roll/80g	208	2.5	260	8.6	48.2	3.1	3.3
Rolls, COU, M & S*	1 Roll/51g	120	1.2	235	9.8	44.0	2.3	3.4
Rolls, Country Grain, Mini, M & S*	1 Roll/31g	85	3.0	275	10.2	38.9	9.7	3.8
Rolls, Crisp, Original, Organic, Kallo*	1 Roll/9g	34	0.5	390	11.0	74.0	5.6	3.0
Rolls, Crusty, Booths*	1 Roll/50g	123	0.6	247	8.7	50.3	1.2	2.6
Rolls, Crusty, French, M & S*	1 Roll/65g	159	0.8	245	8.1	50.5	1.2	3.3
Rolls, Crusty, Part-Baked, Budgens*	1 Roll/50g	148	0.7	296	9.4	61.4	1.4	2.5
Rolls, Finger, Morrisons*	1 Roll/46g	119	0.8	259	10.7	50.0	1.8	2.3
Rolls, Finger, White, Sainsbury's*	1 Roll/40g	96	1.0	240	9.0	45.2	2.6	3.2
Rolls, Focaccia, Tesco*	1 Roll/75g	226	7.0	302	8.7	45.6	9.4	3.8
Rolls, Gluten Free, Antoinette Savill*	1 Roll/70g	157	1.5	224	1.9	48.8	2.2	1.5
Rolls, Granary, Average	1 Roll/70g	176	2.7	251	9.6	45.2	3.9	3.3
Rolls, Granary, Bakers Premium, Tesco*	1 Roll/65g	158	0.8	243	9.9	47.8	1.3	2.3
Rolls, Granary, Original, Hovis*	1 Roll/70g	180	2.9	257	10.7	44.3	4.1	5.3
Rolls, Granary Malted Wheatgrain, Soft, M & S*	1 Roll/80g	208	3.1	260	9.3	47.2	3.9	2.3
Rolls, Green Olive, M & S*	1 Roll/75g	210	4.5	280	11.2	44.0	6.0	1.8
Rolls, Hot Dog, Sliced, Asda*	1 Roll/84g	197	2.8	234	7.0	44.0	3.3	0.0
Rolls, Hot Dog, Tesco*	1 Roll/85g	200	2.8	235	7.3	44.0	3.3	1.9
Rolls, Hot Dog, Value, Tesco*	1 Roll/40g	93	0.8	232	8.7	45.0	1.9	2.2
Rolls, Hot Dog, Warburton's*	1 Roll/60g	137	2.8	228	8.7	37.8	4.7	1.7
Rolls, Malted, Whole Grain Rolls, Batched, Soft, M & S*	1 Roll/80g	180	3.6	225	7.8	38.5	4.5	3.1
Rolls, Malted Grain, Sainsbury's*	1 Roll/68g	190	2.9	280	8.7	51.6	4.3	4.2
Rolls, Malted Grain, Soft, Weight Watchers*	1 Roll/57g	142	1.0	251	11.7	47.1	1.8	4.2
Rolls, Malted Grain, Submarine, M & S*	1 Roll/109g	300	4.7	275	8.9	53.6	4.3	3.0
Rolls, Mini Submarine, M & S*	1 Roll/23g	63	1.1	275	11.4	47.7	4.9	1.1
Rolls, Mixed Seed, Deli, Tesco*	1 Roll/65g	165	2.1	255	9.4	46.8	3.3	5.2
Rolls, Morning, Tesco*	1 Roll/48g	117	1.2	243	10.4	44.8	2.5	4.7
Rolls, Multi Seed, Free From, Free From, Tesco*	1 Roll/70g	213	8.3	305	5.4	44.2	11.8	6.3
Rolls, Multigrain, Torpedo, Sainsbury's*	1 Roll/112g	328	7.5	293	10.5	47.7	6.7	6.3
Rolls, Oatmeal, Ploughmans, GFY, Asda*	1 Roll/72g	181	3.2	252	10.0	43.0	4.4	3.9
Rolls, Oatmeal, Soft, M & S*	1 Roll/80g	224	5.1	280	12.3	43.4	6.4	2.7
Rolls, Panini, Sainsbury's*	1 Roll/90g	249	5.6	276	11.0	44.1	6.2	3.0
Rolls, Panini, White, Tesco*	1 Roll/75g	210	4.6	280	10.1	45.2	6.1	2.7
Rolls, Part Baked, Mini, Tesco*	1 Roll/50g	120	0.6	240	7.8	49.5	1.2	3.4
Rolls, Poppy Seeded Knot, Waitrose*	1 Roll/60g	169	3.2	282	10.3	48.3	5.3	2.2
Rolls, Premium Seeded, Four, Aldi, Village Bakery*	1 Roll/82g	196	3.6	239	9.4	40.5	4.4	7.3
Rolls, Rye, Toasting, Good & Hot*	1 Roll/65g	143	0.7	220	7.3	44.6	1.1	7.1
Rolls, Scottish Morning, Morrisons*	1 Roll/60g	157	1.3	261	11.3	51.4	2.2	2.4
Rolls, Seed Sensations, Deli, Hovis*	1 Roll/70g	184	5.9	263	10.3	36.5	8.5	10.6
Rolls, Seeded, Mixed Mini Loaf Pack, M & S*	1 Roll/76g	220	7.3	290	10.6	39.7	9.6	4.0
Rolls, Seeded, Sandwich, Warburton's*	1 Roll/77g	242	6.7	314	13.3	41.2	8.7	6.0
Rolls, Snack, Mini, Tesco*	1 Roll/35g	95	2.1	271	19.0	43.0	6.0	4.0
Rolls, Soft, Wholemeal, Finger, M & S*	1 Roll/66g	145	1.3	220	12.6	38.0	2.0	5.8
Rolls, Submarine, Sainsbury's*	1 Roll/117g	305	4.6	261	9.1	47.4	3.9	2.4
Rolls, Sun Dried Tomato, Homebake, Tesco*	1 Roll/50g	123	1.5	246	11.3	44.0	3.0	0.0
Rolls, Sunflower Seed, Toasting, Good & Hot*	1 Roll/65g	162	3.2	250	8.5	41.0	5.0	8.0
Rolls, Tomato & Basil, Sub, COU, M & S*	1 Roll/33g	86	0.9	265	11.0	48.7	2.7	2.4
Rolls, White, 50/50, Soft, Kingsmill*	1 Roll/63g	154	2.4	245	9.3	41.2	3.8	4.4
Rolls, White, BGTY, Sainsbury's*	1 Roll/50g	113	0.5	227	9.1	45.3	1.0	3.0
Rolls, White, Cheese Topped, Asda*	1 Roll/46g	121	2.0	264	10.0	46.0	4.4	2.0
Rolls, White, Cheese Topped, Sainsbury's*	1 Roll/75g	218	6.4	291	12.1	41.6	8.5	2.0
Rolls, White, Chunky, Hovis*	1 Roll/73g	173	2.4	237	9.4	41.7	3.3	2.5

BREAD

INFO/WEIGHT	Measure		Nutrition Values per 100g / 100ml				
	KCAL	FAT	KCAL	PROT	CARB	FAT	FIBRE
Rolls, White, Crusty, Average	**1 Roll/50g**	**140**	**1.1**	**280**	**10.9**	**57.6**	**2.3**	**1.5**
Rolls, White, Crusty, Home Bake, Tesco*	1 Roll/69g	185	1.0	270	9.3	54.2	1.4	2.9
Rolls, White, Crusty, Morning, M & S*	1 Roll/65g	175	0.8	270	8.8	53.8	1.3	2.7
Rolls, White, Finger, Smart Price, Asda*	1 Roll/50g	121	0.8	242	9.0	48.0	1.6	2.1
Rolls, White, Finger, Tesco*	1 Roll/68g	170	2.4	250	8.5	45.8	3.5	2.1
Rolls, White, Finger, Value, Tesco*	1 Roll/50g	116	0.9	232	8.7	45.0	1.9	2.2
Rolls, White, Floured, Batch, Tesco*	1 Roll/76g	193	2.5	254	8.8	47.3	3.3	2.2
Rolls, White, Floured, Warburton's*	1 Roll/50g	123	1.9	247	9.8	43.3	3.8	2.7
Rolls, White, Floury, Roberts Bakery*	1 Roll/63g	160	1.6	254	8.4	49.5	2.5	2.0
Rolls, White, Floury Batch, Sainsbury's*	1 Roll/68g	168	1.9	247	8.3	47.2	2.8	2.2
Rolls, White, Good Health, Warburton's*	1 Roll/54g	122	1.1	226	9.6	42.0	2.0	4.1
Rolls, White, Large, Sliced, Warburton's*	1 Roll/89g	230	4.0	258	10.1	44.4	4.5	2.7
Rolls, White, Mini, Submarine, M & S*	1 Roll/30g	85	1.5	285	11.4	47.7	4.9	1.1
Rolls, White, Morning, Co-Op*	1 Roll/47g	134	1.4	285	12.0	53.0	3.0	2.0
Rolls, White, Old Fashioned, Waitrose*	1 Roll/64g	176	2.9	275	8.8	49.8	4.5	2.8
Rolls, White, Organic, Sainsbury's*	1 Roll/65g	170	1.9	262	8.7	49.9	3.0	1.0
Rolls, White, Part Baked, Morrisons*	1 Roll/75g	227	1.0	303	9.6	63.0	1.4	2.6
Rolls, White, Ploughman's, Sainsbury's*	1 Roll/65g	185	2.5	285	8.6	54.1	3.8	2.3
Rolls, White, Premium, Brown Hill Bakery*	1 Roll/74g	206	2.2	279	11.0	51.5	3.0	2.3
Rolls, White, Premium, Hovis*	1 Roll/70g	180	3.1	257	9.5	44.8	4.4	3.0
Rolls, White, Premium Soft, Rathbones*	1 Roll/65g	190	3.9	293	9.3	50.3	6.0	2.7
Rolls, White, Sandwich, Large, Warburton's*	1 Roll/88g	224	3.5	254	10.2	44.3	4.0	2.5
Rolls, White, Sandwich, Regular, Warburton's*	1 Roll/58g	143	2.5	249	9.7	42.6	4.3	2.4
Rolls, White, Scottish, Tesco*	1 Roll/48g	117	1.2	243	10.4	44.8	2.5	4.7
Rolls, White, Seeded, Sainsbury's*	1 Roll/80g	217	4.7	271	10.9	43.4	5.9	4.8
Rolls, White, Seeded, Soft, M & S*	1 Roll/75g	214	4.3	285	11.7	46.2	5.7	2.8
Rolls, White, Snack, Sainsbury's*	1 Roll/67g	159	0.7	237	7.9	49.2	1.0	2.3
Rolls, White, Soft, Average	**1 Roll/45g**	**114**	**1.5**	**253**	**9.2**	**46.5**	**3.3**	**2.2**
Rolls, White, Soft, COU, M & S*	1 Roll/37g	94	1.0	255	10.7	47.1	2.7	1.5
Rolls, White, Soft, Dietary Specials*	1 Roll/75g	130	2.9	172	2.2	29.8	3.8	4.7
Rolls, White, Soft, Farmhouse, Warburton's*	1 Roll/59g	147	2.6	250	9.7	43.0	4.4	2.5
Rolls, White, Soft, Hovis*	1 Roll/60g	154	2.6	257	9.5	44.8	4.4	3.0
Rolls, White, Soft, Kingsmill*	1 Roll/62g	156	1.7	252	8.9	46.7	2.8	2.4
Rolls, White, Submarine, M & S*	1 Roll/109g	300	5.4	275	11.0	47.0	5.0	1.0
Rolls, White, Warburton's*	1 Roll/57g	141	2.4	248	9.7	42.8	4.2	0.0
Rolls, White, Weight Watchers*	1 Roll/54g	135	1.0	251	11.7	47.1	1.8	4.2
Rolls, Wholemeal	**1 Roll/45g**	**108**	**1.3**	**241**	**9.0**	**48.3**	**2.9**	**5.9**
Rolls, Wholemeal, COU, M & S*	1 Roll/110g	225	3.1	205	11.3	33.4	2.8	7.1
Rolls, Wholemeal, Floury Batch, Sainsbury's*	1 Roll/68g	152	2.3	223	9.9	37.8	3.4	6.5
Rolls, Wholemeal, Food Explorers, Waitrose*	1 Roll/32g	74	1.0	231	10.6	40.2	3.1	5.7
Rolls, Wholemeal, Golden, Hovis*	1 Roll/50g	111	1.9	223	10.5	36.5	3.9	6.8
Rolls, Wholemeal, HL, Tesco*	1 Roll/67.5	155	1.4	230	10.4	41.3	2.1	6.6
Rolls, Wholemeal, Kingsmill*	1 Roll/68g	167	2.7	245	10.7	41.5	4.0	5.1
Rolls, Wholemeal, Milk, Warburton's*	1 Roll/22g	51	0.7	231	12.5	38.1	3.2	7.0
Rolls, Wholemeal, Mini, Assorted, Waitrose*	1 Roll/36g	84	1.9	236	9.0	38.1	5.3	5.2
Rolls, Wholemeal, Mini, Tesco*	1 Roll/34g	82	1.9	240	10.9	36.4	5.6	5.8
Rolls, Wholemeal, Oat Topped, Tesco*	1 Roll/65g	166	2.9	255	11.3	42.2	4.5	5.1
Rolls, Wholemeal, Oatbran, HL, Tesco*	1 Roll/56g	115	1.4	205	11.4	33.6	2.5	7.4
Rolls, Wholemeal, Old Fashioned, Waitrose*	1 Roll/57g	135	2.7	236	11.1	37.2	4.8	6.6
Rolls, Wholemeal, Organic, Sainsbury's*	1 Roll/66g	152	1.8	230	10.7	41.0	2.7	6.6
Rolls, Wholemeal, Organic, Tesco*	1 Roll/65g	177	4.0	273	10.3	44.1	6.2	5.5
Rolls, Wholemeal, Ploughman's, Sainsbury's*	1 Roll/67g	153	2.1	229	10.7	39.3	3.2	8.6
Rolls, Wholemeal, Seeded, The Country Miller, Waitrose*	1 Roll/75g	190	7.7	255	13.6	26.9	10.3	7.6

B

BREAD

	Measure INFO/WEIGHT	per Measure		Nutrition Values per 100g / 100ml				
		KCAL	FAT	KCAL	PROT	CARB	FAT	FIBRE
Rolls, Wholemeal, Sliced, Hovis*	1 Roll/60g	150	3.5	250	10.6	38.7	5.9	6.8
Rolls, Wholemeal, Soft, Sainsbury's*	1 Roll/60g	133	2.0	221	9.9	37.8	3.4	6.5
Rolls, Wholemeal, Soft, Seeded, Sainsbury's*	1 Roll/75g	193	5.5	257	11.8	35.6	7.4	6.2
Rolls, Wholemeal, Submarine, Tesco*	1 Roll/100g	221	3.1	221	9.3	39.0	3.1	5.2
Rolls, Wholemeal, Submarine, Warburton's*	1 Roll/94g	231	4.1	246	10.9	40.6	4.4	6.3
Rolls, Wholemeal, Sunflower & Honey, Sainsbury's*	1 Roll/85g	225	4.3	265	9.2	45.4	5.1	4.5
Rolls, Wholemeal, Tasty, Great Everyday, Kingsmill*	1 Roll/68g	158	2.6	232	10.6	38.8	3.8	6.5
Rolls, Wholemeal, Warburton's*	1 Roll/58g	124	2.1	214	10.2	35.1	3.7	6.6
Rolls, Wholemeal & White, Kingsmill*	1 Roll/60g	151	2.5	251	9.5	43.7	4.2	3.5
Rolls, Wholemeal with Cracked Wheat, Allinson*	1 Roll/58g	134	2.3	231	11.0	38.0	3.9	7.0
Rolls, Wholewhite, Kingsmill*	1 Roll/63g	158	2.6	251	9.5	43.7	4.2	3.5
Rolls, Wholmeal, Deli, Tesco*	1 Roll/65g	156	3.1	240	9.0	40.2	4.8	5.7
Roti, Tesco*	1 Bread/95g	256	5.2	269	8.4	46.4	5.5	3.2
Rye, Artisan Bread Organic*	1 Slice/50g	80	0.7	160	5.0	28.4	1.4	7.1
Rye, Average	*1 Slice/25g*	*55*	*0.4*	*219*	*8.3*	*45.8*	*1.7*	*4.4*
Rye, Dark, Sliced, Trianon*	1 Slice/41g	74	0.6	180	6.5	35.0	1.5	0.0
Rye, German Style, Bolletje*	1 Slice/60g	114	1.2	190	6.0	35.0	2.0	9.5
Rye, German Style, Kelderman*	1 Slice/57g	88	0.8	155	5.6	30.2	1.4	7.7
Rye, Light, Finest, Tesco*	1 Slice/20g	47	0.4	237	10.4	44.3	2.0	3.7
Rye, Swedish Style, Kelderman*	1 Slice/50g	92	1.6	185	7.2	31.5	3.2	4.3
Rye, Wheat Free, New York Deli, The Stamp Collection*	1 Slice/33g	61	0.5	184	6.6	43.6	1.4	7.3
Rye, Wholemeal with Sunflower Seeds, Organic, Biona*	1 Slice/72g	150	2.9	210	7.0	36.0	4.0	6.0
Rye with Sunflower Seeds, Organic, Schneider Brot*	1 Slice/72g	138	2.6	191	6.2	33.4	3.6	7.9
Rye with Sunflower Seeds, Organic, Sunnyvale*	1 Slice/25g	49	1.6	198	5.1	30.3	6.3	7.9
Rye with Wholegrain, Sliced, Rivercote*	1 Slice/55g	134	1.1	244	6.7	40.1	2.0	0.0
Seeded, Batch, Finest, Tesco*	1 Slice/65g	168	4.0	259	9.3	41.8	6.1	6.1
Seeded, Farmhouse, Loaf, Extra Special, Asda*	1 Slice/44g	92	0.5	207	11.0	38.0	1.2	8.0
Seeded, Farmhouse, Roberts Bakery*	1 Slice/37g	89	1.1	240	10.6	49.0	2.9	6.7
Seeded, Medium Sliced, Average	1 Slice/44g	116	2.9	262	11.3	38.6	6.5	5.6
Seeded, Rye, Loaf, la Brea Bakery*	1 Slice/55g	120	0.5	218	7.0	42.5	1.0	5.7
Seeded Batch, Toasted Seeds, 800g, Warburton's*	1 Slice/50g	137	3.7	270	11.4	35.1	7.3	10.2
Seeded Farmhouse, Organic, Cranks*	2 Slices/94g	232	3.5	247	10.1	39.9	3.7	6.9
Seriously Seeded, Gold, Kingsmill*	1 Slice/50g	136	3.4	272	10.9	41.6	6.9	6.4
Sesame Seed, la Brea Bakery*	1 Slice/35g	85	0.8	244	8.8	47.1	2.3	2.0
Seven Grain, Hearty, Golden Wonder*	1 Slice/38g	80	1.0	211	10.5	47.4	2.6	7.9
Sliced Fruited Malt Loaf, Weight Watchers*	1 Slice/23g	68	0.4	294	8.9	60.2	1.9	3.6
Soda	*1oz/28g*	*72*	*0.7*	*258*	*7.7*	*54.6*	*2.5*	*2.1*
Soda, Fruit, M & S*	1 Slice/40g	105	1.9	260	5.9	51.3	4.6	2.5
Soda Farls, M & S*	1 Farl/110g	267	3.0	243	9.6	50.1	2.7	2.3
Soda Farls, Tesco*	1 Farl/142g	325	4.5	229	7.1	42.2	3.2	2.6
Sourdough, Average	1 Slice/50g	144	0.9	289	11.7	56.4	1.8	2.4
Sourdough, Solero*	1 Serving/43g	110	2.5	256	9.3	46.5	5.8	2.3
Soya & Linseed, Burgen*	1 Slice/43g	124	4.4	287	15.9	29.8	10.1	6.8
Soya & Linseed, Vogel*	1 Slice/42g	95	2.1	227	11.7	34.1	4.9	6.8
Spelt & Seed, Sliced, Lifefibre*	1 Slice/42g	141	5.8	335	11.6	32.2	13.7	9.2
Sprouted Spelt with Raisins, Everfresh Bakery*	¼ Loaf/100g	230	1.9	230	9.2	43.9	1.9	6.6
Square Wraps, White, Warburton's*	1 Wrap/65g	159	2.9	245	12.5	38.6	4.5	2.1
Sunflower, Multi-Grain, Allinson*	1 Slice/47g	113	2.2	240	9.8	39.6	4.7	3.9
Sunflower & Honey, M & S*	1 Serving/67g	206	9.0	308	12.9	34.0	13.4	5.6
Sunflower & Honey, Organic, Cranks*	1 Slice/30g	64	0.9	215	11.6	37.2	3.0	8.3
Sunflower & Pumpkin Seed, Batched, Organic, Tesco*	1 Slice/30g	73	2.2	243	11.0	33.1	7.4	5.2
Sunflower & Pumpkin Seed, So Organic, Sainsbury's*	1 Slice/30g	76	1.6	254	11.4	40.0	5.4	12.9
Sunflower Seed, Bolletje, Delhaize*	1 Slice/44g	106	3.1	240	7.5	35.0	7.0	6.0

	Measure INFO/WEIGHT	per Measure KCAL	per Measure FAT	Nutrition Values per 100g / 100ml KCAL	PROT	CARB	FAT	FIBRE
BREAD								
Sunflower Seed, Organic, Natural, Mestemacher*	1 Slice/75g	162	3.0	216	5.6	34.7	4.0	9.4
Tiger Loaf, Tesco*	1 Slice/40g	96	0.8	239	8.7	46.6	2.0	2.6
Toaster, White, Rathbones*	1 Slice/38g	92	0.5	243	9.1	48.6	1.3	2.3
Tomato & Chilli, BGTY, Sainsbury's*	¼ Bread/65g	155	3.1	238	11.9	36.9	4.7	2.8
Tomato & Garlic, Flatbread, Italian Style, Iceland*	1 Serving/75g	195	8.8	260	6.3	32.3	11.8	2.4
Tomato & Garlic, Flatbread, Sainsbury's*	1/3 Bread/73g	191	4.9	261	8.4	41.7	6.7	3.4
Tomato & Garlic, Italian Style, Morrisons*	½ Pack/155g	355	12.4	229	5.8	33.4	8.0	2.5
Tomato & Herb, Tear & Share, Tesco*	¼ Pack/73g	164	3.2	226	6.3	40.2	4.4	2.1
Veda Malt, St Michael*	1 Serving/45g	99	0.5	219	7.1	45.3	1.1	2.2
Walnut, Waitrose*	1/8 Loaf/50g	169	7.6	339	10.0	40.6	15.2	5.9
Wheat	**1 Slice/25g**	**65**	**1.0**	**260**	**9.1**	**47.2**	**4.1**	**4.3**
Wheat, Tasty, Kingsmill*	1 Serving/38g	84	1.3	221	10.1	37.6	3.4	6.8
Wheat Rye, Wholemeal, Goldaehren, Aldi*	1 Slice/30g	68	1.2	226	8.0	36.0	4.0	7.0
Wheaten, Big Slice	1 Slice/65g	139	1.7	214	7.5	40.2	2.6	3.6
Wheaten, Loaf, Sliced, Genesis*	1 Slice/40g	86	1.0	214	7.5	40.2	2.6	3.6
Wheaten, M & S*	1 Slice/33g	74	1.2	225	9.3	42.9	3.5	3.9
Wheaten, Sliced, Healthy, Irwin's Bakery*	1 Slice/40g	76	0.8	190	9.0	40.5	1.9	6.2
Wheaten Loaf, Sliced, No Added Sugar, Genesis Crafty*	1 Slice/40g	86	1.0	214	7.5	40.2	2.6	3.6
Wheatgerm, Hovis, Soft, Sliced, M & S*	1 Slice/23g	50	0.7	220	10.1	38.5	3.0	4.6
Wheatgrain, Robertson*	1 Slice/30g	90	1.2	300	9.3	57.3	4.0	4.0
White, Batch, Warburton's*	1 Slice/42g	98	0.9	233	9.8	43.6	2.1	2.7
White, Batch Loaf, Extra Special, Asda*	1 Slice/47g	109	0.9	233	9.0	45.0	1.9	2.2
White, Chopped Roasted Garlic, Loaf, la Brea Bakery*	1 Loaf/400g	1196	16.4	299	9.9	53.0	4.1	2.5
White, Classic, Medium Sliced, Hovis*	1 Slice/38g	91	0.9	240	11.4	40.3	2.3	2.5
White, Classic, Thick Sliced, Hovis*	1 Slice/50g	120	2.2	240	9.2	40.5	4.5	3.1
White, Commercially Prepared, Average	1oz/28g	74	0.9	266	7.6	50.6	3.3	2.4
White, Commercially Prepared, Toasted, Average	1oz/28g	82	1.1	293	9.0	54.4	4.0	2.5
White, COU, M & S*	1 Slice/26g	60	0.6	231	10.6	41.9	2.3	4.6
White, Country Maid*	1 Slice/33g	76	0.7	229	8.5	44.1	2.1	3.0
White, Crusty, Fresh, Finest, Tesco*	1 Slice/52g	130	1.0	250	8.6	48.5	1.9	2.4
White, Crusty, Gold, Kingsmill*	1 Slice/27g	70	0.8	258	9.4	48.5	2.9	2.7
White, Crusty, Hovis*	1 Slice/44g	103	1.0	233	8.8	44.3	2.2	2.1
White, Crusty, Sliced, Premium, Budgens*	1 Slice/50g	121	1.1	242	8.8	46.9	2.2	2.2
White, Crusty, Sliced Loaf, Tesco*	1 Slice/50g	116	1.0	233	7.4	46.0	2.1	2.0
White, Danish, Medium Sliced, BFY, Morrisons*	1 Slice/17g	42	0.3	245	10.2	49.1	1.8	2.2
White, Danish, Sliced, Weight Watchers*	1 Slice/21g	50	0.3	243	9.8	46.5	1.3	2.9
White, Danish, Soft & Light, Thick Cut, Asda*	1 Slice/26g	60	0.4	230	9.0	45.0	1.6	2.1
White, Danish Style, Thick Sliced, Light, Tesco*	1 Slice/22g	55	0.6	255	9.4	47.3	2.9	2.7
White, Extra Thick Sliced, Kingsmill*	1 Slice/58g	135	1.4	232	8.8	43.8	2.4	2.8
White, Farmhouse, Hovis*	1 Slice/44g	103	1.0	234	8.7	44.6	2.3	2.4
White, Farmhouse, Seeded, Waitrose*	1 Serving/75g	192	4.1	256	10.8	40.9	5.5	5.6
White, Farmhouse Crusty, M & S*	1 Slice/34g	82	0.7	240	8.9	46.6	2.2	3.0
White, Farmhouse Gold Premium, Morrisons*	1 Slice/38g	90	0.5	236	8.9	47.4	1.2	2.2
White, Fibre, Morrisons*	1 Slice/40g	96	0.7	240	8.0	48.4	1.7	0.3
White, Fresh, Gluten Free, Glutafin*	1 Slice/35g	80	0.9	228	3.5	43.5	2.7	7.6
White, Fried in Blended Oil	**1 Slice/28g**	**141**	**9.0**	**503**	**7.9**	**48.5**	**32.2**	**1.6**
White, Gluten & Wheat Free, Free From, Sainsbury's*	1 Slice/33g	75	2.8	227	1.9	35.5	8.6	1.0
White, Gluten Free, Bakers Delight*	1 Serving/28g	64	2.4	227	1.9	35.5	8.6	1.0
White, Gluten Free, Genius*	1 Slice/40g	124	5.5	311	7.7	42.3	13.8	13.8
White, Gold Seeded, Kingsmill*	1 Slice/44g	108	2.5	245	9.7	38.8	5.7	3.5
White, Golden, Square Cut, M & S*	1 Slice/40g	85	0.8	215	8.9	40.7	2.1	6.1
White, Good Health, Warburton's*	1 Slice/38g	84	0.7	220	9.4	41.6	1.8	4.1
White, Harvest Crust Premium, Ormo*	1 Slice/40g	92	0.6	229	9.4	47.4	1.5	2.7

B

BREAD

	Measure INFO/WEIGHT	per Measure KCAL	FAT	Nutrition Values per 100g / 100ml KCAL	PROT	CARB	FAT	FIBRE
White, High Fibre, Nimble*	1 Slice/22g	48	0.4	219	10.1	40.6	1.8	7.5
White, Invisible Crust, Hovis*	1 Slice/40g	90	0.6	226	8.8	44.1	1.6	2.4
White, Loaf, Crusty, Premium, Warburton's*	1 Slice/31g	76	0.7	249	10.6	46.5	2.3	2.6
White, Loaf, Danish, Asda*	1 Slice/23g	53	0.5	236	9.0	45.0	2.2	2.0
White, Low Carb, Sliced, Tesco*	1 Slice/16g	35	0.4	211	11.3	36.4	2.2	6.9
White, Medium, Round Top, Kingsmill*	1 Slice/42g	97	1.0	232	8.8	43.8	2.4	2.8
White, Medium, Stayfresh, Tesco*	1 Slice/45g	108	0.7	240	8.2	47.8	1.5	3.0
White, Medium Sliced, Asda*	1 Slice/37g	80	0.6	218	8.0	43.0	1.5	3.3
White, Medium Sliced, Basics, Sainsbury's*	1 Slice/36g	83	0.5	231	8.0	46.4	1.5	2.1
White, Medium Sliced, Brace's*	1 Slice/32g	75	0.4	235	9.5	46.6	1.2	2.6
White, Medium Sliced, Budgens*	1 Slice/36g	82	0.6	229	8.0	45.6	1.6	3.0
White, Medium Sliced, Great Everyday, Kingsmill*	1 Slice/40g	93	0.8	232	9.0	44.6	2.0	2.7
White, Medium Sliced, Long Life, Asda*	1 Slice/36g	82	0.6	228	8.0	45.0	1.8	2.7
White, Medium Sliced, Mother's Pride*	1 Slice/36g	82	0.6	229	8.0	45.6	1.6	3.0
White, Medium Sliced, Sainsbury's*	1 Slice/36g	78	0.7	216	8.7	41.1	1.9	7.1
White, Medium Sliced, Smart Price, Asda*	1 Slice/36g	81	0.5	226	7.0	46.0	1.5	2.8
White, Medium Sliced, Square, Kingsmill*	1 Slice/66g	88	0.9	133	5.0	25.1	1.4	1.7
White, Medium Sliced, Stay Fresh, Tesco*	1 Slice/35g	85	0.7	246	8.9	48.1	2.0	0.8
White, Medium Sliced, Superlife, Morrisons*	1 Slice/30g	79	1.2	263	9.6	47.4	3.9	2.5
White, Medium Sliced, Tesco*	1 Slice/36g	86	0.5	240	8.2	47.8	1.5	3.0
White, Medium Sliced, Value, Tesco*	1 Slice/36g	81	0.4	225	7.9	46.1	1.0	2.1
White, Medium Sliced, Warburton's*	1 Slice/40g	94	0.8	234	9.9	43.8	2.0	2.6
White, Medium Sliced, Weight Watchers*	1 Slice/12g	30	0.2	247	12.5	45.2	1.9	3.2
White, Medium VLH Kitchens	1 Slice/30g	72	6.3	241	8.4	49.3	1.9	1.5
White, Oatmeal, Allinson*	1 Slice/47g	111	1.4	237	9.0	43.5	3.0	2.7
White, Organic, Hovis*	1 Slice/44g	108	1.4	246	8.6	45.8	3.2	2.3
White, Organic, Sainsbury's*	1 Slice/36g	84	0.6	234	8.9	45.5	1.8	2.3
White, Plain, Scottish, Sunblest*	1 Slice/57g	133	1.5	233	10.1	42.3	2.6	2.8
White, Premium, M & S*	1 Slice/40g	95	0.8	235	8.5	45.8	1.9	2.7
White, Soft, Batch Loaf, Sliced, Tesco*	1 Slice/50g	116	1.0	233	7.5	46.1	2.1	2.1
White, Soft, Farmhouse, M & S*	1 Slice/25g	60	0.8	239	9.8	42.6	3.3	2.5
White, Soft, Gold, Kingsmill*	1 Slice/47g	112	1.5	239	8.2	44.5	3.1	2.7
White, Soft, Great Everyday, Thick Sliced, Kingsmill*	1 Slice/44g	102	0.9	232	9.0	44.6	2.0	2.7
White, Soft, Hovis*	1 Slice/40g	94	0.9	234	8.7	44.6	2.3	2.4
White, Soft, M & S*	1 Slice/47g	105	0.8	225	7.3	46.1	1.7	2.4
White, Soft, Organic, Warburton's*	1 Slice/27g	61	0.8	228	9.7	44.6	3.0	2.6
White, Soft Batch, Sliced, Sainsbury's*	1 Slice/44g	102	0.8	232	8.2	45.4	1.9	2.3
White, Soft Crusty, M & S*	1 Slice/25g	64	0.6	256	9.3	49.0	2.5	2.4
White, Square, Extra Thick Sliced, Hovis*	1 Slice/67g	155	1.3	231	8.5	44.7	2.0	2.6
White, Square, Medium Sliced, Hovis*	1 Slice/40g	92	0.8	231	8.5	44.7	2.0	2.6
White, Square, Thick Sliced, Hovis*	1 Slice/50g	116	1.0	231	8.5	44.7	2.0	2.6
White, Stay Fresh, Tesco*	1 Slice/40g	100	1.0	249	8.6	48.3	2.4	1.5
White, Super Toastie, Warburton's*	1 Slice/57g	134	1.0	235	10.1	44.6	1.8	2.7
White, Thick, So Organic, Sainsbury's*	1 Slice/44g	102	1.0	231	8.2	44.6	2.2	3.1
White, Thick, Super Soft, M & S*	1 Slice/48g	115	1.2	240	8.7	45.3	2.6	2.5
White, Thick, Toastie, 800g Loaf, Warburton's*	1 Slice/47g	111	0.9	234	9.9	43.9	1.9	2.5
White, Thick Sliced, Bakers Gold, Asda*	1 Slice/44g	101	0.8	229	8.0	45.0	1.9	2.3
White, Thick Sliced, Brace's*	1 Slice/38g	90	0.5	235	9.5	46.6	1.2	2.6
White, Thick Sliced, Budgens*	1 Slice/40g	89	0.5	223	7.4	45.3	1.3	2.5
White, Thick Sliced, Family Favourite*	1 Slice/37g	83	0.5	225	8.5	44.5	1.4	2.3
White, Thick Sliced, Fine Lady*	1 Slice/44g	113	0.5	254	7.8	53.1	1.2	2.3
White, Thick Sliced, Golden Sun*	1 Slice/44g	100	0.7	228	7.5	46.1	1.5	2.4
White, Thick Sliced, Healthy, Warburton's*	1 Slice/38g	84	0.7	222	10.3	41.2	1.8	4.1

BREAD

	Measure INFO/WEIGHT	per Measure KCAL	FAT	Nutrition Values per 100g / 100ml KCAL	PROT	CARB	FAT	FIBRE
White, Thick Sliced, M & S*	1 Slice/42g	96	0.5	228	7.3	46.7	1.3	2.8
White, Thick Sliced, Organic, Tesco*	1 Slice/44g	108	0.9	245	8.5	46.8	2.1	3.1
White, Thick Sliced, Premium, Tesco*	1 Slice/44g	99	0.3	222	8.7	45.2	0.7	1.5
White, Thick Sliced, Sainsbury's*	1 Slice/44g	95	0.8	216	8.7	41.1	1.9	7.1
White, Thick Sliced, Square Cut, Asda*	1 Slice/44g	101	0.7	230	8.0	46.0	1.5	2.1
White, Thick Sliced, Staysoft, Rathbones*	1 Slice/38g	87	0.5	228	8.5	45.5	1.3	2.7
White, Thick Sliced, Sunblest*	1 Slice/40g	91	0.6	228	8.0	45.7	1.5	2.8
White, Thick Sliced, Super Toastie, Morrisons*	1 Slice/50g	128	1.5	257	8.7	48.9	3.0	2.1
White, Thick Sliced, Tesco*	1 Slice/44g	106	0.7	240	8.2	47.8	1.5	3.0
White, Thick Sliced, Warburton's, Weight Watchers*	1 Slice/29g	69	0.2	237	10.4	48.6	0.8	2.0
White, Thick Sliced, Warburton's*	1 Slice/28g	65	0.6	233	9.8	43.6	2.1	2.7
White, Thin Sliced, Sainsbury's*	1 Slice/29g	66	0.4	228	7.1	46.4	1.5	2.8
White, Thin Sliced, Tesco*	1 Slice/30g	68	0.4	228	9.5	44.5	1.3	3.4
White, Toast, Gamle Mølle*	1 Slice/32g	83	0.6	260	8.0	52.0	2.0	3.0
White, Toasted, Average	*1 Slice/33g*	*87*	*0.5*	*265*	*9.3*	*57.1*	*1.6*	*1.8*
White, Toastie, Thick, Love to Toast, Kingsmill*	1 Slice/50g	116	1.0	232	9.0	44.6	2.0	2.7
White, Toastie, Thick Cut, Hovis*	1 Slice/50g	115	1.0	230	8.5	44.7	2.0	2.5
White, Weight Watchers*	1 Slice/29g	71	0.5	246	12.3	45.1	1.6	3.3
White, Whole, Extra Thick, Kingsmill*	1 Slice/57g	130	1.4	228	9.0	42.3	2.5	4.0
White, Whole, Kingsmill*	1 Slice/38g	87	0.9	230	9.0	42.9	2.5	3.4
White, Wholesome, Loaf, Sainsbury's*	1 Serving/36g	81	0.7	224	9.4	42.5	1.8	4.4
White, Wholesome, Medium Sliced, Asda*	1 Slice/35g	78	0.9	223	7.0	43.0	2.6	5.0
White, Wholesome, Medium Sliced, Premium, Tesco*	1 Slice/37g	85	0.8	232	8.9	43.9	2.3	4.2
White, Wholesome, Thick Sliced, Tesco*	1 Serving/80g	177	1.5	221	10.5	40.5	1.9	4.8
White Loaf, Gluten & Wheat Free, Lovemore*	1 Serving/35g	111	3.8	316	0.0	3.4	10.9	0.0
Whole Grain, Batch, Finest, Tesco*	1 Slice/44g	112	1.2	254	9.8	47.7	2.7	4.2
Whole Grain, Brennans*	1 Slice/39g	79	0.6	203	9.0	40.0	1.5	4.9
Whole Grain & Rye, Schneider Brot*	1 Slice/50g	98	0.6	197	5.9	36.6	1.2	8.2
Whole Grain with Sunflower Seeds, Landgut*	1 Slice/83g	183	4.1	221	7.0	37.0	5.0	29.0
Whole Wheat, 100%, Soft, Farmhouse, Ocean Spray*	1 Slice/43g	110	2.0	256	11.6	44.2	4.7	7.0
Whole Wheat, 100%, Stoneground, Maxwell House*	1 Slice/27g	60	0.5	222	11.1	44.4	1.9	7.4
Whole Wheat, Harvest	1 Slice/42g	90	1.0	214	7.1	45.2	2.4	7.1
Whole Wheat, Nature's Own*	1 Slice/28g	66	1.0	236	14.3	39.3	3.6	10.7
Whole Wheat, Soft, Trader Joe's*	1 Slice/37g	70	1.0	189	10.8	37.8	2.7	5.4
Wholegrain, Average	1 Slice/44g	117	1.9	265	13.4	43.3	4.2	7.4
Wholegrain, Medium Sliced, Irish Pride*	1 Slice/38g	90	0.8	237	9.2	46.6	2.1	7.6
Wholegrain, Soft, M & S*	1 Slice/51g	115	2.8	225	13.0	31.2	5.4	8.2
Wholegrain, Toasted, Average	1 Slice/40g	117	1.9	288	14.5	47.1	4.6	8.1
Wholemeal, & Oat Flakes, Gold, Kingsmill*	1 Slice/47g	103	1.6	220	10.0	37.3	3.4	7.0
Wholemeal, 7 Seeded, Irwin's Bakery*	1 Slice/38g	90	2.0	237	9.5	33.4	5.2	9.4
Wholemeal, Allinson*	1 Slice/47g	102	1.4	216	12.5	34.8	3.0	7.4
Wholemeal, American Sandwich, Harry's*	1 Slice/43g	110	2.1	259	9.0	45.0	5.0	5.0
Wholemeal, Average	*1 Slice/40g*	*88*	*1.0*	*215*	*9.2*	*41.6*	*2.5*	*5.8*
Wholemeal, Baker`s Soft, Medium, Tesco*	1 Slice/40g	94	1.1	235	10.8	37.8	2.8	6.9
Wholemeal, Batch, Allinson*	1 Slice/48g	112	1.5	233	10.5	37.0	3.2	7.1
Wholemeal, Batch, Organic, Waitrose*	1 Slice/40g	88	1.0	219	10.0	38.8	2.6	7.2
Wholemeal, Batch Loaf, Allinson*	1 Slice/47g	110	1.5	233	10.5	37.0	3.2	7.1
Wholemeal, BGTY, Sainsbury's*	1 Slice/20g	41	0.2	207	12.6	36.8	1.0	7.3
Wholemeal, Brennans*	1 Slice/33g	78	1.4	236	11.2	38.4	4.2	7.7
Wholemeal, Brown, Medium Sliced, Hovis*	1 Slice/40g	92	1.1	230	10.0	37.7	2.7	6.7
Wholemeal, COU, M & S*	1 Slice/21g	45	0.5	213	13.6	33.7	2.6	7.0
Wholemeal, Crusty, Finest, Tesco*	1 Slice/50g	103	0.0	206	10.8	37.0	1.7	6.9
Wholemeal, Crusty, Kingsmill*	1 Slice/42g	104	1.8	247	11.2	41.1	4.2	7.0

BREAD

INFO/WEIGHT	Measure	per Measure		Nutrition Values per 100g / 100ml				
		KCAL	FAT	KCAL	PROT	CARB	FAT	FIBRE
Wholemeal, Danish, BFY, Morrisons*	1 Slice/17g	39	0.3	228	11.2	47.9	1.8	6.2
Wholemeal, Danish, Warburton's*	1 Slice/25g	57	0.6	229	13.3	38.5	2.4	7.2
Wholemeal, Economy, Sainsbury's*	1 Slice/28g	61	0.7	217	10.3	38.4	2.5	6.5
Wholemeal, Farmhouse, Hovis*	1 Slice/44g	91	1.0	207	11.0	36.0	2.2	7.1
Wholemeal, Farmhouse Soft Golden, M & S*	1 Slice/30g	64	0.9	215	11.0	35.1	3.1	7.4
Wholemeal, Fh, Stoneground, Batch, Finest, Tesco*	1 Slice/50g	107	1.4	215	10.3	36.1	2.8	6.9
Wholemeal, Fresher for Longer, Sainsbury's*	1 Slice/44g	98	1.6	222	10.9	36.2	3.7	6.5
Wholemeal, Gold, Kingsmill*	1 Slice/44g	95	1.3	217	10.9	36.8	2.9	7.0
Wholemeal, Golden, M & S*	1 Slice/30g	69	1.4	230	10.8	36.6	4.5	7.7
Wholemeal, Golden Crust, Ormo*	1 Slice/38g	83	0.8	218	10.4	36.1	2.0	7.0
Wholemeal, Golden Wheat, Kingsmill*	1 Slice/44g	97	1.3	221	10.9	37.8	2.9	6.0
Wholemeal, Light, Irish Pride*	1 Slice/28g	68	0.4	241	13.3	44.1	1.3	4.5
Wholemeal, Little Brown Loaf, Unsliced, Hovis*	1 Slice/40g	86	1.1	216	10.0	37.8	2.7	6.8
Wholemeal, Loaf, Sliced, Medium, 800g, Hovis*	1 Slice/40g	92	1.1	229	10.0	37.8	2.7	6.8
Wholemeal, Loaf, Sliced, Thick, 800g, Hovis*	1 Slice/50g	115	1.4	229	10.0	37.8	2.7	6.8
Wholemeal, Longer Life, Medium Sliced, Sainsbury's*	1 Slice/35g	78	1.3	222	10.9	36.2	3.7	6.5
Wholemeal, Longer Life, Sainsbury's*	1 Slice/36g	85	1.2	237	10.7	41.0	3.4	6.2
Wholemeal, Longer Life, Thick Slice, Sainsbury's*	1 Slice/45g	101	1.6	224	10.6	37.4	3.6	5.9
Wholemeal, Medium, 800g Loaf, Warburton's*	1 Slice/40g	93	1.0	231	10.2	39.6	2.5	6.5
Wholemeal, Medium Sliced, Great Everyday, Kingsmill*	1 Slice/40g	91	1.5	227	10.5	37.7	3.8	6.2
Wholemeal, Medium Sliced, Little Big Loaf, Kingsmill*	1 Slice/39g	93	1.5	239	10.5	37.7	3.8	6.2
Wholemeal, Medium Sliced, M & S*	1 Slice/40g	80	1.2	200	10.5	32.7	3.1	6.7
Wholemeal, Medium Sliced, Morrisons*	1 Slice/32g	68	0.8	214	9.9	38.0	2.5	5.8
Wholemeal, Medium Sliced, Organic, Tesco*	1 Slice/27g	55	0.7	209	9.2	37.2	2.8	6.0
Wholemeal, Medium Sliced, Premium, Tesco*	1 Slice/36g	71	0.2	196	9.8	37.8	0.6	7.2
Wholemeal, Medium Sliced, Roberts Bakery*	1 Slice/37g	86	0.6	233	10.9	38.1	1.5	6.6
Wholemeal, Medium Sliced, Sainsbury's*	1 Slice/36g	77	0.9	214	10.3	37.8	2.4	7.4
Wholemeal, Medium Sliced, The Village Bakery*	1 Slice/33g	69	0.7	209	9.8	38.0	2.0	6.0
Wholemeal, Medium Sliced, Waitrose*	1 Slice/36g	76	0.9	213	10.1	37.6	2.4	7.0
Wholemeal, Multi Seeded, TTD, Sainsbury's*	1 Slice/47g	110	3.4	234	11.7	30.7	7.2	8.1
Wholemeal, Multigrain, Sliced, Finest, Tesco*	1 Slice/50g	123	2.0	246	10.1	42.1	4.1	6.5
Wholemeal, Multigrain, Soft Batch, Sainsbury's*	1 Slice/44g	106	2.9	242	11.3	34.5	6.5	5.6
Wholemeal, Multiseed, Organic, Sainsbury's*	1 Slice/26g	75	2.5	289	13.8	36.6	9.7	6.0
Wholemeal, Nimble*	1 Slice/22g	48	0.5	219	12.2	37.0	2.5	6.8
Wholemeal, Oat Topped, TTD, Sainsbury's*	1 Slice/47g	109	1.3	232	10.0	38.5	2.8	0.3
Wholemeal, Organic, 400g Loaf, Warburton's*	1 Slice/28g	63	0.9	223	10.3	37.9	3.2	6.7
Wholemeal, Organic, Hovis*	1 Slice/44g	92	1.3	209	10.2	35.6	2.9	7.6
Wholemeal, Premium, Medium Slice, M & S*	1 Slice/33g	65	1.0	200	10.5	32.9	3.1	6.7
Wholemeal, Premium, Thick Slice, M & S*	1 Slice/50g	95	1.5	190	9.8	30.8	3.0	6.4
Wholemeal, Rathbones*	1 Slice/27g	57	0.5	211	9.4	39.2	1.8	7.1
Wholemeal, Rolls, Mini Loaves, Hovis*	1 Loaf/70g	175	4.1	250	10.6	38.7	5.9	6.8
Wholemeal, Rustic, Tin, Tesco*	1 Slice/37g	92	1.3	249	12.2	44.0	3.5	3.1
Wholemeal, Rye, Warburton's*	1 Slice/44g	108	1.1	246	9.9	40.6	2.4	7.5
Wholemeal, Sandwich Loaf, Brennans*	1 Slice/40g	88	0.7	221	9.8	38.5	1.7	8.0
Wholemeal, Seed Sensation, Hovis*	1 Slice/44g	109	2.5	249	11.9	31.4	5.6	12.4
Wholemeal, Seeded, Roll, Love Life, Waitrose*	1 Roll/72g	192	6.3	266	12.6	34.1	8.8	6.4
Wholemeal, Sliced, Gluten Free, Glutano*	1 Slice/56g	107	1.7	191	7.0	34.0	3.0	0.0
Wholemeal, Sliced, McCambridge*	1 Slice/38g	90	0.7	237	7.9	44.7	1.8	0.0
Wholemeal, Sliced, Medium, Tesco*	1 Slice/36g	79	0.8	220	11.0	39.1	2.2	6.6
Wholemeal, Sliced, Organic, Harvestime*	1 Slice/44g	95	1.2	216	9.0	38.7	2.7	5.6
Wholemeal, Small Loaf, Sliced, 400g, Hovis*	1 Slice/25g	57	0.7	229	10.0	37.8	2.7	6.8
Wholemeal, Soft Crusty, M & S*	1 Slice/25g	57	0.8	230	11.4	39.1	3.1	6.5
Wholemeal, Square Cut, Thick Sliced, Asda*	1 Slice/44g	91	1.0	208	10.0	37.0	2.2	6.0

BREAD	Measure INFO/WEIGHT	per Measure KCAL	FAT	Nutrition Values per 100g / 100ml KCAL	PROT	CARB	FAT	FIBRE
Wholemeal, Stayfresh, Tesco*	1 Slice/36g	81	0.8	225	11.0	39.1	2.2	6.0
Wholemeal, Stoneground, 800g Loaf, Warburton's*	1 Slice/45g	95	1.2	210	10.4	35.8	2.6	6.8
Wholemeal, Stoneground, Organic, Sainsbury's*	1 Slice/29g	61	0.6	210	10.2	37.9	1.9	7.8
Wholemeal, Stoneground, Organic, Waitrose*	1 Slice/25g	57	0.9	228	10.8	38.2	3.6	7.1
Wholemeal, Stoneground, Thick Sliced, Sainsbury's*	1 Slice/44g	92	0.8	210	10.2	37.9	1.9	7.8
Wholemeal, Supersoft, Eat Well, M & S*	1 Slice/33g	81	1.1	245	10.9	40.0	3.3	6.7
Wholemeal, Tasty, Medium, Kingsmill*	1 Slice/40g	96	1.5	239	10.5	37.7	3.8	6.2
Wholemeal, Thick Slice, Brennans*	1 Slice/27g	69	0.6	257	9.2	45.4	2.1	6.8
Wholemeal, Thick Sliced, Bakers Gold, Asda*	1 Slice/44g	99	1.4	225	12.0	37.0	3.2	6.0
Wholemeal, Thick Sliced, COU, M & S*	1 Slice/26g	56	0.7	215	13.6	33.7	2.6	7.0
Wholemeal, Thick Sliced, Great Everyday, Kingsmill*	1 Slice/44g	100	1.7	227	10.5	37.7	3.8	6.2
Wholemeal, Thick Sliced, Healthy Living, Co-Op*	1 Slice/44g	95	0.9	215	11.0	38.0	2.0	7.0
Wholemeal, Thick Sliced, Organic, Tesco*	1 Slice/44g	98	1.2	220	8.8	38.8	2.8	5.9
Wholemeal, Thick Sliced, Premium, Tesco*	1 Slice/44g	95	0.7	214	10.0	40.1	1.5	5.7
Wholemeal, Thick Sliced, Sainsbury's*	1 Slice/48g	102	1.2	213	10.1	37.4	2.6	8.5
Wholemeal, Thick Sliced, Stephenson's Bakery*	1 Slice/40g	84	0.8	209	10.7	37.3	1.9	6.2
Wholemeal, Thick Sliced, Tesco*	1 Slice/40g	96	1.1	240	9.5	40.9	2.7	6.8
Wholemeal, Thick Sliced, Waitrose*	1 Slice/44g	94	1.1	213	10.1	37.6	2.4	7.0
Wholemeal, Thick Sliced, with Mustard Seed, Lozzas	1 Slice/26g	56	0.7	215	13.6	33.7	2.6	7.0
Wholemeal, Toasted, Average	*1 Slice/26g*	*58*	*0.6*	*224*	*8.6*	*42.3*	*2.2*	*5.8*
Wholemeal, Toastie, 800g Loaf, Warburton's*	1 Slice/45g	101	1.1	224	9.7	39.3	2.4	6.6
Wholemeal, Unsliced, Organic, Dove's Farm*	1 Slice/35g	77	0.9	221	11.4	37.9	2.6	8.3
Wholemeal & Oat, Loaf, Vogel*	1 Slice/42g	86	0.6	205	8.7	34.3	1.5	9.7
Wholemeal Loaf, British Farmers, Hovis*	1 Slice/47g	108	1.3	229	10.0	37.9	2.8	6.8
Wholemeal Oatbran, Sliced, Tesco*	1 Slice/45g	90	0.7	200	10.1	35.3	1.6	7.4
Wholemeal with Rye, M & S*	1 Slice/33g	79	1.2	240	10.5	37.2	3.5	7.8
Wholemeal with Seeds, Thick Sliced, Love Life, Waitrose*	1 Slice/54g	131	4.5	243	12.7	28.8	8.4	9.7
Wholewheat, No Crusts, Harry's*	1 Slice/25g	58	1.1	233	8.0	40.0	4.5	5.5
BREAD & BUTTER PUDDING								
Average	1 Serving/250g	400	19.5	160	6.2	17.5	7.8	0.3
BGTY, Sainsbury's*	1 Serving/125g	126	2.9	101	6.3	13.4	2.3	5.4
Chilled, Chosen By You, Asda*	¼ Pack/125g	267	13.9	213	5.1	22.0	11.1	2.4
COU, M & S*	1 Pot/140g	161	2.8	115	6.1	18.4	2.0	0.8
Finest, Tesco*	1 Serving/153g	379	22.0	248	4.9	24.6	14.4	0.9
Frozen, Chosen By You, Asda*	1 Serving/125g	275	10.2	220	5.5	30.4	8.2	1.4
GFY, Asda*	1 Serving/125g	152	2.0	122	7.0	20.0	1.6	1.3
Low Fat, Individual, BGTY, Sainsbury's*	1 Pack/125g	125	2.9	100	6.3	13.4	2.3	5.4
Reduced Fat, Waitrose*	1 Serving/205g	299	5.3	146	7.4	23.3	2.6	2.0
Sticky Toffee, M & S*	1oz/28g	83	3.0	295	4.1	46.3	10.6	2.2
BREAD MIX								
Brown, Sunflower, Sainsbury's*	1 Serving/60g	151	3.7	251	10.0	38.9	6.1	4.0
Cheese & Onion, Dry Mix, Sainsbury's*	1 Serving/100g	311	2.8	311	11.9	59.5	2.8	2.6
Crusty White, Made Up, Tesco*	1 Slice/126g	316	2.3	251	9.4	49.3	1.8	2.5
Focaccia, Garlic & Herb, Asda*	1 Serving/125g	385	10.0	308	11.0	48.0	8.0	3.3
Mixed Grain, Sainsbury's*	1 Serving/45g	103	0.7	228	7.7	46.0	1.5	4.4
Multiseed, Baked, Sainsbury's*	1 Slice/44g	112	4.3	252	10.8	30.5	9.6	6.8
Parmesan & Sun Dried Tomato, Made Up, Wrights*	1 Slice/45g	103	0.6	229	9.3	46.0	1.3	2.4
White Loaf, Asda*	1 Slice/60g	150	0.9	250	10.0	49.0	1.5	3.1
Wholemeal, Hovis*	1 Serving/65g	148	3.1	227	10.0	35.8	4.8	6.8
BREADCRUMBS								
Average	*1oz/28g*	*98*	*0.5*	*350*	*10.7*	*74.8*	*1.9*	*2.5*
BREADFRUIT								
Raw	*1oz/28g*	*27*	*0.1*	*95*	*1.3*	*23.1*	*0.3*	*0.0*

	Measure INFO/WEIGHT	per Measure KCAL	FAT	Nutrition Values per 100g / 100ml KCAL	PROT	CARB	FAT	FIBRE
BREADSTICKS								
Grissini, Thin with Olive Oil, Forno Bianco*	1 Stick/5g	21	0.4	420	11.0	77.0	7.5	0.0
Grissini, Waitrose*	1 Stick/6g	25	0.4	397	12.0	72.5	6.2	3.1
Italian Original, Tesco*	1 Stick/6g	23	0.4	410	11.6	72.9	7.8	2.9
Mini, Wheat & Gluten Free, Free From, Tesco*	1 Stick/3g	11	0.3	414	4.0	72.1	12.2	2.2
Olive, Italian, Finest, Tesco*	1 Stick/40g	170	5.4	424	10.5	65.0	13.6	4.8
Onion, M & S*	1 Serving/40g	166	5.6	415	12.6	59.6	14.1	4.8
Original, Italian, Tesco*	1 Stick/6g	23	0.4	410	11.6	72.9	7.8	2.9
Original, Organic, Kallo*	1 Stick/6g	24	0.5	393	11.8	69.5	7.6	4.7
Oven Baked, Mini, Quaker Oats*	1 Pack/35g	145	3.1	415	12.9	71.0	8.8	3.7
Perfectly Balanced, Waitrose*	1 Stick/5g	20	0.1	378	13.7	77.3	1.6	3.8
Plain, Asda*	1 Stick/5g	21	0.4	412	12.0	73.0	8.0	2.9
Rosemary, Asda*	1 Stick/7g	29	1.0	439	12.0	64.0	15.0	3.5
Salted, Asda*	1 Stick/8g	36	1.4	445	13.0	60.0	17.0	4.3
Sesame Seed Grissini, Sainsbury's*	1 Stick/5g	21	0.6	419	12.7	65.5	11.8	3.2
Thin, Healthy Eating, D'oro, Primo*	1 Stick/3g	11	0.2	400	10.0	75.0	6.5	1.1
Torrinesi, TTD, Sainsbury's*	1 Stick/3g	13	0.2	411	11.0	77.0	6.5	1.1
BREAKFAST CEREAL								
3 in One, Raisin & Apple, Jordans*	1 Serving/50g	170	2.2	340	7.6	67.4	4.4	9.8
3 in One, Strawberry, Jordans*	1 Serving/50g	181	2.9	362	9.4	68.0	5.8	11.9
Advantage, Weetabix*	1 Serving/30g	105	0.7	350	10.2	72.0	2.4	9.0
All Bran, Bran Flakes, & Fruit, Kellogg's*	1 Serving/40g	143	2.4	358	8.0	68.0	6.0	9.0
All Bran, Bran Flakes, Chocolate, Kellogg's*	1 Serving/30g	106	1.8	354	10.0	65.0	6.0	13.0
All Bran, Bran Flakes, Kellogg's*	1 Serving/30g	106	0.6	355	10.0	67.0	2.0	15.0
All Bran, Fruit 'n' Fibre, Kellogg's*	1 Serving/30g	114	1.8	380	8.0	69.0	6.0	9.0
All Bran, Fruitful, Kellogg's*	1 Serving/40g	136	3.0	340	12.5	57.5	7.5	0.0
All Bran, Golden Crunch, Kellogg's*	1 Serving/45g	182	4.9	405	8.0	62.0	11.0	13.0
All Bran, Original, High Fibre, Kellogg's*	1 Serving/40g	134	1.4	334	14.0	48.0	3.5	27.0
Almond, Low Carb, Atkins*	1 Serving/30g	100	1.5	333	50.0	26.7	5.0	0.0
Almond, Oats & More, Nestle*	1 Serving/30g	119	2.7	398	10.7	68.7	8.9	5.5
Amaranth, Flakes, Organic, Gillian McKeith*	1 Serving/50g	198	2.0	396	10.0	80.0	4.0	3.0
Apple, Blackberry & Raspberry Flakes, GFY, Asda*	1 Serving/30g	103	0.5	344	9.0	73.0	1.8	11.0
Apple & Cinnamon, Crisp, Sainsbury's*	1 Serving/50g	216	7.3	433	6.2	69.1	14.7	3.4
Apple & Cinnamon Flakes, M & S*	1 Serving/30g	111	0.6	370	6.0	82.7	1.9	3.4
Apricot Wheats, Whole Grain, Tesco*	1 Serving/40g	130	0.6	326	7.6	70.6	1.4	8.0
Balance, Sainsbury's*	1 Serving/30g	111	0.4	370	11.4	77.7	1.5	3.2
Banana & Toffee Crisp, Mornflake*	1 Serving/30g	133	4.8	443	5.7	68.8	16.1	5.4
Barley Flakes, Organic, Infinity Foods*	1 Serving/45g	140	0.8	311	10.0	57.0	1.8	4.0
Berry Burst, Oat So Simple, Quaker Oats*	1 Serving/39g	144	2.3	370	8.0	70.0	6.0	6.5
Berry Crunchy, Sainsbury's*	1 Serving/30g	122	3.6	408	7.7	67.3	12.0	4.8
Biscuit, Baked with Golden Syrup, Weetabix*	2 Biscuits/44g	158	0.8	363	10.3	72.0	1.9	8.2
Bitesize, Weetabix*	1 Serving/40g	135	0.8	338	11.5	68.4	2.0	10.0
Blackberry & Apple, Alpen*	1 Serving/40g	140	1.5	349	9.2	69.4	3.8	8.3
Blueberry Wheats, Tesco*	1 Serving/50g	165	0.7	330	7.5	71.6	1.5	8.5
Bran, Natural, Sainsbury's*	1 Serving/30g	64	1.5	212	14.7	27.0	5.0	36.0
Bran Crunch, Raisin, Kellogg's*	1 Pack/80g	280	1.5	350	6.2	83.7	1.9	7.5
Bran Flakes, Asda*	1 Serving/47g	157	1.5	333	11.0	65.0	3.2	14.0
Bran Flakes, Crunchy Nut, Sainsbury's*	1 Serving/40g	203	3.8	507	19.7	85.7	9.5	11.0
Bran Flakes, Harvest Home, Nestle*	1 Serving/30g	99	0.7	331	10.2	67.1	2.4	14.1
Bran Flakes, Honey Nut, Asda*	1 Serving/50g	180	2.2	360	10.0	70.0	4.4	11.0
Bran Flakes, Honey Nut, Sainsbury's*	1 Serving/40g	143	1.8	358	9.6	70.0	4.4	11.0
Bran Flakes, Kellogg's*	1 Serving/50g	163	1.0	326	10.0	67.0	2.0	15.0
Bran Flakes, Organic, Sainsbury's*	1 Serving/30g	100	0.7	332	10.2	67.4	2.4	14.1
Bran Flakes, Sainsbury's*	1 Serving/30g	100	0.7	333	10.3	67.5	2.5	14.3

B

	Measure INFO/WEIGHT	per Measure KCAL	FAT	Nutrition Values per 100g / 100ml KCAL	PROT	CARB	FAT	FIBRE
BREAKFAST CEREAL								
Bran Flakes, Sultana, Dry, Sainsbury's*	1 Serving/30g	97	0.6	325	8.3	68.6	1.9	12.1
Bran Flakes, Sultana Bran, Kellogg's*	1 Serving/40g	138	0.8	344	8.0	67.0	2.0	13.0
Bran Flakes, Value, Tesco*	1 Serving/50g	167	1.2	335	10.3	67.2	2.4	14.2
Breakfast Biscuits, Aldi*	4 Biscuits/60g	213	1.5	355	13.7	69.5	2.5	7.5
Cheerios, Chocolate, Dry, Nestle*	1 Serving/30g	115	1.0	384	8.0	73.4	3.5	2.2
Cheerios, Honey, Nestle*	1 Serving/50g	184	1.4	369	6.6	79.2	2.8	5.8
Cheerios, Honey Nut, Nestle*	1 Serving/30g	112	1.1	374	7.0	78.3	3.7	5.2
Cheerios, Nestle*	1 Serving/30g	114	1.1	381	8.6	74.5	3.8	7.1
Choc & Nut Crisp, Tesco*	1 Serving/40g	185	8.0	462	8.3	62.5	19.9	4.8
Choco Crackles, Morrisons*	1 Serving/30g	115	0.7	383	5.5	84.8	2.4	1.9
Choco Flakes, Kellogg's*	1 Serving/30g	114	0.9	380	5.0	84.0	3.0	2.5
Choco Flakes, Sainsbury's*	1 Serving/30g	111	0.2	370	5.5	85.4	0.7	3.0
Choco Hoops, Asda*	1 Serving/40g	154	1.8	385	7.0	79.0	4.5	4.0
Choco Hoops, Co-Op*	1 Serving/30g	115	1.2	385	7.0	80.0	4.0	5.0
Choco Snaps, Asda*	1 Serving/30g	115	0.7	382	5.0	85.0	2.4	1.9
Choco Snaps, Sainsbury's*	1 Serving/30g	115	0.7	383	5.5	84.8	2.4	1.9
Choco Squares, Asda*	1 Serving/30g	130	4.2	434	10.0	67.0	14.0	4.0
Chocolate, Granola, Diet Chef Ltd*	1 Serving/40g	195	11.5	487	10.7	45.0	28.7	13.0
Chocolate Crisp, Minis, Weetabix*	1 Serving/36g	134	1.9	371	9.0	71.7	5.3	8.5
Chocolate Wheats, Kellogg's*	1 Serving/40g	148	3.6	369	10.0	62.0	9.0	12.0
Cinnamon, Puffins, Barbara's Bakery*	1 Serving/30g	100	1.0	333	6.7	86.7	3.3	20.0
Cinnamon Grahams, Nestle*	1 Serving/40g	164	3.9	411	4.7	76.1	9.8	4.2
Clusters, Nestle*	1 Serving/30g	111	1.4	371	9.3	72.6	4.8	7.4
Coco Pops, Crunchers, Kellogg's*	1 Serving/30g	114	1.0	380	7.0	81.0	3.5	3.0
Coco Pops, Kellogg's*	1 Serving/30g	116	0.7	387	5.0	85.0	2.5	2.0
Coco Pops, Mega Munchers, Kellogg's*	1 Serving/30g	112	0.7	375	8.0	80.0	2.5	4.5
Coco Snaps, Value, Tesco*	1 Serving/30g	117	0.7	390	7.0	84.1	2.4	2.4
Cocoa Rice, Gluten Free, Organic, Dove's Farm*	1 Serving/30g	114	0.4	379	5.0	85.0	1.5	2.8
Cookie Crunch, Nestle*	1 Serving/40g	154	1.1	385	4.6	85.3	2.8	1.8
Corn Flakes, Asda*	1 Serving/30g	111	0.2	370	7.0	84.0	0.7	3.0
Corn Flakes, Banana Crunch, Kellogg's*	1 Serving/40g	163	3.2	408	6.0	78.0	8.0	3.0
Corn Flakes, Crispy Nut, Asda*	1 Serving/30g	117	1.3	390	7.0	81.0	4.2	2.5
Corn Flakes, Harvest Home, Nestle*	1 Serving/25g	92	0.2	367	7.3	82.7	0.8	3.6
Corn Flakes, Hint of Honey, Kellogg's*	1 Serving/30g	113	0.2	377	6.0	87.0	0.6	2.5
Corn Flakes, Honey Nut, Asda*	1 Serving/30g	119	1.3	397	7.4	81.7	4.5	2.5
Corn Flakes, Honey Nut, Harvest Home, Nestle*	1 Serving/30g	118	1.3	392	7.4	81.1	4.2	2.5
Corn Flakes, Honey Nut, Sainsbury's*	1 Serving/30g	119	1.3	397	7.4	81.7	4.5	2.5
Corn Flakes, Honey Nut, Tesco*	1 Serving/30g	118	1.3	392	7.4	81.2	4.2	2.5
Corn Flakes, Honey Nut & Cranberries, Sainsbury's*	1 Serving/40g	166	4.0	416	7.4	74.4	9.9	3.1
Corn Flakes, Kellogg's*	1 Serving/30g	112	0.3	372	7.0	84.0	0.9	3.0
Corn Flakes, Organic, Lima*	1 Serving/50g	177	0.5	355	8.3	77.7	1.0	6.4
Corn Flakes, Organic, Whole Earth*	1 Serving/40g	154	0.4	386	8.6	84.2	1.0	3.0
Corn Flakes with 125ml Semi Skimmed Milk, Kellogg's*	1 Serving/30g	170	2.5	567	20.0	106.7	8.3	3.0
Country Crisp, & Flakes, Red Berry, Jordans*	1 Serving/50g	203	5.8	407	7.1	68.5	11.6	7.3
Country Crisp, Chocolate Clusters, 70% Cocoa, Jordans*	1 Serving/50g	136	5.3	452	7.4	65.7	17.7	6.1
Country Crisp, Four Nut Combo, Jordans*	1 Serving/50g	240	12.3	480	8.9	55.4	24.7	6.9
Country Crisp, Wild About Berries, Jordans*	1 Serving/50g	221	7.8	443	7.5	68.0	15.7	5.7
Country Crisp with Real Raspberries, Jordans*	1 Serving/50g	214	7.9	429	7.5	64.1	15.8	7.1
Country Crisp with Real Strawberries, Jordans*	1 Serving/50g	214	7.8	428	7.5	64.1	15.7	7.1
Country Honey, Oat So Simple, Quaker Oats*	1 Serving/36g	134	2.3	373	8.5	69.0	6.5	6.0
Cranberry Wheats, Tesco*	1 Serving/50g	160	0.7	320	7.6	72.0	1.5	8.0
Cranberry Wheats, Whole Grain, Sainsbury's*	1 Serving/50g	162	0.7	325	7.3	70.9	1.4	7.7
Crunchy Bran, Weetabix*	1 Serving/40g	122	1.4	306	11.9	56.6	3.6	20.0

	Measure INFO/WEIGHT	per Measure		Nutrition Values per 100g / 100ml				
		KCAL	FAT	KCAL	PROT	CARB	FAT	FIBRE
BREAKFAST CEREAL								
Crunchy Bran Muesli, Diet Chef Ltd*	1 Serving/40g	164	3.8	409	8.1	68.4	9.5	8.9
Crunchy Choco, Crisp & Square, Tesco*	1 Serving/50g	211	7.0	423	8.0	66.3	14.0	6.0
Crunchy Chocolate, Carrefour*	1 Serving/40g	176	6.8	440	9.0	62.0	17.0	8.0
Crunchy Nut, Clusters, Honey & Nut, Kellogg's*	1 Serving/40g	161	2.0	402	6.0	82.0	5.0	2.5
Crunchy Nut, Clusters, Milk Chocolate Curls, Kellogg's*	1 Serving/40g	183	7.2	458	8.0	66.0	18.0	4.0
Crunchy Nut, Clusters, Summer Berries, Kellogg's*	1 Serving/40g	176	6.0	439	8.0	68.0	15.0	5.0
Crunchy Nut, Red, Kellogg's*	1 Serving/40g	138	0.8	346	10.0	72.0	2.0	9.0
Crunchy Oat, Co-Op*	1 Serving/50g	202	6.5	405	8.0	64.0	13.0	10.0
Crunchy Oat, Golden Sun*	1 Serving/50g	205	6.4	411	8.6	65.0	12.9	6.2
Crunchy Oat with Tropical Fruits, Tesco*	1 Serving/35g	146	4.8	417	7.8	65.3	13.8	6.1
Crunchy Oats with Tropical Fruits, Jordans*	1 Serving/75g	319	10.9	425	8.1	65.4	14.6	6.7
Crunchy Rice & Wheat Flakes, Co-Op*	1 Serving/30g	111	0.6	370	11.0	78.0	2.0	3.0
Curiously Cinnamon, Nestle*	1 Serving/30g	124	3.0	412	4.9	75.9	9.9	4.1
Fibre Flakes, Gluten Free, Organic, Dove's Farm*	1 Serving/30g	105	0.4	351	7.1	69.7	1.5	15.0
Fitnesse & Fruits, Nestle*	1 Serving/40g	148	0.4	370	6.6	83.4	1.1	3.4
Flakes, 7 Cereal, De Halm*	1 Serving/40g	139	1.3	347	11.3	66.7	3.4	9.0
Flakes & Grains, Exotic Fruit, BGTY, Sainsbury's*	1 Serving/30g	113	1.5	377	6.8	76.4	4.9	5.9
Flakes & Orchard Fruits, BGTY, Sainsbury's*	1 Serving/40g	154	0.5	385	13.0	80.6	1.2	4.5
Force, Nestle*	1 Serving/40g	138	0.9	344	10.6	70.3	2.3	9.2
Four Berry Crisp, Organic, Jordans*	1 Serving/50g	221	7.9	442	7.7	67.1	15.8	5.4
Frosted Flakes, Sainsbury's*	1 Serving/30g	112	0.1	374	4.9	87.8	0.4	2.4
Frosted Flakes, Tesco*	1 Serving/30g	112	0.1	374	4.9	87.8	0.4	2.4
Frosties, Chocolate, Kellogg's*	1 Serving/40g	158	2.4	394	5.0	80.0	6.0	3.5
Frosties, Kellogg's*	1 Serving/30g	112	0.2	375	4.5	87.0	0.6	2.0
Frosties, Reduced Sugar, Kellogg's*	1 Serving/30g	111	0.2	369	6.0	85.0	0.6	2.5
Fruit, Nuts & Flakes, M & S*	1 Serving/30g	117	2.5	391	9.1	69.6	8.5	3.5
Fruit & Fibre, Asda*	1 Serving/40g	146	2.6	366	8.2	68.4	6.6	8.5
Fruit & Fibre, Flakes, Waitrose*	1 Serving/40g	143	2.5	357	8.2	67.2	6.2	9.9
Fruit & Fibre, Organic, Sainsbury's*	1 Serving/40g	147	1.6	367	10.0	72.4	4.1	7.8
Fruit & Fibre, Tesco*	1 Serving/30g	111	2.0	370	8.0	69.1	6.6	7.7
Fruit & Nut Crisp, Minis, Weetabix*	1 Serving/40g	144	1.8	359	9.3	70.0	4.6	8.9
Fruit 'n' Fibre, Kellogg's*	1 Serving/40g	152	2.4	380	9.0	69.0	6.0	9.0
Golden Balls, Asda*	1 Serving/30g	112	0.4	374	5.0	85.0	1.5	1.5
Golden Grahams, Nestle*	1 Serving/30g	112	0.9	375	6.0	81.0	3.0	3.4
Golden Honey Puffs, Tesco*	1 Serving/30g	115	0.4	382	6.6	86.3	1.2	3.0
Golden Nuggets, Nestle*	1 Serving/40g	152	0.3	381	6.2	87.4	0.7	1.5
Golden Puffs, Sainsbury's*	1 Serving/28g	107	0.3	383	6.6	86.3	1.2	3.0
Granola	1 Serving/45g	194	8.7	430	17.5	48.8	19.4	16.8
Granola, Quaker Oats*	1 Serving/48g	210	7.0	437	10.4	72.9	14.6	6.2
Granola, Quinoa, Organic, Perfekt*	1 Serving/40g	186	6.6	466	12.4	48.5	16.4	8.9
Granola, Superfoods, Jordans*	1 Serving/50g	207	6.7	415	9.0	64.7	13.4	8.6
Grape Nuts, Kraft*	1 Serving/45g	157	0.9	350	10.9	81.9	2.0	11.9
Harvest Crunch, Nut, Quaker Oats*	1 Serving/40g	184	7.8	459	8.0	62.5	19.5	6.0
Harvest Crunch, Real Red Berries, Quaker Oats*	1 Serving/50g	223	8.5	447	7.0	66.0	17.0	4.5
Harvest Crunch, Soft Juicy Raisins, Quaker Oats*	1 Serving/50g	221	8.0	442	6.0	67.0	16.0	4.0
Hawaiian Crunch, Asda*	1 Serving/50g	224	7.6	448	8.0	69.6	15.3	7.0
High Bran, Chosen By You, Asda*	1 Serving/40g	136	1.5	341	13.6	49.5	3.8	27.1
High Fibre, Alpen*	1 Serving/45g	154	3.2	343	7.7	62.1	7.1	14.1
High Fibre Bran, Sainsbury's*	1 Serving/40g	134	1.5	335	14.3	48.4	3.7	25.4
High Fibre Bran, Tesco*	1 Serving/40g	110	1.4	275	14.7	45.5	3.5	27.0
High Fibre Bran, Waitrose*	1 Serving/40g	112	1.5	281	14.4	47.2	3.8	26.0
Honey, Crisp Minis, Weetabix*	1 Serving/40g	150	0.8	375	9.5	75.0	2.0	9.2
Honey, Oats & More, Nestle*	1 Serving/30g	114	1.6	379	9.7	73.1	5.3	5.9

BREAKFAST CEREAL

Measure INFO/WEIGHT	per Measure KCAL	FAT	Nutrition Values per 100g / 100ml KCAL	PROT	CARB	FAT	FIBRE
Honey & Nut Crisp, Mini, Weetabix*	1 Serving/40g	150	0.8	375	9.4	75.1	2.0	9.3
Honey Loops, Kellogg's*	1 Serving/30g	110	0.9	367	8.0	77.0	3.0	6.0
Honey Nut & Flakes, M & S*	1 Serving/40g	164	3.5	411	9.8	73.4	8.7	2.6
Honey Raisin & Almond, Crunchy, Waitrose*	1 Serving/40g	170	4.8	425	10.5	68.8	12.0	5.7
Hooplas, Sainsbury's*	1 Serving/30g	112	1.1	375	6.5	78.6	3.8	4.6
Hoops, Multigrain, Asda*	1 Serving/30g	113	1.2	376	6.5	78.4	4.0	4.6
Just Right, Kellogg's*	1 Serving/40g	145	1.2	362	7.0	77.0	3.0	4.5
Krave, Chocolate & Hazelnut, Kellogg's*	1 Serving/30g	132	4.8	440	8.0	66.0	16.0	4.0
Lion, Nestle*	1 Serving/40g	166	3.1	415	7.2	76.9	7.7	4.3
Lion with 125ml Semi Skimmed Milk, Nestle*	1 Serving/30g	185	4.4	617	21.7	97.3	14.7	4.3
Malt Crunchies, Co-Op*	1 Serving/50g	167	1.0	335	10.0	69.0	2.0	10.0
Malted Wheaties, Asda*	1 Serving/50g	171	1.4	342	10.0	69.0	2.9	10.0
Malted Wheats, Waitrose*	1 Serving/32g	110	0.6	343	9.7	71.7	1.9	9.9
Malties, Sainsbury's*	1 Serving/40g	137	1.2	343	10.0	69.2	2.9	10.0
Malty Flakes, Peach Melba, Tesco*	1 Serving/30g	115	1.1	385	8.0	79.6	3.8	1.7
Malty Flakes, Tesco*	1 Serving/40g	148	0.6	371	11.0	78.4	1.5	4.3
Maple & Pecan, Crisp, Asda*	1 Serving/30g	135	5.7	451	8.0	62.0	19.0	6.0
Maple & Pecan, Sainsbury's*	1 Serving/60g	318	13.2	530	13.3	69.7	22.0	5.3
Maple & Pecan Crisp, Sainsbury's*	1 Serving/50g	226	9.7	452	7.9	61.3	19.5	5.4
Maple & Pecan Crisp, Tesco*	1 Serving/50g	215	7.6	430	10.5	62.5	15.2	10.2
Maple Frosted Flakes, Whole Earth*	1 Serving/30g	112	0.3	375	6.2	85.6	1.0	1.6
Minibix, Weetabix*	1 Serving/40g	134	1.5	335	8.8	71.2	3.8	8.1
Muddles, Kellogg's*	1 Serving/30g	110	1.0	368	8.0	76.0	3.5	8.0
Muesli, Apricot, Traidcraft*	1 Serving/30g	103	1.8	344	8.0	68.0	6.0	5.0
Muesli, Base, Nature's Harvest*	1 Serving/50g	179	2.5	358	11.0	71.2	5.1	7.4
Muesli, Basics, Sainsbury's*	1 Serving/50g	172	3.1	344	11.2	60.6	6.3	10.1
Muesli, Berries & Cherries, Dorset Cereals*	1 Serving/70g	225	1.5	321	6.5	68.8	2.2	6.3
Muesli, Carb Control, Tesco*	1 Serving/35g	154	9.3	439	25.0	25.0	26.6	13.8
Muesli, COU, M & S*	1 Serving/60g	201	1.5	335	7.6	70.2	2.5	8.1
Muesli, Cranberry & Blueberry, Love Life, Waitrose*	1 Serving/50g	164	1.8	329	8.5	65.3	3.7	7.5
Muesli, Creamy Tropical Fruit, Finest, Tesco*	1 Serving/80g	283	4.5	354	7.2	68.8	5.6	6.9
Muesli, Crunchy, Organic, Sainsbury's*	1 Serving/40g	168	5.8	420	10.6	62.0	14.4	9.2
Muesli, De Luxe, No Added Salt or Sugar, Sainsbury's*	1 Serving/40g	161	5.6	403	11.9	57.6	13.9	8.4
Muesli, Fruit, 55%, Asda*	1 Serving/35g	111	1.0	318	6.0	67.0	2.9	7.0
Muesli, Fruit, GFY, Asda*	1 Serving/50g	152	0.9	304	8.0	64.0	1.8	10.0
Muesli, Fruit, Luxury, Weight Watchers*	1 Serving/40g	127	0.8	318	7.2	67.7	2.0	8.1
Muesli, Fruit, Nuts & Seeds, Dorset Cereals*	1 Serving/70g	265	8.0	379	10.6	58.4	11.4	6.1
Muesli, Fruit & Nut, 55%, Asda*	1 Serving/40g	151	5.6	378	9.0	54.0	14.0	7.0
Muesli, Fruit & Nut, COU, M & S*	1 Serving/40g	128	1.1	320	7.4	74.5	2.8	7.4
Muesli, Fruit & Nut, Jordans*	1 Serving/50g	180	4.7	361	8.0	61.2	9.4	7.5
Muesli, Fruit & Nut, Luxury, Co-Op*	1 Serving/40g	150	4.0	375	8.0	64.0	10.0	6.0
Muesli, Fruit & Nut, Luxury, Sainsbury's*	1 Serving/50g	177	4.5	355	10.3	57.9	9.1	11.3
Muesli, Fruit & Nut, M & S*	1 Serving/40g	128	1.1	320	7.4	74.5	2.8	7.4
Muesli, Fruit & Nut, Organic, M & S*	1 Serving/50g	166	3.0	333	8.2	61.6	6.0	7.6
Muesli, Fruit & Nut, Sainsbury's*	1 Serving/30g	121	5.2	402	10.4	51.3	17.2	9.2
Muesli, Fruit & Seeds, Organic, Pertwood Farm*	1 Serving/50g	164	3.3	328	11.4	55.5	6.7	12.6
Muesli, Fruit & Spice, Sainsbury's*	1 Serving/50g	184	3.4	368	7.4	69.4	6.8	7.7
Muesli, Fruit Nut & Seed, Organic, Dorset Cereals*	1 Serving/70g	251	6.9	358	10.8	56.6	9.8	8.4
Muesli, Fruit Sensation, M & S*	1 Serving/50g	157	1.5	315	6.0	66.0	3.0	7.4
Muesli, Fruity Fibre, Jordans*	1 Serving/50g	172	3.1	344	7.7	64.2	6.3	8.5
Muesli, High Fibre, Neal's Yard*	1 Serving/50g	182	0.9	364	7.6	72.7	1.9	12.9
Muesli, High Fibre, You Count, Love Life, Waitrose*	1 Serving/45g	155	1.3	344	7.7	67.4	2.9	8.8
Muesli, HL, Tesco*	1 Serving/40g	126	0.9	315	7.6	64.3	2.3	7.5

BREAKFAST CEREAL

	Measure INFO/WEIGHT	per Measure		Nutrition Values per 100g / 100ml				
		KCAL	FAT	KCAL	PROT	CARB	FAT	FIBRE
Muesli, Light & Crispy, Jordans*	1 Serving/50g	171	2.5	343	7.7	66.7	5.0	9.5
Muesli, Luscious Berries & Cherries, Dorset Cereals*	1 Serving/50g	163	1.1	327	6.5	66.2	2.2	8.4
Muesli, Luxury, Finest, Tesco*	1 Serving/50g	197	6.5	394	8.3	60.8	13.1	5.4
Muesli, Luxury, Jordans*	1 Serving/40g	154	5.0	384	9.6	58.4	12.5	8.2
Muesli, Luxury, Sainsbury's*	1 Serving/40g	144	4.3	359	8.5	57.1	10.7	7.7
Muesli, Luxury Fruit, Perfectly Balanced, Waitrose*	1 Serving/50g	162	1.6	324	7.1	66.4	3.3	7.0
Muesli, Luxury Fruit, Sainsbury's*	1 Serving/50g	162	1.6	324	7.1	66.4	3.3	7.0
Muesli, Natural, No Added Sugar Or Salt, Jordans*	1 Serving/50g	210	4.1	420	16.0	70.4	8.2	8.4
Muesli, No Added Sugar, Waitrose*	1 Serving/40g	146	2.5	364	12.0	64.9	6.3	6.7
Muesli, No Added Sugar Or Salt, Organic, Jordans*	1 Serving/50g	175	4.4	350	9.2	58.4	8.8	9.3
Muesli, Organic, Waitrose*	1 Serving/50g	187	0.8	375	10.3	59.6	1.6	8.3
Muesli, Original, Holland & Barrett*	1 Serving/30g	105	2.5	351	11.1	61.2	8.4	7.1
Muesli, Original, Sainsbury's*	1 Serving/60g	226	5.0	376	9.3	65.7	8.4	7.1
Muesli, Original, Simply, Hubbards*	1 Serving/50g	212	6.7	424	11.8	59.4	13.4	9.2
Muesli, Peach & Vanilla, Sainsbury's*	1 Serving/50g	162	2.6	324	7.6	61.4	5.3	7.6
Muesli, Really Nutty, Dorset Cereals*	1 Serving/70g	253	6.1	362	9.8	61.1	8.7	6.3
Muesli, Rich, Nature's Harvest*	1 Serving/40g	143	3.7	358	10.0	60.5	9.2	7.6
Muesli, Simply Delicious, Dorset Cereals*	1 Serving/70g	256	6.6	366	10.8	59.2	9.5	7.4
Muesli, Simply Fruity, Dorset Cereals*	1 Serving/75g	226	1.9	301	6.8	63.9	2.5	7.7
Muesli, Special, Fruit, Jordans*	1 Serving/50g	161	1.3	323	6.6	68.0	2.7	8.4
Muesli, Special, Jordans*	1 Serving/50g	183	5.3	366	7.9	59.5	10.7	8.5
Muesli, Special, Luxury Fruit & Nut, Goody*	1 Serving/50g	193	6.9	386	8.0	57.6	13.8	8.0
Muesli, Super Berry, Jordans*	1 Serving/50g	174	3.8	348	9.0	60.8	7.6	8.1
Muesli, Super High Fibre, Dorset Cereals*	1 Serving/70g	250	6.6	357	8.0	60.1	9.4	8.4
Muesli, Superfoods, Jordans*	1 Serving/50g	173	3.6	346	9.2	60.9	7.3	10.2
Muesli, Swiss Style, No Added Sugar Or Salt, Asda*	1 Serving/50g	181	3.5	363	11.0	64.0	7.0	8.0
Muesli, Swiss Style, Organic, Whole Earth*	1 Serving/50g	172	3.5	344	9.2	60.8	7.1	11.3
Muesli, Swiss Style, Sainsbury's*	1 Serving/50g	180	2.9	361	9.2	68.1	5.8	7.1
Muesli, Swiss Style with Fruit, Tesco*	1 Serving/40g	144	2.1	360	10.4	67.4	5.3	7.4
Muesli, Toasted Spelt, Barley & Oat Flakes, Dorset Cereals*	1 Serving/40g	148	4.5	371	9.5	57.9	11.3	7.4
Muesli, Tropical, Sainsbury's*	1 Serving/50g	182	3.4	365	6.5	69.4	6.8	6.4
Muesli, Tropical Fruit, Holland & Barrett*	1 Serving/60g	197	1.9	328	7.5	69.8	3.2	5.1
Muesli, Tropical Fruits, Jordans*	1 Serving/50g	164	1.4	329	6.9	68.7	2.9	7.1
Muesli, Twelve Fruit & Nut, Sainsbury's*	1 Serving/50g	166	2.3	332	8.1	64.2	4.7	7.8
Muesli, Unsweetened, M & S*	1 Serving/40g	129	1.1	322	8.1	68.0	2.7	9.4
Muesli, Whole Wheat, Co-Op*	1 Serving/40g	140	2.8	350	11.0	61.0	7.0	7.0
Muesli, Whole Wheat, No Added Sugar & Salt, Tesco*	1 Serving/40g	154	5.0	386	9.5	59.1	12.4	7.4
Muesli Mix, Perfect Start, Organic, The Food Doctor*	1 Serving/50g	196	7.1	392	12.1	55.5	14.2	7.1
Multi Fruit & Flake, COU, M & S*	1 Serving/39g	142	0.4	365	6.5	81.8	1.1	4.0
Multigrain, Balanced Lifestyle, Aldi*	1 Serving/30g	108	0.7	360	7.5	77.1	2.4	4.5
Multigrain, Fitnesse, Nestle*	1 Serving/30g	109	0.4	363	8.0	79.8	1.3	5.1
Nesquik, Chocolatey Corn & Rice, Nestle*	1 Serving/30g	114	1.2	380	7.2	79.1	3.9	5.1
No Added Sugar, Alpen*	1 Serving/40g	142	2.4	354	10.5	64.6	6.0	7.7
Nutty Crunch, Alpen*	1 Serving/40g	159	4.5	398	10.7	63.6	11.2	6.5
Nutty Crunch, Deliciously, M & S*	1 Serving/50g	238	11.2	476	8.8	59.6	22.5	4.4
Oat, Crunchy, Sainsbury's*	1 Serving/50g	226	10.1	453	8.2	59.3	20.3	6.6
Oat, Raisin, Nut & Honey, Crunchy, Dry, Sainsbury's*	1 Serving/50g	201	7.0	402	8.5	60.2	14.1	7.6
Oat & Bran Flakes, Sainsbury's*	1 Serving/30g	97	1.7	324	12.2	56.0	5.7	17.7
Oat Bran, Crispies, Quaker Oats*	1 Serving/40g	153	2.6	383	11.0	69.0	6.5	9.0
Oat Bran, Hodgson Mill*	1 Serving/40g	48	1.2	120	6.0	23.0	3.0	6.0
Oat Crisp, Chocolate, Quaker Oats*	1 Serving/35g	135	3.9	385	10.2	57.5	11.1	12.4
Oat Crunchy, Blueberry & Cranberry, Waitrose*	1 Serving/60g	259	9.1	432	8.0	65.9	15.2	8.5
Oat Granola, Quaker Oats*	1 Serving/50g	205	4.4	411	8.6	73.0	8.8	5.2

BREAKFAST CEREAL

	Measure INFO/WEIGHT	per Measure KCAL	FAT	Nutrition Values per 100g / 100ml KCAL	PROT	CARB	FAT	FIBRE
Oat Krunchies, Quaker Oats*	1 Serving/30g	118	2.1	393	9.5	72.0	7.0	5.5
Oatbran, & Oatgerm, Prewett's*	1 Serving/30g	103	2.9	345	14.8	49.7	9.7	15.2
Oatbran, 100%, Mornflake*	1 Serving/40g	146	3.8	364	13.4	47.3	9.4	18.2
Oatbran Flakes, Nature's Path*	1 Serving/30g	124	1.4	414	8.7	83.0	4.7	6.7
Oatbran Flakes, Original, Mornflake*	1 Serving/40g	149	2.1	372	11.9	63.2	5.2	12.4
Oatbran Sprinkles, Mornflake*	1 Serving/40g	146	3.8	364	13.4	47.3	9.4	18.2
Oatibix, Bitesize, Original, Weetabix*	1 Serving/36g	133	2.4	370	10.6	66.5	6.8	10.1
Oatibix, Flakes, Weetabix*	1 Serving/50g	190	2.8	381	9.5	73.2	5.6	3.5
Oatibix, Weetabix*	2 Biscuits/48g	189	3.8	394	12.5	64.3	8.0	7.3
Oatiflakes with Raisin, Cranberry & Apple, Weetabix*	1 Serving/40g	135	0.5	338	6.7	75.0	1.2	8.6
Oatmeal, Coarse, Prewett's*	1 Serving/40g	137	4.2	343	14.3	47.6	10.6	16.0
Oatmeal, Instant, Heart to Heart, Kashi*	1 Serving/43g	150	2.0	349	7.0	76.7	4.6	9.3
Oatmeal, Scottish, Hamlyns of Scotland*	1 Portion/40g	157	3.7	392	11.2	66.0	9.2	7.1
Oats, Apple Flavour, Instant, Hot, Waitrose*	1 Serving/36g	141	2.2	392	8.1	76.4	6.0	6.7
Oats, Apple Flavour, Micro, Tesco*	1 Sachet/36g	128	1.9	356	6.8	70.1	5.4	5.4
Oats, Free From, Sainsbury's*	1 Serving/40g	155	3.2	388	14.9	64.0	8.0	11.0
Oats, Golden Syrup, Dry, Micro, Tesco*	1 Sachet/39g	144	2.2	370	7.8	71.6	5.7	6.4
Oats, Golden Syrup Flavour, Instant, Hot, Waitrose*	1 Serving/39g	153	2.3	393	7.8	77.4	5.8	6.0
Oats, Jumbo, Organic, Waitrose*	1 Serving/50g	180	4.0	361	11.0	61.1	8.1	7.8
Oats, Original, Instant, Hot, Waitrose*	1 Sachet/27g	97	2.2	359	11.0	60.4	8.1	8.5
Oats, Tesco*	1 Serving/40g	142	3.2	356	11.0	60.0	8.0	8.0
Oats, Wholegrain, Organic, Quaker Oats*	1 Serving/25g	89	2.0	356	11.0	60.0	8.0	9.0
Optimum Power, Nature's Path*	1 Serving/30g	109	2.0	363	15.3	60.0	6.7	12.6
Optivita, Berry Oat Crisp, Kellogg's*	1 Serving/30g	107	1.5	357	10.0	68.0	5.0	9.0
Organic, Spelt Flakes, Queenswood*	1 Tbsp/10g	33	0.3	331	11.0	60.0	3.0	9.0
Organic, Weetabix*	2 Biscuits/38g	134	0.7	358	11.5	68.6	2.0	10.0
Perfect Balance, Weight Watchers*	1 Serving/30g	90	0.5	300	7.8	63.3	1.7	15.6
Perfekt, Granola, Ultimate, Organic, GranoVita*	1 Serving/40g	190	6.6	474	13.3	40.6	16.4	11.8
Pink Apple & Cinnamon, Granola, Diet Chef Ltd*	1 Pack/40g	193	10.7	483	10.1	49.3	26.8	11.2
Pomegranate & Raspberry Wheats, Tesco*	1 Serving/45g	151	0.6	335	7.5	71.8	1.4	8.2
Porridge, Apple, Sultana & Cinnamon, M & S*	1 Sachet/40g	144	3.0	360	10.3	62.3	7.5	8.6
Porridge, Apple & Raspberry, Seriously Oaty, Weetabix*	1 Serving/40g	142	2.4	354	8.3	63.7	6.0	7.8
Porridge, Chocolate, Oatibix, Weetabix*	1 Pack/40g	149	3.9	372	9.9	61.3	9.7	6.2
Porridge, Express, Apple & Cinnamon, Dry, Sainsbury's*	1 Sachet/36g	138	2.1	383	8.6	70.3	5.9	7.2
Porridge, Free From, Sainsbury's*	1 Serving/50g	174	1.5	348	8.6	72.0	3.0	3.4
Porridge, Fruitful, Traditional, Hubbards*	1 Bowl/50g	180	3.8	360	13.4	51.6	7.7	13.3
Porridge, Fruity, Apple & Raisin, Dorset Cereals*	1 Serving/70g	233	3.4	333	9.7	62.7	4.8	8.9
Porridge, Fruity, Cranberry & Raspberry, Dorset Cereals*	1 Sachet/30g	99	1.8	330	10.2	58.7	6.0	12.3
Porridge, Fruity, Fruit & Nut, Dorset Cereals*	1 Serving/70g	242	5.6	346	9.4	59.0	8.0	8.2
Porridge, Fruity, Mixed Berries, Dorset Cereals*	1 Serving/70g	243	4.2	347	10.8	62.6	6.0	7.9
Porridge, Golden Honey, Oatibix, Weetabix*	1 Serving/40g	145	2.6	363	9.2	66.7	6.6	7.0
Porridge, Instant, Quaker Oats*	1 Serving/34g	124	2.9	364	11.0	60.0	8.5	9.0
Porridge, Made with Semi Skimmed Milk, Waitrose*	1 Serving/50g	277	7.5	554	24.6	80.4	15.0	8.6
Porridge, Multigrain, Jordans*	1 Serving/40g	134	2.2	335	10.4	60.9	5.5	10.0
Porridge, Oats, Golden Syrup, Sainsbury's*	1 Sachet/39g	143	2.1	367	6.3	73.6	5.3	6.7
Porridge, Original, Diet Chef Ltd*	1 Sachet/40g	157	2.5	392	12.0	67.0	6.3	9.8
Porridge, Original, Dry, Oat So Simple, Quaker Oats*	1 Serving/27g	98	2.3	364	11.0	60.0	8.5	9.0
Porridge, Original, Oatibix, Weetabix*	1 Sachet/30g	104	2.5	347	12.5	55.6	8.3	10.1
Porridge, Original, Simply Porridge, Asda*	1 Sachet/27g	96	2.2	356	11.0	60.0	8.0	8.0
Porridge, Perfectly, Dorset Cereals*	1 Sachet/30g	107	2.5	356	11.8	58.2	8.4	11.0
Porridge, Porage Oats, Old Fashioned, Dry, Scotts*	1 Serving/40g	142	3.2	355	11.0	60.0	8.0	9.0
Porridge, Porage Oats, Original, Dry, Scotts*	1 Serving/40g	142	3.2	356	11.0	60.0	8.0	9.0
Porridge, Porage Oats, Original, So-Easy, Dry, Scotts*	1 Serving/30g	109	2.5	364	11.0	60.0	8.5	9.0

BREAKFAST CEREAL

	Measure INFO/WEIGHT	per Measure KCAL	FAT	Nutrition Values per 100g / 100ml KCAL	PROT	CARB	FAT	FIBRE
Porridge, Porage Oats, Syrup Swirl, So-Easy, Dry, Scotts*	1 Sachet/37g	135	2.2	366	8.0	70.0	6.0	6.5
Porridge, Ready Made, COU, M & S*	1 Pot/200g	180	4.4	90	3.9	13.3	2.2	0.9
Porridge, Real Fruit, Raisin & Apple, Jordans*	1 Serving/40g	133	2.7	332	9.1	58.8	6.7	7.4
Porridge, Real Fruit, Sultana & Apricot, Jordans*	1 Sachet/40g	127	2.3	317	8.5	57.7	5.8	7.2
Porridge, Spiced Apple, Sultana, Oatibix, Weetabix*	1 Sachet/40g	138	2.3	345	9.7	65.4	5.7	8.5
Porridge, Superfoods, Jordans*	1 Serving/40g	145	3.6	362	10.4	59.8	9.0	8.3
Porridge Oats, Honey Flavour, Paw Ridge, Quaker Oats*	1 Sachet/29g	103	2.0	361	9.6	64.7	7.0	7.9
Porridge Oats, Mornflake*	1 Serving/50g	179	4.0	359	11.0	60.4	8.1	8.5
Porridge Oats, Organic, Evernat*	1 Serving/40g	167	3.8	418	13.0	69.0	9.6	7.4
Porridge Oats, Organic, Jordans*	1 Serving/40g	146	3.7	364	11.7	58.4	9.3	9.0
Porridge Oats, Organic, Tesco*	1 Serving/28g	100	2.3	358	11.0	60.4	8.1	8.5
Porridge Oats, Original, Paw Ridge, Quaker Oats*	1 Sachet/25g	89	2.0	356	11.0	60.0	8.0	9.0
Porridge Oats, Quaker Oats*	1 Serving/45g	160	3.6	356	11.0	60.0	8.0	4.0
Porridge Oats & Bran, Co-Op*	1 Serving/40g	141	2.8	353	12.5	60.0	7.0	12.0
Porridge Oats with Bran, Scottish, Sainsbury's*	1 Serving/50g	190	2.5	380	9.6	74.1	5.0	10.3
Porridge Oats with Wheat Bran, Tesco*	1 Serving/50g	167	3.6	334	12.3	55.0	7.2	13.0
Porridge Oats with Wheat Bran, Waitrose*	1 Serving/50g	168	3.8	336	11.2	55.8	7.6	13.0
Porridge with Apple & Cinnamon, Diet Chef Ltd*	1 Packet/40g	150	1.9	375	8.9	69.5	4.7	9.0
Quaker Oats Crunch, Quaker Oats*	1 Serving/40g	146	2.0	366	9.1	71.1	5.0	7.4
Raisin, Bran Flakes, Asda*	1 Serving/50g	165	1.5	331	7.0	69.0	3.0	10.0
Raisin, Honey & Almond Crunch, Asda*	1 Serving/60g	238	6.8	397	8.8	64.8	11.4	7.4
Raisin, Oats & More, Nestle*	1 Serving/30g	112	1.4	373	8.9	73.7	4.7	5.8
Raisin & Almond, Crunchy, Jordans*	1 Serving/56g	230	7.0	411	8.4	66.0	12.5	5.0
Raisin & Coconut, Crunchy, Organic, Jordans*	1 Serving/50g	206	6.7	412	8.4	64.2	13.5	7.1
Raisin Wheats, Kellogg's*	1 Serving/30g	99	0.6	330	9.0	70.0	2.0	8.0
Raspberry Crisp, Mornflake*	1 Serving/50g	214	7.1	428	6.5	68.2	14.3	6.8
Ready Brek, Banana, Weetabix*	1 Serving/40g	146	2.6	365	8.9	68.0	6.4	6.7
Ready Brek, Chocolate, Porridge Oats, Weetabix*	1 Serving/30g	114	2.4	380	10.0	63.6	8.0	7.0
Ready Brek, Original, Weetabix*	1 Serving/40g	149	3.5	373	11.7	57.9	8.7	7.9
Rice Krispies, Honey, Kellogg's*	1 Serving/30g	114	0.2	380	4.0	89.0	0.7	1.0
Rice Krispies, Kellogg's*	1 Serving/30g	115	0.3	383	6.0	87.0	1.0	1.0
Rice Krispies, Multi-Grain Shapes, Kellogg's*	1 Serving/30g	111	0.7	370	8.0	77.0	2.5	8.0
Rice Pops, Blue Parrot Cafe, Sainsbury's*	1 Serving/30g	111	0.4	370	7.2	82.3	1.3	2.2
Rice Pops, Organic, Dove's Farm*	1 Serving/30g	107	0.2	357	6.8	86.1	0.8	2.0
Rice Pops, Sainsbury's*	1 Serving/30g	114	0.4	381	7.4	84.8	1.3	1.5
Rice Snaps, Asda*	1 Serving/28g	105	0.4	376	7.0	84.0	1.3	1.5
Rice Snaps, Harvest Home, Nestle*	1 Serving/25g	94	0.3	378	7.4	84.2	1.3	1.5
Ricicles, Kellogg's*	1 Serving/30g	114	0.2	381	4.5	89.0	0.8	0.8
Shredded Wheat, 100% Whole Grain, Nestle*	2 Biscuits/45g	153	1.0	340	11.6	68.5	2.2	11.6
Shredded Wheat, Bitesize, Nestle*	1 Serving/45g	155	1.0	344	11.7	69.3	2.2	11.8
Shredded Wheat, Honey Nut, Nestle*	1 Serving/40g	151	2.6	378	11.2	68.8	6.5	9.4
Shredded Wheat, Triple Berry, Nestle*	1 Serving/40g	138	0.8	344	10.6	70.6	2.1	11.1
Shreddies, Coco, Nestle*	1 Serving/45g	161	0.9	358	8.4	76.5	2.0	8.6
Shreddies, Frosted, Kellogg's*	1 Serving/50g	161	0.9	323	0.7	78.5	1.8	4.7
Shreddies, Frosted, Nestle*	1 Serving/45g	164	0.7	365	7.4	80.7	1.5	6.4
Shreddies, Frosted, Variety Pack, Nestle*	1 Pack/45g	163	0.6	363	6.7	81.1	1.3	6.8
Shreddies, Honey, Nestle*	1 Serving/45g	169	0.7	375	8.2	78.1	1.5	8.1
Shreddies, Malt Wheats, Tesco*	1 Serving/45g	169	0.9	375	10.3	73.8	2.0	8.2
Shreddies, Nestle*	1 Serving/45g	185	0.9	371	10.0	73.7	1.9	9.9
Special K, Bliss, Creamy Berry Crunch, Kellogg's*	1 Serving/30g	114	0.7	379	13.0	76.0	2.5	2.5
Special K, Bliss, Strawberry & Chocolate, Kellogg's*	1 Serving/30g	115	0.9	383	13.0	76.0	3.0	2.5
Special K, Choco, Kellogg's*	1 Serving/40g	160	2.8	400	14.0	70.0	7.0	3.5
Special K, Clusters, Honey, Kellogg's*	1 Serving/45g	175	1.3	389	9.0	80.0	3.0	3.5

	Measure INFO/WEIGHT	per Measure KCAL	per Measure FAT	Nutrition Values per 100g / 100ml KCAL	PROT	CARB	FAT	FIBRE
BREAKFAST CEREAL								
Special K, Kellogg's*	1 Serving/30g	114	0.4	379	14.0	76.0	1.5	2.5
Special K, Oats & Honey, Kellogg's*	1 Serving/50g	191	1.2	383	13.0	77.0	2.5	3.0
Special K, Peach & Apricot, Kellogg's*	1 Serving/30g	112	0.3	373	14.0	77.0	1.0	2.5
Special K, Protein Plus, Kellogg's*	1 Serving/29g	100	3.0	345	34.5	31.0	10.3	17.2
Special K, Purple Berries, Kellogg's*	1 Serving/30g	112	0.3	374	13.0	77.0	1.0	3.5
Special K, Red Berries, Kellogg's*	1 Serving/30g	112	0.4	374	14.0	76.0	1.5	3.0
Special K, Yoghurty, Kellogg's*	1 Serving/30g	115	0.9	383	14.0	75.0	3.0	2.5
Sugar Puffs, Quaker Oats*	1 Serving/30g	114	0.5	379	5.3	85.8	1.6	3.7
Sultana Bran, Co-Op*	1 Serving/40g	130	1.2	325	9.0	66.0	3.0	11.0
Sultana Bran, HL, Tesco*	1 Serving/30g	97	0.6	325	8.2	68.0	1.9	12.0
Sultana Bran, Waitrose*	1 Serving/30g	97	0.6	324	8.2	68.6	1.9	11.6
Swiss Muesli with Berries, Dry, Love Life, Waitrose*	1 Serving/45g	172	4.3	383	13.5	55.7	9.6	9.8
Vitality, Asda*	1 Serving/30g	111	0.4	370	11.0	78.0	1.5	3.2
Vitality with Red Fruit, Asda*	1 Serving/30g	110	0.5	366	11.0	77.0	1.6	3.8
Vitality with Tropical Fruit, Asda*	1 Serving/30g	112	1.5	373	9.0	73.0	5.0	4.9
Weetabix, Chocolate, Weetabix*	2 Biscuits/45g	156	1.8	346	10.6	66.6	4.1	10.5
Weetabix*	1 Biscuit/19g	67	0.4	358	11.5	68.6	2.0	10.0
Weetaflakes, Weetabix*	1 Serving/30g	102	0.4	340	8.9	72.9	1.4	11.0
Weetaflakes with Raisin, Cranberry & Apple, Weetabix*	1 Serving/40g	135	0.5	338	6.7	75.0	1.2	8.6
Weetos, Chocolate, Weetabix*	1 Serving/30g	113	1.5	378	8.4	75.1	4.9	5.8
Wheat Biscuits, Sainsbury's*	2 Biscuits/36g	123	0.7	342	11.5	68.4	2.0	10.0
Wheat Biscuits, Whole Grain, Tesco*	2 Biscuits/38g	137	0.8	360	11.5	68.5	2.1	10.1
Wheat Bisks, Banana, Mini, Asda*	1 Serving/50g	190	2.7	380	9.7	73.1	5.4	7.4
Wheat Bisks, Harvest Morn *	2 Biscuits/38g	136	0.8	358	11.5	68.6	2.0	10.0
Wheat Flakes, Alpen*	1 Serving/40g	140	1.0	350	10.2	72.0	2.4	9.0
Wholegrain, Apricot, Wheats, Sainsbury's*	1 Serving/50g	160	0.7	320	7.9	71.6	1.5	8.2
Wholegrain, Fruit & Fibre, Sainsbury's*	1 Serving/30g	109	1.8	363	8.1	69.1	6.0	8.9
Wholegrain, Mini Wheats, Sainsbury's*	1 Serving/40g	139	0.9	348	11.8	69.9	2.3	11.9
Wholegrain, Minis, Weetabix*	1 Serving/40g	149	0.8	372	10.2	73.2	2.0	10.0
Wholegrain, Sultana Bran, Sainsbury's*	1 Serving/30g	97	0.6	325	8.3	68.6	1.9	12.1
Wholewheat Muesli, Asda*	1 Serving/45g	150	3.5	333	8.0	57.9	7.7	9.7
BRESAOLA								
Della Valtellina, Sainsbury's*	1 Slice/14g	23	0.4	163	34.7	0.1	2.6	0.1
Finest, Tesco*	1 Serving/35g	64	1.4	182	36.0	0.5	4.0	0.0
BROCCOLI								
Bellaverde, TTD, Sainsbury's*	1 Serving/100g	33	0.9	33	4.4	1.8	0.9	2.6
Chinese, Kai Lan, Cooked	1 Serving/80g	18	0.6	22	1.4	3.8	0.7	2.5
Florets, Broccoliroosjes, Albert Heijn*	1 Serving/100g	27	0.7	27	3.0	0.8	0.7	3.0
Green, Boiled, Average	***1 Serving/80g***	***19***	***0.6***	***24***	***3.1***	***1.1***	***0.8***	***2.3***
Green, Raw, Average	***1 Serving/80g***	***25***	***0.7***	***31***	***3.9***	***1.7***	***0.9***	***2.6***
Purple Sprouting, Boiled, Average	***1 Serving/80g***	***15***	***0.5***	***19***	***2.1***	***1.3***	***0.6***	***2.3***
Purple Sprouting, Raw	***1oz/28g***	***10***	***0.3***	***35***	***3.9***	***2.6***	***1.1***	***3.5***
Steamed, Average	1 Serving/100g	24	0.8	24	3.1	1.1	0.8	2.3
BROWNIES								
Chocolate, Bites, Mini, Weight Watchers*	1 Brownie/9g	29	0.5	325	5.3	63.7	5.5	2.2
Chocolate, Cadbury*	1 Brownie/36g	145	5.7	403	6.1	59.7	15.8	0.0
Chocolate, Chewy, M & S*	1 Brownie/29g	130	6.0	455	6.5	59.8	21.1	2.0
Chocolate, Sainsbury's*	1 Brownie/60g	265	13.6	442	4.6	55.0	22.6	1.6
Chocolate, Slices, M & S*	1 Brownie/36g	158	8.7	440	5.3	51.1	24.1	1.3
Chocolate, Tray Bake, Tesco*	1 Brownie/37g	155	6.8	420	5.5	57.1	18.4	5.7
Chocolate, Waitrose*	1 Brownie/45g	192	8.9	426	6.3	55.6	19.8	2.7
Chocolate, Weight Watchers*	1 Brownie/47g	143	1.8	304	4.8	62.5	3.8	3.2
Chocolate, Wheat & Gluten Free, Mrs Crimble's*	1 Slice/48g	180	9.6	379	4.2	47.9	20.3	1.5

B

	Measure INFO/WEIGHT	per Measure KCAL	FAT	Nutrition Values per 100g / 100ml KCAL	PROT	CARB	FAT	FIBRE
BROWNIES								
Chocolate & Pecan, Gu*	1 Brownie/45g	200	12.0	444	6.7	44.4	26.6	5.0
BRUSSELS SPROUTS								
Boiled, Average	*1 Serving/90g*	*31*	*1.2*	*35*	*3.1*	*3.2*	*1.3*	*3.5*
Button, & Chestnuts, Tesco*	1 Serving/100g	80	1.8	80	3.1	12.8	1.8	4.1
Button, Raw, Average	*1 Serving/80g*	*30*	*1.1*	*37*	*3.5*	*2.9*	*1.3*	*3.2*
Canned, Drained	*1oz/28g*	*8*	*0.3*	*28*	*2.6*	*2.4*	*1.0*	*2.6*
Raw, Average	*1 Serving/80g*	*29*	*0.9*	*37*	*3.5*	*3.3*	*1.1*	*3.0*
Steamed, Average	1 Serving/100g	35	1.3	35	3.1	3.2	1.3	3.5
BUBBLE & SQUEAK								
Aunt Bessie's*	1 Serving/100g	145	7.1	145	2.7	17.5	7.1	1.3
Fried in Vegetable Oil	1oz/28g	35	2.5	124	1.4	9.8	9.1	1.5
BUCKWHEAT								
Average	*1oz/28g*	*102*	*0.4*	*364*	*8.1*	*84.9*	*1.5*	*2.1*
BUFFALO								
Mince, Raw, Lean, Abel & Cole*	1 Serving/100g	95	0.7	95	21.7	0.4	0.7	0.0
BULGAR WHEAT								
Dry Weight, Average	*1oz/28g*	*99*	*0.5*	*353*	*9.7*	*76.3*	*1.7*	*8.0*
BUNS								
Bath, M & S*	1 Bun/71g	217	5.7	305	8.3	49.8	8.0	1.9
Belgian, Asda*	1 Bun/133g	464	19.9	350	4.8	49.0	15.0	2.2
Belgian, Iced, Chosen By You, Asda*	1 Bun/115g	375	6.8	327	6.1	62.3	5.9	2.9
Belgian, Sainsbury's*	1 Bun/110g	398	11.3	362	6.1	61.3	10.3	1.9
Chelsea	1 Bun/78g	285	10.8	366	7.8	56.1	13.8	1.7
Choux, Caramel, Asda*	1 Bun/189g	745	51.0	394	4.3	33.5	27.0	1.3
Choux, Custard, M & S*	1 Bun/85g	234	18.7	275	4.2	15.0	22.0	0.3
Choux, Fresh Cream, Tesco*	1 Bun/95g	340	23.7	358	4.9	28.5	24.9	0.9
Choux, M & S*	1 Bun/78g	247	17.3	317	5.4	25.6	22.2	0.3
Currant	1 Bun/60g	178	4.5	296	7.6	52.7	7.5	0.0
Currant, HL, Tesco*	1 Bun/63g	159	1.6	252	7.1	50.2	2.5	2.4
Fingers, Sticky, Iced, Chosen By You, Asda*	1 Finger/40g	132	2.4	330	7.1	62.0	5.9	2.7
Fruit, Waitrose*	1 Bun/54g	155	2.3	287	8.1	54.0	4.3	1.6
Hot Cross	1 Bun/50g	156	3.5	312	7.4	58.5	7.0	1.7
Hot Cross, 25% Reduced Fat, Asda*	1 Bun/61g	153	1.4	253	9.0	49.0	2.3	3.0
Hot Cross, Best of Both, Hovis*	1 Bun/65g	185	4.3	285	9.1	47.3	6.6	4.4
Hot Cross, BGTY, Sainsbury's*	1 Bun/70g	160	1.6	229	7.6	44.4	2.3	2.7
Hot Cross, Chocolate, Mini, Sainsbury's*	1 Bun/39g	127	4.4	325	7.7	48.1	11.3	2.5
Hot Cross, Chocolate & Raisin, Mini, Tesco*	1 Bun/40g	127	4.4	318	8.1	47.0	10.9	2.8
Hot Cross, Extra Spicy, M & S*	1 Bun/76g	175	1.4	230	8.6	44.1	1.9	4.2
Hot Cross, Golden Wholemeal, 3% Fat, M & S*	1 Bun/67g	144	1.5	215	8.9	39.6	2.2	6.7
Hot Cross, Golden Wholemeal, Sainsbury's*	1 Bun/65g	180	4.0	277	9.9	45.4	6.2	4.3
Hot Cross, HL, Tesco*	1 Bun/70g	176	1.9	251	6.7	50.3	2.7	2.6
Hot Cross, Less Than 3% Fat, M & S*	1 Bun/70g	175	1.3	250	8.1	49.8	1.8	2.2
Hot Cross, Lightly Fruited, M & S*	1 Bun/64g	165	3.4	260	8.1	45.1	5.4	4.7
Hot Cross, Low Fat, Co-Op*	1 Bun/60g	156	1.8	260	9.0	50.0	3.0	3.0
Hot Cross, Luxury, M & S*	1 Bun/79g	201	3.2	255	8.6	46.2	4.0	2.1
Hot Cross, Mini, M & S*	1 Bun/41g	110	1.4	265	7.8	51.4	3.4	3.7
Hot Cross, Reduced Fat, GFY, Asda*	1 Bun/63g	156	1.6	248	8.4	47.9	2.5	3.7
Hot Cross, Reduced Fat, Waitrose*	1 Bun/67g	171	1.4	255	8.1	54.3	2.1	3.3
Hot Cross, TTD, Sainsbury's*	1 Bun/75g	200	4.2	267	7.2	47.0	5.6	3.8
Hot Cross, White, Light Choices, Tesco*	1 Bun/70g	185	1.4	260	8.3	50.3	1.9	3.8
Hot Cross, Wholemeal, Asda*	1 Bun/70g	182	4.2	262	9.0	43.0	6.0	6.0
Hot Cross, Wholemeal, Organic, Tesco*	1 Bun/55g	140	2.7	254	7.6	44.8	4.9	4.5
Hot Cross, Wholemeal, Waitrose*	1 Bun/64g	177	4.3	276	8.8	45.2	6.7	4.9

B

	Measure INFO/WEIGHT	per Measure KCAL	FAT	Nutrition Values per 100g / 100ml KCAL	PROT	CARB	FAT	FIBRE
BUNS								
Iced, Filled with Raspberry Jam, M & S*	1 Bun/48g	155	3.2	320	6.4	58.9	6.6	1.9
Iced, Finger, Average	1 Bun/40g	130	3.1	325	7.1	57.0	7.7	2.3
Iced, Fingers, Coconut, Genesis Crafty*	1 Bun/64g	210	6.9	328	7.7	52.4	10.8	2.4
Iced, Spiced Fruit, M & S*	1 Bun/90g	270	3.3	300	7.0	60.3	3.7	1.5
Marlborough, M & S*	1 Bun/71g	215	6.3	305	6.2	43.4	8.9	2.2
Swiss, Tesco*	1 Bun/100g	334	11.9	334	4.0	52.8	11.9	1.4
Vanilla Iced, Soft, M & S*	1 Bun/39g	125	3.1	320	7.6	54.9	8.0	2.9
BURGERS								
American Style, Asda*	1 Burger/42g	156	10.8	374	25.0	10.0	26.0	1.1
American Style, Tesco*	1 Burger/125g	250	9.1	200	13.0	20.4	7.3	3.9
Beef, 100%, Average	1 Burger/52g	148	11.6	286	20.5	0.6	22.3	0.1
Beef, 100%, Birds Eye*	1 Burger/41g	120	10.2	292	17.3	0.0	24.8	0.0
Beef, 100%, Mega, Birds Eye*	1 Burger/96g	280	23.8	293	17.3	0.0	24.9	0.0
Beef, 100% Pure, Ross*	1 Burger/56g	128	9.6	229	17.1	1.4	17.1	0.0
Beef, 100% with Seasoning, No Onion, Birds Eye*	1 Burger/41g	134	11.9	326	16.1	0.2	29.0	0.0
Beef, Aberdeen Angus, Asda*	1 Burger/112g	249	13.3	222	22.2	6.7	11.8	0.9
Beef, Aberdeen Angus, Fresh, Waitrose*	1 Burger/113g	269	21.0	238	16.4	1.2	18.6	0.0
Beef, Aberdeen Angus, Frozen, Waitrose*	1 Burger/57g	145	11.6	255	18.1	0.0	20.3	1.1
Beef, Aberdeen Angus, M & S*	1 Burger/142g	298	18.9	210	18.3	4.1	13.3	0.1
Beef, Aberdeen Angus, Mega, Birds Eye*	1 Burger/101g	279	22.6	276	16.3	2.4	22.4	0.1
Beef, Asda*	1 Burger/114g	304	18.6	267	26.8	3.2	16.3	0.7
Beef, Barbecue, Tesco*	1 Burger/114g	295	22.7	260	15.6	3.5	20.0	0.5
Beef, BGTY, Sainsbury's*	1 Burger/110g	177	6.0	161	20.8	7.1	5.5	1.1
Beef, British, Finest, Tesco*	1 Burger/95g	185	11.8	195	17.2	3.3	12.4	0.9
Beef, Chargrill, Tesco*	1 Burger/114g	246	18.4	217	17.0	0.8	16.2	2.5
Beef, Farmfoods*	1 Burger/50g	127	9.8	255	14.4	5.4	19.6	0.1
Beef, Flame Grilled, Dalepak*	1 Burger/44g	134	11.4	304	15.3	2.1	26.0	0.4
Beef, Mega, Birds Eye*	1 Burger/109g	300	25.1	275	14.3	2.7	23.0	0.3
Beef, Morrisons*	1 Burger/57g	169	14.3	298	12.3	5.5	25.2	0.6
Beef, Organic, M & S*	1 Burger/110g	239	17.6	217	18.2	0.0	16.0	0.2
Beef, Original & Best, Birds Eye*	1 Burger/46g	115	8.9	252	14.1	5.1	19.5	0.4
Beef, Original with Onion, Grilled, Birds Eye*	1 Burger/38g	110	9.5	287	13.4	2.6	24.8	0.3
Beef, Quarter Pounder, Chilled, Morrisons*	1 Burger/115g	228	13.9	198	17.2	4.4	12.1	0.2
Beef, Quarter Pounders, Farmfoods*	1 Burger/113g	289	22.1	256	14.4	5.4	19.6	0.1
Beef, Quarter Pounders, Flame Grilled, Rustlers*	1 Burger/190g	557	28.7	293	14.9	24.3	15.1	0.0
Beef, Quarter Pounders, Flame Grilled, Tesco*	1 Burger/88g	246	20.4	280	13.1	4.8	23.2	0.8
Beef, Quarter Pounders, Reduced Fat, Tesco*	1 Burger/95g	171	12.3	180	14.0	1.8	13.0	0.8
Beef, Quarter Pounders, Steak Country*	1 Burger/68g	188	15.1	276	16.3	2.4	22.2	0.1
Beef, Quarter Pounders, Tesco*	1 Burger/113g	292	23.1	258	17.8	0.7	20.4	1.3
Beef, Quarter Pounders with Onion, BGTY, Sainsbury's*	1 Burger/83g	171	7.8	205	26.6	3.8	9.3	0.9
Beef, Quarter Pounders with Onion, Birds Eye*	1 Burger/114g	286	22.1	252	14.1	5.1	19.5	0.4
Beef, Quarter Pounders with Onion, Cooked, Birds Eye*	1 Burger/100g	230	16.0	230	16.0	5.9	16.0	0.4
Beef, Quarter Pounders with Onion, Sainsbury's*	1 Burger/113g	306	22.4	271	18.0	5.1	19.8	1.5
Beef, Sainsbury's*	1 Burger/57g	152	9.1	267	29.6	1.3	15.9	1.5
Beef, Scotch, Quarter Pounder, Moordale*	1 Burger/114g	277	21.2	243	0.0	0.8	18.6	0.0
Beef, Scotch, Ultimate, TTD, Sainsbury's*	1 Burger/142g	284	12.2	200	26.0	4.7	8.6	1.0
Beef, Simply Seasoned, TTD, Sainsbury's*	1 Burger/110g	298	25.0	271	15.3	18.1	22.7	0.5
Beef, Steak, Ultimate, TTD, Sainsbury's*	1 Burger/136g	355	24.1	261	25.3	0.1	17.7	0.5
Beef, Sundried Tomato, Grilled, Finest, Tesco*	1 Burger/99g	170	7.3	172	20.5	5.8	7.4	0.5
Cheeseburger	1 Burger/275g	706	29.0	257	13.7	25.6	10.6	1.8
Cheeseburger, American, Tesco*	1 Burger/275g	660	26.3	240	13.6	24.9	9.6	1.6
Cheeseburger, Bacon with Bun, Chargrilled, Tesco*	1 Burger/265g	726	42.1	274	13.0	19.6	15.9	1.0
Cheeseburger, Micro Snack, Tesco*	1 Burger/115g	309	14.5	269	12.6	26.4	12.6	0.0

B

BURGERS

BURGERS								
Cheeseburger, Smart Price, Asda*	1 Burger/150g	374	14.0	249	13.3	28.0	9.3	1.4
Cheeseburger, with Relish, American Style, Tesco*	1 Burger/61g	132	6.0	215	14.2	17.5	9.8	4.2
Cheeseburger, with Sesame Seed Bun, Tesco*	1 Burger/275g	644	32.2	234	12.2	20.1	11.7	2.0
Chicken, Average	1 Burger/46g	111	5.6	242	14.9	18.7	12.1	1.0
Chicken, Breaded, Value, Tesco*	1 Burger/57g	165	10.8	290	10.5	19.2	19.0	1.4
Chicken, Crispy Crumb, Farmfoods*	1 Burger/242g	707	45.5	292	10.5	20.2	18.8	1.1
Chicken, Crunch Crumb, Tesco*	1 Burger/57g	161	10.8	282	12.3	15.6	18.9	0.0
Chicken, Fresh, Non Coated, Waitrose*	1 Burger/100g	141	4.0	141	16.0	10.4	4.0	0.9
Chicken, Golden Breadcrumbs, Frozen, Birds Eye*	1 Burger/56g	130	6.9	232	13.8	16.4	12.4	0.3
Chicken, in Bun, Morrisons*	1 Burger/110g	250	4.7	228	12.7	38.1	4.3	3.8
Chicken, Quarter Pounders, Birds Eye*	1 Burger/117g	280	16.1	239	13.5	15.2	13.8	0.6
Chicken, Southern Fried, Sainsbury's*	1 Burger/52g	154	10.3	297	12.6	17.2	19.8	1.3
Chicken Cajun, Fillet, Birds Eye*	1 Pack/180g	275	8.8	153	21.5	5.8	4.9	0.3
Chilli, Quarter Pounders, Asda*	1 Burger/88g	221	14.0	252	25.0	2.0	16.0	0.0
Chilli, Quarter Pounders, Farmfoods*	1 Burger/115g	285	23.3	248	13.5	2.9	20.3	0.9
Chilli, Quarter Pounders, Iceland*	1 Burger/84g	265	20.1	316	18.6	6.5	23.9	0.4
Lamb, Minted, Average	1 Burger/56g	125	7.4	223	20.6	5.5	13.1	0.1
Lamb, Quarter Pounders, Average	1 Burger/113g	283	19.3	250	17.4	5.2	17.1	0.7
Lamb, Quarter Pounders, Birds Eye*	1 Burger/112g	232	16.9	207	13.9	3.8	15.1	0.3
Lamb, Waitrose*	1 Burger/67g	99	4.7	148	15.7	5.4	7.0	0.9
Less Than 7% Fat, Sainsbury's*	1 Burger/102g	164	5.6	161	20.8	7.1	5.5	1.1
Mushroom & Wensleydale Cheese, Cauldron Foods*	1 Burger/87g	156	9.6	179	9.0	11.0	11.0	4.0
Nacho, Chicken & Sweetcorn, Asda*	½ Pack/144g	249	13.0	173	14.0	9.0	9.0	2.3
Ostrich, Quarter Pounders, Oslinc*	1 Burger/113g	132	1.5	117	22.9	3.5	1.3	1.1
Pork, Quarter Pounders, Birds Eye*	1 Burger/122g	292	23.2	239	13.9	3.2	19.0	0.2
Pork & Apple, Quarter Pounders, Grilled, Asda*	1 Burger/80g	147	6.4	184	23.9	4.1	8.0	0.5
Quarter Pounder, with Cheese, Flame Grilled, Feasters*	1 Burger/200g	550	19.8	275	17.2	22.1	9.9	0.9
Quarter Pounder, with Cheese & Buns, Sainsbury's*	1 Burger/198g	471	22.8	238	15.6	19.1	11.5	1.4
Quarter Pounder, with Onion, Tesco*	1 Burger/87g	213	16.2	245	16.0	3.0	18.6	0.5
Quarter Pounders, Big Country*	1 Burger/90g	271	20.8	301	22.1	1.8	23.1	0.0
Quarter Pounders, Chargrilled, BGTY, Sainsbury's*	1 Burger/114g	184	6.3	161	20.8	7.1	5.5	1.1
Quarter Pounders, Iceland*	1 Burger/83g	253	18.8	305	20.4	5.1	22.6	0.6
Quarter Pounders, Scotch Beef, Sainsbury's*	1 Burger/114g	255	15.4	225	22.2	3.5	13.6	0.5
Salmon, Quarter Pounders, Morrisons*	1 Burger/110g	235	13.0	214	21.4	5.5	11.8	1.7
Salmon, Quarter Pounders, Tesco*	1 Burger/114g	145	2.7	128	15.9	10.6	2.4	1.2
Spicy Bean, Ainsley Harriott*	1 Burger/200g	302	7.5	151	7.2	23.5	3.7	5.2
Spicy Bean, Cooked, Grassington's Food Co*	1 Burger/108g	201	3.8	186	6.5	32.2	3.5	2.5
Spicy Bean, Sainsbury's*	1 Burger/110g	262	13.5	240	5.0	27.1	12.4	2.0
Spicy Bean & Nacho, Morrisons*	1 Burger/113g	288	17.7	254	5.0	23.3	15.6	3.9
Tuna, Quarter Pounder, Asda*	1 Burger/113g	212	11.3	188	21.0	3.4	10.0	0.0
Tuna, Quarter Pounders, Tesco*	1 Burger/114g	132	1.8	116	18.8	6.7	1.6	0.9
Tuna, Sainsbury's*	1 Serving/105g	194	10.3	185	20.8	3.4	9.8	1.2
Turkey, Cheeseburgers, Tesco*	1 Burger/105g	252	14.8	240	15.4	12.8	14.1	1.3
Turkey, Crispy Crumb, Bernard Matthews*	1 Burger/60g	158	9.5	263	12.6	17.5	15.8	1.8
Turkey, Grilled, Cranberry Foods Ltd*	1 Serving/100g	173	5.9	173	21.1	8.8	5.9	1.4
Turkey, Harvestland*	1 Burger/112g	179	9.0	160	23.0	1.0	8.0	0.0
Value, Farmfoods*	1 Burger/49g	138	10.8	282	11.4	9.6	22.1	0.9
Venison, Finnebrougue Estate*	1 Burger/142g	170	7.0	120	19.9	4.2	4.9	0.5
Venison, TTD, Sainsbury's*	1 Burger/150g	224	6.3	149	20.4	6.5	4.2	3.2
Venison & Sweet Onion, M & S*	1 Burger/142g	163	5.0	115	19.3	1.4	3.5	0.5
BURGERS VEGETARIAN								
Bean, Tesco*	1 Burger/90g	192	10.9	213	4.4	21.6	12.1	5.0
Cheese & Spring Onion, Tesco*	1 Burger/87g	178	10.3	204	4.4	20.0	11.8	3.2

INFO/WEIGHT	Measure	per Measure		Nutrition Values per 100g / 100ml				
		KCAL	FAT	KCAL	PROT	CARB	FAT	FIBRE

BURGERS VEGETARIAN

Chilli, Cauldron Foods*	1 Burger/88g	148	8.1	169	11.5	8.5	9.3	3.3
Flame Grilled, Linda McCartney*	1 Burger/60g	104	3.1	174	17.9	13.8	5.2	3.3
Meat Free, Asda*	1 Burger/60g	138	6.0	230	24.0	11.0	10.0	0.3
Meat Free, Sainsbury's*	1 Burger/57g	92	4.2	161	19.6	3.9	7.4	4.8
Mexican Style, Bean, Meat Free, Tesco*	1 Burger/94g	206	8.7	220	4.9	28.2	9.3	3.9
Mushroom, Cauldron Foods*	1 Burger/88g	125	5.5	143	5.5	16.1	6.3	2.6
Mushroom, Meat Free, Tesco*	1 Burger/87g	151	9.5	173	3.6	15.3	10.8	3.7
Mushroom, Organic, Cauldron Foods*	1 Burger/88g	136	7.3	156	7.1	18.2	8.3	2.3
Quarter Pounder, Average	1 Burger/113g	210	9.8	186	9.1	17.7	8.6	3.2
Savoury, Cauldron Foods*	1 Burger/88g	145	8.0	166	108.0	7.9	9.2	2.4
Spicy Bean, Average	1 Burger/56g	125	6.8	223	5.6	24.3	12.2	4.8
Spicy Bean, BGTY, Sainsbury's*	1 Burger/85g	123	2.3	145	6.9	23.3	2.7	3.1
Spicy Bean, Cauldron Foods*	1 Burger/88g	203	9.8	232	5.4	27.4	11.2	6.2
Spicy Bean, Linda McCartney*	1 Burger/85g	190	9.5	223	4.3	26.2	11.2	2.9
Spicy Bean, Quarter Pounder, Dalepak*	1 Burger/115g	237	12.5	206	4.6	22.3	10.9	2.6
Tesco*	1 Burger/56g	92	4.5	164	16.0	7.0	8.0	2.5
Traditional, Fry's Special Vegetarian*	1 Burger/75g	175	9.0	233	19.2	12.9	12.0	0.2
Vegeburger, Linda McCartney*	1 Burger/59g	79	2.1	134	22.6	2.9	3.6	1.6
Vegeburger, Retail, Grilled	1oz/28g	55	3.1	196	16.6	8.0	11.1	4.2
Vegetable, Average	1 Burger/56g	100	4.5	179	4.4	22.4	8.0	2.3
Vegetable, Captains, Birds Eye*	1 Burger/48g	96	4.2	200	4.7	25.5	8.8	2.0
Vegetable, Organic, Goodlife*	1 Burger/67g	114	3.9	170	3.2	26.3	5.8	2.6
Vegetable, Quarter Pounders, Crunchy, Birds Eye*	1 Burger/114g	240	11.6	211	4.8	24.9	10.2	1.8
Vegetable, Quarter Pounders, Dalepak*	1 Burger/114g	227	9.6	200	4.8	26.3	8.5	1.8
Vegetable, Spicy, Asda*	1 Burger/56g	108	6.2	193	3.4	20.0	11.0	0.0

BUTTER

Brandy, Average	1 Serving/10g	56	3.8	555	0.2	46.2	38.3	0.1
Brandy with Cognac, Sainsbury's*	1/8 Pot/25g	137	9.4	549	0.2	44.1	37.6	0.0
Coconut, Artisana*	2 Tbsp/32g	186	18.0	574	6.2	21.6	55.5	15.4
Creamery, Average	*1 Serving/10g*	*74*	*8.1*	*735*	*0.5*	*0.3*	*81.3*	*0.0*
Fresh, Average	*1 Thin Spread/7g*	*51*	*5.7*	*735*	*0.5*	*0.4*	*81.3*	*0.0*
Granules, Butter Buds*	1 Tsp/1g	5	0.1	368	1.8	77.9	6.5	2.3
Reduced Fat, Fresh, Average	*1 Thin Spread/7g*	*26*	*2.8*	*368*	*2.3*	*1.2*	*39.4*	*0.2*
Salted, Average	*1 Thin Spread/7g*	*51*	*5.7*	*729*	*0.4*	*0.3*	*81.1*	*0.0*
Spreadable, Butterpak, Lighter, Tesco*	1 Serving/10g	54	5.6	545	0.5	0.5	56.0	0.0
Spreadable, Fresh, Average	*1 Thin Spread/7g*	*51*	*5.7*	*730*	*0.4*	*0.3*	*80.8*	*0.0*
Spreadable, Lightest, Lurpak*	1oz/28g	106	11.2	377	3.3	0.9	40.0	0.0
Spreadable, Organic, Lighter, Yeo Valley*	1 Serving/12g	66	7.3	550	0.7	0.9	60.7	0.0
Spreadable, Reduced Fat, Average	*1 Thin Spread/7g*	*38*	*4.2*	*540*	*0.5*	*0.5*	*60.0*	*0.0*
Spreadable, Slightly Salted, Lurpak*	1 Serving/10g	72	8.0	724	0.5	0.6	80.0	0.0
with Crushed Garlic, Lurpak*	1 Serving/10g	70	7.5	700	1.0	4.0	75.0	0.0

BUTTERMILK

Average	*1 Mug/400ml*	*177*	*1.3*	*44*	*4.2*	*5.9*	*0.3*	*0.0*

BUTTONS

Chocolate, Giant, Dairy Milk, Cadbury*	1 Button/3g	15	0.9	525	7.7	56.7	29.9	0.7
Dairy Milk, Milk Chocolate, Cadbury*	1 Pack/32g	170	9.7	525	7.7	56.7	29.9	0.7
Milk Chocolate, Asda*	1 Bag/70g	368	21.0	526	7.0	57.0	30.0	1.5
Milk Chocolate, M & S*	1 Pack/75g	375	19.0	500	8.6	59.8	25.3	1.9
Milk Chocolate, Tesco*	1 Bag/70g	359	19.3	513	7.1	59.1	27.6	2.1
White Chocolate, Cadbury*	1 Pack/32g	180	11.0	555	4.5	58.4	33.8	0.0
White Chocolate, Co-Op*	½ Pack/35g	185	9.8	530	7.0	64.0	28.0	0.0
White Chocolate, Milkybar, Nestle*	1 Bag/30g	164	9.5	546	7.5	58.1	31.6	0.0
White Chocolate, Tesco*	1 Bag/70g	388	23.4	554	5.1	68.0	33.5	0.0

	Measure INFO/WEIGHT	per Measure KCAL	FAT	Nutrition Values per 100g / 100ml KCAL	PROT	CARB	FAT	FIBRE
CABBAGE								
Boiled, Average	*1 Serving/90g*	*14*	*0.3*	*15*	*1.0*	*2.2*	*0.3*	*1.7*
Creamed, Sainsbury's*	½ Pack/150g	88	6.3	59	1.5	3.9	4.2	2.3
Greens, Trimmed, Average	*1oz/28g*	*8*	*0.1*	*28*	*2.9*	*2.9*	*0.5*	*3.4*
Medley, Washed, Ready to Cook, Tesco*	1 Pack/200g	60	1.2	30	2.3	3.7	0.6	2.8
Raw, Average	*1 Serving/100g*	*21*	*0.4*	*21*	*1.3*	*3.1*	*0.4*	*1.8*
Red, Average	*1 Serving/100g*	*19*	*0.2*	*21*	*1.0*	*3.7*	*0.3*	*2.2*
Red, Pickled, Average	*1 Serving/100g*	*26*	*0.1*	*26*	*0.9*	*4.6*	*0.1*	*1.5*
Red, Spiced, Steamer, Sainsbury's*	½ Pack/150g	105	3.3	70	1.0	10.5	2.2	2.9
Red, with Apple, Finest, Tesco*	½ Pack/150g	177	8.8	118	1.6	14.7	5.9	4.6
Red, with Apple, Frozen, Sainsbury's*	1 Serving/75g	37	0.0	50	1.8	10.8	0.0	2.2
Red, with Apples, Onions & Redcurrant Jelly, M & S*	½ Pack/150g	112	3.3	75	0.9	12.4	2.2	2.0
Red, with Bramley Apple, Braised, Sainsbury's*	½ Pack/150g	145	7.2	97	0.9	12.6	4.8	1.7
Savoy, Boiled in Salted Water, Average	*1 Serving/90g*	*15*	*0.4*	*17*	*1.1*	*2.2*	*0.5*	*2.0*
Savoy, Raw, Average	*1 Serving/90g*	*24*	*0.4*	*27*	*2.1*	*3.9*	*0.5*	*3.1*
Steamed, Average	1 Serving/100g	15	0.3	15	1.0	2.2	0.3	1.7
Sweetheart, Raw	*1 Serving/100g*	*26*	*0.6*	*26*	*2.1*	*3.2*	*0.6*	*2.8*
White, Raw, Average	*1oz/28g*	*8*	*0.1*	*27*	*1.4*	*5.0*	*0.2*	*2.1*
CAKE								
Action Man, Birthday, Memory Lane Cakes*	1/12 Cake/83g	322	13.6	388	3.0	57.0	16.4	0.8
Alabama Chocolate Fudge, Morrisons*	1/6 Cake/58g	195	6.4	337	4.5	55.1	11.0	2.3
Almond Slices, GFY, Asda*	1 Slice/25g	67	0.8	268	4.0	56.0	3.1	0.7
Almond Slices, Lyons*	1 Slice/27g	114	6.9	426	7.1	41.3	25.8	1.6
Almond Slices, Mr Kipling*	1 Slice/33g	131	4.5	403	6.3	63.4	14.0	2.0
Almond Slices, Weight Watchers*	1 Slice/26g	95	2.6	365	5.2	63.8	9.9	2.4
Angel, Average	1 Slice/44g	175	7.9	397	4.2	54.9	17.9	0.8
Angel Slices, Mr Kipling*	1 Slice/38g	153	7.0	403	2.9	58.8	18.3	0.6
Angel Slices, Snap Packs, Mr Kipling*	1 Slice/34g	148	6.6	417	2.7	60.1	18.5	0.6
Apple, Bramley & Blackberry Crumble, M & S*	1/8 Cake/56g	221	10.0	395	4.4	54.1	17.9	1.5
Apple & Cinnamon, Oat Break, Go Ahead, McVitie's*	1 Serving/35g	122	2.3	349	5.2	67.2	6.6	2.6
Apple & Cinnamon Mini Popcorn, M & S*	1 Serving/22g	84	0.2	380	5.8	87.4	1.0	2.2
Apple Bakes, Go Ahead, McVitie's*	1 Cake/35g	126	2.7	361	2.6	70.0	7.8	2.0
Apple Crumble, Slices, Weight Watchers*	1 Slice/26g	90	2.0	346	4.5	64.8	7.7	2.3
Apple Slice, Delightful, Mr Kipling*	1 Slice/29g	92	1.1	317	4.4	66.2	3.9	1.3
Apricot & Almond, Bakers Delight*	1oz/28g	106	4.5	379	5.5	53.2	16.0	1.8
Apricot & Apple, Trimlyne*	1 Cake/50g	133	1.3	267	4.3	58.4	2.7	1.9
Bakewell, Lemon, Average	1 Cake/42g	173	6.4	411	3.7	64.6	15.2	1.3
Bakewell, The Handmade Flapjack Company*	1 Cake/75g	311	17.1	415	4.5	47.4	22.8	0.0
Bakewell, Tray Bake, Kate's Cakes Ltd*	1 Serving/100g	475	28.3	475	6.6	46.3	28.3	2.8
Bakewell Slice, Weight Watchers*	1 Slice/26g	84	0.6	324	3.7	71.0	2.4	2.0
Bakewell Slices, Mr Kipling*	1 Slice/36g	163	7.3	454	4.2	63.4	20.4	1.2
Banana, Organic, Loaf, Respect Organics*	¼ Pack/65g	254	13.6	391	3.9	48.6	21.0	1.5
Banana, The Handmade Flapjack Company*	1 Cake/75g	290	10.8	387	5.3	59.2	14.4	0.0
Battenberg, Mini, Mr Kipling*	1 Cake/35g	143	3.8	410	4.6	76.2	11.0	1.3
Battenberg, Mr Kipling*	1 Slice/38g	164	4.8	428	6.1	73.0	12.5	1.4
Birthday, M & S*	1 Serving/60g	240	7.1	400	2.3	70.9	11.9	0.8
Birthday Present, Tesco*	1 Serving/79g	347	13.9	439	3.5	66.6	17.6	0.4
Bites, Caramel, Mr Kipling*	1 Cake/14g	68	3.8	492	5.9	55.3	27.4	0.8
Butterfly, Mr Kipling*	1 Cake/29g	114	6.4	392	4.4	43.4	22.2	0.6
Buttons, Happy Birthday, Cadbury*	1 Slice/50g	235	13.5	470	4.1	52.8	27.1	0.0
Cappuccino, Finest, Tesco*	1oz/28g	105	6.2	374	2.8	40.4	22.3	0.2
Caramel, Milk Chocolate, Holly Lane*	1 Cake/25g	110	5.1	441	6.9	57.6	20.3	1.1
Caramel Crunchy, Devondale*	1 Cake/80g	359	19.2	449	2.9	56.3	24.0	1.3
Caramel Shortcake Slices, McVitie's*	1 Slice/32g	146	7.7	463	4.3	56.5	24.4	1.6

C

CAKE

INFO/WEIGHT	Measure	per Measure KCAL	FAT	Nutrition Values per 100g / 100ml KCAL	PROT	CARB	FAT	FIBRE
Caramel Slice, M & S*	1 Slice/64g	304	16.1	475	4.9	60.4	25.2	2.6
Carrot, Average	1 Slice/56g	211	10.4	377	4.6	47.5	18.6	1.4
Carrot, Entenmann's*	1 Serving/40g	156	8.2	391	4.1	47.4	20.5	1.5
Carrot, Handmade, Delicious, Boots*	1 Slice/75g	292	13.5	389	4.1	53.0	18.0	1.4
Carrot, Mini, Weight Watchers*	1 Cake/31g	120	3.3	388	3.7	68.9	10.8	2.7
Carrot, Organic, Respect Organics*	1 Slice/45g	179	10.1	398	3.1	47.4	22.4	1.5
Carrot, Slices, Inspirations, Mr Kipling*	1 Slice/34g	139	6.3	411	3.5	57.7	18.5	1.3
Carrot, Square, Margaret's Country Kitchen*	1 Cake/80g	307	13.5	384	3.6	54.4	16.9	2.4
Carrot, The Handmade Flapjack Company*	1 Cake/75g	295	13.0	393	6.4	53.0	17.3	0.0
Carrot & Orange, Finest, Tesco*	1/8 Cake/50g	205	10.2	410	4.6	51.2	20.5	2.1
Carrot & Orange, Light Choices, Tesco*	1/6 Cake/63g	227	6.2	360	3.9	64.2	9.8	1.3
Carrot & Walnut, Mini Classics, Mr Kipling*	1 Cake/39g	172	9.8	440	4.5	48.6	25.2	1.0
Carrot Slices, GFY, Asda*	1 Slice/28g	83	0.6	298	2.8	66.4	2.3	2.1
Carrot Slices, Less Than 3% Fat, BGTY, Sainsbury's*	1 Slice/30g	94	0.8	313	3.4	68.7	2.7	2.4
Carrot Slices, Weight Watchers*	1 Slice/27g	84	0.2	311	2.8	73.0	0.8	0.9
Carrot Wedge, Tesco*	1 Pack/175g	532	27.6	304	3.9	36.6	15.8	1.5
Cherry, Asda*	1 Slice/37g	131	4.5	351	4.7	56.0	12.0	0.6
Cherry, Linda Kearns*	1 Serving/100g	265	14.2	265	12.1	29.9	14.2	4.2
Cherry, M & S*	1 Serving/75g	285	9.5	380	5.0	60.6	12.7	0.8
Cherry Bakewell, Gluten Free, Bakers Delight*	1 Cake/50g	211	8.1	422	2.9	66.1	16.3	0.4
Cherry Bakewell, M & S*	1 Cake/44g	185	7.8	420	4.5	61.7	17.7	1.0
Cherry Bakewell, Sainsbury's*	1 Cake/46g	200	8.1	436	3.1	66.3	17.6	1.4
Cherry Bakewell, Sara Lee*	1/5 Slice/70g	228	7.9	326	4.1	51.9	11.3	1.4
Cherry Bakewell, Waitrose*	1 Cake/44g	184	8.5	419	3.8	57.4	19.3	2.1
Cherry Bakewells, Delightful, Mr Kipling*	1 Cake/45g	176	5.8	390	3.9	66.4	12.9	1.2
Chocolate	1oz/28g	128	7.4	456	7.4	50.4	26.4	0.0
Chocolate, Birthday, Tesco*	1 Serving/54g	229	13.2	425	5.9	45.5	24.4	2.1
Chocolate, Caterpillar, Tesco*	1 Serving/53g	248	13.2	468	5.7	55.3	24.9	1.1
Chocolate, Champagne, Sainsbury's*	1 Serving/75g	304	12.1	405	2.5	62.4	16.2	0.5
Chocolate, Fondants, Weight Watchers*	1 Cake/19g	70	2.3	368	6.1	59.0	12.0	3.2
Chocolate, Fudge, The Cake Shop*	1 Cake/37g	178	10.8	480	3.7	50.5	29.2	1.3
Chocolate, Individual with Mini Eggs, Cadbury*	1 Cake/26g	119	6.1	455	4.6	57.5	23.1	1.3
Chocolate, Sara Lee*	1/4 Cake/88g	339	14.8	385	4.1	54.3	16.8	0.0
Chocolate, Smarties, Celebration, Large, Nestle*	1/16 Cake/71g	308	17.4	432	5.4	48.9	24.4	1.2
Chocolate, The Handmade Flapjack Company*	1 Cake/75g	303	16.2	404	12.5	39.8	21.6	0.0
Chocolate, Thorntons*	1 Serving/87g	408	25.1	469	5.2	47.1	28.8	0.6
Chocolate, Triple, Frozen, Majestic*	1/4 Cake/58g	87	5.4	150	2.2	14.1	9.4	0.1
Chocolate, Triple Layer, Celebration, Tesco*	1 Slice/100g	385	18.4	385	5.4	49.0	18.4	6.4
Chocolate, with Butter Icing, Average	1oz/28g	135	8.3	481	5.7	50.9	29.7	0.0
Chocolate & Orange Rolls, M & S*	1 Cake/60g	228	17.0	380	3.6	27.0	28.4	1.3
Chocolate & Orange Slices, GFY, Asda*	1 Serving/30g	95	0.8	315	3.2	70.0	2.5	1.3
Chocolate Box, Asda*	1 Serving/60g	263	13.8	439	5.0	53.0	23.0	0.7
Chocolate Brownie, Gluten & Wheat Free, Lovemore*	1 Slice/36g	127	4.6	352	3.7	56.1	12.8	0.2
Chocolate Button, Cakes for the Connoisseur*	1 Cake/30g	145	9.8	485	5.2	42.1	32.8	2.3
Chocolate Chip, Co-Op*	1/6 Cake/63g	275	16.9	440	5.0	44.0	27.0	0.5
Chocolate Chip, The Cake Shop*	1 Cake/35g	178	11.0	508	4.7	50.2	31.5	1.1
Chocolate Egg, Small, Tesco*	1 Cake/31g	132	6.3	425	5.4	57.2	20.2	1.7
Chocolate Fudge	1 Serving/110g	415	19.1	377	4.4	50.4	17.4	1.4
Chocolate Fudge, & Vanilla Cream, M & S*	1/6 Cake/69g	310	17.9	450	5.2	49.8	26.0	1.3
Chocolate Fudge, Belgian, TTD, Sainsbury's*	1 Slice/66g	278	14.3	423	4.4	52.5	21.7	2.5
Chocolate Fudge, Classics, M & S*	1 Serving/71g	195	7.5	275	2.8	42.8	10.6	1.1
Chocolate Fudge, Entenmann's*	1 Serving/48g	173	7.2	361	4.4	51.8	15.1	0.9
Chocolate Fudge, Maison Blanc*	1/4 Cake/111g	421	22.2	378	1.2	42.5	20.0	2.7

CAKE

	Measure INFO/WEIGHT	per Measure KCAL	per Measure FAT	KCAL	PROT	CARB	FAT	FIBRE
Chocolate Fudge, Tea Time Treats, Asda*	1 Cake/37g	157	8.1	424	3.6	53.0	22.0	1.7
Chocolate Log, Fresh Cream, Finest, Tesco*	1 Slice/85g	301	15.4	354	4.5	43.2	18.1	1.4
Chocolate Orange, Slices, Weight Watchers*	1 Slice/82g	249	2.2	304	4.9	64.9	2.7	2.6
Chocolate Slice, Go Ahead, McVitie's*	1 Slice/32g	94	2.6	293	4.5	49.4	8.2	1.9
Chocolate Slices, Mr Kipling*	1 Slice/33g	132	6.7	406	5.6	50.4	20.6	2.7
Chocolate Tiffin, Devondale*	1 Cake/100g	513	27.0	513	2.8	54.0	27.0	1.7
Christmas, Connoisseur, M & S*	1 Slice/60g	216	5.5	360	4.1	64.7	9.2	3.3
Christmas, Iced Rich Fruit, Finest, Tesco*	1 Serving/100g	345	7.7	345	3.1	65.3	7.7	3.7
Christmas, Knightsbridge*	1 Slice/50g	188	5.4	377	4.3	65.7	10.8	3.2
Christmas, Rich Fruit, All Iced, Sainsbury's*	1/16 Cake/85g	307	7.6	361	4.0	66.4	8.9	1.5
Christmas, Rich Fruit, Free From, Tesco*	1 Serving/100g	340	3.6	340	2.6	73.6	3.6	2.7
Christmas Pudding, Slices, Mr Kipling*	1 Slice/51g	173	3.6	339	3.6	62.1	7.1	1.3
Coconut & Raspberry, M & S*	1 Serving/52g	231	13.9	445	5.0	45.5	26.8	2.3
Coconut Delight, Burton's*	1 Cake/21g	89	3.5	424	4.0	63.0	16.9	2.0
Coconut Snowballs, Tunnock's*	1 Cake/30g	134	6.2	446	4.2	56.7	20.8	3.6
Coffee, Entenmann's*	1 Serving/41g	159	7.1	388	4.0	54.7	17.3	0.6
Coffee, TTD, Sainsbury's*	1 Slice/68g	294	16.4	430	4.3	49.1	24.0	2.6
Coffee & Walnut, Mrs Beeton's*	1 Slice/54g	219	13.5	405	3.7	41.4	25.0	0.3
Colin the Caterpillar, M & S*	1 Slice/60g	234	12.8	390	5.3	57.2	21.3	1.3
Cornflake, Average	1 Cake/18g	83	3.7	464	5.2	64.6	20.4	2.0
Cornflake, Bobby's*	1/6 Cake/45g	207	9.2	461	3.9	65.5	20.4	0.0
Country Farmhouse, Waitrose*	1 Serving/80g	308	12.1	385	4.7	57.5	15.1	1.4
Country Slices, Asda*	1 Serving/27g	111	5.1	411	3.9	56.0	19.0	2.4
Country Slices, Mr Kipling*	1 Slice/31.8	121	4.8	380	4.4	56.7	15.0	1.2
Cranberry, Linda Kearns*	1 Serving/100g	265	14.2	265	12.0	29.9	14.2	5.2
Date, Linda Kearns*	1 Serving/100g	269	16.8	269	12.7	24.4	16.8	4.4
Date & Walnut, Bakers Delight*	1oz/28g	88	2.2	315	5.2	55.5	8.0	1.2
Date & Walnut, Slices, Light Choices, Tesco*	1 Slice/25g	72	0.3	290	5.6	63.7	1.1	1.1
Date & Walnut, Slices, Weight Watchers*	1 Slice/27g	73	0.4	271	3.5	60.6	1.6	4.2
Eccles	1 Cake/45g	214	11.9	475	3.9	59.3	26.4	1.6
Eccles, Weight Watchers*	1 Cake/48g	190	7.9	396	4.4	57.5	16.5	2.0
Fairy, Average	1 Cake/23g	96	4.6	416	5.1	53.0	20.2	1.5
Fairy, Iced, Average	1 Cake/23g	91	3.4	393	4.2	60.8	14.8	0.9
Fairy, Lemon Iced, Average	1 Cake/23g	90	3.1	393	4.4	63.2	13.6	1.1
Fairy, Plain, Average	1 Cake/23g	95	4.6	413	5.5	51.1	20.2	1.5
Fairy, Snowman, Christmas, Tesco*	1 Cake/24g	114	6.8	471	4.6	49.8	28.1	2.9
Farmhouse Loaf, The Handmade Flapjack Company*	1 Cake/75g	274	12.9	365	4.5	48.4	17.2	0.0
Farmhouse Slice, Weight Watchers*	1 Slice/23g	73	0.9	317	5.5	64.9	4.0	1.3
Flake, Cadbury*	1 Cake/20g	90	4.5	445	6.3	54.5	22.3	0.0
Fondant Fancies, Lemon, Waitrose*	1 Cake/40g	176	7.1	441	2.5	67.9	17.7	0.6
French Fancies, Average	1 Cake/27g	100	2.5	371	2.7	69.6	9.1	0.8
French Fancies, Lemon, Average	1 Cake/28g	106	2.7	378	2.5	69.9	9.8	0.5
French Fancies, Lemon, Mr Kipling*	1 Cake/28g	106	2.7	378	2.5	69.9	9.8	0.5
French Fancies, Mr Kipling*	1 Cake/28g	106	2.8	378	2.6	69.7	9.9	0.6
French Fancies, Strawberry, Mr Kipling*	1 Cake/28g	106	2.7	379	2.5	70.6	9.6	0.4
Fruit, Luxury, Fully Iced Slice, The Best, Morrisons*	1 Serving/50g	178	3.8	356	3.7	66.6	7.6	3.1
Fruit, Parisienne, Rich, Finest, Tesco*	1 Serving/69g	262	9.7	380	4.7	55.2	14.1	1.9
Fruit, Plain, Average	1 Slice/90g	319	11.6	354	5.1	57.9	12.9	0.0
Fruit, Rich, Average	1 Slice/70g	225	8.7	322	4.9	50.7	12.5	1.7
Fudge Brownie, The Handmade Flapjack Company*	1 Cake/75g	286	9.2	381	4.9	62.8	12.3	0.0
Genoa, Tesco*	1 Serving/50g	162	3.7	325	3.6	60.9	7.4	4.0
Ginger Orange, The Handmade Flapjack Company*	1 Cake/75g	289	15.2	385	4.3	46.3	20.3	0.0
Granola, Tray Bake, Kate's Cakes Ltd*	1 Serving/100g	425	16.7	425	7.3	58.2	16.7	4.7

CAKE

INFO/WEIGHT	Measure	per Measure KCAL	FAT	Nutrition Values per 100g / 100ml KCAL	PROT	CARB	FAT	FIBRE
Happy Birthday, Sainsbury's*	1 Slice/50g	207	8.0	414	2.8	64.5	16.1	0.6
Holly Hedgehog, Tesco*	1 Serving/55g	227	7.9	413	2.0	69.0	14.3	0.8
Hot Chocolate Fudge, Sainsbury's*	1/8 Cake/91g	343	15.6	376	5.1	50.3	17.1	3.5
Jaffa, Mini Rolls, Weight Watchers*	1 Bar/21g	76	2.6	367	4.3	50.3	12.8	16.8
Jamaica Ginger, McVitie's*	1 Cake/291g	1056	30.6	363	3.7	63.4	10.5	1.6
Jamaica Ginger, with Lemon Filling, McVitie's*	1 Cake/33g	143	8.2	434	4.0	48.3	25.0	0.8
Lemon, Average	1 Slice/81g	320	14.5	396	4.1	54.8	18.0	0.6
Lemon, Half Moon, Bobby's*	1/6 Cake/60g	244	11.0	406	4.1	55.7	18.4	0.0
Lemon, Home Bake, McVitie's*	1oz/28g	108	5.1	384	4.6	53.9	18.2	1.0
Lemon, Mini, Weight Watchers*	1 Cake/27g	90	3.0	333	3.7	66.7	11.1	11.1
Lemon, The Handmade Flapjack Company*	1 Cake/75g	312	16.3	416	4.5	50.5	21.8	0.0
Lemon & Orange, Finest, Tesco*	1 Serving/53g	216	10.7	410	4.5	52.4	20.3	1.1
Lemon Drizzle, Tray Bake, Kate's Cakes Ltd*	1 Serving/100g	324	14.4	324	4.5	44.2	14.4	1.1
Lemon Drizzle Cake, Asda*	1 Serving/50g	149	6.0	299	2.8	45.0	12.0	0.4
Lemon Drizzle Slices, Light Choices, Tesco*	1 Slice/23g	67	0.5	290	4.8	62.7	2.0	2.8
Lemon Slices, Low Fat, Weight Watchers*	1 Slice/26g	79	0.5	303	3.1	68.1	2.0	2.2
Lemon Slices, Mr Kipling*	1 Slice/29g	120	4.8	413	4.2	61.9	16.6	0.7
Madeira	1 Slice/40g	157	6.8	393	5.4	58.4	16.9	0.9
Magic Roundabout, Dougal, Tesco*	1 Serving/50g	214	8.0	428	2.3	68.7	16.0	0.2
Manor House, Mr Kipling*	1 Serving/69g	277	13.8	400	5.3	49.7	20.0	1.4
Marble, Home Bake, McVitie's*	1oz/28g	115	5.3	411	3.7	56.9	18.8	0.9
Marble, Tesco*	1/8 Cake/45g	184	8.4	410	4.4	55.9	18.7	1.5
Mini Rolls, Blackforest, Weight Watchers*	1 Cake/24g	89	3.4	374	5.3	58.9	14.2	4.4
Mini Rolls, Cadbury*	1 Roll/27g	120	6.1	445	4.4	56.4	22.5	1.3
Mini Rolls, Chocolate, Average	1 Cake/27g	122	6.2	453	4.8	56.9	22.9	0.9
Mini Rolls, Jaffa, Average	1 Cake/29g	111	3.3	382	3.5	67.2	11.2	1.3
Mini Rolls, Jam, Average	1 Cake/29g	115	4.5	395	3.8	59.8	15.6	1.8
Mini Rolls, Juicy Orange, Cadbury*	1 Cake/28g	110	4.7	390	5.0	55.0	16.8	0.0
Mini Rolls, Lemon, Average	1 Cake/29g	125	5.8	430	4.8	58.6	19.9	0.9
Mini Rolls, Milk Chocolate, Cadbury*	1 Roll/27g	120	6.0	445	4.4	56.5	22.2	0.0
Mint Aero, Celebration, Nestle*	1 Slice/58g	232	11.8	400	4.0	49.7	20.3	1.7
Panettone, Average	1 Portion/90g	345	15.3	383	8.0	52.0	17.0	0.0
Panettone, Bauli*	1 Serving/75g	313	15.1	418	5.9	53.5	20.1	0.0
Party, Asda*	1 Serving/57g	238	9.0	421	2.3	67.0	16.0	0.4
Perfect Pumpkin & Ginger, Graze*	1 Punnet/34g	101	5.1	298	6.1	38.6	15.0	4.0
Piece of Cake, Birthday, M & S*	1 Serving/85g	395	24.4	465	4.3	39.7	28.7	0.9
Raisin, Dernys*	1 Cake/45g	175	7.6	388	5.0	54.0	17.0	0.0
Raspberry Flavour Sponge, Value, Tesco*	1 Slice/39g	130	4.6	334	3.4	53.4	11.9	0.7
Raspberry Smoothie Bake, Go Ahead, McVitie's*	1 Bar/35g	126	2.6	359	3.0	69.8	7.5	2.2
Rich Choc' Roll, Cadbury*	1/6 Portion/39g	149	6.1	381	4.8	50.2	15.6	1.0
Rich Chocolate, Christmas, Tesco*	1 Slice/82g	300	13.5	367	7.0	47.5	16.5	1.6
Rich Fruit, Devondale*	1 Cake/60g	204	7.8	340	1.3	51.0	13.0	0.6
Rich Fruit Slices, Free From, Sainsbury's*	1 Slice/40g	144	5.0	361	4.5	57.4	12.6	3.7
Rock	1 Cake/40g	158	6.6	396	5.4	60.5	16.4	1.5
Rock, Tesco*	1 Serving/87g	311	8.4	357	7.4	60.1	9.7	1.6
Shrek Birthday, Tesco*	1/16 Cake/72g	248	8.8	344	3.3	64.0	12.2	0.5
Simnel, Slices, Mr Kipling*	1 Slice/47g	177	5.9	379	2.9	63.4	12.6	1.2
Snowballs, Sainsbury's*	1 Snowball/18g	80	4.1	445	2.5	55.6	23.0	3.6
Sponge	1 Slice/53g	243	13.9	459	6.4	52.4	26.3	0.9
Sponge, Fatless	1 Slice/53g	156	3.2	294	10.1	53.0	6.1	0.9
Sponge, Fresh Cream & Strawberry, Asda*	1/12 Cake/60g	170	6.0	284	4.6	44.0	10.0	1.1
Sponge, Jam Filled	1 Slice/65g	196	3.2	302	4.2	64.2	4.9	1.8
Sponge, Victoria, TTD, Sainsbury's*	1 Slice/57g	229	11.0	401	5.0	51.8	19.3	1.4

C

CAKE

INFO/WEIGHT	Measure	per Measure KCAL	FAT	Nutrition Values per 100g / 100ml KCAL	PROT	CARB	FAT	FIBRE
Sponge Roll, Chocolate, M & S*	¼ Cake/66g	251	12.1	380	3.9	50.5	18.4	1.8
Spooky, Birthday, Memory Lane Cakes*	1 Slice/75g	295	14.6	393	3.5	50.8	19.5	0.7
St. Clements, Finest, Tesco*	1 Serving/49g	194	10.5	395	3.1	47.2	21.5	0.4
Stem Ginger, 96% Fat Free, Trimlyne*	¼ Cake/63g	170	2.2	272	4.4	58.1	3.6	1.2
Stem Ginger, Mrs Crimble's*	1 Slice/48g	158	1.1	329	2.7	73.3	2.2	2.7
Stollen, Christmas Range, Tesco*	1oz/28g	99	3.8	355	5.0	52.9	13.7	1.8
Stollen, Slices, Finest, Tesco*	1 Slice/45g	164	5.2	365	6.9	57.3	11.6	4.2
Sultana, Apple & Cranberry, 99% Fat Free, Trimlyne*	1/6 Cake/67g	130	0.6	195	4.6	45.5	0.9	3.3
Sultana, Fair Trade, Co-Op*	1/8 Cake/45g	155	4.0	345	5.0	60.0	9.0	1.0
Sultana & Cherry, Slice, Co-Op*	1oz/28g	87	3.4	310	3.0	48.0	12.0	2.0
Sultana & Cherry, Tesco*	1 Cake/37g	124	4.0	334	4.7	54.4	10.8	2.5
Swiss Roll, Average	1oz/28g	77	1.2	276	7.2	55.5	4.4	0.8
Swiss Roll, Chocolate, Individual	1 Roll/26g	88	2.9	337	4.3	58.1	11.3	0.0
Swiss Roll, Chocolate, Lyons*	1 Serving/50g	189	9.6	379	4.3	47.0	19.3	0.9
Swiss Roll, Chocolate, M & S*	1 Serving/46g	168	11.1	365	4.6	32.6	24.2	1.2
Swiss Roll, Raspberry, Average	1 Slice/35g	107	1.2	305	3.8	64.8	3.5	0.6
Swiss Roll, Raspberry, Lyons*	1 Roll/175g	485	2.4	277	5.2	60.6	1.4	0.0
Swiss Roll, Raspberry Jam, Mr Kipling*	1/6 Cake/52g	184	5.3	355	2.8	63.0	10.2	1.0
Syrup & Ginger, Tesco*	1 Serving/32g	134	7.0	420	4.5	51.4	21.8	0.7
Tangy Lemon Trickle, M & S*	1 Slice/75g	281	14.1	375	4.7	47.4	18.8	1.1
The Ultimate Carrot Passion, Entenmann's*	1 Slice/52g	210	12.6	403	4.6	42.4	24.3	1.0
Tiffin, Chocolate, Sainsbury's*	1 Cake/61g	184	11.6	301	2.7	29.8	19.0	1.3
Toffee, Iced, Tesco*	1 Serving/35g	132	5.2	376	3.3	57.2	14.9	1.6
Toffee, Slices, BGTY, Sainsbury's*	1 Slice/27g	88	0.7	327	4.3	71.7	2.5	1.8
Toffee, Slices, Value, Tesco*	1 Slice/14g	62	3.2	440	4.2	54.9	22.6	0.6
Toffee & Pecan Slices, M & S*	1 Slice/36g	160	8.5	445	4.7	54.0	23.7	1.3
Toffee Apple, McVitie's*	1 Slice/29g	104	3.2	354	3.5	60.2	11.0	1.5
Toffee Bakewell, Tesco*	1 Cake/49g	203	7.9	414	3.9	63.5	16.1	1.4
Toffee Flavour Slices, Low Fat, Weight Watchers*	1 Slice/27g	80	0.7	297	4.2	63.9	2.6	3.2
Toffee Fudge, Entenmann's*	1 Serving/65g	274	14.1	421	3.4	53.0	21.7	0.5
Toffee Snap, The Handmade Flapjack Company*	1 Cake/75g	365	19.6	487	4.6	62.2	26.1	0.0
Turkish Delight, Fry's*	1 Cake/26g	96	2.8	371	4.5	62.4	10.8	0.5
Vanilla Sponge, Fresh Cream, Sainsbury's*	1 Slice/50g	152	5.1	304	7.5	45.6	10.2	0.4
Very Berry, Kate's Cakes Ltd*	1 Serving/100g	346	14.6	346	3.4	50.3	14.6	1.4
Victoria Sandwich, Average	1 Slice/68g	267	12.9	392	4.4	50.9	19.0	1.0
Victoria Slices, Mr Kipling*	1 Slice/28g	122	4.4	432	3.9	68.8	15.7	0.4
Victoria Sponge, Lemon, Co-Op*	1 Slice/42g	151	8.0	360	4.0	44.0	19.0	0.7
Victoria Sponge, Mini, Bobby's*	1 Cake/35g	164	9.6	469	4.0	51.3	27.5	0.2
Victoria Sponge, Mini, Mr Kipling*	1 Cake/36g	152	6.9	420	3.9	58.5	19.0	0.8
Victoria Sponge, Mini, Weight Watchers*	1 Cake/30g	103	2.5	343	5.7	57.2	8.3	8.4
Viennese, M & S*	1 Cake/51g	250	14.1	495	4.1	58.9	28.0	2.8
Viennese Whirl, Average	1 Cake/28g	131	6.9	467	4.1	56.7	24.8	1.1
Viennese Whirl, Chocolate, Mr Kipling*	1 Whirl/28g	134	7.8	484	4.6	53.1	28.0	2.1
Viennese Whirl, Lemon, Mr Kipling*	1 Cake/28g	115	4.5	409	4.2	62.2	15.9	0.7
Viennese Whirl, Mr Kipling*	1 Cake/28g	141	7.8	504	3.9	59.1	28.0	1.4
Walnut, Sandwich, Sainsbury's*	1/8 Cake/48g	182	8.3	379	5.4	53.7	17.3	1.3

CAKE BAR

INFO/WEIGHT	Measure	per Measure KCAL	FAT	Nutrition Values per 100g / 100ml KCAL	PROT	CARB	FAT	FIBRE
Blueberry, Trimlyne*	1 Cake/50g	141	1.1	283	3.9	64.0	2.2	2.2
Bounty, McVitie's*	1 Cake/36g	166	8.8	461	5.1	55.2	24.5	0.0
Caramel, Cadbury*	1 Bar/26g	107	4.4	411	6.4	57.0	16.8	0.0
Caramel, Weight Watchers*	1 Bar/23g	89	3.0	381	5.3	56.2	12.8	9.9
Carrot, Gu*	1 Slice/38g	135	6.6	354	1.4	17.2	17.5	0.9
Carrot, Tesco*	1 Bar/68g	239	12.6	351	4.7	41.4	18.5	2.4

	Measure INFO/WEIGHT	per Measure KCAL	FAT	Nutrition Values per 100g / 100ml KCAL	PROT	CARB	FAT	FIBRE
CAKE BAR								
Choc Chip, Go Ahead, McVitie's*	1 Cake/28g	100	3.5	356	6.4	56.9	12.4	1.0
Choc Chip, Mini, Go Ahead, McVitie's*	1 Bar/27g	93	3.3	343	5.7	55.3	12.1	0.9
Chocolate, Average	1 Cake/28g	125	6.2	446	5.6	56.3	22.1	1.9
Chocolate, High Lights, Cadbury*	1 Bar/25g	95	3.5	380	5.5	58.8	14.0	1.1
Chocolate, Snack Cakes, Penguin, McVitie's*	1 Bar/24g	122	7.2	510	4.8	54.6	30.2	1.6
Chocolate & Orange, Go Ahead, McVitie's*	1 Cake/33g	109	2.0	330	4.3	64.9	6.0	1.0
Chocolate Chip, Average	1 Cake/28g	428	21.6	428	6.3	51.9	21.6	1.6
Chocolate Chip, Mr Kipling*	1 Bar/32g	151	8.4	472	5.3	53.5	26.3	1.2
Chocolate Chip, Sainsbury's*	1 Cake/25g	107	5.6	430	6.1	51.2	22.3	0.6
Chocolate Dream, Go Ahead, McVitie's*	1 Bar/36g	141	4.8	391	4.6	63.2	13.4	0.9
Double Chocolate, Free From, Sainsbury's*	1 Cake/50g	196	7.9	391	4.2	58.2	15.7	1.0
Dream, Cadbury*	1 Cake/38g	170	8.5	450	4.5	57.2	22.6	0.0
Flake, Cadbury*	1 Cake/22g	97	5.1	442	6.5	51.8	23.3	0.5
Fruit & Nut Crisp, Go Ahead, McVitie's*	1 Bar/22g	95	3.0	430	5.3	71.3	13.7	1.7
Fudge, Cadbury*	1 Pack/52g	220	9.2	420	5.7	60.3	17.6	0.0
Galaxy Caramel, McVitie's*	1 Cake/31g	137	6.5	441	5.5	57.4	21.1	0.0
Golden Syrup, McVitie's*	1 Cake/33g	127	4.8	385	3.6	60.2	14.4	1.2
Jaffa, McVitie's*	1 Bar/25g	97	3.5	390	3.2	62.4	14.2	2.4
Jamaica Ginger, McVitie's*	1 Cake/33g	128	4.9	388	3.5	60.2	14.7	1.2
Lemon, with Sugar Pearls, Kate's Cakes Ltd*	1 Serving/100g	325	15.8	325	4.2	43.4	15.8	0.9
Lemon Meringue, Indulgence, Weight Watchers*	1 Bar/24g	21	0.3	86	1.1	7.1	1.3	0.0
Milk Chocolate, Cadbury*	1 Bar/35g	150	7.6	430	5.6	53.3	21.7	1.2
Milk Chocolate & Orange, Crispy, Asda*	1 Bar/22g	91	2.2	413	4.8	75.6	10.2	2.0
Milk Chocolate Orange, Sandwich Bar, Lyons*	1 Bar/28g	142	8.0	516	5.0	62.0	29.0	0.0
Milky Way, McVitie's*	1 Cake/26g	124	6.2	476	5.1	58.5	23.6	1.2
Rich Chocolate, Trimlyne*	1 Serving/40g	115	1.7	287	5.2	59.2	4.2	2.2
Toffee Cake, High Lights, Cadbury*	1 Bar/25g	95	3.5	380	7.6	56.7	14.0	0.9
CAKE MIX								
Carrot Cake, Betty Crocker*	¼ Pack/125g	504	8.4	403	5.8	78.9	6.7	1.4
Cheesecake, Original, Made Up, Asda*	1/6 Cake/85g	228	10.2	268	4.1	36.0	12.0	1.4
Cheesecake, Strawberry, Real, Green's*	1 Serving/100g	254	12.8	253	3.9	30.6	12.8	0.6
Cheesecake, Tesco*	1 Serving/76g	199	7.9	262	4.1	38.0	10.4	1.6
Chocolate Brownie, Chocolate Chips, Weight Watchers*	1 Pack/190g	568	13.5	299	3.2	55.6	7.1	2.1
Dennis, Green's*	1 Cake/17g	55	1.3	319	4.6	57.8	7.7	0.0
Free From, Sainsbury's*	1 Serving/50g	173	0.1	346	1.3	84.4	0.3	2.2
Sponge, Value, Tesco*	1 Slice/55g	181	4.8	329	4.6	57.9	8.8	1.4
Yellow, Super Moist, Betty Crocker*	1 Cake/128g	517	9.5	404	3.3	81.6	7.4	1.1
CALLALOO								
Leaves, Raw, Unprepared	1 Cup/28g	6	0.1	23	2.5	4.0	0.3	0.0
CALZONE								
Bolognese, Weight Watchers*	1 Calzone/88g	178	3.0	202	11.7	31.2	3.4	4.3
Cheese & Tomato, Weight Watchers*	1 Calzone/88g	191	3.8	217	11.3	33.4	4.3	3.4
Ham & Gruyere, Asda*	1 Serving/280g	661	22.4	236	10.0	31.0	8.0	2.7
CANNELLONI								
Beef, Great Value, Asda*	1 Pack/400g	384	10.8	96	6.0	12.0	2.7	1.6
Beef, Italian, Sainsbury's*	1 Pack/400g	498	26.2	124	5.9	10.5	6.5	1.6
Beef, Italian, Tesco*	1 Pack/400g	520	26.8	130	5.3	11.6	6.7	0.9
Beef, Ready Meal	1 Serving/335g	501	21.8	149	8.4	14.1	6.5	1.4
Beef, Ready Meal, Healthy Range, Average	1 Serving/300g	267	7.0	89	5.9	11.0	2.3	1.6
Beef & Red Wine, TTD, Sainsbury's*	½ Pack/180g	448	11.5	249	14.8	32.1	6.4	1.8
Chicken & Pesto, Italian, Sainsbury's*	1 Pack/450g	675	33.7	150	6.1	14.4	7.5	1.1
Mushroom, Italian, Sainsbury's*	1 Pack/450g	598	31.0	133	5.2	12.5	6.9	0.5
Parmesan & Basil, M & S*	1 Pack/360g	504	28.4	140	5.9	11.4	7.9	0.8

C

	Measure INFO/WEIGHT	per Measure		Nutrition Values per 100g / 100ml				
		KCAL	FAT	KCAL	PROT	CARB	FAT	FIBRE
CANNELLONI								
Spinach & Cheese, Finest, Tesco*	1 Pack/350g	532	31.8	152	5.4	12.1	9.1	1.5
Spinach & Ricotta, Frozen, Sainsbury's*	1 Pack/350g	513	25.8	147	6.1	13.9	7.4	1.1
Spinach & Ricotta, Italian Style, Co-Op*	1 Pack/450g	540	27.0	120	5.0	12.0	6.0	2.0
Spinach & Ricotta, Ross*	1 Pack/299g	296	8.1	99	3.3	15.2	2.7	1.6
Spinach & Wild Mushroom, Linda McCartney*	1 Pack/340g	381	13.6	112	4.9	14.1	4.0	1.7
Tubes, Dry, Average	*1oz/28g*	*101*	*1.0*	*361*	*12.5*	*69.1*	*3.6*	*1.2*
Vegetarian, Tesco*	1 Pack/400g	552	34.4	138	5.3	9.8	8.6	1.5
CAPERS								
in Brine, Tesco*	1 Tsp/2g	1	0.0	29	2.4	3.5	0.6	2.7
in Vinegar, Average	1 Tsp/5g	2	0.0	34	1.7	3.0	0.6	2.8
CAPRI SUN								
Orange	1 Pouch/200ml	90	0.0	45	0.0	11.0	0.0	0.0
Orange, 100%, Juice	1 Pouch/200ml	75	0.0	38	0.5	9.2	0.0	0.1
CARAMAC								
Nestle*	1 Bar/30g	173	11.0	567	5.7	54.7	36.1	0.0
CARAMBOLA								
Average	*1oz/28g*	*9*	*0.1*	*32*	*0.5*	*7.3*	*0.3*	*1.3*
CARAWAY								
Seeds, Schwartz*	1 Pack/38g	170	8.1	448	23.3	40.9	21.2	0.0
CARDAMOM								
Ground, Average	*1 Tsp/2g*	*6*	*0.1*	*314*	*10.7*	*53.6*	*7.1*	*28.6*
CAROB POWDER								
Average	*1 Tsp/2g*	*3*	*0.0*	*159*	*4.9*	*37.0*	*0.1*	*0.0*
CARP								
Fillet, Raw, Average	1 Fillet/218g	244	10.2	112	17.5	0.0	4.7	0.0
CARROT & SWEDE								
Diced for Mashing, Average	*½ Pack/250g*	*57*	*0.7*	*23*	*0.6*	*4.7*	*0.3*	*1.9*
Mash, from Supermarket, Average	1 Serving/150g	138	7.5	92	1.3	10.4	5.0	1.3
Mash, Healthy Range, Average	1 Serving/150g	98	4.2	65	1.3	8.6	2.8	2.1
CARROTS								
Baby, Canned, Average	*1 Can/195g*	*40*	*0.5*	*21*	*0.5*	*4.2*	*0.3*	*2.1*
Baby, Fresh, Average	*1 Serving/80g*	*28*	*0.1*	*35*	*0.6*	*8.2*	*0.1*	*2.9*
Baby, with Fine Beans, Tesco*	1 Pack/200g	58	1.0	29	1.3	4.7	0.5	2.3
Batons, Broccoli & Cauliflower, Freshly Frozen, Asda*	1 Bag/156g	39	0.9	25	1.9	2.9	0.6	2.4
Batons, Fresh, Average	*½ Pack/150g*	*41*	*0.4*	*27*	*0.6*	*5.7*	*0.3*	*2.6*
Batons & Sliced Runner Beans, Sainsbury's*	1 Serving/200g	40	1.0	20	1.0	3.2	0.5	3.2
Boiled, Average	*1oz/28g*	*6*	*0.1*	*22*	*0.6*	*4.4*	*0.4*	*2.3*
Canned, Average	*1oz/28g*	*6*	*0.1*	*22*	*0.6*	*4.4*	*0.2*	*2.1*
Raw, Scrubbed, Average	1 Serving/80g	24	0.4	30	0.7	6.0	0.5	2.4
Sliced, Canned, Average	*1 Serving/180g*	*36*	*0.2*	*20*	*0.7*	*4.1*	*0.1*	*1.5*
Sliced, Canned, Drained, Basics, Sainsbury's*	1 Can/160g	30	0.3	19	0.4	3.9	0.2	2.5
Sliced, Fresh, Average	*1 Serving/60g*	*17*	*0.2*	*28*	*0.7*	*5.7*	*0.3*	*2.0*
Sliced, Fresh, Value, Tesco*	1/6 Pack/100g	35	0.3	35	0.6	7.9	0.3	2.4
Whole, Raw, Peeled, Average	*1 Carrot/75g*	*21*	*0.2*	*29*	*0.6*	*6.3*	*0.3*	*2.2*
CASHEW NUTS								
BBQ, Graze*	1 Pack/26g	142	10.8	546	13.9	37.0	41.7	0.0
Ca-shew! Bless You, Graze*	1 Punnet/40g	146	5.8	365	6.1	57.2	14.5	0.0
Cheese Flavour, Graze*	1 Pack/26g	140	10.8	540	15.3	35.7	41.5	0.0
Cracked Black Pepper, Graze*	1 Punnet/35g	196	15.6	560	14.9	33.2	44.5	3.0
Frosted, Graze*	1 Pack/26g	134	8.4	516	10.5	53.0	32.2	0.0
Honey, Graze*	½ Pack/13g	67	4.2	516	10.5	53.0	32.2	0.0
Hot Chilli, Graze*	1 Pack/26g	139	10.9	535	14.5	33.6	41.8	0.0
Mexican Chilli, Graze*	1 Pack/26g	140	10.8	539	14.3	34.9	41.6	0.0

	Measure INFO/WEIGHT	per Measure KCAL	FAT	Nutrition Values per 100g / 100ml KCAL	PROT	CARB	FAT	FIBRE
CASHEW NUTS								
Natural, Roasted, Love Life, Waitrose*	1 Serving/25g	160	12.5	640	22.0	23.6	50.1	4.3
Plain, Average	*¼ Pack/25g*	*146*	*12.2*	*584*	*15.7*	*18.7*	*48.9*	*3.4*
Roasted & Salted, Average	*1 Serving/50g*	*306*	*25.5*	*612*	*18.8*	*19.5*	*51.1*	*3.1*
CASHEWS								
Fiery, Graze*	1 Punnet/35g	198	15.9	566	15.3	29.8	45.3	2.9
Salsa Tossed, Graze*	1 Pack/40g	220	17.4	549	14.7	29.4	43.5	0.0
CASSAVA								
Baked, Average	*1oz/28g*	*43*	*0.1*	*155*	*0.7*	*40.1*	*0.2*	*1.7*
Boiled in Unsalted Water, Average	*1oz/28g*	*36*	*0.1*	*130*	*0.5*	*33.5*	*0.2*	*1.4*
Gari, Average	*1oz/28g*	*100*	*0.1*	*358*	*1.3*	*92.9*	*0.5*	*0.0*
Raw, Average	*1oz/28g*	*40*	*0.1*	*142*	*0.6*	*36.8*	*0.2*	*1.6*
Steamed, Average	*1oz/28g*	*40*	*0.1*	*142*	*0.6*	*36.8*	*0.2*	*1.6*
CASSEROLE								
Bean, Spicy, BGTY, Sainsbury's*	1 Pack/300g	171	2.7	57	3.0	9.1	0.9	4.2
Bean & Lentil, Morrisons*	1 Can/410g	287	1.6	70	4.1	12.5	0.4	0.0
Beef, & Ale, Average	1 Serving/300g	251	6.7	84	9.4	6.5	2.2	1.3
Beef, & Red Wine, Average	1 Serving/350g	290	7.3	83	7.2	8.2	2.1	1.5
Beef, Average	1 Serving/336g	490	23.0	146	16.3	4.6	6.8	0.6
Beef, with Dumplings, Ready Meal, Average	1 Serving/350g	464	21.1	132	9.5	10.1	6.0	1.5
Beef & Onion, Minced, British Classics, Tesco*	1 Pack/340g	367	19.0	108	5.0	9.3	5.6	0.8
Beef & Red Wine, BGTY, Sainsbury's*	1 Pack/300g	192	1.8	64	8.0	6.7	0.6	0.9
Beef & Red Wine, Weight Watchers*	1 Pack/330g	254	9.2	77	4.3	8.6	2.8	0.3
Beef & Red Wine, You Count, Love Life, Waitrose*	1 Pack/381g	297	5.2	78	6.5	9.5	1.4	0.9
Chicken, & Dumplings, HL, Tesco*	1 Pack/450g	441	12.1	98	7.4	11.1	2.7	0.6
Chicken, & Dumplings, Sainsbury's*	1 Serving/450g	612	32.4	136	6.8	11.0	7.2	0.6
Chicken, Carrots, Peas & Potatoes, Weight Watchers*	1 Serving/302g	193	4.2	64	4.3	8.6	1.4	0.5
Chicken, Diet Chef Ltd*	1 Pack/300g	219	2.7	73	9.0	7.2	0.9	2.5
Chicken, Green Isle*	1 Pack/400g	300	6.8	75	5.7	9.2	1.7	1.0
Chicken, Leek & Mushroom, Tesco*	1 Pack/350g	381	22.0	109	4.5	8.6	6.3	1.0
Chicken, Perfectly Balanced, Waitrose*	1 Pack/400g	392	14.4	98	6.6	9.8	3.6	1.2
Chicken, Skinny Chef, All About Weight*	1 Meal/269g	277	0.8	103	11.2	11.9	0.3	3.8
Chicken, You Count, Love Life, Waitrose*	1 Pack/400g	297	4.8	74	7.4	7.9	1.2	1.2
Chicken & Asparagus, HL, Tesco*	1 Serving/450g	342	10.3	76	6.3	8.3	2.3	0.5
Chicken & Asparagus in White Wine, Tesco*	½ Pack/300g	444	23.7	148	11.5	7.7	7.9	0.8
Chicken & Red Wine, Duchy Originals*	½ Pack/175g	187	7.5	107	14.0	5.1	4.3	1.6
Chicken & Vegetable, Apetito*	1 Pack/330g	286	9.9	87	6.3	9.4	3.0	1.6
Chicken & Vegetable, Long Life, Sainsbury's*	1 Pack/300g	186	4.5	62	4.6	7.4	1.5	0.8
Chicken & White Wine, BGTY, Sainsbury's*	1 Serving/300g	216	6.6	72	7.2	5.9	2.2	1.3
Ham Hock & Mash, Tesco*	1 Pack/250g	225	8.0	90	6.1	9.0	3.2	0.8
Lamb, & Rosemary, Eat Well, M & S*	1 Pack/380g	325	11.0	86	7.6	7.0	2.9	2.2
Lamb, BGTY, Sainsbury's*	1 Serving/200g	242	8.6	121	20.7	0.1	4.3	0.1
Lamb, Braised, British Classics, Tesco*	1 Pack/350g	332	18.2	95	7.5	4.6	5.2	1.2
Lamb, COU, M & S*	1 Pack/390g	253	6.6	65	5.9	6.7	1.7	1.6
Lamb, Ready Meal, Healthy Range, Average	1 Serving/220g	200	7.3	91	10.5	4.9	3.3	1.0
Lamb, with Mint Dumplings, Minced, Sainsbury's*	1 Pack/450g	558	30.6	124	5.4	10.4	6.8	1.1
Mediterranean Seafood, HL, Tesco*	1 Pack/344g	292	6.9	85	5.8	10.5	2.0	3.2
Rabbit, Average	1oz/28g	29	1.4	102	11.6	2.6	5.1	0.4
Sausage, & Potato, M & S*	1 Serving/200g	190	11.8	95	3.3	7.5	5.9	0.9
Sausage, 154, Oakhouse Foods Ltd*	1 Meal/400g	484	28.0	121	4.8	10.0	7.0	0.7
Sausage, Chosen By You, Asda*	1 Pot/400g	240	15.2	60	3.6	1.9	3.8	2.1
Sausage, Pork, Diet Chef Ltd*	1 Pack/300g	303	18.3	101	6.6	4.9	6.1	1.4
Sausage, Solo Slim, Rosemary Conley*	1 Pack/300g	312	15.0	104	5.7	9.0	5.0	3.1
Sausage, Wiltshire Farm Foods*	1 Pack/420g	394	20.4	94	3.0	9.7	4.9	1.4

	Measure INFO/WEIGHT	per Measure KCAL	FAT	Nutrition Values per 100g / 100ml KCAL	PROT	CARB	FAT	FIBRE
CASSEROLE								
Steak & Ale, Average	1 Serving/275g	324	14.4	118	9.0	8.8	5.2	1.0
Steak & Kidney, Mini, Favourites, M & S*	1 Pack/200g	240	10.8	120	7.9	9.5	5.4	1.5
Steak & Mushroom, Average	1 Serving/275g	274	15.5	100	6.2	6.0	5.6	1.0
Steak & Mushroom, Wiltshire Farm Foods*	1 Pack/362g	322	16.3	89	5.0	7.2	4.5	1.3
Three Bean, Solo Slim, Rosemary Conley*	1 Pack/300g	195	2.7	65	4.0	10.3	0.9	3.6
Vegetable, Average	1 Serving/275g	77	0.8	28	0.8	5.5	0.3	1.5
Vegetable, with Dumplings, Ready Meal, Average	1 Serving/400g	376	13.8	94	2.1	13.0	3.5	2.7
Vegetable, with Herb Dumplings, COU, M & S*	1 Pack/450g	270	5.4	60	1.6	10.1	1.2	1.0
Vegetable & Lentil, Canned, Granose*	1 Can/400g	272	8.0	68	3.5	9.0	2.0	3.0
Venison, Scottish Wild, & Beaujolais, Tesco*	1 Pack/425g	365	8.9	86	11.9	4.9	2.1	0.6
CASSEROLE MIX								
Beef, Colman's*	1 Pack/40g	123	0.6	308	7.5	66.0	1.5	2.5
Beef, Recipe, Colman's*	1 Pack/42g	142	0.5	338	9.1	13.1	1.1	4.0
Beef, Recipe, Schwartz*	1 Pack/43g	123	0.9	287	7.0	56.6	2.1	6.6
Beef & Ale, Colman's*	1 Pack/45g	144	0.9	320	9.2	66.3	2.0	2.3
Chicken, Authentic, Schwartz*	1 Pack/36g	131	1.5	363	10.4	70.7	4.3	2.0
Chicken, Traditional, Colman's*	1 Pack/40g	124	0.5	311	5.7	69.4	1.3	1.5
Chicken Chasseur, Asda*	1 Pack/80g	273	0.8	341	9.0	74.0	1.0	1.4
Farmhouse Sausage, Schwartz*	1 Pack/39g	124	1.1	317	8.1	64.6	2.9	0.5
Honey Chicken, Colman's*	1 Pack/50g	128	0.5	257	3.4	58.3	1.1	1.8
Lamb, Authentic, Schwartz*	1 Pack/35g	116	1.2	332	7.7	68.0	3.3	1.3
Liver & Bacon, Colman's*	1 Pack/40g	121	0.7	303	10.3	61.6	1.7	4.7
Moroccan Lamb, Schwartz*	1 Pack/35g	124	2.0	354	6.2	74.1	5.7	4.5
Peppered Beef, Schwartz*	1 Pack/40g	129	2.0	323	7.0	62.9	4.9	7.3
Pork, Colman's*	1 Pack/40g	131	0.6	328	6.7	72.0	1.4	2.8
Sausage, Classic, Schwartz*	1 Pack/35g	96	0.9	275	12.4	50.1	2.7	14.9
Sausage, Colman's*	1 Pack/40g	144	0.6	361	8.9	77.7	1.6	1.6
Sausage & Onion, Colman's*	1 Pack/45g	143	1.2	318	9.6	64.2	2.6	2.6
Somerset Pork, Colman's*	1 Pack/45g	144	0.6	321	7.1	70.2	1.3	2.2
Somerset Pork, Schwartz*	1 Pack/36g	115	1.4	320	9.4	61.9	3.8	7.7
Spicy Chicken, Colman's*	1 Pack/45g	151	0.8	336	6.5	73.4	1.8	1.5
Turkey, Colman's*	1 Pack/50g	156	0.9	313	5.9	68.0	1.9	3.5
CATFISH								
Cooked, Steamed, Weighed with Bone, Average	*1 Serving/100g*	*101*	*3.1*	*101*	*18.2*	*0.0*	*3.1*	*0.7*
Raw, Average	*1oz/28g*	*27*	*0.8*	*96*	*17.6*	*0.0*	*2.8*	*0.0*
CAULIFLOWER								
Boiled, Average	*1 Serving/80g*	*22*	*0.7*	*28*	*2.9*	*2.1*	*0.9*	*1.6*
Organic, Tesco*	1 Serving/100g	35	0.9	35	3.6	3.0	0.9	1.8
Raw, Average	*1 Serving/80g*	*25*	*0.7*	*31*	*3.2*	*2.7*	*0.8*	*1.6*
Steamed, Average	1 Serving/100g	28	0.9	28	2.9	2.1	0.9	1.6
CAULIFLOWER CHEESE								
& Bacon, Gastropub, M & S*	1 Pack/300g	318	21.0	106	6.3	4.5	7.0	1.0
& Broccoli, Average	1 Serving/200g	127	6.4	64	3.8	4.6	3.2	2.0
Average	1 Meal/400g	320	19.3	80	4.2	4.9	4.8	1.4
Birds Eye*	1 Pack/329g	355	21.1	108	4.8	7.7	6.4	0.8
Extra Special, Asda*	½ Pack/200g	166	11.6	83	4.0	3.7	5.8	2.1
Frozen, Tesco*	1 Pack/450g	427	30.1	95	4.2	4.3	6.7	1.3
Grills, Grassington's Food Co*	1 Grill/92g	157	4.6	171	6.1	25.3	5.0	2.6
Healthy Range, Average	1 Serving/200g	99	3.9	50	4.1	4.0	1.9	1.3
Less Than 3% fat, BGTY, Sainsbury's*	½ Pack/200g	98	3.4	49	3.3	5.3	1.7	1.0
Made with Half Fat Cheese, HL, Tesco*	1 Pack/500g	285	13.0	57	6.5	2.0	2.6	2.2
Made with Semi-Skimmed Milk	1oz/28g	28	1.8	100	6.0	5.2	6.4	1.3
Made with Skimmed Milk	1oz/28g	27	1.7	97	6.0	5.2	6.0	1.3

	Measure INFO/WEIGHT	per Measure KCAL	per Measure FAT	Nutrition Values per 100g / 100ml KCAL	PROT	CARB	FAT	FIBRE
CAULIFLOWER CHEESE								
Made with Whole Milk	1oz/28g	29	1.9	105	6.0	5.2	6.9	1.3
Ross*	1 Pack/300g	300	19.8	100	4.9	5.5	6.6	0.1
with Crispy Bacon, Finest, Tesco*	1/3 Pack/166g	211	14.1	127	6.5	6.1	8.5	0.4
with Roasted Potatoes, M & S*	1 Pack/200g	500	23.6	250	10.8	24.8	11.8	3.2
CAVATELLI								
Egg, Asda*	1 Serving/100g	203	3.4	203	9.0	34.0	3.4	3.0
King Prawn & Scallop, M & S*	1 Pack/400g	600	22.4	150	6.4	18.0	5.6	1.3
CAVIAR								
Average	*1oz/28g*	*26*	*1.3*	*92*	*11.9*	*0.5*	*4.7*	*0.0*
CELERIAC								
Boiled in Salted Water, Average	*1oz/28g*	*4*	*0.1*	*15*	*0.9*	*1.9*	*0.5*	*3.2*
Raw, Average	*1 Serving/100g*	*42*	*0.3*	*42*	*1.5*	*9.2*	*0.3*	*1.8*
CELERY								
Boiled in Salted Water	*1 Serving/50g*	*4*	*0.1*	*8*	*0.5*	*0.8*	*0.3*	*1.2*
Raw, Trimmed	*1 Stalk/40g*	*3*	*0.1*	*7*	*0.5*	*0.9*	*0.2*	*1.1*
CHAMPAGNE								
Average	*1 Glass/120ml*	*91*	*0.0*	*76*	*0.3*	*1.4*	*0.0*	*0.0*
CHANNA MASALA								
Indian, Sainsbury's*	1 Serving/149g	165	7.3	111	4.2	12.4	4.9	3.3
M & S*	1 Pack/225g	360	23.7	160	5.6	11.2	10.5	8.2
Waitrose*	1 Pack/300g	300	18.3	100	3.7	7.4	6.1	7.9
CHAPATIS								
Brown Wheat Flour, Waitrose*	1 Chapati/42g	128	3.4	305	8.6	49.4	8.0	4.6
Elephant Atta*	1 Chapati/45g	129	2.9	287	7.5	53.1	6.4	3.2
Indian Style, Asda*	1 Chapati/43g	95	0.4	221	8.0	45.0	1.0	2.9
Made with Fat	1 Chapati/60g	197	7.7	328	8.1	48.3	12.8	0.0
Made without Fat	1 Chapati/55g	111	0.5	202	7.3	43.7	1.0	0.0
Plain, Wraps, Original, Patak's*	1 Chapati/42g	115	3.1	273	9.4	48.8	7.5	0.0
Wholemeal, Patak's*	1 Chapati/42g	130	4.0	310	11.2	44.9	9.5	9.0
CHAR								
Arctic, Whole, Raw	1 Serving/100g	137	6.0	137	20.8	0.0	6.0	0.0
CHARD								
Average	1 Serving/80g	15	0.2	19	1.4	3.3	0.2	0.8
Swiss, Boiled in Unsalted Water	*1oz/28g*	*6*	*0.0*	*20*	*1.9*	*4.1*	*0.1*	*2.1*
Swiss, Raw	*1oz/28g*	*5*	*0.1*	*19*	*1.8*	*3.7*	*0.2*	*1.6*
CHEDDARS								
Baked, Mini, Cheese & Ham Flavour, McVitie's*	1 Bag/30g	160	8.9	534	11.0	55.5	29.8	2.0
Baked, Mini, Original, Cheddar Cheese, McVitie's*	1 Bag/26g	130	7.5	522	10.6	51.4	29.9	2.5
Baked, Mini, Peperami, McVitie's*	1 Bag/30g	160	9.1	532	9.7	55.2	30.2	2.0
Baked, Mini, Tangy Salsa, McVitie's*	1 Bag/50g	266	14.9	532	11.0	54.7	29.9	2.1
Branston Pickle, McVitie's*	1 Bag/30g	155	8.9	517	9.1	53.1	29.8	2.7
Mini, Average	1 Bag/26g	134	7.8	516	11.2	50.7	29.9	2.4
CHEESE								
Appenzellar, Sainsbury's*	1 Serving/25g	96	7.9	386	25.4	0.0	31.6	0.0
Babybel, Emmental, Fromageries Bel*	1 Serving/20g	63	4.9	316	23.0	1.0	24.5	0.0
Babybel, Mini, Light, Fromageries Bel*	1 Cheese/20g	42	2.4	210	25.5	0.2	12.0	0.0
Babybel, Original, Mini, Fromageries Bel*	1 Cheese/20g	61	4.8	304	22.0	0.1	24.0	0.0
Bavarian, Smoked, Slices, Asda*	1 Slice/18g	50	4.1	277	17.0	0.4	23.0	0.0
Bavarian, Smoked with Ham, Sainsbury's*	1 Serving/30g	89	7.2	298	19.4	0.8	24.1	0.0
Blue, Castello, Soft, Castello*	1/4 Pack/38g	162	15.6	432	14.0	0.5	41.5	0.0
Blue, Saint Agur*	1 Serving/30g	109	9.9	363	16.0	0.2	33.0	0.0
Brie, Average	*1 Serving/25g*	*74*	*6.0*	*296*	*19.7*	*0.3*	*24.0*	*0.0*
Brie, Reduced Fat, Average	*1 Serving/50g*	*99*	*5.7*	*198*	*23.0*	*0.8*	*11.4*	*0.0*

CHEESE

	Measure INFO/WEIGHT	per Measure KCAL	FAT	Nutrition Values per 100g / 100ml KCAL	PROT	CARB	FAT	FIBRE
Caerphilly, Average	**1 Serving/50g**	**187**	**15.6**	**374**	**23.0**	**0.1**	**31.3**	**0.0**
Camembert, Average	**1 Serving/50g**	**141**	**11.1**	**283**	**20.5**	**0.1**	**22.2**	**0.0**
Camembert, Breaded, Average	1 Serving/90g	307	20.9	341	16.6	14.2	23.2	0.4
Cantal, French, Sainsbury's*	1 Serving/30g	106	8.7	353	23.0	0.1	29.0	0.0
Cantenaar, M & S*	1 Serving/28g	84	5.4	300	32.2	0.1	19.2	0.0
Cheddar, Canadian, Average	**1 Serving/30g**	**123**	**10.3**	**409**	**25.0**	**0.1**	**34.3**	**0.0**
Cheddar, Davidstow, Mature, Average	**1 Serving/28g**	**115**	**9.6**	**410**	**25.0**	**0.1**	**34.4**	**0.0**
Cheddar, Extra Mature, Average	**1 Serving/30g**	**123**	**10.3**	**410**	**25.1**	**0.1**	**34.3**	**0.0**
Cheddar, Grated, Average	**1 Serving/50g**	**206**	**17.1**	**413**	**24.4**	**1.5**	**34.3**	**0.0**
Cheddar, Mature, Average	**1 Serving/30g**	**123**	**10.3**	**410**	**25.0**	**0.1**	**34.4**	**0.0**
Cheddar, Mature, Grated, Average	**1 Serving/28g**	**113**	**9.3**	**404**	**24.7**	**1.6**	**33.2**	**0.0**
Cheddar, Mature, Reduced Fat, Average	**1 Serving/25g**	**68**	**4.2**	**271**	**30.0**	**0.1**	**16.7**	**0.0**
Cheddar, Medium, Average	**1 Serving/30g**	**123**	**10.3**	**411**	**24.9**	**0.1**	**34.5**	**0.0**
Cheddar, Mild, Average	**1 Serving/30g**	**123**	**10.3**	**409**	**25.0**	**0.1**	**34.3**	**0.0**
Cheddar, Reduced Fat, Average	**1 Serving/30g**	**76**	**4.2**	**255**	**32.1**	**0.1**	**13.9**	**0.0**
Cheddar, Smoked, Average	**1 Serving/30g**	**123**	**10.3**	**411**	**25.2**	**0.1**	**34.4**	**0.0**
Cheddar, Wexford, Average	**1 Serving/20g**	**82**	**6.9**	**410**	**25.0**	**0.1**	**34.4**	**0.0**
Cheddar & Mozzarella, Spicy, Grated, Tesco*	1 Serving/40g	140	10.5	350	26.0	2.5	26.2	0.0
Cheddar with Caramelised Onion, Sainsbury's*	1 Serving/28g	109	8.7	391	22.8	5.1	31.0	0.0
Cheddar with Onion & Chives, Davidson*	1 Serving/25g	100	8.3	400	24.3	0.6	33.3	0.0
Cheddar with Pickled Onion Relish, Christmas, Tesco*	¼ Cheese/50g	191	15.5	382	23.0	2.7	31.0	0.1
Cheestrings, Cheddar, Original, Golden Vale*	1 Stick/21g	69	5.0	328	28.0	0.0	24.0	0.0
Cheestrings, Double Cheese Flavour, Golden Vale*	1 Stick/21g	69	5.0	328	28.0	0.0	24.0	0.0
Cheshire	**1oz/28g**	**106**	**8.8**	**379**	**24.0**	**0.1**	**31.4**	**0.0**
Cottage, Natural, COU, M & S*	½ Pot/125g	100	2.2	80	11.9	3.3	1.8	0.3
Cottage, Natural, GFY, Asda*	1 Serving/113g	95	2.0	84	13.0	3.9	1.8	0.3
Cottage, Natural, Longley Farm*	1 Pot/125g	130	7.5	104	10.3	2.2	6.0	0.0
Cottage, Natural, Plain, Average	**1oz/28g**	**27**	**1.1**	**98**	**11.8**	**3.9**	**3.8**	**0.1**
Cottage, Natural with Creme Fraiche, Tesco*	½ Pack/125g	131	6.0	105	12.1	2.7	4.8	0.6
Cottage, Virtually Fat Free, Average	1 Tbsp/20g	16	0.2	79	13.0	4.5	1.0	0.0
Cottage, Virtually Fat Free, Eden Vale*	1oz/28g	22	0.1	80	12.9	6.5	0.3	0.0
Cottage, Virtually Fat Free, Longley Farm*	½ Pot/125g	84	0.1	67	13.4	3.0	0.1	0.0
Cottage, Whole Milk, Natural, Average	1 Serving/75g	77	3.4	103	12.5	2.7	4.5	0.0
Cottage, with Chargrilled Vegetables, BGTY, Sainsbury's*	1oz/28g	25	0.3	88	12.1	7.8	0.9	0.6
Cottage, with Chives, Low Fat, Westacre*	1 Pot/100g	81	1.4	81	13.7	3.5	1.4	1.2
Cottage, with Chives, M & S*	1oz/28g	28	1.1	100	11.9	3.5	3.9	0.0
Cottage, with Chives, Virtually Fat free, Longley Farm*	½ Pot/125g	87	0.1	70	14.3	2.9	0.1	0.0
Cottage, with Coronation Chicken, BGTY, Sainsbury's*	1oz/28g	25	0.3	91	11.3	8.7	1.2	0.1
Cottage, with Cucumber & Mint, COU, M & S*	1 Pot/113g	85	1.7	75	11.6	3.1	1.5	0.2
Cottage, with Mango & Pineapple, BGTY, Sainsbury's*	½ Pot/125g	112	0.9	90	10.7	10.4	0.7	0.2
Cottage, with Onion & Chive, GFY, Asda*	¼ Tub/75g	49	1.0	66	9.3	3.8	1.4	0.5
Cottage, with Onion & Chive, Low Fat, Sainsbury's*	1oz/28g	28	1.1	99	11.6	4.4	4.0	0.1
Cottage, with Onion & Chive, M & S*	¼ Pot/65g	88	5.5	135	10.4	4.0	8.5	0.1
Cottage, with Peach & Mango, COU, M & S*	1 Pot/113g	96	1.1	85	9.1	9.7	1.0	0.4
Cottage, with Pineapple, Asda*	1oz/28g	31	1.1	109	10.0	8.0	3.9	0.0
Cottage, with Pineapple, BGTY, Sainsbury's*	1 Serving/125g	105	0.9	84	10.5	8.9	0.7	0.1
Cottage, with Pineapple, Shape, Danone*	1oz/28g	20	0.1	73	9.8	8.0	0.2	0.1
Cottage, with Prawn, GFY, Asda*	1oz/28g	22	0.5	79	10.0	6.0	1.7	0.3
Cottage, with Prawn Cocktail, BGTY, Sainsbury's*	1oz/28g	25	0.3	91	12.3	8.3	0.9	0.1
Cottage, with Smoked Cheese & Onion, GFY, Asda*	1 Serving/50g	39	0.8	78	12.0	3.9	1.6	0.4
Cottage, with Tomato & Cracked Black Pepper, Asda*	½ Pot/113g	86	2.4	76	10.0	3.1	2.1	1.3
Cottage, with Tuna & Sweetcorn, BGTY, Sainsbury's*	1oz/28g	25	0.3	91	12.1	8.4	0.9	0.2
Cream, Average	**1 Portion/30g**	**132**	**14.2**	**439**	**3.1**	**0.0**	**47.4**	**0.0**

CHEESE

INFO/WEIGHT	Measure	per Measure KCAL	FAT	Nutrition Values per 100g / 100ml KCAL	PROT	CARB	FAT	FIBRE
Cream, Garlic & Herbs, Light, Boursin*	1 Portion/20g	28	1.8	140	12.0	2.5	9.0	0.0
Cream, Reduced Fat, Average	*1 Serving/20g*	*23*	*1.1*	*117*	*13.0*	*4.0*	*5.3*	*0.1*
Creme de Saint Agur, Saint Agur*	1 Serving/10g	28	2.5	285	13.5	2.3	24.7	0.0
Dairylea, Light, Slices, Kraft*	1 Slice/25g	51	2.6	205	17.0	8.6	10.5	0.0
Dairylea, Rippers, Straight, Kraft*	1 Ripper/21g	60	3.9	285	28.0	1.0	18.5	0.0
Dairylea, Slices, Kraft*	1 Slice/25g	69	5.1	275	13.0	8.6	20.5	0.0
Danish Blue, Average	*1 Serving/30g*	*106*	*8.7*	*352*	*20.7*	*0.0*	*29.1*	*0.0*
Demi Pont L'eveque, Finest, Tesco*	1 Serving/46g	138	10.6	301	21.1	0.4	23.0	0.0
Dolcelatte, Average	*1 Serving/30g*	*110*	*9.7*	*366*	*17.8*	*0.4*	*32.3*	*0.4*
Double Gloucester, Average	*1 Serving/30g*	*121*	*10.2*	*404*	*24.5*	*0.1*	*34.0*	*0.0*
Doux De Montagne, Average	*1 Serving/25g*	*88*	*7.1*	*352*	*22.9*	*1.5*	*28.3*	*0.0*
Edam, Average	*1 Serving/10g*	*33*	*2.5*	*326*	*25.3*	*0.0*	*24.9*	*0.0*
Edam, Dutch, Garlic & Herb Wedge, Asda*	1 Serving/60g	197	15.0	329	26.0	0.0	25.0	0.0
Edam, Reduced Fat, Average	*1 Serving/30g*	*69*	*3.3*	*230*	*32.4*	*0.1*	*11.1*	*0.0*
Edam, Slices, Average	*1 Slice/30g*	*96*	*7.2*	*320*	*25.0*	*0.4*	*24.1*	*0.0*
Emmental, Average	*1 Serving/10g*	*37*	*2.8*	*368*	*28.3*	*0.0*	*28.3*	*0.0*
Emmental, Grated, President*	1 Pack/200g	728	56.0	364	28.0	0.0	28.0	0.0
Emmental, Light, Slices, President*	1 Slice/20g	60	3.6	298	34.0	0.0	18.0	0.0
Feta, Average	*1 Serving/30g*	*79*	*6.4*	*262*	*16.3*	*1.0*	*21.5*	*0.0*
Feta, Lemon, Asda*	1 Serving/25g	75	6.8	302	13.2	1.0	27.2	0.6
Fondue, Original, Fromalp*	1 Pack/400g	888	68.0	222	15.0	2.5	17.0	0.0
Fondue, Swiss, Easy Cook, Tesco*	¼ Pack/100g	235	17.0	235	15.5	4.0	17.0	0.0
Fondue, Traditionnelle, Co-Op*	1 Serving/100g	409	34.0	409	26.0	0.9	34.0	0.0
Fontina, Average	*1 Serving/28g*	*109*	*9.0*	*389*	*25.0*	*0.0*	*32.1*	*0.0*
Goats, Average	*1 Tsp/10g*	*26*	*2.1*	*262*	*13.8*	*3.8*	*21.2*	*0.0*
Goats, French, Mild, Average	*1 Serving/30g*	*49*	*3.5*	*163*	*11.2*	*3.0*	*11.8*	*0.0*
Goats, Premium, Average	*1 Serving/30g*	*98*	*7.8*	*327*	*20.5*	*0.6*	*26.1*	*0.0*
Gorgonzola, Average	*1 Serving/30g*	*100*	*8.1*	*334*	*20.0*	*0.0*	*27.0*	*0.0*
Gouda, Average	*1 Serving/30g*	*113*	*9.4*	*375*	*24.0*	*0.0*	*31.5*	*0.0*
Grana Padano, Italian Cheese, Waitrose*	1 Serving/14g	54	4.0	388	33.0	0.0	28.4	0.0
Gruyere	*1oz/28g*	*115*	*9.3*	*409*	*27.2*	*0.0*	*33.3*	*0.0*
Halloumi, Average	*1 Serving/80g*	*253*	*19.7*	*316*	*20.8*	*1.6*	*24.7*	*0.0*
Halloumi, Light Average	1 Serving/100g	245	15.3	245	24.7	1.7	15.3	0.0
Italian, Grated, Average	*1 Serving/30g*	*144*	*10.0*	*481*	*44.0*	*1.1*	*33.4*	*0.0*
Italian Hard, Basics, Sainsbury's*	1 Portion/30g	122	9.6	408	28.1	1.8	32.0	0.1
Jarlsberg, Slices, Average	*1 Slice/15g*	*54*	*4.0*	*360*	*27.0*	*0.0*	*27.0*	*0.0*
Lactose Free, Arla*	1 Serving/30g	103	8.1	344	25.3	1.0	27.0	0.0
Lancashire	*1oz/28g*	*104*	*8.7*	*373*	*23.3*	*0.1*	*31.0*	*0.0*
Manchego	*1 Serving/70g*	*339*	*30.8*	*485*	*22.2*	*0.1*	*44.0*	*0.0*
Marscapone, Lighter, Tesco*	½ Tub/125g	306	26.9	245	9.5	3.0	21.5	0.0
Mascarpone, 25% Less Fat, Sainsbury's*	1 Portion/30g	95	9.0	316	6.7	4.8	30.0	0.0
Mascarpone, Average	*1 Serving/30g*	*131*	*13.1*	*437*	*5.6*	*4.1*	*43.6*	*0.0*
Mature, Full Flavoured, LowLow, Kerry*	1 Serving/30g	91	6.6	302	26.0	0.2	22.0	0.0
Mature, Half Fat, Average	1 Serving/25g	66	3.9	265	29.9	0.4	15.6	0.1
Mature, Reduced Fat, Weight Watchers*	1 Serving/30g	65	3.1	217	31.0	0.1	10.3	0.0
Mild, Reduced Fat, Grated, Average	*1 Serving/30g*	*70*	*3.3*	*235*	*31.5*	*2.2*	*11.1*	*0.0*
Monterey Jack, Iga*	1 Serving/28g	110	9.0	393	25.0	0.0	32.1	0.0
Monterey Jack, Shredded, Kraft*	¼ Cup/28g	101	8.1	360	22.0	3.6	28.8	0.0
Morbier, Sainsbury's*	1 Serving/10g	33	2.4	330	28.0	0.1	24.2	0.0
Mozzarella, Average	*½ Ball/63g*	*172*	*12.9*	*275*	*21.2*	*1.2*	*20.6*	*0.0*
Mozzarella, Reduced Fat, Average	*½ Ball/63g*	*115*	*6.4*	*184*	*21.1*	*1.0*	*10.2*	*0.0*
Ossau-Iraty, Average	*1 Serving/30g*	*120*	*10.2*	*400*	*22.3*	*0.2*	*34.0*	*0.0*
Parmesan, Average	*1 Tbsp/10g*	*40*	*2.9*	*401*	*35.2*	*0.0*	*29.4*	*0.0*

CHEESE

INFO/WEIGHT	Measure	per Measure KCAL	FAT	Nutrition Values per 100g / 100ml KCAL	PROT	CARB	FAT	FIBRE
Parmigianino Reggiano, TTD, Sainsbury's*	1 Serving/30g	116	8.5	388	33.0	0.0	28.4	0.0
Pecorino, Italian, Tesco*	1 Serving/30g	119	9.9	397	22.0	0.0	33.0	0.0
Poivre, Boursin*	1oz/28g	116	11.8	414	7.0	2.0	42.0	0.0
Port Salut, M & S*	1oz/28g	90	7.3	322	21.0	1.0	26.0	0.0
Provolone Piccante, Sainsbury's*	1 Serving/30g	119	9.9	398	25.0	0.2	33.0	0.0
P'tit Louis, St Moret*	1 Serving/20g	49	4.6	247	5.0	5.0	23.0	0.0
Quark, Average	*1 Serving/20g*	*13*	*0.0*	*66*	*11.9*	*4.0*	*0.2*	*0.0*
Raclette, Richsmonts*	1 Slice/28g	100	8.0	357	25.0	0.0	28.6	0.0
Reblochon	*1 Serving/30g*	*95*	*8.0*	*318*	*19.7*	*0.0*	*26.6*	*0.0*
Red Leicester, Average	*1 Serving/30g*	*120*	*10.1*	*400*	*23.8*	*0.1*	*33.7*	*0.0*
Red Leicester, Reduced Fat, Average	*1 Serving/30g*	*78*	*4.6*	*261*	*30.2*	*0.1*	*15.4*	*0.0*
Ricotta, Average	*1 Serving/50g*	*67*	*4.7*	*134*	*9.3*	*2.9*	*9.5*	*0.0*
Roquefort, Average	*1oz/28g*	*105*	*9.2*	*375*	*19.7*	*0.0*	*32.9*	*0.0*
Roule, French, Sainsbury's*	1 Serving/30g	96	9.1	321	8.5	3.0	30.5	0.0
Roule, Garlic & Parsley, Light, BGTY, Sainsbury's*	1 Serving/30g	51	3.2	171	16.4	2.6	10.6	0.0
Sage Derby	*1oz/28g*	*113*	*9.5*	*402*	*24.2*	*0.1*	*33.9*	*0.0*
Sheeps, Hard, Parlick Fell, Sainsbury's*	1 Serving/30g	109	9.1	364	22.6	0.0	30.4	0.0
Shropshire, Blue, Average	*1 Serving/50g*	*195*	*17.1*	*391*	*21.0*	*0.0*	*34.2*	*0.0*
Soft, Blue, Philadelphia, Kraft*	1 Serving/28g	76	7.1	270	6.8	3.4	25.5	0.2
Soft, Extra Light, Average	*1 Serving/20g*	*25*	*1.2*	*125*	*14.3*	*3.5*	*5.9*	*0.1*
Soft, Fruit & Rum Halo, Discover*	1 Serving/25g	103	8.5	414	8.6	11.7	34.1	0.0
Soft, Full Fat, Average	*1 Serving/50g*	*156*	*15.2*	*312*	*8.2*	*1.7*	*30.3*	*0.0*
Soft, Full Fat, Original, Philadelphia, Kraft*	1 Serving/30g	76	7.2	253	6.0	3.3	24.0	0.3
Soft, Goats Milk	*1oz/28g*	*55*	*4.4*	*198*	*13.1*	*1.0*	*15.8*	*0.0*
Soft, Light, Average	*1 Tbsp/30g*	*54*	*3.9*	*179*	*12.1*	*3.2*	*13.1*	*0.0*
Soft, Light, Philadelphia, Kraft*	1 Serving/30g	47	3.5	157	8.7	4.0	11.7	0.3
Soft, Light with Grilled Peppers, Philadelphia*	1 Portion/30g	44	3.1	147	7.0	5.4	10.5	0.7
Soft, Medium Fat, Average	*1 Serving/30g*	*62*	*5.4*	*207*	*8.4*	*3.0*	*17.9*	*0.0*
Soft, Onion & Chives, Extra Light, Light Choices, Tesco*	1 Serving/30g	37	1.8	125	11.7	5.6	6.0	0.2
Soft, Onion & Chives, Less Than 5% Fat, M & S*	1 Serving/30g	30	1.4	100	10.7	4.4	4.7	1.2
Soft, Philadelphia, Extra Light, Kraft*	1 Serving/30g	33	1.4	110	11.7	5.0	4.7	0.3
Soft, Philadelphia, Garlic & Herb, Light, Kraft*	1 Serving/30g	47	3.5	157	8.3	4.0	11.7	0.3
Soft, Philadelphia, Light, Basil, Philadelphia, Kraft*	1 Serving/35g	51	3.7	146	8.0	4.0	10.5	0.5
Soft, Philadelphia, Mini Tubs, Cracked Pepper, Kraft*	1 Tub/35g	56	4.5	161	7.7	2.5	13.0	0.4
Soft, Philadelphia, Mini Tubs, Extra Light, Kraft*	1 Tub/35g	38	1.7	108	11.0	4.2	5.0	0.6
Soft, Philadelphia, Mini Tubs, Light, Kraft*	1 Tub/35g	55	4.0	158	8.7	4.0	11.5	0.4
Soft, Philadelphia with Chives, Light, Kraft*	1 Serving/30g	48	3.6	160	8.3	4.3	12.0	0.7
Soft, Pineapple Halo, Discover*	1 Serving/25g	101	8.1	404	7.2	16.6	32.6	1.2
Soft, Sun Dried Tomato & Basil, Light, Philadelphia*	1/8 Pack/25g	39	2.7	157	8.3	4.8	11.0	0.4
Soft, White, Lactofree, Arla*	1 Serving/30g	59	4.9	197	8.6	3.0	16.5	0.0
Soya	*1oz/28g*	*89*	*7.6*	*319*	*18.3*	*0.0*	*27.3*	*0.0*
Stilton, Average	*1 Serving/30g*	*123*	*10.6*	*410*	*22.4*	*0.1*	*35.5*	*0.0*
Stilton, Blue, Average	*1 Serving/30g*	*124*	*10.7*	*412*	*22.8*	*0.1*	*35.7*	*0.0*
Stilton, White, Average	*1oz/28g*	*101*	*8.8*	*362*	*19.9*	*0.1*	*31.3*	*0.0*
Stilton, White & Apricot, M & S*	1oz/28g	94	6.5	337	13.8	18.5	23.1	0.0
Stilton, White with Cranberries, Tesco*	1 Serving/50g	184	14.8	368	15.8	9.5	29.7	0.7
Stilton, White with Mango & Ginger, Tesco*	1/3 Pack/65g	227	14.0	350	13.1	25.8	21.6	0.6
Taleggio D.o.p., Finest, Tesco*	1 Serving/30g	89	7.5	297	18.0	0.0	25.0	0.0
Wedge, Leerdammer*	1 Serving/30g	112	8.6	373	28.3	0.0	28.6	0.0
Wedges, Camembert, Breaded, Morrisons*	1 Wedge/25g	88	5.5	352	15.1	22.9	22.2	2.0
Wensleydale, Average	*1 Serving/25g*	*92*	*7.8*	*369*	*22.4*	*0.1*	*31.0*	*0.0*
Wensleydale, Cranberry & Mustard, Lozzas	1 Block/50g	179	13.9	359	20.7	6.4	27.8	0.0
Wensleydale with Blueberries, M & S*	1 Portion/30g	111	7.9	370	18.7	13.4	26.4	0.9

	Measure INFO/WEIGHT	per Measure KCAL	FAT	Nutrition Values per 100g / 100ml KCAL	PROT	CARB	FAT	FIBRE
CHEESE								
Wensleydale with Cranberries, Sainsbury's*	1 Serving/50g	179	13.9	359	20.7	6.4	27.8	0.0
CHEESE ALTERNATIVE								
Cheezly, Cream, Original Flavour, The Redwood Co*	1 Pack/113g	357	34.5	316	5.6	4.8	30.5	0.0
Cheezly, Feta Style in Oil, The Redwood Co*	1 Serving/25g	119	11.7	475	2.5	10.6	47.0	0.0
Cheezly, Grated Cheddar Style, The Redwood Co*	1 Pack/150g	241	11.2	161	3.1	21.5	7.5	0.0
Cheezly, Mozzarella Style, The Redwood Co*	1 Portion/25g	69	6.3	274	5.4	5.9	25.4	1.0
Cheezly, Nacho Style, The Redwood Co*	1 Serving/25g	42	2.0	169	3.3	21.1	7.9	0.0
Mozzarella, Slices, Dairy Free	1 Slice/19g	80	6.0	420	10.5	10.5	31.5	0.0
Vegetarian, Average	1 Serving/30g	110	8.4	368	28.2	0.0	28.1	0.0
CHEESE ON TOAST								
Average	1 Slice/130g	494	34.2	380	13.8	23.8	26.3	0.7
CHEESE PUFFS								
Average	1 Bag/25g	129	7.4	517	7.7	54.8	29.5	1.5
Healthy Range, Average	1 Bag/25g	113	3.8	454	7.5	71.1	15.0	2.1
CHEESE SINGLES								
American, 2% Milk, Kraft*	1 Slice/19g	45	3.0	237	21.0	5.3	15.8	0.0
Healthy Range, Average	1 Slice/20g	39	2.1	197	20.6	5.2	10.4	0.0
Kraft*	1 Single/20g	52	3.7	260	13.5	7.6	18.5	0.0
CHEESE SPREAD								
60% Less Fat, Asda*	1 Serving/30g	52	2.7	174	16.0	7.3	9.0	0.0
Average	1 Serving/30g	76	6.4	254	9.4	5.9	21.4	0.1
Cheese & Garlic, Primula*	1 Serving/20g	49	3.7	247	15.7	4.3	18.6	0.0
Cheese & Ham, Primula*	1 Serving/20g	40	3.0	200	12.3	3.1	15.0	4.9
Cheese & Salmon with Dill, Primula*	1 Serving/30g	78	5.8	261	17.6	3.8	19.5	0.0
Cheez Whiz, Original, Light, 41% Less Fat, Kraft*	1 Tbsp/15g	31	1.7	210	15.7	11.7	11.3	0.0
Dairylea, Light, Tub, Kraft*	1 Serving/30g	44	2.1	147	14.5	6.1	7.0	0.0
Dairylea, Tub, Kraft*	1 Serving/25g	60	4.9	240	11.0	5.3	19.5	0.0
Flavoured	1oz/28g	72	5.7	258	14.2	4.4	20.5	0.0
Garlic & Herbs, Light, Benecol*	1 Serving/20g	35	2.8	174	7.8	4.2	14.0	0.7
Healthy Range, Average	1 Serving/30g	31	1.0	102	14.3	3.8	3.2	0.9
Light, Primula*	1 Serving/20g	30	1.8	149	15.2	3.0	8.9	3.6
Low Fat, Weight Watchers*	1 Serving/50g	56	1.4	112	18.1	3.4	2.9	1.2
Plain, Original, Primula*	1 Serving/30g	60	4.6	200	12.1	3.3	15.3	4.4
Squeeze, Light, The Laughing Cow, Fromageries Bel*	1 Portion/30g	42	2.1	139	12.0	7.0	7.0	5.0
Triangles, 50% Less Fat, Morrisons*	1 Portion/18g	29	1.4	166	15.0	8.5	8.0	0.0
with Chives, Primula*	1 Serving/30g	57	4.3	190	12.5	2.9	14.2	4.5
with Garlic & Herb, Soft, Free From, Sainsbury's*	1 Serving/30g	91	9.0	302	2.5	5.5	30.0	0.1
with Prawn, Primula*	1 Squeeze/25g	47	3.6	190	12.5	3.3	14.4	3.6
CHEESE STRAWS								
& Bacon, Party, Tesco*	1 Straw/13g	40	2.5	321	10.5	23.8	20.4	2.1
Cheddar, M & S*	1 Straw/11g	59	3.8	535	14.9	40.1	34.9	2.4
Cheese Twists, Tesco*	1 Straw/10g	99	5.6	494	14.0	46.4	28.0	4.2
Fudges*	1 Serving/10g	53	3.5	534	14.9	40.1	34.9	0.0
Homemade or Bakery, Average	1 Straw/41g	173	12.6	422	11.9	24.1	30.7	0.7
Selection, Sainsbury's*	1 Straw/7g	41	2.9	558	16.6	34.5	39.3	2.8
CHEESE TRIANGLES								
Average	1 Triangle/14g	33	2.2	238	10.3	14.1	15.6	0.2
Dairylea, Light, Kraft*	1 Triangle/20g	31	1.4	154	15.0	7.0	7.0	0.0
Extra Light, The Laughing Cow, Fromageries Bel*	1 Triangle/18g	20	0.5	116	15.0	6.5	3.0	0.0
Original, The Laughing Cow, Fromageries Bel*	1 Triangle/18g	42	3.3	239	11.0	6.0	19.0	0.0
Reduced Fat, Average	1 Triangle/18g	27	1.2	154	15.4	7.0	7.0	0.0
Tri-Bites, Dairylea, Kraft*	1 Triangle/20g	60	4.6	300	20.0	3.2	23.0	0.0

	Measure INFO/WEIGHT	per Measure KCAL	FAT	Nutrition Values per 100g / 100ml KCAL	PROT	CARB	FAT	FIBRE
CHEESE TWISTS								
Pre Packed, Average	1 Twist/8g	41	2.2	515	13.7	47.9	27.7	2.3
CHEESECAKE								
Apple & Cinnamon, Baked, M & S*	1 Serving/116g	390	22.0	335	3.7	39.7	18.9	2.1
Apricot, Co-Op*	1 Cake/100g	230	11.0	230	4.0	29.0	11.0	0.9
Autumn Berry, Waitrose*	1 Slice/92g	316	20.3	343	4.4	31.5	22.1	2.0
Average	1 Slice/115g	490	40.8	426	3.7	24.6	35.5	0.4
Belgian Chocolate, M & S*	1 Slice/100g	385	23.9	385	5.3	39.2	23.9	2.5
Blackcurrant, Average	1 Serving/90g	237	11.9	263	3.6	32.3	13.2	2.3
Blackcurrant, Healthy Range, Average	1 Serving/90g	182	4.7	203	4.7	33.6	5.3	2.1
Blackcurrant, VLH Kitchens	1 Serving/120g	341	13.7	285	3.4	32.0	16.4	0.9
Blackcurrant, Weight Watchers*	1 Cake/103g	191	2.9	185	4.6	35.4	2.8	3.5
Blackcurrant Devonshire, McVitie's*	1/6 Cake/67g	193	11.5	288	3.8	29.7	17.1	1.7
Blackcurrant Swirl, Heinz*	1/5 Cake/87g	241	13.4	277	4.1	30.3	15.4	3.6
Blueberry & Lemon Flavour Wedges, Sainsbury's*	1 Serving/80g	262	16.9	327	5.1	29.2	21.1	1.2
Caramel Swirl, Cadbury*	1 Slice/91g	373	23.5	410	6.0	40.1	25.8	0.0
Cherry, BGTY, Sainsbury's*	1 Serving/91g	181	3.9	199	4.6	35.5	4.3	0.5
Cherry, Healthy Range, Average	1 Serving/90g	172	3.0	191	3.7	36.4	3.3	1.1
Chocolate, Baked, Ultimate, Entenmann's*	1 Serving/100g	331	19.0	331	5.7	34.2	19.0	2.8
Chocolate, Pure Indulgence, Thorntons*	1 Serving/75g	307	17.5	410	5.6	44.3	23.4	0.6
Chocolate, Tesco*	1 Serving/91g	317	17.4	348	6.2	37.8	19.1	1.5
Chocolate, Weight Watchers*	1 Cake/95g	143	3.8	151	7.5	20.7	4.0	0.7
Chocolate & Hazelnut, Sara Lee*	1 Serving/65g	224	13.9	345	6.5	31.2	21.4	1.2
Chocolate & Irish Cream Liqueur, Tesco*	1 Serving/93g	385	28.0	414	5.0	30.7	30.1	0.8
Chocolate & Vanilla, Gu*	1 Cake/90g	323	22.4	359	4.1	29.6	24.9	1.4
Chocolate & Vanilla, Reduced Fat, M & S*	1 Serving/114g	319	13.7	280	7.0	37.9	12.0	1.5
Chocolate Swirl, Deeply Delicious, Heinz*	1/5 Cake/82g	221	9.4	271	4.6	37.4	11.5	4.7
Chocolate Truffle, HL, Tesco*	1 Slice/96g	250	13.2	260	10.3	23.7	13.8	6.5
Commercially Prepared	1/6 Cake/80g	257	18.0	321	5.5	25.5	22.5	0.4
Fudge, Tesco*	1 Serving/102g	384	23.6	376	4.6	37.5	23.1	0.5
Irish Cream, McVitie's*	¼ Slice/190g	616	36.9	324	4.4	33.0	19.4	0.4
Lemon, Average	1 Serving/90g	307	19.5	341	4.1	33.0	21.6	1.8
Lemon, Carb Control, Tesco*	1 Serving/85g	269	23.0	316	8.6	9.6	27.1	11.1
Lemon, Healthy Range, Average	1 Serving/90g	185	4.0	205	5.3	33.5	4.4	1.1
Lemon, Swirl, Asda*	1 Pack/125g	445	29.9	356	3.1	32.1	23.9	1.8
Lemon, Weight Watchers*	1 Serving/100g	211	5.0	211	6.3	30.1	5.0	1.8
Lemon Meringue, Tesco*	1 Slice/94g	352	25.0	375	3.8	30.1	26.6	0.3
Mandarin, Co-Op*	1 Slice/99g	297	16.8	300	4.0	32.0	17.0	0.3
Mandarin, GFY, Asda*	1/6 Cake/92g	178	4.0	194	3.6	35.0	4.4	1.2
Mandarin, Low Fat, Tesco*	1 Serving/70g	145	3.3	207	3.3	37.0	4.7	1.4
Mandarin, Weight Watchers*	1 Cake/103g	180	2.9	175	4.6	32.9	2.8	1.5
Raspberry, BGTY, Sainsbury's*	1 Pot/95g	154	2.5	163	6.6	28.2	2.6	2.8
Raspberry, Creamy, Tesco*	1 Serving/100g	365	23.4	365	5.9	32.1	23.4	0.9
Raspberry, Light Choices, Tesco*	1 Cake/95g	185	4.1	195	4.3	34.7	4.3	1.3
Raspberry, M & S*	1 Slice/105g	331	21.5	315	5.0	32.2	20.5	1.0
Raspberry, Perfectly Balanced, Waitrose*	1 Serving/106g	212	3.7	200	4.0	36.2	3.5	1.7
Raspberry, Weight Watchers*	1 Serving/100g	213	4.3	213	5.9	29.7	4.3	1.9
Raspberry Swirl, Heinz*	1 Serving/100g	266	14.5	266	3.9	30.1	14.5	2.8
Rhubarb Crumble, Sainsbury's*	1 Serving/114g	268	10.6	235	3.1	34.8	9.3	2.4
Strawberries & Cream, Finest, Tesco*	1 Serving/104g	325	22.4	312	4.3	25.3	21.5	0.5
Strawberries & Devonshire Cream, Heinz*	1/6 Cake/66g	184	10.1	279	3.9	31.4	15.3	3.7
Strawberry, Baked New York, Sara Lee*	1 Serving/100g	248	9.9	248	4.7	34.9	9.9	0.7
Strawberry, Creamy, Weight Watchers*	1 Cake/105g	187	2.6	178	4.7	34.2	2.5	2.2
Strawberry, Finest, Tesco*	1 Slice/113g	383	25.1	339	4.8	30.1	22.2	0.9

	Measure INFO/WEIGHT	per Measure KCAL	FAT	Nutrition Values per 100g / 100ml KCAL	PROT	CARB	FAT	FIBRE
CHEESECAKE								
Strawberry, Fresh, M & S*	¼ Cake/125g	300	19.2	240	2.8	23.1	15.4	1.1
Strawberry, Heinz*	1 Pack/245g	588	31.1	240	3.4	28.1	12.7	2.4
Strawberry, Tesco*	1 Serving/100g	254	12.0	254	3.9	32.5	12.0	0.0
Strawberry Shortcake, Sara Lee*	1/6 Slice/68g	230	15.7	337	4.9	27.6	23.0	0.5
Strawberry Swirl, Chosen By You, Asda*	1 Serving/100g	329	15.9	329	4.5	41.5	15.9	1.0
Toffee, American Style, Asda*	1 Serving/75g	269	15.7	359	4.5	38.0	21.0	3.8
Toffee, Asda*	1 Cake/87g	295	19.1	339	4.3	31.0	22.0	3.5
Toffee, M & S*	1 Serving/105g	357	22.6	340	5.2	37.2	21.5	0.9
Toffee, Mini, Asda*	1 Cake/20g	57	2.4	286	4.6	40.0	12.0	2.1
Toffee & Pecan, Wedge, Sainsbury's*	1 Serving/75g	296	21.7	395	5.4	28.1	29.0	3.1
Toffee Swirl, Chosen By You, Asda*	1 Serving/100g	334	16.1	334	5.5	41.4	16.1	0.9
Vanilla	1 Serving/100g	395	26.2	395	5.3	42.8	26.2	1.1
Vanilla, Tesco*	1 Serving/115g	417	28.4	363	5.7	29.4	24.7	0.6
CHERRIES								
Black, Fresh, Average	*1 Serving/80g*	*41*	*0.1*	*51*	*0.9*	*11.5*	*0.1*	*1.6*
Black in Syrup, Average	*1 Serving/242g*	*160*	*0.0*	*66*	*0.6*	*16.0*	*0.0*	*0.7*
Dried, Love Life, Waitrose*	1 Portion/10g	35	0.1	348	0.2	84.3	1.1	2.1
Glace, Average	*1oz/28g*	*79*	*0.0*	*280*	*0.3*	*71.2*	*0.1*	*1.1*
Picota, Average	1 Serving/80g	42	0.1	52	0.9	11.4	0.1	1.2
Raw, Average	*1oz/28g*	*14*	*0.0*	*49*	*0.9*	*11.2*	*0.1*	*1.4*
Stewed with Sugar, Average	*1oz/28g*	*23*	*0.0*	*82*	*0.7*	*21.0*	*0.1*	*0.7*
Stewed without Sugar, Average	*1oz/28g*	*12*	*0.0*	*42*	*0.8*	*10.1*	*0.1*	*0.8*
CHESTNUTS								
Roasted, Peeled, Average	*1 Nut/10g*	*17*	*0.3*	*170*	*2.0*	*36.6*	*2.7*	*4.1*
CHEWING GUM								
Airwaves, Sugar Free, Wrigleys*	1 Pack/15g	23	0.0	155	0.0	62.0	0.0	0.0
Extra, Cool Breeze, Wrigleys*	1 Piece/2g	3	0.0	153	0.0	64.0	0.0	0.0
Extra, Peppermint, Sugar Free, Wrigleys*	1 Piece/2g	3	0.0	155	0.0	39.0	0.0	0.0
Peppermint, Soft, Sugar Free, Trident*	1 Stick/3g	4	0.0	155	0.4	62.3	0.4	0.0
Peppermint, Sugar Free, Active, Aldi*	2 Pieces/3g	4	0.0	146	0.0	61.0	0.0	0.0
Spearmint, Extra, Wrigleys*	1 Piece/1g	1	0.0	143	0.0	64.3	0.0	0.0
Spearmint, Wrigleys*	1 Piece/3g	9	0.0	295	0.0	73.0	0.0	0.0
Splash, Raspberry & Peach, Trident*	1 Piece/2g	4	0.0	180	1.6	68.5	0.5	0.0
Sugar Free, Pulse, Crisp Tropical Flavour, Wrigleys*	1 Stick/1g	2	0.0	161	0.0	65.0	0.0	0.0
CHICK PEAS								
Canned, Drained, Asda*	½ Can/120g	125	1.2	104	7.6	12.6	1.0	7.2
Canned in Water, Drained, Tesco*	1 Can/120g	144	3.5	120	7.2	16.1	2.9	4.1
Dried, Average	*1 Serving/100g*	*319*	*5.4*	*319*	*21.7*	*47.4*	*5.4*	*8.0*
Dried, Boiled, Average	*1 Serving/75g*	*85*	*1.7*	*114*	*7.3*	*16.4*	*2.2*	*2.5*
in Mediterranean Tomato Sauce, Branston*	½ Can/210g	189	2.1	90	4.8	15.5	1.0	3.2
in Salted Water, Canned, Average	*1 Can/179g*	*204*	*5.2*	*114*	*7.2*	*14.9*	*2.9*	*4.1*
in Salted Water, KTC*	1 Can/400g	304	6.0	76	5.0	13.0	1.5	0.0
in Water, Canned, Average	*1 Can/250g*	*282*	*6.5*	*113*	*7.2*	*15.3*	*2.6*	*4.8*
in Water, Canned, Essential, Waitrose*	1 Can/410g	451	9.4	110	6.6	15.5	2.3	4.8
CHICKEN								
Bites, Battered, Tesco*	1 Pack/200g	440	28.6	220	15.2	7.6	14.3	2.0
Bites, Hot & Spicy, Tesco*	1 Pack/110g	143	1.8	130	18.9	9.6	1.6	2.5
Bites, Southern Fried, Tesco*	1 Pack/300g	720	33.3	240	18.1	16.9	11.1	2.1
Bites, Tikka, Average	1 Serving/50g	96	5.3	193	20.7	3.8	10.5	1.9
Bites in Light Batter, Captain Birds Eye, Birds Eye*	1 Piece/15g	31	1.9	210	18.6	5.8	12.5	0.2
Breast, Chargrilled, Lemon & Herb, Bernard Matthews*	1 Serving/100g	154	4.5	154	23.7	4.7	4.5	0.0
Breast, Chargrilled, Premium, Average	1 Piece/10g	20	1.1	197	21.6	1.5	11.2	0.3
Breast, Chargrilled, Sliced, Average	1 Slice/19g	24	0.5	124	24.4	0.5	2.7	0.4

C

CHICKEN

	Measure INFO/WEIGHT	per Measure KCAL	FAT	Nutrition Values per 100g / 100ml KCAL	PROT	CARB	FAT	FIBRE
Breast, Chinese Style, Cooked, Sliced, Sainsbury's*	½ Pack/65g	96	1.2	148	28.3	4.7	1.8	0.1
Breast, Diced, Average	**1 Serving/188g**	**242**	**4.4**	**129**	**26.9**	**0.1**	**2.3**	**0.1**
Breast, Eastern Spices, Birds Eye*	1 Portion/175g	308	20.8	176	13.5	3.8	11.9	1.5
Breast, Escalope, Plain, Average	**1 Serving/100g**	**110**	**2.2**	**110**	**22.3**	**0.7**	**2.2**	**0.5**
Breast, Fillet, Mesquite, KP Snacks*	1 Serving/85g	130	7.0	153	20.0	1.2	8.2	0.0
Breast, Fillets, Breaded, Average	1 Fillet/112g	246	11.6	220	17.5	14.0	10.4	1.3
Breast, Fillets, Breaded, Lemon & Pepper, Average	1 Fillet/89g	133	2.0	150	22.0	10.1	2.3	1.3
Breast, Fillets, Cajun, Average	1 Fillet/93g	124	2.6	134	23.6	3.5	2.8	0.3
Breast, Fillets, Chargrilled, Average	1 Serving/100g	120	1.1	120	27.3	0.3	1.1	0.3
Breast, Fillets, Free Range, TTD, Sainsbury's*	1 Fillet/146g	186	1.8	127	29.1	0.0	1.2	0.0
Breast, Fillets, Frozen, Value, Tesco*	1 Fillet/125g	125	2.1	100	20.4	0.7	1.7	0.0
Breast, Fillets, Garlic & Herb, Tesco*	1 Fillet/135g	290	12.1	215	18.9	14.4	9.0	1.3
Breast, Fillets, Korma Style, Average	1 Serving/100g	131	2.7	131	27.4	0.8	2.7	0.5
Breast, Fillets, Lemon Parsley, M & S*	½ Pack/145g	232	3.5	160	14.3	20.7	2.4	4.3
Breast, Fillets, Mini, Raw, Average	**1oz/28g**	**34**	**0.4**	**121**	**26.9**	**0.2**	**1.5**	**0.1**
Breast, Fillets, Organic, Average	**1 Serving/150g**	**153**	**1.1**	**102**	**23.9**	**0.0**	**0.7**	**0.0**
Breast, Fillets, Skinless & Boneless, Raw, Average	**1 Breast/100g**	**129**	**2.0**	**129**	**27.8**	**0.0**	**2.0**	**0.0**
Breast, Grilled, Average	**1 Breast/130g**	**174**	**2.8**	**134**	**28.9**	**0.1**	**2.2**	**0.0**
Breast, Joint, Lemon & Tarragon, Finest, Tesco*	1 Serving/175g	247	11.0	141	18.8	2.3	6.3	0.2
Breast, Latino Style, Asda*	1 Breast/65g	99	2.0	152	27.0	4.1	3.1	0.5
Breast, Lemon Pepper, Cooked, Birds Eye*	1 Piece/101g	261	14.1	260	15.0	19.0	14.0	0.9
Breast, Meat & Skin, Raw, Average	**1 Serving/145g**	**249**	**13.4**	**172**	**20.8**	**0.0**	**9.2**	**0.0**
Breast, Meat & Skin, Weighed with Bone, Raw, Average	**1oz/28g**	**48**	**2.6**	**172**	**20.8**	**0.0**	**9.2**	**0.0**
Breast, Meat Only, Fried	**1 Portion/50g**	**93**	**2.4**	**187**	**33.4**	**0.5**	**4.7**	**0.0**
Breast, Pieces, Tikka, Average	1 Serving/100g	154	3.3	154	28.2	2.7	3.3	0.4
Breast, Roast, Sliced, From Supermarket, Average	**1 Slice/13g**	**17**	**0.4**	**139**	**25.0**	**1.8**	**3.5**	**0.2**
Breast, Roast, without Skin, Average	**1oz/28g**	**42**	**1.3**	**149**	**25.4**	**1.0**	**4.7**	**0.2**
Breast, Roll, Average	**1 Slice/10g**	**17**	**1.0**	**167**	**16.1**	**3.2**	**10.0**	**0.2**
Breast, Smoked, Sliced, Average	**1 Slice/20g**	**22**	**0.5**	**110**	**20.7**	**0.9**	**2.6**	**0.1**
Breast, Southern Fried, Premium, Bernard Matthews*	1 Serving/60g	70	1.7	117	19.6	3.1	2.9	0.6
Breast, Strips, Raw, Average	**1 Serving/280g**	**358**	**5.7**	**128**	**27.1**	**0.3**	**2.0**	**0.3**
Breast, Tandoori Style, Average	1 Serving/180g	237	6.7	131	22.3	2.3	3.7	1.0
Breast, Tikka, Sliced, Average	1oz/28g	34	0.5	120	24.9	2.0	1.7	0.6
Chargrills, Garlic, Weight After Cooking, Birds Eye*	1 Chargrill/95g	182	10.4	192	19.0	4.0	11.0	0.1
Chargrills, Garlic, Weight Before Cooking, Birds Eye*	1 Chargrill/95g	190	10.7	200	20.3	4.2	11.3	0.1
Chargrills, Original, Weight Before Cooking, Birds Eye*	1 Chargrill/95g	156	8.5	164	17.5	3.2	9.0	0.1
Chargrills, Weight After Cooking, Baked, Birds Eye*	1 Chargrill/90g	160	8.7	178	18.9	3.4	9.7	0.1
Drumsticks, BBQ Flavour, Average	1 Serving/200g	348	16.0	174	22.6	3.1	8.0	0.4
Drumsticks, Breaded, Fried, Average	1oz/28g	70	4.1	248	19.6	9.9	14.6	0.6
Drumsticks, Chinese Style, Average	1 Stick/100g	177	8.1	177	22.5	3.5	8.1	0.7
Drumsticks with Skin, Average	**1 Piece/125g**	**268**	**16.6**	**215**	**22.1**	**1.8**	**13.3**	**0.3**
Escalope, Breaded, Average	1 Piece/128g	361	21.6	282	13.4	19.1	16.9	0.7
Fillets, Battered, Average	1 Fillet/90g	199	10.4	221	16.1	13.3	11.5	0.5
Fillets, Breaded, Average	1 Piece/98g	214	10.5	219	14.2	15.9	10.7	1.9
Fillets, Chilli & Mango, Tesco*	1 Serving/100g	130	0.7	130	27.1	3.7	0.7	1.0
Fillets, Chinese Style, Average	1oz/28g	37	0.5	131	24.4	4.6	1.7	0.5
Fillets, Coronation, BGTY, Sainsbury's*	1 Fillet/100g	136	2.6	136	27.1	2.4	2.6	1.0
Fillets, Hickory Barbecue & Chilli, BGTY, Sainsbury's*	1 Fillet/100g	133	1.2	133	26.9	3.6	1.2	0.9
Fillets, Hickory Style BBQ, Tesco*	1 Fillet/80g	112	1.8	140	28.4	1.5	2.2	0.5
Fillets, Honey & Mustard, Average	1 Serving/100g	138	3.7	138	18.4	7.5	3.7	0.8
Fillets, Hot & Spicy, Average	1oz/28g	58	3.1	206	16.4	10.5	11.0	1.1
Fillets, Lime & Coriander, Mini, Average	1 Fillet/42g	49	0.5	118	24.3	2.6	1.3	0.6
Fillets, Red Thai, Mini, Average	1oz/28g	36	0.6	127	21.7	5.4	2.0	0.6

CHICKEN

INFO/WEIGHT	Measure	per Measure		Nutrition Values per 100g / 100ml				
		KCAL	FAT	KCAL	PROT	CARB	FAT	FIBRE
Fillets, Southern Fried, Meat Only, Average	1 Piece/100g	222	12.0	222	16.4	12.2	12.0	1.1
Fillets, Tandoori Style, Mini, Average	1 Serving/100g	127	2.0	127	24.7	2.5	2.0	0.3
Fillets, Tikka, Average	1 Serving/100g	141	5.0	141	22.4	1.7	5.0	1.1
Fillets, Tikka, Mini, Average	1oz/28g	35	0.6	124	25.1	1.3	2.1	1.1
Fillets, Tomato & Basil, Mini, Average	1oz/28g	34	0.6	123	23.4	2.5	2.1	0.3
Fingers, Average	1 Serving/75g	187	9.9	250	13.7	18.7	13.2	1.1
Garlic, Frozen, Tesco*	1 Serving/95g	182	8.3	192	15.6	12.9	8.7	1.0
Garlic Basted, Morrisons*	1 Serving/100g	231	13.1	231	23.3	0.7	13.1	0.4
Goujons, Breaded, Average	1 Serving/114g	293	17.1	258	15.8	15.2	15.0	1.0
Goujons, Breast, Fresh, Average	1oz/28g	36	0.5	127	28.0	0.0	1.6	0.0
Goujons, Cracked Black Pepper, American, Asda*	1 Serving/150g	333	21.0	222	16.0	8.0	14.0	2.5
Goujons, Garlic & Herb, Breaded, American, Asda*	½ Pack/150g	376	22.5	251	17.0	12.0	15.0	2.1
Goujons, Hot & Spicy, Sainsbury's*	½ Pack/125g	252	9.6	202	20.0	13.1	7.7	1.2
Leg, Meat Only, Raw, Average	*1oz/28g*	*34*	*1.1*	*120*	*20.1*	*0.0*	*3.8*	*0.0*
Leg, Meat Only, Raw with Skin & Bone, Average	*1oz/28g*	*38*	*1.2*	*134*	*22.5*	*0.0*	*4.3*	*0.0*
Leg, Meat Only, Stewed with Bone & Skin, Average	*1oz/28g*	*52*	*2.3*	*185*	*26.3*	*0.0*	*8.1*	*0.0*
Leg or Thigh, Hot & Spicy, Average	1oz/28g	50	3.0	179	19.4	1.0	10.8	0.4
Leg Portion, Roast, weighed with Bone, without Skin	1 Portion/114g	246	15.5	216	43.5	0.0	13.6	0.0
Leg with Skin, Raw, Average	*1oz/28g*	*48*	*2.9*	*172*	*19.1*	*0.0*	*10.4*	*0.0*
Leg with Skin, Roasted, Average	*1oz/28g*	*66*	*4.6*	*234*	*21.5*	*0.1*	*16.4*	*0.0*
Light Meat, Raw	*1oz/28g*	*30*	*0.3*	*106*	*24.0*	*0.0*	*1.1*	*0.0*
Light Meat, Roasted	*1oz/28g*	*43*	*1.0*	*153*	*30.2*	*0.0*	*3.6*	*0.0*
Meat, Roasted, Average	*1oz/28g*	*50*	*2.1*	*177*	*27.3*	*0.0*	*7.5*	*0.0*
Meat & Skin, Raw, Average	*1oz/28g*	*64*	*5.0*	*230*	*17.6*	*0.0*	*17.7*	*0.0*
Meat & Skin, Roasted, Average	*1oz/28g*	*60*	*3.9*	*216*	*22.6*	*0.0*	*14.0*	*0.0*
Meat & Skin Portions, Deep Fried, Average	1oz/28g	73	4.7	259	26.9	0.0	16.8	0.0
Mince, Average	*1oz/28g*	*39*	*1.7*	*140*	*20.9*	*0.1*	*6.0*	*0.2*
Nuggets, Battered, Average	1 Nugget/20g	50	2.9	251	13.5	16.9	14.4	0.9
Nuggets, Breaded, Average	1 Nugget/14g	37	2.0	263	14.8	19.8	13.8	1.9
Skewers, BBQ, George Foreman's Lean Mean Grillers*	1 Skewer/60g	68	0.8	114	20.0	5.5	1.4	0.4
Skewers, Marinated, Asda*	1 Skewer/35g	50	0.4	142	24.9	8.0	1.2	0.9
Skewers with Chorizo, Bighams*	1 Skewer/95g	129	6.5	136	17.1	1.5	6.9	0.5
Spatchcock, Poussin, Sainsbury's*	1 Serving/122g	168	6.6	138	21.1	0.1	5.4	0.2
Spatchcock, Salt & Cracked Pepper, Sainsbury's*	1 Serving/122g	168	6.6	138	21.1	0.1	5.4	0.2
Spicy, Fried, Sainsbury's*	1 Serving/150g	414	24.9	276	28.8	2.9	16.6	2.1
Steaks, Average	*1 Serving/100g*	*205*	*9.4*	*205*	*21.1*	*9.0*	*9.4*	*0.7*
Steaks, Garlic & Herb, Tesco*	1 Serving/138g	354	23.2	257	14.1	12.2	16.9	1.7
Sticks, Chilli, Southern Fried, Tesco*	5 Sticks/52g	167	11.4	322	13.4	17.8	21.9	1.1
Strips, Breast, Grilled, KP Snacks*	1 Serving/84g	90	1.5	107	25.0	0.0	1.8	0.0
Strips, Mexican, Sliced, M & S*	½ Pack/70g	77	0.4	110	24.3	2.3	0.6	0.5
Strips or Tenders, Chinese Style, Average	1oz/28g	41	1.1	145	19.6	7.9	4.1	1.0
Thigh, Meat & Skin, Average	*1 Serving/100g*	*218*	*14.7*	*218*	*21.4*	*0.0*	*14.7*	*0.0*
Thigh, Meat & Skin, Casseroled, Average	*1oz/28g*	*65*	*4.6*	*233*	*21.5*	*0.0*	*16.3*	*0.0*
Thigh, Meat Only, Diced, Casseroled	*1oz/28g*	*50*	*2.4*	*180*	*25.6*	*0.0*	*8.6*	*0.0*
Thigh, Meat Only, Raw, Average	*1 Thigh/90g*	*113*	*4.9*	*126*	*19.4*	*0.0*	*5.4*	*0.0*
Thigh, Roast, Average	*1 Serving/100g*	*238*	*15.6*	*238*	*23.8*	*0.4*	*15.6*	*0.0*
Wafer Thin, Average	1 Slice/10g	12	0.4	120	19.0	2.8	3.6	0.1
Wafer Thin, Coronation, Sainsbury's*	½ Pack/50g	67	2.2	135	19.1	4.5	4.5	0.1
Whole, Roast, Average	*1oz/28g*	*59*	*3.7*	*211*	*21.2*	*1.5*	*13.4*	*0.2*
Whole, Roasted, Brown Sugar Marinade, Tesco*	1 Serving/100g	195	11.3	195	22.1	0.1	11.3	0.1
Wing, Breaded, Fried, Average	1oz/28g	82	5.2	294	18.4	14.0	18.5	0.4
Wing, Meat & Skin, Cooked, Average	*1oz/28g*	*67*	*4.4*	*241*	*23.3*	*1.9*	*15.6*	*0.3*
Wing Quarter, Meat Only, Casseroled	*1oz/28g*	*46*	*1.8*	*164*	*26.9*	*0.0*	*6.3*	*0.0*

C

	Measure INFO/WEIGHT	per Measure KCAL	FAT	Nutrition Values per 100g / 100ml KCAL	PROT	CARB	FAT	FIBRE

CHICKEN

	Measure INFO/WEIGHT	per Measure KCAL	FAT	KCAL	PROT	CARB	FAT	FIBRE
Wings, BBQ Flavour, Average	1oz/28g	61	3.5	219	20.3	6.5	12.4	0.6
Wings, Chinese Style, Average	1oz/28g	72	4.3	256	24.2	5.1	15.5	0.6
Wings, Hot & Spicy, Average	1oz/28g	65	3.8	231	21.8	5.1	13.6	0.8
Wings, Meat & Skin, Raw, Average	*1oz/28g*	*52*	*3.3*	*184*	*19.0*	*0.5*	*11.8*	*0.2*

CHICKEN &

	Measure INFO/WEIGHT	per Measure KCAL	FAT	KCAL	PROT	CARB	FAT	FIBRE
Apricot Rice, COU, M & S*	1 Pack/400g	360	3.6	90	9.4	10.6	0.9	0.7
Asparagus in a Champagne Sauce, Finest, Tesco*	1 Pack/500g	615	33.5	123	8.8	7.0	6.7	0.9
Asparagus with Rice, Frozen, Low Fat, Waitrose*	1 Pack/380g	403	7.6	106	8.5	13.6	2.0	0.6
Bacon, Easy Steam, Tesco*	1 Pack/400g	728	36.4	182	11.7	13.6	9.1	0.8
Bacon Parcels, Sainsbury's*	½ Pack/170g	406	28.6	239	21.9	0.1	16.8	0.0
Black Bean, Chinese, Tesco*	1 Pack/350g	381	17.2	109	8.9	7.4	4.9	0.7
Black Bean, Chinese Takeaway, Tesco*	1 Serving/200g	190	6.6	95	8.3	8.0	3.3	0.5
Black Bean, Special Fried Rice, HL, Tesco*	1 Pack/450g	360	6.3	80	6.8	9.5	1.4	0.9
Black Bean, with Noodles, Tesco*	1 Pack/475g	470	7.6	99	7.6	13.6	1.6	0.2
Black Bean, with Rice, Chinese, Tesco*	1 Serving/450g	459	9.5	102	5.3	15.4	2.1	0.5
Black Bean, with Rice, HL, Tesco*	1 Pack/450g	463	7.2	103	6.9	19.6	1.6	0.6
Black Bean Noodles, Sainsbury's*	1 Serving/130g	155	0.9	119	4.3	23.9	0.7	0.8
Cashew Nuts, Chinese, Cantonese, Sainsbury's*	½ Pack/175g	171	8.7	98	8.4	4.9	5.0	1.3
Cashew Nuts, Chinese, Ready Meal, Average	1 Serving/400g	497	24.0	124	9.2	7.5	6.0	1.2
Cashew Nuts, Chinese, Tesco*	1 Pack/350g	378	19.6	108	9.5	4.9	5.6	0.6
Cashew Nuts, Easy Steam, Tesco*	1 Serving/400g	460	19.2	115	8.7	9.2	4.8	1.0
Cashew Nuts, Oriental, HL, Tesco*	1 Pack/450g	436	4.5	97	7.0	15.1	1.0	0.7
Chorizo Paella, Go Cook, Asda*	½ Pack/475g	591	10.5	124	10.2	15.9	2.2	2.6
Cranberry, Perfectly Balanced, Waitrose*	1 Pack/240g	161	1.0	67	11.8	4.1	0.4	1.1
Fries, Southern Fried, Sainsbury's*	½ Pack/250g	562	21.7	225	10.5	26.2	8.7	0.8
Gravy, COU, M & S*	1 Pack/300g	216	3.9	72	7.2	7.8	1.3	1.6
Herb Pasta with Lemon, HL, Tesco*	1 Pack/400g	520	8.0	130	8.2	18.8	2.0	1.6
King Prawn Special Fried Rice, Finest, Tesco*	1 Pack/450g	733	31.9	163	7.7	17.0	7.1	0.7
Mushroom, Chinese, Sainsbury's*	½ Pack/175g	115	3.5	66	7.6	4.4	2.0	0.9
Mushroom, Chinese, Tesco*	1 Pack/460g	474	12.9	103	5.7	13.8	2.8	1.0
Peppers, M & S*	1 Serving/240g	264	10.8	110	14.7	2.3	4.5	0.6
Pineapple, Chilled, Tesco*	1 Pack/350g	364	8.4	104	9.6	11.1	2.4	5.5
Pineapple, with Egg Fried Rice, HL, Tesco*	1 Pack/450g	414	3.1	92	6.0	15.4	0.7	0.6
Pineapple, with Egg Fried Rice, Tesco*	1 Pack/450g	450	10.8	100	7.6	12.1	2.4	1.2
Pineapple, with Rice, HL, Tesco*	1 Pack/450g	400	7.2	89	6.6	12.0	1.6	1.0
Pineapple, with Vegetable Rice, M & S*	1 Pack/400g	400	7.6	100	7.2	13.0	1.9	1.6
Roasted Peppers, 655, Oakhouse Foods Ltd*	1 Meal/440g	356	11.4	81	6.6	8.0	2.6	0.9
Stuffing, Roast, HL, Tesco*	1 Serving/17g	19	0.2	111	23.3	1.3	1.4	0.2
Tomato Saag, with Pilau Rice, BGTY, Sainsbury's*	1 Pack/400g	404	4.0	101	7.3	15.6	1.0	1.0

CHICKEN ALFREDO

	Measure INFO/WEIGHT	per Measure KCAL	FAT	KCAL	PROT	CARB	FAT	FIBRE
Average	1 Pack/400g	416	10.0	104	12.2	8.2	2.5	0.8
BGTY, Sainsbury's*	1 Serving/200g	208	5.4	104	18.0	1.9	2.7	0.5

CHICKEN ARRABBIATA

	Measure INFO/WEIGHT	per Measure KCAL	FAT	KCAL	PROT	CARB	FAT	FIBRE
Al Forno, Sainsbury's*	1 Pack/900g	1026	22.5	114	6.5	16.4	2.5	1.4
Bistro, Waitrose*	½ Pack/175g	156	5.2	89	12.9	2.5	3.0	0.5
Easy Steam, HL, Tesco*	1 Pack/400g	284	3.2	71	8.4	7.6	0.8	1.2
GFY, Asda*	1 Pack/448g	394	3.1	88	5.2	15.1	0.7	1.1
Weight Watchers, Heinz*	1 Serving/300g	222	1.8	74	5.4	11.5	0.6	0.8

CHICKEN BANG BANG

	Measure INFO/WEIGHT	per Measure KCAL	FAT	KCAL	PROT	CARB	FAT	FIBRE
Oriental Express*	½ Pack/200g	170	3.4	85	6.4	11.0	1.7	3.2
Waitrose*	1 Pack/350g	367	17.2	105	9.4	5.9	4.9	1.2

CHICKEN BARBECUE

	Measure INFO/WEIGHT	per Measure KCAL	FAT	KCAL	PROT	CARB	FAT	FIBRE
with Potato Wedges, Eat Smart, Morrisons*	1 Pack/350g	367	4.9	105	8.5	14.5	1.4	1.5

	Measure INFO/WEIGHT	per Measure		Nutrition Values per 100g / 100ml				
		KCAL	FAT	KCAL	PROT	CARB	FAT	FIBRE
CHICKEN BUTTER								
with Rice, Average	1 Serving/400g	561	27.6	140	10.5	8.9	6.9	1.4
CHICKEN CAJUN								
& Potato Hash, HL, Tesco*	1 Pack/450g	427	6.3	95	6.5	14.1	1.4	1.5
Breast, Chargrilled, Iceland*	1 Serving/80g	114	1.5	142	27.4	3.9	1.9	0.0
Breast, Morrisons*	½ Pack/180g	328	16.9	182	16.6	7.7	9.4	2.0
CHICKEN CANTONESE								
& Rice, Sizzler, Tesco*	1 Serving/450g	639	25.6	142	7.7	14.9	5.7	0.9
Breast, Fillets, Sainsbury's*	1 Serving/154g	168	2.3	109	20.3	3.6	1.5	0.6
Chinese, Tesco*	½ Pack/175g	196	6.5	112	10.3	9.4	3.7	0.4
Honey, Sesame, Sainsbury's*	1/3 Pack/135g	116	3.6	86	9.8	5.5	2.7	0.8
Honey Pepper, Sainsbury's*	½ Pack/175g	124	3.9	71	6.6	6.1	2.2	0.9
CHICKEN CARIBBEAN								
Fruity with Rice & Peas, New, BGTY, Sainsbury's*	1 Pack/400g	352	3.6	88	6.9	13.1	0.9	2.2
Style, Breasts, COU, M & S*	1 Serving/205g	205	3.1	100	14.6	7.3	1.5	1.3
CHICKEN CHASSEUR								
Average	1 Serving/400g	363	9.2	91	12.2	4.9	2.3	0.9
BGTY, Sainsbury's*	1 Pack/320g	243	3.5	76	6.8	9.5	1.1	1.0
Breast Fillets, Morrisons*	1 Pack/380g	384	11.4	101	15.7	2.9	3.0	0.8
Mix, Colman's*	1 Pack/38g	120	0.4	316	8.6	68.2	1.0	3.7
CHICKEN CHILLI								
Sweet, Findus*	1 Pack/350g	420	12.2	120	6.0	15.0	3.5	1.5
Sweet, Just Cook, Sainsbury's*	½ Pack/191g	200	1.3	105	15.2	9.4	0.7	0.5
Sweet, With Noodles, Ready Meal, Average	1 Serving/400g	404	5.8	101	6.5	15.5	1.4	1.4
Sweet & Egg Fried Rice, HL, Tesco*	1 Serving/450g	446	8.1	99	5.7	15.0	1.8	0.4
Sweet with Noodles, Frozen, HL, Tesco*	1 Pack/369g	340	5.1	92	6.7	13.1	1.4	1.0
with Lime, Breast, Simple Solutions, Tesco*	1 Pack/400g	564	21.2	141	22.5	0.8	5.3	1.4
CHICKEN CHINESE								
Balls, M & S*	1 Ball/16g	45	2.2	280	10.8	29.2	13.6	2.1
Battered with Plum Sauce, Tesco*	1 Pack/350g	647	20.3	185	6.7	26.5	5.8	0.8
Crispy Aromatic, Half, Tesco*	1 Serving/233g	524	24.2	225	16.3	16.7	10.4	1.2
Fillets with Sweet Chilli Sauce, Tesco*	1 Serving/350g	591	22.0	169	8.8	19.2	6.3	0.7
Stir Fry, Morrisons*	1 Serving/319g	341	5.4	107	5.7	17.0	1.7	1.5
Style Sauce, Breast Fillets, Morrisons*	½ Pack/200g	162	2.0	81	13.5	4.6	1.0	1.2
with Ginger & Spring Onion, Tesco*	1 Serving/350g	299	10.1	85	7.6	7.3	2.9	0.6
CHICKEN CIDER								
COU, M & S*	1 Pack/400g	300	9.2	75	7.2	6.7	2.3	0.8
with Colcannon, Perfectly Balanced, Waitrose*	1 Pack/401g	353	12.4	88	6.2	8.9	3.1	1.1
CHICKEN CORDON BLEU								
Breast, Fillets, Sainsbury's*	1 Serving/150g	304	14.3	203	17.5	11.5	9.5	1.6
Waitrose*	1 Serving/160g	325	15.4	203	20.1	9.1	9.6	2.4
CHICKEN CORONATION								
COU, M & S*	1oz/28g	34	0.6	120	16.3	8.6	2.2	0.7
M & S*	1 Serving/200g	420	26.4	210	12.6	10.6	13.2	1.3
CHICKEN DINNER								
Breast with Pork, Sage & Onion Stuffing, Tesco*	1 Serving/180g	277	14.8	154	19.4	0.7	8.2	0.5
Kershaws*	1 Pack/350g	210	3.5	60	4.3	8.4	1.0	1.2
Tesco*	1 Serving/400g	388	7.2	97	9.2	10.9	1.8	1.2
with Gravy, The Crafty Cook*	1 Serving/320g	330	6.7	103	5.6	15.3	2.1	1.9
CHICKEN EN CROUTE								
Asda*	½ Pack/174g	393	17.4	226	14.0	20.0	10.0	1.5
Breast, Tesco*	1 Serving/215g	555	33.1	258	9.4	20.4	15.4	0.6
Just Cook, Sainsbury's*	1 Serving/180g	481	27.2	267	16.8	15.9	15.1	0.4

	Measure INFO/WEIGHT	per Measure KCAL	FAT	Nutrition Values per 100g / 100ml KCAL	PROT	CARB	FAT	FIBRE
CHICKEN ESCALOPE								
Creamy Peppercorn, Sainsbury's*	1 Serving/150g	367	24.5	245	13.3	11.2	16.3	1.1
Lemon & Herb, Waitrose*	1 Serving/200g	242	6.4	121	22.0	1.0	3.2	0.6
Topped with Cheese, Ham & Mushrooms, Asda*	½ Pack/149g	217	9.0	145	22.0	0.8	6.0	0.4
CHICKEN FLORENTINE								
Asda*	1 Serving/200g	322	18.0	161	18.0	2.1	9.0	0.9
Finest, Tesco*	½ Pack/225g	358	19.1	159	11.0	9.7	8.5	1.3
HL, Tesco*	1 Pack/400g	340	10.8	85	12.1	3.0	2.7	0.9
CHICKEN FORRESTIERE								
COU, M & S*	1 Serving/220g	187	3.7	85	14.5	2.2	1.7	0.6
CHICKEN FU YUNG								
Chinese Takeaway, Tesco*	1 Pack/350g	315	3.5	90	5.6	14.5	1.0	0.8
CHICKEN GINGER								
& Plum with Rice, Perfectly Balanced, Waitrose*	1 Pack/400g	492	2.0	123	6.3	23.5	0.5	1.0
& Spring Onion, with Rice, Sharwood's*	1 Pack/375g	347	6.4	93	5.1	14.2	1.7	1.7
CHICKEN GLAZED								
Balsamic, HL, Tesco*	1 Pack/400g	288	3.6	72	5.1	10.8	0.9	0.9
CHICKEN HARISSA								
BGTY, Sainsbury's*	1 Serving/250g	211	3.0	84	10.4	8.0	1.2	1.5
with Cous Cous, Perfectly Balanced, Waitrose*	1 Pack/400g	348	8.0	87	7.6	9.5	2.0	1.7
CHICKEN HAWAIIAN								
with Rice, Birds Eye*	1 Pack/350g	406	5.2	116	5.5	20.2	1.5	0.6
CHICKEN IN								
Bacon, Mushroom & Red Wine Sauce, Asda*	1 Serving/151g	145	3.9	96	16.0	2.2	2.6	0.5
Barbecue Sauce, COU, M & S*	1 Pack/352g	370	5.6	105	8.6	13.8	1.6	1.2
Barbeque Sauce, Breasts, COU, M & S*	1 Pack/350g	420	6.7	120	8.5	20.6	1.9	0.6
BBQ Sauce, Breast, Sainsbury's*	1 Serving/170g	199	1.2	117	14.5	13.1	0.7	1.3
BBQ Sauce, Chargrilled, Breast, GFY, Asda*	1 Serving/166g	214	6.1	129	19.0	5.0	3.7	1.0
BBQ Sauce, GFY, Asda*	1 Pack/380g	494	2.7	130	18.0	13.0	0.7	0.2
BBQ Sauce, Weight Watchers*	1 Pack/339g	332	11.9	98	5.8	10.8	3.5	0.9
Black Bean Sauce, Budgens*	1 Pack/350g	332	14.0	95	9.9	4.9	4.0	0.9
Black Bean Sauce, Canned, BGTY, Sainsbury's*	1 Can/400g	308	3.6	77	9.3	7.9	0.9	0.7
Black Bean Sauce, Frozen, BGTY, Sainsbury's*	1 Pack/400g	380	4.4	95	4.5	16.6	1.1	0.5
Black Bean Sauce, M & S*	1 Pack/350g	297	7.0	85	8.7	8.0	2.0	1.1
Black Bean Sauce, Sainsbury's*	1 Pack/465g	484	7.9	104	5.0	17.3	1.7	0.3
Black Bean Sauce, Waitrose*	1 Pack/300g	243	3.6	81	10.9	6.6	1.2	0.8
Chilli & Lemon Grass with Rice, Sainsbury's*	1 Pack/450g	526	11.2	117	6.2	17.4	2.5	0.7
Coconut, Sizzler, HL, Tesco*	1 Pack/350g	280	7.7	80	9.8	4.5	2.2	2.1
Creamy Madeira Sauce, HL, Tesco*	1 Pack/400g	320	6.8	80	12.8	2.3	1.7	1.0
Creamy Mushroom Sauce, HL, Tesco*	1 Pack/400g	296	6.0	74	13.2	1.8	1.5	0.5
Creamy Mushroom Sauce, Weight Watchers*	1 Pack/330g	343	9.6	104	7.0	12.5	2.9	0.6
Creamy Tomato & Mascarpone Sauce, Waitrose*	1 Serving/400g	492	23.2	123	7.9	9.9	5.8	0.8
Creamy White Wine Sauce, Sainsbury's*	1 Pack/324g	285	12.0	88	8.9	4.7	3.7	1.0
Garlic & Cream Sauce, Breast Fillet, Morrisons*	1 Serving/180g	262	15.8	146	14.9	1.8	8.8	0.6
Garlic & Herbs, Breast, Sainsbury's*	1 Serving/200g	316	5.2	158	28.3	5.4	2.6	0.1
Gravy, Chunky, M & S*	1 Can/489g	465	19.1	95	13.6	1.4	3.9	0.8
Honey Mustard & Parsnip Mash, Light Choices, Tesco*	1 Pack/400g	340	6.8	85	8.0	9.0	1.7	2.0
Hunter's BBQ Sauce, Asda*	½ Pack/190g	348	14.1	183	19.1	10.3	7.4	0.0
Leek & Bacon Sauce, Chilled, Co-Op*	1 Pack/400g	460	20.0	115	15.0	2.0	5.0	0.2
Leek & Bacon Sauce with Mash, HL, Tesco*	1 Pack/450g	337	8.1	75	6.7	8.0	1.8	1.6
Lemon & Garlic Marinade, Thighs, Go Cook, Asda*	½ Pack/265g	493	30.2	186	19.7	1.2	11.4	0.8
Lemon Sauce with Rice, Sainsbury's*	1 Pack/450g	513	6.7	114	8.1	17.0	1.5	0.7
Madeira Sauce with Mushrooms, Finest, Tesco*	½ Pack/200g	210	8.3	105	13.8	2.9	4.1	0.9
Masala with Spiced Indian Lentils, M & S*	1 Pack/330g	297	8.2	90	10.3	6.1	2.5	5.9

	Measure INFO/WEIGHT	per Measure KCAL	FAT	Nutrition Values per 100g / 100ml KCAL	PROT	CARB	FAT	FIBRE
CHICKEN IN								
Mediterranean Sauce, Iceland*	1 Pack/500g	640	6.0	128	7.4	21.8	1.2	0.5
Mexican Salsa, Tesco*	1 Pack/320g	368	8.6	115	19.5	3.1	2.7	0.6
Mexican Style Sauce, Tesco*	1 Serving/180g	128	1.4	71	13.3	2.6	0.8	0.7
Mushroom & Red Wine Sauce, Breast Fillets, Morrisons*	1 Serving/177g	184	4.4	104	15.7	4.6	2.5	0.7
Mushroom Sauce, 124, Oakhouse Foods Ltd*	1 Meal/380g	334	8.0	88	8.5	9.7	2.1	1.7
Mushroom Sauce, Diet Chef Ltd*	1 Pack/300g	225	6.9	75	7.9	5.7	2.3	0.1
Oyster Sauce & Mushrooms, Tesco*	1 Pack/350g	252	5.6	72	8.0	6.3	1.6	0.7
Peppercorn Sauce, GFY, Asda*	1 Serving/399g	431	7.2	108	6.0	17.0	1.8	0.5
Peppers, Fillets, Sainsbury's*	1 Pack/360g	378	13.3	105	13.7	4.2	3.7	1.1
Pesto Style Dressing, Asda*	1 Serving/150g	210	10.0	140	18.7	1.3	6.7	0.0
Red Pepper Dressing, Tesco*	1 Serving/140g	228	13.3	163	19.2	0.1	9.5	0.5
Red Wine with Mash, Morrisons*	1 Serving/400g	288	5.2	72	9.1	6.1	1.3	1.4
Reggae Reggae Sauce, Drumsticks, Levi Roots*	1 Serving/100g	165	7.3	165	21.5	3.4	7.3	0.0
Smoky Barbecue Sauce, Breast, Fresh Tastes, Asda*	1 Breast/160g	258	6.2	161	21.9	9.6	3.9	0.9
Smoky Barbeque Sauce, Tesco*	1 Serving/185g	229	3.9	124	16.3	9.9	2.1	1.0
Sweet Chilli Sauce, Breast, Fresh Tastes, Asda*	½ Pack/180g	288	9.0	160	18.4	10.3	5.0	0.5
Tarragon Sauce, Lean Cuisine*	1 Pack/338g	270	6.7	80	4.0	11.0	2.0	1.5
Tomato & Basil Sauce, Breast, Fresh Tastes, Asda*	½ Pack/130g	136	2.7	105	19.3	2.3	2.1	0.7
Tomato & Basil Sauce, Breast, GFY, Asda*	1 Pack/392g	447	13.3	114	12.0	9.0	3.4	1.5
Tomato & Basil Sauce, Eat Smart, Morrisons*	1 Pack/375g	300	6.4	80	8.3	7.8	1.7	2.4
Tomato & Basil Sauce, HL, Tesco*	1 Breast/200g	154	2.4	77	12.4	4.2	1.2	0.6
Tomato & Basil Sauce, Oven Baked, Asda*	½ Pack/143g	153	3.0	107	19.3	2.3	2.1	0.7
Tomato & Herb Sauce, Breasts, Tesco*	½ Pack/173g	155	2.4	90	15.0	3.6	1.4	0.5
White Sauce, BGTY, Sainsbury's*	1 Can/200g	162	4.2	81	1.2	2.4	2.1	1.1
White Sauce, Canned, Asda*	½ Can/400g	644	44.0	161	12.0	3.5	11.0	0.0
White Sauce, Canned, HL, Tesco*	½ Can/200g	180	5.8	90	14.3	1.3	2.9	5.4
White Wine & Asparagus Panzerotti, Asda*	½ Pack/150g	238	2.5	159	8.0	28.0	1.7	0.0
White Wine & Tarragon Sauce, Waitrose*	½ Pack/225g	281	17.3	125	10.7	3.1	7.7	0.3
White Wine Sauce, Breasts, Tesco*	1 Serving/370g	388	14.1	105	16.9	0.8	3.8	0.6
White Wine Sauce, Wild Rice, Pub Specials, Birds Eye*	1 Pack/450g	335	5.9	74	7.1	8.4	1.3	2.1
White Wine with Pasta, Perfectly Balanced, Waitrose*	1 Pack/400g	400	10.0	100	8.2	12.1	2.5	2.5
Wild Mushroom Sauce, Breasts, HL, Tesco*	1 Serving/212g	191	5.1	90	15.1	2.1	2.4	1.5
Wild Mushroom Sauce, Extra Special, Asda*	1 Serving/225g	319	19.0	142	14.2	2.2	8.4	0.3
Zesty Orange Sauce, Asda*	1 Serving/200g	340	12.0	170	16.0	13.0	6.0	0.4
CHICKEN INDIAN								
Style, Fillets, Sainsbury's*	1 Pack/200g	224	8.8	112	13.7	4.4	4.4	1.2
CHICKEN ITALIAN								
Style, BGTY, Sainsbury's*	1 Pack/400g	364	4.4	91	6.0	14.5	1.1	0.9
Style, Dinner, Asda*	1 Pack/400g	244	4.0	61	6.0	7.0	1.0	1.1
Style, Sainsbury's*	½ Pack/190g	222	7.6	117	16.3	3.9	4.0	0.1
CHICKEN JEERA								
Sainsbury's*	½ Pack/201g	247	14.1	123	10.5	4.6	7.0	1.8
CHICKEN KUNG PO								
Sainsbury's*	½ Pack/175g	131	4.4	75	9.2	4.0	2.5	1.0
Waitrose*	1 Pack/350g	318	3.9	91	8.2	12.1	1.1	1.2
with Egg Fried Rice, Asda*	1 Pack/450g	688	22.5	153	6.0	21.0	5.0	1.0
CHICKEN LEMON								
Balls, Asda*	1 Ball/15g	42	2.5	279	14.0	19.0	17.0	1.6
Battered, Cantonese, Sainsbury's*	1 Pack/350g	560	19.6	160	10.7	16.6	5.6	0.9
Breast, Fillets, BGTY, Sainsbury's*	1 Fillet/113g	195	2.4	173	18.4	19.9	2.1	1.9
Cantonese, Sainsbury's*	½ Pack/140g	218	8.8	156	11.0	13.9	6.3	0.6
Cantonese Style with Egg Fried Rice, Farmfoods*	1 Pack/324g	486	15.6	150	4.9	21.8	4.8	0.1
Chinese, Tesco*	1 Serving/350g	563	11.2	161	7.0	26.0	3.2	0.3

	Measure INFO/WEIGHT	per Measure		Nutrition Values per 100g / 100ml				
		KCAL	FAT	KCAL	PROT	CARB	FAT	FIBRE
CHICKEN LEMON								
COU, M & S*	1 Pack/150g	150	1.3	100	17.9	5.6	0.9	0.8
Tesco*	½ Pack/175g	213	7.3	122	11.0	10.1	4.2	0.6
with Vegetable Rice, BGTY, Sainsbury's*	1 Pack/400g	428	6.4	107	6.5	16.8	1.6	0.8
CHICKEN LUNCH								
French Style, Light, John West*	1 Pack/240g	194	6.5	81	7.2	6.9	2.7	2.1
Italian Style, Light, John West*	1 Pack/240g	209	6.2	87	6.9	9.0	2.6	0.7
CHICKEN MEAL								
American, Fillets, Asda*	1 Pack/345g	838	37.9	243	9.0	27.0	11.0	2.3
Breast Fillets, Meal For One, Eat Well, M & S*	1 Pack/400g	340	10.4	85	7.0	7.9	2.6	1.5
Roast, M & S*	1 Pack/280g	294	9.2	105	6.6	11.6	3.3	1.9
CHICKEN MEXICAN								
Style, BGTY, Sainsbury's*	1 Serving/260g	255	6.5	98	6.9	12.1	2.5	2.2
Style, Combo, Asda*	1 Pack/380g	562	16.7	148	21.0	6.0	4.4	2.0
Style Sauce, Breast, Tesco*	1 Serving/180g	128	1.4	71	13.3	2.6	0.8	0.7
CHICKEN MOROCCAN								
Style, Sainsbury's*	½ Pack/269g	334	7.0	124	14.7	10.4	2.6	3.1
Style with Spicy Cous Cous, BGTY, Sainsbury's*	1 Serving/225g	304	3.8	135	9.2	20.6	1.7	0.0
with Cous Cous, GFY, Asda*	1 Serving/450g	414	5.8	92	8.0	12.0	1.3	0.8
with Cous Cous & Fruity Sauce, BGTY, Sainsbury's*	1 Pack/400g	440	8.0	110	10.0	13.1	2.0	2.6
CHICKEN ORIENTAL								
with Noodles, SteamFresh, Birds Eye*	1 Pack/400g	336	8.8	84	7.1	9.0	2.2	0.3
CHICKEN PAPRIKA								
COU, M & S*	1 Pack/400g	380	6.4	95	9.0	11.7	1.6	2.0
with Savoury Rice & Vegetables, BGTY, Sainsbury's*	1 Pack/400g	383	2.4	96	7.1	15.5	0.6	1.1
CHICKEN PARMESAN								
& Sun Dried Tomato, Fillets, Mini, Sainsbury's*	1 Pack/200g	278	5.8	139	22.1	6.0	2.9	0.5
Sun Dried Tomato, Fillets, BGTY, Sainsbury's*	½ Pack/100g	138	2.9	138	22.1	6.0	2.9	0.5
CHICKEN PENANG								
Waitrose*	1 Pack/400g	364	10.8	91	10.1	6.6	2.7	0.8
CHICKEN PEPPER								
Fry, Sainsbury's*	1 Pack/400g	508	24.8	127	15.0	2.9	6.2	1.6
CHICKEN PIRI PIRI								
Breast, Fillets, Mini, Tesco*	½ Pack/100g	135	1.1	135	22.7	7.6	1.1	0.0
GFY, Asda*	1 Pack/400g	406	2.8	102	5.8	18.0	0.7	1.4
M & S*	1 Pack/300g	420	23.1	140	10.0	7.3	7.7	1.3
Sainsbury's*	½ Pack/200g	248	10.8	124	14.0	4.8	5.4	0.5
CHICKEN ROAST								
in a Pot, Sainsbury's*	1 Pack/450g	477	13.0	106	9.6	10.3	2.9	0.7
Meal, Blue Parrot Cafe, Sainsbury's*	1 Pack/285g	259	9.7	91	6.9	8.1	3.4	1.5
CHICKEN SIZZLER								
GFY, Asda*	1 Pack/350g	289	5.0	83	12.9	4.6	1.4	1.4
HL, Tesco*	1 Serving/350g	273	7.0	78	11.1	3.8	2.0	4.3
CHICKEN SPANISH								
Style, Asda*	½ Pack/275g	322	13.5	117	14.0	4.1	4.9	0.7
CHICKEN STUFFED								
Asparagus & Ricotta with Herb Rice, BGTY, Sainsbury's*	1 Pack/400g	444	10.4	111	8.1	13.8	2.6	0.3
with Moroccan Style Cous Cous, GFY, Asda*	½ Pack/180g	259	4.9	144	20.0	10.0	2.7	0.0
with Mushrooms, Finest, Tesco*	1 Serving/150g	177	7.6	118	15.9	2.0	5.1	0.6
CHICKEN SUPREME								
BGTY, Sainsbury's*	1 Pack/350g	416	4.9	119	9.4	17.2	1.4	0.5
Breast, Sainsbury's*	1 Serving/187g	421	29.5	225	20.6	0.3	15.8	0.6
with Rice, Asda*	1 Pack/450g	616	31.5	137	15.0	3.4	7.0	1.1
with Rice, Birds Eye*	1 Pack/376g	470	9.8	125	6.6	18.8	2.6	0.5

	Measure INFO/WEIGHT	per Measure KCAL	FAT	Nutrition Values per 100g / 100ml KCAL	PROT	CARB	FAT	FIBRE
CHICKEN SUPREME								
with Rice, Oakhouse Foods Ltd*	1 Meal/400g	520	16.8	130	6.7	16.5	4.2	0.5
with Rice, Weight Watchers*	1 Pack/300g	255	4.8	85	5.6	11.9	1.6	0.5
CHICKEN SZECHUAN								
Chilli & Peppercorn, Sainsbury's*	1 Pack/400g	352	16.0	88	9.9	3.2	4.0	0.5
Tesco*	1 Pack/350g	385	10.5	110	7.2	13.6	3.0	0.3
with Noodles, Sainsbury's*	1 Pack/450g	423	13.9	94	6.0	10.4	3.1	0.9
CHICKEN TAGINE								
with Cous Cous, BGTY, Sainsbury's*	1 Pack/450g	625	17.5	139	10.1	15.9	3.9	1.5
CHICKEN TANDOORI								
Fresh Tastes, Asda*	1 Pack/400g	356	5.6	89	6.4	12.7	1.4	2.1
GFY, Asda*	1 Pack/400g	324	9.6	81	7.5	7.3	2.4	1.7
Masala, Asda^	1 Pack/400g	580	20.0	145	7.0	18.0	5.0	1.3
Masala, Sainsbury's*	1 Pack/400g	536	27.2	134	13.2	5.0	6.8	0.5
Masala & Rice, HL, Tesco*	1 Serving/450g	409	7.6	91	6.6	12.9	1.7	0.6
Sizzler, HL, Tesco*	1 Pack/350g	275	7.0	79	11.1	3.8	2.0	4.3
Sizzler, Sainsbury's*	1 Pack/400g	536	29.2	134	12.8	4.3	7.3	1.7
Sizzler, Tesco*	1 Serving/175g	243	11.5	139	10.0	10.0	6.6	1.0
CHICKEN TERIYAKI								
& Noodles, Asda*	½ Pack/340g	445	8.8	131	9.0	18.0	2.6	0.9
Asda*	1 Pack/360g	299	5.0	83	9.1	8.6	1.4	0.8
CHICKEN TIKKA								
& Coriander Rice, Weight Watchers*	1 Pack/400g	348	2.4	87	6.2	14.3	0.6	1.6
& Cous Cous, Boots*	1 Pack/160g	307	17.6	192	6.2	17.0	11.0	1.3
& Lemon Rice, Deli Meal, M & S*	1 Pack/360g	342	7.2	95	9.8	10.2	2.0	0.7
BGTY, Sainsbury's*	1 Serving/188g	265	3.0	141	10.5	21.2	1.6	0.0
Creamy, Breast, Tesco*	1 Breast/190g	215	10.4	113	15.1	0.7	5.5	0.8
Masala, & Pilau Rice, Asda*	1 Serving/500g	720	20.0	144	6.2	20.7	4.0	0.9
Masala, & Rice, 231, Oakhouse Foods Ltd*	1 Meal/400g	528	18.0	132	5.5	17.2	4.5	0.6
Masala, Canned, Chosen By You, Asda*	½ Can/200g	222	10.6	111	10.9	4.0	5.3	1.7
Masala, COU, M & S*	½ Pack/175g	245	12.9	140	12.5	5.6	7.4	1.6
Masala, with Pilau Rice, Hot, Tesco*	1 Pack/550g	797	31.9	145	7.4	15.0	5.8	1.4
Masala, with Rice, Ready Meal, Healthy Range, Average	1 Serving/400g	390	6.4	98	6.6	14.3	1.6	1.1
Masala, with Rice & Naan, Big Dish, Tesco*	1 Pack/600g	960	40.4	160	6.7	18.1	6.7	1.2
Masala, with Yellow Rice, Light Choices, Tesco*	1 Pack/441g	485	8.8	110	4.9	17.4	2.0	1.0
with Basmati Rice, GFY, Asda*	1 Pack/400g	592	7.2	148	9.0	24.0	1.8	1.6
with Pilau Rice, GFY, Asda*	1 Pack/450g	382	2.7	85	7.0	13.0	0.6	1.8
CHICKEN VINDALOO								
Average	1 Serving/410g	787	51.2	192	18.5	2.6	12.5	0.3
CHICKEN WITH								
Asparagus & Rice, BGTY, Sainsbury's*	1 Pack/400g	428	5.6	107	9.1	14.5	1.4	0.9
Bacon & Leeks, GFY, Asda*	1 Pack/400g	328	8.0	82	13.0	3.0	2.0	0.6
Basil, Puy Lentils & Spelt, Roasted, The Food Doctor*	1 Pack/350g	210	7.3	60	9.6	0.7	2.1	10.2
Broccoli & Pesto Pasta, BGTY, Sainsbury's*	1 Pack/301g	328	5.1	109	10.3	13.2	1.7	2.5
Caramelised Peppers, Chargrilled, M & S*	½ Pack/237g	225	9.0	95	12.9	2.1	3.8	1.3
Cheddar & Bacon Filling, Breast, Just Cook, Sainsbury's*	1 Serving/180g	346	14.6	192	23.2	6.5	8.1	0.1
Cheese, Leek & Ham, Breast, Fresh Tastes, Asda*	1 Pack/430g	658	30.5	153	18.9	3.4	7.1	0.7
Cheese & Bacon, Tesco*	½ Pack/175g	262	11.9	150	18.9	2.6	6.8	0.4
Cheese Croutons & Onion, Asda*	1 Serving/200g	200	6.4	100	16.0	2.0	3.2	0.9
Cherrywood Barbecue Sauce, Simply Cook, Tesco*	1 Serving/147g	165	2.5	112	16.6	7.6	1.7	0.4
Chorizo & Patatas Bravas, COU, M & S*	1 Pack/400g	380	9.2	95	7.8	10.8	2.3	1.7
Chorizo & Tomato Sauce, Catalan, Bighams*	1 Pack/479g	407	15.8	85	10.9	2.8	3.3	0.7
Cous Cous, Lemon & Herb, Finest, Tesco*	1 Pack/370g	492	18.5	133	10.5	11.5	5.0	0.9
Cranberry & Orange Stuffing, Sainsbury's*	1 Serving/100g	201	10.3	201	23.0	4.1	10.3	0.8

CHICKEN WITH

	Measure INFO/WEIGHT	per Measure KCAL	FAT	Nutrition Values per 100g / 100ml KCAL	PROT	CARB	FAT	FIBRE
Cranberry Stuffing, Breast, Finest, Tesco*	½ Pack/200g	252	4.8	126	16.2	9.9	2.4	0.9
Creamy Spinach & Parmesan, M & S*	1 Pack/390g	468	17.2	120	10.8	12.3	4.4	2.5
Fusilli & Courgette, Sainsbury's*	1 Pack/450g	675	28.8	150	8.6	14.6	6.4	0.5
Garlic & Chilli Balti, Tesco*	1 Pack/400g	320	7.6	80	11.0	4.4	1.9	0.8
Garlic Mushrooms, Asda*	1 Serving/320g	342	16.0	107	13.7	1.7	5.0	2.2
Grapes & Asparagus, Sainsbury's*	½ Pack/200g	240	13.2	120	13.3	1.8	6.6	1.0
Gravy & Stuffing, Breasts, Tesco*	½ Pack/173g	257	11.1	149	14.4	8.3	6.4	2.2
Gruyere Cheese & Parma Ham, Breast, COOK!, M & S*	1 Breast/194g	349	21.3	180	18.0	2.5	11.0	0.9
Honey & Ginger Sauce, 125, Oakhouse Foods Ltd*	1 Dinner/365g	339	8.0	93	8.7	9.8	2.2	1.2
Honey & Mustard Sauce, Breasts, Simply Cook, Tesco*	½ Pack/219g	230	1.3	105	16.3	8.0	0.6	0.3
Honey & Sesame with Rice, Light Choices, Tesco*	1 Pack/400g	432	12.0	108	5.3	14.9	3.0	2.2
Leek & Bacon, 119, Oakhouse Foods Ltd*	1 Meal/400g	340	13.6	85	7.0	6.6	3.4	1.2
Lemon Grass, Thai Greens & Baby Corn, Sainsbury's*	1 Serving/200g	196	6.8	98	10.0	6.9	3.4	1.4
Lime & Coriander, Chargrilled, Asda*	1 Serving/190g	351	17.1	185	24.0	2.0	9.0	1.1
Lime & Coriander, Easy, Waitrose*	½ Pack/168g	203	7.9	121	18.9	0.7	4.7	0.5
Lime & Tequila, Asda*	1 Serving/150g	193	2.7	129	24.0	4.3	1.8	0.5
Lyonnaise Potatoes, M & S*	½ Pack/260g	286	8.1	110	12.6	8.0	3.1	0.9
Mango, Lime & Coriander, Asda*	1 Pack/400g	416	6.0	104	6.6	15.9	1.5	1.4
Mango Salsa & Potato Wedges, BGTY, Sainsbury's*	1 Pack/400g	336	6.4	84	7.0	10.4	1.6	1.5
Mozzarella & Pancetta, Breast, Finest, Tesco*	½ Pack/225g	326	13.9	145	14.4	7.9	6.2	1.1
Mozzarella & Pesto Melt, Breasts, COOK!, M & S*	½ Pack/165g	206	10.2	125	16.4	1.3	6.2	0.7
Mushroom & Garlic Butter, Breasts, Sainsbury's*	½ Pack/195g	388	20.1	199	20.0	4.6	10.3	0.1
Mushroom Pilaff, BGTY, Sainsbury's*	1 Serving/400g	320	2.0	80	8.0	10.5	0.5	1.4
Mushroom Risotto, M & S*	1 Pack/400g	480	11.6	120	6.9	16.7	2.9	0.8
Mushroom Sauce & Herby Rice, Fillets, M & S*	1 Pack/380g	475	19.4	125	7.7	12.0	5.1	1.3
Pasta, Chianti & Balsamic, BGTY, Sainsbury's*	1 Pack/400g	372	7.6	93	9.4	9.5	1.9	1.9
Pesto & Linguine Pasta, Meal, SteamFresh, Birds Eye*	1 Pack/400g	440	16.0	110	8.5	10.0	4.0	1.3
Plum Sauce, Battered, Tesco*	1 Serving/175g	324	10.2	185	6.7	26.5	5.8	0.8
Pork, Parsnip Herb Stuffing, Sainsbury's*	1 Serving/100g	181	9.0	181	22.9	2.1	9.0	0.7
Pork Stuffing, Breast, Roast, M & S*	1 Serving/100g	165	6.5	165	24.1	3.0	6.5	0.0
Pork Stuffing & Chipolatas, Breast Joint, Tesco*	½ Pack/340g	524	27.9	154	16.7	3.4	8.2	0.5
Potato & Smoked Bacon Topping, M & S*	1 Serving/175g	227	8.4	130	17.8	3.2	4.8	1.2
Potato Wedges, Tomato & Basil, Weight Watchers*	1 Pack/330g	247	6.9	75	4.7	9.3	2.1	1.3
Sage & Onion Stuffing & Chipolatas, Breast Joint, Tesco*	½ Pack/280g	507	32.8	181	16.2	2.8	11.7	1.9
Soured Cream, Cajun Spiced, Breast, COOK!, M & S*	½ Pack/200g	230	10.2	115	14.7	2.1	5.1	1.1
Soy & Ginger Noodles, Love Life, Waitrose*	1 Pot/360g	212	4.7	59	5.0	6.7	1.3	2.3
Spinach, Honey Mustard, American Style, Asda*	1 Serving/240g	394	24.0	164	14.0	4.4	10.0	0.3
Spirelli, Steam Meal, Tesco*	1 Serving/400g	400	10.8	100	6.6	12.0	2.7	1.2
Spring Vegetables, Chargrilled, COU, M & S*	1 Pack/414g	290	3.7	70	8.8	7.3	0.9	1.8
Stilton & Port Sauce, Breasts, Finest, Tesco*	1 Serving/400g	668	34.4	167	18.5	3.9	8.6	0.7
Sun Dried Tomato & Basil Butter, Sainsbury's*	1 Breast/185g	363	17.6	196	25.0	2.5	9.5	0.2
Sun Dried Tomato & Basil Sauce, Bistro, Waitrose*	½ Pack/175g	254	14.2	145	14.2	3.7	8.1	0.3
Sweet Chilli & Garlic, Chinese, Asda*	1 Serving/400g	436	2.4	109	8.0	18.0	0.6	2.1
Sweet Chilli Sauce & Egg Fried Rice, Tesco*	1 Pack/380g	494	10.3	130	7.5	18.2	2.7	1.3
Sweet Potato Mash, Jerk, Super Naturals, Sainsbury's*	1 Pack/400g	284	4.4	71	6.1	9.2	1.1	2.2
Tagine, Cous Cous, Perfectly Balanced, Waitrose*	1 Pack/400g	516	14.0	129	8.2	16.2	3.5	1.0
Tangy Lemon Sauce, Breasts, Just Cook, Sainsbury's*	1 Serving/164g	244	3.0	149	16.2	16.9	1.8	0.1
Tomato & Basil, GFY, Sainsbury's*	1 Pack/400g	300	3.2	75	13.6	3.4	0.8	1.4
Tomato & Basil, Steam Cuisine, M & S*	1 Pack/400g	460	13.6	115	9.6	11.6	3.4	2.0
Tomato & Basil Sauce, Breast, Light Choices, Tesco*	½ Pack/200g	150	2.3	77	12.0	3.9	1.2	0.6

CHICORY

	Measure INFO/WEIGHT	per Measure KCAL	FAT	Nutrition Values per 100g / 100ml KCAL	PROT	CARB	FAT	FIBRE
Fresh, Raw, Average	1 Head/150g	30	0.9	20	0.6	2.8	0.6	0.9

CHILLI	Measure INFO/WEIGHT	per Measure KCAL	FAT	Nutrition Values per 100g / 100ml KCAL	PROT	CARB	FAT	FIBRE
& Lemon Grass Prawns with Noodles, BGTY, Sainsbury's*	1 Pack/400g	328	2.8	82	5.0	13.8	0.7	1.3
& Potato Wedges, Good Choice, Iceland*	1 Pack/400g	368	13.6	92	5.5	9.8	3.4	1.2
& Potato Wedges, Sainsbury's*	1 Pack/371g	393	15.2	106	7.2	10.1	4.1	2.2
& Rice, Birds Eye*	1 Serving/285g	305	7.7	107	3.4	17.2	2.7	1.0
& Rice, Frozen, Sainsbury's*	1 Pack/400g	436	7.6	109	4.8	18.4	1.9	0.6
& Rice, GFY, Asda*	1 Pack/400g	352	1.6	88	5.0	16.0	0.4	1.8
& Rice, Morrisons*	1 Serving/500g	630	15.5	126	5.7	18.9	3.1	1.1
& Wedges, BBQ, HL, Tesco*	1 Pack/420g	391	10.9	93	5.4	12.2	2.6	1.9
& Wedges, GFY, Asda*	1 Pack/400g	364	10.0	91	7.0	10.1	2.5	2.5
Beef, Asda*	½ Pack/200g	190	7.8	95	7.0	8.0	3.9	1.2
Beef, with Potato Wedges, Naturally Good Food, Tesco*	1 Pack/440g	352	12.3	80	7.2	6.2	2.8	1.8
Beef, with Rice, GFY, Asda*	1 Serving/402g	354	6.0	88	4.7	14.0	1.5	0.9
Beef, with Rice, Sainsbury's*	1 Serving/300g	360	5.1	120	5.6	20.6	1.7	1.1
Beef & Mushrooms, GFY, Asda*	1 Pack/400g	364	6.0	91	9.1	10.2	1.5	1.2
Beef & Potato Crush, Weight Watchers*	1 Pack/400g	232	6.0	58	5.0	5.9	1.5	3.4
Beef & Rice Pot, Shapers, Boots*	1 Pot/301g	250	4.5	83	4.0	12.0	1.5	2.1
Con Carne, 2 Minute Meals, Sainsbury's*	1 Pouch/200g	146	3.2	73	6.0	8.6	1.6	2.7
Con Carne, Asda*	1 Can/392g	376	13.7	96	7.0	9.0	3.5	0.0
Con Carne, Baked Bean, Heinz*	1 Can/390g	324	5.8	83	7.0	10.3	1.5	2.8
Con Carne, Beef, North Yorkshire, Look What We Found*	1 Pack/270g	194	7.6	72	7.6	2.9	2.8	2.3
Con Carne, BGTY, Sainsbury's*	1 Serving/400g	384	8.8	96	5.3	13.8	2.2	2.8
Con Carne, Canned, la Caldera*	¼ Can/200g	240	12.8	120	6.9	8.6	6.4	0.0
Con Carne, Canned, Sainsbury's*	½ Can/200g	162	4.2	81	6.6	8.9	2.1	2.5
Con Carne, Diet Chef Ltd*	1 Pack/300g	306	14.4	102	8.6	6.2	4.8	4.4
Con Carne, Dynamite Hot, Stagg*	1 Serving/250g	310	15.5	124	7.6	9.6	6.2	2.5
Con Carne, From Restaurant, Average	1 Serving/253g	256	8.3	101	9.7	8.7	3.3	0.0
Con Carne, Frozen, Co-Op*	1 Pack/340g	306	3.4	90	6.0	15.0	1.0	1.0
Con Carne, Homepride*	1 Can/390g	234	2.3	60	2.5	11.2	0.6	0.0
Con Carne, M & S*	1 Pack/285g	285	10.5	100	8.7	7.4	3.7	2.0
Con Carne, Recipe Mix, Colman's*	1 Pack/50g	158	1.2	316	10.4	62.9	2.5	6.8
Con Carne, Restaurant, Sainsbury's*	1 Serving/100g	80	2.7	80	6.9	7.0	2.7	1.5
Con Carne, Slim Fast*	1 Pack/375g	394	7.1	105	5.5	16.2	1.9	1.5
Con Carne, Tex Mex, Recipe Mix, Schwartz*	1 Sachet/35g	97	2.3	277	12.9	66.6	6.6	24.6
Con Carne & Rice, Everyday, Value, Tesco*	1 Pack/400g	455	11.1	115	5.0	15.5	2.8	3.3
Con Carne & Rice, Healthy Living, Co-Op*	1 Pack/400g	400	6.8	100	7.8	13.9	1.7	2.1
Con Carne & Rice, Meal for One, M & S*	1 Pack/450g	495	12.1	110	6.4	13.6	2.7	1.6
Con Carne with Rice, Birds Eye*	1 Pack/285g	291	7.1	102	3.3	16.6	2.5	0.8
Con Carne with Rice, GFY, Asda*	1 Serving/400g	456	6.4	114	6.0	19.0	1.6	0.9
Con Carne with Rice, Healthy Choice, Asda*	1 Pack/400g	412	8.4	103	6.0	15.0	2.1	0.9
Con Carne with Rice, Organic, Sainsbury's*	1 Pack/400g	472	10.8	118	5.0	18.5	2.7	1.8
Con Carne with Rice, Perfectly Balanced, Waitrose*	1 Pack/400g	404	7.2	101	5.8	15.3	1.8	1.7
Con Carne with Rice, Weight Watchers*	1 Serving/301g	262	3.3	87	4.6	14.7	1.1	0.4
Mealpack, Flavoured, All About Weight*	1 Pack/35g	120	2.8	343	31.4	34.9	8.0	9.1
Three Bean, Diet Chef Ltd*	1 Pack/300g	195	2.7	65	4.0	10.3	0.9	3.6
Uncle Ben's*	1oz/28g	17	0.2	59	1.8	11.1	0.8	0.0
Vegetable	1oz/28g	16	0.2	57	3.0	10.8	0.6	2.6
Vegetable, Canned, Heated, Asda*	½ Can/200g	158	1.0	79	3.2	14.1	0.5	2.5
Vegetable, Canned, Sainsbury's*	1 Can/400g	230	1.6	58	3.1	10.4	0.4	3.2
Vegetable, Diet Chef Ltd*	1 Pack/300g	258	4.8	86	3.4	14.5	1.6	4.4
Vegetable, Retail	1oz/28g	20	0.6	70	4.0	9.4	2.1	0.0
Vegetable & Rice, BGTY, Sainsbury's*	1 Pack/450g	409	4.9	91	3.5	16.7	1.1	3.5
Vegetable Garden, Stagg*	1 Can/410g	254	2.0	62	3.6	10.8	0.5	2.3
Vegetarian with Rice, Ready Meal, Average	1 Serving/400g	434	6.0	108	3.8	20.0	1.5	1.3

	Measure INFO/WEIGHT	per Measure		Nutrition Values per 100g / 100ml				
		KCAL	FAT	KCAL	PROT	CARB	FAT	FIBRE
CHINESE LEAF								
Fresh, Raw, Average	*1oz/28g*	*4*	*0.1*	*14*	*1.5*	*1.5*	*0.2*	*1.7*
CHIPS								
11mm Fresh, Deep Fried, McCain*	1oz/28g	66	3.0	235	3.2	31.8	10.6	0.0
14mm Fresh, Deep Fried, McCain*	1oz/28g	59	1.9	209	2.7	34.2	6.8	0.0
14mm Friers Choice, Deep Fried, McCain*	1oz/28g	56	2.2	199	3.5	29.3	8.0	0.0
9/16" Straight Cut Caterpack, Deep Fried, McCain*	1oz/28g	63	2.6	225	3.1	32.1	9.4	0.0
American Style, Oven, Sainsbury's*	1 Serving/165g	313	13.7	190	5.4	23.6	8.3	1.3
American Style, Thin, Oven, Tesco*	1 Serving/125g	210	8.1	168	2.7	24.6	6.5	2.1
Beefeater, Deep Fried, McCain*	1oz/28g	71	2.8	253	3.3	37.7	9.9	0.0
Beefeater, Oven Baked, McCain*	1oz/28g	55	1.6	195	4.0	32.2	5.6	0.0
British Classics, HL, Tesco*	½ Pack/200g	250	1.6	125	2.6	26.9	0.8	1.3
Chippy, Microwave, McCain*	1oz/28g	49	2.0	176	2.6	25.2	7.2	1.7
Chunky, Baked, Organic, M & S*	1 Serving/100g	150	3.7	150	1.7	27.1	3.7	2.2
Chunky, Crisp & Golden, Waitrose*	½ Pack/225g	259	7.0	115	2.1	17.7	3.1	3.9
Chunky, Fresh, Chilled, Finest, Tesco*	1 Pack/450g	607	18.0	135	2.1	22.3	4.0	2.7
Chunky, Gastropub, M & S*	1 Pack/400g	520	12.4	130	2.6	22.4	3.1	2.3
Chunky Oven, Harry Ramsden's*	1 Serving/150g	184	5.4	123	2.8	19.9	3.6	1.6
Crinkle Cut, Frozen, Fried in Corn Oil	1oz/28g	81	4.7	290	3.6	33.4	16.7	2.2
Crinkle Cut, M & S*	1 Serving/150g	270	8.1	180	3.3	29.5	5.4	2.4
Crinkle Cut, Oven, Asda*	1 Serving/100g	134	3.8	134	2.0	23.0	3.8	8.0
Crinkle Cut, Oven Baked, Aunt Bessie's*	1 Serving/100g	206	9.2	206	2.9	28.0	9.2	3.2
Fine Cut, Frozen, Fried in Blended Oil	1oz/28g	102	6.0	364	4.5	41.2	21.3	2.4
Fine Cut, Frozen, Fried in Corn Oil	1oz/28g	102	6.0	364	4.5	41.2	21.3	2.7
Fried, Average	1 Serving/130g	266	10.9	204	3.2	29.6	8.4	1.2
Fried, Chip Shop, Average	1 Serving/100g	239	12.4	239	3.2	30.5	12.4	2.2
Frozen, Crinkle Cut, Aunt Bessie's*	1 Serving/100g	163	7.3	163	3.1	21.3	7.3	2.2
Homemade, Fried in Blended Oil, Average	1oz/28g	53	1.9	189	3.9	30.1	6.7	2.2
Homemade, Fried in Corn Oil, Average	1oz/28g	53	1.9	189	3.9	30.1	6.7	2.2
Homemade, Fried in Dripping, Average	1oz/28g	53	1.9	189	3.9	30.1	6.7	2.2
Homestyle, Frozen, Aunt Bessie's*	1 Serving/200g	260	11.2	130	2.2	17.6	5.6	2.7
Homestyle, Oven Cooked, Aunt Bessie's*	1 Serving/100g	191	7.8	191	3.1	27.0	7.8	2.9
Homestyle Oven, Sainsbury's*	1 Serving/125g	206	5.4	165	2.4	29.2	4.3	2.1
Micro, Asda*	1 Serving/112g	221	7.8	197	3.5	30.0	7.0	4.0
Micro, Crinkle Cut, Tesco*	1 Serving/100g	203	8.0	203	3.3	29.5	8.0	1.8
Micro Chips, Crinkle Cut, Cooked, McCain*	1 Pack/100g	166	4.2	166	2.9	28.9	4.2	2.4
Micro Chips, Straight Cut, Cooked, McCain*	1 Pack/100g	163	4.8	163	2.3	27.7	4.8	2.0
Oven, 5% Fat, Frozen, McCain*	1 Serving/200g	238	6.0	119	1.9	21.0	3.0	1.6
Oven, American Style, Champion*	1 Serving/200g	372	14.4	186	2.2	28.2	7.2	2.0
Oven, Best in the World, Iceland*	1 Serving/175g	332	11.7	190	3.4	28.9	6.7	3.5
Oven, Chunky, Ross*	1 Serving/100g	177	6.5	177	3.1	26.6	6.5	3.9
Oven, Cooked, Weight Watchers*	1 Serving/100g	150	3.0	150	2.8	33.7	3.0	5.9
Oven, Crinkle Cut, 5% Fat, Weighed Baked, McCain*	1 Serving/100g	163	4.3	163	3.1	27.9	4.3	3.0
Oven, Crinkle Cut, 5% Fat, Weighed Frozen, McCain*	1 Serving/100g	134	3.6	134	2.4	23.2	3.6	2.4
Oven, Frozen, Baked	1 Portion/80g	130	3.4	162	3.2	29.8	4.2	2.0
Oven, Homefries, McCain*	1 Serving/100g	134	4.6	134	2.2	21.0	4.6	1.7
Oven, Original, McCain*	1 Serving/100g	158	3.8	158	2.5	28.5	3.8	2.3
Oven, Original, Straight Cut, 5% Fat, Cooked, McCain*	1 Serving/100g	172	4.9	172	3.4	32.4	4.9	2.3
Oven, Original, Straight Cut, 5% Fat, Frozen, McCain*	1 Serving/100g	138	4.0	138	2.5	26.2	4.0	1.9
Oven, Straight Cut, Reduced Fat, Tesco*	1 Serving/100g	127	3.0	127	2.3	22.7	3.0	2.1
Oven, Straight Cut, Waitrose*	1 Serving/165g	219	6.1	133	2.0	23.0	3.7	1.7
Oven, Stringfellows, McCain*	1oz/28g	72	2.9	256	4.1	37.0	10.2	0.0
Oven, Sweet Potato, Tesco*	¼ Pack/125g	169	6.5	135	2.6	18.9	5.2	5.0
Oven, Thick Cut, Frozen, Baked	1oz/28g	44	1.2	157	3.2	27.9	4.4	1.8

	Measure INFO/WEIGHT	per Measure KCAL	FAT	Nutrition Values per 100g / 100ml KCAL	PROT	CARB	FAT	FIBRE
CHIPS								
Oven, Thin & Crispy, Tesco*	1 Portion/100g	205	4.9	205	2.7	37.6	4.9	5.8
Oven, Thin Cut, American Style, Asda*	1 Serving/100g	240	10.0	240	3.4	34.0	10.0	3.0
Oven, Thin Fries, Morrisons*	1 Serving/100g	161	6.1	161	2.9	23.6	6.1	1.2
Steak Cut, Frying, Asda*	1 Serving/97g	181	6.8	187	2.9	28.0	7.0	2.8
Steak Cut, Oven, Tesco*	1 Serving/165g	233	6.4	141	2.0	24.4	3.9	2.0
Steakhouse, Fry, Tesco*	1 Serving/125g	278	15.1	222	3.1	25.2	12.1	2.0
Straight Cut, Frozen, Fried in Blended Oil	1oz/28g	76	3.8	273	4.1	36.0	13.5	2.4
Straight Cut, Frozen, Fried in Corn Oil	1oz/28g	76	3.8	273	4.1	36.0	13.5	2.4
Straight Cut, Low Fat, Tesco*	1 Serving/125g	159	3.7	127	2.3	22.7	3.0	2.1
Straight Cut, Microwave Baked, McCain*	1oz/28g	70	3.0	251	3.5	35.0	10.7	0.0
Straight Cut, Oven, BGTY, Sainsbury's*	1 Portion/165g	226	3.5	137	2.7	26.8	2.1	4.1
The Big Chip, Frozen, Tesco^	1 Serving/200g	220	4.8	110	1.8	20.3	2.4	2.1
Thick Cut, Caterpack, Deep Fried, McCain*	1oz/28g	60	2.7	215	3.1	28.8	9.7	0.0
Thick Cut, Frozen, Fried in Corn Oil, Average	1oz/28g	66	2.9	234	3.6	34.0	10.2	2.4
CHIVES								
Fresh, Average	*1 Tsp/2g*	*0*	*0.0*	*23*	*2.8*	*1.7*	*0.6*	*1.9*
CHOC ICES								
Chocolate, Dark, Seriously Creamy, Waitrose*	1 Ice/82g	195	12.9	238	2.6	21.6	15.7	1.7
Chocolate, Real Milk, Sainsbury's*	1 Ice/48g	151	9.5	312	3.5	30.3	19.7	0.8
Chunky, Wall's Ice Cream*	1 Ice/81g	162	10.6	200	2.6	18.9	13.1	0.0
Dark, Sainsbury's*	1 Ice/43g	136	9.5	315	3.8	25.5	22.0	0.4
Dark, Tesco*	1 Ice/43g	141	9.1	325	2.8	30.2	21.0	0.1
Everyday, Value, Tesco*	1 Ice/31g	95	6.3	300	2.3	26.7	19.9	1.0
Mini Mix, Eis Stern*	1 Ice/39g	129	8.9	334	4.2	29.0	23.0	0.0
Morrisons*	1 Ice/31g	86	6.0	279	3.0	24.7	19.3	0.4
Neapolitan Chocolate, Co-Op*	1 Ice/62g	120	8.2	194	2.0	16.9	13.2	0.4
Smart Price, Asda*	1 Ice/31g	81	5.9	262	2.8	20.0	19.0	0.0
White Chocolate, Sainsbury's*	1 Ice/48g	140	8.9	292	3.8	27.3	18.6	0.1
CHOCOLATE								
Advent Calendar, Dairy Milk, Cadbury*	1 Chocolate/4g	22	1.3	525	7.5	56.6	30.1	0.7
Advent Calendar, Maltesers, Mars*	1 Chocolate/4g	21	1.2	537	6.8	57.9	30.9	0.0
Advent Calendar, Pirates of the Caribbean, Kinnerton*	1 Chocolate/4g	19	1.0	525	5.4	61.2	28.6	1.6
Advent Calendar, The Simpsons, Kinnerton*	1 Chocolate/4g	20	1.1	526	5.3	63.2	28.9	1.6
Advent Calendar, The Snowman, M & S*	1 Chocolate/4g	21	1.2	550	6.6	60.4	31.0	0.0
Almond & Honey, Dairy Milk, Cadbury*	1 Sm Bar/54g	281	15.6	520	8.0	57.1	28.9	1.0
Animal Bar, Nestle*	1 Bar/19g	97	5.0	513	5.8	63.6	26.1	0.0
Baking, Belgian, Milk for Cakes, Luxury, Sainsbury's*	1 Chunk/8g	44	2.7	556	7.6	56.5	33.3	1.5
Baking, Continental for Home Baking, Luxury, Tesco*	1 Pack/150g	822	67.6	548	2.7	27.7	45.1	0.9
Baking, Milk for Home Baking, Luxury, Tesco*	1 Pack/150g	838	54.3	559	7.0	51.4	36.2	1.7
Bar, Apricot & Raisin, Thorntons*	1 Bar/40g	185	10.9	462	8.0	46.0	27.3	3.5
Bar, Bubbles, Galaxy, Mars*	1 Bar/31g	172	10.6	555	6.5	54.7	34.2	1.5
Bar, Cappuccino, Thorntons*	1 Bar/38g	201	13.2	529	5.2	49.7	34.7	0.5
Bar, Chocolate, Cherry, Lindt*	1 Bar/100g	470	22.8	470	4.5	61.7	22.8	0.0
Bar, Chocolate, Pistacho, Lindt*	1 Bar/100g	585	40.5	585	7.1	48.2	40.5	0.0
Bar, Chocolate, Strawberry, Lindt*	1 Bar/100g	470	22.8	470	4.5	61.6	22.8	0.0
Bar, Dark, 60% Cocoa with Macadamia, Thorntons*	1 Bar/70g	183	12.8	523	6.5	42.3	36.5	12.6
Bar, Dark, Thorntons*	1 Sm Bar/48g	250	17.7	521	7.3	39.9	36.9	10.9
Bar, Dark Chocolate, Diabetic, Thorntons*	1 Bar/75g	345	26.8	460	5.4	28.5	35.8	8.1
Bar, Dark with Ginger, Thorntons*	1 Bar/100g	509	35.1	509	5.8	44.3	35.1	8.8
Bar, Extra Dark, 60% Cocoa, Lindor, Lindt*	1 Bar/150g	900	73.5	600	5.0	35.0	49.0	2.0
Bar, Flake Allure, Cadbury*	1 Bar/30g	170	10.9	567	6.7	51.0	36.3	0.7
Bar, Hazel Nut & Cashew, Dairy Milk, Cadbury*	3 Chunks/18g	96	6.0	540	8.8	50.6	33.5	1.8
Bar, Milk Chocolate, Galaxy, Mars*	1 Bar/46g	250	14.9	544	6.6	56.3	32.5	1.5

CHOCOLATE

	Measure INFO/WEIGHT	per Measure KCAL	FAT	Nutrition Values per 100g / 100ml KCAL	PROT	CARB	FAT	FIBRE
Bar, Milk Chocolate, Gold, Lindt*	1 Bar/300g	1605	92.9	535	6.6	58.7	31.0	0.0
Bar, Milk Chocolate, Lindt*	1 Bar/100g	535	31.0	535	6.6	57.6	31.0	0.0
Bar, Milk Chocolate, Raisin & Hazelnut, Lindt*	1 Bar/100g	530	31.6	530	3.1	54.7	31.6	0.0
Bar, Twisted, Creme Egg, Cadbury*	1 Bar/45g	210	9.4	465	5.2	64.6	20.8	0.5
Bar, Very Peculiar, Milk with Marmite Flavour, Marmite*	4 Squares/13g	70	4.2	540	6.9	54.9	32.1	2.0
Bar, White, Thorntons*	1 Bar/50g	273	15.6	547	6.5	59.5	31.3	0.0
Beans, Coffee, Dark, Solid, M & S*	1 Serving/10g	53	3.8	532	4.7	42.4	37.6	11.6
Beans, Non Dairy, Graze*	1 Pack/40g	196	8.8	491	3.3	70.0	22.0	0.0
Beans, Plain, Carl Brandt*	4 Beans/5g	25	1.4	501	5.7	54.6	28.9	0.0
Bear, Lindt*	1 Bear/11g	60	3.6	572	7.5	57.7	34.6	0.0
Belgian, Kschocolat*	4 Pieces/40g	212	12.2	530	6.0	57.5	30.5	2.3
Belgian, Milk, Mini Eggs, M & S*	1 Egg/8g	43	2.5	535	7.0	55.8	31.7	2.7
Black Magic, Nestle*	1oz/28g	128	5.8	456	4.4	62.6	20.8	1.6
Breakaway, Nestle*	1 Bar/20g	100	5.0	499	6.5	61.1	25.2	0.0
Bubbly, Dairy Milk, Cadbury*	1 Bar/35g	185	10.5	525	7.7	56.9	29.7	0.7
Bubbly Santa, M & S*	1 Santa/23g	124	7.3	540	7.0	55.8	31.7	2.7
Bunny, Easter, Mars*	1 Bunny/29g	155	9.2	535	6.2	56.2	31.7	0.0
Bunny, Lindt*	1 Bunny/11g	60	3.6	572	7.5	57.5	34.6	0.0
Cappuccino, Nestle*	1 Serving/20g	109	6.6	545	6.1	56.0	32.9	0.0
Cappuccino Mountain Bar, M & S*	1oz/28g	149	9.1	533	8.4	52.0	32.5	2.6
Caramel, Chunk, Dairy Milk, Cadbury*	1 Chunk/33g	158	7.6	480	5.0	63.0	23.0	0.0
Caramel, Dairy Milk, Cadbury*	1 Bar/47g	225	10.9	479	4.9	62.8	23.2	0.4
Choco Swing, Kraft*	1 Square/16g	89	5.5	555	5.7	54.0	34.5	0.0
Chocolat Noir, Lindt*	1/6 Bar/17g	87	5.4	510	6.0	50.0	32.0	0.0
Chomp, Cadbury*	1 Bar/24g	112	4.8	465	3.3	67.9	20.0	0.2
Christmas Tree Decoration, Cadbury*	1 Piece/12g	60	3.4	525	7.6	56.2	29.9	0.0
Coconut, White, Excellence, Lindt*	1 Square/10g	61	4.4	610	6.0	48.0	44.0	0.0
Coins, Milk, Sainsbury's*	1 Coin/5g	26	1.4	502	5.5	58.8	27.1	2.5
Cool & Delicious, Dairy Milk, Cadbury*	1 Bar/21g	110	6.3	525	7.6	56.1	30.1	0.0
Counters, Galaxy, Mars*	4 Counters/10g	53	2.9	529	6.8	59.4	29.1	1.4
Crispies, Chunk, Dairy Milk, Cadbury*	1 Chunk/31g	158	8.5	510	7.6	58.6	27.4	0.0
Crispies, Dairy Milk, Cadbury*	1 Bar/49g	250	13.4	510	7.6	58.6	27.4	0.0
Crispy, Sainsbury's*	4 Squares/19g	99	5.4	521	9.1	56.9	28.5	2.1
Dairy Milk, Cadbury*	1 Bar/49g	260	14.8	525	7.5	57.0	29.8	0.7
Dairy Milk, Toffee Popcorn, Dairy Milk, Cadbury*	1 Bar/150g	765	39.7	510	7.0	59.5	26.5	1.7
Dark, 70% Cocoa Solida, Extra Fine, Lindt*	1 Square/10g	54	4.1	537	8.0	33.0	41.0	0.0
Dark, 70% Cocoa Solids, Organic, Morrisons*	½ Bar/50g	265	20.5	531	7.9	31.6	41.1	11.0
Dark, 75% Cacao, Rausch*	1 Row/31g	163	12.9	522	8.8	28.5	41.1	15.0
Dark, 85% Cocoa, Excellence, Lindt*	1 Serving/40g	212	18.4	530	11.0	19.0	46.0	0.0
Dark, 85% Cocoa, TTD, Sainsbury's*	1 Serving/25g	142	12.8	569	9.7	17.0	51.4	14.1
Dark, Belgian, Extra Special, Asda*	2 Squares/20g	102	8.0	508	11.0	26.0	40.0	16.0
Dark, Belgian, Luxury Continental, Sainsbury's*	1 Bar/100g	490	38.7	490	11.1	24.2	38.7	7.4
Dark, Bittersweet with Cherries, Organic, Green & Black's*	1 Bar/100g	477	28.2	477	7.9	48.0	28.2	8.7
Dark, Chilli, Excellence, Lindt*	1 Serving/40g	202	12.8	506	5.4	49.0	32.0	0.0
Dark, Classic, Bourneville, Cadbury*	4 Squares/25g	125	6.8	505	4.7	58.8	27.3	2.0
Dark, Espresso with Coffee, Organic, Green & Black's*	1 Bar/150g	823	62.4	549	9.8	33.8	41.6	11.7
Dark, Feuilles with Orange, Nestle*	1 Piece/8g	42	2.6	524	4.6	54.4	32.0	0.0
Dark, Luxury Continental, Sainsbury's*	½ Bar/50g	252	20.0	504	10.7	25.5	40.0	16.1
Dark, Mint, Intense, Lindt*	1 Square/10g	51	3.2	510	5.0	50.0	32.0	0.0
Dark, Orange with Slivered Almonds, Excellence, Lindt*	1 Square/10g	50	3.1	500	6.0	49.0	31.0	0.0
Dark, Plain, Average	*1oz/28g*	*143*	*7.8*	*510*	*5.0*	*63.5*	*28.0*	*2.5*
Dark, Raspberry, Ruffles, Jameson's*	1oz/28g	123	5.3	441	1.9	65.9	18.9	4.4
Dark, Raw Organic, Loving Earth*	1 Serving/20g	99	7.9	495	9.3	46.4	39.5	0.0

CHOCOLATE

	Measure INFO/WEIGHT	per Measure KCAL	FAT	Nutrition Values per 100g / 100ml KCAL	PROT	CARB	FAT	FIBRE
Dark, Smooth, Bar, Galaxy, Mars*	1 Bar/125g	651	42.0	521	6.2	48.0	33.6	9.3
Dark, Special, Hershey*	1 Pack/41g	180	12.0	439	4.9	61.0	29.3	7.3
Dark, Whole Nut, Tesco*	1 Serving/13g	67	4.5	539	6.1	48.3	35.7	6.5
Dark, with a Soft Mint Centre, Organic, Green & Black's*	1 Bar/100g	478	27.3	478	7.4	50.5	27.3	8.6
Diet, Ritter Sport*	1 Square/6g	25	1.8	412	6.0	44.0	30.0	0.0
Drops, Plain, Sainsbury's*	1 Serving/125g	637	34.5	510	5.3	60.1	27.6	4.0
Egg, Double Cream, Nestle*	1 Egg/28g	163	11.1	582	6.9	49.2	39.7	0.4
Egg, Mars*	1 Egg/38g	183	9.4	482	5.3	59.7	24.7	0.0
Egg, Truffle Filled, Dark Chocolate, Black Magic, Nestle*	1 Egg/28g	144	8.9	522	5.8	52.0	32.3	3.4
Ferrero Rocher, Ferrero*	1 Choc/13g	74	5.1	593	7.0	49.0	41.0	0.0
Freddo, Caramel, Dairy Milk, Cadbury*	1 Bar/20g	95	4.8	485	5.5	60.2	24.6	0.0
Freddo, Dairy Milk, Cadbury*	1 Freddo/18g	95	5.4	525	7.5	57.0	29.8	0.7
Fruit & Nut, Belgian, Waitrose*	1 Serving/50g	254	14.6	508	8.6	54.6	29.2	3.4
Fruit & Nut, Dark, Tesco*	4 Squares/25g	123	7.0	494	5.8	54.8	27.9	6.5
Ginger, Traidcraft*	1 Bar/50g	212	7.4	424	3.9	68.2	14.8	0.0
Golf Balls, Milk Chocolate, Lindt*	1 Pack/110g	619	39.5	563	6.5	53.6	35.9	0.0
Hazelnut & Walnut, Dark, Organic, Seeds of Change*	1 Bar/100g	559	41.7	559	8.4	37.5	41.7	9.2
Kinder, Bueno Bar, Ferrero*	1 Bar/22g	121	8.1	563	9.8	46.6	37.5	0.0
Kinder, Riegel, Ferrero*	1 Bar/21g	117	7.1	558	10.0	53.0	34.0	0.0
Kinder Maxi, Ferrero*	1 Bar/21g	115	7.1	550	10.0	51.0	34.0	0.0
Kinder Surprise, Ferrero*	1 Egg/20g	110	6.8	550	10.0	51.0	34.0	0.4
Kitten, Milk Chocolate, Lindt*	1 Kitten/11g	60	3.6	572	7.5	57.7	34.6	0.0
Macadamia Nut, Excellence, Lindt*	1 Bar/100g	560	37.0	560	7.0	51.0	37.0	0.0
Matchmakers, Mint, Nestle*	1 Stick/4g	20	0.8	477	4.3	69.7	20.1	0.9
Milk, A Darker Shade of Milk Chocolate, Green & Black's*	1 Sm Bar/35g	183	10.4	523	9.9	54.0	29.7	3.7
Milk, Average	*1oz/28g*	*146*	*8.6*	*520*	*7.7*	*56.9*	*30.7*	*0.8*
Milk, Bubbly, Swiss, M & S*	1 Serving/40g	218	13.7	545	8.0	52.0	34.3	2.5
Milk, Creamy, Organic, Green & Black's*	6 Pieces/20g	110	7.0	560	9.1	50.3	35.5	1.6
Milk, Extra Au Lait, Milch Extra, Lindt*	½ Bar/50g	267	15.5	535	6.5	57.0	31.0	0.0
Milk, Extra Creamy, Excellence, Lindt*	1 Bar/100g	560	37.1	560	6.0	51.1	37.1	0.0
Milk, Extra Fine, Swiss, M & S*	1 Serving/25g	141	9.2	565	7.2	50.9	36.7	2.3
Milk, Figures, Hollow, Dairyfine, Aldi*	1 Serving/11g	58	3.2	523	5.5	59.9	29.0	3.1
Milk, Fimbles Bar, Kinnerton*	1 Bar/12g	65	3.8	539	5.8	57.0	31.8	1.9
Milk, Honey, Traidcraft*	1 Bar/50g	272	16.5	545	6.0	54.0	33.0	0.0
Milk, Italian, Low Sugar, Groder*	1 Serving/40g	199	14.6	498	6.9	51.2	36.5	1.9
Milk, Less Than 99 Calories, M & S*	1 Bar/16g	85	4.6	531	7.5	61.2	28.7	0.6
Milk, Lindor, Lindt*	1 Square/11g	68	5.2	615	4.7	43.0	47.0	0.0
Milk, Organic, Tesco*	1 Serving/25g	139	9.1	558	6.3	51.4	36.3	2.3
Milk, Ryelands*	4 Squares/29g	155	8.2	520	7.3	60.7	27.6	1.7
Milk, Sainsbury's*	4 Squares/25g	133	7.7	533	9.2	54.6	30.8	2.2
Milk, Santas, Tesco*	1 Bag/90g	433	21.8	481	4.5	61.4	24.2	1.4
Milk, Super Naturals, Sainsbury's*	4 Pieces/40g	85	4.9	212	2.4	23.0	12.2	0.9
Milk, Swiss, Diabetic with Fruit & Nuts, Boots*	½ Bar/21g	97	6.7	462	7.0	55.0	32.0	2.7
Milk, Swiss Made, Organic, Traidcraft*	4 Squares/17g	91	5.6	550	7.0	50.0	34.0	0.0
Milk, Whole Nut, Tesco*	1 Serving/25g	129	8.4	517	8.7	53.4	33.8	9.0
Milk, Winnie the Pooh, Solid Shapes, M & S*	1 Chocolate/6g	32	1.9	540	8.1	54.1	32.4	1.3
Milk, with Crisped Rice, Dubble*	1 Bar/40g	211	11.8	528	6.4	59.6	29.4	0.0
Milk, with Crunchy Butterscotch, Organic, Green & Black's*	1 Bar/100g	810	47.1	540	9.3	52.5	31.4	2.9
Milk, with Honey & Almond Nougat, Swiss, Toblerone*	1 Piece/8g	42	2.4	525	5.4	59.0	29.5	2.2
Milk, with Peanut Butter Filling, Ghirardelli*	1 Serving/45g	250	17.0	556	8.9	48.9	37.8	2.2
Milk, with Raisins & Hazelnuts, Green & Black's*	1 Bar/100g	556	36.9	556	9.2	46.8	36.9	3.2
Milk, with Whole Almonds, Organic, Green & Black's*	1 Bar/100g	578	42.2	578	11.8	37.7	42.2	6.2
Milk & Hazelnut, Bar, Swiss, M & S*	1oz/28g	156	10.1	556	6.4	51.9	36.0	3.3

CHOCOLATE

	Measure INFO/WEIGHT	per Measure KCAL	FAT	Nutrition Values per 100g / 100ml KCAL	PROT	CARB	FAT	FIBRE
Milk Chips, Silver Spoon*	1oz/28g	148	8.4	529	6.9	58.0	30.1	0.3
Milky Bar, Giant Buttons, Mars*	1 Sweet/2g	11	0.6	546	7.5	57.7	31.6	0.0
Mini Bites, Chunky, Moments, Fox's*	1 Roll/20g	90	4.9	450	5.7	52.4	24.6	2.2
Mini Eggs, Cadbury*	1 Egg/3g	16	0.7	485	4.6	67.8	21.9	1.3
Mini Eggs, Caramel, Cadbury*	1 Mini Egg/11g	55	2.9	485	5.7	59.0	25.7	0.4
Mini Eggs, Lindor, Lindt*	3 Eggs/15g	90	6.3	600	6.7	46.7	42.0	0.0
Mini Eggs with Soft White Truffle Centre, M & S*	1 Egg/6g	33	2.0	550	6.5	56.3	33.9	1.4
Mint, Lamb, Aero, Nestle*	1 Lamb/27g	147	8.3	543	5.3	60.2	30.7	0.0
Mint Chips, Chunk, Dairy Milk, Cadbury*	1 Chunk/32g	162	8.4	505	6.5	61.2	26.1	0.0
Mint Chips, Dairy Milk, Cadbury*	1 Bar/49g	247	12.8	505	6.6	61.6	26.1	0.6
Mint Creme, Sainsbury's*	1 Serving/20g	93	4.9	467	2.8	62.7	24.5	2.1
Mistletoe Kisses, Mars*	1 Pack/42g	209	11.5	498	5.3	57.0	27.3	0.0
Mountain Bar, Swiss, M & S*	1 Bar/100g	555	35.3	555	6.5	55.2	35.3	0.2
Mountain Bar with Orange, Swiss, M & S*	½ Bar/50g	267	16.4	535	8.0	52.2	32.8	3.2
Natural Orange, Excellence, Lindt*	1 Bar/100g	560	37.0	560	7.0	50.0	37.0	0.0
Natural Vanilla, Excellence, Lindt*	1 Bar/100g	590	40.0	590	6.0	51.0	40.0	0.0
Neapolitans, Terry's*	1oz/28g	146	8.3	522	6.0	57.3	29.7	4.1
Nibs, Raw, Cacao, Organic, Navitas Naturals*	1 Serving/28g	130	12.0	464	14.3	35.7	42.9	32.1
Noir, Special, Frey*	1 Bar/35g	197	15.7	562	8.0	30.0	45.0	0.0
NutRageous, Reese's, Hershey*	1 Bar/51g	260	16.0	510	11.8	54.9	31.4	3.9
Nuts About Caramel, Cadbury*	1 Bar/55g	272	15.1	495	5.8	56.6	27.4	0.0
Nutty Nougat, Bite Sized, Sainsbury's*	1 Bar/23g	111	5.5	481	7.6	59.0	23.8	0.6
Old Jamaica, Bournville, Cadbury*	4 Chunks/23g	107	5.4	465	4.2	59.6	23.4	2.0
Orange, Bar, Terry's*	1 Bar/40g	210	11.7	530	7.3	58.0	29.5	2.1
Orange, Fair Trade, Divine Foods*	4 Squares/17g	92	5.4	541	6.5	57.7	31.5	0.0
Orange, Sainsbury's*	4 Squares/19g	100	5.8	531	9.2	54.3	30.7	2.2
Orange Cream, Cadbury*	1 Bar/51g	217	7.9	425	2.6	68.6	15.4	0.0
Orange Cream, Fry's*	1 Bar/50g	210	6.8	420	2.8	72.3	13.7	0.0
Panna Cotta & Raspberry, M & S*	1 Bar/36g	190	12.1	528	4.7	51.4	33.6	0.3
Peppermint, Ritter Sport*	1 Bar/100g	483	26.0	483	3.0	60.0	26.0	0.0
Peppermint Cream, Fry's*	1 Bar/51g	217	7.9	425	2.6	68.8	15.4	0.0
Plain, 50% Cocoa Solids Minimum, Tesco*	4 Squares/22g	115	6.2	523	7.4	60.0	28.1	1.8
Planets, Mars*	1 Pack/37g	178	8.3	481	4.9	65.4	22.4	0.0
Praline, M & S*	1 Bar/34g	185	12.0	545	7.3	49.6	35.2	3.1
Probiotic, Bar, Ohso*	1 Bar/14g	72	5.0	514	5.0	47.0	36.0	15.5
Rafaello, Roche, Ferrero*	1 Sweet/10g	60	4.7	600	9.7	35.4	46.6	0.0
Rocky Road, Clusters, Tesco*	1 Serving/32g	160	9.5	500	7.1	51.0	29.7	6.7
Shots, Cadbury*	1 Pack/160g	752	37.1	470	5.9	59.7	23.2	0.0
Snack Bar, Kinder*	1 Bar/21g	116	7.1	554	10.0	52.0	34.0	0.0
Snack Size, Dairy Milk, Cadbury*	1 Bar/30g	159	9.0	530	7.8	57.1	29.9	0.0
Snaps, Hazelnut, Cadbury*	1 Curl/4g	20	1.1	520	6.8	57.8	28.8	0.0
Snaps, Milk, Cadbury*	1 Snap/3g	15	0.8	505	6.3	60.5	27.0	1.0
Snaps, Orange, Cadbury*	1 Snap/3g	15	0.8	505	6.3	60.4	27.0	1.0
Snickers, More Nuts, Snickers*	1 Bar/58g	299	17.3	515	10.1	52.8	29.8	0.0
Speckled Eggs, M & S*	1 Egg/6g	25	1.0	440	6.6	63.1	18.2	1.5
Tasters, Dairy Milk, Cadbury*	1 Bag/45g	238	13.7	530	7.6	56.4	30.5	0.0
Taz Chocolate Bar, Cadbury*	1 Bar/25g	121	6.0	485	4.8	62.0	24.0	0.0
Teddy Bear, Milk Chocolate, Thorntons*	1 Teddy/250g	1357	83.7	543	7.6	52.6	33.5	1.0
Toblerone, Mini*	1 Serving/6g	31	1.8	525	5.6	57.5	30.0	3.5
Toffifee, Storck*	1 Sweet/6g	32	1.9	535	6.0	58.0	31.0	0.0
Treatsize, Dairy Milk, Cadbury*	1 Bar/14g	73	4.2	525	7.5	57.0	29.8	0.7
Truffle, Dark Chocolate, Balls, Lindor, Lindt*	1 Ball/12g	76	6.2	630	3.4	38.5	51.4	0.0
Turkish Delight, Large Bar, Dairy Milk, Cadbury*	1 Square/8g	35	1.6	470	5.6	63.2	21.4	0.5

	Measure INFO/WEIGHT	per Measure		Nutrition Values per 100g / 100ml				
		KCAL	FAT	KCAL	PROT	CARB	FAT	FIBRE
CHOCOLATE								
Wafer, Dairy Milk, Cadbury*	1 Bar/46g	235	12.9	510	7.7	57.0	28.0	0.0
White, Average	*1oz/28g*	*148*	*8.7*	*529*	*8.0*	*58.3*	*30.9*	*0.0*
White, Belgian, Sugar Less, Sweet' N Low*	1 Piece/25g	128	9.6	512	5.8	63.1	38.3	0.0
White, Creamy Vanilla, Green & Black's*	1 Sm Bar/35g	201	12.8	573	7.4	53.5	36.6	0.1
White, Crispy, Fair Trade, Co-Op*	½ Bar/50g	277	17.5	555	9.0	51.0	35.0	0.1
White, Double Berry, Nestle*	¼ Bar/30g	167	10.3	556	6.6	54.9	34.5	0.0
White, Nestle*	4 Pieces/40g	220	13.0	550	7.5	55.0	32.5	0.0
White, No Added Sugar, Belgian, Boots*	1 Serving/30g	146	10.8	488	6.0	47.8	36.0	7.0
White, with Honey & Almond Nougat, Toblerone*	1 Serving/25g	132	7.2	530	6.2	60.5	29.0	0.2
White, with Strawberries, Divine*	1 Piece/3g	16	0.9	534	7.6	59.9	29.3	0.1
White, with Strawberry Pieces, Under 99 Cals, M & S*	1 Bar/16g	86	4.9	540	6.6	60.4	30.4	0.3
Whole Nut, Dairy Milk, Cadbury*	1 Bar/49g	270	17.4	550	8.9	49.5	35.4	1.7
Whole Nut, Sainsbury's*	4 Chunks/25g	141	9.4	566	8.5	48.5	37.6	2.6
Whole Nut, Smart Price, Asda*	½ Bar/16g	92	6.2	562	8.0	47.0	38.0	3.3
Wildlife Bar, Cadbury*	1 Bar/21g	109	6.2	520	7.8	56.8	29.3	0.0
CHOCOLATE DROPS								
Plain, Asda*	1 Serving/100g	489	29.0	489	7.0	50.0	29.0	10.0
CHOCOLATE NUTS								
Almonds, Dark Chocolate Covered, Bolero*	2 Almonds/3g	15	1.0	510	2.6	48.8	33.5	0.0
Peanuts, Assorted, Thorntons*	1 Bag/140g	785	57.1	561	13.8	34.8	40.8	3.6
Peanuts, Belgian Coated, M & S*	1 Serving/20g	109	7.6	545	14.7	35.6	38.0	5.8
Peanuts, Milk, Tesco*	1 Bag/227g	1221	86.0	538	17.5	31.8	37.9	4.4
CHOCOLATE ORANGE								
Crunchball, Terry's*	1 Segment/9g	45	2.4	520	6.9	59.8	28.1	2.0
Dark, Terry's*	1 Segment/9g	45	2.6	511	4.3	57.0	29.3	6.2
Egg & Spoon, Terry's*	1 Egg/34g	195	12.9	575	5.5	51.6	38.0	1.7
Goes Minty, Terry's*	3 Slices/26g	133	7.7	510	4.3	57.0	29.5	6.2
Milk, Mini Segments, Terry's*	1 Segment/8g	42	2.4	527	7.7	57.9	29.4	2.1
Milk, Terry's*	1 Orange/175g	931	51.6	532	7.4	57.8	29.5	2.1
Plain, Terry's*	1 Orange/175g	889	51.4	508	3.8	56.8	29.4	6.2
Segsations, Terry's*	1 Segsation/8g	43	2.3	520	6.9	58.5	28.5	2.8
White, Terry's*	1 Segment/11g	61	3.4	535	6.3	60.9	29.4	0.0
CHOCOLATE RAISINS								
Assorted, Thorntons*	1 Bag/140g	601	27.6	429	4.2	58.8	19.7	2.9
Bonds Sweetstars*	1 Serving/28g	109	4.5	391	4.7	57.0	16.0	0.0
Californian, Belgian White Chocolate, M & S*	1 Pack/100g	450	20.9	450	4.3	60.6	20.9	0.8
Californian, Tesco*	¼ Bag/57g	268	11.7	472	5.2	66.2	20.7	1.3
Coated, Californian, M & S*	1 Bag/130g	520	19.1	400	4.3	63.2	14.7	1.9
Jameson's*	1 Serving/23g	96	3.8	418	4.7	62.7	16.5	1.4
Milk Chocolate Coated, Average	1 Serving/50g	207	7.7	415	4.4	64.6	15.4	2.0
CHOCOLATE SPREAD								
& Caramel, Chosen By You, Asda*	1 Serving/100g	564	34.7	564	2.5	60.1	34.7	0.8
Average	*1 Tsp/12g*	*68*	*4.5*	*569*	*4.1*	*57.1*	*37.6*	*0.0*
Hazelnut, Nutella, Ferrero*	1oz/28g	149	8.7	533	6.6	56.4	31.0	3.5
Snickers, Mars*	1 Serving/7g	38	2.6	548	8.7	43.3	37.8	0.0
with Nuts	*1 Tsp/12g*	*66*	*4.0*	*549*	*6.2*	*60.5*	*33.0*	*0.8*
CHOCOLATES								
All Gold, Dark, Terry's*	1 Serving/30g	151	8.7	505	4.0	57.5	29.0	4.3
All Gold, Milk, Terry's*	1 Serving/30g	157	9.1	525	4.8	58.0	30.5	1.5
Assortment, Belgian, Waitrose*	1oz/28g	127	7.6	453	6.3	45.5	27.3	3.8
Bites, Galaxy*	1 Pack/40g	197	9.7	492	5.0	63.0	24.2	0.8
Bittermint, Bendicks*	1 Mint/18g	80	3.0	440	4.3	60.9	16.3	2.4
Brandy Liqueurs, Asda*	1 Chocolate/8g	34	1.4	409	4.0	60.0	17.0	0.8

CHOCOLATES

	Measure INFO/WEIGHT	per Measure KCAL	FAT	Nutrition Values per 100g / 100ml KCAL	PROT	CARB	FAT	FIBRE
Caramels, Sainsbury's*	1 Sweet/12g	57	2.6	490	3.5	69.0	22.2	0.2
Celebrations, Mars*	1 Sweet/8g	41	2.2	512	5.7	61.5	27.0	1.7
Country Caramel, Milk, Thorntons*	1 Chocolate/9g	45	2.4	500	4.6	62.2	26.7	0.0
Dairy Box, Milk, Nestle*	1 Piece/11g	50	2.1	456	4.4	65.9	19.4	0.7
Dark, Elegant, Elizabeth Shaw*	1 Chocolate/8g	38	1.8	469	2.9	62.5	23.1	0.0
Dark, Swiss Thins, Lindt*	1 Pack/125g	681	46.2	545	4.7	49.2	37.0	0.0
Eclipse, Truffle, Plain, Dark, Montezuma*	1 Truffle/16g	93	8.5	581	0.6	21.9	53.1	0.0
Gorgeous, Bendicks*	3 Sweets/15g	82	5.0	550	6.6	55.3	33.3	1.1
Italian Collection, Cappuccino, M & S*	1 Bag/100g	545	37.0	545	6.3	46.7	37.0	1.8
Milk, Mini Eggs, Green & Black's*	1 Mini Egg/8g	42	2.7	562	8.6	48.3	35.5	3.8
Milk, Swiss Thins, Lindt*	1 Pack/125g	687	43.3	550	5.8	53.6	34.6	0.0
Milk Tray, Cadbury*	1 Chocolate/9g	47	2.4	495	4.7	61.5	25.8	0.7
Mingles, Bendicks*	1 Chocolate/5g	27	1.6	540	6.5	58.6	31.3	0.1
Mint Creams, Dark, Smooth & Fragrant, Waitrose*	1 Sweet/10g	42	0.9	410	3.0	77.9	9.1	2.4
Mint Crisp, Bendicks*	1 Mint/8g	38	2.3	494	5.2	55.0	29.9	0.0
Mint Crisp, Dark, Elizabeth Shaw*	1 Chocolate/6g	27	1.2	458	1.9	68.0	20.7	0.0
Mint Crisp, Milk, Elizabeth Shaw*	1 Chocolate/6g	30	1.3	493	4.0	70.9	21.4	0.0
Mint Crisp, Thorntons*	1 Chocolate/7g	34	2.2	486	7.7	40.0	31.4	4.3
Mints, After Eight, Dark, Nestle*	1 Sweet/7g	32	0.9	461	5.0	63.0	12.9	2.0
Mints, After Eight, Orange, Nestle*	1 Sweet/7g	29	0.9	417	2.5	72.6	12.9	1.1
Mints, After Eight, Straws, Nestle*	1 Sweet/5g	24	1.4	526	5.1	56.6	31.0	4.0
Misshapes, Assorted, Cadbury*	1 Chocolate/8g	41	2.3	515	5.2	57.5	29.1	0.0
Moments, Thorntons*	1 Chocolate/7g	37	2.0	511	5.4	59.9	27.8	1.9
Orange Crisp, Elizabeth Shaw*	1 Chocolate/6g	29	1.3	478	2.9	68.2	21.5	0.0
Praline, Coffee, Thorntons*	1 Chocolate/7g	37	2.4	529	7.0	47.1	34.3	2.9
Praline, Hazelnut, Thorntons*	1 Chocolate/5g	27	1.8	540	7.0	48.0	36.0	4.0
Quality Street, Nestle*	1 Sweet/9g	44	1.9	470	3.5	67.3	20.5	1.5
Roses, Cadbury*	1 Chocolate/9g	42	2.2	495	4.8	62.6	25.3	0.7
Sea Shells, Belgian, Guylian*	1 Shell/11g	65	4.4	574	8.0	49.0	39.0	0.0
Seashells, Milk & White, Belgian, Waitrose*	1 Serving/15g	77	4.6	511	5.0	53.1	31.0	2.8
Stars, Mini Wishes, Truffle Centre, Cadbury*	1 Star/13g	70	4.1	540	6.9	55.6	31.8	1.3
Swiss Tradition, De Luxe, Lindt*	1 Pack/250g	1387	90.7	555	6.3	51.9	36.3	0.0
Swiss Tradition, Mixed, Lindt*	1 Pack/392g	2215	149.4	565	6.1	49.8	38.1	0.0
Truffle, Belgian, Flaked, Tesco*	1 Truffle/14g	80	5.4	575	4.4	52.7	38.5	2.3
Truffle, Belgian Milk, Waitrose*	1 Truffle/14g	73	4.8	525	5.8	52.9	34.1	1.2
Truffle, Caramel, Thorntons*	1 Choc/14g	67	3.6	479	4.2	57.9	25.7	2.1
Truffle, Champagne, Petit, Thorntons*	1 Choc/6g	31	1.9	517	7.5	48.3	31.7	3.3
Truffle, Champagne, Premier, Thorntons*	1 Choc/17g	88	5.6	518	6.9	45.3	32.9	2.4
Truffle, Cherry, Thorntons*	1 Choc/14g	58	3.0	414	4.2	50.7	21.4	1.4
Truffle, Continental Champagne, Thorntons*	1 Choc/16g	78	4.5	488	6.1	51.3	28.0	0.6
Truffle, French Cocoa Dusted, Sainsbury's*	1 Truffle/10g	57	4.5	570	4.0	37.0	45.0	0.0
Truffle, Grand Marnier, Thorntons*	1 Choc/15g	77	5.1	513	7.2	40.7	34.0	4.0
Truffle, Hazelnut, Balls, Lindor, Lindt*	1 Ball/12g	76	6.1	632	5.0	39.1	50.6	0.0
Truffle, Irish Milk Chocolate Cream, Elizabeth Shaw*	1 Choc/12g	57	2.7	477	3.9	63.4	22.8	0.0
Truffle, Lemon, White, Thorntons*	1 Choc/14g	63	3.5	450	4.6	64.3	25.0	0.7
Truffle, Milk Chocolate, Balls, Lindor, Lindt*	1 Ball/12g	73	6.0	611	5.6	41.7	50.0	2.7
Truffle, Rum, Average	1 Truffle/11g	57	3.7	521	6.1	49.7	33.7	1.9
Truffle, Rum, Thorntons*	1 Choc/13g	63	3.2	485	4.8	58.5	24.6	4.8
Truffle, Selection, Tesco*	1 Choco/14g	75	4.2	539	5.1	62.0	29.8	0.5
Truffle, Seville, Thorntons*	1 Choc/14g	76	4.7	543	7.1	53.6	33.6	1.4
Truffle, Thorntons*	1 Choc/7g	33	1.9	471	6.0	48.6	27.1	1.4
Truffle, Vanilla, Thorntons*	1 Choc/13g	64	3.5	492	4.8	57.7	26.9	1.5
Truffle, Viennese, Dark, Thorntons*	1 Choc/10g	53	3.6	530	5.9	47.0	36.0	3.0

	Measure INFO/WEIGHT	per Measure KCAL	FAT	Nutrition Values per 100g / 100ml KCAL	PROT	CARB	FAT	FIBRE
CHOCOLATES								
Truffle, Viennese, Milk, Thorntons*	1 Choc/10g	56	3.6	560	4.9	54.0	36.0	0.0
Truffle, White Chocolate, Balls, Lindor, Lindt*	1 Ball/12g	78	6.2	649	5.2	40.2	51.9	0.0
Truffle Filled, Swiss, Balls, Finest, Tesco*	3 Balls/37g	240	19.0	640	5.0	40.7	50.8	1.5
Truffle Hearts, Baileys*	1 Choco/15g	76	4.3	506	5.2	52.6	28.9	1.3
Truffles, Mini Milk Chocolate Balls, Lindor, Lindt*	3 Balls/15g	90	7.0	600	6.7	40.0	46.7	0.0
Twilight, Dark with Mint, Terry's*	1 Chocolate/6g	33	1.9	530	3.1	59.5	30.5	4.2
Valentine, Thorntons*	1 Choc/11g	60	3.8	542	5.7	52.0	34.5	2.1
Winter Selection, Thorntons*	1 Choc/10g	51	3.1	506	6.2	51.3	30.6	3.8
CHOP SUEY								
Chicken, with Noodles, Sainsbury's*	1 Pack/300g	300	7.5	100	5.7	13.6	2.5	1.2
Chinese, Vegetable, Stir Fry, Sharwood's*	1 Pack/310g	223	3.4	72	1.5	13.9	1.1	0.6
Vegetable, M & S*	½ Pack/150g	90	6.1	60	2.0	3.1	4.1	2.9
CHOW MEIN								
Beef, Ready Meal, Average	1 Serving/400g	422	12.2	105	6.0	13.4	3.0	0.9
Beef, Sainsbury's*	1 Pack/450g	499	11.2	111	6.6	15.5	2.5	0.8
Char Sui, Cantonese, Sainsbury's*	½ Pack/225g	205	7.0	91	5.7	10.0	3.1	1.1
Chicken, & Vegetable, Simply Fuller Longer, M & S*	1 Pack/380g	266	4.9	70	6.3	8.7	1.3	2.1
Chicken, Ainsley Harriott*	1 Serving/250g	447	11.8	179	14.0	21.2	4.7	2.0
Chicken, Ready Meal, Average	1 Serving/400g	375	9.4	94	6.5	11.5	2.4	1.2
Chicken, Ready Meal, Healthy Range, Average	1 Serving/400g	329	8.5	82	5.9	9.9	2.1	1.3
Chicken, with Vegetable Spring Roll, Oriental Express*	1 Pack/300g	213	1.8	71	5.5	12.4	0.6	1.9
Pork, Perfectly Balanced, Waitrose*	½ Pack/310g	332	2.8	107	7.6	17.2	0.9	1.6
Special, COU, M & S*	1 Pack/400g	400	15.2	100	6.6	10.3	3.8	1.4
Special, HL, Tesco*	1 Pack/450g	351	5.4	78	6.3	10.6	1.2	0.6
Special, Perfectly Balanced, Waitrose*	1 Pack/400g	316	4.4	79	7.4	10.0	1.1	0.9
Special, Ready Meal, Average	1 Serving/400g	383	9.7	96	6.5	12.1	2.4	1.0
Stir Fry, Asda*	1 Pack/350g	269	17.5	77	2.1	6.0	5.0	0.0
Stir Fry, Tesco*	½ Pack/240g	180	3.4	75	2.8	12.0	1.4	1.6
Vegetable, Ready Meal, Average	1 Serving/400g	337	6.7	84	4.2	12.8	1.7	2.0
Vesta*	1 Pack/433g	594	17.3	137	4.8	20.4	4.0	3.3
CHRISTMAS PUDDING								
Average	1oz/28g	81	2.7	291	4.6	49.5	9.7	1.3
BGTY, Sainsbury's*	1 Serving/114g	302	2.8	266	2.8	58.2	2.5	4.6
Luxury	1 Serving/114g	416	18.8	365	2.5	48.5	16.4	1.0
Retail	1oz/28g	92	3.3	329	3.0	56.3	11.8	1.7
Rich Fruit, Laced with Brandy, Tesco*	1 Serving/100g	305	9.7	305	3.7	50.8	9.7	1.3
Rich Fruit, Tesco*	1 Serving/114g	331	6.7	290	2.4	55.0	5.9	0.0
VLH Kitchens	1 Serving/114g	310	2.2	272	3.1	59.3	2.5	4.6
Wheat Free, Gluten Free, Tesco*	1oz/28g	84	2.0	295	1.9	60.4	7.1	4.5
with Cider, Value, Tesco*	1 Serving/100g	312	7.0	312	2.7	59.6	7.0	3.3
with Cider & Sherry, Waitrose*	¼ Pud/113g	344	7.2	303	2.5	59.0	6.3	3.2
CHUTNEY								
Albert's Victorian, Baxters*	1 Serving/25g	40	0.1	159	1.1	37.9	0.3	1.5
Apple, Tomato & Sultana, Tesco*	1 Serving/50g	88	0.1	176	1.1	42.4	0.2	1.3
Apple & Pear, TTD, Sainsbury's*	1 Serving/20g	38	0.2	190	0.6	45.2	0.8	1.7
Apple & Walnut, Waitrose*	1 Serving/20g	49	0.5	243	12.0	53.8	2.6	3.8
Apricot, Sharwood's*	1 Tsp/16g	21	0.0	131	0.6	32.0	0.1	2.3
Bengal Hot, Sharwood's*	1oz/28g	56	0.1	200	0.5	48.7	0.3	1.1
Bengal Spice Mango, Sharwood's*	1 Tsp/5g	12	0.0	236	0.5	58.0	0.2	1.2
Caramelised Onion, Sainsbury's*	1 Serving/25g	28	0.3	111	1.1	23.5	1.4	1.1
Caramelised Onion, TTD, Sainsbury's*	1 Serving/20g	31	0.1	157	0.8	37.3	0.5	2.1
Caramelised Red Onion, Loyd Grossman*	1 Serving/10g	11	0.0	111	0.5	27.2	0.0	0.5
Cranberry & Caramelised Red Onion, Baxters*	1 Serving/20g	31	0.0	154	0.3	38.0	0.1	0.3

	Measure INFO/WEIGHT	per Measure KCAL	FAT	Nutrition Values per 100g / 100ml KCAL	PROT	CARB	FAT	FIBRE
CHUTNEY								
Fruit, Spiced, Baxters*	1 Tsp/16g	23	0.0	143	6.0	34.8	0.1	0.0
Indian Appetisers, Pot, Waitrose*	1 Pot/158g	330	2.2	209	1.8	47.3	1.4	1.8
Lime & Chilli, Geeta's*	1 Serving/25g	69	0.3	277	2.0	64.0	1.4	1.9
Mango, Green Label, Sharwood's*	1 Tsp/10g	23	0.0	234	0.3	57.8	0.2	0.9
Mango, Hot, Patak's*	1 Jar/340g	877	0.7	258	0.4	67.1	0.2	0.7
Mango, Hot & Spicy, Waitrose*	1 Serving/20g	46	0.1	230	0.6	51.6	0.3	1.8
Mango, Indian Takeaway, Asda*	1 Pack/70g	145	0.1	207	0.3	50.9	0.2	1.0
Mango, Major Grey, Patak's*	1 Tbsp/15g	38	0.0	255	0.4	66.0	0.2	0.7
Mango, Sensations, Walkers*	¼ Jar/57g	122	0.1	214	0.3	53.0	0.1	0.6
Mango, Spiced, M & S*	1 Serving/15g	26	0.1	175	1.2	42.3	0.4	3.2
Mango, Spicy, Sainsbury's*	1 Tbsp/15g	24	0.1	160	0.7	37.0	0.7	1.3
Mango, Sweet	*1 Serving/16g*	*30*	*0.0*	*189*	*0.7*	*48.3*	*0.1*	*0.0*
Mango, Tesco*	1 Serving/20g	45	0.0	224	0.4	55.5	0.1	1.3
Mango, Waitrose*	1 Serving/20g	43	0.3	215	1.0	49.0	1.5	2.0
Mango & Ginger, Baxters*	1 Jar/320g	598	0.6	187	5.0	45.7	0.2	0.9
Mango & Lime, Sharwood's*	1oz/28g	58	0.1	206	0.4	50.5	0.3	0.8
Mango & Mint, Cofresh*	1 Tbsp/20g	31	0.1	155	1.7	36.4	0.3	2.0
Mango with Hint of Chilli & Ginger, Waitrose*	1 Serving/20g	52	0.0	259	0.5	64.2	0.0	0.7
Mixed Fruit	*1 Serving/16g*	*25*	*0.0*	*155*	*0.6*	*39.7*	*0.0*	*0.0*
Peach, Spicy, Waitrose*	1 Serving/20g	43	0.3	215	1.0	49.0	1.5	1.5
Ploughman's Plum, The English Provender Co.*	1 Tsp/10g	16	0.0	160	1.3	38.1	0.2	1.6
Red Onion & Sherry Vinegar, Sainsbury's*	1 Serving/10g	24	0.1	236	0.5	57.1	0.6	1.4
Spicy Fruit, Baxters*	1 Serving/15g	22	0.0	146	0.6	35.4	0.2	0.0
Spicy Onion, Organic, The English Provender Co*	1 Serving/10g	24	0.0	245	1.2	59.0	0.5	3.5
Tomato	*1 Serving/16g*	*20*	*0.0*	*128*	*1.2*	*31.0*	*0.2*	*1.3*
Tomato, Waitrose*	1 Pot/100g	195	0.3	195	1.3	46.8	0.3	0.0
Tomato & Red Pepper, Baxters*	1 Jar/312g	512	1.2	164	2.0	38.0	0.4	1.5
CIDER								
Cyder, Organic, Aspall*	1 Glass/200ml	120	0.2	60	0.1	3.1	0.1	0.0
Cyder, Perronelle's Blush, Aspall*	1 Glass/200ml	122	0.2	61	0.1	5.4	0.1	0.5
Cyder, Premier Cru, Aspall*	1 Glass/200ml	120	0.0	60	0.0	3.1	0.0	0.0
Cyder, Suffolk, Medium, Aspall*	1 Glass/200ml	134	0.0	67	0.1	4.4	0.0	0.0
Diamond White*	1 fl oz/30ml	11	0.0	36	0.0	2.6	0.0	0.0
Dry, Average	*1 Pint/568ml*	*205*	*0.0*	*36*	*0.0*	*2.6*	*0.0*	*0.0*
Dry, Strongbow*	1 Bottle/375ml	161	0.0	43	0.0	3.4	0.0	0.0
Frosty Jacks, Strong, Aston Manor Brewery Company Ltd*	1 Pint/568ml	250	0.0	44	0.0	0.0	0.0	0.0
Gold, Thatchers*	1 Bottle/500ml	230	0.0	46	0.0	4.5	0.0	0.0
Light, Bulmers*	1 Can/500ml	140	0.0	28	0.0	0.8	0.0	0.0
Low Alcohol	*1 Pint/568ml*	*97*	*0.0*	*17*	*0.0*	*3.6*	*0.0*	*0.0*
Low Carb, Stowford*	1 Bottle/500ml	140	0.0	28	0.0	0.2	0.0	0.0
Magner's*	½ Pint/284ml	105	0.0	37	0.0	2.0	0.0	0.0
Organic, Westons*	1 Glass/200ml	96	0.0	48	0.0	3.1	0.0	0.0
Original, Bulmers*	1 Glass/250ml	105	0.0	42	0.0	4.0	0.0	0.0
Original, Gaymers*	1 Bottle/330ml	148	0.0	45	0.0	4.7	0.0	0.0
Pear, Average	*1 Glass/200ml*	*86*	*0.0*	*43*	*0.0*	*3.6*	*0.0*	*0.0*
Pear, Bulmers*	1 Glass/200ml	86	0.0	43	0.0	3.6	0.0	0.0
Pear, Gaymers*	1 Bottle/330ml	168	0.0	51	0.0	6.2	0.0	0.0
Pear, Magner's*	1 Bottle/568ml	179	0.0	31	0.0	0.0	0.0	0.0
Pear, Non Alcoholic, Kopparberg*	1 Bottle/500ml	170	0.5	34	0.0	8.4	0.1	0.0
Pear, Organic, Westons*	1 Glass/200ml	106	0.0	53	0.0	5.1	0.0	0.0
Scrumpy, Average	*1 Glass/200ml*	*93*	*0.0*	*46*	*0.0*	*2.3*	*0.0*	*0.0*
Scrumpy, Westons*	1 Glass/200ml	94	0.0	47	0.0	1.8	0.0	0.0
Sweet, Average	*1 Pint/568ml*	*239*	*0.0*	*42*	*0.0*	*4.3*	*0.0*	*0.0*

	INFO/WEIGHT	KCAL	FAT	KCAL	PROT	CARB	FAT	FIBRE
CIDER								
Vintage	*1 Pint/568ml*	*574*	*0.0*	*101*	*0.0*	*7.3*	*0.0*	*0.0*
CINNAMON								
Ground, Average	*1 Tsp/3g*	*8*	*0.1*	*261*	*3.9*	*55.5*	*3.2*	*0.0*
Stick, Schwartz*	1 Stick/2g	7	0.0	339	4.7	79.3	0.3	0.0
CLAMS								
in Brine, Average	*1oz/28g*	*22*	*0.2*	*79*	*16.0*	*2.4*	*0.6*	*0.0*
Raw, Average	*20 Sm/180g*	*133*	*1.7*	*74*	*12.8*	*2.6*	*1.0*	*0.0*
CLEMENTINES								
Raw, Weighed with Peel, Average	*1 Med/60g*	*28*	*0.1*	*46*	*1.1*	*10.9*	*0.1*	*2.1*
Raw, Weighed without Peel, Average	*1 Med/46g*	*17*	*0.0*	*37*	*0.9*	*8.7*	*0.1*	*1.7*
COCKLES								
Boiled	*1 Cockle/4g*	*2*	*0.0*	*53*	*12.0*	*0.0*	*0.6*	*0.0*
Bottled in Vinegar, Drained	*1oz/28g*	*17*	*0.2*	*60*	*13.3*	*0.0*	*0.7*	*0.0*
COCKTAIL								
Alcoholic, Juice Based, Average	1 Glass/200ml	464	29.2	232	6.4	18.7	14.6	1.4
Bucks Fizz, Premixed, M & S*	1 Glass/250ml	152	0.0	61	0.0	9.0	0.0	0.0
Cosmopolitan, Canned, M & S*	1 Can/200ml	456	0.0	228	0.0	22.0	0.0	0.0
Grenadine, Orange Juice, Pineapple Juice	1 Glass/200ml	158	0.3	79	0.5	19.2	0.1	0.2
Mai Tai, Average	1 Glass/200ml	209	0.1	105	0.2	13.9	0.1	0.1
Pina Colada	1 Glass/250ml	592	20.0	237	1.0	28.0	8.0	0.0
COCOA BUTTER								
Average	*1oz/28g*	*251*	*27.9*	*896*	*0.0*	*0.0*	*99.5*	*0.0*
COCOA POWDER								
Cadbury*	1 Tbsp/16g	52	3.3	322	23.1	10.5	20.8	0.0
Dry, Unsweetened, Average	1 Tbsp/5g	12	0.7	229	19.6	54.3	13.7	33.2
Organic, Green & Black's*	1 Tbsp/15g	52	3.4	345	22.5	12.5	22.6	30.5
Valrhona*	1 Tsp/5g	22	1.0	450	25.0	45.0	20.0	30.0
COCONUT								
Chips, Organic, Infinity Foods*	1 Serving/100g	604	62.0	604	5.6	6.4	62.0	13.7
Creamed, Average	*1oz/28g*	*186*	*19.2*	*665*	*6.0*	*6.7*	*68.4*	*7.0*
Desiccated, Average	*1oz/28g*	*169*	*17.4*	*604*	*5.6*	*6.4*	*62.0*	*13.7*
Desiccated, Whitworths*	1oz/28g	170	17.4	606	5.6	6.4	62.0	13.7
Fresh, Flesh Only, Average	*1oz/28g*	*98*	*10.1*	*351*	*3.2*	*3.7*	*36.0*	*7.3*
Ice, Average	*1oz/28g*	*104*	*3.6*	*371*	*1.7*	*66.7*	*12.7*	*2.6*
Milk, Average	*1 Can/400ml*	*698*	*69.7*	*174*	*1.4*	*2.9*	*17.4*	*2.9*
Milk, KTC*	1 Can/400g	776	73.2	194	0.9	1.2	18.3	0.0
Milk, Reduced Fat, Average	*1 Serving/100g*	*103*	*10.0*	*103*	*0.9*	*2.4*	*10.0*	*0.4*
Water with Pineapple, Vita Coco*	1 Carton/330ml	82	0.0	25	0.0	6.0	0.0	0.0
COD								
Baked, Average	*1oz/28g*	*27*	*0.3*	*96*	*21.4*	*0.0*	*1.2*	*0.0*
Beer Battered, Crispy, Finest, Tesco*	1 Portion/250g	575	35.0	230	12.0	13.4	14.0	1.3
Dried, Salted, Average	*1oz/28g*	*82*	*0.7*	*290*	*62.8*	*0.0*	*2.4*	*0.0*
Dried, Salted, Boiled, Average	*1oz/28g*	*39*	*0.3*	*138*	*32.5*	*0.0*	*0.9*	*0.0*
Fillets, Battered, Average	1 Serving/90g	158	7.3	175	12.5	12.9	8.1	1.0
Fillets, Breaded, Average	1 Serving/97g	200	9.4	206	13.0	16.7	9.7	1.0
Fillets, Breaded, Chunky, Average	1 Piece/135g	204	8.0	151	13.7	10.9	5.9	1.4
Fillets, Breaded, Light, Healthy Range, Average	1 Fillet/135g	209	6.9	154	13.6	13.3	5.1	1.2
Fillets, Chunky, Average	*1 Fillet/198g*	*267*	*7.3*	*135*	*17.1*	*8.2*	*3.7*	*0.8*
Fillets, Skinless & Boneless, Raw, Average	*1 Portion/92g*	*90*	*1.6*	*98*	*17.8*	*2.7*	*1.7*	*0.4*
Fillets, Smoked, Average	*1 Serving/150g*	*151*	*2.4*	*101*	*21.6*	*0.0*	*1.6*	*0.0*
Fillets with a Red Pepper Salsa, Love Life, Waitrose*	½ Pack/170g	92	1.5	54	9.0	2.5	0.9	0.5
Loins, Average	*1 Serving/145g*	*116*	*1.2*	*80*	*17.9*	*0.1*	*0.8*	*0.2*
Loins, Beer Battered, TTD, Sainsbury's*	1 Fillet/93g	182	10.8	196	14.4	8.5	11.6	2.7

C

	Measure INFO/WEIGHT	per Measure KCAL	FAT	Nutrition Values per 100g / 100ml KCAL	PROT	CARB	FAT	FIBRE
COD								
Loins, Steaks, Skinless & Boneless, TTD, Sainsbury's*	1 Steak/100g	105	0.4	105	25.2	0.1	0.4	0.1
Poached, Average	*1oz/28g*	*26*	*0.3*	*94*	*20.9*	*0.0*	*1.1*	*0.0*
Smoked, Raw, Average	*1oz/28g*	*22*	*0.2*	*79*	*18.3*	*0.0*	*0.6*	*0.0*
Steaks, Battered, Chip Shop Style, Average	1 Serving/150g	321	18.0	214	12.5	14.3	12.0	1.1
Steamed, Average	*1oz/28g*	*23*	*0.3*	*83*	*18.6*	*0.0*	*0.9*	*0.0*
COD IN								
Butter Sauce, Ross*	1 Serving/150g	126	5.8	84	9.1	3.2	3.9	0.1
Butter Sauce, Sainsbury's*	1 Serving/170g	224	15.3	132	10.6	2.0	9.0	0.1
Butter Sauce, Steaks, Birds Eye*	1 Pack/170g	185	9.3	109	9.8	5.0	5.5	0.1
Butter Sauce, Steaks, Frozen, Asda*	1 Pouch/152g	163	4.0	107	16.0	5.0	2.6	0.8
Butter Sauce, Steaks, Youngs*	1 Pack/139g	107	3.2	77	9.7	4.1	2.3	0.4
Butter Sauce, Tesco*	1 Pack/150g	123	5.4	82	9.4	2.9	3.6	0.5
Cheese Sauce, BGTY, Sainsbury's*	1 Serving/170g	144	4.1	85	12.8	3.1	2.4	0.0
Cheese Sauce, Pre Packed, Average	1 Serving/150g	136	4.4	90	11.8	4.1	2.9	0.0
Cheese Sauce, Steaks, Birds Eye*	1 Pack/182g	175	6.4	96	10.9	5.2	3.5	0.1
Mushroom Sauce, BGTY, Sainsbury's*	1 Serving/170g	112	2.9	66	9.9	2.8	1.7	0.1
Parsley Sauce, COU, M & S*	1 Pack/185g	129	4.6	70	10.6	1.4	2.5	0.6
Parsley Sauce, Portions, Ocean Trader*	1 Serving/120g	112	4.7	93	9.4	4.0	3.9	0.1
Parsley Sauce, Pre Packed, Average	1 Serving/150g	123	4.7	82	10.1	3.3	3.1	0.5
Parsley Sauce, Steaks, Birds Eye*	1 Steak/172g	155	4.8	90	10.5	5.6	2.8	0.1
Red Pepper Sauce, SteamFresh, Birds Eye*	1 Serving/125g	115	2.4	92	14.4	4.7	1.9	0.3
Rich Butter Sauce, Steaks, Ocean Trader*	1 Pouch/150g	136	6.1	91	10.3	3.3	4.1	0.1
Sweet Red Pepper Sauce, Fillets, GFY, Asda*	½ Pack/170g	143	2.7	84	15.0	2.3	1.6	0.1
COD WITH								
Chips & Peas, 240, Oakhouse Foods Ltd*	1 Meal/300g	510	18.6	170	6.4	22.3	6.2	2.2
Chunky Chips, M & S*	1 Serving/340g	510	20.4	150	6.5	17.5	6.0	1.5
Fish Pesto, Fillets, COOK!, M & S*	½ Pack/165g	210	5.1	127	16.4	8.4	3.1	4.2
Mediterranean Butter, Sainsbury's*	1 Pack/170g	196	8.9	115	17.0	0.1	5.2	0.1
Parma Ham & Sardinian Chick Peas, M & S*	½ Pack/255g	268	12.5	105	9.8	5.3	4.9	0.5
Roasted Vegetables, M & S*	1 Serving/280g	238	10.6	85	8.0	4.9	3.8	1.7
Salsa & Rosemary Potatoes, BGTY, Sainsbury's*	1 Pack/450g	355	4.0	79	4.7	13.1	0.9	1.6
Sunblush Tomato Sauce, GFY, Asda*	½ Pack/177g	117	2.7	66	13.0	0.1	1.5	1.0
Sweet Chilli, COU, M & S*	1 Pack/400g	360	2.0	90	7.7	13.1	0.5	1.6
Tomato Sauce, Fillets, Asda*	1 Serving/181g	210	10.9	116	13.0	2.6	6.0	2.3
Vegetables, Haches, Steaks, Peche Ocean*	1 Serving/200g	184	7.8	92	12.0	2.1	3.9	0.0
COFFEE								
Alternative, Wake Up, Whole Earth*	1 Cup/5g	19	0.0	377	5.5	88.4	0.2	0.0
Black, Average	1 Mug/270ml	5	0.0	2	0.2	0.3	0.0	0.0
Cafe Caramel, Cafe Range, Nescafe*	1 Sachet/17g	72	2.4	423	9.2	64.6	14.1	1.3
Cafe Hazelnut, Nescafe*	1 Sachet/17g	73	2.4	428	9.3	66.0	14.1	0.0
Cafe Irish Cream, Cafe Range, Nescafe*	1 Sachet/23g	98	3.2	425	8.2	65.2	14.1	1.2
Cafe Latte, Dry, Douwe Egberts*	1 Serving/12g	58	2.6	480	10.0	60.0	22.0	0.0
Cafe Latte, Instant, Maxwell House*	1 Serving/16g	67	3.0	420	17.0	45.5	18.9	0.1
Cafe Mocha, Cafe Range, Nescafe*	1 Sachet/22g	92	2.9	418	8.5	66.6	13.1	0.0
Cafe Vanilla, Cafe Range, Nescafe*	1 Sachet/19g	79	2.8	429	9.3	64.6	14.9	1.2
Cappuccino, Cafe Mocha, Dry, Maxwell House*	1 Serving/23g	100	2.5	434	4.3	78.2	10.8	0.0
Cappuccino, Cappio, Iced, Kenco*	1 Can/200ml	138	6.0	69	3.0	7.0	3.0	0.0
Cappuccino, Cappio, Kenco*	1 Sachet/18g	79	1.9	439	11.7	73.9	10.6	0.6
Cappuccino, Decaff, Instant, Made Up, Nescafe*	1 Mug/200ml	68	2.3	34	0.9	5.0	1.1	0.0
Cappuccino, Decaff, Nescafe*	1 Sachet/16g	68	2.3	428	11.6	62.6	14.6	0.0
Cappuccino, Decaff, Unsweetened, Nescafe*	1 Sachet/16g	70	3.1	437	14.5	51.2	19.4	4.3
Cappuccino, Dreamy, Cafe, Options*	1 Serving/30g	77	5.1	256	12.9	58.1	16.9	0.0
Cappuccino, Dry, Maxwell House*	1 Mug/15g	52	1.4	350	12.0	64.0	9.6	0.4

COFFEE

	Measure INFO/WEIGHT	per Measure KCAL	FAT	Nutrition Values per 100g / 100ml KCAL	PROT	CARB	FAT	FIBRE
Cappuccino, for Filter Systems, Kenco*	1 Sachet/6g	22	0.8	375	19.0	44.0	13.5	0.0
Cappuccino, Instant, Unsweetened, Douwe Egberts*	1 Serving/12g	48	1.9	400	11.0	53.0	16.0	0.0
Cappuccino, Italian, Nescafe*	1 Cup/150ml	60	2.9	40	1.2	4.4	1.9	0.0
Cappuccino, Made Up, Dolce Gusto, Nescafe*	1 Serving/240g	84	3.7	35	1.1	4.0	1.5	0.3
Cappuccino, Organic Chocolate, Traidcraft*	1 Serving/25g	139	9.5	555	7.0	43.0	38.0	0.0
Cappuccino, Original, Sachets, Nescafe*	1 Sachet/18g	80	3.1	444	11.7	60.3	17.4	0.0
Cappuccino, Original Mugsticks, Maxwell House*	1 Serving/18g	73	2.8	406	14.4	52.8	15.6	0.0
Cappuccino, Premium Quality, Ernesto*	1 Sachet/13g	46	0.4	372	12.0	71.0	3.0	1.0
Cappuccino, Semi Skimmed Milk, Average	1 Mug/200ml	63	2.3	31	2.2	3.2	1.1	0.0
Cappuccino, Skinny, Nescafe*	1 Sachet/16g	51	0.7	318	23.6	43.9	4.4	10.6
Cappuccino, Swiss Chocolate, Nescafe*	1 Sachet/20g	81	2.3	404	10.5	65.3	11.5	2.9
Cappuccino, to Go, Original, Nescafe*	1 Serving/19g	84	3.3	444	11.7	60.3	17.4	0.0
Cappuccino, to Go, Unsweetened, Nescafe*	1 Serving/17g	79	4.0	464	15.0	47.3	23.8	0.0
Cappuccino, Unsweetened, Cappio, Kenco*	1 Serving/18g	73	1.8	406	12.2	66.7	10.0	0.6
Cappuccino, Unsweetened, Nescafe*	1 Sachet/16g	74	3.8	464	15.0	47.3	23.8	0.0
Cappuccino, Unsweetened Taste, Maxwell House*	1 Serving/15g	65	2.9	434	17.4	47.6	19.3	0.3
Chococino, Made Up, Dolce Gusto, Nescafe*	1 Serving/210g	147	5.4	70	2.3	9.4	2.6	0.7
Columbian, Nescafe*	1 Serving/2g	2	0.0	111	16.7	11.1	0.0	5.6
Compliment*	1 Serving/14ml	20	1.8	143	1.4	6.4	12.9	0.0
Espresso, Double Shot, McDonald's*	1 Double/60ml	0	0.0	0	0.0	0.0	0.0	0.0
Espresso, Made Up, Dolce Gusto, Nescafe*	1 Serving/60ml	1	0.1	2	0.1	0.0	0.1	0.3
Frappe Iced, Nestle*	1 Sachet/24g	92	1.0	384	15.0	72.0	4.0	0.5
Gold Blend, Decaffinated, Nescafe*	1 Tsp/5g	3	0.0	63	7.0	9.0	0.2	27.0
Gold Blend, Nescafe*	1 Cup/200ml	3	0.0	63	7.0	9.0	0.2	27.0
Infusion, Average with Semi-Skimmed Milk	1 Cup/220ml	15	0.4	7	0.6	0.7	0.2	0.0
Infusion, Average with Single Cream	1 Cup/220ml	31	2.6	14	0.4	0.3	1.2	0.0
Infusion, Average with Whole Milk	1 Cup/220ml	15	0.9	7	0.5	0.5	0.4	0.0
Instant, Alta Rica, Nescafe*	1 Tsp/2g	2	0.0	98	13.8	10.0	0.3	21.0
Instant, Decaffeinated, Nescafe*	1 Tsp/2g	2	0.0	101	14.9	10.0	0.2	8.4
Instant, Made with Skimmed Milk	1 Mug/270ml	15	0.0	6	0.6	0.8	0.0	0.0
Instant, Made with Water & Semi-Skimmed Milk	1 Mug/350ml	24	1.4	7	0.4	0.5	0.4	0.0
Instant, Original, Nescafe*	1 Tsp/2g	1	0.0	63	7.0	9.0	0.2	27.0
Instant, with Skimmed Milk, Costa Rican, Kenco*	1 Mug/300ml	17	0.1	6	0.6	0.8	0.0	0.0
Latte, Instant, Skinny, Douwe Egberts*	1 Serving/12g	35	1.3	290	11.0	38.0	11.0	29.0
Latte, Luscious, Options*	1 Serving/14g	62	2.4	443	14.3	57.9	17.1	3.6
Latte, Macchiato, Tassimo*	1 Cup/275ml	135	7.7	49	2.3	3.6	2.8	0.0
Latte, Nescafe*	1 Sachet/22g	110	6.3	498	14.5	45.7	28.5	0.0
Latte, No Sugar, In Cup, From Machine, Kenco*	1 Cup/4g	17	0.9	400	7.6	44.0	22.0	0.0
Latte, Skinny, Nescafe*	1 Sachet/20g	72	1.1	359	24.1	54.3	5.3	1.1
Latte Macchiato, Made Up, Dolce Gusto, Nescafe*	1 Serving/220g	89	4.2	40	1.9	4.1	1.9	0.3
Mocha, Instant, Skinny, Douwe Egberts*	1 Serving/12g	37	1.3	308	10.8	40.8	10.8	5.0
Mocha, Made Up, Dolce Gusto, Nescafe*	1 Serving/210g	117	5.1	56	2.4	6.1	2.4	0.6
Mocha, Skinny, Made Up, Nescafe*	1 Sachet/21g	77	0.7	367	13.6	70.3	3.5	4.3
Regular, Ground or Instant	1 Cup/177g	6	0.0	4	0.2	0.7	0.0	0.0
Skinny Cappuccino, Made Up, Dolce Gusto, Nescafe*	1 Mug/15g	49	0.1	337	33.3	48.8	0.9	2.3

COFFEE MATE

	Measure INFO/WEIGHT	per Measure KCAL	FAT	Nutrition Values per 100g / 100ml KCAL	PROT	CARB	FAT	FIBRE
Original, Nestle*	1 Tsp/4g	19	1.2	547	2.4	56.7	34.4	0.0
Virtually Fat Free, Nestle*	1 Tsp/5g	10	0.1	200	1.0	42.0	3.0	0.0

COFFEE SUBSTITUTE

	Measure INFO/WEIGHT	per Measure KCAL	FAT	Nutrition Values per 100g / 100ml KCAL	PROT	CARB	FAT	FIBRE
Bambu, Vogel*	1 Tsp/3g	10	0.0	320	3.5	75.3	0.5	0.0

COFFEE WHITENER

	Measure INFO/WEIGHT	per Measure KCAL	FAT	Nutrition Values per 100g / 100ml KCAL	PROT	CARB	FAT	FIBRE
Half Fat, Co-Op*	1 Tsp/5g	21	0.6	430	0.9	78.0	13.0	0.0
Light, Asda*	1 Serving/3g	13	0.4	433	0.9	78.0	13.0	0.0

C

	Measure INFO/WEIGHT	per Measure KCAL	FAT	Nutrition Values per 100g / 100ml KCAL	PROT	CARB	FAT	FIBRE
COFFEE WHITENER								
Morrisons*	1 Serving/10g	53	3.3	535	2.6	57.5	32.8	0.0
COGNAC								
40% Volume	**1 Shot/35ml**	**78**	**0.0**	**222**	**0.0**	**0.0**	**0.0**	**0.0**
French, All Flavours, Alize*	1 fl oz/30ml	69	0.0	230	0.0	6.7	0.0	0.0
COLA								
Average	1 Can/330ml	135	0.0	41	0.0	10.9	0.0	0.0
Coke, Cherry, Coca-Cola*	1 Bottle/500ml	225	0.0	45	0.0	11.2	0.0	0.0
Coke, Coca-Cola*	1 Can/330ml	142	0.0	43	0.0	10.7	0.0	0.0
Coke, Diet, Caffeine Free, Coca-Cola*	1 Can/330ml	1	0.0	0	0.0	0.1	0.0	0.0
Coke, Diet, Coca-Cola*	1 Can/330ml	1	0.0	0	0.0	0.0	0.0	0.0
Coke, Diet with Cherry, Coca-Cola*	1 Bottle/500ml	5	0.0	1	0.0	0.0	0.0	0.0
Coke, Vanilla, Coca-Cola*	1 Bottle/500ml	215	0.0	43	0.0	10.7	0.0	0.0
Coke, with Lemon, Diet, Coca-Cola*	1 Can/330ml	5	0.0	1	0.0	0.0	0.0	0.0
Coke, with Vanilla, Diet, Coca-Cola*	1 Glass/200ml	1	0.0	0	0.0	0.1	0.0	0.0
Curiosity, Fentiman's*	1 Bottle/275ml	129	0.0	47	0.1	11.6	0.0	0.0
Diet, Classic, Sainsbury's*	1 Can/330ml	1	0.0	0	0.0	0.0	0.0	0.0
Diet, Pepsi*	1 Can/330ml	1	0.0	0	0.0	0.0	0.0	0.0
Diet, Tesco*	1 Glass/200ml	2	0.2	1	0.1	0.1	0.1	0.0
Diet, Virgin Trains*	1 Glass/250ml	1	0.2	0	0.1	0.1	0.1	0.0
Max, Pepsi*	1 Can/330ml	2	0.0	1	0.1	0.1	0.0	0.0
Pepsi*	1 Can/330ml	145	0.0	44	0.0	11.1	0.0	0.0
Twist, Light, Pepsi*	1 Bottle/500ml	4	0.0	1	0.0	0.1	0.0	0.0
Twist, Pepsi*	1 Bottle/500ml	235	0.0	47	0.0	11.7	0.0	0.0
Zero, Caffeine Free, Coca-Cola*	1 Glass/200ml	0	0.0	0	0.0	0.0	0.0	0.0
Zero, Coca-Cola*	1 Can/330ml	2	0.0	0	0.0	0.0	0.0	0.0
COLCANNON								
Chosen By You, Asda*	1 Serving/100g	90	4.2	90	1.5	11.5	4.2	0.0
COLESLAW								
20% Less Fat, Asda*	1 Serving/100g	88	6.0	88	1.5	7.0	6.0	1.7
50% Less Fat, Asda*	1oz/28g	17	0.8	61	2.1	6.8	2.8	0.9
99% Fat Free, Kraft*	1 Serving/40ml	50	0.4	126	1.0	28.9	1.0	0.0
Apple, M & S*	1oz/28g	53	4.6	190	1.4	9.2	16.6	1.4
BFY, Morrisons*	1oz/28g	17	1.0	62	1.5	6.7	3.5	0.0
Cheese, Asda*	1 Serving/100g	242	22.0	242	4.8	6.3	22.0	1.6
Cheese, M & S*	1 Serving/57g	185	19.1	325	4.2	2.0	33.5	1.7
Cheese, Sainsbury's*	1 Serving/75g	174	16.3	232	3.4	5.6	21.8	0.6
Cheese, Supreme, Waitrose*	¼ Pack/88g	197	18.2	225	4.5	5.0	20.8	1.2
Chunky, Asda*	1oz/28g	54	5.0	194	1.0	7.1	18.0	1.6
Coronation, Sainsbury's*	¼ Pot/75g	135	10.6	180	1.2	11.9	14.2	2.4
COU, M & S*	½ Pack/125g	75	3.4	60	1.3	7.4	2.7	1.7
Creamy, 30% Less Fat, Sainsbury's*	1 Tub/300g	378	33.0	126	1.0	5.5	11.0	1.4
Creamy, Asda*	1 Serving/25g	62	6.0	248	0.9	7.0	24.0	1.8
Creamy, GFY, Asda*	1 Serving/100g	163	14.9	163	0.7	6.5	14.9	0.8
Creamy, Light Choices, Tesco*	1/3 Pot/100g	105	8.8	105	1.2	4.9	8.8	1.6
Crunchy, Premium, Millcroft*	1 Pack/400g	756	69.6	189	0.9	7.3	17.4	1.5
Deli Style, BGTY, Sainsbury's*	1 Serving/75g	64	4.6	85	1.5	6.0	6.1	1.7
Deli Style, Creamy, Sainsbury's*	1 Serving/75g	133	12.7	178	0.8	5.4	17.0	1.5
Deli Style, M & S*	1 Serving/50g	110	10.6	220	1.0	4.8	21.2	1.9
Deli Style, Sainsbury's*	½ Pot/150g	291	28.2	194	0.9	5.2	18.8	1.5
Finest, Tesco*	1 Serving/51g	145	15.0	285	0.8	4.1	29.4	1.3
Fruity, Asda*	½ Pot/125g	101	6.1	81	1.3	8.0	4.9	1.7
Fruity, M & S*	1 Serving/63g	151	14.3	240	1.1	8.3	22.7	3.1
Garlic & Herb, Asda*	1 Tbsp/15g	22	2.0	147	0.9	5.8	13.3	1.7

	Measure INFO/WEIGHT	per Measure KCAL	FAT	Nutrition Values per 100g / 100ml KCAL	PROT	CARB	FAT	FIBRE
COLESLAW								
GFY, Asda*	1 Serving/50g	27	1.4	55	1.3	6.0	2.9	2.3
Half Fat, Waitrose*	1 Serving/100g	64	4.5	64	1.0	4.8	4.5	2.0
Heinz*	1oz/28g	38	2.9	135	1.6	9.4	10.2	1.2
Light, Reduced Fat, Morrisons*	1 Serving/30g	37	3.1	125	0.8	7.4	10.2	0.0
Low Fat Mayonnaise, Tesco*	1oz/28g	18	1.2	64	1.4	4.7	4.4	1.4
Luxury, Asda*	1 Serving/50g	108	10.5	217	0.9	6.0	21.0	0.0
Luxury, M & S*	1oz/28g	43	3.9	152	1.0	6.0	13.8	1.0
M & S*	1oz/28g	50	4.6	180	1.7	6.1	16.5	1.1
Organic, M & S*	1oz/28g	41	3.5	145	1.1	7.3	12.4	1.0
Prawn, Asda*	1oz/28g	54	4.8	192	2.4	6.6	17.3	1.4
Premium, Co-Op*	1 Serving/50g	160	17.0	320	1.0	3.0	34.0	2.0
Reduced Calorie, Budgens*	½ Pot/125g	124	8.6	99	1.0	8.3	6.9	2.3
Reduced Calorie, Iceland*	1 Serving/50g	51	3.7	102	0.7	7.8	7.5	1.6
Reduced Fat, Average	1 Tbsp/20g	23	1.9	113	1.0	6.4	9.3	2.0
Standard Range, From Supermarket, Average	1oz/28g	72	7.4	258	1.2	4.2	26.4	1.4
Supreme, Waitrose*	1oz/28g	53	5.1	190	1.8	4.9	18.1	1.7
Three Cheese, Asda*	1 Serving/78g	203	18.7	260	5.0	6.0	24.0	1.7
Three Cheese, Finest, Tesco*	1/3 Pack/100g	255	22.7	255	6.4	5.8	22.7	1.1
TTD, Sainsbury's*	¼ Pot/75g	218	22.5	291	1.5	3.5	30.1	2.8
with 60% Less Fat, GFY, Asda*	1 Serving/41g	36	2.5	88	1.5	7.0	6.0	1.7
with Free Range Egg Mayonnaise, Reduced Fat, M & S*	1oz/28g	62	5.9	220	1.0	7.0	21.1	1.8
with Reduced Calorie Dressing, Retail	1 Serving/40g	27	1.8	67	0.9	6.1	4.5	1.4
COLEY								
Portions, Raw, Average	*1 Serving/92g*	*75*	*0.7*	*81*	*18.4*	*0.0*	*0.7*	*0.0*
Steamed, Average	*1oz/28g*	*29*	*0.4*	*105*	*23.3*	*0.0*	*1.3*	*0.0*
CONCHIGLIE								
Cooked, Average	*1 Serving/185g*	*247*	*1.6*	*133*	*4.8*	*26.6*	*0.8*	*0.5*
Dry Weight, Average	*1 Serving/100g*	*352*	*1.7*	*352*	*12.5*	*71.6*	*1.7*	*2.6*
Whole Wheat, Dry Weight, Average	*1 Serving/75g*	*237*	*1.5*	*316*	*12.6*	*62.0*	*2.0*	*10.7*
CONCHIGLIONI								
Dry, Waitrose*	1 Serving/75g	256	1.0	341	12.5	69.8	1.3	3.7
CONSERVE								
Apricot, Average	*1 Tbsp/15g*	*37*	*0.0*	*244*	*0.5*	*59.3*	*0.2*	*1.5*
Apricot, Reduced Sugar, Streamline*	1 Tbsp/20g	37	0.0	184	0.5	45.0	0.2	0.0
Black Cherry with Amaretto, Finest, Tesco*	1 Serving/10g	26	0.0	261	0.5	64.4	0.1	0.8
Blackcurrant, Average	*1 Tbsp/15g*	*37*	*0.0*	*245*	*0.6*	*60.0*	*0.1*	*1.9*
Blueberry, M & S*	1 Tsp/8g	15	0.0	206	0.3	51.1	0.1	1.3
Hedgerow, TTD, Sainsbury's*	1 Tbsp/15g	41	0.0	276	0.5	68.2	0.1	0.5
Morello Cherry, Waitrose*	1 Tbsp/15g	39	0.0	258	0.4	64.2	0.0	1.4
Plum, TTD, Sainsbury's*	1 Tbsp/15g	44	0.0	295	0.3	73.1	0.1	0.5
Raspberry, Average	*1 Tbsp/15g*	*37*	*0.1*	*249*	*0.6*	*61.0*	*0.3*	*1.3*
Red Cherry, TTD, Sainsbury's*	1 Tbsp/15g	43	0.0	283	0.4	70.2	0.1	0.5
Rhubarb & Ginger, M & S*	1 Tbsp/15g	29	0.0	194	0.3	47.9	0.1	1.0
Strawberry, 60% Fruit, Reduced Sugar, M & S*	1 Tsp/7g	9	0.0	135	0.4	30.1	0.2	1.9
Strawberry, Average	*1 Tbsp/15g*	*37*	*0.0*	*250*	*0.4*	*61.6*	*0.1*	*0.5*
CONSOMME								
Average	*1oz/28g*	*3*	*0.0*	*12*	*2.9*	*0.1*	*0.0*	*0.0*
Beef, Canned, Sainsbury's*	1 Can/415g	46	0.0	11	2.0	0.7	0.0	0.0
Beef, Luxury, Baxters*	1 Can/415g	54	0.0	13	2.6	0.7	0.0	0.0
COOKIES								
All Butter, Almond, Italian Style, M & S*	1 Cookie/23g	120	6.4	515	6.7	59.4	27.6	3.6
All Butter, Ginger Bread, M & S*	1 Cookie/23g	102	5.0	445	4.3	57.5	21.8	2.4
All Butter, Italian Style Sorrento Lemon, M & S*	1 Cookie/24g	120	6.4	500	4.9	60.4	26.7	2.1

C

COOKIES

INFO/WEIGHT	Measure	per Measure KCAL	FAT	KCAL	PROT	CARB	FAT	FIBRE
All Butter, Melting Moment, M & S*	1 Cookie/23g	110	6.4	470	4.5	51.5	27.5	3.4
All Butter, Sultana, TTD, Sainsbury's*	1 Cookie/17g	79	3.8	476	5.4	62.7	22.6	2.0
Almond, Ose*	1 Cookie/10g	46	1.4	456	8.4	74.0	14.0	0.0
Apple & Raisin, Go Ahead, McVitie's*	1 Cookie/15g	66	1.9	443	5.3	76.8	12.7	3.4
Blueberry & Oatmeal, M & S*	1 Cookie/100g	90	3.5	90	1.1	13.4	3.5	0.5
Brazil Nut, Organic, Traidcraft*	1 Cookie/17g	91	5.4	547	5.8	57.7	32.6	2.1
Brazil Nut, Prewett's*	1 Cookie/50g	122	7.4	244	2.6	25.2	14.8	1.0
Butter & Sultana, Sainsbury's*	1 Cookie/13g	61	2.6	473	4.5	68.4	20.1	1.6
Cherry Bakewell, COU, M & S*	1 Cookie/25g	90	0.6	355	6.0	77.2	2.5	3.4
Choc Chip, Bonte Fudge, Paterson's*	1 Cookie/6g	28	1.5	503	6.2	60.1	26.4	2.2
Choc Chip, Bronte*	1 Cookie/17g	79	3.6	474	5.8	64.0	21.6	0.0
Choc Chip, Cadbury*	1 Cookie/11g	55	2.8	503	5.9	62.2	25.6	0.0
Choc Chip, Giant, Paterson's*	1 Cookie/60g	296	15.2	493	0.1	61.3	25.3	3.2
Choc Chip, Lyons*	1 Cookie/11g	57	2.7	499	5.2	68.3	23.4	1.7
Choc Chip, Maryland*	1 Cookie/11g	56	2.6	511	6.2	68.0	23.9	1.3
Choc Chip, Parkside*	1 Cookie/11g	56	2.7	495	5.3	64.5	23.7	0.0
Choc Chip, Reduced Fat, Maryland*	1 Cookie/11g	51	1.9	478	5.9	73.0	18.0	0.0
Choc Chip, Sainsbury's*	1 Cookie/11g	55	2.6	508	6.2	67.0	23.9	1.3
Choc Chip & Coconut, Maryland*	1 Cookie/10g	55	2.5	512	5.1	62.9	23.7	0.0
Choc Chip & Hazelnut, Maryland*	1 Cookie/11g	55	2.7	513	6.3	65.3	25.0	0.0
Choc Chip 'n' Chunk, McVitie's*	1 Cookie/11g	55	2.9	498	5.8	59.2	26.4	3.5
Choc Chunk, Fabulous Bakin' Boys*	1 Cookie/60g	270	12.6	450	5.0	59.0	21.0	3.0
Choc Chunk, Finest, Tesco*	1 Cookie/80g	355	14.1	445	5.7	65.3	17.7	1.8
Choc Chunk & Hazelnut, Co-Op*	1 Cookie/17g	89	5.3	525	6.0	56.0	31.0	3.0
Chocolate, Belgian, Extra Special, Asda*	1 Cookie/26g	138	8.0	535	6.0	58.0	31.0	2.0
Chocolate, Milk, Free From, Tesco*	1 Cookie/20g	100	6.1	500	5.6	50.4	30.7	4.1
Chocolate, Quadruple, Sainsbury's*	1 Cookie/20g	117	6.6	585	6.0	66.5	33.0	1.5
Chocolate, Soft, American Style, Budgens*	1 Cookie/50g	215	9.3	431	5.1	60.8	18.6	2.2
Chocolate, Triple, Half Coated, Finest, Tesco*	1 Cookie/25g	131	7.3	525	5.7	58.7	29.3	2.3
Chocolate & Nut, Organic, Evernat*	1 Cookie/69g	337	15.6	489	7.2	64.1	22.6	0.0
Chocolate & Orange, COU, M & S*	1 Cookie/26g	90	0.7	350	5.7	77.2	2.6	3.2
Chocolate Chip, Average	1 Cookie/10g	49	2.5	489	5.5	64.1	24.7	2.9
Chocolate Chip, BGTY, Sainsbury's*	1 Cookie/17g	72	2.0	428	4.5	75.6	11.9	2.5
Chocolate Chip, Carb Check, Heinz*	1 Cookie/20g	91	5.0	457	7.2	43.1	24.9	7.2
Chocolate Chip, Chips Ahoy*	1 Cookie/11g	55	2.7	500	6.0	65.0	25.0	3.0
Chocolate Chip, GFY, Asda*	1 Cookie/10g	48	2.0	463	5.0	68.0	19.0	3.5
Chocolate Chip, Gluten & Wheat Free, Lovemore*	1 Cookie/17g	81	4.5	483	3.8	57.8	26.8	3.5
Chocolate Chip, Gluten Free, Organic, Dove's Farm*	1 Cookie/17g	77	3.1	451	4.3	66.9	18.5	0.0
Chocolate Chip, Handbaked, Border*	1 Cookie/15g	72	3.4	480	5.9	67.4	22.6	0.0
Chocolate Chip, Low Price, Sainsbury's*	1 Cookie/11g	54	2.3	500	7.0	70.1	21.3	2.5
Chocolate Chip, Lyons*	1 Cookie/12g	56	2.5	483	5.6	66.5	21.6	1.7
Chocolate Chip, McVitie's*	1 Cookie/11g	54	2.8	496	5.8	60.2	25.8	3.0
Chocolate Chip, Mini, McVitie's*	1 Bag/40g	196	9.2	491	5.5	65.1	23.1	2.8
Chocolate Chip, Mini, Tesco*	1 Bag/30g	148	7.1	493	5.4	64.6	23.7	1.7
Chocolate Chip, The Decadent, President's Choice*	1 Cookie/16g	79	4.1	513	6.1	61.3	26.4	3.5
Chocolate Chip, Weight Watchers*	1 Cookie/11g	49	1.9	443	7.6	65.4	17.2	4.6
Chocolate Chip & Hazelnut, Extra Special, Asda*	1 Cookie/25g	130	8.1	516	6.0	51.0	32.0	2.5
Chocolate Chunk, All Butter, M & S*	1 Cookie/24g	120	6.0	500	5.2	62.4	25.2	2.9
Chocolate Chunk, Cadbury*	1 Cookie/22g	119	6.9	540	6.5	58.0	31.2	0.0
Chocolate Chunk, Devondale*	1 Cookie/65g	308	16.3	474	4.6	59.2	25.1	2.8
Chocolate Chunk & Hazelnut, Tesco*	1 Cookie/22g	118	6.7	538	6.2	60.2	30.3	1.9
Chocolate Chunk & Hazelnut, TTD, Sainsbury's*	1 Cookie/17g	88	5.2	528	6.5	54.8	31.4	2.8
Chocolate Chunk & Orange, So Good, Somerfield*	1 Cookie/22g	117	6.5	525	5.3	60.0	29.3	1.8

COOKIES

INFO/WEIGHT	Measure	per Measure KCAL	FAT	Nutrition Values per 100g / 100ml KCAL	PROT	CARB	FAT	FIBRE
Chocolate Fruit & Nut, Extra Special, Asda*	1 Cookie/25g	125	7.1	509	6.0	56.0	29.0	2.0
Chocolate Orange, Half Coated, Finest, Tesco*	1 Cookie/22g	107	5.6	488	4.9	59.6	25.5	1.2
Cocoa, Organic, Bites, No Junk, Organix*	1 Bag/25g	105	3.2	421	7.0	69.0	13.0	5.5
Coconut, Gluten-Free, Sainsbury's*	1 Cookie/20g	103	6.1	516	5.6	54.4	30.7	4.1
Coconut & Raspberry, Gluten Free, Sainsbury's*	1 Cookie/20g	102	5.9	511	5.9	56.0	29.3	6.7
Cranberry & Orange, Finest, Tesco*	1 Cookie/26g	125	5.8	490	4.1	67.4	22.6	3.2
Cranberry & Orange, Go Ahead, McVitie's*	1 Cookie/17g	77	2.2	452	5.3	78.0	13.2	2.4
Danish Butter, Tesco*	1 Cookie/26g	133	6.6	516	4.7	66.7	25.6	1.3
Dark Treacle, Weight Watchers*	1 Cookie/11g	49	1.7	423	5.2	66.7	15.1	1.7
Double Choc, Cadbury*	1 Cookie/11g	55	2.5	485	7.3	64.3	22.2	0.0
Double Choc, Maryland*	1 Cookie/10g	51	2.6	510	5.2	64.4	25.7	0.0
Double Choc Chip, Giant, Paterson's*	1 Cookie/60g	293	15.2	489	0.3	61.3	25.3	3.7
Double Choc Chip, Mini, M & S*	1 Cookie/22g	108	5.2	490	5.3	63.6	23.7	1.8
Double Choc Chip, Tesco*	1 Cookie/11g	55	2.7	500	4.2	65.3	24.7	3.0
Double Choc Chip, Weight Watchers*	1 Cookie/11g	49	1.9	443	7.6	65.4	17.2	4.6
Double Chocolate, Organic, Dove's Farm*	1 Cookie/17g	80	3.4	468	4.5	67.5	20.1	0.3
Double Chocolate, Premium, Co-Op*	1 Cookie/17g	86	4.6	505	5.0	62.0	27.0	2.0
Double Chocolate & Walnut, Soft, Tesco*	1 Cookie/25g	116	6.4	463	5.8	52.1	25.7	4.7
Double Chocolate Chip, Co-Op*	1 Cookie/17g	87	4.6	510	5.0	63.0	27.0	2.0
Double Chocolate Chip, Organic, Waitrose*	1 Cookie/18g	96	5.6	535	5.1	58.6	31.0	1.9
Double Chocolate Chip, Somerfield*	1 Cookie/11g	56	2.8	513	5.2	64.9	25.8	1.3
Double Chocolate Chip, Traidcraft*	1 Cookie/22g	114	5.9	520	5.8	64.1	26.7	2.4
Double Fudge & Chocolate, Sugar Free, Murray*	1 Cookie/12g	47	2.3	400	5.7	65.7	20.0	5.7
Fortune, Average	1 Cookie/8g	30	0.2	378	4.2	84.0	2.7	1.6
Fruit, Giant, Cookie Coach*	1 Cookie/60g	280	13.2	466	4.9	62.0	22.0	0.0
Fruit & Oat, Soft, Diet Chef*	1 Cookie/45g	198	8.8	439	4.8	58.8	19.6	4.0
Fruity Shrewsbury, Giant, Paterson's*	1 Cookie/60g	298	15.2	496	4.8	62.6	25.4	1.7
Fudge Brownie, Maryland*	1 Cookie/11g	56	2.7	510	5.8	63.0	25.0	0.0
Ginger, Gluten Free, Barkat*	1 Cookie/17g	85	4.4	501	3.2	63.8	25.9	0.0
Ginger, Half Coated, Finest, Tesco*	1 Cookie/25g	124	6.1	495	4.7	64.2	24.4	3.8
Ginger, Low Fat, M & S*	1 Cookie/23g	82	1.0	358	5.1	74.9	4.3	2.4
Ginger & Brazil Nut, Organic, Dove's Farm*	1 Cookie/17g	79	3.5	464	5.0	65.0	20.5	4.8
Ginger & Choc Chip, BGTY, Sainsbury's*	1 Cookie/17g	69	3.2	415	5.8	55.3	19.0	12.1
Glace Cherry, Border*	1 Cookie/15g	74	3.8	493	5.4	64.3	25.6	0.0
Gman, Gingerbread, Gluten Free, Barkat*	2 Cookies/34g	167	9.3	490	15.8	49.5	27.3	6.0
Hazelnut, Gluten Free, Organic, Dove's Farm*	1 Cookie/17g	79	3.7	463	4.8	61.5	21.9	1.8
Hazelnut & Choc Chip 'n' Chunk, McVitie's*	1 Cookie/11g	55	3.0	505	6.1	57.8	27.7	3.5
Lemon & Currant, Weight Watchers*	2 Cookies/19g	86	3.4	451	5.1	63.6	17.7	8.4
Lemon & Ginger, Weight Watchers*	1 Cookie/11g	49	2.0	450	6.4	65.0	18.2	5.0
Lemon Meringue, COU, M & S*	1 Cookie/25g	89	0.6	355	5.6	77.6	2.6	3.0
Milk Chocolate, Classic, Millie's Cookies*	1 Cookie/45g	190	10.2	422	5.1	49.3	22.7	1.3
Milk Chocolate Chunk, Average	1 Cookie/25g	129	6.9	515	6.5	60.0	27.6	1.6
Oat, Giant Jumbo, Paterson's*	1 Cookie/60g	299	16.2	499	0.4	58.4	27.0	3.2
Oat & Cranberry, BGTY, Sainsbury's*	1 Cookie/28g	126	5.0	449	6.8	65.0	18.0	5.1
Oat & Raisin, Health Matters*	1 Cookie/8g	33	0.7	414	7.0	76.6	8.8	3.3
Oat & Treacle, TTD, Sainsbury's*	1 Cookie/25g	121	5.9	482	5.7	61.8	23.6	3.7
Oatflake & Honey, Organic, Sainsbury's*	1 Cookie/17g	82	3.6	480	6.3	66.0	21.2	2.6
Oatmeal, Chocolate Chip, Chewy, Dad's*	1 Cookie/15g	70	3.0	467	6.7	66.7	20.0	3.3
Oreo, Nabisco*	1 Cookie/11g	52	2.3	471	5.9	70.6	20.6	2.9
Raspberry & White Choc, Weight Watchers*	2 Cookies/19g	87	3.7	458	6.9	59.0	19.4	9.8
Raspberry Spritz, Heaven Scent*	1 Cookie/19g	90	6.0	474	5.3	52.6	31.6	0.0
Rolo, Nestle*	1 Cookie/73g	242	11.1	331	3.4	46.0	15.2	0.6
Spiced Apple, M & S*	1 Cookie/25g	90	0.7	360	5.2	75.6	2.8	2.0

C

	Measure INFO/WEIGHT	per Measure KCAL	FAT	Nutrition Values per 100g / 100ml KCAL	PROT	CARB	FAT	FIBRE
COOKIES								
Stem Ginger, BGTY, Sainsbury's*	1 Cookie/17g	73	2.0	431	4.5	76.5	11.9	1.7
Stem Ginger, Free From, Sainsbury's*	1 Cookie/17g	84	4.8	489	6.5	58.0	28.0	6.8
Stem Ginger, Half Coated, Finest, Tesco*	1 Cookie/25g	127	6.7	508	4.4	62.4	26.8	3.6
Stem Ginger, Less Than 5% Fat, M & S*	1 Cookie/22g	79	0.9	360	6.2	73.9	4.3	3.0
Stem Ginger, Reduced Fat, Waitrose*	1 Cookie/17g	75	2.7	448	4.5	71.0	16.2	1.6
Stem Ginger, TTD, Sainsbury's*	1 Cookie/17g	79	3.7	476	5.2	64.3	22.0	2.3
Sultana, All Butter, Reduced Fat, M & S*	1 Cookie/17g	70	2.4	420	4.9	68.6	14.2	2.6
Sultana, Soft & Chewy, Sainsbury's*	1 Cookie/25g	103	3.5	414	4.4	67.8	13.9	2.5
Sultana & Cinnamon, Weight Watchers*	1 Cookie/12g	46	1.4	398	5.0	67.1	12.1	1.8
Toffee, Weight Watchers*	1 Cookie/12g	52	1.9	456	5.2	71.1	16.8	2.9
Triple Chocolate Chunk, Bakery, Finest, Tesco*	1 Cookie/80g	360	15.9	450	7.4	59.2	19.9	2.1
White Chocolate, Asda*	1 Cookie/54g	256	11.9	474	5.0	64.0	22.0	2.1
White Chocolate, Maryland*	1 Cookie/10g	51	2.5	512	5.7	64.0	25.0	0.0
White Chocolate, TTD, Sainsbury's*	1 Cookie/25g	126	6.4	504	5.5	62.5	25.8	1.2
White Chocolate & Cranberry, Devondale*	1 Cookie/65g	300	15.3	462	4.7	60.7	23.5	2.1
White Chocolate & Raspberry, Finest, Tesco*	1 Cookie/76g	304	9.6	400	5.2	66.3	12.6	2.4
White Chocolate & Raspberry, McVitie's*	1 Cookie/17g	87	4.4	512	4.7	64.1	25.9	1.8
COQ AU VIN								
Diet Chef Ltd*	1 Pack/300g	285	13.2	95	7.7	6.1	4.4	2.2
Finest, Tesco*	1 Serving/273g	251	9.8	92	14.3	0.7	3.6	1.8
HL, Tesco*	½ Pack/200g	172	3.8	86	15.2	2.1	1.9	0.4
M & S*	1 Serving/295g	398	22.7	135	14.2	1.5	7.7	1.0
Perfectly Balanced, Waitrose*	1 Pack/500g	445	15.5	89	12.6	2.7	3.1	0.6
Sainsbury's*	1 Pack/400g	484	17.6	121	16.8	3.5	4.4	0.2
with Potatoes, Diet Chef Ltd*	1 Pack/300g	285	13.2	95	7.7	6.1	4.4	2.2
CORDIAL								
Blackcurrant, New Zealand Honey Co*	1 Serving/30ml	109	0.3	363	1.0	88.0	1.0	0.0
Cox's Apple & Plum, Diluted, Bottle Green*	1 Serving/10ml	3	0.0	29	0.0	7.2	0.0	0.0
Elderflower, Made Up, Bottle Green*	1 Glass/200ml	46	0.0	23	0.0	5.6	0.0	0.0
Elderflower, Undiluted, Waitrose*	1 Serving/20ml	22	0.0	110	0.0	27.5	0.0	0.0
Honey & Lemonbalm with Chamomile, Bottle Green*	1 fl oz/30ml	8	0.0	27	0.0	6.8	0.0	0.0
Lemon & Lime, High Juice, M & S*	1 Glass/250ml	75	0.0	30	0.0	7.0	0.0	0.0
Lime, Juice, Concentrated	1 Serving/20ml	22	0.0	112	0.1	29.8	0.0	0.0
Lime, Juice, Diluted	1 Glass/250ml	55	0.0	22	0.0	6.0	0.0	0.0
Lime, Juice, Diluted, Rose's*	1 Glass/250ml	60	0.0	24	0.0	5.7	0.0	0.0
Lime, with Aromatic Bitters & Ginger, Sainsbury's*	1 Serving/40ml	12	0.1	29	0.0	6.9	0.3	0.3
Pomegreat, Original, Pomegreat*	1 Serving/50ml	16	0.0	32	0.0	7.6	0.0	0.0
Sicilian Lemon & Elderflower, Diluted, Weight Watchers*	1 Glass/250ml	3	0.1	1	0.0	0.3	0.0	0.0
CORIANDER								
Leaves, Dried, Average	*1oz/28g*	*78*	*1.3*	*279*	*21.8*	*41.7*	*4.8*	*0.0*
Leaves, Fresh, Average	*1 Bunch/20g*	*5*	*0.1*	*23*	*2.1*	*3.7*	*0.5*	*2.8*
Seeds, Ground, Schwartz*	1 Tsp/5g	22	0.9	446	14.2	54.9	18.8	0.0
CORN MEAL								
Yellow, Enriched & Degerminated, Quaker Oats*	1 Tbsp/9g	30	0.2	333	7.4	77.8	1.8	7.4
CORNED BEEF								
Average	*1 Slice/35g*	*75*	*4.3*	*214*	*25.9*	*0.7*	*12.1*	*0.0*
Lean, Healthy Range, Average	*1 Slice/30g*	*57*	*2.6*	*191*	*27.0*	*1.0*	*8.7*	*0.0*
Sliced, Premium, Average	*1 Slice/31g*	*69*	*3.9*	*222*	*26.6*	*0.5*	*12.6*	*0.0*
Slices, Value, Tesco*	1 Slice/31g	66	3.7	213	26.0	0.8	11.8	0.0
CORNFLOUR								
Average	*1 Tsp/5g*	*18*	*0.1*	*355*	*0.6*	*86.9*	*1.2*	*0.1*
COURGETTE								
& Sweetcorn, Fresh 'n' Ready, Sainsbury's*	1oz/28g	12	0.3	42	2.3	6.7	0.9	1.3

	Measure INFO/WEIGHT	per Measure KCAL	per Measure FAT	Nutrition Values per 100g / 100ml KCAL	PROT	CARB	FAT	FIBRE
COURGETTE								
Boiled in Unsalted Water, Average	*1oz/28g*	*5*	*0.1*	*19*	*2.0*	*2.0*	*0.4*	*1.2*
Fried, Average	*1oz/28g*	*18*	*1.3*	*63*	*2.6*	*2.6*	*4.8*	*1.2*
Raw, Average	*1 Fruit/224g*	*40*	*0.9*	*18*	*1.8*	*1.8*	*0.4*	*0.9*
Stuffed, Round, Lovely Vegetables, M & S*	½ Pack/200g	110	2.6	55	1.8	7.7	1.3	1.8
COUS COUS								
& Chargrilled Vegetables, M & S*	1 Serving/200g	200	3.0	100	3.9	17.3	1.5	1.6
& Chickpeas, TTD, Sainsbury's*	¼ Pot/72g	121	6.8	167	4.7	15.8	9.4	1.4
& Wok Oriental, Findus*	½ Pack/300g	510	25.5	170	4.5	19.0	8.5	0.0
Chargrilled Red & Yellow Pepper, Tesco*	1 Pack/200g	212	3.6	106	4.6	17.8	1.8	0.5
Chargrilled Vegetable, Morrisons*	1 Serving/225g	227	5.4	101	3.3	16.5	2.4	1.3
Chargrilled Vegetables & Olive Oil, Delphi*	½ Pot/75g	105	2.9	140	3.8	22.5	3.9	1.9
Cooked, Average	*1 Tbsp/15g*	*24*	*0.3*	*158*	*4.3*	*31.4*	*1.9*	*1.3*
Coriander & Lemon, Morrisons*	1 Serving/100g	159	3.4	159	4.4	27.7	3.4	1.4
Coriander & Lemon, Sainsbury's*	½ Pack/137g	205	5.9	150	4.3	23.4	4.3	2.7
Dry, Average	*1 Serving/50g*	*178*	*0.7*	*356*	*13.7*	*72.8*	*1.5*	*2.6*
Garlic & Coriander, Dry, Waitrose*	1 Serving/70g	235	2.5	336	11.7	64.2	3.6	6.2
Giant, Tesco*	1 Pack/220g	350	14.4	160	4.1	20.7	6.6	1.2
Harissa Style Savoury, Sainsbury's*	1 Serving/260g	434	12.0	167	4.7	26.8	4.6	1.3
Hot & Spicy Flavour, Dry, Amazing Grains, Haldane's*	1 Serving/50g	182	2.1	365	12.5	67.0	4.2	3.1
Indian Style, Sainsbury's*	½ Pack/143g	204	3.9	143	4.5	25.1	2.7	1.0
Israeli & Sardinian, TTD, Sainsbury's*	¼ Pot/55g	69	2.6	126	3.2	17.7	4.7	1.6
Lemon & Coriander, Cooked, Tesco*	1 Serving/137g	207	3.3	151	4.0	28.3	2.4	2.0
Lemon & Coriander, Dry, Tesco*	1 Pack/110g	375	3.0	341	11.0	68.2	2.7	6.1
Mediterranean Style, Cooked, Tesco*	1 Serving/146g	215	3.8	147	4.4	26.5	2.6	1.3
Mediterranean Style, Dry, Tesco*	1 Pack/110g	368	3.3	335	11.9	65.1	3.0	5.6
Mint & Coriander Flavour, Dry, Amazing Grains*	1 Sachet/99g	349	2.7	353	12.2	70.0	2.7	3.2
Moroccan, Roast Chicken, Delicious, Shapers, Boots*	1 Pack/250g	247	3.7	99	9.2	12.0	1.5	2.6
Moroccan Style, Break, GFY, Asda*	1 Pack/150g	215	2.7	143	5.6	26.1	1.8	1.8
Moroccan Style, Finest, Tesco*	1 Tub/225g	292	5.6	130	4.3	22.6	2.5	3.7
Moroccan Style, Fruity, M & S*	1 Serving/200g	370	5.4	185	3.4	36.7	2.7	3.4
Moroccan Style, Sainsbury's*	½ Pack/150g	195	4.0	130	5.0	21.5	2.7	1.0
Moroccan Style, TTD, Sainsbury's*	1 Pot/200g	364	7.2	182	4.4	30.3	3.6	5.5
Moroccan Sultana & Pine Nuts, Dry, Sammy's*	1 Serving/50g	171	1.5	343	12.0	72.0	3.0	6.0
Mushroom & Garlic, Cooked, Morrisons*	1 Serving/100g	164	3.0	164	5.7	28.7	3.0	1.7
Mushrooms, Onion, Garlic & Herbs, Dry, Tesco*	½ Pack/50g	166	1.3	333	11.3	66.2	2.6	4.9
Plain, Dry Weight, Tesco*	1 Serving/50g	182	0.5	365	15.1	73.1	1.1	0.8
Red Pepper & Chilli, Waitrose*	1 Pack/200g	344	13.8	172	4.5	23.0	6.9	1.3
Roasted Vegetable, Cooked, Ainsley Harriott*	1 Serving/130g	180	2.0	138	5.6	25.5	1.5	2.6
Roasted Vegetable, Dry, Ainsley Harriott*	½ Sachet/50g	180	2.0	360	14.6	66.4	4.0	6.8
Roasted Vegetable, Snack Salad Pot, HL, Tesco*	1 Pack/60g	213	2.4	355	15.1	64.6	4.0	4.2
Roasted Vegetables, Waitrose*	1 Serving/200g	328	13.2	164	3.9	22.0	6.6	0.9
Spice Fusion, Lyttos*	1 Serving/100g	134	1.5	134	4.3	23.9	1.5	3.4
Spice Sensation, Dry, Ainsley Harriott*	½ Sachet/50g	166	1.2	332	11.6	66.2	2.4	9.2
Spicy Moroccan Chicken & Veg, COU, M & S*	1 Pack/400g	380	6.8	95	9.1	10.3	1.7	1.9
Spicy Vegetable, GFY, Asda*	½ Pack/55g	71	0.6	129	4.7	25.0	1.1	2.0
Spicy Vegetable, Morrisons*	1 Pack/110g	187	5.5	170	5.1	26.2	5.0	2.9
Spicy Vegetable, Morrisons*	½ Pack/55g	69	0.7	126	5.5	23.2	1.2	3.5
Sweet Vegetable, Chosen By You, Asda*	1 Serving/100g	120	0.0	120	2.9	14.8	0.0	0.0
Tangy Tomato, Cooked, Ainsley Harriott*	1 Serving/133g	166	0.8	125	4.6	25.3	0.6	3.3
Tangy Tomato, Dry, Ainsley Harriott*	½ Sachet/50g	166	0.8	332	12.2	67.2	1.6	8.8
Tomato & Basil, Made Up, Tesco*	1 Serving/200g	348	16.6	174	3.9	21.0	8.3	3.4
Tomato & Onion, Dry Weight, Waitrose*	1 Pack/110g	376	4.0	342	12.6	64.9	3.6	5.1
Tomato & Vegetable, Snack Pack, Dry, Sammy's*	1 Serving/70g	228	2.4	326	12.0	67.9	3.5	6.3

	Measure INFO/WEIGHT	per Measure		Nutrition Values per 100g / 100ml				
		KCAL	FAT	KCAL	PROT	CARB	FAT	FIBRE
COUS COUS								
Vegetable, Roasted, Veg Pot, Summer Special, Innocent*	1 Pot/400g	460	9.2	115	3.6	17.5	2.3	4.3
Wholewheat, Tesco*	1 Serving/50g	177	1.0	355	12.0	72.0	2.0	5.0
Zesty Lemon & Coriander, Dry, Sammy's*	1 Serving/50g	171	1.4	342	13.0	74.0	2.8	6.0
CRAB								
Blue, Soft Shelled, Raw, Average	1 Crab/84g	73	0.9	87	18.1	0.0	1.1	0.0
Boiled, Meat Only, Average	**1 Tbsp/40g**	**51**	**2.2**	**128**	**19.5**	**0.0**	**5.5**	**0.0**
Brown, Cornish, Seafood & Eat It*	1 Pack/100g	171	10.7	171	17.9	1.9	10.7	0.0
Claws, Asda*	1oz/28g	25	0.3	89	11.0	9.0	1.0	0.2
Cocktail, Waitrose*	1 Serving/100g	217	17.6	217	10.8	3.8	17.6	0.4
Cornish 50/50, Seafood & Eat It*	1 Pot/100g	144	5.8	144	21.6	1.2	5.8	0.5
Cornish Potted, Seafood & Eat It*	1 Pack/100g	235	17.5	235	15.0	5.1	17.5	0.8
Dressed, Average	**1 Can/43g**	**66**	**3.4**	**154**	**16.8**	**4.1**	**7.9**	**0.2**
Meat, Raw, Average	**1oz/28g**	**28**	**0.2**	**100**	**20.8**	**2.8**	**0.6**	**0.0**
Meat in Brine, Average	**½ Can/60g**	**46**	**0.3**	**76**	**17.2**	**0.9**	**0.4**	**0.1**
White Cornish, Seafood & Eat It*	1 Pack/100g	81	0.5	81	19.0	0.1	0.5	0.0
White Meat, See Food & Eat It*	1 Pack/100g	81	0.5	81	19.0	0.1	0.5	0.0
CRAB CAKES								
Goan, M & S*	1 Pack/190g	228	7.6	120	8.0	12.9	4.0	1.8
Iceland*	1 Serving/18g	52	3.2	288	7.2	25.6	18.0	1.3
Tesco*	1 Serving/130g	281	16.0	216	11.0	15.4	12.3	1.1
Thai, TTD, Sainsbury's*	½ Pack/106g	201	9.5	189	9.5	17.8	8.9	1.4
CRAB STICKS								
Average	1 Stick/15g	14	0.0	94	9.1	13.9	0.3	0.0
CRACKERBREAD								
Original, Ryvita*	1 Slice/5g	21	0.2	380	10.3	76.9	3.5	3.5
Rice, Asda*	1 Slice/5g	19	0.1	374	9.1	79.4	2.2	1.9
Sainsbury's*	1 Slice/5g	19	0.2	380	10.0	80.0	4.0	2.0
Wholegrain, Ryvita*	1 Slice/6g	20	0.2	360	12.4	68.7	3.9	9.8
CRACKERS								
Bath Oliver, Jacob's*	1 Cracker/12g	52	1.6	432	9.6	67.6	13.7	2.6
Bean Mix, Habas Tapas, Graze*	1 Punnet/30g	131	3.8	438	11.7	68.9	12.8	1.5
Black Olive, M & S*	1 Cracker/4g	20	1.0	485	8.3	59.4	23.5	4.3
Black Pepper for Cheese, Ryvita*	1 Cracker/7g	27	0.2	384	13.2	72.9	2.9	6.8
Bran, Jacob's*	1 Cracker/7g	32	1.3	454	9.7	62.8	18.2	3.2
Butter Puff, Sainsbury's*	1 Cracker/10g	54	2.7	523	10.4	60.7	26.5	2.5
Chapati Chips, Tikka, Medium Spicy, Patak's*	1 Serving/25g	127	7.0	508	8.0	56.0	28.0	4.0
Cheddars, McVitie's*	1 Cracker/4g	22	1.3	543	10.0	55.1	31.3	2.6
Cheese, Cheddar, Crispies, TTD, Sainsbury's*	1 Thin/4g	21	1.5	576	14.2	39.0	40.4	2.2
Cheese, Cheese Heads, Walkers*	1 Pack/27g	128	6.0	475	10.8	58.0	22.3	2.8
Cheese, Mini, Heinz*	1 Pack/25g	108	3.6	433	9.4	68.6	14.6	0.6
Cheese, Mini, Shapers, Boots*	1 Serving/23g	97	3.2	421	9.4	65.0	14.0	4.6
Cheese, Puff Pastry, Somerfield*	1 Cracker/4g	21	1.5	500	10.6	36.1	34.8	2.1
Cheese, Ritz*	1 Cracker/4g	17	0.9	486	10.1	55.9	24.7	2.2
Cheese, Trufree*	1 Cracker/8g	42	2.6	524	9.0	50.0	32.0	0.5
Cheese Thins, Asda*	1 Cracker/4g	21	1.3	532	12.0	49.0	32.0	0.0
Cheese Thins, Cheddar, The Planet Snack Co*	1 Serving/30g	153	8.8	509	11.5	50.1	29.2	2.1
Cheese Thins, Co-Op*	1 Cracker/4g	21	1.3	530	12.0	49.0	32.0	3.0
Cheese Thins, Mini, Snack Rite*	1 Bag/30g	144	6.8	480	12.9	55.9	22.7	2.5
Cheese Thins, Waitrose*	1 Cracker/4g	21	1.2	545	11.9	52.6	31.9	2.5
Chinese, Pop Pan*	1 Cracker/8g	40	2.5	533	13.3	53.3	33.3	0.0
Chives, Jacob's*	1 Cracker/6g	28	1.0	457	9.5	67.5	16.5	2.7
Choice Grain, Jacob's*	1 Cracker/8g	32	1.1	427	9.0	65.5	14.3	5.4
Corn Thins, 97% Fat Free, Real Foods*	1 Cracker/6g	23	0.2	378	10.2	81.7	3.0	8.6

C

CRACKERS

	Measure INFO/WEIGHT	per Measure KCAL	FAT	Nutrition Values per 100g / 100ml KCAL	PROT	CARB	FAT	FIBRE
Corn Thins, Real Foods*	1 Cracker/6g	22	0.2	378	10.2	81.7	3.0	8.6
Cream, 45% Less Fat, Morrisons*	1 Cracker/8g	32	0.6	403	10.5	74.2	7.1	3.3
Cream, Average	1 Cracker/7g	31	1.1	440	9.5	68.3	16.3	2.2
Cream, BFY, Morrisons*	1 Cracker/8g	32	0.6	406	10.9	74.4	7.2	2.8
Cream, BGTY, Sainsbury's*	1 Cracker/8g	32	0.6	400	10.9	71.7	7.7	3.1
Cream, Choice Grain, Jacob's*	1 Cracker/7g	30	0.9	400	9.0	64.5	11.8	7.0
Cream, Jacob's*	1 Cracker/8g	34	1.1	431	10.0	67.5	13.5	3.8
Cream, Light, Jacob's*	1 Cracker/8g	31	0.5	388	10.6	72.2	6.3	4.1
Cream, Lower Fat, Tesco*	1 Cracker/5g	20	0.3	393	11.0	72.4	6.6	3.1
Cream, Reduced Fat, Tesco*	1 Cracker/8g	31	0.5	406	10.9	74.4	7.2	2.8
Cream, Roasted Onion, Jacob's*	1 Cracker/8g	35	1.2	441	10.2	66.8	14.8	2.9
Cream, Sun Dried Tomato Flavour, Jacob's*	1 Cracker/8g	35	1.1	434	10.2	66.7	14.0	3.0
Crispy Cheese, M & S*	1 Cracker/4g	20	1.0	470	9.4	58.1	22.1	3.0
Garden Herbs, Jacob's*	1 Cracker/6g	28	1.0	457	9.5	67.5	16.5	2.7
Garlic, Chosen By You, Asda*	2 Crackers/12g	58	2.6	483	7.0	63.3	21.5	4.2
Garlic & Herb, Jacob's*	1 Cracker/100g	450	16.7	450	10.0	68.3	16.7	3.3
Glutafin*	1 Serving/11g	52	2.2	470	2.4	70.0	20.0	0.7
Goan Curry, Graze*	1 Pack/15g	80	4.2	532	4.5	65.5	28.0	0.9
Golden Rye for Cheese, Ryvita *	1 Cracker/7g	27	0.2	384	13.2	72.9	2.9	6.5
Harvest Grain, Sainsbury's*	1 Cracker/6g	27	1.1	458	8.5	64.5	18.4	4.1
Herb & Onion, 99% Fat Free, Rakusen's*	1 Cracker/5g	18	0.0	360	9.1	82.6	1.0	3.9
Herb & Onion, Trufree*	1 Cracker/6g	25	0.7	418	2.5	75.0	12.0	10.0
Herb & Spice, Jacob's*	1 Cracker/6g	27	1.0	457	9.5	67.5	16.5	2.7
Herbs & Spice Selection, Jacob's*	1 Cracker/6g	27	0.9	451	9.5	68.0	15.7	2.7
Krackawheat, McVitie's*	1 Cracker/7g	33	1.4	446	9.7	60.0	18.6	5.8
Light & Crispy, Sainsbury's*	1 Cracker/11g	42	1.2	384	11.3	61.0	10.5	13.0
Lightly Salted, Crispy, Sainsbury's*	1 Cracker/5g	25	1.3	533	7.8	62.6	27.9	2.1
Lightly Salted, Italian, Jacob's*	1 Cracker/6g	26	0.8	429	10.3	67.6	13.0	2.9
Mediterranean, Jacob's*	1 Cracker/6g	27	1.0	450	9.7	66.5	16.1	2.7
Mix, Yaki Soba, Graze*	1 Punnet/26g	131	8.0	504	24.5	33.9	30.8	6.8
Mixed Seed, Multi Grain, Asda*	1 Cracker/6g	28	1.1	445	11.0	62.0	17.0	4.4
Multi-grain, Aldi, Savour Bakes, Aldi*	1 Cracker/5g	20	0.8	404	8.3	55.0	16.8	5.1
Multigrain, Corn Thins, Real Foods*	1 Cracker/6g	23	0.2	388	10.9	71.0	3.7	10.3
Multigrain, Snack Crackers, Special K, Kellogg's*	1 Pack/30g	120	3.0	400	10.0	73.3	10.0	6.7
Multigrain, Tesco*	1 Cracker/6g	27	1.1	458	8.5	64.5	18.4	4.1
Oat & Wheat, Weight Watchers*	4 Crackers/20g	74	0.4	368	8.3	78.9	2.1	3.5
Olive Oil & Oregano, Mediterreaneo, Jacob's*	1 Cracker/6g	25	0.7	412	12.4	65.5	11.2	6.0
Oriental, Asda*	1 Serving/30g	115	6.0	383	1.7	49.0	20.0	4.3
Passionately Pizza, Jacobites, Jacob's*	1 Pack/150g	708	38.1	472	5.7	55.3	25.4	1.7
Peanut, Wasabi, Graze*	1 Pack/26g	125	5.6	479	15.2	53.8	21.4	5.4
Peking Dynasty, Graze*	1 Punnet/26g	130	7.3	498	19.8	43.1	27.9	4.6
Peking Spare Rib & 5 Spice, Oriental, Sensations, Walkers*	1 Bag/24g	116	6.2	485	1.3	62.0	26.0	3.5
Pesto, Jacob's*	1 Cracker/6g	27	1.0	450	9.7	66.5	16.1	2.7
Poppy & Sesame Seed, Sainsbury's*	1 Cracker/4g	21	1.1	530	9.6	58.9	28.4	3.4
Ritz, Mini, Kraft*	1 Bag/25g	126	6.0	504	7.9	63.0	24.0	2.0
Ritz, Original, Jacob's*	1 Cracker/3g	17	1.0	509	6.9	55.6	28.8	2.0
Rye, Organic, Dove's Farm*	1 Cracker/7g	28	1.0	393	7.0	58.4	14.6	8.7
Salt & Black Pepper, Eat Well, M & S*	1 Pack/25g	105	3.7	422	9.6	62.9	14.7	5.1
Salt & Black Pepper, Jacob's*	1 Cracker/6g	27	1.0	457	9.5	67.5	16.5	2.7
Salted, Ritz, Nabisco*	1 Cracker/3g	17	0.9	493	7.0	57.5	26.1	2.9
Selection, Finest, Tesco*	1 Serving/30g	136	4.3	452	9.6	71.0	14.4	0.0
Sesame & Poppy Thins, Tesco*	1 Cracker/4g	20	1.0	485	9.9	57.6	23.5	4.4
Spicy, Trufree*	1 Cracker/6g	25	0.8	412	3.8	70.0	13.0	12.5

CRACKERS

	Measure INFO/WEIGHT	per Measure KCAL	per Measure FAT	KCAL	PROT	CARB	FAT	FIBRE
Spicy Indonesian Vegetable, Waitrose*	1 Pack/60g	295	16.3	492	1.2	60.6	27.2	2.2
Spicy Vegetable, Tesco*	1 Serving/60g	340	23.0	566	2.6	52.4	38.4	1.2
Sweet Chilli, Thins, Savours, Jacob's*	1 Cracker/4g	21	0.9	472	8.0	62.3	21.2	3.6
Tangy Malaysian Chutney, Oriental, Sensations, Walkers*	1 Serving/35g	170	9.1	485	0.9	62.0	26.0	3.5
Tarallini with Fennel Seeds, Crosta & Mollica*	1 Cracker/4g	21	0.9	529	8.2	67.5	22.0	4.2
Thai Spicy Vegetable, Sainsbury's*	1 Pack/50g	231	10.4	462	7.2	61.5	20.8	2.6
The British Barbecue, Graze*	1 Punnet/23g	117	7.4	508	17.4	36.5	32.2	7.4
Tom Yum Yum, Graze*	1 Pack/23g	90	0.6	390	7.2	84.8	2.4	1.4
Tuc, Cheese Sandwich, Jacob's*	1 Cracker/14g	72	4.3	531	8.4	53.8	31.4	0.0
Tuc, Jacob's*	1 Cracker/5g	24	1.3	522	7.0	60.5	28.0	2.9
Tuc, Mini with Sesame Seeds, Jacob's*	1 Cracker/2g	10	0.5	523	9.7	63.1	25.8	3.9
Unsalted, Tops, Premium Plus, Impress*	1 Cracker/3g	13	0.3	448	10.3	75.9	10.3	0.0
Vegetable, Oriental Snack Selection, Sainsbury's*	1 Cracker/20g	42	1.9	209	4.5	26.2	9.6	3.4
Veggie, Heinz, Heinz*	1 Pack/25g	110	3.0	440	7.0	76.0	12.0	3.6
Wasapeas, Graze*	1 Pack/32g	128	2.5	406	14.8	65.2	7.8	7.1
Waterthins, Wafers, Philemon*	1 Crackers/2g	7	0.1	392	10.6	77.9	3.6	5.0
Wheaten, M & S*	1 Cracker/4g	20	0.9	450	10.2	57.0	20.2	5.0
Whole Wheat, 100%, Oven Baked, Master Choice*	1 Cracker/4g	17	0.4	429	10.0	75.0	9.6	12.1
Wholemeal, Tesco*	1 Cracker/7g	29	1.0	414	9.4	60.6	14.9	10.4
Wholewheat, Saiwa*	1 Pack/31g	128	3.9	414	12.5	62.9	12.5	7.9
Wholmeal, Organic, Nairn's*	1 Cracker/14g	58	2.0	413	9.0	61.4	14.6	8.7

CRANBERRIES

Dried, Sweetened, Average	**1 Serving/10g**	**34**	**0.1**	**335**	**0.3**	**81.1**	**0.8**	**4.4**
Dried, Wholesome, Love Life, Waitrose*	¼ Pack/25g	92	0.2	370	0.3	86.8	0.8	4.6
Fresh, Raw, Average	**1oz/28g**	**4**	**0.0**	**15**	**0.4**	**3.4**	**0.1**	**3.0**
Organic, Infinity Foods*	1 Serving/100g	334	0.6	334	0.9	80.3	0.6	7.2

CRAYFISH

Raw	**1oz/28g**	**19**	**0.2**	**67**	**14.9**	**0.0**	**0.8**	**0.0**
Tails, Chilli & Garlic, Asda*	1 Serving/140g	133	4.3	95	16.0	1.1	3.1	0.8
Tails in Brine, Luxury, The Big Prawn Co*	½ Tub/90g	46	0.6	51	10.1	1.0	0.7	0.0

CREAM

Aerosol, Average	**1oz/28g**	**87**	**8.7**	**309**	**1.7**	**6.2**	**30.9**	**0.0**
Aerosol, Reduced Fat, Average	**1 Serving/55ml**	**33**	**3.0**	**59**	**0.6**	**1.9**	**5.4**	**0.0**
Brandy, Pourable with Remy Martin*, Finest, Tesco*	½ Pot/125ml	460	35.5	368	2.7	19.8	28.4	0.0
Brandy, Really Thick, Finest, Tesco*	½ Pot/125ml	579	49.5	463	1.3	19.7	39.6	0.0
Brandy, Really Thick, Tesco*	1 Pot/250ml	1162	98.2	465	1.4	21.3	39.3	0.0
Chantilly, TTD, Sainsbury's*	2 Tbsp/30g	136	14.0	455	1.4	6.9	46.8	0.0
Clotted, Fresh, Average	**1 Serving/28g**	**162**	**17.5**	**579**	**1.6**	**2.3**	**62.7**	**0.0**
Double, Average	**1 Serving/25ml**	**113**	**12.1**	**452**	**1.6**	**2.4**	**48.4**	**0.0**
Double, Reduced Fat, Average	**1 Serving/30g**	**73**	**7.0**	**243**	**2.7**	**5.6**	**23.3**	**0.1**
Extra Thick, 99% Real Dairy Cream, Anchor*	1 Serving/13g	51	5.4	409	1.7	3.9	43.0	0.0
Extra Thick, Reduced Fat, Weight Watchers*	1 Serving/30g	42	3.4	140	2.5	6.7	11.5	0.8
Oat Alternative, Dairy Free, Oatly*	1 Carton/250ml	375	32.5	150	1.0	6.0	13.0	0.8
Single, Average	**1 Tbsp/15ml**	**28**	**2.7**	**188**	**2.6**	**3.9**	**18.0**	**0.1**
Single, Extra Thick, Average	**1 Serving/38ml**	**72**	**6.9**	**192**	**2.7**	**4.1**	**18.4**	**0.0**
Sour, Avonmore*	1 Tub/200ml	440	50.0	220	2.4	4.0	25.0	0.5
Sour, Eat Smart, Morrisons*	2 Tbsp/30g	37	2.7	124	3.9	7.0	9.0	0.0
Soured, Fresh, Average	**1 Tsp/5ml**	**10**	**0.9**	**191**	**2.7**	**3.9**	**18.4**	**0.0**
Soured, Reduced Fat, Average	**1 Tsp/5g**	**6**	**0.4**	**119**	**5.2**	**6.7**	**8.6**	**0.4**
Strawberry, Light, Real Dairy, Uht, Anchor*	1 Serving/13g	25	2.1	198	2.6	8.7	17.0	0.0
Thick, Sterilised, Average	**1 Tbsp/15ml**	**35**	**3.5**	**233**	**2.6**	**3.6**	**23.1**	**0.0**
Uht, Double, Average	**1 Tbsp/15g**	**41**	**3.9**	**274**	**2.2**	**7.3**	**26.3**	**0.0**
Uht, Reduced Fat, Average	**1 Serving/25ml**	**15**	**1.4**	**62**	**0.5**	**2.2**	**5.6**	**0.0**

	Measure INFO/WEIGHT	per Measure KCAL	per Measure FAT	Nutrition Values per 100g / 100ml KCAL	PROT	CARB	FAT	FIBRE
CREAM								
Uht, Single, Average	*1 Tbsp/15ml*	*29*	*2.8*	*194*	*2.6*	*4.0*	*18.8*	*0.0*
Whipping, Average	*1 Tbsp/15ml*	*52*	*5.5*	*348*	*2.1*	*3.2*	*36.4*	*0.0*
CREAM HORN								
Fresh, Tesco*	1 Horn/57g	244	15.8	428	4.1	40.3	27.8	0.3
CREAM SODA								
American with Vanilla, Tesco*	1 Glass/313ml	75	0.0	24	0.0	5.9	0.0	0.0
Diet, Sainsbury's*	1 Glass/250ml	2	0.0	1	0.0	0.0	0.0	0.0
No Added Sugar, Sainsbury's*	1 Can/330ml	2	0.3	0	0.1	0.1	0.1	0.1
Shapers, Boots*	1 Bottle/300ml	3	0.0	1	0.0	0.0	0.0	0.0
Traditional Style, Tesco*	1 Can/330ml	139	0.0	42	0.0	10.4	0.0	0.0
CREME BRULEE								
Average	1 Serving/100g	313	26.0	313	3.8	15.7	26.0	0.2
Gastropub, M & S*	1 Brulee/84g	285	24.6	340	3.1	15.7	29.3	0.7
CREME CARAMEL								
Average	1 Serving/128g	140	2.8	109	3.0	20.6	2.2	0.0
Carmelle, Green's*	1 Pack/70g	82	2.8	117	3.0	17.0	4.0	0.0
La Laitiere*	1 Pot/100g	135	4.0	135	5.0	20.0	4.0	0.0
CREME EGG								
Cadbury*	1 Egg/39g	180	6.3	462	4.1	73.0	16.1	0.5
Minis, Cadbury*	1 Egg/11g	50	1.8	445	4.1	67.5	16.4	0.4
CREME FRAICHE								
Average	*1 Tbsp/15g*	*54*	*5.7*	*362*	*2.2*	*2.6*	*38.0*	*0.0*
Cucumber & Mint, Triangles, Sainsbury's*	1 Serving/25g	105	2.4	421	11.0	72.3	9.7	2.5
Extra Light, President*	1 Tub/200g	182	10.0	91	2.7	8.7	5.0	0.0
Half Fat, Average	*1 Serving/30g*	*54*	*4.9*	*181*	*3.1*	*5.5*	*16.2*	*0.0*
Lemon & Rocket, Sainsbury's*	1 Serving/150g	187	17.2	125	2.2	3.0	11.5	0.5
Low Fat, Average	1 Tbsp/30ml	43	3.6	143	3.3	5.6	12.1	0.1
Low Fat, Weight Watchers*	1 Tbsp/20g	15	0.5	76	5.1	7.7	2.7	0.5
CREPES								
Chocolate Filled, Tesco*	1 Crepe/32g	140	5.8	437	5.9	62.5	18.1	1.6
Lobster, Finest, Tesco*	1 Serving/160g	250	10.2	156	10.7	14.0	6.4	1.2
Mushroom, M & S*	1 Pack/186g	195	4.5	105	5.7	17.1	2.4	2.5
CRISPBAKES								
Broccoli & Leek, Asda*	1 Bake/132g	263	13.2	199	6.3	21.0	10.0	2.0
Bubble & Squeak, M & S*	1 Bake/47g	79	4.1	170	2.7	19.6	8.8	1.5
Cheese, Spring Onion & Chive, Sainsbury's*	1 Bake/114g	287	16.8	253	7.1	24.5	14.8	1.7
Cheese & Onion, Dalepak*	1 Bake/98g	239	12.6	243	7.2	24.1	12.8	1.7
Cheese & Onion, M & S*	1 Bake/114g	285	18.5	250	6.4	19.4	16.2	1.7
Cheese & Onion, Tesco*	1 Bake/109g	275	17.2	252	7.9	19.6	15.8	2.1
Dutch, Asda*	1 Bake/8g	31	0.3	388	14.7	74.9	3.3	4.2
Dutch, Co-Op*	1 Bake/10g	37	0.3	375	16.0	69.6	3.5	6.5
Dutch, HL, Tesco*	1 Bake/8g	30	0.2	385	14.7	74.9	2.7	4.2
Dutch, Sainsbury's*	1 Bake/10g	38	0.5	392	14.5	72.3	5.0	5.8
Minced Beef, M & S*	1 Bake/113g	226	12.3	200	10.0	15.6	10.9	1.5
Mushroom, Uncooked, Dalepak*	1 Bake/84g	141	7.4	168	3.8	18.5	8.8	2.1
Roast Vegetable & Basil, Cauldron Foods*	1 Bake/115g	241	11.0	210	3.5	26.0	9.6	2.9
Spinach, Cheese & Sweetcorn, Cauldron Foods*	1 Bake/115g	233	12.2	203	5.6	21.3	10.6	2.1
Vegetable, M & S*	1 Bake/114g	200	10.3	175	2.5	19.2	9.0	2.6
Vegetable, Sainsbury's*	1 Bake/114g	246	13.0	216	2.0	26.2	11.4	2.0
CRISPBREAD								
3 Seed, Classic, Gourmet, Dr Karg*	1 Bread/25g	107	4.9	430	16.5	46.6	19.7	10.9
3 Seed, Organic, Gourmet	1 Bread/25g	101	4.7	405	15.8	48.8	18.8	14.6
Bran, Scandinavian, Gg*	1 Bake/8g	18	0.4	223	14.9	29.0	5.3	42.1

	Measure INFO/WEIGHT	per Measure KCAL	FAT	Nutrition Values per 100g / 100ml KCAL	PROT	CARB	FAT	FIBRE
CRISPBREAD								
Corn, Orgran*	1 Bread/5g	18	0.1	360	7.5	83.0	1.8	3.0
Cracked Black Pepper, Ryvita*	1 Slice/11g	38	0.2	344	8.8	66.6	1.6	14.5
Crisp 'n' Light, Wasa*	1 Bread/7g	24	0.1	360	12.0	73.0	2.2	5.3
Dark Rye, Morrisons*	1 Bake/13g	39	0.4	300	11.5	61.5	3.1	16.9
Dark Rye, Ryvita*	1 Bread/10g	34	0.1	342	8.5	66.5	1.2	15.2
Emmental Cheese & Pumpkin Seed, Gourmet, Dr Karg*	1 Bread/25g	100	4.1	402	17.7	45.5	16.6	12.3
Fibre Plus, Wholegrain with Sesame, Wasa*	1 Bread/10g	35	0.7	350	13.0	47.0	7.0	24.0
Fruit Crunch, Ryvita*	1 Slice/15g	54	0.8	358	8.3	61.8	5.4	14.9
Gluten Free	1 Serving/8g	25	0.1	331	6.4	72.9	1.5	0.0
Hint of Chilli, Ryvita*	1 Slice/12g	42	0.2	349	8.6	66.6	1.9	16.8
Light Rye, Leksands Knacke*	4 Slices/50g	158	1.1	317	10.4	62.7	2.2	16.0
Mildly Seasoned, Gourmet, Dr Karg*	1 Bread/25g	101	4.0	405	16.2	48.8	16.1	11.6
Mini, Sesame & Linseed, Dr Karg*	1 Slice/3g	13	0.4	424	12.1	57.6	12.1	9.1
Multigrain, Ryvita*	1 Slice/11g	41	0.8	370	11.2	56.0	7.2	18.3
Multigrain, Wasa*	1 Bread/13g	43	0.3	320	12.0	62.0	2.6	14.0
Original, Ryvita*	1 Bread/10g	35	0.2	350	8.5	66.9	1.7	16.5
Original Rye, Thin, Finn Crisp*	1 Slice/6g	20	0.1	360	11.0	60.0	2.4	19.0
Original Rye, Wasa*	1 Bread/11g	35	0.2	315	9.0	67.0	1.4	14.0
Poppyseed, Wasa*	1 Bread/13g	45	1.0	350	13.0	56.0	8.0	14.0
Provita*	1 Bread/6g	26	0.6	416	12.5	68.4	9.9	0.0
Pumpkin Seeds & Oats, Ryvita*	1 Slice/13g	46	0.9	370	11.2	56.0	7.2	18.3
Rice, Original, Sakata*	1 Bread/25g	102	0.6	410	6.9	88.0	2.6	1.3
Rice, Sakata*	1 Bread/25g	25	0.2	102	1.7	22.0	0.7	0.3
Rice & Cracked Pepper, Orgran*	1 Bread/5g	18	0.1	388	8.4	81.9	1.8	2.0
Roasted Onion, Gourmet, Dr Karg*	1 Bread/25g	100	4.1	399	15.9	46.6	16.5	11.1
Roasted Onion, Organic, Dr Karg*	1 Bread/25g	97	3.7	390	15.8	48.5	14.8	12.9
Rounds, Multigrain, Finn Crisp*	1 Bread/13g	41	0.7	330	13.0	56.0	6.0	18.0
Rounds, Wholegrain Wheat, Finn Crisp*	1 Bread/13g	45	0.7	360	11.0	66.0	5.9	10.0
Rustikal, Wasa*	1 Bread/15g	51	0.2	340	9.0	6.4	1.5	16.0
Scan Bran, Slimming World*	1 Slice/10g	31	0.5	310	14.9	29.0	5.3	42.1
Seeded, Spelt, Organic, Dr Karg*	1 Bread/25g	107	4.5	430	17.2	44.4	18.0	11.2
Sesame, Ryvita*	1 Bread/10g	37	0.7	373	10.5	58.3	7.0	17.5
Sesame, Savour Bakes, Aldi*	1 Bread/9g	33	0.5	366	12.3	57.2	5.2	20.6
Spelt, Cheese, Sunflower Seeds, Organic, Dr Karg*	1 Bread/25g	103	4.5	411	19.2	42.8	18.1	10.4
Spelt, Muesli, Organic, Dr Karg*	1 Bread/25g	94	2.8	375	14.2	54.4	11.2	10.6
Spelt, Sesame, Sunflower, Amisa*	1 Bread/29g	85	4.3	297	11.7	28.5	15.1	5.0
Sport, Wasa*	1 Bread/15g	46	0.2	310	9.0	64.0	1.5	16.0
Sunflower Seeds & Oats, Ryvita*	1 Bread/12g	46	1.1	384	9.7	58.4	9.0	15.3
Sweet Onion, Ryvita*	1 Bread/12g	43	0.2	356	9.0	70.6	1.4	12.6
Thin Crisps, Original Taste, Finn Crisp*	1 Bread/6g	20	0.2	320	11.0	63.0	2.4	19.0
Trufree*	1 Bread/6g	22	0.1	370	6.0	82.0	2.0	1.0
Wheat with Poppy Seeds, Morrisons*	1 Serving/12g	45	0.9	390	11.0	68.0	8.0	8.0
Whole Grain, Classic, Organic, Dr Karg*	1 Bread/25g	89	4.1	355	13.4	38.2	16.5	10.2
Whole Grain, Crispy, Thin, Kavli*	3 Breads/15g	50	0.3	333	10.0	70.0	1.7	12.7
Wholemeal, Light, Allinson*	1 Bread/5g	17	0.1	349	11.7	69.7	2.6	11.0
Wholemeal, Organic, Allinson*	1 Bread/5g	17	0.1	336	14.2	66.0	1.7	12.2
Wholemeal, Rye with Milk, Grafschafter*	1 Bread/9g	29	0.1	316	11.4	64.0	1.6	15.0
Wholemeal Rye, Organic, Kallo*	1 Bread/10g	31	0.2	314	9.7	65.0	1.7	15.4
CRISPS								
Apple, Dried, Snapz*	1 Packet/15g	52	0.0	344	2.0	77.0	0.0	14.7
Apple, The Fruit Factory*	1 Packet/10g	33	0.0	334	1.3	81.1	0.5	12.4
Apple, Thyme & Sage, M & S*	1 Bag/55g	253	13.4	460	5.5	55.3	24.3	6.1
Argentinean Flame Grilled Steak, Walkers*	1 Bag/35g	182	11.3	520	6.5	50.7	32.4	4.2

	Measure INFO/WEIGHT	per Measure KCAL	FAT	Nutrition Values per 100g / 100ml KCAL	PROT	CARB	FAT	FIBRE

CRISPS

	Measure INFO/WEIGHT	KCAL	FAT	KCAL	PROT	CARB	FAT	FIBRE
Bacon, Shapers, Boots*	1 Bag/23g	99	3.4	431	8.0	66.0	15.0	3.0
Bacon & Cheddar, Baked, Walkers*	1 Pack/38g	149	3.2	397	6.5	73.7	8.5	4.7
Bacon Crispies, Sainsbury's*	1 Bag/25g	117	5.7	468	19.9	45.8	22.8	4.8
Bacon Flavour Rashers, BGTY, Sainsbury's*	1 Pack/10g	34	0.2	340	10.8	70.3	1.6	3.5
Bacon Pillows, Light, Shapers, Boots*	1 Pack/12g	44	0.3	367	3.7	83.0	2.3	4.0
Bacon Rashers, Blazin, Tesco*	1 Bag/25g	121	6.6	485	16.5	45.7	26.3	3.8
Bacon Rashers, COU, M & S*	1 Pack/20g	72	0.6	360	9.4	77.5	2.9	3.5
Bacon Rashers, Tesco*	1 Bag/25g	125	6.4	500	7.1	59.8	25.5	4.0
Bacon Rice Bites, Asda*	1 Bag/30g	136	4.8	452	7.0	70.0	16.0	0.4
Bacon Sizzler, Ridge Cut, McCoys*	1 Bag/32g	165	9.7	516	7.1	53.6	30.3	3.9
Baked, Average	1 Bag/25g	93	1.5	374	6.5	73.5	5.9	5.8
Baked, Ready Salted, Walkers*	1 Packet/38g	146	3.0	390	6.0	74.0	8.0	5.5
Baked, Sour Cream & Chive, Walkers*	1 Packet/38g	148	3.2	395	7.0	73.0	8.5	5.0
Baked Bean Flavour, Walkers*	1 Bag/35g	184	11.5	525	6.5	50.0	33.0	4.0
Banging BBQ, Shots, Walkers*	1 Pack/18g	87	4.5	485	5.5	60.0	25.0	1.3
Barbecue, Handcooked, Tesco*	1 Bag/40g	187	10.0	468	6.6	53.8	25.1	5.2
Barbecue, Savoury Snacks, Weight Watchers*	1 Pack/22g	81	1.9	366	18.6	61.0	8.7	6.1
Barbecue, Snack Rite*	1 Bag/25g	131	8.3	524	5.1	51.3	33.2	0.0
Barbecue, Sunseed Oil, Walkers*	1 Pack/33g	171	10.7	525	6.5	50.0	33.0	4.0
Barbecue Beef, Select, Tesco*	1 Pack/25g	134	8.7	536	6.4	49.2	34.8	4.4
Barbecue Flavour Waffles, American Style, Shapers, Boots*	1 Pack/20g	95	4.4	476	4.5	65.0	22.0	3.7
BBQ Rib, Sunseed, Walkers*	1 Bag/25g	131	8.2	525	6.5	50.0	33.0	4.0
Beef, Squares, Walkers*	1 Bag/25g	105	4.5	420	6.0	59.0	18.0	4.6
Beef & Onion, Tayto*	1 Bag/35g	184	11.9	526	7.6	47.3	34.0	4.5
Beef & Onion, Walkers*	1 Bag/33g	171	10.7	525	6.5	50.0	33.0	4.0
Beef & Onion Flavour, Average	1 Bag/32g	168	10.6	524	6.5	50.0	33.1	4.3
Beefy, Smiths, Walkers*	1 Bag/25g	133	9.2	531	4.3	45.2	37.0	0.0
Beetroot, Seasoned In Salt, Glennans*	1 Bag/27g	130	8.9	480	8.2	36.0	32.8	13.2
Beetroot Chips, Crunchy, Apple Snapz*	1 Bag/20g	52	0.2	260	14.7	76.0	1.0	28.0
Big Snak, Crisp 'n Tasty Potato Chips, Herrs*	1 Pack/43g	212	12.1	494	7.1	56.5	28.2	3.6
Bread, Baked, Sweet Chilli Flavour, Seabrook*	1 Serving/100g	416	10.5	416	12.2	65.2	10.5	6.1
Bread, Baked, Tangy Barbeque Flavour, Seabrook*	1 Serving/100g	405	8.8	405	12.9	65.5	8.8	6.5
Buffalo Mozzarella & Herbs, Walkers*	1 Serving/35g	171	9.1	490	6.1	57.0	26.0	4.2
Builders Breakfast, Walkers*	1 Sm Bag/25g	131	8.3	524	5.6	50.8	33.2	4.0
Butter & Chive, COU, M & S*	1 Bag/26g	95	0.5	365	7.7	77.3	1.9	4.6
Cajun Squirrel, Walkers*	1 Sm Bag/25g	130	8.2	522	5.8	51.2	32.7	4.2
Canadian Ham Flavour, Seabrook*	1 Pack/30g	159	9.8	531	5.7	50.9	32.7	5.1
Chargrilled Chicken, Ridge Cut, McCoys*	1 Pack/32g	167	10.0	521	7.0	52.9	31.3	4.0
Chargrilled Chicken Crinkles, Shapers, Boots*	1 Bag/20g	96	4.8	482	6.6	60.0	24.0	4.0
Chargrilled Steak, Max, Walkers*	1 Bag/55g	289	18.1	525	6.5	50.0	33.0	4.0
Cheddar & Onion, Ridge Cut, McCoys*	1 Bag/32g	165	9.8	516	7.0	53.2	30.6	3.9
Cheddar & Red Onion Chutney, Sensations, Walkers*	1 Bag/40g	198	11.2	495	6.5	54.0	28.0	4.5
Cheddar & Spring Onion, 35% Less Fat, Sainsbury's*	1 Pack/20g	93	4.2	463	6.3	62.4	20.9	0.9
Cheese, Space Raiders, KP Snacks*	1 Bag/16g	76	3.5	473	7.1	61.6	22.0	3.1
Cheese & Branston Pickle, Walkers*	1 Bag/35g	181	11.4	525	6.5	50.0	33.0	4.0
Cheese & Chive Flavour, GFY, Asda*	1 Bag/25g	119	6.0	476	6.0	59.0	24.0	6.0
Cheese & Chives, Walkers*	1 Bag/33g	172	10.7	530	6.5	50.0	33.0	4.1
Cheese & Onion, 30% Less Fat, Sainsbury's*	1 Pack/25g	115	5.4	459	7.5	58.1	21.8	5.4
Cheese & Onion, Baked, Walkers*	1 Bag/25g	99	2.1	396	6.5	73.8	8.3	4.7
Cheese & Onion, Crinkle Cut, Low Fat, Waitrose*	1 Bag/25g	122	5.8	490	7.7	62.6	23.2	4.7
Cheese & Onion, Flavour Crinkles, Shapers, Boots*	1 Bag/20g	96	4.8	482	6.6	60.0	24.0	4.0
Cheese & Onion, GFY, Asda*	1 Pack/26g	122	5.7	470	7.0	61.0	22.0	4.2
Cheese & Onion, Golden Wonder*	1 Bag/25g	129	7.9	516	5.8	52.4	31.5	3.8

CRISPS

INFO/WEIGHT	Measure	per Measure KCAL	FAT	Nutrition Values per 100g / 100ml KCAL	PROT	CARB	FAT	FIBRE
Cheese & Onion, KP Snacks*	1 Bag/25g	133	8.7	534	6.6	48.7	34.8	4.8
Cheese & Onion, Lights, Walkers*	1 Bag/24g	113	5.0	470	7.5	62.0	21.0	5.0
Cheese & Onion, M & S*	1 Bag/25g	134	8.9	535	5.5	48.8	35.5	5.0
Cheese & Onion, Max, Walkers*	1 Pack/50g	262	16.0	525	6.8	52.0	32.0	5.2
Cheese & Onion, Organic, Tesco*	1 Bag/25g	128	8.1	514	5.2	49.9	32.6	7.0
Cheese & Onion, Oven Baked, Asda*	1 Bag/25g	95	2.0	380	5.1	72.0	8.0	3.3
Cheese & Onion, Oven Baked, Tesco*	1 Bag/25g	102	1.6	410	5.3	74.7	6.6	7.7
Cheese & Onion, Potato Heads, Walkers*	1 Pack/23g	108	5.3	470	6.0	60.0	23.0	5.5
Cheese & Onion, Sainsbury's*	1 Bag/25g	132	8.7	527	4.6	48.8	34.8	3.9
Cheese & Onion, Seabrook*	1 Pack/30g	159	9.8	530	7.0	50.8	32.6	3.9
Cheese & Onion, Snack Rite*	1 Pack/25g	132	8.3	527	5.3	51.3	33.4	0.0
Cheese & Onion, Sprinters*	1 Bag/25g	137	9.1	549	5.4	49.4	36.6	0.0
Cheese & Onion, Squares, Walkers*	1 Bag/25g	107	4.5	430	6.5	61.0	18.0	5.5
Cheese & Onion, Sunseed Oil, Walkers*	1 Bag/33g	171	10.7	525	7.0	50.0	33.0	4.0
Cheese & Onion, Tayto*	1 Bag/25g	131	8.5	526	7.6	47.3	34.0	4.5
Cheese & Onion, Tesco*	1 Pack/25g	132	8.3	530	5.8	51.6	33.2	4.4
Cheese & Onion, Value, Tesco*	1 Bag/20g	108	7.2	541	6.0	48.3	36.0	4.8
Cheese & Onion Flavour, Asda*	1 Bag/25g	130	7.8	519	5.6	53.6	31.4	3.7
Cheese & Onion Rings, Crunchy, Shapers, Boots*	1 Bag/15g	56	0.4	374	5.9	81.0	2.9	2.0
Cheese Bites, Weight Watchers*	1 Pack/18g	73	1.0	406	13.9	71.1	5.6	2.2
Cheese Curls, Morrisons*	1 Bag/14g	71	4.5	510	4.5	51.0	32.0	2.6
Cheese Curls, Red Mill*	½ Bag/50g	276	18.0	553	6.6	50.6	36.0	2.0
Cheese Curls, Shapers, Boots*	1 Pack/14g	68	3.8	489	4.5	57.0	27.0	2.7
Cheese Curls, Sprinters*	1 Bag/14g	68	3.8	483	4.1	56.4	26.8	0.0
Cheese Curls, Tesco*	1 Bag/14g	75	4.5	520	4.5	54.4	31.1	1.9
Cheese Curls, Weight Watchers*	1 Pack/20g	78	1.7	392	5.0	73.8	8.6	3.4
Cheese Moments, Smiths*	1 Pack/28g	148	9.2	530	8.0	50.0	33.0	2.0
Cheese Puffs, Weight Watchers*	1 Pack/18g	80	1.9	444	7.8	77.2	10.6	3.3
Cheese Twirls, Boulevard, Simply Delicious*	1 Pack/25g	137	8.7	550	12.1	46.7	35.0	0.0
Cheese Xl, Golden Wonder*	1 Bag/30g	155	9.6	516	6.2	50.6	32.1	4.2
Cheeses with Onion, Soulmates, Kettle Chips*	1 Pack/40g	195	11.6	488	7.7	50.2	29.0	5.4
Cheesy & Oniony, Potato, Tasty Little Numbers*	1 Pack/19g	100	6.1	527	7.9	51.6	32.1	2.6
Cheesy Curls, Bobby's*	1 Bag/40g	225	14.8	563	7.6	50.1	36.9	0.0
Cheesy Curls, Tesco*	1 Pack/17g	90	5.4	530	3.5	56.0	32.0	1.9
Cheesy Puffs, Co-Op*	1 Bag/60g	321	20.4	535	3.0	54.0	34.0	2.0
Chicken, Firecracker, McCoys*	1 Bag/35g	177	10.3	506	6.2	54.0	29.5	4.0
Chicken, Oven Roasted with Lemon & Thyme, Walkers*	1 Bag/40g	200	11.2	500	6.5	55.0	28.0	4.5
Chicken, Potato Heads, Walkers*	1 Pack/23g	106	4.8	460	8.5	58.0	21.0	6.0
Chicken & Thyme, Oven Roasted, Tesco*	1 Pack/150g	727	40.5	485	6.5	54.0	27.0	4.5
Chilli & Chocolate, Walkers*	1 Pack/25g	131	8.3	523	6.1	50.1	33.1	4.2
Chilli & Lemon, Walkers*	1 Pack/25g	131	8.2	525	6.3	51.0	33.0	3.8
Chinese Sizzling Beef, McCoys*	1 Bag/35g	178	10.6	506	6.9	51.8	30.2	4.0
Chinese Spare Rib, Walkers*	1 Bag/25g	131	8.2	525	6.5	50.0	33.0	4.0
Cider Vinegar & Sea Salt, Tyrrells*	1 Pack/40g	192	9.8	481	7.2	60.1	24.6	2.4
Cool Cheese Curly, Tesco*	1 Bag/14g	71	4.5	510	4.5	51.0	32.0	2.6
Corn Chips, Fritos*	1 Pack/43g	240	15.0	565	4.7	56.5	35.3	0.0
Coronation Chicken, Walkers*	1 Bag/25g	131	8.2	525	6.5	50.0	33.0	4.0
Crinkle Cut, Lower Fat, No Added Salt, Waitrose*	1 Bag/40g	193	10.0	483	6.5	58.0	25.0	3.9
Crinkles, Cheddar & Onion, Walkers*	1 Bag/28g	150	9.3	537	6.0	51.5	33.3	3.5
Crispy Duck & Hoi Sin, Walkers*	1 Bag/25g	131	8.1	523	5.8	51.5	32.6	4.0
Crushed Natural Sea Salt, Darling Spuds*	1 Bag/40g	195	12.0	488	5.6	53.4	30.0	4.5
Curls, Cheesy, Asda*	1 Pack/17g	87	4.9	511	3.8	59.7	28.6	1.7
D'lites, Cheddar & Red Onion Bites, The Real Crisp Co.*	1 Pack/20g	83	2.0	414	2.1	78.8	10.0	2.7

	Measure INFO/WEIGHT	per Measure KCAL	FAT	Nutrition Values per 100g / 100ml KCAL	PROT	CARB	FAT	FIBRE

CRISPS

	Measure INFO/WEIGHT	KCAL	FAT	KCAL	PROT	CARB	FAT	FIBRE
Double Gloucester & Red Onion, Kettle Chips*	1 Serving/40g	188	9.9	471	6.6	55.5	24.7	4.8
Dutch Edam Cheese, Walkers*	1 Bag/25g	131	8.3	523	6.1	50.2	33.1	4.0
English Cheddar & Red Onion, Red Sky*	1 Pack/40g	183	8.4	457	6.9	60.2	21.0	5.1
English Roast Beef & Yorkshire Pudding, Walkers*	1 Bag/35g	180	11.3	522	6.6	50.4	32.7	4.0
Extra Crunchy, Salt & Malt Vinegar, Walkers*	1 Pack/30g	139	6.2	463	6.6	59.9	20.8	4.8
Feta Cheese Flavour, Mediterranean, Walkers*	1 Pack/25g	127	8.2	510	6.5	49.0	33.0	4.5
Flame Grilled Steak, Extra Crunchy, Walkers*	1 Bag/150g	702	31.6	468	6.9	60.0	21.1	5.0
Flame Grilled Steak, Ridge Cut, McCoys*	1 Bag/32g	165	9.8	516	7.0	53.0	30.7	4.0
Flamed Grilled Steak, Deep Ridge, Walkers*	1 Pack/28g	144	8.4	515	6.4	52.6	30.1	4.3
Four Cheese & Red Onion, Sensations, Walkers*	1 Bag/40g	194	10.8	485	6.5	54.0	27.0	4.5
French Garlic Baguette, Walkers*	1 Packet/25g	131	8.2	523	5.9	50.8	32.9	4.1
Greek Kebab, Mediterranean, Walkers*	1 Pack/25g	127	8.2	510	6.0	49.0	33.0	4.5
Grilled Chicken Flavour, Golden Lights, Golden Wonder*	1 Bag/21g	93	3.8	444	4.4	66.2	18.0	4.3
Ham & Mustard, Salty Dog*	1 Pack/40g	192	10.8	480	7.5	54.5	27.1	4.2
Heinz Tomato Ketchup, Sunseed, Walkers*	1 Bag/35g	179	11.0	520	6.5	51.0	32.0	4.0
Honey & BBQ, Wholgrain, Snacks, M & S*	1 Serving/30g	145	7.5	485	7.8	57.6	24.9	5.2
Honey Roast Gammon & English Mustard, Sainsbury's*	1 Serving/50g	236	12.4	472	7.2	55.0	24.8	5.0
Honey Roasted Ham, Sensations, Walkers*	1 Bag/40g	196	10.8	490	6.5	55.0	27.0	4.0
Hoops, Ready Salted, Weight Watchers*	1 Bag/20g	73	0.3	365	3.4	82.7	1.4	4.1
Hot & Spicy Salami, Tesco*	1 Bag/50g	215	17.9	431	26.2	0.7	35.9	0.0
Irish Cheddar with Onion Chutney, Philleas Fogg*	1 Pack/38g	195	11.2	512	7.1	54.3	29.6	4.3
Jalapeno Peppers, Fire Roasted, Darling Spuds*	1 Pack/40g	191	11.4	478	6.3	53.4	28.5	4.5
Lamb & Mint, Slow Roasted, Sensations, Walkers*	1 Bag/35g	170	9.4	485	6.5	54.0	27.0	4.5
Lamb & Mint, Sunseed Oil, Walkers*	1 Pack/33g	171	10.7	525	6.5	50.0	33.0	4.0
Lant Chips, Ikea*	1 Serving/25g	126	6.9	505	8.3	55.9	27.6	4.5
Lightly Salted, Baked, COU, M & S*	1 Bag/25g	87	0.6	350	8.5	76.4	2.3	5.7
Lightly Salted, Crinkle Cut, Low Fat, Waitrose*	1 Pack/35g	163	8.0	466	5.2	60.1	22.8	5.1
Lightly Salted, Crinkles, Shapers, Boots*	1 Pack/20g	96	4.8	482	6.6	60.0	24.0	4.0
Lightly Salted, Handcooked, Finest, Tesco*	1 Bag/40g	206	11.5	515	5.1	58.6	28.8	2.5
Lightly Salted, Hoops, Mini, Weight Watchers*	1 Pack/20g	71	0.2	355	4.0	82.0	1.0	3.5
Lightly Salted, Kettle Chips*	1 Serving/50g	241	12.9	482	6.3	56.0	25.8	5.1
Lightly Salted, Low Fat, Waitrose*	1 Bag/25g	125	6.2	500	7.5	61.3	25.0	4.8
Lightly Salted, Organic, Kettle Chips*	1 Serving/40g	198	11.4	495	5.5	54.1	28.5	4.4
Lightly Salted, Potato Bakes, Weight Watchers*	1 Pack/20g	78	1.8	392	5.0	72.0	9.0	5.0
Lightly Salted, Reduced Fat, Crinkles, Eat Well, M & S*	1 Pack/30g	140	6.6	460	6.7	59.4	21.8	4.5
Lightly Sea Salted, Jonathan Crisp*	1 Bag/35g	176	10.1	503	6.5	52.0	29.0	5.4
Lightly Sea Salted, Potato Chips, Hand Fried, Burts*	¼ Bag/50g	252	13.8	504	6.4	57.4	27.7	0.0
Lightly Sea Salted, Tyrrells*	1 Pack/40g	204	10.2	510	5.9	49.0	25.4	5.3
Lime & Thai Spices, Gently Infused, Sensations, Walkers*	1 Pack/40g	200	11.6	500	6.5	54.0	29.0	4.0
Lincolnshire Sausage, Tyrrells*	1 Pack/100g	530	28.2	530	8.6	60.8	28.2	3.0
Mango & Chilli, Baked, Walkers*	1 Packet/38g	147	3.0	392	6.4	74.0	8.0	4.8
Mango Chilli, Kettle Chips*	1 Serving/40g	190	9.6	475	6.3	53.9	24.0	6.1
Marmite, Sunseed, Walkers*	1 Bag/33g	169	10.7	520	6.5	49.0	33.0	4.0
Marmite*	1 Pack/25g	130	7.7	519	6.2	52.6	30.7	3.7
Mature Cheddar & Chive, Kettle Chips*	1 Serving/50g	239	12.7	478	8.1	54.4	25.4	5.0
Mature Cheddar & Chive, Tyrrells*	1 Bag/40g	194	10.0	485	8.4	58.7	25.1	2.4
Mature Cheddar & Onion, Deep Ridge, Walkers*	1 Pack/28g	145	8.6	518	6.4	51.8	30.7	4.3
Mature Cheddar & Red Onion, Kettle Chips*	1 Bag/40g	187	10.2	467	7.5	52.2	25.4	6.2
Mature Cheddar & Shallot, Temptations, Tesco*	1/6 Bag/25g	131	8.5	524	6.6	47.4	34.2	4.4
Mediterranean Baked Potato, COU, M & S*	1 Pack/25g	90	0.6	360	7.6	74.0	2.4	6.8
Mexican Chilli, Ridge Cut, McCoys*	1 Bag/32g	164	9.8	514	6.9	53.0	30.5	4.5
Mexican Chilli & Cheese, Golden Wonder*	1 Pack/45g	230	14.1	511	6.6	50.7	31.3	0.0
Mexican Lime with a Hint of Chilli, Kettle Chips*	1 Serving/50g	242	13.7	484	5.0	54.1	27.5	5.4

CRISPS

INFO/WEIGHT	Measure	per Measure KCAL	FAT	Nutrition Values per 100g / 100ml KCAL	PROT	CARB	FAT	FIBRE
Mexy Tex, Smoked BBQ Corn Snacks, Tasty Little Numbers*	1 Pack/21g	100	4.5	475	6.8	64.3	21.2	1.9
Mild Cheese & Sweet Onion, Crispy Bakes, Kettle Chips*	1 Bag/24g	91	1.9	379	10.6	66.7	7.8	4.3
Mixed Pepper Flavour Burst, M & S*	1 Bag/55g	286	18.4	520	6.0	50.1	33.5	4.0
Mystery Dairy Flavour A, Walkers*	1 Pack/25g	132	8.1	529	6.0	51.0	32.6	4.1
Mystery Meaty Flavour B, Walkers*	1 Pack/25g	132	8.1	527	5.9	51.2	32.3	4.1
Mystery Spicy Flavour C, Walkers*	1 Pack/25g	132	8.1	528	6.0	51.3	32.3	4.2
Naked, Tyrrells*	1 Pack/150g	748	41.2	499	7.7	56.5	27.5	0.0
New York Cheddar, Kettle Chips*	1 Bag/50g	241	13.3	483	6.7	53.9	26.7	4.5
Olive Oil, Mozzarella & Oregano, Walkers*	1 Serving/30g	151	8.7	505	6.5	54.0	29.0	4.0
Onion Bhaji, Walkers*	1 Pack/25g	130	8.2	522	6.1	50.7	32.7	4.3
Onion Rings, Corn Snacks, Average	1 Bag/25g	122	6.1	486	5.8	60.9	24.2	2.7
Onion Rings, Crunchy, Shapers, Boots*	1 Bag/12g	61	3.4	507	2.5	62.0	28.0	2.6
Onion Rings, M & S*	1 Pack/40g	186	8.6	465	5.2	62.1	21.5	4.3
Onion Rings, Tayto*	1 Pack/17g	82	4.1	484	3.0	63.4	24.0	2.4
Onion Rings, Tesco*	1 Serving/30g	148	7.6	495	8.4	57.8	25.5	2.5
Oriental Ribs, Ridge Cut, McCoys*	1 Pack/50g	255	15.0	511	7.3	52.7	30.1	4.2
Paprika, Handcooked, Shapers, Boots*	1 Bag/20g	99	4.8	493	7.2	62.0	24.0	5.0
Paprika, Max, Walkers*	1 Bag/50g	260	15.9	520	6.5	52.0	31.9	5.1
Paprika, Mini Hoops, Shapers, Boots*	1 Bag/13g	64	3.5	494	8.7	54.0	27.0	2.2
Parsnip, Passions, Snack Rite*	1 Serving/25g	123	9.4	494	4.5	34.5	37.6	18.8
Parsnip & Black Pepper, Sainsbury's*	1 Serving/35g	166	11.1	473	3.2	43.6	31.8	15.2
Pastrami & Cheese, Crinkle, M & S*	1 Bag/25g	120	5.9	485	6.5	61.0	24.0	3.5
Peri Peri Chicken, Nando's*	½ Bag/75g	410	20.2	547	5.1	57.4	27.0	3.4
Pickled Onion, Beastie Bites, Asda*	1 Bag/20g	100	5.2	498	6.0	60.0	26.0	0.0
Pickled Onion, Golden Wonder*	1 Bag/25g	131	8.5	524	5.6	49.0	34.0	2.0
Pickled Onion, Monster Bites, Sainsbury's*	1 Bag/20g	107	6.7	535	5.2	53.5	33.3	1.0
Pickled Onion, Stompers, Morrisons*	1 Pack/25g	129	7.9	518	6.1	52.2	31.6	1.3
Pickled Onion, Sunseed, Walkers*	1 Bag/33g	171	10.7	525	6.5	50.0	33.0	4.0
Pickled Onion Flavour, Average	1 Bag/25g	132	8.2	527	6.6	52.5	32.6	3.5
Pickled Onion Flavour Rings, BGTY, Sainsbury's*	1 Serving/10g	34	0.1	345	5.0	81.7	1.5	3.7
Pickled Onion Rings, COU, M & S*	1 Bag/20g	69	0.3	345	5.0	81.7	1.5	3.7
Potato, Average	1oz/28g	148	9.6	530	5.7	53.3	34.2	5.3
Potato, Baked, COU, M & S*	1 Bag/25g	87	0.6	350	8.5	76.4	2.3	5.7
Potato, Cheddar & Onion, Hand Cooked, Aldi*	1 Pack/150g	753	41.8	502	7.7	54.9	27.9	4.0
Potato, Low Fat	1oz/28g	128	6.0	458	6.6	63.5	21.5	5.9
Potato, Tyrrells*	1 Pack/261g	1362	72.8	522	6.1	56.5	27.9	0.0
Potato Chips, Anglesey Sea Salt, Red Sky*	1 Serving/40g	185	8.7	463	6.8	59.8	21.8	5.0
Potato Chips, Popped, Cheeses & Onion Flavour, M & S*	1 Bag/23g	95	3.2	413	7.4	60.9	13.9	4.3
Potato Chips, Roasted Red Pepper & Lime, Red Sky*	1 Serving/40g	187	9.0	467	6.8	59.5	22.4	4.8
Potato Chips, Sour Cream & Green Herbs, Red Sky*	1 Pack/40g	188	9.4	471	6.8	58.4	23.4	4.8
Potato Squares, Ready Salted, Sainsbury's*	1 Bag/50g	192	7.9	384	6.5	53.8	15.9	7.8
Potato Thins, Lightly Salted, Light Choices, Tesco*	1 Pack/20g	72	0.4	360	5.1	79.5	2.0	4.2
Potato Triangles, Ready Salted, Sainsbury's*	½ Pack/50g	243	11.7	486	9.4	59.7	23.4	3.4
Potato Zoo, Crispy Potato Animals, Kids, Tesco*	1 Bag/30g	57	1.9	190	2.5	24.5	6.3	2.1
Prawn Cocktail, 30% Less Fat, Sainsbury's*	1 Pack/25g	117	5.9	470	6.3	58.9	23.6	5.7
Prawn Cocktail, BGTY, Sainsbury's*	1 Bag/25g	118	5.9	473	6.3	58.6	23.7	5.7
Prawn Cocktail, Boots*	1 Pack/21g	99	4.6	470	6.8	60.0	22.0	4.3
Prawn Cocktail, Golden Wonder*	1 Bag/25g	130	8.4	521	5.8	49.0	33.5	2.0
Prawn Cocktail, KP Snacks*	1 Bag/25g	133	8.7	531	5.9	48.4	34.9	4.7
Prawn Cocktail, Lites, Advantage, Tayto*	1 Pack/21g	96	4.1	455	5.3	65.1	19.3	3.8
Prawn Cocktail, Lites, Shapers, Boots*	1 Bag/21g	92	3.8	438	5.1	64.0	18.0	4.1
Prawn Cocktail, Snack Rite*	1 Bag/25g	129	8.3	516	5.0	49.2	33.2	0.0
Prawn Cocktail, Sunseed Oil, Walkers*	1 Bag/33g	171	10.7	525	6.5	50.0	33.0	4.0

C

CRISPS

	Measure INFO/WEIGHT	per Measure KCAL	FAT	Nutrition Values per 100g / 100ml KCAL	PROT	CARB	FAT	FIBRE
Prawn Cocktail, Tayto*	1 Bag/35g	185	12.3	526	7.5	46.6	35.0	4.5
Prawn Cocktail Flavour, Seabrook*	1 Bag/30g	163	10.1	544	5.7	49.2	33.7	4.5
Prawn Crackers, Tesco*	1 Bag/60g	316	17.5	527	3.2	62.8	29.2	0.8
Ready Salted, 30% Less Fat, Sainsbury's*	1 Serving/25g	121	5.6	486	7.3	63.7	22.4	8.2
Ready Salted, Average	1 Bag/25g	127	7.4	508	6.1	53.4	29.7	4.0
Ready Salted, BGTY, Sainsbury's*	1 Bag/25g	121	6.5	486	6.8	55.7	26.2	6.6
Ready Salted, Deep Ridge, Walkers*	1 Pack/28g	148	9.0	529	6.4	51.1	32.1	4.6
Ready Salted, GFY, Asda*	1 Bag/23g	109	5.3	475	7.0	60.0	23.0	4.3
Ready Salted, Golden Wonder*	1 Bag/25g	135	8.8	539	5.5	49.9	35.3	2.0
Ready Salted, KP Snacks*	1 Bag/24g	131	8.8	545	5.6	47.9	36.8	4.9
Ready Salted, Lower Fat, Asda*	1 Bag/25g	120	6.2	481	6.0	58.0	25.0	4.8
Ready Salted, Lower Fat, Sainsbury's*	1 Bag/25g	111	5.4	444	7.0	55.0	21.8	5.1
Ready Salted, Reduced Fat, Tesco*	1 Pack/25g	114	6.2	456	6.3	52.0	24.7	5.9
Ready Salted, Ridge Cut, McCoys*	1 Bag/49g	257	15.6	524	6.6	52.6	31.9	4.1
Ready Salted, Select, Tesco*	1 Bag/25g	136	9.1	544	6.2	47.9	36.6	4.5
Ready Salted, Snack Rite*	1 Bag/25g	136	9.0	545	4.9	50.3	36.0	0.0
Ready Salted, Squares, M & S*	1 Bag/35g	150	6.3	430	6.8	63.5	18.1	3.9
Ready Salted, Squares, Walkers*	1 Pack/25g	109	4.7	435	6.5	60.0	19.0	6.0
Ready Salted, Sunseed Oil, Walkers*	1 Bag/33g	175	11.1	537	5.9	49.7	34.1	4.2
Red Leicester & Spring Onion, Handcooked, M & S*	1 Pack/40g	194	10.6	485	6.8	55.0	26.4	5.1
Ridge, Thick & Chunky, Ready Salted, Eastmans*	1 Pack/30g	155	9.2	515	5.9	53.5	30.6	4.1
Roast Beef, KP Snacks*	1 Bag/25g	133	8.8	534	6.6	47.5	35.3	4.7
Roast Beef & Horseradish, Walkers*	1oz/28g	147	9.2	524	6.0	51.2	32.8	4.0
Roast Beef & Mustard, Thick Cut, Brannigans*	1 Bag/40g	203	12.0	507	7.6	51.7	30.0	3.7
Roast Chicken, 30% Less Fat, Sainsbury's*	1 Pack/25g	115	5.5	460	7.4	58.3	21.9	5.2
Roast Chicken, Golden Wonder*	1 Bag/25g	130	8.4	522	6.2	48.6	33.6	2.0
Roast Chicken, Highlander*	1 Bag/25g	138	9.7	554	5.3	46.0	38.9	5.1
Roast Chicken, Select, Tesco*	1 Bag/25g	134	8.7	536	6.6	48.6	35.0	4.4
Roast Chicken, Snack Rite*	1 Bag/25g	131	8.3	526	5.3	51.3	33.3	0.0
Roast Chicken, Sunseed Oil, Walkers*	1 Bag/33g	171	10.7	525	6.5	50.0	33.0	4.0
Roast Chicken, Tayto*	1 Bag/35g	184	11.9	526	7.6	47.3	34.0	4.5
Roast Chicken & Sage Flavour, M & S*	1 Bag/25g	135	8.6	540	5.9	50.6	34.6	4.6
Roast Chicken Flavour, Average	1 Bag/25g	132	8.6	528	6.1	48.8	34.2	3.9
Roast Chicken Flavour, BGTY, Sainsbury's*	1 Bag/25g	118	5.9	473	6.2	58.9	23.6	5.7
Roast Chicken Flavour, Crinkle, Weight Watchers*	1 Pack/16g	76	3.3	475	5.6	63.1	20.6	6.2
Roast Ham & Mustard, Ridge Cut, McCoys*	1 Pack/35g	181	10.7	518	7.1	53.5	30.6	3.9
Roast Pork & Apple Sauce, Select, Tesco*	1 Bag/25g	136	8.8	544	6.5	50.0	35.3	3.7
Roasted Lamb, Moroccan Spices, Sensations, Walkers*	1 Bag/40g	198	11.6	495	6.0	53.0	29.0	4.5
Salsa with Mesquite, Kettle Chips*	1 Serving/50g	231	12.1	462	5.8	55.2	24.2	5.7
Salt & Balsamic Vinegar, Perfectly Balanced, Waitrose*	1 Bag/20g	69	0.5	347	4.2	76.4	2.7	5.2
Salt & Black Pepper, Handcooked, M & S*	1 Bag/40g	180	9.2	450	5.7	55.0	22.9	5.2
Salt & Cracked Black Pepper, Shapers, Boots*	1 Bag/20g	91	4.4	453	7.2	57.0	22.0	5.0
Salt & Malt Vinegar, Deep Ridge, Walkers*	1 Pack/28g	143	8.6	511	6.1	50.7	30.7	4.3
Salt & Malt Vinegar, Ridge Cut, McCoys*	1 Bag/32g	165	9.8	515	6.7	53.3	30.6	3.9
Salt & Shake, Walkers*	1 Bag/30g	162	10.5	540	6.5	50.0	35.0	4.0
Salt & Vinegar, 30% Less Fat, Sainsbury's*	1 Bag/25g	114	5.4	458	7.2	58.3	21.8	5.1
Salt & Vinegar, Average	1 Bag/25g	130	8.2	519	5.5	50.3	32.9	3.4
Salt & Vinegar, Baked, Walkers*	1 Packet/38g	150	3.0	400	6.0	73.5	8.1	4.6
Salt & Vinegar, BGTY, Sainsbury's*	1 Bag/25g	120	6.3	482	6.5	57.3	25.2	5.2
Salt & Vinegar, Crinkle, M & S*	1 Pack/25g	120	5.9	485	6.5	61.0	24.0	3.5
Salt & Vinegar, Crinkle Cut, Seabrook*	1 Bag/32g	181	11.7	569	5.4	54.4	36.7	3.9
Salt & Vinegar, Crinkles, Shapers, Boots*	1 Pack/20g	96	4.8	482	6.6	60.0	24.0	4.0
Salt & Vinegar, Crispy Discs, Shapers, Boots*	1 Bag/92g	404	17.5	439	4.8	63.0	19.0	4.9

CRISPS

Measure INFO/WEIGHT		per Measure		Nutrition Values per 100g / 100ml				
		KCAL	FAT	KCAL	PROT	CARB	FAT	FIBRE
Salt & Vinegar, Fish Shapes, Food Explorers, Waitrose*	1 Bag/20g	86	3.2	430	2.4	69.1	16.0	1.3
Salt & Vinegar, GFY, Asda*	1 Bag/26g	120	5.7	466	6.0	61.0	22.0	4.1
Salt & Vinegar, Golden Lights, Golden Wonder*	1 Bag/21g	94	3.9	446	4.2	65.7	18.5	3.7
Salt & Vinegar, Golden Wonder*	1 Bag/25g	130	8.5	522	5.4	48.5	34.0	2.0
Salt & Vinegar, KP Snacks*	1 Bag/25g	133	8.7	532	5.5	48.7	35.0	4.7
Salt & Vinegar, Lights, Walkers*	1 Bag/28g	133	6.2	475	7.0	62.0	22.0	4.5
Salt & Vinegar, Lower Fat, Asda*	1 Bag/25g	120	6.2	481	5.0	58.0	25.0	4.8
Salt & Vinegar, Oven Baked, Asda*	1 Bag/25g	95	2.0	380	5.1	72.0	8.0	2.9
Salt & Vinegar, Potato Bakes, Weight Watchers*	1 Bag/20g	81	1.8	404	5.3	76.0	8.8	2.3
Salt & Vinegar, Red Mill*	1 Bag/40g	174	7.0	436	3.9	65.8	17.5	2.4
Salt & Vinegar, Rough Cuts, Tayto*	1 Bag/30g	152	9.2	506	4.6	56.8	30.8	0.0
Salt & Vinegar, Snack Rite*	1 Bag/25g	127	8.2	508	4.7	48.1	33.0	0.0
Salt & Vinegar, Space Raiders, KP Snacks*	1 Bag/17g	81	3.8	478	6.9	61.7	22.6	2.2
Salt & Vinegar, Squares, Walkers*	1 Bag/25g	107	4.5	430	6.5	61.0	18.0	5.5
Salt & Vinegar, Sunseed Oil, Walkers*	1 Bag/33g	171	10.7	525	6.5	50.0	33.0	4.0
Salt & Vinegar, Tayto*	1 Bag/35g	184	11.9	526	7.6	47.3	34.0	4.5
Salt & Vinegar, Tubes, HL, Tesco*	1 Bag/17g	61	0.3	357	3.2	82.4	1.6	3.0
Salt & Vinegar, Walkers*	1 Pack/25g	131	8.3	524	6.4	50.0	33.2	4.0
Salt & Vinegar Chiplets, M & S*	1 Pack/50g	220	9.4	440	5.7	61.3	18.9	4.7
Salt & Vinegar Flavour, Half Fat, M & S*	1 Bag/40g	168	6.8	420	5.8	61.0	17.0	7.7
Salt & Vinegar Flavour, Sprinters*	1 Bag/25g	133	8.8	532	4.8	49.1	35.2	0.0
Salt & Vinegar Fries, COU, M & S*	1 Bag/25g	85	0.4	340	5.0	80.0	1.6	4.0
Salt & Vinegar in Sunflower Oil, Sainsbury's*	1 Serving/25g	131	8.4	524	5.2	49.7	33.8	3.7
Salt & Vinegar Spirals, Shapers, Boots*	1 Pack/15g	71	3.4	475	3.1	64.0	23.0	1.7
Salt Your Own, Excluding Salt, Aldi*	1 Pack/24g	130	8.1	536	6.0	52.6	33.5	4.5
Salt Your Own, Jacket, 35% Less Fat, Sainsbury's*	1 Bag/20g	98	4.5	490	7.5	64.5	22.5	9.5
Salt Your Own, Sainsbury's*	1 Pack/24g	127	7.9	520	5.0	52.2	32.3	3.7
Sausage & Tomato, Sainsbury's*	1 Pack/25g	131	8.4	525	6.0	49.3	33.8	3.8
Sausage & Tomato Flavour, Golden Wonder*	1 Bag/35g	174	10.6	505	6.1	51.3	30.6	4.5
Scotch Bonnet Flavour, Mackies Of Scotland*	1 Pack/150g	732	369.0	488	78.0	574.0	246.0	42.0
Sea Salt, Golden Lights, Golden Wonder*	1 Bag/21g	94	3.9	448	3.9	66.4	18.5	4.4
Sea Salt, Gourmet, TTD, Sainsbury's*	1/3 Pack/50g	249	15.0	498	5.7	51.4	30.0	6.4
Sea Salt, Handcooked, Extra Special, Asda*	1 Pack/31g	149	7.8	477	7.0	56.0	25.0	4.1
Sea Salt, Original, Crinkle Cut, Seabrook*	1 Bag/30g	155	9.3	517	5.7	53.7	31.1	4.2
Sea Salt & Balsamic Vinegar, Kettle Chips*	1 Bag/40g	190	10.0	476	5.9	56.8	25.0	4.5
Sea Salt & Balsamic Vinegar, Low Fat, Peak*	1 Serving/25g	87	0.3	348	7.4	76.6	1.4	6.7
Sea Salt & Black Pepper, GFY, Asda*	1 Bag/100g	476	24.0	476	6.0	59.0	24.0	6.0
Sea Salt & Black Pepper, Highlander*	1 Serving/25g	141	9.6	564	5.6	44.0	38.4	4.8
Sea Salt & Black Pepper, Shapers, Boots*	1 Bag/20g	96	4.8	482	6.6	60.0	24.0	4.0
Sea Salt & Black Pepper, Tyrrells*	¼ Pack/38g	182	9.3	480	7.3	59.9	24.5	2.4
Sea Salt & Cider Vinegar, TTD, Sainsbury's*	1/3 Pack/50g	245	14.3	489	5.5	52.7	28.5	6.1
Sea Salt & Cracked Black Pepper, Lights, Walkers*	1 Bag/24g	115	5.3	480	7.0	63.0	22.0	5.0
Sea Salt & Cracked Black Pepper, Sensations, Walkers*	1 Bag/40g	196	10.8	490	6.5	55.0	27.0	4.0
Sea Salt & Indian Black Pepper, Pipers Crisps*	1 Pack/40g	195	11.6	487	6.6	49.9	29.0	0.0
Sea Salt & Malt Vinegar, Sensations, Walkers*	1 Bag/40g	194	10.8	485	6.5	54.0	27.0	4.5
Sea Salt & Malt Vinegar Flavour, Potato Fries, GFY, Asda*	1 Bag/15g	54	0.3	358	6.3	79.6	1.7	2.1
Sea Salt & Modena Balsamic Vivegar, Darling Spuds*	1 Bag/40g	190	11.4	475	5.4	54.3	28.5	4.2
Sea Salt with Crushed Black Peppercorns, Kettle Chips*	1 Serving/40g	193	10.7	482	6.5	53.8	26.7	4.9
Shells, Prawn Cocktail, Asda*	1 Bag/18g	90	5.3	501	4.6	54.9	29.2	6.2
Simply Salted, Extra Crunchy, Walkers*	1 Bag/30g	142	6.5	473	6.8	59.8	21.8	5.0
Simply Salted, Lights, Walkers*	1 Bag/24g	113	5.3	470	7.0	61.0	22.0	5.0
Sizzling Beef, Spice, McCoys*	1 Bag/35g	175	10.4	501	6.4	51.7	29.8	4.0
Sizzling King Prawn, Ridge Cut, McCoys*	1 Packet/50g	259	15.1	518	6.6	54.7	30.3	4.0

CRISPS

INFO/WEIGHT	Measure		per Measure		Nutrition Values per 100g / 100ml				
			KCAL	FAT	KCAL	PROT	CARB	FAT	FIBRE
Smoked Ham & Pickle, Thick Cut, Brannigans*	1 Bag/40g		203	11.9	507	7.0	52.8	29.8	3.8
Smokey Bacon, Budgens*	1 Bag/25g		130	8.2	519	6.2	49.3	33.0	4.8
Smokey Bacon, Crinkle, Shapers, Boots*	1 Pack/20g		96	4.8	482	6.6	60.0	24.0	4.0
Smokey Bacon, Seabrook*	1 Bag/32g		181	11.7	569	5.4	54.4	36.7	3.9
Smokey Bacon, Select, Tesco*	1 Bag/25g		134	8.7	536	6.4	49.0	34.9	4.3
Smokey Bacon Potato Hoops, COU, M & S*	1 Pack/16g		58	0.4	360	5.6	78.7	2.7	4.5
Smoky Bacon, 30% Lower Fat, Sainsbury's*	1 Bag/25g		118	5.9	471	6.5	58.4	23.6	5.7
Smoky Bacon, BGTY, Sainsbury's*	1 Bag/25g		118	5.9	472	6.5	58.5	23.6	5.7
Smoky Bacon, Golden Wonder*	1 Bag/25g		131	8.4	523	5.9	49.1	33.7	2.0
Smoky Bacon, Snack Rite*	1 Bag/25g		131	8.3	525	5.5	51.2	33.1	0.0
Smoky Bacon, Sunseed Oil, Walkers*	1 Bag/35g		183	11.4	530	6.5	51.0	33.0	4.0
Smoky Bacon, Tayto*	1 Bag/35g		184	11.9	526	7.6	47.3	34.0	4.5
Smoky Bacon Flavour, Average	1 Bag/25g		132	8.4	527	6.2	49.7	33.7	3.2
Snaps, Spicy Tomato Flavour, Walkers*	1 Bag/18g		91	4.8	508	1.5	65.5	26.8	0.0
Snax, Tayto*	1 Pack/17g		82	3.7	483	2.4	70.0	21.5	1.6
Sour Cream & Chive, Crinkle, Reduced Fat, M & S*	1 Bag/40g		178	8.2	445	5.6	58.8	20.6	5.6
Sour Cream & Chive, Lights, Walkers*	1 Bag/24g		114	5.3	475	7.5	62.0	22.0	5.0
Sour Cream & Chive, Perfectly Balanced, Waitrose*	1 Pack/20g		69	0.5	347	4.4	76.3	2.7	5.2
Sour Cream & Chive, Potato Bakes, Weight Watchers*	1 Bag/20g		83	1.8	417	3.8	80.7	8.8	3.6
Sour Cream & Chive, Potato Bites, BGTY, Sainsbury's*	1 Pack/20g		73	0.6	365	7.2	77.8	2.8	3.9
Sour Cream & Chive Baked Potato, COU, M & S*	1 Pack/24g		84	0.7	350	7.5	73.2	2.8	7.9
Sour Cream & Chive Crispy Discs, Shapers, Boots*	1 Bag/21g		94	4.0	448	5.7	61.9	19.0	4.3
Sour Cream & Chives, Jordans*	1 Bag/30g		125	3.6	417	7.3	69.9	12.0	2.7
Sour Cream & Onion, Golden Lights, Golden Wonder*	1 Bag/21g		93	3.8	442	4.1	66.0	17.9	4.4
Sour Cream with a Hint of Mexican Chilli, Darling Spuds*	1 Packet/40g		192	11.4	479	6.2	53.8	28.6	4.3
Space Raiders, Pickled Onion, KP Snacks*	1 Bag/16g		77	3.7	480	6.7	61.3	23.3	4.0
Spare Rib Flavour, Chinese, Walkers*	1 Bag/35g		181	11.4	525	6.5	50.0	33.0	4.0
Spiced Chilli, McCoys*	1 Bag/35g		175	10.1	500	6.1	54.2	28.8	4.2
Spicy Chilli, Sunseed, Walkers*	1 Pack/35g		183	11.4	530	6.5	51.0	33.0	4.0
Spring Onion, Seabrook*	1 Bag/32g		182	11.7	569	5.4	54.4	36.7	3.9
Spring Onion Flavour, M & S*	1 Bag/40g		210	13.7	525	5.9	48.7	34.3	5.1
Spring Onion Flavour, Tayto*	1 Bag/35g		184	11.9	526	7.6	47.3	34.0	4.5
Steak & Onion, Walkers*	1 Pack/33g		169	10.7	520	6.5	49.0	33.0	4.0
Sun Bites, Wholegrain, Lightly Sea Salted, Walkers*	1 Bag/25g		120	5.4	481	7.5	60.7	21.7	6.6
Sun Dried Tomato & Basil, Jonathan Crisp*	1 Pack/35g		176	10.1	503	5.6	52.0	29.0	5.4
Sun Dried Tomato & Chilli, Asda*	1 Pack/150g		700	34.5	467	7.0	58.0	23.0	4.1
Sunbites, Cheddar & Caramelised Onion, Walkers*	1 Bag/25g		120	5.4	480	7.6	60.8	21.6	6.4
Sunbites, Sweet Chilli, Sun Ripened, Walkers*	1 Bag/25g		120	5.4	480	7.6	60.8	21.6	6.4
Superbly Spiced, Cassava, Gluten Free, Hale & Hearty*	1 Bag/30g		136	7.0	453	3.3	56.7	23.3	6.7
Sweet Chill, Mexican, Phileas Fogg*	1 Bag/38g		193	11.0	507	6.7	54.8	29.0	4.2
Sweet Chilli, Baked Potato, COU, M & S*	1 Bag/26g		91	0.7	350	7.6	73.9	2.8	8.5
Sweet Chilli, Crinkle Cut, Weight Watchers*	1 Bag/20g		94	4.1	470	5.6	62.9	20.6	5.8
Sweet Chilli, Hand Cooked, Asda*	1 Pack/25g		120	7.1	479	5.7	54.5	28.3	4.5
Sweet Chilli & Red Peppers, Fusion, Tayto*	1 Bag/28g		140	8.3	500	4.9	52.2	29.8	4.6
Sweet Chilli Chicken, Extra Crunchy, Walkers*	1 Bag/30g		143	6.7	477	6.5	59.9	22.5	4.8
Sweet Chilli Flavour, Average	1 Bag/25g		115	5.6	461	5.1	59.9	22.6	4.5
T Bone Steak, Roysters*	1 Pack/28g		148	9.0	530	5.2	55.3	32.0	3.0
Tangy Malaysian Chutney, Sensations, Walkers*	1 Bag/24g		116	6.2	485	0.9	62.0	26.0	0.0
Tangy Tomato & Red Pepper Salsa, Sensations, Walkers*	1 Bag/35g		168	9.4	480	6.5	53.0	27.0	4.5
Tangy Toms, Red Mill*	1 Bag/15g		76	4.1	507	6.0	60.0	27.3	0.7
Thai Curry & Coriander, Tyrrells*	1 Pack/50g		261	13.9	522	6.1	56.5	27.9	5.4
Thai Sweet Chicken, Ridge Cut, McCoys*	1 Bag/50g		257	15.0	514	7.0	54.0	30.0	4.1
Thai Sweet Chilli, Sensations, Walkers*	1 Bag/40g		194	10.4	485	6.0	57.0	26.0	4.2

	Measure INFO/WEIGHT	per Measure KCAL	FAT	Nutrition Values per 100g / 100ml KCAL	PROT	CARB	FAT	FIBRE
CRISPS								
Thai Sweet Chilli Flavour, Velvet Crunch, King*	1 Pack/20g	81	1.9	404	1.6	77.5	9.7	2.0
Tomato & Basil, Mediterranean, Walkers*	1 Pack/25g	127	8.2	510	6.5	49.0	33.0	4.5
Tomato & Herb, Shapers, Boots*	1 Bag/20g	94	4.2	468	3.7	66.0	21.0	3.9
Tomato Ketchup Flavour, Golden Wonder*	1 Bag/25g	135	8.0	521	5.1	54.0	30.8	3.6
Tortillas, Nacho Cheese Flavour, Weight Watchers*	1 Pack/18g	78	2.9	433	6.1	66.7	16.1	3.9
Traditional, Hand Cooked, Finest, Tesco*	1 Bag/150g	708	39.1	472	6.4	52.9	26.1	5.1
Turkey & Paxo, Walkers*	1 Bag/35g	181	11.4	525	6.4	50.1	33.0	4.1
Unsalted, Potato Heads, Walkers*	1 Serving/23g	106	5.1	460	5.0	61.0	22.0	5.0
Unsalted, Seabrook*	1 Bag/30g	163	10.7	544	5.7	47.9	35.8	4.1
Vegetable, Average	1 Bag/25g	118	7.4	470	4.1	46.5	29.6	12.1
Waffles, Bacon Flavour, BGTY, Sainsbury's*	1 Serving/12g	41	0.2	345	6.4	79.7	1.4	2.9
Wild Chilli, McCoys*	1 Bag/50g	255	15.1	510	6.0	53.2	30.3	4.8
Wild Paprika Flavour, Croky*	1 Pack/45g	234	13.0	521	6.0	58.0	29.0	0.0
Worcester Sauce, Sunseed Oil, Walkers*	1 Bag/35g	183	11.4	530	6.5	52.0	33.0	4.0
Worcester Sauce Flavour, Hunky Dorys*	1 Bag/45g	211	12.9	469	6.3	49.3	28.7	0.0
Yoghurt & Green Onion, Kettle Chips*	1 Serving/50g	236	13.0	473	6.6	54.1	26.1	5.4
CRISPY PANCAKE								
Beef Bolognese, Findus*	1 Pancake/65g	104	2.6	160	6.5	25.0	4.0	1.0
Chicken, Bacon & Sweetcorn, Findus*	1 Pancake/63g	101	2.5	160	5.5	26.0	4.0	1.1
Minced Beef, Findus*	1 Pancake/63g	100	2.5	160	6.5	25.0	4.0	1.0
Three Cheeses, Findus*	1 Pancake/62g	118	4.0	190	7.0	25.0	6.5	0.9
CROISSANT								
All Butter, BGTY, Sainsbury's*	1 Roll/44g	151	6.5	343	9.3	42.7	14.8	1.8
All Butter, Budgens*	1 Roll/45g	185	11.1	412	7.9	39.7	24.6	3.3
All Butter, Finest, Tesco*	1 Roll/77g	328	18.2	426	8.6	44.9	23.6	1.9
All Butter, M & S*	1 Roll/54g	222	12.8	415	7.4	45.2	23.8	1.6
All Butter, Mini, Sainsbury's*	1 Roll/35g	150	8.6	428	9.2	42.6	24.5	1.2
All Butter, Mini, Tesco*	1 Roll/35g	150	8.2	430	9.3	45.2	23.5	2.0
All Butter, Reduced Fat, Tesco*	1 Roll/52g	164	5.5	315	7.5	47.4	10.6	1.8
All Butter, Sainsbury's*	1 Roll/44g	188	10.8	428	9.2	42.6	24.5	1.2
All Butter, Tesco*	1 Roll/48g	192	10.4	400	8.5	41.7	21.6	2.6
Asda*	1 Roll/47g	190	9.9	405	9.0	45.0	21.0	0.0
Average	1 Roll/50g	180	10.1	360	8.3	38.3	20.3	1.6
Butter, Asda*	1 Roll/46g	191	11.0	416	8.0	42.0	24.0	1.9
Butter, GFY, Asda*	1 Roll/44g	153	7.0	352	6.0	46.0	16.0	2.0
Butter, Morrisons*	1 Roll/44g	196	12.5	446	9.3	38.2	28.4	2.0
Butter, Part Bake, Morrisons*	1 Roll/45g	179	8.5	397	7.3	49.6	18.8	1.9
Butter, Part Baked, De Graaf*	1 Roll/45g	170	8.4	378	7.3	45.2	18.7	0.0
Cheese & Ham, Mini, Waitrose*	1 Roll/17g	64	4.1	383	13.2	28.1	24.5	3.0
Continental, Mini, Chosen By You, Asda*	1 Roll/35g	150	8.9	427	9.2	40.6	25.3	1.6
Flaky Pastry with a Plain Chocolate Filling, Tesco*	1 Roll/78g	318	19.0	408	6.5	41.0	24.3	2.0
French Butter, You Count, Love Life, Waitrose*	1 Roll/44g	168	7.4	382	9.8	46.4	16.8	3.1
Heart Shaped, Breakfast in Bed, M & S*	1 Roll/54g	230	13.6	430	8.2	43.7	25.5	1.2
Homebake, Long Life, Stay Fresh Range, Harvestime*	1 Roll/44g	159	6.0	362	7.6	51.9	13.7	1.9
Low Fat, M & S*	1 Roll/45g	180	9.1	400	8.2	46.0	20.2	1.8
Mini, Lidl*	1 Roll/30g	112	5.0	373	7.8	48.0	16.6	0.0
Organic, Tesco*	1 Roll/45g	195	11.6	433	8.2	42.0	25.8	2.2
Reduced Fat, Asda*	1 Roll/44g	159	6.5	361	9.7	47.2	14.8	2.0
Reduced Fat, Sainsbury's*	1 Roll/44g	173	7.7	393	9.8	49.2	17.5	2.2
TTD, Sainsbury's*	1 Roll/70g	289	16.1	413	8.1	43.4	23.0	2.5
Wholesome, Sainsbury's*	1 Roll/44g	192	12.1	436	8.8	38.3	27.5	4.0
CROQUETTES								
Morrisons*	1 Serving/150g	231	8.1	154	3.3	23.1	5.4	1.1

	Measure INFO/WEIGHT	per Measure KCAL	FAT	Nutrition Values per 100g / 100ml KCAL	PROT	CARB	FAT	FIBRE
CROQUETTES								
Potato, Asda*	3 Pieces/81g	144	5.7	177	2.0	26.5	7.0	2.2
Potato, Birds Eye*	1 Piece/29g	44	1.7	152	2.6	22.6	5.7	1.2
Potato, Chunky, Aunt Bessie's*	1 Serving/41g	62	2.5	152	2.3	23.9	6.1	1.8
Potato, Crispy, Chilled, Sainsbury's*	3 Pieces/125g	245	11.5	196	2.5	25.7	9.2	1.9
Potato, Fried in Blended Oil, Average	1 Piece/80g	171	10.5	214	3.7	21.6	13.1	1.3
Potato, M & S*	1 Piece/41g	68	3.6	165	2.4	19.3	8.8	2.2
Potato, Sainsbury's*	1 Piece/28g	50	2.4	180	2.8	22.6	8.6	2.5
Potato, Waitrose*	1 Piece/30g	47	2.4	157	3.0	17.9	8.1	1.5
Potato & Parsnip, Finest, Tesco*	2 Pieces/74g	155	7.3	210	6.0	23.2	9.9	3.9
Vegetable, Sainsbury's*	1 Serving/175g	392	20.8	224	5.8	23.3	11.9	2.2
CROUTONS								
Fresh, M & S*	1 Scrving/10g	53	3.3	530	11.4	50.0	32.8	3.2
Garlic, Waitrose*	1 Serving/40g	209	12.0	522	10.8	52.1	30.0	2.7
Herb, Sainsbury's*	1 Serving/15g	64	1.7	429	13.4	68.2	11.4	2.8
Herb & Garlic, La Rochelle*	¼ Pack/18g	106	7.2	587	6.9	49.8	40.0	2.1
Italian Salad, Sainsbury's*	1 Pack/40g	204	10.0	510	8.5	62.7	25.0	2.5
La Rochelle*	1 Bag/70g	400	28.0	572	7.0	49.0	40.0	0.0
Lightly Sea Salted, Asda*	1 Serving/20g	83	1.9	414	12.9	69.7	9.3	4.3
Migros*	1 Serving/15g	56	0.4	375	14.0	72.0	3.0	3.5
Sun Dried Tomato, Sainsbury's*	¼ Pack/15g	75	3.8	497	11.7	55.2	25.5	2.5
CRUDITE								
Platter, Sainsbury's*	1 Pack/275g	96	0.8	35	1.4	6.6	0.3	1.6
Selection, Prepared, M & S*	1 Serving/250g	75	1.0	30	1.4	5.8	0.4	2.0
Vegetable Sticks, Average	1 Serving/100g	24	0.2	24	0.7	4.5	0.2	1.9
CRUMBLE								
Almond & Apricot, Devondale*	1 Cake/80g	314	13.2	392	3.6	57.0	16.5	9.8
Apple, Average	1 Serving/240g	497	12.0	207	0.9	40.5	5.0	1.1
Apple, Fresh, Chilled, Tesco*	¼ Pack/150g	367	13.3	245	2.8	38.0	8.9	1.4
Apple, Frozen, Iceland*	1 Serving/97g	240	9.8	247	2.1	36.9	10.1	1.8
Apple, Frozen, Tesco*	¼ Pack/150g	345	16.3	230	2.1	30.7	10.9	3.9
Apple, Sara Lee*	1 Serving/200g	606	18.0	303	2.3	53.3	9.0	1.2
Apple, with Custard, Green's*	1 Serving/79g	171	5.3	216	1.9	37.0	6.7	1.2
Apple, with Sultanas, Weight Watchers*	1 Dessert/110g	196	4.3	178	1.4	34.2	3.9	1.3
Apple & Blackberry, Asda*	1 Serving/175g	427	15.7	244	2.7	38.0	9.0	1.2
Apple & Blackberry, M & S*	1 Serving/135g	398	15.1	295	3.5	44.9	11.2	1.6
Apple & Blackberry, Sainsbury's*	1 Serving/110g	232	6.2	211	3.0	37.1	5.6	2.1
Apple & Blackberry, with Custard, Somerfield*	1 Serving/120g	324	15.0	270	2.3	36.3	12.5	1.1
Apple & Custard, Asda*	1 Serving/125g	250	8.7	200	2.3	32.0	7.0	0.0
Apple & Toffee, Weight Watchers*	1 Pot/98g	190	4.5	194	1.6	36.6	4.6	0.0
Blackcurrant & Apple, Devondale*	1 Cake/80g	314	13.2	393	3.6	57.0	16.5	9.8
Bramley Apple, Chosen By You, Asda*	1 Serving/100g	257	8.4	257	2.5	41.8	8.4	2.3
Bramley Apple, Favourites, M & S*	1 Serving/140g	390	13.8	279	4.6	43.2	9.9	1.2
Bramley Apple, M & S*	1 Serving/149g	387	13.7	260	4.3	40.3	9.2	1.1
Bramley Apple, Tesco*	1/3 Pack/155g	378	14.9	244	2.8	36.7	9.6	1.8
Cauliflower & Camembert, Sainsbury's*	1 Pack/400g	588	43.2	147	5.5	6.9	10.8	0.7
Christmas, Devondale*	1 Cake/100g	359	12.4	359	3.3	58.7	12.4	2.4
Fish & Prawn, Youngs*	1 Pie/375g	476	27.0	127	5.8	9.7	7.2	1.3
Fruit	1 Portion/170g	337	11.7	198	2.0	34.0	6.9	1.7
Fruit, Wholemeal	1oz/28g	54	2.0	193	2.6	31.7	7.1	2.7
Fruit with Custard	1 Serving/270g	463	17.6	171	2.4	27.0	6.5	1.3
Gooseberry, M & S*	1 Serving/133g	379	14.2	285	3.5	43.3	10.7	1.7
Rhubarb, Average	1 Portion/150g	330	11.1	220	2.7	35.5	7.4	1.9
Rhubarb, Devondale*	1 Cake/80g	316	13.2	395	3.5	57.0	16.5	9.0

INFO/WEIGHT	Measure	per Measure		Nutrition Values per 100g / 100ml				
		KCAL	FAT	KCAL	PROT	CARB	FAT	FIBRE
CRUMBLE								
Rhubarb with Custard, Sainsbury's*	1 Serving/120g	288	13.9	240	2.4	31.4	11.6	2.3
Salmon, Youngs*	1 Pie/360g	367	14.4	102	5.4	11.1	4.0	1.0
CRUMBLE MIX								
Luxury, Tesco*	¼ Pack/55g	243	9.0	441	5.7	67.9	16.3	3.2
Luxury, Wholegrain, Gluten Free, Hale & Hearty*	1 Serving/100g	447	17.0	447	2.5	71.0	17.0	3.6
CRUMBLE TOPPING								
Morrisons*	1 Serving/40g	179	6.6	448	5.4	69.5	16.5	2.8
Sainsbury's*	1 Serving/47g	188	9.2	401	5.9	50.3	19.6	5.3
CRUMPETS								
Asda*	1 Crumpet/45g	85	0.4	188	6.0	39.0	0.9	2.1
Co-Op*	1 Crumpet/40g	70	0.3	175	7.0	35.0	0.7	2.0
Essential, Waitrose*	1 Crumpet/41g	77	0.4	187	5.9	38.8	0.9	2.3
Fruit from Bakery, Tesco*	1 Crumpet/73g	161	1.7	220	6.2	43.2	2.3	1.1
Gluten, Wheat & Milk Free, Free From, Livwell*	1 Crumpet/55g	83	1.7	151	3.6	26.9	3.1	2.0
Golden Sun*	1 Crumpet/43g	83	0.7	193	7.8	37.1	1.6	1.6
Kingsmill*	1 Crumpet/55g	99	0.4	180	5.8	37.5	0.8	1.7
Less Than 2% Fat, M & S*	1 Crumpet/61g	116	0.8	190	8.0	36.9	1.3	2.1
Morning Fresh*	1 Crumpet/20g	36	0.3	180	7.3	34.8	1.3	5.2
Mother's Pride*	1 Crumpet/43g	80	0.4	185	5.6	38.3	1.0	2.3
Perfectly Balanced, Waitrose*	1 Crumpet/55g	94	0.2	171	6.1	36.1	0.3	4.4
Premium, Sainsbury's*	1 Crumpet/50g	95	0.7	191	6.1	38.6	1.4	1.7
Rowan Hill Bakery, Lidl*	1 Crumpet/44g	78	0.5	178	5.5	34.5	1.2	0.0
Sainsbury's*	1 Crumpet/46g	86	0.3	186	5.8	39.1	0.7	2.5
Scottish, Nick Nairn's*	1 Serving/100g	186	9.6	186	5.3	43.0	9.6	1.5
Somerfield*	1 Crumpet/41g	79	0.4	192	5.9	39.9	1.0	2.5
Square, Spongebob Squarepants*	1 Crumpet/50g	93	0.5	186	7.0	37.2	1.0	1.0
Square, Tesco*	1 Crumpet/60g	101	0.5	168	6.3	33.8	0.8	2.7
Toasted, Average	1 Crumpet/40g	80	0.4	199	6.7	43.4	1.0	2.0
Warburton's*	1 Crumpet/55g	98	0.4	178	5.6	36.1	0.7	2.3
CRUNCHIE								
Blast, Cadbury*	1 Serving/42g	199	8.3	480	4.7	69.6	20.1	0.7
Cadbury*	1 Bar/40g	185	7.5	465	4.0	69.5	18.9	0.5
Nuggets, Cadbury*	1 Bag/125g	569	20.5	455	3.8	73.1	16.4	0.0
Treat Size, Cadbury*	1 Bar/17g	80	3.1	470	4.0	71.5	18.4	0.0
CRUNCHY STICKS								
Ready Salted, M & S*	1 Pack/75g	397	24.7	530	5.6	52.2	33.0	3.8
Ready Salted, Tesco*	1 Serving/25g	119	5.9	475	5.6	60.3	23.5	3.0
Salt & Vinegar, Sainsbury's*	1 Bag/25g	118	6.1	474	5.9	58.0	24.3	2.4
Salt & Vinegar, Shapers, Boots*	1 Pack/21g	96	3.8	457	5.7	66.7	18.1	2.4
Salt & Vinegar, Tesco*	1 Serving/25g	117	6.1	470	6.9	55.7	24.4	2.7
Salt & Vinegar, Value, Tesco*	1 Bag/22g	113	5.9	512	5.7	62.1	26.8	0.7
CUCUMBER								
Average	*1 Serving/80g*	*8*	*0.1*	*10*	*0.7*	*1.5*	*0.1*	*0.6*
CUMIN								
Seeds, Ground, Schwartz*	1 Tsp/5g	22	1.2	446	19.0	40.3	23.2	0.0
Seeds, Whole, Average	*1 Tsp/2g*	*7*	*0.5*	*375*	*17.8*	*44.2*	*22.7*	*10.5*
CUPCAKES								
Assorted, Sainsbury's*	1 Cake/38g	130	2.3	341	2.2	69.3	6.1	0.4
Carrot, Average	1 Cake/40g	157	8.6	391	3.6	45.4	21.6	0.6
Chocolate, 5% Fat, Sainsbury's*	1 Cake/38g	133	1.7	349	2.5	74.8	4.4	1.7
Chocolate, Average	1 Cake/40g	159	6.4	398	3.5	59.9	16.0	1.2
Chocolate, BGTY, Sainsbury's*	1 Cake/38g	121	1.7	318	2.5	66.5	4.6	0.8
Chocolate, COU, M & S*	1 Cake/45g	130	1.3	290	4.6	62.2	2.8	4.3

	Measure INFO/WEIGHT	per Measure KCAL	FAT	Nutrition Values per 100g / 100ml KCAL	PROT	CARB	FAT	FIBRE
CUPCAKES								
Chocolate, Fabulous Bakin' Boys*	1 Cake/34g	152	8.1	448	4.0	54.0	24.0	1.0
Chocolate, Healthy Option, Average	1 Cake/40g	128	1.6	319	3.2	67.8	3.9	2.3
Chocolate, Lyons*	1 Cake/39g	125	1.8	321	2.4	67.5	4.6	0.8
Chocolate, Mini, Weight Watchers*	1 Cake/20g	87	4.3	426	6.1	52.0	21.1	1.8
Cookies & Cream, Secret Chocolate Centre, Tesco*	1 Cake/69g	335	20.0	485	2.7	52.2	29.0	1.0
Jam Splatter, Tesco*	1 Cake/47g	221	10.2	470	2.3	65.6	21.8	0.5
Lemon, Average	1 Cake/40g	184	10.1	461	3.0	55.5	25.3	1.1
Lemon, Healthy Option, Average	1 Cake/40g	131	1.5	328	2.7	68.9	3.7	5.2
Lemon, Mini, Weight Watchers*	1 Cake/17g	56	0.8	333	2.4	63.3	4.9	12.1
Pink, M & S*	1 Cake/39g	160	3.3	410	2.5	81.3	8.5	0.6
CURACAO								
Average	*1 Shot/35ml*	*109*	*0.0*	*311*	*0.0*	*28.3*	*0.0*	*0.0*
CURLY WURLY								
Cadbury*	1 Bar/26g	115	4.5	442	3.5	69.2	17.3	0.8
Squirlies, Cadbury*	1 Squirl/3g	13	0.5	442	3.5	69.2	17.3	0.8
CURRANTS								
Average	*1oz/28g*	*75*	*0.1*	*267*	*2.3*	*67.8*	*0.4*	*1.9*
CURRY								
Aubergine	1oz/28g	33	2.8	118	1.4	6.2	10.1	1.5
Beef, Hot, Canned, M & S*	1 Can/425g	446	21.7	105	12.2	2.8	5.1	1.0
Beef, Sainsbury's*	1 Serving/400g	552	32.8	138	10.7	5.4	8.2	0.9
Beef, Smart Price, Asda*	1 Serving/392g	223	2.0	57	4.0	9.0	0.5	1.0
Beef, Thai, Finest, Tesco*	1 Serving/500g	770	29.0	154	9.0	16.5	5.8	1.2
Beef, with Rice, Asda*	1 Pack/406g	548	15.8	135	6.0	19.0	3.9	1.2
Beef, with Rice, Asda*	1 Pack/400g	476	10.4	119	6.0	18.0	2.6	0.9
Beef, with Rice, Birds Eye*	1 Pack/388g	524	10.9	135	6.9	20.8	2.8	0.8
Beef, with Rice, Iceland*	1 Pack/400g	404	6.8	101	6.7	14.7	1.7	1.0
Beef, with Rice, Morrisons*	1 Serving/400g	480	20.0	120	6.0	12.6	5.0	0.6
Beef, with Rice, Tesco*	1 Pack/400g	595	18.0	149	2.8	23.1	4.5	1.9
Beef, with Rice, Weight Watchers*	1 Pack/328g	249	3.3	76	4.2	12.5	1.0	0.3
Blackeye Bean, Gujerati	1oz/28g	36	1.2	127	7.2	16.1	4.4	2.8
Bombay, Butternut Squash, Veg Pot, Innocent*	1 Pot/380g	296	4.2	78	2.6	12.5	1.1	4.1
Cabbage, Average	1oz/28g	23	1.4	82	1.9	8.1	5.0	2.1
Cauliflower & Chickpea, Lovely Vegetables, M & S*	1 Serving/390g	351	13.6	90	2.9	11.2	3.5	3.7
Cauliflower & Potato	1oz/28g	17	0.7	59	3.4	6.6	2.4	1.8
Chana Dahl, Curry Special*	1 Pack/350g	434	22.7	124	6.0	10.5	6.5	5.9
Chick Pea, Whole, Average	1oz/28g	50	2.1	179	9.6	21.3	7.5	4.5
Chicken, & Rice, 267, Oakhouse Foods Ltd*	1 Meal/400g	528	16.4	132	7.0	16.9	4.1	0.9
Chicken, & Rice, International Cuisine*	1 Serving/400g	420	11.6	105	3.3	16.4	2.9	0.8
Chicken, & Vegetable, Big Eat, Heinz*	1 Pot/350g	392	18.2	112	5.4	10.9	5.2	4.3
Chicken, Asda*	1 Can/200g	210	10.0	105	10.0	5.0	5.0	0.0
Chicken, Canned, Sainsbury's*	1 Serving/100g	136	6.1	136	11.1	9.1	6.1	1.0
Chicken, Chinese with Rice, Ready Meal, Average	1 Serving/450g	490	11.5	109	7.2	14.1	2.5	1.3
Chicken, Diet Chef Ltd*	1 Portion/300g	342	13.2	114	9.1	9.5	4.4	1.0
Chicken, Green Thai, BGTY, Sainsbury's*	1 Pack/400g	316	10.4	79	10.6	3.4	2.6	1.9
Chicken, Green Thai, Birds Eye*	1 Pack/450g	535	19.8	119	4.7	15.2	4.4	0.3
Chicken, Green Thai, Breasts, Finest, Tesco*	1 Serving/200g	292	16.0	146	16.5	2.0	8.0	0.7
Chicken, Green Thai, Jasmine Rice, Weight Watchers*	1 Pack/320g	291	3.2	91	6.1	14.3	1.0	0.5
Chicken, Green Thai, Sainsbury's*	½ Pack/200g	264	13.6	132	13.0	4.8	6.8	0.9
Chicken, Green Thai Style & Sticky Rice, Asda*	1 Pack/450g	585	10.8	130	7.0	20.0	2.4	0.1
Chicken, Healthy Options, Birds Eye*	1 Pack/350g	336	3.1	96	5.1	16.8	0.9	0.5
Chicken, Hot, Can, Tesco*	1 Can/418g	514	26.3	123	9.7	6.9	6.3	0.9
Chicken, Hot, Canned, Asda*	1 Can/398g	501	23.9	126	11.0	7.0	6.0	0.5

	Measure INFO/WEIGHT	per Measure KCAL	FAT	Nutrition Values per 100g / 100ml KCAL	PROT	CARB	FAT	FIBRE
Chicken, Hot, Iceland*	1 Can/392g	492	20.4	126	9.9	9.8	5.2	0.7
Chicken, Kashmiri, Waitrose*	1 Serving/400g	640	36.4	160	14.5	5.0	9.1	0.6
Chicken, Medium Hot, M & S*	1 Serving/200g	310	14.2	155	7.8	14.3	7.1	0.8
Chicken, Mild, Asda*	½ Can/190g	239	11.4	126	11.0	7.0	6.0	0.5
Chicken, Mild, BGTY, Sainsbury's*	1 Serving/200g	184	5.2	92	10.0	7.2	2.6	0.5
Chicken, Mild, Canned, Bilash*	½ Can/200g	180	7.6	90	9.5	4.5	3.8	0.7
Chicken, Mild, Iceland*	½ Can/200g	234	9.0	117	10.6	8.5	4.5	0.7
Chicken, Mild, Sainsbury's*	1 Can/400g	472	27.6	118	10.5	3.5	6.9	1.3
Chicken, Mild, Tinned, Sainsbury's*	1 Serving/200g	214	7.0	107	12.7	6.1	3.5	1.1
Chicken, Red Thai, 97% Fat Free, Birds Eye*	1 Pack/366g	425	7.0	116	5.7	19.0	1.9	0.5
Chicken, Red Thai, Asda*	1 Pack/360g	461	27.7	128	9.1	5.5	7.7	1.0
Chicken, Red Thai, COU, M & S*	1 Pack/400g	420	9.2	105	7.1	13.4	2.3	1.4
Chicken, Red Thai, Tesco*	1 Serving/175g	215	11.5	123	10.5	5.5	6.6	1.4
Chicken, Red Thai with Fragrant Rice, Somerfield*	1 Pack/340g	503	17.0	148	8.0	18.0	5.0	0.0
Chicken, Red Thai with Jasmine Rice, Weight Watchers*	1 Pack/400g	344	3.2	86	6.5	12.9	0.8	0.8
Chicken, Red Thai with Rice, Tesco*	1 Serving/475g	746	32.3	157	7.2	16.8	6.8	1.1
Chicken, Reduced Fat, Asda*	1 Pack/400g	476	10.4	119	6.0	18.0	2.6	0.9
Chicken, Smart Price, Asda*	1 Can/392g	282	5.1	72	4.0	11.0	1.3	1.0
Chicken, with Naan Bread, Iceland*	1 Portion/260g	484	16.4	186	10.1	22.3	6.3	1.4
Chicken, with Potatoes, Diet Chef Ltd*	1 Pack/300g	291	13.2	97	7.5	6.9	4.4	2.8
Chicken, with Rice, Average	1 Serving/400g	465	11.0	116	5.1	17.8	2.7	0.8
Chicken, with Rice, Birds Eye*	1 Pack/400g	468	11.2	117	4.5	18.4	2.8	0.6
Chicken, with Rice, Dunnes Stores*	1 Pack/375g	400	6.3	107	4.2	20.2	1.7	0.8
Chicken, with Rice, Fresh, Co-Op*	1 Pack/300g	270	9.0	90	3.0	13.0	3.0	1.0
Chicken, with Rice, Frozen, Tesco*	1 Pack/400g	488	15.6	122	4.6	17.2	3.9	0.7
Chicken, with Rice, Fruity, HL, Tesco*	1 Pack/450g	495	5.4	110	6.5	18.2	1.2	1.2
Chicken, with Rice, Malaysian, Bernard Matthews*	1 Pack/400g	512	15.6	128	6.1	17.0	3.9	0.0
Chicken, with Rice, Ready Meal, Average	1 Serving/450g	502	11.8	112	5.2	16.8	2.6	1.0
Chicken, with Rice, Ross*	1 Serving/320g	275	3.8	86	3.7	14.8	1.2	0.5
Chicken, with White Rice, Weight Watchers*	1 Pack/320g	306	4.8	96	5.3	15.4	1.5	0.1
Chicken, Yellow Thai Style, HL, Tesco*	1 Pack/450g	504	12.1	112	9.3	12.6	2.7	0.5
Chicken Biryani, Recipe Mix, Schwartz*	1 Pack/30g	75	2.4	249	14.6	58.1	8.1	28.6
Chicken Katsu, City Kitchen, Tesco*	1 Pack/385g	465	13.2	121	6.0	16.3	3.4	1.3
Chicken Korma, Diet Chef Ltd*	1 Pack/300g	324	15.0	108	11.1	4.6	5.0	0.6
Cod, Red Thai with Rice, Perfectly Balanced, Waitrose*	1 Pack/400g	360	7.2	90	7.5	11.0	1.8	1.0
Courgette & Potato	1oz/28g	24	1.5	86	1.9	8.7	5.2	1.2
Dudhi, Kofta	1oz/28g	32	2.1	113	2.6	9.4	7.4	2.8
Fish, & Vegetable, Bangladeshi, Average	1oz/28g	33	2.4	117	9.1	1.4	8.4	0.5
Fish, Bangladeshi, Average	1oz/28g	35	2.2	124	12.2	1.5	7.9	0.3
Fish, Red Thai, Waitrose*	1 Pack/500g	275	11.0	55	5.2	3.7	2.2	1.0
Gobi Aloo Sag, Retail	1oz/28g	27	1.9	95	2.2	7.1	6.9	1.4
Green Thai, & Rice, GFY, Asda*	1 Pack/400g	356	7.6	89	7.0	11.0	1.9	1.6
Green Thai, with Sticky Rice, HL, Tesco*	1 Pack/450g	517	12.1	115	7.7	14.9	2.7	0.6
Indian Daal, Tasty Veg Pot, Innocent*	1 Pot/380g	319	9.9	84	2.8	9.7	2.6	5.3
Indian Vegetable, Sainsbury's*	½ Pack/200g	206	14.6	103	2.5	6.8	7.3	4.6
King Prawn, Coconut & Lime, Sainsbury's*	½ Pack/351g	207	8.8	59	3.7	5.4	2.5	1.0
King Prawn, Goan, M & S*	1 Pack/400g	680	44.4	170	5.1	11.6	11.1	1.5
King Prawn, Malay with Rice, Sainsbury's*	1 Pack/400g	608	20.4	152	5.0	21.5	5.1	1.4
King Prawn, Red Thai, City Kitchen, Tesco*	1 Pack/385g	460	14.4	119	4.5	16.7	3.7	1.0
King Prawn Malay, Waitrose*	1 Pack/350g	364	19.2	104	6.6	7.1	5.5	0.9
Lamb, Extra Strong, M & S*	1oz/28g	35	1.9	125	11.5	4.6	6.9	0.9
Lamb, Hot, M & S*	½ Can/213g	320	19.6	150	14.9	6.0	9.2	2.3
Lamb, Kefthedes, Waitrose*	½ Pack/200g	294	17.6	147	9.0	8.0	8.8	2.1

CURRY

	Measure INFO/WEIGHT	per Measure KCAL	FAT	Nutrition Values per 100g / 100ml KCAL	PROT	CARB	FAT	FIBRE
Masala, Aubergine, TTD, Sainsbury's*	½ Pack/115g	135	11.4	117	2.9	4.1	9.9	5.8
Masala, Indian, Veg Pot, Innocent*	1 Pot/380g	331	10.3	87	2.9	11.6	2.7	3.6
Masala, with Babycorn & Asparagus, Waitrose*	½ Pack/125g	92	5.6	74	3.1	5.3	4.5	5.0
Matar Paneer, Peas & Cheese, Ashoka*	½ Pack/150g	183	10.0	122	5.3	10.0	6.7	2.0
Medium, with Rice, Rice Time, Uncle Ben's*	1 Pot/300g	396	9.0	132	2.3	23.2	3.0	1.2
Mushroom & Pea, Masala, Indian, Sainsbury's*	1 Pack/300g	264	14.7	88	3.3	5.2	4.9	5.1
Potato & Pea	1oz/28g	26	1.1	92	2.9	13.0	3.8	2.4
Prawn, Red Thai, Sainsbury's*	1 Pack/300g	546	39.6	182	6.3	9.4	13.2	1.7
Prawn, Red Thai Sauce, Youngs*	1 Pack/255g	197	8.7	77	4.8	6.5	3.4	0.8
Prawn, Thai with Jasmine Rice, BGTY, Sainsbury's*	1 Serving/401g	353	6.0	88	4.2	14.5	1.5	2.0
Prawn, with Rice, Asda*	1 Pack/400g	420	10.4	105	3.5	17.0	2.6	1.1
Prawn, with Rice, Birds Eye^	1 Pack/375g	442	0.0	118	3.5	20.6	0.0	0.0
Prawn, with Rice, Frozen, Sainsbury's*	1 Pack/400g	552	7.6	138	3.9	26.4	1.9	2.1
Prawn, with Rice, Iceland*	1 Pack/450g	468	14.4	104	3.2	16.4	3.2	1.5
Prawn, with Rice, Light & Easy, Youngs*	1 Pack/310g	248	3.4	80	3.3	14.2	1.1	0.9
Prawn, with Rice, Morrisons*	1 Serving/400g	484	9.2	121	3.2	21.9	2.3	0.9
Prawn & Mushroom	1oz/28g	47	4.0	168	7.3	2.5	14.4	1.0
Red Kidney Bean, Punjabi	1oz/28g	30	1.6	106	4.7	10.1	5.6	3.8
Red Thai, Vegetarian, Tesco*	1 Pack/429ml	588	21.9	137	5.4	17.3	5.1	1.6
Red Thai, with Rice, Finest, Tesco*	1 Pack/500g	660	15.5	132	8.0	17.8	3.1	0.6
Salmon, Green, Waitrose*	1 Pack/401g	581	40.5	145	9.1	4.5	10.1	2.7
Spicy Paneer, Lovely Vegetables, M & S*	1 Pot/300g	330	12.0	110	4.3	11.9	4.0	4.0
Vegetable, Asda*	1 Pack/350g	329	21.0	94	1.9	8.0	6.0	1.9
Vegetable, Budgens*	1 Pack/350g	248	14.0	71	1.8	6.9	4.0	2.2
Vegetable, Canned, Sainsbury's*	½ Can/200g	200	12.2	100	1.4	9.8	6.1	1.8
Vegetable, Canned, Savers, Morrisons*	1 Can/400g	208	1.2	52	2.2	9.3	0.3	1.9
Vegetable, Diet Chef Ltd*	1 Pack/300g	153	3.6	51	2.0	8.0	1.2	2.1
Vegetable, Frozen, Mixed Vegetables, Average	1oz/28g	25	1.7	88	2.5	6.9	6.1	0.0
Vegetable, Indian, Canned, Tesco*	1 Can/400g	320	18.0	80	2.0	6.7	4.5	1.1
Vegetable, Indian, Tesco*	1 Serving/225g	257	17.8	114	2.1	8.6	7.9	1.6
Vegetable, Indian Meal for One, Tesco*	1 Serving/200g	218	14.4	109	2.0	9.0	7.2	1.2
Vegetable, Light Choices, Tesco*	1 Pack/350g	350	4.2	100	2.3	19.4	1.2	1.5
Vegetable, Medium, Tesco*	1 Pack/350g	325	21.7	93	2.3	7.1	6.2	1.9
Vegetable, Mild, Tesco*	1 Can/425g	314	10.6	74	2.1	10.7	2.5	1.7
Vegetable, Mixed, Organic, Pure & Pronto*	1 Pack/400g	368	11.6	92	4.2	12.4	2.9	4.8
Vegetable, Pakistani, Average	1oz/28g	17	0.7	60	2.2	8.7	2.6	2.2
Vegetable, Sabzi Tarkari, Patak's*	1 Pack/400g	500	31.2	125	2.5	11.1	7.8	2.2
Vegetable, Smart Price, Asda*	½ Can/203g	132	1.0	65	2.0	13.0	0.5	1.7
Vegetable, Solo Slim, Rosemary Conley*	1 Pack/300g	153	3.6	51	2.0	8.0	1.2	2.1
Vegetable, Takeaway, Average	1 Serving/330g	346	24.4	105	2.5	7.6	7.4	0.0
Vegetable, Tinned, Asda*	½ Can/200g	206	12.0	103	2.2	10.0	6.0	2.5
Vegetable, Way to Five, Sainsbury's*	½ Pack/344g	227	3.8	66	2.5	11.6	1.1	1.4
Vegetable, with Pilau Rice, Linda McCartney*	1 Pack/339g	224	2.0	66	1.6	13.5	0.6	0.5
Vegetable, with Pilau Rice, Weight Watchers*	1 Pack/400g	296	3.2	74	1.6	15.1	0.8	1.9
Vegetable, with Rice, Asda*	1 Pack/393g	432	12.2	110	2.6	18.0	3.1	1.4
Vegetable, with Rice, Birds Eye*	1 Pack/414g	455	9.5	110	2.3	19.6	2.3	1.1
Vegetable, with Rice, Co-Op*	1 Pack/340g	289	3.4	85	2.0	17.0	1.0	0.7
Vegetable, with Rice, Healthy Range, Average	1 Serving/400g	351	4.6	88	2.3	16.8	1.1	1.9
Vegetable, with Rice, Ready Meal, Average	1 Serving/330g	337	9.9	102	3.3	16.4	3.0	0.0
Vegetable, with Rice, Tesco*	1 Pack/400g	440	12.0	110	2.1	18.7	3.0	1.0
Vegetable, with Yoghurt, Average	1oz/28g	17	1.1	62	2.6	4.6	4.1	1.4
Vegetable, Yellow, Tocco*	1 Pack/356g	324	17.4	91	1.9	9.9	4.9	1.4
Vegetable, Yellow Thai, Sainsbury's*	1 Pack/400g	624	48.8	156	2.2	9.4	12.2	1.1

C

CURRY	Measure INFO/WEIGHT	per Measure KCAL	FAT	Nutrition Values per 100g / 100ml KCAL	PROT	CARB	FAT	FIBRE
CURRY								
Vegetable Masala, Light Choices, Tesco*	1 Pack/350g	297	5.9	85	3.8	13.6	1.7	3.4
CURRY LEAVES								
Fresh	*1oz/28g*	*27*	*0.4*	*97*	*7.9*	*13.3*	*1.3*	*0.0*
CURRY PASTE								
Balti, Asda*	1 Tube/100g	164	9.8	164	4.2	11.6	9.8	6.3
Balti, Sharwood's*	¼ Pack/73g	328	28.7	453	5.0	19.2	39.6	3.1
Balti, Tomato & Coriander, Original, Patak's*	1 Tbsp/15g	58	5.1	388	4.0	14.6	34.0	3.7
Bhuna, Tomato & Tamarind, Patak's*	1 Serving/10g	40	5.6	397	4.3	17.5	56.2	6.3
Garam Masala, Cinnamon & Ginger, Hot, Patak's*	1 Serving/30g	121	10.6	403	3.2	17.9	35.4	0.6
Green Thai, Average	1 Tsp/5g	6	0.4	128	2.1	11.7	7.9	3.1
Hot, Sharwood's*	1oz/28g	123	10.7	439	5.1	18.6	38.3	2.6
Jalfrezi, Patak's*	1 Serving/30g	96	8.1	320	3.7	14.2	26.9	5.6
Korma, Asda*	1 Tube/100g	338	23.5	338	5.1	26.6	23.5	1.2
Korma, Coconut & Coriander, Original, Patak's*	1 Serving/30g	124	11.7	415	3.5	11.6	39.0	5.2
Madras, Cumin & Chilli, Hot, Patak's*	¼ Jar/70g	202	18.1	289	4.7	7.6	25.9	10.8
Medium, Asda*	1 Tsp/5ml/5g	18	1.6	364	5.0	14.0	32.0	5.0
Medium, Barts Spices*	1 Serving/30g	88	6.4	295	4.5	19.2	21.5	5.5
Medium, M & S*	1oz/28g	64	5.5	230	2.5	10.7	19.5	4.9
Medium, Sharwood's*	1oz/28g	122	10.9	434	4.5	16.8	38.8	2.7
Mild, Asda*	¼ Jar/46g	206	18.9	448	3.8	16.0	41.0	7.0
Mild, Coriander & Cumin, Original, Patak's*	1 Serving/35g	99	8.6	283	4.8	9.1	24.6	10.7
Mild, Sharwood's*	1oz/28g	78	6.0	279	3.6	17.7	21.5	3.4
Red, Thai, Average	1 Tsp/5g	7	0.5	132	2.3	9.5	9.1	3.0
Rogan Josh, Tomato & Paprika, Patak's*	1 Serving/30g	119	11.0	397	4.1	12.7	36.7	5.9
Tamarind & Ginger, Original, Patak's*	1 Tbsp/15g	20	0.3	133	3.4	23.1	2.0	2.9
Tandoori, Sharwood's*	1oz/28g	64	4.4	228	5.9	15.5	15.8	1.9
Tandoori, Tamarind & Ginger, Patak's*	1 Serving/30g	33	0.5	110	3.1	20.4	1.8	2.6
Tikka, Asda*	½ Tube/50g	117	8.5	235	4.5	16.1	17.0	1.6
Tikka Masala, Coriander & Lemon, Medium, Patak's*	1 Serving/30g	111	9.5	369	3.8	16.9	31.8	2.9
Tikka Masala, Sharwood's*	1oz/28g	53	4.3	191	3.2	9.9	15.4	2.6
Tom Yum, Thai Taste*	1 Tsp/13g	35	2.0	269	5.4	30.8	15.4	7.7
CURRY POWDER								
Average	*1 Tsp/2g*	*6*	*0.3*	*325*	*12.7*	*41.8*	*13.8*	*0.0*
CURRY SAUCE								
Asda*	1 Tbsp/15g	62	2.1	414	13.0	59.0	14.0	1.3
Balti, Asda*	¼ Jar/125g	155	12.5	124	1.6	7.0	10.0	1.7
Balti, Loyd Grossman*	½ Jar/175g	173	11.7	99	1.3	8.4	6.7	1.7
Basics, Sainsbury's*	¼ Jar/110g	70	2.7	64	0.7	9.7	2.5	0.9
Chinese Style, Cooking, Asda*	1 Jar/560g	465	24.1	83	1.5	9.6	4.3	1.7
Dopiaza, Finest, Tesco*	1 Jar/350g	234	10.5	67	1.3	8.5	3.0	3.7
Green Curry, Thai, Stir Fry, Blue Dragon*	1 Sachet/120g	74	4.8	62	0.9	5.7	4.0	0.5
Green Thai, Asda*	1 Jar/340g	309	27.2	91	0.5	4.3	8.0	0.2
Green Thai, Express, Uncle Ben's*	1 Pack/170g	131	9.9	77	1.1	5.4	5.8	0.0
Jalfrezi, Loyd Grossman*	½ Jar/213g	270	20.2	127	2.1	8.2	9.5	1.2
Jalfrezi, Piri Piri, Finest, Tesco*	1 Serving/175g	145	10.8	83	1.2	5.7	6.2	1.5
Jalfrezi, Tesco*	1 Jar/500g	450	32.5	90	1.3	6.6	6.5	2.4
Korma, Loyd Grossman*	½ Jar/175g	259	17.1	145	2.3	12.3	9.6	1.7
Korma, Uncle Ben's*	1 Jar/500g	630	42.0	126	1.4	11.1	8.4	0.0
Madras, Aldi*	1 Serving/113g	68	2.3	60	1.5	9.0	2.0	0.0
Madras, Cooking, Asda*	¼ Jar/142g	109	6.2	77	1.3	8.0	4.4	1.0
Madras, Cooking, Sharwood's*	1 Tsp/2g	2	0.1	86	1.5	6.9	5.8	1.3
Madras, Cooking, Tesco*	1/3 Jar/161g	145	9.2	90	1.9	6.9	5.7	2.5
Madras, Cumin & Chilli, Original, in Glass Jar, Patak's*	1 Jar/540g	648	38.3	120	2.1	11.9	7.1	1.8

	Measure INFO/WEIGHT	per Measure		Nutrition Values per 100g / 100ml				
		KCAL	FAT	KCAL	PROT	CARB	FAT	FIBRE
CURRY SAUCE								
Madras, Curry, Somerfield*	1 Serving/110g	106	6.7	96	1.7	8.3	6.1	0.7
Madras, Indian, Sharwood's*	1 Jar/420g	433	26.5	103	1.8	9.7	6.3	1.9
Madras, Sharwood's*	1 Jar/420g	521	38.2	124	1.7	8.9	9.1	1.4
Madras, Tesco*	½ Jar/200g	168	13.0	84	1.1	5.2	6.5	1.3
Makhani, Sharwood's*	1 Jar/420g	399	29.0	95	0.9	7.2	6.9	0.4
Malaysian Rendang, Loyd Grossman*	1 Serving/100g	143	10.1	143	2.6	10.4	10.1	1.4
Masala, Red Pepper & Mango, Sainsbury's*	½ Jar/175g	142	8.6	81	1.4	7.8	4.9	1.1
Medium, Uncle Ben's*	1 Jar/500g	330	10.0	66	0.9	10.9	2.0	0.0
Moglai Pasanda, Asda*	½ Jar/170g	277	21.0	163	2.9	10.0	12.3	1.1
Oven Bake Biryani, Medium & Aromatic, Patak's*	½ Jar/175g	135	9.3	77	1.1	6.1	5.3	1.7
Red Curry, Thai, Stir Fry, Blue Dragon*	1 Sachet/120g	112	9.6	93	0.9	4.4	8.0	0.5
Rogan Josh, Loyd Grossman*	1 Serving/106g	206	16.7	194	2.4	10.5	15.8	1.5
Rogan Josh, Worldwide Sauces*	1 Jar/500g	255	1.5	51	1.1	11.0	0.3	0.0
Smart Price, Asda*	¼ Jar/110g	73	2.0	66	1.4	11.0	1.8	0.6
Sri Lankan Devil Curry, Sharwood's*	1 Jar/380g	220	11.4	58	0.5	7.2	3.0	2.1
Tikka, Cooking, Tesco*	1 Std Jar/500g	617	42.1	123	1.7	10.1	8.4	2.0
Tikka Masala, Cooking, HL, Tesco*	¼ Jar/125g	94	3.7	75	2.6	8.2	3.0	1.2
Tikka Masala, COU, M & S*	½ Pack/100g	80	2.6	80	4.5	9.9	2.6	1.7
Tikka Masala, Loyd Grossman*	½ Jar/213g	438	34.4	206	2.6	12.5	16.2	1.0
Vindaloo, Cooking, Chosen By You, Asda*	½ Jar/160g	128	5.4	80	1.5	10.4	3.4	1.0
Vindaloo, Hot, Patak's*	1 Jar/540g	643	46.4	119	1.7	8.5	8.6	2.1
CUSTARD								
Banana Flavour, Ambrosia*	1 Sm Pot/135g	139	3.9	103	2.9	16.1	2.9	0.0
Banana Flavour, Pot, Average	1 Pot/135g	138	3.9	102	2.9	16.0	2.9	0.0
Chocolate, COU, M & S*	1 Pot/140g	147	3.1	105	3.1	18.6	2.2	1.0
Chocolate Flavour, Ambrosia*	1 Pot/150g	177	4.3	118	3.0	20.0	2.9	0.7
Chocolate Flavour, Pot, Average	1 Pot/125g	138	3.4	111	3.1	18.2	2.7	0.6
Dairy Free, Sainsbury's*	1 Serving/250g	210	4.2	84	3.0	14.2	1.7	0.2
Low Fat, Average	*1/3 Pot/141g*	*116*	*1.6*	*82*	*2.9*	*15.0*	*1.2*	*0.0*
Powder	*1 Tsp/5g*	*18*	*0.0*	*354*	*0.6*	*92.0*	*0.7*	*0.1*
Ready to Eat, Chocolate, Tesco*	1 Pot/150g	150	3.4	100	3.2	16.2	2.3	0.3
Ready to Serve, Average	*1 Serving/50g*	*59*	*2.3*	*118*	*3.3*	*16.1*	*4.6*	*0.2*
Ready to Serve, Tinned, Value, Tesco*	1 Serving/99g	75	0.7	76	3.1	14.4	0.7	0.0
Strawberry Flavour, Pot, Average	1 Pot/125g	130	3.3	104	2.7	17.3	2.7	0.0
Strawberry Flavoured, Ambrosia*	1 Serving/135g	139	3.8	103	2.8	16.7	2.8	0.0
Strawberry Style, Shapers, Boots*	1 Pot/148g	83	1.2	56	4.0	8.2	0.8	0.1
Summer, Ambrosia*	1 Pack/500g	490	15.0	98	2.7	15.0	3.0	0.0
Toffee Flavour, Ambrosia*	1 Pot/150g	156	4.2	104	2.8	17.0	2.8	0.0
Vanilla, COU, M & S*	1 Pot/140g	147	3.5	105	4.3	16.6	2.5	0.6
Vanilla, Fresh, Waitrose*	1 Serving/100g	214	15.3	214	3.2	15.8	15.3	1.1
Vanilla, TTD, Sainsbury's*	1 Pot/150g	312	23.2	208	2.5	14.7	15.5	0.1
Vanilla Flavour, Pot, Average	1 Pot/125g	127	3.5	102	2.8	16.4	2.8	0.0
Vanilla with Apple Crunch, Ambrosia*	1 Pack/193g	276	8.7	143	3.4	22.4	4.5	0.8
CUSTARD APPLE								
Cherimoya, Weighed without Skin & Seeds, Average	1 Apple/312g	234	2.1	75	1.6	17.7	0.7	3.0
CUTLETS								
Nut, Goodlife*	1 Cutlet/88g	283	19.4	322	9.1	21.8	22.0	3.4
Nut, Meat Free, Tesco*	1 Cutlet/70g	235	16.4	330	8.0	22.7	23.0	3.8
Nut, Retail, Fried in Vegetable Oil, Average	1 Cutlet/90g	260	20.1	289	4.8	18.7	22.3	1.7
Nut, Retail, Grilled, Average	1 Cutlet/90g	191	11.7	212	5.1	19.9	13.0	1.8
Vegetable & Nut, Asda*	1 Cutlet/88g	296	20.3	335	10.0	22.0	23.0	4.6
CUTTLEFISH								
Raw	*1oz/28g*	*20*	*0.2*	*71*	*16.1*	*0.0*	*0.7*	*0.0*

	Measure INFO/WEIGHT	per Measure KCAL	FAT	Nutrition Values per 100g / 100ml KCAL	PROT	CARB	FAT	FIBRE
DAB								
Fillets, Lightly Dusted, M & S*	1 Fillet/112g	190	9.7	170	12.8	9.7	8.7	0.5
Raw	*1oz/28g*	*21*	*0.3*	*74*	*15.7*	*0.0*	*1.2*	*0.0*
DAIRYLEA DUNKERS								
Baked Crisps, Dairylea, Kraft*	1 Pack/45g	101	4.0	225	9.2	26.0	9.0	1.1
Jumbo Munch, Dairylea, Kraft*	1 Serving/50g	150	9.2	300	7.2	26.5	18.5	1.2
Salt & Vinegar, Dairylea, Kraft*	1 Tub/42g	115	8.2	275	6.7	17.5	19.5	0.3
with Jumbo Tubes, Kraft*	1 Pack/43g	108	5.1	255	9.1	27.0	12.0	0.9
with Ritz Crackers, Dairylea, Kraft*	1 Tub/46g	122	6.4	265	9.6	25.0	13.9	0.6
DAIRYLEA LUNCHABLES								
Ham & Cheese Pizza, Dairylea, Kraft*	1 Pack/97g	247	10.7	255	11.5	26.0	11.0	1.6
Harvest Ham, Dairylea, Kraft*	1 Pack/110g	313	18.7	285	16.5	16.5	17.0	0.3
Tasty Chicken, Dairylea, Kraft*	1 Pack/110g	313	18.1	285	17.0	17.5	16.5	0.3
DAMSONS								
Raw, Weighed with Stones, Average	*1oz/28g*	*10*	*0.0*	*34*	*0.5*	*8.6*	*0.0*	*1.6*
Raw, Weighed without Stones, Average	*1oz/28g*	*11*	*0.0*	*38*	*0.5*	*9.6*	*0.0*	*1.8*
DANDELION & BURDOCK								
Fermented, Botanical, Fentiman's*	1 Bottle/275ml	130	0.0	47	0.0	11.6	0.0	0.0
Original, Ben Shaws*	1 Can/440ml	128	0.0	29	0.0	7.0	0.0	0.0
Sparkling, Diet, Morrisons*	1 Glass/200ml	2	0.0	1	0.0	0.3	0.0	0.0
DANISH PASTRY								
Apple, Fresh Cream, Sainsbury's*	1 Pastry/67g	248	14.6	368	3.1	40.2	21.6	0.4
Apple & Cinnamon, Danish Twist, Entenmann's*	1 Serving/52g	150	1.0	288	5.6	62.0	1.9	1.5
Average	1 Pastry/110g	411	19.4	374	5.8	51.3	17.6	1.6
Cherry, Bar, Sainsbury's*	¼ Bar/88g	220	10.0	252	4.2	33.2	11.4	1.7
Cherry & Custard, Bar, Tesco*	1 Bar/350g	910	49.0	260	3.5	29.9	14.0	7.7
Custard, Bar, Sara Lee*	¼ Bar/100g	228	6.4	228	6.6	36.1	6.4	0.8
Fruit Filled, Average	1 Pastry/94g	335	15.9	356	5.1	47.9	16.9	0.0
Pecan, M & S*	1 Serving/67g	287	17.4	428	6.2	45.0	26.0	1.3
Toasted Pecan, Danish Twist, Entenmann's*	1 Slice/48g	171	7.6	351	7.0	47.2	15.6	1.4
DATES								
Bite Size, Snack Pack, Whitworths*	1 Pack/35g	119	0.6	340	2.0	74.7	1.8	8.2
Deglet Nour, Graze*	1 Pack/60g	181	0.3	301	2.1	72.0	0.5	0.0
Deglet Nour, Love Life, Waitrose*	1 Portion/50g	143	0.1	287	3.3	68.0	0.2	8.0
Dried, Average	*1 Date/20g*	*54*	*0.1*	*272*	*2.8*	*65.4*	*0.4*	*4.2*
Dried, Medjool, Average	*1 Date/20g*	*56*	*0.1*	*279*	*2.2*	*69.3*	*0.3*	*4.3*
Fresh, Raw, Yellow, Average	*1 Date/20g*	*23*	*0.0*	*115*	*1.4*	*29.1*	*0.1*	*1.6*
Hadrawi, Love Life, Waitrose*	5 Dates/50g	144	0.1	288	3.4	68.0	0.2	8.0
Halawi, Tesco*	6 Dates/60g	165	0.1	275	2.3	65.5	0.2	4.3
Medjool, Love Life, Waitrose*	1 Date/20g	58	0.0	291	3.3	68.0	0.2	6.7
Medjool, Stuffed with Walnuts, Tesco*	2 Dates/40g	98	2.3	245	4.4	44.0	5.7	3.4
Medjool, TTD, Sainsbury's*	1 Serving/50g	148	0.0	296	1.9	72.0	0.1	6.7
Milk Chocolate Coated, Julian Graves*	1 Pack/200g	768	22.6	384	4.5	66.0	11.3	2.6
Organic, Medjool, Pitted, Love Life, Waitrose*	1 Date/18g	52	0.0	292	3.3	68.0	0.2	6.7
Soft, Whitworths*	1 Serving/25g	85	0.4	340	2.0	74.7	1.8	8.2
Stoned, Wholefoods, Tesco*	1 Pack/500g	1600	13.0	320	4.4	69.2	2.6	8.4
DELIGHT								
Butterscotch Flavour, No Added Sugar, Tesco*	1 Pack/49g	225	10.0	460	4.8	63.3	20.5	0.0
Chocolate Flavour, Dry, Tesco*	1 Pack/49g	220	9.0	450	6.2	64.2	18.4	2.3
Ravishing Raspberry, Made Up, Asda*	1/3 Pack/100g	112	3.9	112	3.2	16.0	3.9	0.0
Strawberry, No Added Sugar, Dry, Tesco*	1 Pack/49g	51	1.8	105	3.4	13.7	3.7	0.1
Strawberry, Shapers, Boots*	1 Pot/122g	96	1.2	79	4.5	13.0	1.0	0.1
Vanilla, No Added Sugar, Dry, Tesco*	1 Pack/49g	51	1.8	105	3.4	13.7	3.7	0.1

DESSERT

	Measure INFO/WEIGHT	per Measure KCAL	FAT	Nutrition Values per 100g / 100ml KCAL	PROT	CARB	FAT	FIBRE
After Dark, Black Forest, Gateaux, Gu*	1 Pot/85g	258	18.5	303	3.0	24.7	21.8	1.3
Almond, Naturgreen*	1 Serving/130g	143	6.2	110	2.3	14.5	4.8	0.2
Apple Crumble, Sainsbury's*	1 Pot/136g	291	10.5	214	3.2	33.0	7.7	2.7
Baked Lemon, COU, M & S*	1 Serving/100g	140	2.5	140	6.8	22.0	2.5	0.8
Banana Split	1 Serving/175g	368	25.5	210	2.2	18.0	14.6	0.1
Banoffee, Sainsbury's*	1 Pot/140g	360	19.1	257	2.7	30.9	13.6	1.3
Banoffee, Shape, Danone*	1 Pot/120g	175	2.8	146	3.3	28.0	2.3	0.5
Banoffee, Weight Watchers*	1 Dessert/81g	170	3.6	210	4.9	37.7	4.4	1.4
Banoffee Layered, Sainsbury's*	1 Pot/115g	270	14.7	235	2.2	27.8	12.8	1.0
Black Cherry, Dragana, Waitrose*	1 Pot/125g	236	11.4	189	2.1	24.7	9.1	0.5
Black Cherry & Chocolate, COU, M & S*	1 Pack/115g	132	1.6	115	3.6	22.6	1.4	1.2
Black Forest, Light Choices, Tesco*	1 Pot/145g	188	2.3	130	3.2	25.8	1.6	0.9
Black Forest, Tesco*	1 Pot/100g	287	14.4	287	3.5	35.8	14.4	2.4
Bounty, Mars*	1 Pot/110g	253	15.0	230	5.3	23.2	13.6	0.0
Butterscotch Flavour Whip, Co-Op*	1 Pack/64g	241	0.1	377	0.6	93.4	0.1	0.0
Buttons, Milk Chocolate, Cadbury*	1 Pot/100g	280	14.9	280	6.2	30.8	14.9	0.0
Caramel, Delights, Shape, Danone*	1 Pot/110g	109	2.5	99	3.3	16.3	2.3	0.1
Caramel Crunch, Weight Watchers*	1 Serving/89g	174	2.6	196	4.6	37.9	2.9	1.7
Caramel Flavour, Soya, Dairy Free, Organic, Provamel*	1 Pot/125g	125	2.2	100	3.0	17.8	1.8	0.5
Caramel Shortcake, Luxury, Weight Watchers*	1 Pot/100ml	103	3.5	103	1.9	17.9	3.5	0.8
Cheeky & Saucy Little Pots Au Chocolat, Gu*	1 Pot/45g	199	16.6	443	3.3	24.1	36.9	2.3
Chocolate, Campina*	1 Pot/125g	186	8.6	149	3.2	18.5	6.9	0.0
Chocolate, Custardz, Chosen By You, Asda*	1 Pot/90g	97	2.0	108	3.2	18.8	2.2	0.0
Chocolate, Delights, Shape, Danone*	1 Pot/110g	109	2.4	99	3.3	16.3	2.2	0.6
Chocolate, HL, Tesco*	1 Pot/95g	87	2.2	92	3.7	14.1	2.3	1.1
Chocolate, M & S*	1 Serving/120g	168	2.5	140	5.6	26.4	2.1	1.1
Chocolate, Triple Delight, Weight Watchers*	1 Dessert/110g	183	2.9	166	4.9	30.8	2.6	2.6
Chocolate, Value, Tesco*	1 Pot/115g	112	3.0	97	2.8	15.7	2.6	0.0
Chocolate, Weight Watchers*	1 Serving/82g	145	2.5	177	5.2	32.3	3.0	2.9
Chocolate & Coconut, COU, M & S*	1 Pot/125g	169	2.7	135	3.6	25.6	2.2	0.7
Chocolate Banoffee, Gu*	1 Pot/85g	325	21.5	382	3.9	35.0	25.3	1.0
Chocolate Brownie, M & S*	¼ Pack/144g	610	39.5	425	4.7	39.6	27.5	1.0
Chocolate Buttons, Cadbury*	1 Pack/100g	275	14.5	275	5.0	30.5	14.5	0.0
Chocolate Desire, Magnum, Wall's Ice Cream*	1 Dessert/85g	374	24.0	440	5.3	40.0	28.2	0.0
Chocolate Dream, Co-Op*	1 Pot/110g	184	7.7	167	4.1	22.0	7.0	0.0
Chocolate Duetto, Weight Watchers*	1 Pot/85g	99	2.4	117	4.4	18.4	2.8	0.0
Chocolate Flavour, Soya, Dairy Free, Organic, Provamel*	1 Pot/125g	111	3.0	89	3.0	13.6	2.4	1.0
Chocolate Fudge Brownie, Tesco*	1 Pot/125g	374	16.6	299	4.6	40.2	13.3	1.3
Chocolate Honeycomb Crisp, COU, M & S*	1 Serving/71g	110	2.1	155	4.6	27.6	2.9	1.0
Chocolate Marshmallow, Weight Watchers*	1 Serving/50g	97	2.3	194	3.2	34.5	4.7	1.3
Chocolate Mint Torte, Weight Watchers*	1 Dessert/88g	174	4.1	198	4.7	34.3	4.7	5.2
Chocolate Mocha, BGTY, Sainsbury's*	1 Pot/100g	115	2.6	115	3.8	19.2	2.6	2.8
Chocolate Mousse Cake, Weight Watchers*	1 Dessert/75g	148	2.2	198	5.9	37.1	2.9	1.0
Chocolate Muffin, COU, M & S*	1 Pot/110g	154	2.7	140	6.1	26.1	2.5	1.5
Chocolate Muffin, Light Choices, Tesco*	1 Pot/108g	140	2.4	130	4.3	22.6	2.2	1.3
Chocolate Toffee, Weight Watchers*	1 Dessert/89g	177	4.0	197	4.3	34.9	4.5	2.2
Chocolate Top, Weight Watchers*	1 Pot/75g	162	7.4	216	4.2	29.3	9.9	2.8
Creme Caramel, Sainsbury's*	1 Pot/100g	116	1.6	116	2.6	22.9	1.6	0.0
Crunchie, Dairy Milk, Cadbury*	1 Pot/100g	260	12.2	260	4.4	33.4	12.2	0.0
Fruit & Nut, Cadbury*	1 Pot/100g	285	12.5	285	6.4	36.3	12.5	0.0
Fudge, Cadbury*	1 Pot/90g	216	11.2	240	4.1	28.5	12.4	0.0
Galaxy, Mars*	1 Pot/75g	166	9.2	221	4.9	22.7	12.3	0.0
Jaffa Cake, COU, M & S*	1 Serving/120g	138	3.1	115	2.4	20.1	2.6	1.0

D

	Measure INFO/WEIGHT	per Measure KCAL	FAT	Nutrition Values per 100g / 100ml KCAL	PROT	CARB	FAT	FIBRE
DESSERT								
Key Lime Pie	1 Serving/125g	431	25.0	344	4.1	37.9	20.0	1.4
Lemon & Sultana Sponge, COU, M & S*	1 Pot/130g	169	1.6	130	2.8	26.5	1.2	0.5
Lemon Meringue, Weight Watchers*	1 Pot/85g	161	0.4	189	2.4	43.1	0.5	0.6
Lemon Mousse Cake, Weight Watchers*	1 Serving/90g	130	2.4	144	3.2	26.7	2.7	0.5
Lemoncello, Italian, Co-Op*	1 Pot/90g	265	14.4	295	3.0	34.0	16.0	0.1
Maple & Pecan, American Style, Sainsbury's*	1 Pot/110g	287	15.6	261	2.6	30.6	14.2	1.2
Mars, Mars*	1 Pot/110g	214	7.4	195	6.0	28.2	6.7	0.7
Millionaire's Shortbread, M & S*	1 Dessert/120g	425	25.7	355	2.6	38.3	21.5	1.4
Mississippi Mud Pie	1 Serving/125g	480	32.0	384	5.3	33.1	25.6	1.8
Peach & Raspberry, COU, M & S*	1 Pot/90g	135	1.4	150	2.6	30.5	1.6	1.0
Pineapple & Passionfruit, M & S*	1 Pot/100g	130	3.8	130	0.8	21.7	3.8	0.3
Raspberry, Frappe, Skinny, COU, M & S*	1 Pot/95g	109	1.3	115	3.1	22.0	1.4	0.5
Raspberry & Blackcurrant, Afternoon, Mini Pots, Fru, Gu*	1 Pot/50g	145	11.1	290	1.2	22.5	22.2	0.6
Raspberry Royale, Finest, Tesco*	½ Pack/170g	314	15.8	185	1.7	22.8	9.3	1.4
Raspberry with Light Lemon Sponge, Weight Watchers*	1 Dessert/85g	152	3.7	178	4.1	30.4	4.4	2.8
Rocky Road, Sainsbury's*	1 Pot/110g	328	21.6	298	3.6	26.8	19.6	2.1
Rolo, Nestle*	1 Pot/77g	187	9.5	243	3.1	30.0	12.3	0.5
Strawberry, HL, Tesco*	1 Pot/122g	94	2.3	77	2.7	12.3	1.9	1.1
Strawberry, Value, Tesco*	1 Pot/115g	113	2.6	98	2.4	16.9	2.3	0.0
Strawberry & Rhubarb, COU, M & S*	1 Pot/110g	104	0.8	95	1.5	20.1	0.7	0.9
Strawberry Meringue, Iced, Luxury, Weight Watchers*	1 Pot/100ml	86	0.7	162	2.4	34.2	1.4	1.0
Strawberry Mousse Cake, Weight Watchers*	1 Serving/90g	124	2.4	138	3.0	25.5	2.7	0.5
Summer Berry, HL, Tesco*	1 Pot/93g	120	2.1	130	2.8	24.5	2.3	1.5
Summer Fruits, COU, M & S*	1 Serving/105g	110	1.2	105	2.1	21.6	1.1	1.2
Summer Fruits, Marbled Cream, Waitrose*	1 Serving/125g	214	11.4	171	2.1	20.2	9.1	1.1
Tiramisu	1 Serving/150g	420	20.8	280	4.4	34.0	13.9	0.8
Toffee & Vanilla, Weight Watchers*	1 Pot/67g	107	0.5	159	3.1	34.8	0.8	3.9
Toffee Chocolate, Weight Watchers*	1 Pot/100g	197	4.5	197	4.3	34.9	4.5	2.2
Toffee Flavour Custard, Ambrosia*	1 Pack/135g	139	3.9	103	2.7	16.4	2.9	0.1
Toffee with Biscuit Pieces, Iced, Weight Watchers*	1 Pot/57g	93	2.7	163	2.7	26.2	4.8	0.2
Toffee with Biscuit Pieces, Weight Watchers*	1 Pot/57g	93	2.7	163	2.7	26.2	4.8	0.2
Trifle, Chocolate, Light, Cadbury*	1 Pot/93g	130	4.0	140	4.6	20.4	4.3	0.0
Vanilla & Caramel, Little Desserts, Petits Filous, Yoplait*	1 Pot/50g	75	2.6	150	4.7	21.0	5.3	0.2
Vanilla & Chocolate Twist, Desira, Aldi*	1 Pack/150g	182	7.2	121	0.0	15.0	4.8	0.0
Vanilla & Strawberry Compote, Weight Watchers*	1 Pot/57g	81	2.2	142	2.5	23.4	3.9	0.2
Vanilla & Toffee, Heavenly Swirls, Tesco*	1 Pot/73g	106	1.8	145	2.5	28.1	2.5	0.5
Vanilla Creamed Rice, Weight Watchers*	1 Pot/130g	112	0.6	86	3.2	16.9	0.5	0.4
Vanilla Flavour, Soya, Dairy Free, Organic, Provamel*	1 Pot/125g	105	2.2	84	3.2	13.4	1.8	0.5
Vanilla Supreme, Sainsbury's*	1 Pot/95g	116	3.8	122	3.0	18.0	4.0	0.0
Vanilla with Strawberries Swirl, Weight Watchers*	1 Pot/57g	46	1.3	81	1.5	13.3	2.2	0.2
White Chocolate & Raspberry, Tesco*	1 Dessert/88g	180	8.9	204	3.4	25.0	10.1	3.1
Zabaglione	1 Serving/100g	278	18.3	278	3.6	24.3	18.3	2.3
DHAL								
Black Gram, Average	1oz/28g	21	1.0	74	4.2	7.0	3.4	1.7
Blackeye Bean, Patak's*	1oz/28g	29	1.3	102	3.6	12.4	4.6	1.8
Chick Pea	1oz/28g	42	1.7	149	7.4	17.7	6.1	3.8
Chickpea, Canned, Sainsbury's*	½ Can/432g	933	39.3	216	10.8	22.7	9.1	7.1
Chickpea, Mazadar*	1 Can/400g	360	11.2	90	4.5	11.6	2.8	4.5
Lentil, Patak's*	1 Can/283g	156	2.8	55	2.8	9.3	1.0	1.0
Lentil, Red, Way to Five, Sainsbury's*	½ Pack/273g	254	4.1	93	5.5	14.4	1.5	1.4
Lentil, Red Masoor, Punjabi, Average	1oz/28g	39	1.3	139	7.2	19.2	4.6	2.0
Lentil, Red Masoor & Tomato with Butter, Average	1oz/28g	26	1.4	94	4.0	9.7	4.9	0.9
Lentil, Red Masoor & Vegetable, Average	1oz/28g	31	1.1	110	5.8	14.7	3.8	1.8

	Measure INFO/WEIGHT	per Measure		Nutrition Values per 100g / 100ml				
		KCAL	FAT	KCAL	PROT	CARB	FAT	FIBRE
DHAL								
Lentil, Red Masoor with Vegetable Oil, Average	1oz/28g	48	2.2	172	7.6	19.2	7.9	1.8
Lentil, Red Masoorl & Mung Bean, Average	1oz/28g	32	1.9	114	4.8	9.9	6.7	1.6
Lentil, Tesco*	1 Serving/200g	248	13.2	124	5.1	10.6	6.6	2.5
Makhani, Curry Collection, Veetee*	1 Pack/300g	306	17.4	102	4.2	11.1	5.8	2.8
Mung Bean, Bengali	1oz/28g	20	0.9	73	4.2	7.4	3.3	1.7
Mung Beans, Dried, Boiled in Unsalted Water	1oz/28g	26	0.1	92	7.8	15.3	0.4	0.0
Mung Beans, Dried, Raw	1oz/28g	81	0.3	291	26.8	46.3	1.1	0.0
Regular, Eastern Essence*	1 Serving/113g	105	4.0	93	7.1	19.5	3.5	2.6
Split Peas, Yellow, Chana, Asda*	1 Serving/275g	300	19.2	109	2.6	9.0	7.0	1.8
Tarka, Asda*	½ Pack/150g	216	12.0	144	6.0	12.0	8.0	6.0
DHANSAK								
Vegetable, Sainsbury's*	1 Serving/200g	148	5.6	74	3.1	8.9	2.8	2.8
DILL								
Dried, Average	*1 Tsp/1g*	*3*	*0.0*	*253*	*19.9*	*42.2*	*4.4*	*13.6*
Fresh, Average	*1 Tbsp/3g*	*1*	*0.0*	*25*	*3.7*	*0.9*	*0.8*	*2.5*
DIM SUM								
From Restaurant, Average	1 Piece/12g	50	2.4	433	28.9	31.3	20.4	0.0
DIME								
Terry's*	1oz/28g	154	9.5	550	4.6	68.5	33.8	0.6
DIP								
Cheddar & Onion, M & S*	1oz/28g	88	8.3	315	5.1	7.5	29.5	0.5
Cheddar & Spring Onion, M & S*	1 Pack/125g	581	60.4	465	3.6	4.7	48.3	0.5
Cheese & Chive, 50% Less Fat, Asda*	1 Pot/125g	261	21.5	209	4.5	9.0	17.2	0.0
Cheese & Chive, Asda*	1 Serving/43g	190	19.5	447	4.9	3.4	46.0	0.0
Cheese & Chive, Fresh, Sainsbury's*	1oz/28g	109	11.3	390	3.9	2.7	40.4	0.0
Cheese & Chive, M & S*	1oz/28g	120	12.3	430	4.5	3.9	44.1	0.5
Chilli, M & S*	1 Pot/35g	103	0.1	295	0.4	73.2	0.2	0.4
Chilli Cheese, Asda*	1 Serving/50g	131	11.0	262	8.0	8.0	22.0	1.1
Chilli Cheese, Max, Walkers*	1 Jar/300g	390	27.3	130	3.3	9.4	9.1	0.3
Cucumber & Mint, Fresh, Sainsbury's*	1oz/28g	34	2.8	123	4.5	3.7	10.0	0.0
Garlic, Olive Oil & Butter, Pizza Express*	½ Pot/17g	106	11.5	621	1.5	2.8	67.4	0.5
Garlic & Herb	1 Serving/100g	583	62.3	583	1.3	4.1	62.3	0.2
Garlic & Herb, Big Dipper, Morrisons*	¼ Pot/75g	277	28.1	370	1.3	6.9	37.5	0.4
Garlic & Herb, Reduced Fat, M & S*	1 Serving/10g	9	0.4	95	6.0	8.1	4.0	0.5
Garlic & Herb, Tesco*	¼ Pack/43g	257	27.8	604	0.9	3.2	65.4	0.3
Guacamole, Reduced Fat, BGTY, Sainsbury's*	½ Pot/65g	75	7.2	116	1.3	2.7	11.1	4.0
Guacamole, Supreme, Waitrose*	½ Pot/85g	105	10.3	124	1.6	2.1	12.1	4.3
Guacamole Style, Topping, Discovery*	1 Seving/37g	29	2.1	79	1.2	6.0	5.6	1.2
Hot Salsa, Doritos, Walkers*	1 Jar/300g	87	0.6	29	0.9	5.8	0.2	1.6
Mature Cheddar Cheese & Chive, Fresh, Waitrose*	½ Pot/85g	393	40.5	462	5.8	2.4	47.7	1.7
Mexican Bean, Doritos, Walkers*	1 Tbsp/20g	18	0.7	89	2.7	12.1	3.3	2.4
Mild Salsa, Doritos, Walkers*	1 Tbsp/30g	9	0.1	30	0.8	6.0	0.3	1.5
Mustard & Honey, Fresh, Sainsbury's*	1oz/28g	100	10.2	356	2.2	5.1	36.3	0.0
Nacho Cheese, Average	1 Serving/50g	175	17.2	350	6.3	3.4	34.4	0.9
Nacho Cheese, from Tex-Mex Multipack Selection, Tesco*	1 Tub/125g	619	62.0	495	5.9	5.8	49.6	0.0
Nacho Cheese, M & S*	1oz/28g	76	6.6	270	9.8	3.8	23.7	0.4
Nacho Cheese, Primula*	1 Serving/57g	144	14.2	253	2.7	3.6	24.9	2.1
Nacho Cheese, Sainsbury's*	1 Serving/50g	243	25.1	487	4.8	3.9	50.2	0.0
Nuoc Cham from Selection, Modern Asian, M & S*	1 Pot/60g	85	0.1	140	1.3	32.9	0.2	0.7
Onion & Garlic, Average	1 Serving/50g	205	21.3	410	1.7	4.8	42.7	0.4
Onion & Garlic, Fresh, BGTY, Sainsbury's*	1oz/28g	56	5.1	201	4.4	4.8	18.2	0.8
Onion & Garlic, GFY, Asda*	1/5 Pot/34g	56	4.8	166	2.1	8.0	14.0	0.2
Onion & Garlic, Healthy Selection, Somerfield*	1oz/28g	62	5.9	222	3.0	5.0	21.0	0.0

D

D

DIP

	Measure INFO/WEIGHT	per Measure KCAL	FAT	Nutrition Values per 100g / 100ml KCAL	PROT	CARB	FAT	FIBRE
Onion & Garlic, HL, Tesco*	1 Serving/43g	80	7.2	188	2.5	6.3	17.0	0.1
Pea, Yogurt & Mint, Sainsbury's*	¼ Pack/50g	119	10.8	238	3.4	7.5	21.6	2.1
Pecorino, Basil & Pine Nut, Fresh, Waitrose*	½ Pot/85g	338	33.7	398	5.1	5.1	39.7	0.0
Raita, Indian, Asda*	1 Pot/70g	120	11.5	172	2.6	3.6	16.4	0.5
Red Pepper, Nando's*	1 Serving/260g	550	13.2	211	5.2	36.3	5.1	1.8
Red Pepper, Sainsbury's*	1 Pot/100g	103	4.0	103	2.3	14.6	4.0	0.0
Roast Onion, Garlic & Rocket, Reduced Fat, Waitrose*	1 Serving/25g	50	4.7	202	2.7	5.4	18.8	1.5
Salsa, Chunky, Fresh, Sainsbury's*	1 Serving/100g	51	1.7	51	1.1	7.8	1.7	1.2
Salsa, Chunky Tomato, Tesco*	1 Pot/170g	68	2.2	40	1.1	5.9	1.3	1.1
Salsa, GFY, Asda*	1 Pot/170g	68	0.7	40	1.2	8.0	0.4	1.5
Salsa Mild, Asda*	1 Portion/100g	47	0.3	47	1.4	8.7	0.3	1.8
Smoked Salmon & Dill, Fresh, Waitrose*	½ Pot/85g	373	38.0	439	5.1	4.1	44.7	0.1
Smoked Salmon & Dill, Reduced Fat, Waitrose*	½ Pot/85g	184	16.7	217	3.9	6.1	19.7	1.1
Sour Cream, Co-Op*	1oz/28g	137	14.6	490	2.0	3.0	52.0	0.0
Sour Cream, Tesco*	1 Serving/38g	111	11.2	297	3.4	3.9	29.8	0.2
Sour Cream & Chive, Average	1 Serving/50g	158	16.0	317	3.1	4.0	32.0	0.3
Sour Cream & Chive, BGTY, Sainsbury's*	1oz/28g	46	4.1	165	4.9	3.4	14.6	0.7
Sour Cream & Chive, Doritos, Walkers*	1 Tbsp/20g	52	4.9	258	1.9	6.9	24.7	1.9
Sour Cream & Chive, Half Fat, Waitrose*	½ Pot/85g	133	9.9	157	5.5	7.6	11.6	0.1
Sour Cream & Chive, Primula*	1 Serving/57g	169	17.4	297	4.3	1.3	30.5	1.0
Soured Cream & Chive, 95% Fat Free, M & S*	1oz/28g	25	0.8	90	6.5	9.6	2.8	0.5
Soured Cream & Chive, BGTY, Sainsbury's*	1 Serving/170g	253	17.5	149	4.2	9.9	10.3	0.1
Soured Cream & Chive, HL, Tesco*	1 Serving/31g	45	3.3	145	3.8	7.5	10.6	0.2
Soured Cream & Chive, Light Choices, Tesco*	¼ Pot/50g	65	4.5	130	4.3	7.4	9.0	0.1
Spiced Mango, Ginger & Chilli Salsa, Weight Watchers*	1 Serving/56g	48	0.1	85	1.0	19.9	0.2	2.6
Spicy Moroccan, BGTY, Sainsbury's*	½ Pot/85g	56	1.7	66	2.1	10.0	2.0	1.7
Sweet & Sour, M & S*	1oz/28g	36	0.0	130	0.7	31.4	0.1	0.5
Sweet & Sour, Primula*	1 Serving/57g	76	0.1	133	0.4	32.8	0.2	0.0
Sweet Chilli, Chinese Snack Selection, Morrisons*	½ Pot/20g	64	0.0	320	0.1	79.4	0.2	0.6
Sweet Chilli, Oriental Selection, Waitrose*	½ Pot/35g	88	0.3	250	1.3	59.4	0.8	0.4
Sweet Chilli Mango, Encona*	1 Tbsp/15ml	22	0.1	148	0.4	35.4	0.6	0.0
Thai Sweet Chilli, Primula*	1 Serving/57g	126	0.1	221	0.6	54.4	0.1	0.2
Thousand Island, HL, Tesco*	1 Serving/31g	57	4.6	183	2.5	9.6	14.9	0.3
Thousand Island, M & S*	1oz/28g	69	6.2	245	2.1	9.4	22.2	0.7
Tomato Ketchup, Asda*	1 Pack/25g	18	0.0	71	1.6	16.0	0.1	1.0
Tortilla Chips, Cool Flavour, Big, Morrisons*	½ Pack/100g	453	22.0	453	6.4	57.4	22.0	8.1
Yoghurt & Cucumber Mint, Tesco*	1oz/28g	34	2.0	121	7.0	7.2	7.1	0.6

DISCOS

	Measure INFO/WEIGHT	per Measure KCAL	FAT	Nutrition Values per 100g / 100ml KCAL	PROT	CARB	FAT	FIBRE
Beef, KP Snacks*	1 Pack/28g	145	8.2	518	5.1	58.7	29.3	2.4
Cheese & Onion, KP Snacks*	1 Pack/28g	146	8.2	520	5.1	59.1	29.3	2.5
Salt & Vinegar, KP Snacks*	1 Bag/28g	145	8.3	517	4.7	58.3	29.5	2.3

DOLLY MIXTURES

	Measure INFO/WEIGHT	per Measure KCAL	FAT	Nutrition Values per 100g / 100ml KCAL	PROT	CARB	FAT	FIBRE
M & S*	1 Pack/115g	431	1.6	375	1.8	89.2	1.4	0.0
Sainsbury's*	1 Serving/10g	40	0.2	401	1.4	94.4	1.9	0.1
Smart Price, Asda*	1 Sweet/3g	11	0.0	380	0.5	91.0	1.6	0.0
Tesco*	1 Pack/100g	376	1.5	376	1.6	88.9	1.5	0.0

DOPIAZA

	Measure INFO/WEIGHT	per Measure KCAL	FAT	Nutrition Values per 100g / 100ml KCAL	PROT	CARB	FAT	FIBRE
Chicken, M & S*	1 Pack/350g	402	21.3	115	11.5	3.7	6.1	2.5
Chicken, Sainsbury's*	½ Pack/200g	272	15.8	136	13.2	3.1	7.9	0.8
Chicken, Tesco*	1 Pack/350g	448	24.8	128	10.8	5.3	7.1	0.6
Chicken, with Pilau Rice, Sharwood's*	1 Pack/375g	472	17.2	126	5.3	15.8	4.6	0.8
Chicken, with Pilau Rice, Tesco*	1 Pack/400g	424	15.2	106	5.7	12.3	3.8	1.5
Mushroom, Retail	1oz/28g	19	1.6	69	1.3	3.7	5.7	1.1

	Measure INFO/WEIGHT	per Measure KCAL	FAT	Nutrition Values per 100g / 100ml KCAL	PROT	CARB	FAT	FIBRE
DOPIAZA								
Mushroom, Waitrose*	½ Pack/150g	81	4.6	54	2.2	4.3	3.1	2.3
DORADA								
Whole	1 Serving/100g	92	5.9	92	18.0	1.0	5.9	0.0
DORITOS								
Chargrilled BBQ, Walkers*	1 Bag/35g	170	8.7	485	5.5	59.0	25.0	3.5
Cheesy 3d's, Doritos, Walkers*	1 Pack/20g	89	3.2	445	7.0	68.0	16.0	3.0
Chilli Heatwave, Walkers*	1 Bag/35g	175	9.1	500	7.0	60.0	26.0	3.0
Cool, Ranch Chips, Walkers*	1 Pack/50g	250	13.0	504	8.1	64.5	26.2	4.0
Cool Original, Walkers*	1 Bag/40g	200	10.8	500	7.5	58.0	27.0	3.0
Cool Spice 3ds, Walkers*	1 Bag/24g	108	4.3	450	8.0	64.0	18.0	4.4
Dippas, Hint of Chilli, Dipping Chips, Walkers*	1 Bag/35g	173	8.7	495	7.0	61.0	25.0	3.5
Dippas, Hint of Garlic, Dipping Chips, Walkers*	1 Serving/35g	175	8.7	500	7.0	61.0	25.0	3.5
Dippas, Hint of Lime, Walkers*	1 Bag/35g	173	8.7	495	7.0	60.0	25.0	3.5
Dippas, Lightly Salted, Dipping Chips, Walkers*	1 Serving/35g	178	9.4	510	6.5	60.0	27.0	3.0
Latinos, Chargrilled BBQ, Walkers*	1 Serving/35g	170	8.7	485	5.5	59.0	25.0	3.5
Latinos, Mexican Grill, Walkers*	1 Serving/35g	170	8.7	485	6.5	59.0	25.0	3.5
Latinos, Sour Cream & Sweet Pepper, Walkers*	1 Pack/40g	194	10.0	485	5.5	60.0	25.0	3.5
Lightly Salted Dippas, Doritos, Walkers*	1 Serving/40g	204	10.8	510	6.5	60.0	27.0	3.0
Mexican Hot, Walkers*	1 Bag/40g	202	10.8	505	8.0	57.0	27.0	3.5
Tangy Cheese, Walkers*	1 Bag/40g	200	10.8	500	7.0	57.0	27.0	3.0
DOUBLE DECKER								
Cadbury*	1 Bar/60g	276	11.3	460	4.4	68.4	18.9	0.6
Snack Size, Cadbury*	1 Bar/36g	165	7.4	465	4.8	64.5	20.9	0.0
with Nuts, Cadbury*	1 Bar/60g	291	14.7	485	7.9	58.6	24.5	0.0
DOUGH BALLS								
Cheese & Garlic, Occasions, Sainsbury's*	1 Ball/12g	41	2.2	341	10.3	33.4	18.5	2.1
Garlic, GFY, Asda*	1 Ball/8g	21	0.2	250	9.0	49.0	2.0	2.0
Garlic, HL, Tesco*	1 Serving/40g	110	3.2	274	8.8	42.0	7.9	2.3
Garlic, Tesco*	1 Serving/10g	40	2.3	400	7.0	40.0	23.0	1.0
Garlic, Waitrose*	1 Ball/11g	38	1.8	347	8.5	41.4	16.4	3.3
Garlic & Herb, Asda*	4 Balls/48g	173	8.5	361	9.2	40.9	17.8	3.6
Garlic & Herb, Occasions, Sainsbury's*	1 Ball/12g	41	2.1	343	8.4	38.7	17.2	2.2
Sainsbury's*	1 Ball/12g	41	2.1	343	8.4	38.7	17.2	2.2
Supermarket, Pizza Express*	8 Balls/100g	363	1.7	363	14.3	72.9	1.7	3.3
DOUGHNUTS								
Apple & Custard, Finger, Sainsbury's*	1 Serving/65g	136	6.0	210	4.4	27.5	9.2	1.9
Apple & Fresh Cream, Sainsbury's*	1 Doughnut/79g	216	11.4	273	5.4	30.5	14.4	1.9
Baked, HL, Tesco*	1 Doughnut/67g	166	3.9	248	6.4	42.2	5.9	1.4
Chocolate, Somerfield*	1 Doughnut/57g	203	9.5	356	7.8	43.8	16.6	1.7
Cream & Jam, Assorted Box, Sainsbury's*	1 Doughnut/71g	229	12.7	322	6.2	34.2	17.9	2.2
Cream & Jam, Tesco*	1 Doughnut/90g	288	14.1	320	5.4	39.4	15.7	2.0
Custard & Bramley Apple, Sainsbury's*	1 Doughnut/91g	256	12.6	282	4.5	34.6	13.9	1.0
Custard Filled, Average	1 Doughnut/75g	268	14.2	358	6.2	43.3	19.0	0.0
Dairy Cream & Jam, Somerfield*	1 Doughnut/80g	296	18.5	370	4.6	35.8	23.1	1.3
Finger, Co-Op*	1 Doughnut/82g	299	14.8	365	4.0	45.0	18.0	2.0
Jam, American Style, Budgens*	1 Doughnut/46g	126	3.1	275	7.1	46.5	6.7	0.0
Jam, American Style, Sainsbury's*	1 Doughnut/65g	220	20.6	339	4.9	49.6	31.8	3.5
Jam, Fresh Cream, Sweet Fresh, Tesco*	1 Doughnut/74g	248	12.1	335	5.5	40.7	16.4	1.9
Jam Filled, Average	1 Doughnut/75g	252	10.9	336	5.7	48.8	14.5	0.0
Mini, Chocolate Topped, Chosen By You, Asda*	1 Serving/100g	393	19.5	393	5.2	49.1	19.5	2.0
Mini, Sainsbury's*	1 Doughnut/14g	53	2.7	379	5.2	47.9	18.9	2.1
Original, Glazed, Krispy Kreme*	1 Doughnut/52g	217	13.0	417	6.0	43.0	25.0	4.0
Plain, Ring, Average	1 Doughnut/60g	238	13.0	397	6.1	47.2	21.7	0.0

D

	Measure INFO/WEIGHT	per Measure		Nutrition Values per 100g / 100ml				
		KCAL	FAT	KCAL	PROT	CARB	FAT	FIBRE
DOUGHNUTS								
Ring, Iced, Average	1 Doughnut/70g	268	12.2	383	4.8	55.1	17.5	0.0
Strawberry Jam & Cream, Sainsbury's*	1 Doughnut/80g	299	18.5	374	5.3	36.2	23.2	1.3
Toffee, Tesco*	1 Doughnut/75g	235	8.7	313	8.0	44.2	11.6	1.6
Yum Yums, Glazed, Sweet, Waitrose*	1 Doughnut/45g	172	10.0	382	4.0	41.6	22.2	2.0
Yum Yums, M & S*	1 Doughnut/37g	155	8.9	420	4.9	45.7	23.9	1.6
Yum Yums, Tesco*	1 Doughnut/61g	232	10.1	380	6.1	51.6	16.6	1.7
DOVER SOLE								
Fillet, Raw, Average	*1oz/28g*	*25*	*0.5*	*89*	*18.1*	*0.0*	*1.8*	*0.0*
DR PEPPER*								
Coca-Cola*	1 Bottle/500ml	210	0.0	42	0.0	10.9	0.0	0.0
Z, Coca-Cola*	1 Serving/250ml	10	0.0	4	0.0	0.0	0.0	0.0
Zero, Coca-Cola*	1 Can/330ml	2	0.0	0	0.0	0.0	0.0	0.0
DRAGON FRUIT								
Raw, Edible Portion, Average	1 Serving/100g	41	0.5	41	0.7	9.6	0.5	3.6
DRAMBUIE								
39% Volume	*1 Shot/35ml*	*95*	*0.0*	*272*	*0.0*	*23.0*	*0.0*	*0.0*
DREAM								
Double Fudge, Cadbury*	1oz/28g	139	7.1	495	6.3	61.4	25.2	0.0
Snowbites, Cadbury*	1 Serving/31g	170	10.2	545	3.1	59.7	32.7	0.0
White Chocolate, Cadbury*	1 Piece/8g	44	2.7	555	4.5	59.7	33.3	0.0
DREAM TOPPING								
Dry, Bird's*	1oz/28g	193	16.4	690	6.7	32.5	58.5	0.5
Made Up, Skimmed Milk, Bird's*	1oz/28g	21	1.5	75	2.0	4.8	5.3	0.0
Sugar Free, Dry, Bird's*	1oz/28g	195	16.9	695	7.3	30.5	60.5	0.5
DRESSING								
Balsamic, Fresh Olive Co*	1 Tbsp/15g	42	0.1	282	1.5	67.8	0.5	0.6
Balsamic, Schwartz*	1 Tbsp/15ml	12	0.3	77	0.5	14.2	2.0	0.0
Balsamic, Vinaigrette, Newman's Own*	1 Tbsp/15g	49	5.0	326	0.1	6.4	33.3	0.5
Balsamic, Weight Watchers*	1 Serving/15ml	12	0.3	81	0.1	16.0	1.8	0.5
Balsamic Vinegar, Light, Kraft*	1 Serving/15ml	15	0.9	100	0.3	9.6	6.3	0.5
Balsamic with Olive Oil, Pizza Express*	1 Serving/10g	42	4.1	421	0.3	10.3	41.2	0.0
Basil & Pesto, COU, M & S*	1 Serving/50ml	30	1.1	60	0.6	8.3	2.2	0.8
Blue Cheese, Hellmann's*	1 Tbsp/15g	69	7.1	459	0.7	6.3	47.2	1.1
Blue Cheese, Low Fat, Weight Watchers*	1oz/28g	17	1.0	59	1.5	5.8	3.4	0.0
Caesar, Fat Free, Average	1 Tsp/5g	4	0.2	84	4.5	10.9	4.1	0.1
Caesar, Fresh, Asda*	1 Dtsp/10ml	45	4.8	454	2.4	3.2	48.0	0.0
Caesar, Fresh, M & S*	1 Tsp/6g	31	3.4	525	2.0	1.8	56.4	0.2
Caesar, Hellmann's*	1 Tsp/6g	30	3.1	499	2.5	4.5	51.7	0.3
Caesar, Light, Kraft*	1 Serving/15g	14	0.5	95	1.7	13.0	3.6	0.2
Caesar, Low Fat, Average	1 Tsp/5g	4	0.1	77	2.3	11.1	2.6	0.2
Caesar, Loyd Grossman*	1 Dtsp/10g	34	3.4	342	2.1	7.0	33.9	0.0
Caesar, Luxury, Hellmann's*	1 Tsp/4g	20	2.1	498	2.5	4.4	51.7	0.3
Caesar, Mary Berry*	1 Serving/100g	573	56.9	573	2.4	12.8	56.9	0.1
Caesar, Original, Cardini's*	1 Serving/10g	55	6.0	555	2.3	1.5	60.0	0.2
Citrus Salad, BGTY, Sainsbury's*	1 Tbsp/15ml	13	0.5	90	0.3	14.4	3.1	0.3
Classic French, Fresh, M & S*	1 Serving/10ml	51	5.3	515	0.6	8.2	53.1	0.2
Classic Italian, Get Dressed, Kraft*	1 Serving/25ml	30	2.6	120	0.1	5.6	10.3	0.5
Cream Cheese & Chive, Creamy Ranch, Kraft*	1 Serving/15ml	31	2.5	205	1.2	11.0	17.0	0.0
Creamy, Waistline, 93% Fat Free, Crosse & Blackwell*	1 Tsp/6g	7	0.4	120	1.0	14.4	6.4	0.2
Creme Fraiche, Salad, Kraft*	1 Tbsp/15ml	12	0.4	78	0.8	12.5	2.5	0.0
Dijon Honey Mustard, Briannas*	1 Tbsp/15ml	65	6.0	433	0.0	20.0	40.0	0.0
Fat Free, Vinegar & Oil Based, Average	1 Tsp/5g	2	0.0	37	0.4	7.9	0.2	0.4
Fire Roasted Garlic & Thyme, Tesco*	1 Serving/10ml	45	4.7	447	0.9	4.7	47.2	0.0

DRESSING

	Measure INFO/WEIGHT	per Measure KCAL	FAT	Nutrition Values per 100g / 100ml KCAL	PROT	CARB	FAT	FIBRE
Fire Roasted Red Pepper, M & S*	1 Serving/30g	13	0.0	45	0.5	10.7	0.1	0.9
Fire Roasted Tomato Basil, COU, M & S*	1 Serving/30g	13	0.3	45	0.6	8.1	0.9	1.1
Fragrant Thai, Love Life, Waitrose*	1 Serving/16ml	9	0.0	57	1.8	12.0	0.1	0.6
French, BGTY, Organic, Sainsbury's*	1 Tbsp/15ml	11	0.6	71	0.2	8.3	4.1	0.5
French, BGTY, Sainsbury's*	1 Tbsp/15ml	12	0.7	79	1.1	8.8	4.4	0.5
French, Chilled, Tesco*	1 Tbsp/15ml	63	5.9	421	1.1	15.1	39.6	0.0
French, Cider Vinegar & Mustard, Tesco*	1 Tbsp/15ml	45	4.2	300	0.7	9.9	28.1	0.3
French, Classic, Fat Free, Kraft*	1 Tsp/5ml	2	0.0	39	0.1	8.7	0.0	0.5
French, Classic, Sachet, The English Provender Company*	1 Sachet/25g	21	0.6	84	0.8	14.7	2.4	0.0
French, Classic, Sainsbury's*	1 Tbsp/15ml	71	7.4	473	1.0	5.7	49.6	0.5
French, Classics, M & S*	1 Tbsp/15ml	77	8.0	516	0.6	8.2	53.1	0.2
French, Fresh, Morrisons*	1 Tbsp/15ml	75	7.3	499	1.5	13.6	48.7	0.0
French, Fresh, Organic, Sainsbury's*	1 Tbsp/15ml	45	4.6	301	0.4	5.5	31.0	0.4
French, Fresh, Sainsbury's*	1 Tbsp/15ml	64	6.7	429	0.6	6.6	44.6	0.6
French, Fresh, Somerfield*	1 Tbsp/15ml	73	7.6	490	1.0	7.0	51.0	0.0
French, Less Than 3% Fat, M & S*	1 Tbsp/15ml	10	0.4	68	0.7	11.5	2.6	0.7
French, Light, Heinz*	1 Sachet/12g	13	0.6	111	0.7	15.4	5.4	0.0
French, Light Choices, Tesco*	1 Tbsp/16g	8	0.3	50	0.8	7.6	1.6	1.1
French, Luxury, Hellmann's*	1 Tbsp/15g	45	3.9	297	0.4	14.9	25.9	0.3
French, Oil Free, French, Waitrose*	1 Tsp/5ml	4	0.1	76	1.5	13.1	2.0	0.6
French, Oil Free, Perfectly Balanced, Waitrose*	1 Serving/15ml	11	0.2	72	2.2	12.2	1.6	1.1
French, Organic, Tesco*	1 Tsp/5ml	23	2.2	451	0.6	11.0	44.9	0.2
French, Sainsbury's*	1 Tbsp/15ml	33	2.9	219	0.6	9.8	19.1	0.5
French, Tesco*	1 Serving/25ml	110	11.2	441	0.7	7.2	44.9	0.2
French Salad, M & S*	1 Serving/25ml	156	16.8	625	0.5	3.8	67.3	0.1
French Style Calorie-Wise Salad, Kraft*	1 Tbsp/15ml	24	1.6	160	0.0	18.7	10.7	0.0
Garlic & Herb, Reduced Calorie, Hellmann's*	1 Tbsp/15ml	35	2.9	232	0.6	12.8	19.3	0.4
Garlic & Herb, Tesco*	1 Tbsp/15g	31	3.0	210	0.9	5.8	20.2	0.8
Green Thai, Finest, Tesco*	1 Bottle/250ml	940	81.8	376	0.3	19.1	32.7	0.3
Herb & Garlic, Light, 5% Fat, Get Dressed, Kraft*	1 Serving/25ml	29	1.3	116	1.3	15.5	5.1	0.2
Honey, Orange & Mustard, BGTY, Sainsbury's*	1 Tbsp/15ml	16	0.4	105	1.8	18.6	2.5	1.8
Honey & Mustard, GFY, Asda*	1 Tbsp/15g	13	0.5	89	1.5	13.0	3.4	0.8
Honey & Mustard, Hellmann's*	1 Serving/15ml	27	0.2	182	0.7	13.7	1.6	0.3
Honey & Mustard, M & S*	1 Tbsp/15ml	64	6.4	427	1.7	9.7	42.4	0.6
Honey & Mustard, Sainsbury's*	1 Serving/10ml	37	3.3	366	1.0	15.4	33.0	0.1
Honey & Mustard, Tesco*	1 Serving/10ml	38	3.6	378	0.8	13.1	35.8	0.6
Honey & Mustard, The English Provender Co.*	1 Tbsp/15ml	17	0.2	111	2.5	21.8	1.5	1.0
Hot Lime & Coconut, BGTY, Sainsbury's*	1 Tbsp/15ml	8	0.4	51	0.7	5.7	2.9	1.2
Italian, Light, Low Fat, Newman's Own*	1 Serving/15g	9	0.4	57	0.1	6.7	2.8	0.5
Italian, Low Fat, Heinz*	1 Pot/30ml	26	1.9	86	0.9	6.3	6.3	2.7
Italian, M & S*	1 Tbsp/15ml	62	6.2	415	0.9	8.9	41.5	1.0
Italian, Reduced Calorie, Hellmann's*	1 Serving/25ml	67	5.2	269	0.5	19.5	20.8	0.3
Italian Balsamic, Loyd Grossman*	1 Serving/10g	36	3.3	357	0.9	13.1	33.5	0.1
Italian Balsamic, The English Provender Co.*	1 Serving/30ml	20	0.8	67	0.8	9.9	2.7	0.2
Lemon, Feta & Oregano, M & S*	1 Tbsp/15ml	24	2.0	160	1.3	8.2	13.4	0.6
Lemon & Black Pepper, Good Intentions, Somerfield*	1 Tbsp/15ml	36	3.1	241	2.6	10.5	21.0	0.4
Lemon & Cracked Black Pepper, GFY, Asda*	1 Tbsp/15g	9	0.0	57	0.2	14.0	0.0	0.3
Lemon & Watercress, COU, M & S*	1 Serving/28g	14	0.5	50	0.4	8.5	1.8	0.5
Lime & Coriander, Oil Free, Waitrose*	1 Tsp/5ml	3	0.1	65	1.5	11.9	1.3	0.4
Lime & Coriander, Sainsbury's*	1 Tbsp/15ml	61	6.1	409	0.4	10.0	40.8	0.5
Lime & Coriander, The English Provender Co.*	1 Serving/50g	28	0.1	57	0.3	13.3	0.3	0.0
Mild Mustard, Low Fat, Weight Watchers*	1 Tbsp/10g	6	0.4	63	2.0	5.7	3.6	0.0
Mint & Tomato, Mary Berry*	1 Serving/100g	399	37.1	399	0.8	14.8	37.1	0.3

DRESSING

	Measure INFO/WEIGHT	per Measure KCAL	per Measure FAT	Nutrition Values per 100g / 100ml KCAL	PROT	CARB	FAT	FIBRE
Mustard & Dill, Perfectly Balanced, Waitrose*	1 Tbsp/15ml	24	0.5	159	1.1	31.5	3.2	1.1
Oil & Lemon	1 Tbsp/15g	97	10.6	647	0.3	2.8	70.6	0.0
Olive Oil, Pizza Express*	1 Tbsp/15g	86	9.4	573	1.4	3.4	63.0	0.0
Olive Oil & Balsamic Vinegar, Sainsbury's*	1 Serving/25ml	104	10.4	415	0.9	9.4	41.8	0.2
Orange & Cracked Pepper, Tesco*	1 Tbsp/15ml	17	0.0	114	0.5	27.8	0.1	0.3
Orange & Honey, Luxury, Hellmann's*	1 Serving/15ml	16	0.5	110	0.8	17.5	3.5	0.8
Ranch Style, Asda*	1 Serving/44ml	37	1.7	85	3.5	9.0	3.9	0.0
Red Pepper, BGTY, Sainsbury's*	1 Bottle/250g	107	0.7	43	0.2	9.8	0.3	0.2
Red Pepper, M & S*	1 Tbsp/15ml	58	5.9	385	0.6	7.6	39.2	0.5
Red Pepper & Chilli, Less Than 1% Fat, BGTY, Sainsbury's*	1 Serving/20g	9	0.0	45	0.1	10.6	0.2	0.5
Salad, Caesar, Light, Fry Light*	1 Spray/0.2ml	1	0.1	321	0.4	9.2	30.7	0.1
Salad, Catalina, Kraft*	1 Serving/34g	100	6.0	294	0.0	29.4	17.6	0.0
Salad, Honey & Mustard, Light, Kraft*	1 Tbsp/15ml	19	0.7	126	1.2	19.0	4.6	1.1
Salad, Italian, Light, Kraft*	1 Tbsp/15ml	5	0.0	31	0.1	6.8	0.0	0.6
Salad, Italian, Newman's Own*	1 Tbsp/15g	82	9.0	545	0.2	1.0	59.8	0.0
Salad, Kickin' Mango, Oil Free, Ainsley Harriott*	1 Tbsp/15ml	14	0.0	92	0.1	21.1	0.1	0.0
Salad, Light, Heinz*	1 Serving/10g	24	2.0	244	1.8	13.5	19.9	0.0
Salad, Low Fat, Weight Watchers*	1 Tbsp/10g	10	0.4	106	1.5	15.4	4.3	0.0
Salad, Mary Berry*	1 Serving/15g	77	6.6	513	0.8	28.5	44.0	0.1
Salad, Oil Free, Caper & Hot Peppercorn, Righteous*	1 Tbsp/15ml	8	0.1	53	1.3	7.3	0.7	0.1
Salad, Pizza Express*	1 Serving/5g	29	3.1	573	1.4	3.4	63.0	0.0
Salad, Raspberry Balsamic, GFY, Asda*	1 Tbsp/15ml	6	0.1	40	0.7	9.3	0.7	1.3
Salad, Sun Dried Tomato & Chilli, Loyd Grossman*	1 Tsp/5g	18	1.9	361	0.9	5.3	37.3	0.9
Salad, Thousand Island, 95% Fat Free, Asda*	1 Tsp/6g	6	0.3	99	1.6	12.6	4.7	0.5
Salad, Vinaigrette Style, 95% Fat Free, Asda*	1 Tbsp/15ml	6	0.0	42	0.1	10.6	0.4	0.3
Seafood, M & S*	1 Tsp/7g	39	4.2	555	0.9	4.9	59.3	0.9
Sicilian Lemon, M & S*	1 Tbsp/15ml	73	7.4	485	0.1	10.5	49.1	0.0
Sweet Chilli, COU, M & S*	1 Tbsp/15ml	9	0.1	60	0.5	14.5	0.5	0.4
Sweet Chilli & Mango, Love Life, Waitrose*	1 Serving/16ml	10	0.0	64	1.6	14.0	0.1	0.6
Texas Ranch, Frank Cooper*	1 Pot/28g	128	12.8	457	1.9	9.4	45.8	0.2
Thousand Island	1 Tsp/6g	19	1.8	323	1.1	12.5	30.2	0.4
Thousand Island, BGTY, Sainsbury's*	1 Serving/20g	19	1.4	95	0.4	7.3	7.2	0.5
Thousand Island, COU, M & S*	1 Serving/30g	25	0.8	85	1.4	14.2	2.6	1.1
Thousand Island, Eat Smart, Morrisons*	1 Tbsp/15ml	38	3.2	253	0.0	0.0	21.3	0.0
Thousand Island, Light, Kraft*	1 Tbsp/15ml	16	0.0	105	0.6	23.0	0.2	3.0
Thousand Island, Reduced Calorie	1 Tsp/6g	12	0.9	195	0.7	14.7	15.2	0.0
Thousand Island, Tesco*	1 Tbsp/15g	55	4.7	360	1.1	19.5	30.5	0.3
Tomato & Basil, Fresh, Somerfield*	1 Tbsp/15ml	52	5.2	348	2.0	7.0	35.0	0.0
Tomato & Basil, HL, Tesco*	½ Pot/75ml	41	1.1	55	0.8	9.0	1.5	0.5
Tomato & Herb, Less Than 1% Fat, Asda*	1 Tbsp/15g	6	0.1	43	0.7	8.0	0.9	0.4
Tomato & Red Pepper, BGTY, Sainsbury's*	1 Serving/50ml	41	2.1	83	1.1	10.0	4.3	0.6
True Blue Cheese, Briannas*	2 Tbsp/30ml	120	11.0	400	3.3	16.7	36.7	0.0
Vinaigrette, BGTY, Sainsbury's*	1 Dtsp/20g	13	0.5	64	1.1	9.3	2.4	2.5
Yoghurt & Mint, HL, Tesco*	1 Serving/50g	31	1.2	62	4.1	6.9	2.5	0.2
Yoghurt & Mint Dressing Less Than 3% Fat, Asda*	1 Serving/16g	12	0.3	76	2.8	11.7	2.0	0.4
Yoghurt Mint Cucumber, M & S*	1 Tsp/5ml	6	0.4	115	1.0	8.7	8.0	0.0

DRIED FRUIT

	Measure INFO/WEIGHT	per Measure KCAL	per Measure FAT	Nutrition Values per 100g / 100ml KCAL	PROT	CARB	FAT	FIBRE
Banana, Bites, Kiddylicious, Babylicious*	1 Serving/15g	43	2.9	285	10.8	43.6	19.3	6.1
Beach Bum, Graze*	1 Pack/33g	121	4.1	363	3.3	61.5	12.4	9.7
Exotic, Ready to Eat, Sainsbury's*	1/3 Pack/85g	241	0.1	284	0.2	70.6	0.1	2.4
Figgy Pop, Graze*	1 Pack/40g	100	0.4	251	2.5	61.6	1.1	0.0
Honey Coated Banana Chips, Whitworths*	1 Serving/25g	131	7.8	526	1.0	59.9	31.4	1.7
Jewel of the Nile, Graze*	1 Pack/45g	112	0.4	248	2.5	61.3	0.8	0.0

	Measure INFO/WEIGHT	per Measure		Nutrition Values per 100g / 100ml				
		KCAL	FAT	KCAL	PROT	CARB	FAT	FIBRE
DRIED FRUIT								
Juicy Sprinkle, Nature's Harvest*	1 Serving/20g	79	2.0	397	4.9	71.9	10.0	4.2
Jus Fruit, Mango Pieces, Yu!*	1 Pack/24g	87	0.1	364	1.0	84.7	0.4	0.0
Jus Fruit Blueberry Pieces, Yu!*	1 Pack/24g	84	0.1	350	0.8	80.8	0.4	0.0
Mixed, Value, Tesco*	1 Serving/25g	71	0.2	285	2.1	67.5	0.7	2.3
Strawberry, Banana & Cherry, Sunshine Mix, Graze*	1 Pack/50g	78	0.2	157	9.7	37.2	0.4	0.0
Top Banana, Graze*	1 Serving/40g	115	0.4	287	2.6	70.1	0.9	0.0
Trail Mix, Kick Start, Wholefoods, Asda*	1 Serving/50g	193	10.2	387	10.9	40.0	20.4	10.7
DRIED FRUIT MIX								
5 Fruits, Ready to Eat, Sundora*	½ Pack/100g	233	0.4	233	1.6	58.4	0.4	6.8
Agadoo, Pineapple, Jumbo & Green Raisins, Graze*	1 Pack/40g	110	0.4	275	2.1	69.0	0.9	0.0
Albert Heijn*	1 Serving/50g	110	0.2	220	2.1	51.0	0.5	0.0
Apple Strudel, Graze*	1 Pack/40g	99	0.3	247	2.2	58.7	0.7	5.9
Average	1 Tbsp/25g	67	0.1	268	2.3	68.1	0.4	2.2
Berry, Love Life, Waitrose*	1 Serving/30g	89	0.3	296	1.9	70.0	0.9	3.0
Berry, Whole Foods, Tesco*	1 Serving/25g	66	0.2	265	3.3	60.0	0.7	7.5
Dates, Raisins & Apricots, Wholefoods, Tesco*	1 Serving/20g	52	0.1	260	3.1	59.0	0.4	4.0
Eden, Graze*	1 Punnet/25g	69	0.2	275	2.0	63.7	1.0	8.1
Festival Fruits, Graze*	1 Punnet/32g	87	0.1	271	1.4	70.5	0.4	7.0
Fig & Cherry Preserve, Graze*	1 Pack/44g	116	0.4	263	2.9	64.6	0.9	7.6
Fruit & Oat Bites, Mixed Berry, Planet Lunch*	1 Bar/20g	53	0.6	265	3.9	56.0	2.8	8.0
Fruit & Oat Bites, Strawberry, Planet Lunch*	1 Bar/20g	54	0.5	270	4.0	57.0	2.5	7.2
Fruit Salad, Whitworths*	1 Serving/62g	113	0.3	183	2.9	41.8	0.5	6.6
Fruit Sangria, Graze*	1 Punnet/36g	110	0.6	306	3.8	70.3	1.8	2.6
Fruit Sundae, Graze*	1 Punnet/34g	98	0.3	287	2.1	70.1	1.0	4.1
Garden of England, Graze*	1 Punnet/25g	72	0.1	290	0.7	74.5	0.6	6.0
Hanging Gardens of Babylon, Graze*	1 Punnet/49g	114	0.2	232	3.2	57.1	0.5	7.6
Little Figgy Went to Market, Graze*	1 Punnet/37g	103	0.3	273	1.8	63.9	0.7	7.9
Medley, Shapers, Boots*	1 Serving/50g	131	0.3	262	3.2	61.0	0.6	5.5
Pear Tatin, Graze*	1 Punnet/35g	143	6.3	408	7.0	57.2	18.1	5.9
Raisins Mix, Wholesome, Love Life, Waitrose*	1 Serving/30g	88	0.3	293	2.1	69.0	0.9	3.7
Scrumptious Blueberry Swirl, Graze*	1 Punnet/39g	149	2.7	381	1.2	78.8	6.9	3.5
Sultanas, Currants, Raisins & Citrus Peel, Asda*	1 Serving/100g	283	0.5	283	2.6	67.0	0.5	1.7
Taste of Hawaii, Extra Special, Asda*	1 Serving/100g	314	0.8	314	1.7	75.0	0.8	4.4
Tropical, Morrisons*	1 Pack/200g	368	1.0	184	1.7	50.6	0.5	6.3
Tropical, Somerfield*	1 Bag/50g	305	2.9	611	71.1	68.4	5.9	3.7
Tropical Sundae, Graze*	1 Punnet/29g	86	0.3	299	2.7	72.7	1.0	8.5
Vine Fruit, Wholesome, Waitrose*	1 Serving/30g	87	0.1	289	2.1	69.3	0.4	5.3
DRIFTER								
Nestle*	1 Finger/20g	98	4.8	488	4.8	62.7	24.2	0.7
DRINKING CHOCOLATE								
Cadbury*	1 Tbsp/16g	64	0.4	402	4.4	89.3	2.4	0.0
Dry, Asda*	1 Serving/30g	111	1.8	370	6.0	73.0	6.0	0.0
Dry, Tesco*	3 Tsp/25g	92	1.4	368	6.4	72.6	5.8	4.2
Dry, Waitrose*	3 Tsp/12g	48	0.7	403	7.2	79.9	6.1	2.9
Dry Powder, Cocodirect*	1 Serving/18g	67	1.5	372	8.9	65.1	8.4	0.0
Fairtrade, Truly Irresistible, Co-Op*	1 Serving/20g	73	1.9	365	10.0	60.3	9.4	13.8
Hot Chocolate, Light Choices, Tesco*	1 Cup/11g	38	0.8	345	13.8	54.9	7.7	13.1
Made Up, BGTY, Sainsbury's*	1 Serving/178g	114	0.4	64	3.9	11.4	0.2	0.7
Made Up with Semi-Skimmed Milk, Average	1 Mug/227ml	129	4.3	57	3.5	7.0	1.9	0.2
Made Up with Skimmed Milk, Average	1 Mug/227ml	100	1.1	44	3.5	7.0	0.5	0.0
Made Up with Whole Milk, Average	1 Mug/227ml	173	9.5	76	3.4	6.8	4.2	0.2
Maxpax, Light, Suchard*	1 Serving/11g	37	0.6	355	20.0	56.0	5.5	9.3
Powder, Made Up with Skimmed Milk	1 Mug/227ml	134	1.4	59	3.5	10.8	0.6	0.0

	Measure INFO/WEIGHT	per Measure KCAL	FAT	Nutrition Values per 100g / 100ml KCAL	PROT	CARB	FAT	FIBRE
DRINKING CHOCOLATE								
Powder, Made Up with Whole Milk	1 Mug/227ml	204	9.3	90	3.4	10.6	4.1	0.0
DRIPPING								
Beef	**1oz/28g**	**249**	**27.7**	**891**	**0.0**	**0.0**	**99.0**	**0.0**
DUCK								
Breast, Meat Only, Cooked, Average	**1oz/28g**	**48**	**2.0**	**172**	**25.3**	**1.8**	**7.0**	**0.0**
Breast, Meat Only, Raw, Average	**1 Serving/160g**	**206**	**6.8**	**128**	**22.5**	**0.0**	**4.2**	**0.2**
Fillets, Gressingham, Mini, TTD, Sainsbury's*	½ Pack/90g	127	2.4	141	29.0	0.0	2.7	0.6
Leg, Meat & Skin, Average	**1oz/28g**	**80**	**5.6**	**286**	**17.2**	**9.5**	**20.0**	**0.4**
Raw, Meat, Fat & Skin	**1oz/28g**	**109**	**10.4**	**388**	**13.1**	**0.0**	**37.3**	**0.0**
Raw, Meat Only, Weighed with Fat, Skin & Bone	1 Serving/100g	38	1.8	38	5.5	0.0	1.8	0.0
Roasted, Meat, Fat & Skin	**1oz/28g**	**118**	**10.7**	**423**	**20.0**	**0.0**	**38.1**	**0.0**
Roasted, Meat Only, Weighed with Fat, Skin & Bone	1 Serving/100g	41	2.2	41	5.3	0.0	2.2	0.0
Shredded & Spring Onion Rice Paper Rolls, Waitrose*	1 Pack/95g	101	0.7	104	6.6	17.7	0.7	0.7
DUCK &								
Plum Sauce, Roasted, Sainsbury's*	½ Pack/150g	174	3.7	116	6.9	16.0	2.5	1.8
DUCK A L' ORANGE								
Roast, M & S*	½ Pack/270g	553	42.1	205	12.5	4.1	15.6	0.6
DUCK AROMATIC								
Crispy, Asda*	1/3 Pack/166g	469	24.9	283	19.0	18.0	15.0	0.8
Crispy, Half Duck & Pancakes, M & S*	½ Pack/311g	590	26.7	190	13.9	14.0	8.6	2.1
Crispy, Half with Hoisin Sauce & 12 Pancakes, Tesco*	1/6 Pack/70g	162	7.4	232	18.3	15.9	10.6	1.1
Crispy, Quarter with Hoisin Sauce & 6 Pancakes, Tesco*	1/6 Pack/40g	100	4.2	250	12.3	25.3	10.6	2.0
Crispy, Somerfield*	1 Serving/265g	782	49.0	295	18.1	14.0	18.5	0.7
Crispy, Whole with Hoisin Sauce & 18 Pancakes, Tesco*	1/9 Pack/100g	280	17.2	280	18.9	12.0	17.2	0.4
with Plum Sauce, Finest, Tesco*	1 Serving/250g	400	14.0	160	16.1	11.3	5.6	4.6
DUCK CANTONESE								
Style, Roast, Tesco*	1 Pack/300g	375	6.9	125	8.2	17.9	2.3	0.5
DUCK IN								
Chinese Barbecue, Wings, Sainsbury's*	1 Serving/175g	430	25.0	246	19.4	9.7	14.3	0.0
Orange Sauce, Iceland*	1 Serving/200g	336	20.8	168	11.3	7.4	10.4	1.2
Orange Sauce, Legs, Extra Special, Asda*	1oz/28g	39	1.6	141	18.0	4.3	5.7	1.3
Oriental Sauce, Iceland*	1 Pack/201g	352	22.7	175	12.0	6.3	11.3	1.5
Plum & Chilli Sauce, Legs, Aldi*	½ Pack/200g	342	11.6	171	5.7	24.0	5.8	0.6
Plum Sauce, Crispy, M & S*	1 Pack/325g	569	31.2	175	10.7	11.2	9.6	0.9
Plum Sauce, Legs, Asda*	1 Leg/200g	452	23.0	226	24.1	6.4	11.5	0.5
Red Wine Sauce, Free Range Fillets, Waitrose*	½ Pack/250g	377	19.2	151	16.4	4.1	7.7	2.2
DUCK PEKING								
Crispy, Aromatic, Sainsbury's*	½ Pack/300g	1236	110.7	412	19.5	0.6	36.9	0.1
Crispy, Cherry Valley*	1 Serving/270g	702	35.9	260	17.5	17.8	13.3	0.7
DUCK WITH								
Hoisin & Noodles, Fuller for Longer, M & S*	1 Pack/370g	335	7.4	91	8.2	10.0	2.0	2.0
Noodles, Shanghai Roast, Sainsbury's*	1 Pack/450g	580	17.1	129	5.6	18.0	3.8	1.2
Pancakes, Shredded, Iceland*	1 Pack/220g	471	5.9	214	20.4	27.0	2.7	1.5
Pancakes & Hoisin Sauce, M & S*	1 Pack/80g	136	3.2	170	13.0	19.9	4.0	0.9
DUMPLINGS								
Average	1oz/28g	58	3.3	208	2.8	24.5	11.7	0.9
Dried Mix, Tesco*	1 Pack/137g	404	16.7	295	5.4	39.9	12.2	2.8
Homestyle, Baked Weight, Frozen, Aunt Bessie's*	1 Dumpling/49g	188	8.6	384	9.7	44.4	17.6	2.8
Pork & Garlic Chive, Waitrose*	1 Pack/115g	215	8.1	187	9.4	20.4	7.0	1.1
Prawn, Cantonese, Crispy, Sainsbury's*	1 Dumpling/11g	27	1.5	241	9.3	20.9	13.4	1.1
Prawn, Siu Mai, Chinese, M & S*	8 Dumplings/170g	170	2.9	100	7.8	13.1	1.7	1.3

	Measure INFO/WEIGHT	per Measure		Nutrition Values per 100g / 100ml				
		KCAL	FAT	KCAL	PROT	CARB	FAT	FIBRE
EASTER EGG								
Aero Bubbles, Nestle*	1 Egg/235g	1264	72.4	538	6.6	57.6	30.8	2.2
Buttons, Chocolate Egg Shell Only, Cadbury*	1 Egg/162g	850	48.6	525	7.5	56.8	30.0	0.7
Caramel, Chocolate Egg Shell Only, Cadbury*	1 Egg/343g	1801	102.9	525	7.5	56.8	30.0	0.7
Chick, Dairy Milk, Chocolate Egg Shell Only, Cadbury*	1 Egg/167g	877	50.1	525	7.5	56.8	30.0	0.7
Chocolate Egg Shell Only, Dairy Milk, Cadbury*	1 Egg/178g	934	53.4	525	7.5	56.8	30.0	0.7
Chocolate Orange, Terry's*	1 Egg/120g	636	36.6	530	7.4	57.0	30.5	2.4
Creme Egg, Chocolate Egg Shell Only, Cadbury*	1 Egg/178g	943	53.4	530	7.5	56.8	30.0	0.7
Crunchie, Cadbury*	1 Egg/167g	885	50.1	530	7.5	56.8	30.0	0.7
Dark Chocolate, 70%, Green & Black's*	1 Egg/180g	992	74.0	551	9.3	36.0	41.1	11.5
Dark Chocolate, Thorncroft's*	1 Egg/360g	1890	134.6	525	6.8	39.4	37.4	9.8
Disney, Nestle*	1 Egg/65g	342	18.9	526	6.3	59.7	29.1	0.6
Flake, Chocolate Egg Shell Only, Cadbury*	1 Shell/153g	803	45.9	525	7.5	56.8	30.0	0.7
Kit Kat, Chunky, Nestle*	1 Egg/235g	1250	67.7	532	5.5	61.7	28.8	1.7
Mars*	1 Serving/63g	281	10.9	449	4.2	69.0	17.4	0.0
Milk Chocolate, Nestle*	½ Egg/42g	205	9.7	489	5.0	65.2	23.1	0.5
Milky Bar, Nestle*	1 Egg/40g	182	6.9	454	4.2	70.8	17.2	0.0
Roses, Chocolate Egg Shell Only, Cadbury*	1 Egg/200g	1060	60.0	530	7.5	56.8	30.0	0.7
Smarties, Nestle*	1 Egg/258g	1367	74.0	530	5.3	62.2	28.7	1.7
Twirl, Chocolate Egg Shell Only, Cadbury*	1 Egg/325g	1722	97.5	530	7.5	56.8	30.0	0.7
White Chocolate, Thorntons*	1 Egg/360g	1958	109.1	544	5.5	62.2	30.3	2.1
Wispa, Chocolate Egg Shell Only, Cadbury*	1 Egg/313g	1643	93.9	525	7.5	56.8	30.0	0.7
ECLAIR								
Belgian Chocolate, Weight Watchers*	1 Eclair/30g	81	3.5	271	3.9	37.6	11.7	6.6
Chocolate, 25% Less Fat, Sainsbury's*	1 Eclair/58g	171	9.3	295	6.8	31.1	16.0	1.2
Chocolate, Cream, Fresh, Tesco*	1 Eclair/66g	285	20.5	430	6.0	31.1	30.9	1.8
Chocolate, Cream filled, VLH Kitchens	1 Serving/66g	286	44.2	434	7.0	36.4	29.2	1.8
Chocolate, Fresh Cream, M & S*	1 Eclair/44g	170	12.2	390	6.3	28.4	27.9	2.0
Chocolate, Fresh Cream, Sainsbury's*	1 Eclair/59g	212	13.9	360	4.2	32.7	23.6	0.5
Chocolate, Frozen, Morrisons*	1 Eclair/31g	116	9.6	374	5.0	18.8	31.0	1.3
Chocolate, HL, Tesco*	1 Serving/77g	192	9.7	249	6.8	27.1	12.6	0.9
Chocolate & Fresh Cream, Tempting, Tesco*	1 Eclair/39g	158	11.2	405	6.5	29.1	28.8	1.1
Double Chocolate with Fresh Cream, Tesco*	1 Eclair/69g	275	18.6	400	5.9	33.4	27.0	1.6
EEL								
Cooked or Smoked, Dry Heat, Average	*1 Serving/100g*	*236*	*14.9*	*236*	*23.6*	*0.0*	*14.9*	*0.0*
Jellied, Average	*1oz/28g*	*27*	*2.0*	*98*	*8.4*	*0.0*	*7.1*	*0.0*
Raw, Average	*1oz/28g*	*47*	*3.2*	*168*	*16.6*	*0.0*	*11.3*	*0.0*
EGG SUBSTITUTE								
99% Real Eggs, The Crafty Cook*	¼ Cup/61g	30	0.0	49	10.0	2.0	0.0	0.0
Original, The Crafty Cook*	¼ Cup 1oz/28g	30	0.0	107	21.4	3.6	0.0	0.0
EGG WHITE								
Free Range, Liquid, Two Chicks*	3 Tbsp/45g	23	0.0	50	10.5	1.0	0.0	0.0
Liquid, Myprotein*	1 Serving/32g	16	0.0	50	11.2	0.0	0.0	0.0
EGGS								
Dried, White, Average	*1 Tbsp/14g*	*41*	*0.0*	*295*	*73.8*	*0.0*	*0.0*	*0.0*
Dried, Whole, Average	*1oz/28g*	*159*	*11.6*	*568*	*48.4*	*0.0*	*41.6*	*0.0*
Duck, Boiled & Salted, Average, Weight with Shell	1 Egg/75g	169	13.2	225	16.6	0.0	17.6	0.0
Duck, Whole, Raw, Average, Weight with Shell	*1 Egg/75g*	*139*	*10.0*	*185*	*16.2*	*0.0*	*13.4*	*0.0*
Free Range, Large, Average, Weight with Shell	*1 Egg/68g*	*109*	*7.6*	*161*	*14.1*	*0.9*	*11.2*	*0.0*
Free Range, Medium, Average, Weight with Shell	1 Egg/58g	93	6.5	161	14.1	0.9	11.2	0.0
Fried in Veg Oil, Average	1 Med/60g	107	8.3	179	13.6	0.0	13.9	0.0
Fried without Fat, Average	1 Med/60g	104	7.6	174	15.0	0.0	12.7	0.0
Goose, Whole, Fresh, Raw, Average, Weight with Shell	*1 Egg/144g*	*267*	*19.1*	*185*	*13.9*	*1.3*	*13.3*	*0.0*
Large, Average, Weight with Shell	1oz/28g	37	2.5	131	12.6	0.1	9.0	0.0

E

	Measure INFO/WEIGHT	per Measure KCAL	FAT	Nutrition Values per 100g / 100ml KCAL	PROT	CARB	FAT	FIBRE
EGGS								
Medium, Average, Weight with Shell	1oz/28g	37	2.5	131	12.6	0.1	9.0	0.0
Medium, Boiled, Average, Weight with Shell	1 Egg/50g	83	6.1	165	14.0	0.6	12.1	0.1
Poached, Weight with Shell	1 Med/50g	83	6.1	165	14.0	0.6	12.1	0.6
Quail, Whole, Raw, Weight with Shell	*1 Egg/13g*	*21*	*1.6*	*164*	*14.0*	*0.4*	*12.1*	*0.0*
Scrambled, Average	1 Egg/68g	109	7.9	160	13.8	0.0	11.6	0.0
Scrambled with Milk, Average	1 Egg/60g	154	14.0	257	10.9	0.7	23.4	0.0
Turkey, Whole, Raw, Weight with Shell	*1 Egg/79g*	*154*	*10.9*	*194*	*15.5*	*1.3*	*13.9*	*0.0*
Very Large, Average, Weight with Shell	1 Egg/78g	125	8.7	161	14.1	0.9	11.2	0.0
Whites Only, Raw, Average	*1 Lg Egg/33g*	*12*	*0.2*	*36*	*10.9*	*0.3*	*0.6*	*0.0*
Whole, Raw, Weight with Shell	*1 Small/48g*	*79*	*5.8*	*165*	*14.0*	*0.0*	*12.1*	*0.0*
Yolks, Raw	*1 Yolk/14g*	*47*	*4.3*	*339*	*16.1*	*0.0*	*30.5*	*0.0*
ELDERBERRIES								
Average	*1oz/28g*	*10*	*0.1*	*35*	*0.7*	*7.4*	*0.5*	*0.0*
ELICHE								
Dry Weight, Buitoni*	1 Serving/80g	282	1.5	352	11.2	72.6	1.9	0.0
ELK								
Raw, Meat only	1 Serving/100g	111	1.4	111	22.9	0.0	1.4	0.0
Roasted, Meat only	1 Serving/100g	146	1.9	146	30.2	0.0	1.9	0.0
ENCHILADAS								
3 Bean, Ready Meal, Average	1 Pack/400g	505	16.6	126	4.4	16.9	4.2	3.2
Beef, Light Choices, Tesco*	1 Pack/400g	440	11.2	110	5.4	13.4	2.8	3.1
Chicken, American, HL, Tesco*	1 Serving/240g	353	4.3	147	10.4	22.5	1.8	1.2
Chicken, Average	1 Serving/295g	483	18.8	164	11.6	16.0	6.4	1.7
Chicken, Diner Specials, M & S*	½ Pack/227g	340	12.0	150	9.9	15.4	5.3	2.0
Chicken, in a Spicy Salsa & Bean Sauce, Asda*	½ Pack/212g	373	17.0	176	10.0	16.0	8.0	0.0
Chicken, Perfectly Balanced, Waitrose*	1 Pack/450g	481	14.4	107	6.9	12.7	3.2	1.1
Chicken, Suiza, Smart Ones, Weight Watchers*	1 Pack/255g	290	5.0	114	4.3	18.0	2.0	1.2
Spicy, Three Bean, Cooked, Chosen By You, Asda*	1 Pack/400g	466	15.9	117	4.4	13.7	4.0	4.1
Three Bean, Vegetarian, Tesco*	1 Pack/440g	572	24.6	130	4.9	14.1	5.6	3.3
Vegetable, GFY, Asda*	1 Pack/350g	399	15.7	114	4.4	14.0	4.5	1.3
Vegetable, Morrisons*	1 Pack/400g	468	18.4	117	4.5	14.4	4.6	1.8
Vegetable & Bean, Eat Smart, Morrisons*	1 Pack/380g	475	9.9	125	4.7	20.7	2.6	3.2
ENDIVE								
Raw	*1oz/28g*	*4*	*0.1*	*13*	*1.8*	*1.0*	*0.2*	*2.0*
ENERGY DRINK								
Cherry, Lucozade*	1 Bottle/500ml	345	0.0	69	0.0	17.1	0.0	0.0
Citrus, Isotonic, Umbro*	1 Bottle/500ml	139	0.0	28	0.0	6.5	0.0	0.0
Coffee & Guarana, Self Heat Can, Rocket Fuel*	1 Can/200ml	70	1.0	35	1.4	4.1	0.5	0.1
Isostar Sport, Isostar*	1 Glass/250ml	74	0.0	30	0.0	7.0	0.0	0.0
Juiced Berry, Relentless*	1 Can/500g	230	0.0	46	0.0	10.7	0.0	0.0
Juiced Orange & Tropical Fruit, Relentless*	1 Can/500ml	230	0.0	46	0.0	10.4	0.0	0.0
Libertus, Blue, Sugar Free, Relentless*	1 Can/500ml	20	0.0	4	0.0	0.0	0.0	0.0
Monster*	1 Can/500ml	240	0.0	48	0.0	12.0	0.0	0.0
Orange, Isotonic, Myprotein*	1 Bottle/500ml	147	0.0	29	0.0	6.9	0.0	0.0
Original, Rockstar*	1 Can/500ml	290	0.0	60	0.4	13.6	0.0	0.0
Red Devil, Britvic*	1 Can/250ml	160	0.0	64	0.4	15.1	0.0	0.0
Redcard, Britvic*	1 Can/330ml	96	0.0	29	0.1	7.0	0.0	0.0
Relentless, Original, Relentless*	1 Can/500ml	230	0.0	46	0.0	10.4	0.0	0.0
Relentless, Sugar Free, Coca-Cola*	1 Can/500ml	20	0.0	4	0.0	0.0	0.0	0.0
Revive, Cranberry with Acai, Light Sparkling, Lucozade*	1 Bottle/380ml	50	0.0	13	0.0	2.8	0.0	0.0
SoBe, Appleberry Burst, Britvic*	1 Can/250ml	135	0.0	54	0.4	12.0	0.0	0.0
Sugar Free, Diet, Mountain Dew, Britvic*	1 Can/440ml	3	0.0	1	0.0	0.0	0.0	0.0

	Measure INFO/WEIGHT	per Measure KCAL	FAT	Nutrition Values per 100g / 100ml KCAL	PROT	CARB	FAT	FIBRE
FAGGOTS								
in Rich Gravy, Iceland*	1 Faggot/81g	116	5.2	143	6.5	15.9	6.4	1.1
Mushy Peas & Mash, Sainsbury's*	1 Pack/450g	576	19.3	128	6.0	16.3	4.3	1.6
Pork & Onion Gravy, 222, Oakhouse Foods Ltd*	1 Meal/360g	299	9.0	83	4.9	10.9	2.5	1.6
FAJITA								
Beef, GFY, Asda*	½ Pack/208g	354	9.8	170	11.0	21.0	4.7	1.6
Chicken, Average	1 Serving/275g	409	14.7	149	10.1	15.0	5.3	2.3
Chicken, COU, M & S*	1 Pack/230g	287	5.3	125	10.0	16.5	2.3	1.5
Chicken, GFY, Asda*	½ Pack/225g	233	4.1	104	9.3	12.9	1.8	2.0
Crispy Chicken, Old El Paso*	1 Fajita/70g	183	5.4	263	7.6	41.0	7.8	1.8
Gammon Steaks, Tesco*	1 Serving/250g	367	15.5	147	17.5	5.3	6.2	0.0
Meal Kit, Tesco*	1 Serving/100g	210	3.4	210	6.1	38.2	3.4	2.1
Mini Chicken, Tesco*	1 Fajita/18g	37	1.1	205	8.7	27.8	6.3	3.4
Steak, M & S*	1oz/28g	53	2.5	190	8.9	17.2	9.1	0.6
Vegetable	1 Serving/275g	472	14.9	171	4.9	25.5	5.4	1.9
Vegetable, Somerfield*	1 Pack/500g	640	25.0	128	3.0	17.0	5.0	0.0
Vegetable, Tesco*	1 Fajita/112g	133	5.6	119	4.2	14.3	5.0	1.1
FALAFEL								
Asda*	½ Pack/50g	140	9.5	281	8.3	18.9	19.1	8.2
Falafel, Mix, Organic, Wheat & Gluten Free, Hale & Hearty*	1 Falafel/11g	75	1.4	301	19.2	43.8	5.5	10.7
Fried in Vegetable Oil, Average	1 Falafel/25g	45	2.8	179	6.4	15.6	11.2	3.4
Gourmet, Meat Free, Vegideli, The Redwood Co*	1 Patty/17g	26	1.4	159	6.1	20.5	8.5	8.1
Mini, M & S*	1 Falafel/14g	43	2.5	310	7.9	28.1	18.4	2.6
Mini, Sainsbury's*	1 Serving/168g	499	29.6	297	8.0	26.8	17.6	3.2
Mix, Authentic, Al'fez*	1 Serving/100g	235	13.8	235	7.1	26.3	13.8	8.8
Mix, Lebanese Style, Al'fez*	½ Pack/200g	470	27.6	235	7.1	26.3	13.8	0.0
Mix, Organic, Quick & Easy, Hale & Hearty*	1 Pack/200g	646	11.0	323	19.2	43.8	5.5	10.7
Organic, Cauldron Foods*	1 Falafel/25g	51	2.4	203	8.4	20.3	9.8	7.2
Vegab Mat Ab, Vegab*	1 Falafel/20g	62	3.4	309	11.0	28.0	17.0	0.0
Vegetarian, Organic, Waitrose*	1 Falafel/25g	55	2.6	220	8.0	23.3	10.5	7.6
FANTA								
Apple, Z, Coca-Cola*	1 Can/330ml	13	0.0	4	0.0	0.6	0.0	0.0
Icy Lemon, Coca-Cola*	1 Can/330ml	165	0.0	50	0.0	12.2	0.0	0.0
Icy Lemon, Zero, Coca-Cola*	1 Can/330ml	7	0.0	2	0.0	0.2	0.0	0.0
Lemon, Coca-Cola*	1 Can/330ml	165	0.0	50	0.0	12.0	0.0	0.0
Light, Coca-Cola*	1 Glass/250ml	5	0.0	2	0.0	0.5	0.0	0.0
Orange, Coca-Cola*	1 Glass/250ml	75	0.0	30	0.0	7.1	0.0	0.0
Orange, Zero, Coca-Cola*	1 Can/330ml	11	0.0	3	0.0	0.5	0.0	0.0
Peach, Singapore, Coca-Cola*	1 Bottle/500ml	230	0.0	46	0.0	11.0	0.0	0.0
Summer Fruits, Z, Coca-Cola*	1 fl oz/30ml	1	0.0	3	0.0	0.6	0.0	0.0
FARFALLE								
Bows, Dry, Average	*1 Serving/75g*	*265*	*1.4*	*353*	*11.4*	*72.6*	*1.9*	*1.9*
FENNEL								
Florence, Boiled in Salted Water	*1oz/28g*	*3*	*0.1*	*11*	*0.9*	*1.5*	*0.2*	*2.3*
Florence, Raw, Unprepared, Average	*1 Bulb/250g*	*30*	*0.5*	*12*	*0.9*	*1.8*	*0.2*	*2.4*
Florence, Steamed	*1 Serving/80g*	*9*	*0.2*	*11*	*9.0*	*1.5*	*0.2*	*2.3*
FENUGREEK								
Leaves, Raw, Fresh, Average	*1 Serving/80g*	*28*	*0.2*	*35*	*4.6*	*4.8*	*0.2*	*1.1*
FETTUCINI								
Cajun Chicken, Chosen By You, Asda*	1 Pack/400g	360	5.2	90	6.3	12.6	1.3	1.4
Chicken, Cajun, GFY, Asda*	1 Pack/400g	384	7.6	96	8.9	9.7	1.9	2.4
Chicken, Cajun Spiced, COU, M & S*	1 Pack/400g	400	8.0	100	8.0	12.3	2.0	1.3
Chicken Mushroom, GFY, Asda*	1 Pack/400g	359	7.0	90	7.2	11.2	1.7	0.7
Dry Weight, Buitoni*	1 Serving/90g	326	1.5	362	12.2	74.4	1.7	0.0

F

	Measure INFO/WEIGHT	per Measure KCAL	FAT	Nutrition Values per 100g / 100ml KCAL	PROT	CARB	FAT	FIBRE
FIG ROLLS								
Asda*	1 Biscuit/19g	71	1.7	372	4.8	68.0	9.0	0.0
Bolands*	1 Biscuit/18g	60	1.3	333	3.3	63.9	7.2	3.9
Go Ahead, McVitie's*	1 Biscuit/15g	55	0.7	365	4.2	76.8	4.6	2.9
Jacob's*	1 Biscuit/18g	68	1.5	380	4.0	71.4	8.5	3.3
Sainsbury's*	1 Biscuit/19g	70	1.7	377	4.8	68.3	9.4	2.6
Vitalinea, Jacob's*	1 Biscuit/18g	61	1.0	339	3.7	68.2	5.8	3.8
FIGS								
Dried, Average	***1 Fig/14g***	***32***	***0.1***	***232***	***3.6***	***53.2***	***1.1***	***8.6***
Fresh, Black Bursa, Morrisons*	1 Fig/54g	119	0.8	221	3.3	48.6	1.5	6.9
in Light Syrup, Asda*	1 Serving/100g	75	0.1	75	0.4	18.0	0.1	0.7
Raw, Fresh, Average	***1 Fig/35g***	***16***	***0.1***	***45***	***1.3***	***9.8***	***0.2***	***1.5***
FISH								
Balls, Gefilte, M & S*	1 Pack/200g	280	7.8	140	14.1	11.9	3.9	1.0
Breaded, Asda*	1 Serving/150g	351	21.0	234	15.0	12.0	14.0	0.5
Crumbed, Pak-N-Save*	2 Pieces/140g	298	17.8	213	10.8	13.9	12.7	0.0
Dried, Small, Ogura*	1 Serving/10g	32	0.3	320	69.0	0.3	3.0	0.0
Fillet, Dinner, Light & Easy, Youngs*	1 Pack/385g	362	15.8	94	6.2	8.2	4.1	1.4
Fillets, Garlic & Herb, Youngs*	1 Fillet/118g	261	14.8	222	11.0	16.2	12.6	1.4
Fillets, Lemon & Pepper, Youngs*	1 Fillet/130g	283	16.7	218	10.3	15.3	12.9	4.3
Fillets, Lime & Chilli, Fish Fusions, Birds Eye*	1 Portion/160g	270	10.1	169	15.0	12.9	6.3	0.5
Fillets, White, Breaded, Tesco*	1 Piece/95g	198	10.4	208	10.6	16.9	10.9	1.0
Fillets, White, Breaded, Value, Tesco*	1 Serving/100g	192	9.7	192	10.6	15.6	9.7	2.2
Fillets, White, Natural, Tesco*	1 Fillet/100g	72	0.6	72	16.6	0.0	0.6	0.0
Goujons, Asda*	1 Serving/125g	240	8.0	192	12.8	20.8	6.4	0.2
Nuggets, Battered, Farmfoods*	1oz/28g	60	3.3	214	10.9	16.0	11.8	0.7
Portion, Chip Shop, Youngs*	1 Portion/135g	315	19.7	233	11.0	15.1	14.6	0.6
Portion, in Oven Crisp Batter, Value, Tesco*	1 Serving/100g	209	11.0	209	11.0	16.4	11.0	2.6
Salted, Chinese, Steamed	1oz/28g	43	0.6	155	33.9	0.0	2.2	0.0
Seaside Shapes, Birds Eye*	2 Pieces/80g	197	11.2	246	11.0	19.0	14.0	1.1
Steaks, Chip Shop, Youngs*	1 Serving/100g	198	10.4	198	11.0	14.9	10.4	0.9
White, Battered, Skinless & Boneless, Farmfoods*	1 Serving/122g	238	12.3	195	9.3	16.7	10.1	2.3
White, Breaded, Fillets, Ocean Pure*	1 Fillet/113g	276	11.5	245	20.8	16.9	10.2	1.2
White, Smoked, Average	1 Serving/100g	108	0.9	108	23.4	0.0	0.9	0.0
White, Tesco*	1 Fillet/100g	78	0.6	78	16.6	0.0	0.6	0.0
FISH & CHIPS								
Breaded, Budgens*	1 Pack/340g	544	18.0	160	8.6	19.3	5.3	1.5
Budgens*	1 Pack/284g	625	28.4	220	8.0	24.5	10.0	2.3
Cod, Asda*	1 Serving/280g	450	14.0	161	8.0	21.0	5.0	1.1
Cod, HL, Tesco*	1 Pack/400g	492	7.2	123	5.3	21.4	1.8	1.7
Co-Op*	1 Pack/250g	387	15.0	155	6.0	18.0	6.0	2.0
Ross*	1 Serving/250g	415	19.0	166	6.2	18.1	7.6	1.6
Somerfield*	1 Serving/283g	495	17.0	175	8.0	22.0	6.0	0.0
Tesco*	1 Serving/300g	489	18.6	163	5.5	21.2	6.2	1.6
with Mushy Peas, Kershaws*	1 Pack/315g	450	18.3	143	6.4	16.4	5.8	1.6
FISH CAKES								
Cod, Birds Eye*	1 Cake/51g	93	4.4	182	10.0	16.0	8.7	1.1
Cod, Chunky, Breaded, Chilled, Youngs*	1 Cake/90g	192	11.5	213	9.5	14.9	12.8	1.2
Cod, Homemade, Average	1 Cake/50g	120	8.3	241	9.3	14.4	16.6	0.7
Cod, Macfisheries*	1 Cake/85g	164	7.0	192	7.6	22.1	8.2	1.1
Fried in Blended Oil	1 Cake/50g	109	6.7	218	8.6	16.8	13.4	0.0
Frozen, Average	1 Cake/85g	112	3.3	132	8.6	16.7	3.9	0.0
Grilled, Average	1 Cake/50g	77	2.2	154	9.9	19.7	4.5	0.0
Haddock, Smoked, Breaded, Asda*	1 Cake/90g	202	11.7	225	9.0	18.0	13.0	1.6

FISH CAKES

	Measure INFO/WEIGHT	KCAL	FAT	KCAL	PROT	CARB	FAT	FIBRE
Haddock, Smoked, Frozen, Waitrose*	1 Cake/85g	186	10.3	219	9.6	17.8	12.1	0.8
Haddock, Smoked, M & S*	1 Cake/85g	153	8.0	180	10.6	13.4	9.4	2.6
Haddock, Smoked, Sainsbury's*	1 Cake/63g	127	6.0	201	11.0	17.8	9.5	2.1
Prawn, Battered, Asda*	1 Cake/90g	182	10.0	202	10.0	15.6	11.1	1.0
Prawn, Sainsbury's*	1 Cake/90g	184	7.8	204	9.6	21.7	8.7	1.2
Salmon, & Broccoli, Morrisons*	1 Cake/60g	126	7.1	210	9.8	17.2	11.9	1.3
Salmon, Birds Eye*	1 Cake/50g	84	4.5	168	9.5	12.2	9.0	1.4
Salmon, Breaded, Crispy, Frozen, Sainsbury's*	1 Cake/60g	140	8.7	234	12.2	13.7	14.5	1.9
Salmon, Chunky, Sainsbury's*	1 Cake/84g	192	10.5	228	13.2	15.8	12.5	2.9
Salmon, Coated in a Light & Crispy Breadcrumb, Tesco*	1 Cake/90g	211	10.8	235	9.7	21.0	12.0	1.2
Salmon, Homemade, Average	1 Cake/50g	136	9.8	273	10.4	14.4	19.7	0.7
Salmon, in Crunch Crumb, Birds Eye*	1 Cake/50g	107	6.4	216	9.7	15.0	13.0	1.4
Salmon, VLH Kitchens	1 Cake/56g	155	35.7	278	10.5	14.4	20.0	0.6
Salmon & Dill, Cook*	1 Cake/95g	144	5.3	152	11.3	14.2	5.6	1.5
Salmon & Tarragon, Waitrose*	1 Cake/85g	179	10.0	211	11.9	14.3	11.8	2.2
Smoked Haddock, with Cheddar & Leek, TTD, Sainsbury's*	1 Cake/145g	123	6.1	85	0.0	0.0	4.2	0.0
Thai, Finest, Tesco*	1 Cake/65g	149	8.6	230	7.5	20.3	13.2	1.6
Thai, Frozen, Sainsbury's*	1 Cake/15g	28	1.1	187	21.3	9.3	7.3	0.7
Thai Prawn, Morrisons*	1 Cake/90g	211	9.6	234	7.9	26.4	10.7	0.3
Thai Style, Sainsbury's*	1 Cake/49g	69	2.1	141	12.0	13.8	4.2	1.7
Tuna, Asda*	1 Cake/75g	185	10.1	247	14.9	16.5	13.5	1.4
Tuna, Lime & Coriander, BGTY, Sainsbury's*	1 Cake/91g	200	10.7	220	10.7	17.7	11.8	2.6
Tuna, Sainsbury's*	1 Cake/90g	183	7.5	203	13.7	18.4	8.3	2.1
Tuna, Tesco*	1 Cake/90g	222	9.4	247	12.8	25.4	10.5	0.2
Tuna & Red Pepper, Waitrose*	1 Cake/85g	175	10.0	206	9.5	15.4	11.8	1.6

FISH FINGERS

	Measure INFO/WEIGHT	KCAL	FAT	KCAL	PROT	CARB	FAT	FIBRE
Chip Shop, Youngs*	1 Finger/30g	75	4.9	251	9.3	16.6	16.4	1.2
Cod, 100% Cod Fillet, Tesco*	1 Finger/30g	53	2.2	177	12.4	14.9	7.5	1.4
Cod, Chunky, Tesco*	1 Finger/40g	70	3.0	175	12.3	14.3	7.6	1.6
Cod, Fillet, Asda*	1 Finger/31g	66	3.1	214	13.0	18.0	10.0	0.0
Cod, Fillet, Chunky, M & S*	1 Finger/40g	70	2.4	175	12.0	17.2	6.0	1.0
Cod, Fillet, Waitrose*	1 Finger/30g	55	2.2	183	11.9	16.9	7.5	0.7
Cod, Fried in Blended Oil, Average	1 Finger/28g	67	3.9	238	13.2	15.5	14.1	0.6
Cod, Frozen, Average	1 Finger/28g	48	2.2	170	11.6	14.2	7.8	0.6
Cod, Grilled, Average	1 Finger/28g	56	2.5	200	14.3	16.6	8.9	0.7
Cod, Morrisons*	1 Finger/30g	54	2.2	180	11.7	16.4	7.5	1.1
Cod, Sainsbury's*	1 Finger/28g	53	2.1	190	12.5	17.7	7.7	1.0
Economy, Sainsbury's*	1 Finger/26g	51	2.2	198	12.6	17.7	8.5	1.3
Farmfoods*	1 Finger/27g	49	2.2	183	12.2	15.6	8.0	1.2
Free From, Sainsbury's*	1 Finger/30g	56	2.3	188	11.4	18.0	7.8	0.7
Haddock, Fillet, Asda*	1 Finger/30g	61	2.7	205	14.0	17.0	9.0	0.0
Haddock in Crispy Batter, Birds Eye*	1 Finger/30g	56	2.3	188	14.3	15.1	7.8	0.7
Haddock in Crunchy Crumb, Morrisons*	1 Finger/30g	57	2.4	190	13.1	16.3	8.0	1.1
Hoki, Fillet, Birds Eye*	1 Finger/30g	58	2.7	193	12.6	15.6	8.9	0.7
Ross*	1 Finger/26g	50	2.3	193	10.7	17.7	8.8	0.8
Sainsbury's*	1 Finger/27g	52	2.3	194	13.4	16.0	8.5	0.7
Salmon, Birds Eye*	1 Finger/28g	63	2.7	225	13.2	21.7	9.5	0.9

FISH IN

	Measure INFO/WEIGHT	KCAL	FAT	KCAL	PROT	CARB	FAT	FIBRE
Batter, Morrisons*	1 Fish/140g	235	8.1	168	14.0	15.0	5.8	0.2
Batter, Youngs*	1 Serving/100g	315	19.7	315	14.9	20.4	19.7	0.8
Butter Sauce, Steaks, Youngs*	1 Steak/150g	115	4.2	77	10.2	2.8	2.8	0.8
Butter Sauce, Value, Tesco*	1 Portion/150g	127	3.7	85	10.5	5.2	2.5	1.5
Parsley Sauce, Steaks, Ross*	1 Serving/150g	123	5.5	82	9.1	3.1	3.7	0.1

F

	Measure INFO/WEIGHT	per Measure KCAL	FAT	Nutrition Values per 100g / 100ml KCAL	PROT	CARB	FAT	FIBRE
FIVE SPICE								
Powder, Sharwood's*	1 Tsp/2g	3	0.2	172	12.2	11.6	8.6	23.4
FLAKE								
Cadbury*	1 Bar/32g	170	9.9	530	8.1	55.6	30.8	0.7
Dipped, Cadbury*	1 Bar/41g	215	12.5	530	7.6	56.1	30.8	0.8
Luxury, Cadbury*	1 Bar/45g	240	13.6	533	7.3	57.8	30.2	0.0
Praline, Cadbury*	1 Bar/38g	201	12.9	535	7.7	49.5	34.3	0.0
Snow, Cadbury*	1 Bar/36g	198	11.1	550	7.2	60.1	30.9	0.0
FLAN								
Cauliflower, Cheese & Broccoli, Hot, Sainsbury's*	¼ Flan/100g	303	19.8	303	6.4	24.7	19.8	1.2
Cheese & Onion, M & S*	1oz/28g	81	5.2	290	6.1	25.1	18.7	1.4
Cheese & Potato, Hot, Tesco*	¼ Flan/100g	282	19.7	282	6.0	20.0	19.7	2.3
Chicken & Smoked Bacon, Hot, Sainsbury's*	¼ Flan/100g	293	18.5	293	10.2	21.5	18.5	1.2
Mediterranean Vegetable, Co-Op*	¼ Flan/88g	188	10.5	215	4.0	22.0	12.0	3.0
Pastry with Fruit	1oz/28g	33	1.2	118	1.4	19.3	4.4	0.7
Sponge with Fruit	1oz/28g	31	0.4	112	2.8	23.3	1.5	0.6
FLAN CASE								
Sponge, Average	***1oz/28g***	***90***	***1.5***	***320***	***7.0***	***62.5***	***5.4***	***0.7***
FLAPJACK								
7 Fruits, Graze*	1 Punnet/55g	223	10.5	406	5.1	54.9	19.1	4.3
90% Fat Free, Cookie Coach*	1 Flapjack/75g	287	7.4	383	7.0	66.2	9.9	0.0
All Butter, Organic, Sainsbury's*	1 Flapjack/35g	156	8.0	446	5.3	54.5	23.0	2.7
All Butter, Sainsbury's*	1 Flapjack/35g	156	8.0	446	5.7	54.5	22.8	2.7
All Butter, Squares, M & S*	1 Flapjack/34g	150	7.2	441	6.2	56.2	21.2	4.4
All Butter, Waitrose*	1 Flapjack/34g	126	9.0	376	3.8	52.4	26.8	1.2
Almond, Hazlenut & Almond, Seriously Nutty, Waitrose*	1 Square/26g	133	8.4	517	9.2	46.7	32.6	3.1
Apple & Raspberry, Fox's*	1 Flapjack/26g	105	5.0	403	4.8	52.5	19.4	3.7
Apple & Sultana, Mr Kipling*	1 Flapjack/27g	123	6.0	456	4.6	59.0	22.4	3.6
Banana, The Handmade Flapjack Company*	1 Flapjack/90g	379	13.1	421	5.3	67.2	14.6	0.0
Banoffee, Iced, Devondale*	1 Flapjack/95g	427	24.7	450	3.6	51.0	26.0	2.5
Bite Sized Honeyjack, Kate's Cakes Ltd*	1 Serving/100g	436	23.9	436	5.5	49.9	23.9	4.1
Black Cherry, Blackfriars*	1 Serving/110g	529	25.3	481	5.0	63.0	23.0	0.0
Butter, Mr Kipling*	1 Flapjack/75g	337	15.9	450	5.4	59.6	21.2	3.2
Chocolate, McVitie's*	1 Flapjack/85g	422	23.0	496	6.6	56.6	27.1	3.2
Chocolate, The Handmade Flapjack Company*	1 Flapjack/90g	391	17.6	435	6.0	58.6	19.5	0.0
Chocolate & Hazelnut, M & S*	1 Flapjack/71g	330	18.1	465	7.3	55.6	25.5	3.8
Chocolate Chip, Boots*	1 Flapjack/75g	313	11.2	417	5.6	65.0	15.0	3.5
Chocolate Chip, Happy Shopper*	1 Flapjack/35g	163	8.2	467	5.7	58.7	23.3	0.0
Chocolate Dipped, M & S*	1 Flapjack/96g	442	21.5	460	6.1	61.3	22.4	3.0
Chocolate Special, The Handmade Flapjack Company*	1 Flapjack/90g	392	17.8	436	5.7	58.7	19.8	0.0
Chunky Chocolate, M & S*	1 FlapJack/80g	348	15.1	435	5.8	59.9	18.9	2.2
Co-Op*	1 Flapjack/38g	175	9.4	465	5.0	54.0	25.0	4.0
Cranberry, Apple & Raisin, Light Choices, Tesco*	1 Flapjack/30g	97	1.7	325	5.7	63.1	5.6	5.7
Date & Walnut, The Handmade Flapjack Company*	1 Flapjack/90g	360	13.5	400	6.1	60.2	14.9	0.0
Fruit, GFY, Asda*	1 Flapjack/45g	173	3.6	384	6.0	72.0	8.0	3.4
Fruit, Mr Kipling*	1 Flapjack/75g	306	13.6	408	4.8	56.7	18.1	3.0
Fruit, Somerfield*	1 Flapjack/45g	182	7.4	405	6.3	57.9	16.5	5.0
Fruit, Tesco*	1 Flapjack/33g	136	5.2	412	5.7	62.0	15.7	4.0
Hob Nobs, Milk Chocolate, McVitie's*	1 Flapjack/35g	155	6.0	443	5.8	64.2	17.2	4.2
Honey & Clotted Cream, Devondale*	1 Flapjack/95g	419	23.7	441	4.6	48.0	25.0	3.5
Honey Almond, Multigrain, Devondale*	1 Flapjack/80g	352	20.5	440	4.7	49.0	25.6	3.2
Lemon, Multigrain, Devondale*	1 Flapjack/80g	341	18.2	426	3.9	51.0	22.8	2.9
M & S*	1 Flapjack/53g	228	10.1	430	6.0	59.1	19.0	3.5
Milk Chocolate Digestive, McVitie's*	1 Flapjack/65g	293	13.8	451	5.4	59.7	21.2	3.4

F

	Measure INFO/WEIGHT	per Measure KCAL	FAT	Nutrition Values per 100g / 100ml KCAL	PROT	CARB	FAT	FIBRE
FLAPJACK								
Millionaire, Gu, Naughties*	1 Flapjack/19g	87	4.8	465	4.9	54.2	25.4	2.2
Plain, The Handmade Flapjack Company*	1 Flapjack/90g	398	19.2	442	5.4	57.1	21.3	0.0
Raspberry, Devondale*	1 Flapjack/95g	406	21.7	427	4.0	51.0	22.8	3.0
Snickers, McVitie's*	1 Flapjack/65g	315	18.5	484	7.9	49.0	28.5	6.0
Strawberries & Cream, Iced, Devondale*	1 Flapjack/95g	427	24.1	449	3.3	53.2	25.4	2.3
Strawberry, Multigrain, Devondale*	1 Flapjack/80g	341	18.2	426	3.9	51.6	22.8	2.9
Sultana, Tesco*	1 Flapjack/50g	173	10.0	346	5.0	36.2	20.1	3.7
Sunflower & Raisin, Devondale*	1 Flapjack/95g	426	25.0	448	5.2	47.9	26.3	3.2
Toffee, Finest, Tesco*	1 Flapjack/35g	156	6.7	446	4.9	63.6	19.1	1.3
Toffee Apple, Iced, Devondale*	1 Flapjack/95g	427	24.1	449	3.6	53.2	25.4	2.7
Toffeemac, The Handmade Flapjack Company*	1 Flapjack/90g	411	19.7	457	6.1	59.0	21.9	0.0
Triple Choc, Iced, Devondale*	1 Flapjack/95g	439	23.7	462	3.8	51.0	25.0	3.2
Tropical Mix, Reduced Fat, Fabulous Bakin' Boys*	1 Flapjack/90g	346	10.8	385	6.0	63.0	12.0	3.0
Walnut & Maple, Devondale*	1 Flapjack/95g	445	27.5	468	4.0	45.2	29.0	3.2
Yoghurt & Apricot, Iced, Devondale*	1 Flapjack/95g	443	25.6	466	4.5	51.0	27.0	3.3
FLATBREAD								
BBQ Chicken, Improved, Shapers, Boots*	1 Pack/165g	268	3.8	162	10.0	25.0	2.3	1.2
Chargrilled Chicken, COU, M & S*	1 Pack/163g	245	3.1	150	10.8	23.0	1.9	5.2
Cheese & Onion, Swedish Style, Shapers, Boots*	1 Bread/127g	265	10.3	209	10.0	24.0	8.1	1.3
Chicken & Mango Salad, Sainsbury's*	1 Pack/100g	251	2.5	251	16.9	40.4	2.5	2.5
Chicken Tikka, BGTY, Sainsbury's*	1 Bread/188g	241	2.6	128	10.3	18.5	1.4	2.0
Chicken Tikka, Shapers, Boots*	1 Bread/164g	269	4.1	164	11.0	24.0	2.5	1.5
Chinese Chicken, COU, M & S*	1 Bread/156g	281	4.4	180	13.9	24.3	2.8	2.2
Chinese Chicken, Shapers, Boots*	1 Pack/159g	274	2.1	172	11.0	29.0	1.3	1.8
Feta Cheese, Shapers, Boots*	1 Pack/166g	255	6.5	154	6.7	23.0	3.9	1.4
Gluten, Wheat & Milk Free, 4 Pack, Free From, Livwell*	1 Bread/55g	148	2.9	269	6.4	53.6	5.3	4.5
Greek Feta Salad, Boots*	1 Pack/158g	241	5.7	153	6.4	24.0	3.6	1.2
Greek Style, GFY, Asda*	1 Bread/165g	256	7.1	155	7.0	22.0	4.3	2.1
Greek Style Salad, Waitrose*	1 Pack/172g	280	8.4	163	7.4	22.3	4.9	3.3
Italian Chicken, Improved, Shapers, Boots*	1 Pack/151g	263	6.8	174	11.0	22.0	4.5	1.8
King Prawn Tikka, Waitrose*	1 Pack/165g	257	3.3	156	9.4	25.1	2.0	1.5
Mediterranean Chicken, Ginsters*	1 Pack/168g	302	6.7	180	10.6	25.5	4.0	0.0
Mediterranean Tuna, Ginsters*	1 Pack/167g	297	6.3	178	10.3	25.6	3.8	0.0
Mexican, Chicken, Stonebaked, Finest, Tesco*	1 Pack/155g	280	5.1	180	11.7	25.1	3.3	1.6
Mexican Style Chicken, GFY, Asda*	1 Pack/161g	241	3.2	150	13.0	20.0	2.0	2.5
Peking Duck, Less Than 3% Fat, Shapers, Boots*	1 Pack/156g	246	3.7	158	7.2	27.0	2.4	1.9
Rancher's Chicken, COU, M & S*	1 Pack/174g	270	3.5	155	10.9	23.0	2.0	1.5
Ranchers Chicken, Shapers, Boots*	1 Pack/194g	303	4.3	156	12.0	22.0	2.2	1.5
Salsa Chicken, Shapers, Boots*	1 Pack/191g	328	8.4	172	11.0	22.0	4.4	1.6
Spiced Chicken & Mango, Love Life, Waitrose*	1 Pack/174g	298	4.7	171	9.7	26.1	2.7	1.9
Spicy Chicken, Shapers, Boots*	1 Pack/181g	292	4.5	161	11.0	23.0	2.5	0.0
Spicy Mexican, New, Shapers, Boots*	1 Pack/184g	281	5.0	153	8.0	24.0	2.7	1.9
Spicy Mexican, Shapers, Boots*	1 Pack/190g	296	7.6	156	7.0	23.0	4.0	3.7
Sticky BBQ Style Chicken, Shapers, Boots*	1 Pack/158g	274	7.3	173	10.0	23.0	4.6	2.8
Tomato & Chilli, Sainsbury's*	¼ Bread/65g	155	3.1	238	11.9	36.9	4.7	2.8
FLAXSEED								
Milled, Organic, Linwoods*	2 Dtsp/30g	153	13.9	510	21.9	1.7	46.2	28.9
Organic, Premium Ground, Prewett's*	1 Tbsp/15g	73	6.0	489	24.0	2.0	40.0	23.0
FLORENTINES								
Mince Tarts, Gluten & Wheat Free, Lovemore*	1 Tart/45g	183	8.3	407	4.5	55.7	18.4	2.5
FLOUR								
00 Grade, Pasta, TTD, Sainsbury's*	1 Bag/1000g	3390	13.0	339	11.5	70.3	1.3	3.0
Arrowroot, Average	**_1oz/28g_**	**_100_**	**_0.0_**	**_357_**	**_0.3_**	**_88.1_**	**_0.1_**	**_3.4_**

	Measure INFO/WEIGHT	per Measure KCAL	FAT	Nutrition Values per 100g / 100ml KCAL	PROT	CARB	FAT	FIBRE
FLOUR								
Bread, Brown, Strong, Average	*1 Serving/100g*	*311*	*1.8*	*311*	*14.0*	*61.0*	*1.8*	*6.4*
Bread, White, Strong, Average	*1oz/28g*	*94*	*0.4*	*336*	*11.8*	*68.4*	*1.5*	*3.4*
Brown, Chapati, Average	*1 Tbsp/20g*	*67*	*0.2*	*333*	*11.5*	*73.7*	*1.2*	*0.0*
Brown, Wheat	*1oz/28g*	*90*	*0.5*	*323*	*12.6*	*68.5*	*1.8*	*6.4*
Chakki Wheat Atta, Whole Wheat, Pillsbury*	1 Portion/30g	98	0.5	327	12.0	65.0	1.7	0.0
Chick Pea	*1oz/28g*	*88*	*1.5*	*313*	*19.7*	*49.6*	*5.4*	*10.7*
Gluten Free, Alternative, Wellfoods*	1 Serving/100g	351	1.3	351	1.5	83.1	1.3	2.1
Gram, Stoneground, Gluten & Wheat Free, Dove's Farm*	1 Serving/100g	336	5.0	336	12.8	60.0	5.0	9.7
Millet	*1oz/28g*	*99*	*0.5*	*354*	*5.8*	*75.4*	*1.7*	*0.0*
Peanut, Protein Plus*	¼ Cup/30g	110	4.0	367	53.3	26.7	13.3	13.3
Plain, Average	*1oz/28g*	*98*	*0.4*	*349*	*10.3*	*73.8*	*1.5*	*2.2*
Potato	*1oz/28g*	*92*	*0.3*	*328*	*9.1*	*75.6*	*0.9*	*5.7*
Quinoa	1 Serving/100g	349	5.2	349	14.1	61.4	5.2	3.4
Rice	*1 Tsp/5g*	*18*	*0.0*	*366*	*6.4*	*80.1*	*0.8*	*2.0*
Rye, Whole	*1oz/28g*	*94*	*0.6*	*335*	*8.2*	*75.9*	*2.0*	*11.7*
Sauce, Dry, Sainsbury's*	1 Serving/20g	69	0.3	343	9.8	73.0	1.3	3.0
Soya, Full Fat, Average	*1oz/28g*	*118*	*6.1*	*421*	*37.9*	*19.7*	*21.7*	*11.6*
Soya, Low Fat, Average	*1oz/28g*	*99*	*2.0*	*352*	*45.3*	*28.2*	*7.2*	*13.5*
Speciality Gluten Free, Dove's Farm*	1 Serving/100g	353	1.8	353	4.7	85.2	1.8	2.7
Spelt, Average	*1 Serving/57g*	*216*	*1.7*	*381*	*14.3*	*74.5*	*2.9*	*6.3*
Strong, Wholemeal, Average	*1 Serving/100g*	*315*	*2.2*	*315*	*13.2*	*60.5*	*2.2*	*9.0*
Unbleached, All Purpose, King Arthur Flour*	¼ Cup/30g	110	0.0	367	13.3	73.3	0.0	0.0
White, Average	*1oz/28g*	*89*	*0.3*	*319*	*9.8*	*66.8*	*1.0*	*2.9*
White, Chapati, Average	*1 Tbsp/20g*	*67*	*0.1*	*335*	*9.8*	*77.6*	*0.5*	*0.0*
White, Plain, Value, Tesco*	1oz/28g	94	0.4	335	10.3	70.6	1.3	3.1
White, Self Raising, Average	*1oz/28g*	*94*	*0.4*	*336*	*9.9*	*71.8*	*1.3*	*2.9*
White, Self Raising, Gluten & Wheat Free, Dove's Farm*	1 Serving/100g	344	1.0	344	5.5	78.1	1.0	1.4
White, Wheat, Average	*1oz/28g*	*95*	*0.4*	*341*	*10.4*	*76.5*	*1.3*	*3.1*
Wholemeal, Average	*1oz/28g*	*87*	*0.6*	*312*	*12.6*	*61.9*	*2.2*	*9.0*
Wholemeal, Self Raising, Tesco*	1oz/28g	89	0.6	317	11.5	62.9	2.2	9.0
FLYTE								
Mars*	1 Bar/23g	99	3.2	441	3.4	74.8	14.2	0.0
Snacksize, Mars*	1 Bar/23g	98	3.3	436	3.8	72.5	14.5	0.0
FOOL								
Blackcurrant, BGTY, Sainsbury's*	1 Pot/113g	89	2.9	79	3.5	10.4	2.6	0.6
Fruit, Average	1 Pot/120g	196	11.2	163	1.0	20.2	9.3	1.2
Gooseberry, BFY, Morrisons*	1 Pot/114g	99	3.9	87	3.4	10.7	3.4	0.4
Gooseberry, Perfectly Balanced, Waitrose*	1 Pot/113g	125	2.9	111	3.6	18.3	2.6	0.7
Gooseberry, Sainsbury's*	1 Pot/113g	214	12.9	189	2.6	19.1	11.4	1.1
Gooseberry, Tesco*	1 Pot/112g	225	14.1	200	3.0	17.8	12.5	0.7
Lemon, Fruit, BGTY, Sainsbury's*	1 Pot/113g	94	3.8	83	3.4	9.7	3.4	0.3
Lemon, Fruit, Morrisons*	1 Pot/114g	226	12.9	198	0.0	20.5	11.3	0.0
Raspberry, Fruit, Tesco*	1 Pot/113g	234	12.8	207	2.6	23.6	11.3	0.3
Rhubarb, Fruit, BGTY, Sainsbury's*	1 Pot/120g	91	3.1	76	3.5	9.5	2.6	0.3
Rhubarb, Fruit, Waitrose*	1 Pot/114g	182	12.9	160	2.7	11.9	11.3	0.3
Rhubarb, Perfectly Balanced, Waitrose*	1 Pot/113g	101	2.9	89	3.5	13.0	2.6	0.3
Rhubarb, Sainsbury's*	1 Pot/113g	180	12.9	159	2.6	11.5	11.4	0.4
Strawberry, Fruit, BGTY, Sainsbury's*	1 Pot/120g	100	3.1	83	3.7	11.1	2.6	0.8
Strawberry, GFY, Asda*	1 Pot/114g	95	3.0	83	3.8	11.0	2.6	0.8
FRANKFURTERS								
Average	*1 Frankfurter/42g*	*123*	*11.2*	*292*	*12.0*	*1.3*	*26.6*	*0.0*
FRANKFURTERS VEGETARIAN								
Asda*	1 Frankfurter/27g	54	3.4	199	18.0	3.5	12.5	2.5

	Measure INFO/WEIGHT	per Measure KCAL	FAT	Nutrition Values per 100g / 100ml KCAL	PROT	CARB	FAT	FIBRE
FRANKFURTERS VEGETARIAN								
Tivall*	1 Sausage/30g	73	4.8	244	18.0	7.0	16.0	3.0
FRAZZLES								
Bacon, Smith's, Walkers*	1 Bag/23g	112	5.3	485	6.5	62.0	23.0	1.3
FRENCH FRIES								
Cheese & Onion, Walkers*	1 Pack/22g	95	3.5	430	5.0	66.0	16.0	5.0
Ready Salted, Walkers*	1 Bag/22g	83	3.0	377	4.5	56.4	13.6	4.5
Salt & Vinegar, BGTY, Sainsbury's*	1 Bag/15g	51	0.2	340	6.0	80.1	1.5	4.1
Salt & Vinegar, Walkers*	1 Bag/22g	95	3.5	430	5.0	66.0	16.0	5.0
Worcester Sauce, Walkers*	1 Bag/22g	93	3.7	425	4.5	64.0	17.0	4.1
FRENCH TOAST								
Asda*	1 Toast/8g	30	0.4	381	10.0	74.0	5.0	4.0
Co-Op*	1 Toast/8g	31	0.5	385	10.0	72.0	6.0	5.0
Morrisons*	1 Toast/8g	31	0.5	393	11.0	72.5	6.6	3.0
Sainsbury's*	1 Toast/8g	31	0.5	382	10.0	72.0	6.6	5.0
FRIES								
9/16" Straight Cut Home, Deep Fried, McCain*	1oz/28g	65	2.8	233	3.2	32.7	9.9	0.0
9/16" Straight Cut Home, Oven Baked, McCain*	1oz/28g	53	1.5	188	3.2	31.5	5.5	0.0
American, 3 Way Cook, Somerfield*	1oz/28g	43	1.4	155	3.0	25.0	5.0	0.0
American, Somerfield*	1 Serving/100g	165	5.0	165	2.1	28.0	5.0	4.6
American Style, Frozen, Thin, Tesco*	1 Serving/125g	207	10.1	166	2.2	21.1	8.1	1.9
American Style, Slim, Iceland*	1 Serving/100g	187	6.1	187	2.4	30.6	6.1	2.4
Crispy French, Weighed Deep Fried, McCain*	1 Serving/100g	193	8.5	193	1.9	27.4	8.5	0.9
Curly, Cajun, Weighed Frozen, McCain*	1 Portion/100g	156	8.7	156	1.6	17.7	8.7	1.8
Curly, Southern Style, Tesco*	1 Serving/50g	124	3.6	248	3.8	41.7	7.3	3.8
Curly, Twisters, Frozen, Conagra Foods*	1 Serving/150g	273	13.9	182	2.5	22.0	9.3	2.2
Extra Chunky, Oven Baked, Homefries, McCain*	1 Serving/200g	306	6.2	153	3.2	28.0	3.1	2.3
Oven, American Style, Frozen, Asda*	1 Serving/180g	407	14.4	226	3.9	34.6	8.0	4.0
Oven, Straight Cut, Morrisons*	1 Serving/100g	149	4.3	149	2.8	24.6	4.3	2.6
Seasoned, Conagra Foods*	1 Serving/150g	247	12.0	165	2.4	20.8	8.0	1.9
Southern, Oven Cook, Baked, Potato Winners, McCain*	1 Serving/100g	232	8.3	232	3.6	35.7	8.3	2.4
Southern, Oven Cook, Frozen, Potato Winners, McCain*	1 Serving/100g	176	6.7	176	2.4	26.5	6.7	1.6
Southern Spicy Spiral, Deep Fried, McCain*	1oz/28g	58	2.9	208	2.7	26.4	10.2	0.0
Southern Spicy Spiral, Oven Baked, McCain*	1oz/28g	46	1.8	165	1.7	24.6	6.6	0.0
FRISPS								
Tangy Salt & Vinegar, KP Snacks*	1 Bag/30g	160	10.0	532	5.0	52.6	33.5	2.9
Tasty Cheese & Onion, KP Snacks*	1 Bag/28g	150	9.4	537	5.5	53.2	33.6	3.2
FRITTATA								
Vegetable, Chosen By You, Asda*	1 Frittata/150g	183	7.8	122	6.2	12.1	5.2	1.0
FROG								
Legs, Raw, Meat Only	*1oz/28g*	*20*	*0.1*	*73*	*16.4*	*0.0*	*0.3*	*0.0*
FROMAGE FRAIS								
Apple Pie, Low Fat, Sainsbury's*	1 Pot/90g	108	2.3	120	6.7	17.3	2.6	0.3
Apricot, Layered, Weight Watchers*	1 Pot/100g	46	0.1	46	5.4	5.8	0.1	0.2
Apricot, Tesco*	1 Pot/100g	77	3.0	77	6.5	6.0	3.0	1.3
Bakewell Tart Flavour, BGTY, Sainsbury's*	1 Pot/100g	54	0.2	54	7.6	5.5	0.2	1.1
Banana, Organic, Yeo Valley*	1 Pot/90g	118	5.4	131	6.6	12.6	6.0	0.2
Black Cherry, Asda*	1 Pot/100g	113	5.0	113	4.1	13.0	5.0	0.0
Blackberry, Layered, Weight Watchers*	1 Pot/100g	49	0.2	49	5.5	5.7	0.2	0.4
Blackcurrant, GFY, Asda*	1 Pot/100g	43	0.2	43	6.0	4.2	0.2	0.0
Danone*	1 Pot/100g	73	3.1	73	7.2	3.9	3.1	0.0
Fat Free, Average	*1 Pot/60g*	*35*	*0.1*	*58*	*7.7*	*6.8*	*0.2*	*0.0*
Forest Fruits, Layered, Weight Watchers*	1 Pot/100g	47	0.2	47	5.5	5.7	0.2	0.4
Fruit, Balanced Lifestyle, Aldi*	1 Pot/100g	52	0.2	52	5.4	7.1	0.2	0.7

F

	Measure INFO/WEIGHT	per Measure KCAL	per Measure FAT	Nutrition Values per 100g / 100ml KCAL	PROT	CARB	FAT	FIBRE
FROMAGE FRAIS								
Fruit on the Bottom, BFY, Morrisons*	1 Pot/100g	66	0.1	66	5.6	10.6	0.1	0.0
Lemon Pie, Low Fat, Sainsbury's*	1 Pot/90g	108	2.4	120	6.7	17.3	2.7	0.2
Mandarin & Orange, HL, Tesco*	1 Pot/100g	55	0.2	55	6.2	7.0	0.2	0.3
Mandarin & Orange, Tesco*	1 Pot/100g	75	3.0	75	6.5	5.6	3.0	2.3
Munch Bunch, Nestle*	1 Pot/42g	44	1.3	105	6.7	12.6	3.0	0.0
Natural, Creamy, Co-Op*	1 Pot/200g	204	14.6	102	6.1	2.9	7.3	0.0
Natural, Virtually Fat Free, French, Waitrose*	1 Tub/500g	260	1.5	52	7.3	5.0	0.3	0.0
Normandy, Light Choices, Tesco*	1 Serving/100g	46	0.2	46	7.8	3.3	0.2	0.0
Organic, Vrai*	1 Serving/100g	83	3.6	83	8.1	4.5	3.6	0.0
Peach, BGTY, Sainsbury's*	1 Pot/100g	53	0.2	53	7.2	5.5	0.2	0.5
Peach, Layered, Weight Watchers*	1 Pot/100g	46	0.1	46	5.0	8.0	0.1	0.0
Petit Dessert, Co-Op*	1 Pot/60g	74	2.6	123	6.3	14.5	4.4	0.0
Pineapple & Passion Fruit, HL, Tesco*	1 Pot/100g	55	0.2	55	6.2	7.1	0.2	0.1
Plain, Average	*1oz/28g*	*32*	*2.0*	*113*	*6.8*	*5.7*	*7.1*	*0.0*
Raspberry, COU, M & S*	1 Pot/100g	60	0.2	60	7.0	8.1	0.2	0.5
Raspberry, Healthy Choice, Asda*	1 Pot/100g	41	0.2	41	6.0	3.8	0.2	0.0
Raspberry, Layered, Weight Watchers*	1 Pot/100g	47	0.2	47	5.5	5.7	0.2	0.4
Raspberry, Little Stars, Muller*	1 Pot/60g	66	2.4	110	5.0	12.7	4.0	0.4
Raspberry, Low Fat, Sainsbury's*	1 Pot/90g	96	2.3	107	5.8	15.1	2.6	0.1
Raspberry, Organic, Yeo Valley*	1 Pot/100g	127	6.5	127	6.1	11.1	6.5	0.4
Raspberry & Redcurrant, BGTY, Sainsbury's*	1 Pot/100g	51	0.1	51	7.4	5.4	0.1	1.6
Real Fruit, Tesco*	1 Pot/100g	54	0.1	54	5.6	7.6	0.1	0.1
Red Cherry, Tesco*	1 Pot/100g	75	3.0	75	6.5	5.5	3.0	2.3
Rhubarb & Crumble, Low Fat, Sainsbury's*	1 Pot/90g	96	2.3	107	6.7	14.1	2.6	0.4
Strawberry, 0% Fat, Vitalinea, Danone*	1 Pot/150g	82	0.2	55	6.0	7.4	0.1	1.6
Strawberry, 99.9% Fat Free, Onken*	1 Pot/50g	45	0.0	91	6.9	15.3	0.1	0.0
Strawberry, Balanced Lifestyle, Aldi*	1 Serving/100g	52	0.2	52	5.4	7.1	0.2	0.7
Strawberry, COU, M & S*	1 Pot/100g	60	0.2	60	6.5	8.0	0.2	0.5
Strawberry, GFY, Asda*	1 Pot/100g	58	0.2	58	6.0	8.0	0.2	0.0
Strawberry, Langley Farm*	1 Pot/125g	189	9.7	151	7.0	13.3	7.8	0.0
Strawberry, Low Fat, St Ivel*	1 Pot/100g	69	1.2	69	6.9	6.8	1.2	0.0
Strawberry, Organic, Yeo Valley*	1 Pot/90g	116	5.4	129	6.3	12.5	6.0	0.2
Strawberry, Thomas the Tank Engine, Yoplait*	1 Pot/50g	50	0.6	101	6.8	15.4	1.3	0.0
Strawberry, Value, Tesco*	1 Pot/60g	55	0.8	92	7.2	13.0	1.3	0.0
Strawberry & Raspberry, Organic, Yeo Valley*	1 Pot/90g	118	5.4	131	6.3	12.9	6.0	0.2
Strawberry Cheesecake, Dessert Selection, Sainsbury's*	1 Pot/90g	95	2.2	106	5.8	15.3	2.5	0.1
Strawberry Tart, Sainsbury's*	1 Pot/100g	54	0.2	54	7.6	5.5	0.2	1.1
Toffee & Pecan Pie, Smooth & Creamy, Tesco*	1 Pot/100g	148	6.8	148	6.9	14.8	6.8	0.2
Tropical Fruit, COU, M & S*	1 Pot/100g	60	0.2	60	6.5	8.4	0.2	0.5
Virtually Fat Free, Tesco*	1 Pot/100g	56	0.1	56	5.6	8.2	0.1	0.0
Wildlife, Strawberry, Raspberry Or Peach, Yoplait*	1 Pot/50g	46	0.6	93	7.1	13.2	1.3	0.2
with Fruit, Average	1 Pot/90g	74	2.2	83	6.1	9.0	2.5	0.8
with Fruit, Healthy Range, Average	1 Pot/90g	40	0.1	45	5.8	5.1	0.2	0.3
FROZEN YOGHURT								
Angelmoo, Yoomoo*	1 Pot/150ml	150	2.5	100	2.4	17.7	1.7	2.3
Black Cherry, M & S*	1 Pot/125g	164	1.4	131	3.1	27.1	1.1	0.5
Chocmoo, Yoomoo*	1 Pot/150ml	108	1.3	72	1.8	13.3	0.9	2.1
Chocolate, Average	1 Serving/100g	120	1.9	120	4.3	22.0	1.9	2.1
Chocolate, Snog*	1 Serving/100g	109	1.6	109	4.5	19.9	1.6	1.7
Chocolate Fudge Brownie, Low Fat, Ben & Jerry's*	1 Serving/100g	180	3.0	180	4.0	34.0	3.0	1.5
Devilmoo, Yoomoo*	1 Pot/150ml	151	2.3	101	2.1	18.3	1.5	2.3
Green Tea, Pinkberry*	1 Pot/100g	110	0.0	110	4.0	25.0	0.0	0.0
Lychee, Pinkberry*	1 Pot/140g	154	0.0	110	3.0	23.0	0.0	0.0

	Measure INFO/WEIGHT	per Measure KCAL	FAT	Nutrition Values per 100g / 100ml KCAL	PROT	CARB	FAT	FIBRE
FROZEN YOGHURT								
Nakedmoo, Yoomoo*	1 Serving/76g	102	1.2	134	3.3	24.5	1.6	4.1
Natural, Average	1 Serving/100g	101	0.8	101	3.8	19.9	0.8	0.9
Natural, Snog*	1 Serving/100g	89	0.2	89	3.3	18.4	0.2	0.5
Original, Pinkberry*	1 Pot/140g	140	0.0	100	3.0	21.0	0.0	0.0
Passionfruit, Pinkberry*	1 Pot/140g	140	0.0	100	3.0	22.0	0.0	0.0
Peanut Butter, Pinkberry*	1 Pot/140g	238	9.8	170	7.0	23.0	7.0	1.0
Peppermint, Pinkberry*	1 Pot/140g	154	0.0	110	4.0	24.0	0.0	0.0
Phish Food, Lower Fat, Ben & Jerry's*	½ Pot/211g	464	10.5	220	4.0	40.0	5.0	1.5
Pomegranate, Pinkberry*	1 Pot/140g	168	0.0	120	3.0	26.0	0.0	0.0
Pumpkin, Pinkberry*	1 Pot/140g	154	0.0	110	3.0	23.0	0.0	0.0
Raspberry, Handmade Farmhouse, Sainsbury's*	1 Serving/100g	132	3.8	132	2.7	21.8	3.8	2.2
Raspberry, Orchard Maid*	1 Scrving/80ml	89	1.7	111	2.8	19.9	2.1	0.0
Salted Caramel, Pinkberry*	1 Pot/140g	168	0.0	120	4.0	26.0	0.0	0.0
Strawberry, Average	1 Serving/100g	114	2.2	114	2.6	21.2	2.2	0.5
Strawberry, Tesco*	1 Pot/60g	82	1.3	136	2.6	26.5	2.2	0.8
Strawberry Cheesecake, Low Fat, Ben & Jerry's*	1 Serving/100g	170	3.0	170	4.0	31.0	3.0	1.0
Strawbmoo, Yoomoo*	1 Serving/125ml	102	1.0	82	1.9	17.7	0.8	2.3
Tropicoolmoo, Yoomoo*	1 Pot/92g	136	1.2	148	2.8	29.4	1.3	3.6
Vanilla, Less Than 5% Fat, Tesco*	1 Pot/120g	179	2.9	149	8.1	23.8	2.4	0.7
Watermelon, Pinkberry*	1 Pot/140g	140	0.0	100	3.0	22.0	0.0	0.0
FRUIT								
Apple, Pineapple & Grape, Ready to Eat, Sainsbury's*	1 Pack/180g	94	0.2	52	0.5	8.3	0.1	1.3
Apple & Grape, Bites, Food Explorers, Waitrose*	1 Pack/80g	44	0.1	55	0.4	13.2	0.1	1.4
Apple & Pear, Snack Pack, Great Stuff, Asda*	1 Pack/80g	42	0.1	52	0.4	11.0	0.1	2.6
Berry Medley, Freshly Prepared, M & S*	1 Pack/180g	90	0.4	50	0.7	10.9	0.2	2.9
Black Forest, Frozen, Tesco*	1 Serving/80g	37	0.0	46	0.7	10.5	0.0	1.7
Citrus Selection, Fresh, Sainsbury's*	1 Pack/240g	79	0.2	33	0.9	7.1	0.1	1.6
Deluxe, Fresh, Rindless, Shapers, Boots*	1 Pack/168g	64	0.3	38	0.7	8.3	0.2	0.7
Exotic, M & S*	1 Pack/425g	212	1.3	50	0.7	11.8	0.3	0.0
Exotic Fruit Frenzy, Freshly Prepared, Tesco*	1 Pack/300g	132	0.6	44	0.6	9.8	0.2	1.6
Fingers, Sunmaid*	1 Pack/50g	162	2.1	325	3.5	68.3	4.3	4.3
Garden, Frozen, M & S*	1 Serving/30g	7	0.1	25	0.7	4.6	0.2	1.8
Grapefruit & Orange Segments, Breakfast, Del Monte*	1 Can/411g	193	0.4	47	1.0	10.2	0.1	1.0
Juicy Twist, Tesco*	1 Pack/170g	71	0.3	42	0.4	9.6	0.2	1.2
Mango, Slices, in Juice, SPC Nature's Finest*	1 Pot/400g	224	0.8	56	5.0	12.3	0.2	1.5
Melon, Kiwi, & Strawberry, Fully Prepared, Sainsbury's*	1 Pack/245g	73	0.5	30	0.8	6.3	0.2	1.3
Melon, Pineapple & Mango Fingers, Good to Go, Waitrose*	1 Pot/160g	82	0.3	51	0.7	11.6	0.2	1.2
Melon, Wedges, Snack Pack, Goodness for Kids, Tesco*	1 Pack/90g	17	0.1	19	0.4	4.1	0.1	0.6
Melon & Grape, Sainsbury's*	½ Pack/200g	66	0.2	33	0.5	7.1	0.1	0.7
Melon & Grape Munchies, Eat Well, M & S*	½ Pack/200g	70	0.2	35	0.5	8.3	0.1	0.7
Melon & Grape Pot, Co-Op*	1 Pot/125g	44	0.1	35	0.6	7.0	0.1	0.9
Melon & Mango, Fabulous Fruity Fingers, M & S*	1 Pack/240g	96	0.5	40	0.6	8.2	0.2	1.0
Melon & Pineapple, Fingers, Sainsbury's*	1 Pack/240g	74	0.2	31	0.5	6.5	0.1	0.8
Mixed, Fresh, 5 a Day, Tesco*	1 Pack/400g	136	0.8	34	0.8	7.4	0.2	1.4
Mixed, Fresh, Tesco*	1 Pack/200g	70	0.4	35	0.8	7.4	0.2	1.4
Mixed, Fruitime, Pieces, Tesco*	1 Can/140g	84	0.0	60	0.4	14.0	0.0	1.0
Mixed, in Fruit Juice, Pieces, Fruitini, Del Monte*	1 Serving/120g	61	0.1	51	0.4	12.0	0.1	0.5
Mixed, Pieces, in Orange Jelly, Fruitini, Del Monte*	1 Can/140g	94	0.1	67	0.3	15.8	0.1	0.0
Mixed, Tropical, Fruit Express, Del Monte*	1 Pot/185g	89	0.2	48	0.2	11.2	0.1	1.2
Mixed, Vine, Crazy Jack*	1 Serving/10g	31	0.0	309	2.8	74.0	0.3	4.7
Mount Pleasant, Graze*	1 Pack/21g	87	5.1	415	2.5	46.9	24.2	9.2
Outrageously Orange Melon, M & S*	1 Pack/180g	36	0.2	20	0.6	4.2	0.1	0.8
Peach, Slices, Frozen, Sainsbury's*	1 Serving/80g	30	0.0	37	1.0	7.6	0.0	1.5

	Measure INFO/WEIGHT	per Measure KCAL	FAT	Nutrition Values per 100g / 100ml KCAL	PROT	CARB	FAT	FIBRE
FRUIT								
Pineapple, Grape & Kiwi, Asda*	1 Serving/200g	98	0.6	49	0.6	11.0	0.3	1.7
Pineapple, Grape & Kiwi, Fresh Tastes, Asda*	1 Pack/200g	106	0.6	53	0.6	11.0	0.3	1.8
Pineapple, Mango & Nectarine, Fresh Tastes, Asda*	1 Pack/240g	127	0.5	53	0.8	11.0	0.2	2.1
Pineapple & Mango Tango, Eat Well, M & S*	1 Pack/200g	100	0.8	50	1.0	22.2	0.4	2.6
Pineapple Pot, Chosen By You, Asda*	1 Pot/200g	106	0.0	53	0.4	12.5	0.0	0.7
Pink Lady Apple & Grape, Snack Pack, On The Go, Tesco*	1 Pack/80g	44	0.1	55	0.3	12.3	0.1	2.6
Raspberry, Mini, Bites, HL, Tesco*	1 Bag/25g	87	0.7	350	4.5	76.8	2.7	4.4
Strawberries, Apple & Grapes, Fresh Tastes, Asda*	1 Pot/190g	91	0.2	48	0.5	10.6	0.1	0.0
Summer Berries, M & S*	1 Pack/160g	80	0.3	50	0.7	10.0	0.2	3.0
to Go, Del Monte*	1 Can/113g	80	0.0	71	0.0	17.7	0.0	0.0
Topper, Frozen, Sainsbury's*	1 Bag/400g	168	0.4	42	0.7	8.8	0.1	1.5
Tropical, Tesco*	1 Pack/180g	85	0.4	47	0.6	10.8	0.2	1.9
Tropical in Juice, Dole*	1 Pot/113g	59	0.0	52	0.3	14.2	0.0	1.8
Tropical Shaker with Coulis, Morrisons*	1 Pot/250g	167	1.0	67	0.8	14.6	0.4	0.9
Tutti Frutti Collection, Freshly Prepared, Tesco*	1 Pack/200g	86	0.4	43	0.6	9.1	0.2	1.4
FRUIT & NUT MIX								
After Dinner Mint, Graze*	1 Pack/42g	202	12.9	478	9.8	41.0	30.4	5.6
Almonds & Raisins, Love Life, Waitrose*	1 Pack/150g	681	42.6	454	11.6	38.1	28.4	4.7
Bakewell Tart, Graze*	1 Pack/37g	154	8.1	416	8.9	48.3	21.8	4.7
Banoffee Pie, Graze*	1 Punnet/33g	154	9.1	468	6.9	48.0	27.6	6.6
Billionaire's Shortbread, Graze*	1 Punnet/38g	177	9.5	465	7.8	53.0	24.9	4.3
Born In The USA, Graze*	1 Pack/50g	285	21.9	570	10.6	33.8	43.8	0.0
Bounty Hunter, Graze*	1 Punnet/31g	145	8.2	473	4.0	54.4	26.8	5.6
Cacao Vine, Graze*	1 Punnet/45g	187	9.4	416	8.5	51.4	20.8	0.0
Cherish, Graze*	1 Punnet/40g	148	9.3	369	4.4	35.8	23.2	6.6
Cherries, Raisins & Nuts, Love Life, Waitrose*	1 Serving/30g	132	7.5	439	7.7	45.8	25.0	3.4
Cinnamon & Prailine, Christmas, Finest, Tesco*	¼ Pot/106g	470	26.7	442	8.2	45.9	25.1	11.5
Date & Banana Loaf, Graze*	1 Punnet/41g	132	1.8	327	3.3	68.3	4.4	6.3
Dried, Bear Necessities, Graze*	1 Pack/35g	126	8.1	361	4.6	34.9	23.2	6.5
Dried, Selection, Wholesome, Love Life, Waitrose*	1 Serving/30g	144	9.6	479	9.8	38.0	32.0	4.4
Eleanor's Apple Crumble, Graze*	1 Pack/31g	108	3.9	349	6.3	56.2	12.6	6.7
Fajita, Graze*	1 Box/55g	255	17.0	463	15.1	38.0	30.9	0.0
Flapjack, Fruit & Seed, Graze*	1 Punnet/55g	229	11.2	417	5.2	54.7	20.4	4.3
Fruit & Nut Case, Graze*	1 Punnet/40g	168	8.8	420	5.8	52.1	22.1	2.9
Fruit Squash, Graze*	1 Pack/41g	183	9.7	451	13.4	47.5	23.8	6.4
Fruitabulous, You Are What You Eat*	1 Bag/40g	155	7.8	388	7.2	46.0	19.5	5.5
Grandma's Apple Crumble, Graze*	1 Punnet/40g	154	7.8	385	0.0	48.9	19.6	4.0
Hazelnut Espresso, Natural Treats, Graze*	1 Punnet/39g	191	12.3	490	8.4	42.9	31.6	4.2
Himalayas & Beyond, Graze*	1 Pack/30g	139	9.2	465	5.0	44.1	30.7	6.7
Honeycomb Crunch, Graze*	1 Punnet/40g	181	10.2	452	9.8	48.0	25.4	3.2
Jaffa Cake, Graze*	1 Punnet/44g	210	13.7	476	6.8	43.1	31.0	5.1
Johnny Come Lately, Graze*	1 Pack/65g	262	14.8	403	10.0	41.4	22.8	0.0
Jungle Fever, Graze*	1 Pack/30g	135	8.3	449	7.4	42.3	27.8	6.8
Lemon Meringue Pie, Graze*	1 Punnet/45g	177	6.0	393	5.0	66.3	13.4	2.0
Limoncello, Graze*	1 Punnet/41g	162	8.4	396	6.3	50.6	20.6	4.3
Lost, Coconut, Banana & Raisins, Graze*	1 Punnet/30g	115	5.8	382	3.5	51.0	19.2	5.8
Luxury, Asda*	1 Serving/50g	225	15.2	451	9.0	33.5	30.5	7.4
M & S*	1 Serving/30g	135	7.6	450	12.4	44.3	25.3	6.0
Macadamias & Dried Cranberries, Love Life, Waitrose*	1 Serving/30g	143	9.2	477	3.3	47.1	30.8	6.2
Marvellous Macaroon, Graze*	1 Pack/28g	158	11.4	566	10.7	37.4	40.9	4.7
Mayan Mocha, Graze*	1 Punnet/40g	185	11.1	462	10.4	46.4	27.8	6.0
New World, Graze*	1 Serving/50g	206	11.7	413	16.8	45.2	23.4	0.0
Nuts & Raisins, Mixed, Natural, Love Life, Waitrose*	1 Serving/50g	257	16.4	515	16.5	38.4	32.8	7.2

	Measure INFO/WEIGHT	per Measure KCAL	per Measure FAT	Nutrition Values per 100g / 100ml KCAL	PROT	CARB	FAT	FIBRE
FRUIT & NUT MIX								
Ooh La La, Graze*	1 Punnet/45g	181	7.2	402	5.0	63.6	15.9	1.0
Organic, Love Life, Waitrose*	1 Serving/30g	115	6.1	383	9.8	40.4	20.2	5.8
Organic, Waitrose*	1 Pack/100g	489	32.6	489	15.0	33.8	32.6	5.4
Papaya, Banana & Brazil Nut, Shipwrecked, Dried, Graze*	1 Punnet/50g	259	11.9	518	5.4	48.8	23.8	0.0
Papaya & Cranberry, Sainsbury's*	1 Serving/75g	300	10.9	400	4.1	63.1	14.6	7.3
Peanuts, Cashews & Mango, Fair Trade, Tesco*	1/6 Pack/25g	130	8.7	520	16.4	33.2	34.8	4.8
Port & Winter Spice, Perenium, Christmas, Finest, Tesco*	¼ Pot/90g	379	23.8	421	7.8	37.9	26.5	13.9
Seed, Nut & Sultana Sprinkle, Love Life, Waitrose*	1 Serving/30g	177	15.4	591	17.2	15.4	51.2	4.3
Shangri-la, Graze*	1 Punnet/29g	133	8.3	459	13.9	36.4	28.7	7.4
Strawberry Milkshake, Graze*	1 Pack/35g	135	4.0	385	3.6	66.6	11.3	5.2
Sun Dance, Graze*	1 Punnet/38g	136	3.8	358	4.3	67.2	9.9	4.5
Swallows & Amazons, Graze*	1 Pack/60g	252	11.8	420	6.3	56.3	19.7	0.0
The Mix, Whitworths*	1 Pot/90g	341	13.1	379	4.1	63.1	14.6	7.3
The Waldorf, Graze*	1 Punnet/28g	109	6.2	389	6.0	43.5	22.1	5.7
Trail Mix, Average	1oz/28g	121	8.0	432	9.1	37.2	28.5	4.3
Tropical Praline, Graze*	1 Punnet/35g	121	4.2	347	4.2	59.2	12.1	2.0
Unsalted, Tesco*	1 Serving/25g	112	4.6	449	12.6	58.1	18.5	12.2
Vanilla, Cherry, Frangipane, Graze*	1 Punnet/38g	196	13.0	516	14.8	37.7	34.3	5.6
Walnut & Vanilla Truffle, Graze*	1 Punnet/38g	187	12.1	496	10.0	43.9	32.2	6.0
Walnut Whip, Graze*	1 Pack/38g	187	12.2	495	10.0	43.9	32.2	6.0
White Chocolate & Raspberry Cheesecake, Graze*	1 Punnet/39g	204	13.7	524	7.5	44.7	35.1	4.5
Ying & Yang, Graze*	1 Pack/60g	296	19.5	493	6.8	41.2	32.5	0.0
FRUIT COCKTAIL								
Fresh, Morrisons*	1oz/28g	12	0.1	44	0.6	11.3	0.2	1.0
Fresh & Ready, Sainsbury's*	1 Pack/300g	117	0.3	39	0.6	9.0	0.1	1.2
in Apple Juice, Asda*	1/3 Can/80g	40	0.1	50	0.3	12.0	0.1	1.6
in Fruit Juice, Heinz*	1 Pot/125g	77	0.0	62	0.5	15.0	0.0	1.0
in Fruit Juice, Morrisons*	1 Can/140g	64	0.0	46	0.4	11.0	0.0	0.0
in Fruit Juice, Sainsbury's*	1 Serving/198g	97	0.2	49	0.3	11.9	0.1	1.3
in Fruit Juice, Waitrose*	1 Can/142g	71	0.0	50	0.4	12.0	0.0	1.0
in Grape Juice, Tesco*	1oz/28g	12	0.0	43	0.4	10.0	0.0	1.0
in Juice, Del Monte*	1 Can/415g	203	0.4	49	0.4	11.2	0.1	0.0
in Light Syrup, Princes*	1 Serving/206g	64	0.0	31	0.4	7.3	0.0	1.0
in Light Syrup, Sainsbury's*	½ Can/125g	72	0.1	58	0.4	14.0	0.1	1.3
in Light Syrup, Valfrutta*	1 Serving/206g	95	0.0	46	0.2	11.4	0.0	1.5
in Pear Juice, Kwik Save*	1 Can/411g	189	0.0	46	0.5	11.0	0.0	1.0
in Syrup, Del Monte*	1 Can/420g	315	0.4	75	0.4	18.0	0.1	0.0
in Syrup, Morrisons*	½ Can/205g	129	0.2	63	0.3	14.9	0.1	0.0
in Syrup, Smart Price, Asda*	1 Can/411g	173	0.4	42	0.3	10.0	0.1	1.6
in Syrup, Tesco*	1 Serving/135g	85	0.0	63	0.4	15.0	0.0	1.0
in Syrup, Very Light, Value, Tesco*	1 Can/410g	123	0.0	30	0.4	7.3	0.0	1.0
No Added Sugar, Asda*	1 Serving/134g	67	0.1	50	0.3	12.0	0.1	1.6
Tropical, Asda*	½ Can/135g	81	0.0	60	0.0	15.0	0.0	1.6
Tropical, Canned, Asda*	½ Can/200g	120	0.0	60	0.0	15.0	0.0	1.6
Tropical, Heinz*	1 Pot/113g	61	0.0	54	0.5	13.0	0.0	1.0
Tropical, in Juice, Morrisons*	1 Serving/100g	56	0.0	56	0.0	14.0	0.0	0.0
Tropical, in Syrup, Sainsbury's*	½ Can/130g	95	0.1	73	0.5	17.6	0.1	1.4
FRUIT COMPOTE								
Apple, Strawberry & Blackberry, Organic, Yeo Valley*	½ Pot/112g	73	0.1	65	0.5	15.5	0.1	1.9
Apricot & Prune, Yeo Valley*	1 Pot/225g	207	0.2	92	0.6	22.3	0.1	1.6
Black Cherry & Creme Fraiche, Extra Special, Asda*	1 Pot/118g	188	9.4	159	1.7	20.0	8.0	0.8
Hartley's*	1 Serving/95g	63	0.1	66	0.8	15.5	0.1	2.4
Orchard Fruits, GFY, Asda*	1 Pot/180g	113	0.2	63	0.5	15.0	0.1	0.0

	Measure INFO/WEIGHT	per Measure KCAL	FAT	Nutrition Values per 100g / 100ml KCAL	PROT	CARB	FAT	FIBRE
FRUIT COMPOTE								
Spiced, Tesco*	1 Serving/112g	122	0.6	109	1.7	24.4	0.5	3.1
Strawberry & Raspberry, M & S*	1 Serving/80g	72	0.1	90	0.7	23.5	0.1	2.3
Summerfruit, M & S*	¼ Pot/125g	119	0.7	95	0.9	22.7	0.6	0.8
FRUIT DRINK								
Alive Tropical Torrent, Coca-Cola*	1 Glass/200ml	88	0.0	44	0.0	11.0	0.0	0.0
Cherryade, No Added Sugar, Morrisons*	1 Glass/250ml	2	0.0	1	0.0	0.1	0.0	0.0
Lemon & Lime, Diet, Carbonated, M & S*	1 Glass/250ml	5	0.0	2	0.0	0.2	0.0	0.0
Multivitamin, Rejuvenation, Active Life, Purdy's*	1 Bottle/330ml	125	0.0	38	0.0	9.5	0.0	0.0
Pineapple, Sparkling, KA, Barr's*	1 Can/330ml	168	0.0	51	0.0	12.5	0.0	0.0
FRUIT FILLING								
Cherry & Amaretto, Asda*	¼ Pack/100g	105	0.2	105	0.9	23.0	0.2	0.0
Red Cherry, Morton*	1 Serving/70g	69	0.0	98	0.4	23.9	0.0	0.0
FRUIT FLAKES								
Blackcurrant with Yoghurt Coating, Fruit Bowl*	1 Bag/25g	112	5.1	449	1.7	64.2	20.6	0.0
Raisins with Yoghurt Coating, Fruit Bowl*	1 Pack/30g	133	5.5	444	2.9	66.6	18.4	0.0
Raspberry with Yoghurt Coating, Fruit Bowl*	1 Serving/25g	112	5.1	449	1.7	64.2	20.6	0.0
Strawberry, Fruit Bowl*	1 Pack/20g	66	0.4	330	1.0	78.0	2.0	2.0
Strawberry with Yoghurt Coating, Fruit Bowl*	1 Serving/25g	112	5.1	449	1.7	64.2	20.6	0.0
FRUIT GUMS								
Fruit Salad, Tesco*	6 Sweets/30g	100	0.1	335	8.3	73.4	0.5	0.3
No Added Sugar, Boots*	1 Sweet/2g	1	0.0	88	0.0	22.0	0.0	0.0
Rowntree's*	1 Tube/49g	170	0.1	344	4.8	81.3	0.2	0.0
Sugar Free, Sainsbury's*	1 Serving/30g	63	0.1	209	7.7	71.3	0.2	0.1
FRUIT MIX								
Apple Cosmo, Graze*	1 Punnet/34g	100	0.2	292	1.5	69.8	0.7	4.6
Apple Strudel, Graze*	1 Pack/55g	172	0.4	312	2.6	63.5	0.7	0.0
Banana, Coconut & Mango, Dried, Graze*	1 Punnet/45g	144	3.7	320	18.7	57.1	8.2	0.0
Banana Coins, Graze*	1 Serving/20g	49	0.1	245	2.4	54.0	0.6	0.0
Berry, Sainsbury's*	1 Serving/20g	64	0.4	319	1.0	78.1	1.9	5.5
Caribbean, Dried, Graze*	1 Box/50g	187	6.4	374	1.2	67.6	12.8	0.0
Cherish, Graze*	1 Pack/50g	221	10.0	443	5.2	52.5	20.0	0.0
Date to Remember, Graze*	1 Punnet/40g	131	1.8	327	3.3	68.3	4.4	6.3
Fig & Cherry Fruit Bake, Graze*	1 Punnet/44g	116	0.4	263	2.9	64.6	0.9	7.6
Fig Roll, Graze*	1 Punnet/35g	110	0.6	313	1.6	23.1	1.7	2.0
Forest Fruit, Dried, Graze*	1 Pack/50g	159	0.4	319	1.8	76.0	0.8	0.0
Frozen, Blueberries & Strawberries, Sainsbury's*	1 Portion/75g	25	0.1	34	0.7	6.5	0.2	1.5
Go Goji Go Go Go, Graze*	1 Punnet/40g	112	0.3	279	2.2	69.0	0.8	0.0
Golden Pineapple Rings, Graze*	1 Punnet/20g	53	0.1	263	0.6	72.0	0.6	8.1
Italian Stallion, Graze*	1 Punnet/40g	118	0.4	296	1.7	71.0	0.9	2.6
Juicy Orange Raisins, Graze*	1 Pack/40g	110	0.4	275	2.1	69.0	0.9	0.0
Loco in Acapulco, Graze*	1 Pack/30g	123	6.4	410	4.0	53.2	21.4	0.0
Love Mix, Graze*	1 Pack/40g	99	0.4	245	4.0	58.0	0.9	5.9
Luxury, Sainsbury's*	1 Serving/30g	78	0.1	261	1.8	62.3	0.5	2.7
Mango & Cranberry, Way to Five, Sainsbury's*	1 Serving/50g	165	0.3	331	1.8	79.4	0.7	4.8
Melon, Strawberry & Grape, Sainsbury's*	1 Pack/180g	58	0.4	32	0.5	7.0	0.2	0.4
Muffin, Dried, Graze*	1 Box/60g	221	6.8	368	1.7	65.8	11.3	1.7
Nectarine, Raspberry & Blueberry, Seasonal, M & S*	1 Pack/160g	72	0.3	45	1.3	8.3	0.2	2.7
Pineapple, Kiwi, Mango & Blueberry, Waitrose*	1 Pack/330g	208	1.0	63	0.7	14.5	0.3	1.9
Pineapple, Melon, Mango, Tesco*	1 Pack/440g	242	0.9	55	1.1	11.4	0.2	1.3
Pumpkin Pie, Graze*	1 Pack/65g	274	11.2	422	11.4	48.2	17.2	0.0
Raisins & Apricots, Great Stuff, Asda*	1 Pack/40g	112	0.1	281	2.6	66.9	0.3	6.0
Rocky Mountain, Graze*	1 Pack/50g	264	19.3	529	3.2	38.2	38.6	0.0
Scandi Berries, Graze*	1 Punnet/23g	61	0.1	270	1.6	65.3	0.6	6.6

F

	Measure INFO/WEIGHT	per Measure KCAL	FAT	Nutrition Values per 100g / 100ml KCAL	PROT	CARB	FAT	FIBRE
FRUIT MIX								
Sour Mango Tangtastic, Graze*	1 Pack/34g	110	0.2	323	1.3	79.8	0.6	2.0
Strawberries & Cream, Graze*	1 Pack/70g	303	11.4	433	3.7	66.9	16.3	0.0
Strawberry Fields Forever, Graze*	1 Punnet/40g	117	0.4	292	1.9	70.9	0.9	2.5
Summer Fruits, British, Frozen, Waitrose*	1 Pack/380g	99	0.8	26	1.0	5.2	0.2	5.5
Summer Pudding, Graze*	1 Punnet/32g	109	0.4	342	1.6	81.2	1.2	4.2
Super Berry Detox, Graze*	1 Punnet/43g	129	0.3	299	1.7	73.9	0.7	3.4
Super Dried, Graze*	1 Pack/55g	176	0.9	320	5.6	76.4	1.6	0.0
Tropical, Fresh, Waitrose*	1 Pack/240g	122	0.5	51	0.6	11.6	0.2	1.9
Tutti Frutti, Graze*	1 Punnet/41g	120	0.4	293	1.9	72.3	0.9	4.0
FRUIT SALAD								
Autumn, Fresh, M & S*	½ Pack/160g	64	0.2	40	0.7	9.4	0.1	2.9
Chunky in Fruit Juice, Canned, John West*	1 Can/411g	193	0.8	47	0.4	11.0	0.2	0.8
Citrus, Fresh, M & S*	½ Pack/225g	79	0.2	35	0.9	7.7	0.1	1.5
Classic, Fresh, Sainsbury's*	1 Pack/400g	148	0.8	37	0.6	8.6	0.2	1.8
Classic, Shapers, Boots*	1 Pack/200g	75	0.2	37	0.7	8.5	0.1	1.3
Exotic, Waitrose*	1 Pack/300g	126	0.6	42	0.6	9.5	0.2	1.1
Fresh, Sweet, Ripe & Moist, Tesco*	1 Serving/750g	345	0.7	46	0.7	10.6	0.1	1.6
Frozen, Basics, Sainsbury's*	1 Serving/100g	38	0.1	38	0.5	8.8	0.1	1.1
Golden, Fresh, Asda*	1 Pot/147g	69	0.1	47	0.6	11.0	0.1	1.6
Grapefruit & Orange, Fresh, M & S*	1 Serving/250g	87	0.2	35	0.9	7.4	0.1	1.6
Homemade, Unsweetened, Average	1 Serving/140g	77	0.1	55	0.7	13.8	0.1	1.5
Luxury, Frozen, Boylans*	1 Serving/100g	54	0.2	54	0.7	12.7	0.2	0.0
Mango, Kiwi, Blueberry & Pomegranate, Fresh, M & S*	1 Pack/350g	210	1.0	60	0.9	13.4	0.3	2.4
Mediterranean Style, Budgens*	1 Serving/250g	95	0.5	38	0.6	8.5	0.2	0.8
Melon, Kiwi, Grapes & Pomegranate Seeds, Morrisons*	1 Pack/400g	152	1.2	38	0.7	8.2	0.3	1.2
Melon, Kiwi, Strawberry, Way to Five, Sainsbury's*	1 Pack/245g	73	0.5	30	0.8	6.3	0.2	1.3
Melon, Pineapple & Grapes, Fresh, Tesco*	1 Pack/300g	120	0.3	40	0.5	9.2	0.1	1.0
Melon & Grapes, Shapers, Boots*	1 Pack/220g	75	0.2	34	0.6	7.7	0.1	0.8
Melon & Mango, Shapers, Boots*	1 Pack/80g	29	0.1	36	0.6	7.7	0.1	1.2
Melon & Red Grape, Freshly Prepared, M & S*	1 Pack/450g	157	0.4	35	0.5	8.4	0.1	0.7
Mixed, Average	1 Bowl/100g	42	0.1	42	0.6	9.4	0.1	1.5
Oranges, Apple, Pineapple & Grapes, Fresh, Asda*	1 Pack/260g	120	0.3	46	0.6	10.5	0.1	2.1
Peaches & Pears, Fruit Express, Del Monte*	1 Serving/185g	87	0.2	47	0.4	10.8	0.1	0.9
Pineapple, Apple, Melon & Grape, Shapers, Boots*	1 Serving/100g	49	0.1	49	0.4	10.5	0.1	1.2
Pineapple, Apple & Strawberries, Tesco*	1 Pack/190g	80	0.2	42	0.4	9.8	0.1	1.4
Pineapple, Mandarin & Grapefruit, Asda*	1 Serving/200g	86	0.2	43	0.6	10.0	0.1	0.0
Pineapple, Mango, Apple & Grape, Waitrose*	1 Pack/300g	186	0.6	62	0.5	14.7	0.2	1.7
Pineapple, Mango & Passion Fruit, Prepared, M & S*	1 Pack/400g	200	0.8	50	0.7	10.8	0.2	1.8
Pineapple, Melon, Kiwi & Blueberry, Shapers, Boots*	1 Pack/179g	75	0.4	42	0.6	8.7	0.2	1.4
Radiant Rainbow, Layered, Eat Well, M & S*	1 Pack/350g	140	0.7	40	0.5	9.1	0.2	0.9
Rainbow, Asda*	1 Pack/350g	140	1.0	40	0.6	8.8	0.3	1.4
Rainbow Layers, Tesco*	1 Pack/270g	121	0.5	45	0.5	9.8	0.2	1.1
Seasonal, Fresh, Asda*	1 Pack/125g	55	0.1	44	0.5	10.4	0.1	1.2
Seasonal, M & S*	1 Serving/200g	100	0.4	50	0.5	11.8	0.2	2.1
Seasonal Melon & Grapes, Asda*	½ Pack/200g	66	1.0	33	0.5	7.5	0.5	0.4
Shapers, Boots*	1 Pack/140g	55	0.3	39	0.7	8.6	0.2	1.0
Strawberry & Blueberry, Asda*	1 Pack/240g	86	0.2	36	0.9	7.0	0.1	1.5
Summer, Red, Fresh, M & S*	1 Pack/400g	160	0.8	40	0.0	10.0	0.2	1.2
Summer, Sainsbury's*	1 Pack/240g	84	0.5	35	0.7	7.8	0.2	1.3
Tropical, Fruit Snacks, Frozen, Sainsbury's*	1 Serving/175g	79	0.2	45	0.7	10.4	0.1	1.6
Tropical, Tropical Harvest*	1 Serving/100g	52	0.0	52	0.3	12.8	0.0	1.4
Tropical in Light Syrup, Passion Fruit Juice, Tesco*	½ Can/216g	130	0.2	60	0.3	14.1	0.1	1.1
Virgin Trains*	1 Serving/140g	56	0.1	40	0.4	10.0	0.1	0.8

F

	Measure INFO/WEIGHT	per Measure KCAL	FAT	Nutrition Values per 100g / 100ml KCAL	PROT	CARB	FAT	FIBRE
FRUIT SALAD								
Weight Watchers*	1 Serving/135g	50	0.1	37	0.2	9.0	0.1	0.7
FRUIT SHOOT								
Apple, Low Sugar, Robinson's*	1 Bottle/200ml	14	0.0	7	0.0	1.2	0.0	0.0
Apple & Blackcurrant, Robinson's*	1 Bottle/200ml	10	0.0	5	0.1	0.8	0.0	0.0
Hydro Orange & Pineapple, Spring Water, Robinson's*	1 Bottle/350ml	3	0.0	1	0.0	0.0	0.0	0.0
Orange, Pure, Robinson's*	1 Bottle/250ml	115	0.2	46	0.5	9.9	0.1	0.2
FRUIT SPREAD								
Apricot, Pure, Organic, Whole Earth*	1 Serving/20g	33	0.1	167	0.8	40.0	0.4	0.9
Blackcurrant, Carb Check, Heinz*	1 Tbsp/15g	8	0.0	54	0.5	12.8	0.1	2.7
Blackcurrant, Weight Watchers*	1 Tsp/6g	6	0.0	106	0.2	26.3	0.0	0.9
Cherries & Berries, Organic, Meridian Foods*	1 Tbsp/15g	16	0.0	109	0.5	26.0	0.3	1.1
Cherry & Berry, Meridian Foods*	1 Serving/10g	14	0.1	138	0.7	33.7	0.6	3.2
High, Blueberry, St Dalfour*	1 Tsp/15g	34	0.0	228	0.5	56.0	0.2	2.2
Raspberry, Weight Watchers*	1 Tsp/6g	7	0.0	111	0.4	27.1	0.1	0.9
Raspberry & Cranberry, No Added Sugar, Superjam*	1 Spread/10g	22	0.0	216	2.1	47.0	0.3	0.0
Seville Orange, Weight Watchers*	1 Tsp/15g	17	0.0	111	0.2	27.5	0.0	0.3
Strawberry, Weight Watchers*	1 Tbsp/15g	23	0.0	156	0.7	39.8	0.1	1.8
FU YUNG								
Egg, Average	1oz/28g	67	5.8	239	9.9	2.2	20.6	1.3
FUDGE								
All Butter, Finest, Tesco*	1 Sweet/10g	43	1.4	429	1.3	73.4	14.5	0.0
Butter, Milk, Thorntons*	1 Sweet/13g	60	2.5	462	3.7	68.5	19.2	0.0
Cadbury*	1 Bar/25g	115	4.0	440	2.3	73.7	15.3	0.4
Cherry & Almond, Thorntons*	1 Bag/100g	464	19.1	464	3.2	70.5	19.1	0.4
Chocolate, Average	1 Sweet/30g	132	4.1	441	3.3	81.1	13.7	0.0
Chocolate, Thorntons*	1 Bag/100g	459	19.1	459	3.1	69.0	19.1	0.6
Chunks, Home Cooking, Asda*	1 Portion/10g	45	1.3	446	1.5	79.7	13.2	1.1
Chunks for Baking	1 Serving/100g	427	12.2	427	1.7	77.2	12.2	0.5
Clotted Cream, Sainsbury's*	1 Sweet/8g	35	0.9	430	1.9	81.5	10.7	0.7
Dairy, Co-Op*	1 Sweet/9g	39	1.2	430	2.0	76.0	13.0	0.0
Devon, Somerfield*	1 Pack/250g	1060	27.7	424	2.0	78.9	11.1	0.0
Double Chocolate Bar, M & S*	1 Bar/43g	202	9.0	470	4.2	66.9	21.0	0.7
Mini Chunks, Sainsbury's*	1 Pack/100g	409	11.3	409	1.9	74.8	11.3	0.0
Pure Indulgence, Thorntons*	1 Bar/45g	210	9.9	466	1.8	65.9	21.9	0.0
Vanilla, Bar, Diabetic, Thorntons*	1 Bar/34g	121	6.7	356	3.2	69.7	19.7	0.6
Vanilla, Bar, M & S*	1 Bar/43g	205	10.0	476	3.7	63.0	23.3	0.4
Vanilla, Thorntons*	1 Bag/100g	465	21.9	465	1.8	65.9	21.9	0.0
Vanilla, Whipped, M & S*	1 Serving/43g	210	10.3	490	3.8	65.4	23.9	0.3
FUSE								
Cadbury*	1 Bar/49g	238	12.2	485	7.6	58.2	24.8	0.0
FUSILLI								
Carb Check, Heinz*	1 Serving/75g	219	1.7	292	52.7	15.2	2.3	20.8
Chickpea, Dell'ugo*	1 Serving/100g	275	2.4	275	19.2	38.1	2.4	12.1
Cooked, Average	*1 Serving/210g*	*248*	*1.4*	*118*	*4.1*	*23.8*	*0.6*	*1.1*
Dry, Average	*1 Serving/90g*	*316*	*1.4*	*351*	*12.3*	*72.0*	*1.6*	*2.2*
Fresh, Cooked, Average	*1 Serving/200g*	*329*	*3.6*	*164*	*6.4*	*30.6*	*1.8*	*1.7*
Fresh, Dry, Average	*1 Serving/75g*	*208*	*2.0*	*277*	*10.9*	*53.4*	*2.7*	*2.1*
Tricolore, Dry, Average	*1 Serving/75g*	*264*	*1.3*	*351*	*12.2*	*71.8*	*1.7*	*2.7*
Whole Wheat, Dry Weight, Average	*1 Serving/90g*	*290*	*2.1*	*322*	*13.1*	*62.3*	*2.3*	*9.0*
FYBOGEL								
Lemon, Reckitt Benckiser*	1 Serving/4g	4	0.0	95	2.4	11.3	1.1	64.8
Orange, Reckitt Benckiser*	1 Serving/4g	5	0.0	106	2.3	12.7	1.1	64.3

	Measure INFO/WEIGHT	per Measure		Nutrition Values per 100g / 100ml				
		KCAL	FAT	KCAL	PROT	CARB	FAT	FIBRE
GALANGAL								
Raw, Root, Average	1 Portion/100g	71	0.6	71	1.2	15.3	0.6	2.3
GALAXY								
Amicelli, Mars*	1 Serving/13g	66	3.5	507	6.2	59.7	27.1	0.0
Bubbles Filled, Chocolate Egg, Galaxy, Mars*	1 Egg/28g	155	9.5	555	6.5	54.7	34.1	1.5
Caramel, Mars*	1 Bar/49g	254	13.0	518	5.8	64.2	26.4	0.0
Caramel Crunch, Promises, Mars*	1 Bar/100g	540	31.8	540	6.1	57.5	31.8	0.0
Cookie Crumble, Mars*	1 Bar/119g	658	40.5	553	6.0	55.0	34.0	2.0
Fruit & Hazelnut, Milk, Mars*	1 Bar/47g	235	13.2	501	7.1	55.2	28.0	0.0
Hazelnut, Mars*	1 Piece/6g	37	2.5	582	7.8	49.4	39.2	0.0
Hazelnut, Roast, Promises, Mars*	1 Bar/100g	544	32.9	544	6.4	55.6	32.9	0.0
Liaison, Mars*	1 Bar/48g	233	11.9	485	5.4	60.3	24.7	0.0
Swirls, Mars*	1 Bag/150g	747	39.7	498	4.9	60.2	26.5	0.0
GAMMON								
Breaded, Average	1oz/28g	34	0.9	120	22.5	1.0	3.0	0.0
Dry Cured, Ready to Roast, M & S*	½ Joint/255g	255	3.8	100	20.5	0.5	1.5	0.5
Honey & Mustard, Average	½ Pack/190g	294	13.5	155	19.1	3.6	7.1	0.1
Joint, Applewood Smoked, Tesco*	1 Serving/100g	152	9.0	152	17.5	0.2	9.0	0.0
Joint, Boiled, Average	*1 Serving/60g*	*122*	*7.4*	*204*	*23.3*	*0.0*	*12.3*	*0.0*
Joint, Raw, Average	*1 Serving/100g*	*138*	*7.5*	*138*	*17.5*	*0.0*	*7.5*	*0.0*
Joint, Unsmoked, Tesco*	2 Slices/150g	247	15.6	165	16.8	0.2	10.4	0.0
Roast, Toby Carvery*	1 Serving/100g	193	9.5	193	25.9	1.0	9.5	0.0
Steaks, Average	*1 Steak/97g*	*157*	*7.1*	*161*	*23.3*	*0.4*	*7.4*	*0.0*
Steaks, Healthy Range, Average	*1 Serving/110g*	*107*	*3.5*	*97*	*18.0*	*0.4*	*3.2*	*0.2*
Steaks, Honey Roast, Average	*1 Steak/100g*	*142*	*5.3*	*142*	*21.5*	*2.3*	*5.3*	*0.0*
Steaks, Smoked, Average	*1 Steak/110g*	*150*	*5.5*	*137*	*22.7*	*0.1*	*5.0*	*0.1*
Unsmoked, Dry Cured, TTD, Sainsbury's*	1 Serving/100g	214	11.2	214	27.7	0.5	11.2	0.8
GAMMON &								
Parsley Sauce, Steak, Tesco*	½ Pack/140g	217	7.3	155	23.7	2.9	5.2	0.5
Pineapple, 228, Oakhouse Foods Ltd*	1 Meal/360g	284	4.0	79	7.1	10.9	1.1	1.7
Pineapple, Roast, Dinner, Iceland*	1 Pack/400g	360	6.4	90	6.2	12.7	1.6	1.7
GAMMON IN								
Creamy Cheddar Sauce, Steaks, Fresh Tastes, Asda*	½ Pack/143g	270	14.4	189	19.1	5.4	10.1	1.5
GAMMON WITH								
Cheese Sauce & Crumb, Steaks, Simply Cook, Tesco*	½ Pack/156g	218	12.0	140	14.2	3.1	7.7	1.0
Egg & Fries, Steaks	1 Serving/540g	684	26.9	127	10.3	10.1	5.0	0.0
Pineapple, Steaks, Asda*	½ Pack/195g	253	2.7	130	17.8	11.5	1.4	0.7
Sweet Maple Syrup Glaze, Joint, Waitrose*	1 Serving/100g	211	12.6	211	14.1	10.2	12.6	0.9
Three Cheese & Mustard Crust, Joint, Asda*	1 Serving/270g	351	11.6	130	21.7	1.2	4.3	0.0
GARAM MASALA								
Dry, Ground, Average	*1 Tbsp/15g*	*57*	*2.3*	*379*	*15.6*	*45.2*	*15.1*	*0.0*
GARGANELLI								
Egg, Dry, Waitrose*	1 Serving/125g	450	5.2	360	13.5	66.9	4.2	3.5
GARLIC								
Crushed, Frozen, Taj*	1 Block/18g	18	0.1	102	7.5	14.0	0.6	4.0
Minced, Nishaan*	1 Tsp/5g	5	0.0	97	6.0	16.2	0.9	0.0
Pickled, Bevellini*	1 Serving/12g	5	0.0	42	2.5	0.8	0.1	0.0
Powder, Average	*1 Tsp/3g*	*7*	*0.0*	*246*	*18.7*	*42.7*	*1.2*	*9.9*
Raw, Asda*	1 Clove/3g	3	0.0	98	5.0	10.0	0.6	2.0
Raw, Average	*1 Clove/3g*	*3*	*0.0*	*98*	*7.9*	*16.3*	*0.6*	*2.1*
Very Lazy, The English Provender Co.*	1 Tsp/3g	3	0.0	111	6.0	20.9	0.4	3.0
Wild	1 Clove/3g	1	0.0	23	2.8	1.7	0.6	1.9
GARLIC PUREE								
Average	*1 Tbsp/18g*	*68*	*6.0*	*380*	*3.5*	*16.9*	*33.6*	*0.0*

G

	Measure INFO/WEIGHT	per Measure KCAL	FAT	Nutrition Values per 100g / 100ml KCAL	PROT	CARB	FAT	FIBRE
GARLIC PUREE								
in Vegetable Oil, GIA*	1 Tsp/5g	12	0.9	248	3.6	18.8	17.7	0.0
with Tomato, GIA*	1 Tsp/10g	7	0.1	70	5.1	0.5	1.2	0.0
GATEAU								
Au Fromage Blanc, Ligne Et Plaisir*	1 Serving/80g	128	2.1	160	8.0	26.0	2.6	0.0
Black Forest, 500g Size, Tesco*	1 Cake/500g	1125	55.0	225	4.0	27.1	11.0	1.8
Black Forest, Family Size, 860g, Tesco*	1 Cake/860g	1978	113.5	230	3.4	24.8	13.2	0.9
Black Forest, Mini, Tesco*	1 Serving/55g	136	5.1	247	5.7	35.3	9.2	1.0
Black Forest, Sainsbury's*	1/8 Cake/63g	163	10.8	259	3.9	27.7	17.1	3.5
Black Forest, Sara Lee*	1 Serving/80g	221	9.8	276	3.6	37.9	12.3	1.2
Chocolate, Asda*	1 Serving/100g	176	10.0	176	2.4	19.0	10.0	0.4
Chocolate, Swirl, Tesco*	1 Serving/83g	230	13.3	277	3.8	29.3	16.0	0.2
Chocolate Layer, M & S*	1 Serving/86g	278	15.7	323	4.2	35.9	18.3	0.9
Chocolate Orange, Co-Op*	1 Serving/97g	320	17.5	330	5.0	37.0	18.0	1.0
Coffee, Tesco*	1 Serving/100g	300	17.0	300	4.2	32.5	17.0	0.6
Double Chocolate, Light, Sara Lee*	1/5 Cake/59g	139	2.7	237	5.7	43.3	4.6	2.0
Double Chocolate, Tesco*	1 Serving/45g	124	6.5	276	4.4	32.1	14.4	2.2
Double Strawberry, Sara Lee*	1/8 Cake/199g	533	24.3	268	3.2	36.2	12.2	0.6
Ice Cream, Chocolate & Vanilla, Iceland*	1 Serving/130g	252	12.2	194	3.3	24.1	9.4	0.6
Lemon & Lime, M & S*	1 Serving/100g	295	15.6	295	3.2	35.0	15.6	0.3
Orange & Lemon, Iceland*	1 Serving/90g	220	9.9	245	2.6	33.8	11.0	0.3
Strawberry, Co-Op*	1 Serving/77g	222	12.9	288	5.1	29.2	16.7	1.0
Strawberry, Family Size, Tesco*	1 Serving/84g	197	11.4	235	2.9	25.2	13.6	0.6
Swiss, Cadbury*	1/6 Cake/60g	228	10.1	380	5.2	52.0	16.8	0.9
Triple Chocolate, Heinz*	1/4 Cake/85g	209	9.5	245	5.1	31.2	11.1	2.4
GELATINE								
Average	*1oz/28g*	*95*	*0.0*	*338*	*84.4*	*0.0*	*0.0*	*0.0*
GEMELLI								
Durum Wheat, Tesco*	1 Serving/100g	354	2.0	354	13.2	68.5	2.0	2.9
GHEE								
Butter	*1oz/28g*	*251*	*27.9*	*898*	*0.0*	*0.0*	*99.8*	*0.0*
Palm	*1oz/28g*	*251*	*27.9*	*897*	*0.0*	*0.0*	*99.7*	*0.0*
Vegetable	*1oz/28g*	*251*	*27.8*	*895*	*0.0*	*0.0*	*99.4*	*0.0*
GHERKINS								
Pickled, Average	*1 Gherkin/36g*	*5*	*0.0*	*14*	*0.9*	*2.5*	*0.1*	*1.2*
Pickled with Dill Flower, Drained, Waitrose*	1 Serving/25g	9	0.1	38	1.7	6.0	0.5	1.1
GIN								
& Diet Tonic, Can, Greenalls*	1 Can/250ml	95	0.0	38	0.0	0.0	0.0	0.0
37.5% Volume	*1 Shot/35ml*	*72*	*0.0*	*207*	*0.0*	*0.0*	*0.0*	*0.0*
40% Volume	*1 Shot/35ml*	*78*	*0.0*	*222*	*0.0*	*0.0*	*0.0*	*0.0*
Gordons & Bitter Lemon, Premixed, Canned, Gordons*	1 Can/250ml	170	0.0	68	0.0	7.1	0.0	0.0
Gordons & Schweppes Tonic, Premixed, Canned, Diageo*	1 Can/250ml	152	0.0	61	0.0	6.2	0.0	0.0
London Dry, Bombay Sapphire*	1 Serving/25ml	59	0.0	236	0.0	0.0	0.0	0.0
GINGER								
Chunks, Crystallised, Julian Graves*	1 Serving/10g	28	0.0	283	0.2	70.1	0.2	1.5
Crystalised, Graze*	1 Pack/25g	61	0.1	243	2.9	58.0	0.3	0.0
Crystallised, Suma*	1 Serving/30g	104	0.0	348	0.2	82.0	0.1	0.3
Ground, Average	*1 Tsp/2g*	*5*	*0.1*	*258*	*7.4*	*60.0*	*3.3*	*0.0*
Lazy, Minced, The English Provender Co.*	1 Tsp/5g	1	0.0	15	0.2	3.2	0.2	1.5
Root, Raw, Pared, Average	*1 Tsp/2g*	*2*	*0.0*	*86*	*2.0*	*19.1*	*0.8*	*2.1*
Root, Raw, Unprepared, Average	*1oz/28g*	*22*	*0.2*	*80*	*1.8*	*17.8*	*0.7*	*2.0*
Stem in Sugar Syrup, Sainsbury's*	1oz/28g	76	0.0	271	0.2	67.3	0.1	1.4
Stem in Syrup, Waitrose*	1 Jar/350g	1071	7.7	306	0.1	70.4	2.2	0.7

G

	Measure INFO/WEIGHT	per Measure KCAL	per Measure FAT	Nutrition Values per 100g / 100ml KCAL	PROT	CARB	FAT	FIBRE
GINGER ALE								
American, Finest, Tesco*	1 Glass/150ml	68	0.0	45	0.0	11.0	0.0	0.0
American, Low Calorie, Tesco*	1 fl oz/30ml	0	0.0	1	0.0	0.0	0.0	0.0
American, Tesco*	1 Glass/250ml	57	0.0	23	0.0	5.5	0.0	0.0
Dry	1 Glass/250ml	37	0.0	15	0.0	3.9	0.0	0.0
Dry, Asda*	1 Glass/150ml	55	0.0	37	0.0	9.0	0.0	0.0
Dry, Sainsbury's*	1 Glass/250ml	95	0.2	38	0.1	9.1	0.1	0.1
GINGER BEER								
Alcoholic, Crabbies*	1 Bottle/500ml	254	0.0	51	0.0	7.1	0.0	0.0
Asda*	1 Can/330ml	144	0.0	44	0.0	10.9	0.0	0.0
Classic, Schweppes*	1 Can/330ml	115	0.0	35	0.0	8.4	0.0	0.0
D & G Old Jamaican*	1 Can/330ml	211	0.0	64	0.0	16.0	0.0	0.0
Diet, Crabbies*	1 Bottle/700ml	7	0.0	1	0.0	0.0	0.0	0.0
Fiery, Canned, Waitrose*	1 Can/330ml	178	0.0	54	0.0	13.3	0.0	0.0
Fiery, Low Calorie, Waitrose*	1 Can/330ml	3	0.0	1	0.1	0.0	0.0	0.0
Jamaican, Boots*	1 Bottle/500ml	5	0.0	1	0.0	0.0	0.0	0.0
Light, Waitrose*	1 Glass/250ml	2	0.2	1	0.0	0.0	0.1	0.1
No Added Sugar, Aldi*	1 Glass/250ml	5	0.0	2	0.0	0.0	0.0	0.0
Sainsbury's*	1 Can/330ml	69	0.0	21	0.0	5.1	0.0	0.0
Sparkling, Organic, Whole Earth*	1 Can/330ml	115	0.0	35	0.0	8.2	0.0	0.0
Traditional, Fentiman's*	1 Bottle/275ml	130	0.0	47	0.0	11.3	0.0	0.0
Traditional Style, Tesco*	1 Can/330ml	218	0.0	66	0.0	16.1	0.0	0.0
GINGER WINE								
Green Ginger Wine & Scotch Whisky, Crabbies*	1 Glass/125ml	192	0.0	153	14.3	14.3	0.0	0.0
GINGERBREAD								
Average	1oz/28g	106	3.5	379	5.7	64.7	12.6	1.2
Decorate Your Own, Chosen By You, Asda*	1 Serving/100g	414	12.6	414	4.8	70.4	12.6	2.3
Men, Mini, Asda*	1 Biscuit/11g	46	1.4	433	5.0	74.0	13.0	1.8
Men, Mini, M & S*	1 Biscuit/17g	78	3.1	470	6.2	63.9	18.6	1.7
Men, Mini, Sainsbury's*	1 Biscuit/12g	56	1.4	463	5.7	83.4	11.8	1.5
GNOCCHI								
Aldi*	1 Serving/100g	160	0.3	160	3.8	35.6	0.3	0.0
Di Patate, Italfresco*	½ Pack/200g	296	0.4	148	3.3	33.2	0.2	0.0
Fresh, Italian, Chilled, Sainsbury's*	¼ Pack/125g	190	0.4	152	3.8	33.6	0.3	1.4
Potato, Average	*1 Serving/150g*	*199*	*0.0*	*133*	*0.0*	*33.2*	*0.0*	*0.0*
GOAT								
Meat, Uncooked	1 Portion/100g	109	2.3	109	20.0	0.0	2.3	0.0
Raw	*1oz/28g*	*31*	*0.6*	*109*	*20.6*	*0.0*	*2.3*	*0.0*
GOJI BERRIES								
Average	*1 Serving/100g*	*287*	*0.7*	*287*	*6.6*	*65.1*	*0.7*	*6.8*
GOOSE								
Leg, with Skin, Fire Roasted	*1 Leg/174g*	*482*	*29.8*	*277*	*28.8*	*0.0*	*17.1*	*0.0*
Meat, Fat & Skin, Raw	*1oz/28g*	*101*	*9.2*	*361*	*16.5*	*0.0*	*32.8*	*0.0*
Meat, Raw	*1 Portion/185g*	*298*	*12.9*	*161*	*23.0*	*0.0*	*7.0*	*0.0*
Meat, Roasted	*1 Portion/143g*	*340*	*18.6*	*238*	*29.0*	*0.0*	*13.0*	*0.0*
Meat & Skin, Roasted	*½ Goose/774g*	*2361*	*169.5*	*305*	*25.2*	*0.0*	*21.9*	*0.0*
GOOSEBERRIES								
Dessert, Raw, Tops & Tails Removed	*1oz/28g*	*11*	*0.1*	*40*	*0.7*	*9.2*	*0.3*	*2.4*
Stewed with Sugar	*1 Serving/25g*	*13*	*0.1*	*54*	*0.7*	*12.9*	*0.3*	*4.2*
Stewed without Sugar	*1 Serving/25g*	*4*	*0.1*	*16*	*0.9*	*2.5*	*0.3*	*4.4*
GOULASH								
Beef, 114, Oakhouse Foods Ltd*	1 Meal/380g	410	20.1	108	7.5	7.4	5.3	1.7
Beef, Average	1 Serving/300g	310	9.5	103	8.1	10.4	3.2	0.9
Beef, Weight Watchers*	1 Pack/330g	241	5.6	73	4.8	9.5	1.7	0.6

G

	Measure INFO/WEIGHT	per Measure KCAL	FAT	Nutrition Values per 100g / 100ml KCAL	PROT	CARB	FAT	FIBRE
GRAPEFRUIT								
in Juice, Average	*1oz/28g*	*13*	*0.0*	*46*	*0.5*	*10.6*	*0.0*	*0.4*
in Syrup, Average	*1oz/28g*	*19*	*0.0*	*69*	*0.5*	*16.8*	*0.1*	*0.5*
Raw, Flesh Only, Average	*½ Fruit/160g*	*48*	*0.2*	*30*	*0.8*	*6.8*	*0.1*	*1.3*
Raw, Weighed with Skin & Seeds, Average	*1 Lge/340g*	*109*	*0.3*	*32*	*0.6*	*8.1*	*0.1*	*1.1*
Ruby Red in Juice, Average	*1 Serving/135g*	*54*	*0.1*	*40*	*0.5*	*9.3*	*0.0*	*0.5*
GRAPES								
Green, Average	*1 Grape/5g*	*3*	*0.0*	*61*	*0.4*	*15.2*	*0.1*	*0.7*
Red, Average	*1 Grape/5g*	*3*	*0.0*	*65*	*0.4*	*15.8*	*0.1*	*0.6*
Red & Green Selection, Average	*1 Grape/5g*	*3*	*0.0*	*62*	*0.4*	*15.2*	*0.1*	*0.8*
GRATIN								
Cauliflower, Findus*	1 Pack/400g	340	20.0	85	3.5	7.0	5.0	0.0
Dauphinoise, Budgens*	½ Pack/218g	277	15.7	127	3.0	12.5	7.2	2.5
Leek & Carrot, Findus*	1 Pack/400g	440	26.0	110	3.5	9.5	6.5	0.0
Potato, Creamy, M & S*	½ Pack/225g	360	25.0	160	2.2	11.9	11.1	0.9
Potato, HL, Tesco*	1 Serving/225g	169	4.9	75	2.3	11.4	2.2	0.6
Potato, Sainsbury's*	½ Pack/225g	448	34.0	199	4.4	11.4	15.1	1.0
Potato, Somerfield*	½ Pack/225g	355	27.0	158	2.0	11.0	12.0	0.0
Vegetable, Somerfield*	1 Pack/300g	417	39.0	139	1.0	5.0	13.0	0.0
GRAVLAX								
Salmon, Cured with Salt, Sugar & Herbs	1 Serving/100g	119	3.3	119	18.3	3.1	3.3	0.4
GRAVY								
Beef, Aunt Bessie's*	1 Serving/100g	73	5.3	73	1.0	5.3	5.3	0.5
Beef, Home Style, Savoury, Heinz*	¼ Cup/60g	30	1.0	50	1.7	6.7	1.7	0.0
Beef, Rich, Ready to Heat, Schwartz*	½ Pack/100g	31	1.6	31	0.8	3.4	1.6	0.5
Chicken, Granules For, Dry Weight, Bisto*	1 Serving/20g	80	3.2	400	1.9	62.5	15.8	0.2
Chicken, Rich, Ready to Heat, Schwartz*	½ Pack/100g	27	1.2	27	0.8	3.3	1.2	0.5
Favourite, Granules, Made Up, Bisto*	1 Serving/50ml	15	0.6	30	0.2	4.4	1.2	0.0
Granules, Chicken, Dry, Average	1 Tsp/4g	17	0.9	428	4.5	49.4	23.6	1.2
Granules, Chicken, Dry, Oxo*	1oz/28g	83	1.4	296	11.1	54.2	4.9	0.7
Granules, Chicken, Made Up, Oxo*	1 fl oz/30ml	5	0.1	18	0.7	3.3	0.3	0.0
Granules, Chicken & Hint of Sage & Onion, Oxo*	1 Serving/30g	95	1.8	316	11.1	54.2	6.1	0.7
Granules, Dry, Bisto*	1 Serving/10g	38	1.6	384	3.1	56.4	16.2	1.5
Granules, Dry, Value, Tesco*	1oz/28g	111	5.2	397	3.2	54.4	18.5	1.0
Granules, Instant, Dry	**1oz/28g**	**129**	**9.1**	**462**	**4.4**	**40.6**	**32.5**	**0.0**
Granules, Instant, Made Up	**1oz/28g**	**10**	**0.7**	**34**	**0.3**	**3.0**	**2.4**	**0.0**
Granules, Lamb, Dry, Average	1 Tsp/4g	14	0.3	343	10.8	56.1	8.4	2.8
Granules, Made Up, Bisto*	1 Serving/50ml	15	0.6	30	0.2	4.4	1.2	0.2
Granules, Made Up, Oxo*	1 Serving/150ml	28	0.4	19	0.6	3.4	0.3	0.0
Granules, Onion, Dry, Oxo*	1oz/28g	92	1.3	328	8.2	62.3	4.8	0.8
Granules, Onion, Made Up, Oxo*	1 fl oz/30ml	6	0.1	20	0.5	3.7	0.3	0.0
Granules, Original, Dry, Oxo*	1oz/28g	88	1.3	313	10.2	57.2	4.8	1.0
Granules, Vegetable, Dry, Oxo*	1oz/28g	88	1.4	316	8.4	59.5	4.9	0.9
Granules, Vegetable, Dry, Tesco*	½ Pint/20g	94	6.7	470	3.8	38.5	33.4	3.7
Granules for Vegetarian Dishes, Dry Weight, Bisto*	1 Serving/28g	100	3.7	356	2.7	56.0	13.3	4.5
Onion, Granules, Made Up, Bisto*	1 Serving/50ml	14	0.3	28	0.2	5.6	0.6	0.0
Onion, Granules For, Dry Weight, Bisto*	4 Tsp/20g	78	2.9	391	2.4	62.3	14.7	2.3
Onion, Rich, Ready to Heat, Schwartz*	½ Sachet/100g	24	0.6	24	0.4	4.3	0.6	0.5
Paste, Beef, Antony Worrall Thompson's*	1 Portion/31g	104	5.7	334	11.8	30.3	18.4	0.6
Paste, Onion, Antony Worrall Thompson's*	1 Tsp/10g	26	0.4	262	7.0	48.7	4.4	1.4
Poultry, Fresh, Sainsbury's*	1 Serving/100g	46	1.2	46	3.5	4.9	1.2	0.5
Powder, Gluten Free, Dry, Allergycare*	1 Tbsp/10g	26	0.0	260	0.3	63.8	0.4	0.0
Powder, Vegetarian, Organic, Marigold*	1 Serving/22g	79	1.7	361	10.6	61.5	7.7	1.3
Roast Beef, Best, in Glass Jar, Made Up, Bisto*	1 Serving/70ml	21	0.3	30	0.3	6.1	0.4	0.0

G

	Measure INFO/WEIGHT	per Measure KCAL	FAT	Nutrition Values per 100g / 100ml KCAL	PROT	CARB	FAT	FIBRE
GRAVY								
Roast Lamb, Bisto*	1 Serving/20g	60	0.9	302	3.4	62.3	4.3	0.0
Roast Pork, Best, in Glass Jar, Dry Weight, Bisto*	4 Tsp/20g	63	0.9	314	4.3	64.1	4.5	0.0
Turkey, Granules, Made Up, Bisto*	1 Serving/50ml	14	0.6	28	0.2	4.0	1.2	0.2
Turkey, Granules For, Dry Weight, Bisto*	4 Tsp/20g	75	3.1	377	2.4	57.2	15.5	1.0
Turkey, Pour Over, Bisto*	1 Pack/100g	23	0.6	23	0.4	4.1	0.6	0.1
Turkey, Rich, Ready to Heat, Schwartz*	1 Pack/200g	62	2.4	31	1.9	3.1	1.2	0.5
Vegetable, Granules For, Dry Weight, Bisto*	1 Tsp/4g	15	0.5	380	2.1	63.0	13.3	4.5
Vegetable, Granules For, Made Up, Bisto*	1 Serving/50ml	14	0.2	28	0.2	5.6	0.4	0.2
GREENGAGES								
Raw, Average	*1 Fruit/23g*	*9*	*0.0*	*38*	*0.7*	*9.4*	*0.1*	*2.0*
GREENS								
Spring, Boiled, Average	*1 Serving/80g*	*16*	*0.6*	*20*	*1.9*	*1.6*	*0.7*	*2.6*
Spring, Raw, Average	*1 Serving/80g*	*26*	*0.8*	*33*	*3.0*	*3.1*	*1.0*	*3.4*
Spring, Sliced, Fresh, Tesco*	1 Serving/100g	33	1.0	33	0.0	2.7	1.0	2.6
GRILLS								
Bacon & Cheese, Tesco*	1 Grill/78g	222	14.7	284	15.0	13.4	18.9	1.2
Cheese & Bacon, Danepak*	1 Grill/85g	241	16.0	284	15.0	13.4	18.9	1.2
Tikka, Organic, Waitrose*	1 Grill/100g	185	9.3	185	6.9	18.5	9.3	3.4
Vegetable, Dalepak*	1 Grill/83g	125	4.1	151	4.0	22.5	5.0	1.6
Vegetable, Mediterranean, Cauldron Foods*	1 Grill/88g	145	10.4	166	5.3	15.8	11.9	6.5
Vegetable, Ross*	1 Grill/114g	252	12.9	221	4.3	25.5	11.3	0.9
Vegetable, Tesco*	1 Grill/72g	129	7.2	179	4.2	18.0	10.0	2.2
Vegetarian, Mushroom & Oregano, Organic, Waitrose*	1 Grill/100g	200	10.0	200	7.9	19.5	10.0	4.3
GROUSE								
Meat Only, Roasted	*1oz/28g*	*36*	*0.6*	*128*	*27.6*	*0.0*	*2.0*	*0.0*
GUACAMOLE								
Average	1 Tbsp/17g	22	2.2	128	1.4	2.2	12.7	2.5
Avocado, Reduced Fat, The Fresh Dip Company*	1 Serving/113g	128	9.8	113	2.5	6.1	8.7	2.3
Doritos, Walkers*	1 Tbsp/20g	32	3.2	159	1.2	2.6	16.0	0.1
Fresh, VLH Kitchens	1 Serving/17g	27	85.9	158	1.5	3.0	14.6	2.5
GFY, Asda*	1 Pack/113g	144	12.4	127	2.8	4.3	11.0	2.2
Mexican Style, Dip Selection, Morrisons*	½ Pack/50g	102	10.2	204	1.5	3.7	20.4	0.9
Reduced Fat, Tesco*	1 Pack/200g	280	22.8	140	2.7	5.7	11.4	3.0
Reduced Fat Average	1 Serving/100g	129	10.8	129	2.4	5.2	10.8	3.0
GUAVA								
Canned in Syrup	*1oz/28g*	*17*	*0.0*	*60*	*0.4*	*15.7*	*0.0*	*3.0*
Raw, Flesh Only, Average	*1 Fruit/55g*	*37*	*0.5*	*68*	*3.0*	*14.0*	*1.0*	*5.0*
GUINEA FOWL								
Boned & Stuffed, Fresh, Fayrefield Foods*	1 Serving/325g	650	39.3	200	19.1	3.3	12.1	0.5
Fresh, Free Range, Waitrose*	1 Portion/193g	258	11.9	134	19.5	0.0	6.2	0.3
GUMBO								
Cajun Vegetable, Sainsbury's*	1 Serving/450g	265	11.2	59	1.4	7.7	2.5	1.5
Louisiana Chicken, Perfectly Balanced, Waitrose*	1 Serving/235g	207	6.6	88	12.2	3.5	2.8	1.3
GUMS								
American Hard, Sainsbury's*	1 Sweet/6g	22	0.0	360	0.1	90.0	0.1	0.0
American Hard, Tesco*	1 Serving/200g	646	0.0	323	0.0	80.8	0.0	0.0
Milk Bottles, Bassett's*	1 Pack/25g	88	0.4	353	6.2	78.3	1.6	0.0
Milk Bottles, Milk Flavour, Asda*	1 Pack/100g	369	2.3	369	7.0	80.0	2.3	0.4

G

	Measure INFO/WEIGHT	per Measure KCAL	FAT	Nutrition Values per 100g / 100ml KCAL	PROT	CARB	FAT	FIBRE
HADDOCK								
Fillet, Smoked, in Mustard & Dill, The Saucy Fish Co.*	2 Fillets/270g	262	9.7	97	15.5	0.1	3.6	0.0
Fillets, Battered, Average	1oz/28g	64	3.4	228	13.4	16.3	12.2	1.1
Fillets, in Breadcrumbs, Average	1oz/28g	57	2.8	203	13.5	14.9	9.9	1.2
Fillets, Raw, Average	*1oz/28g*	*22*	*0.2*	*80*	*18.0*	*0.2*	*0.8*	*0.0*
Fillets, Smoked, Cooked, Average	*1 Pack/300g*	*337*	*7.7*	*112*	*21.9*	*0.4*	*2.6*	*0.1*
Fillets, Smoked, Raw, Average	*1 Pack/227g*	*194*	*1.0*	*86*	*20.3*	*0.1*	*0.5*	*0.2*
Flour, Fried in Blended Oil	1oz/28g	39	1.1	138	21.1	4.5	4.1	0.2
Goujons, Batter, Crispy, M & S*	1 Serving/100g	250	14.1	250	11.7	18.5	14.1	0.8
Loins, Beer Battered, Chunky, TTD, Sainsbury's*	1 Fillet/93g	177	8.8	191	15.8	10.5	9.5	2.3
Loins, Skinless, Frozen, TTD, Sainsbury's*	1 Serving/100g	116	0.2	116	28.5	0.1	0.2	0.1
Loins, TTD, Sainsbury's*	1 Serving/100g	108	0.7	108	25.5	0.0	0.7	0.0
HADDOCK &								
Cauliflower Crunchies, Iceland*	1 Serving/111g	222	13.1	200	8.0	15.5	11.8	2.0
HADDOCK IN								
Butter Sauce, Steaks, Youngs*	1 Serving/150g	133	5.5	89	9.9	4.0	3.7	0.5
Cheese & Chive Sauce, Fillets, Go Cook, Asda*	1 Pack/360g	400	19.1	111	14.8	1.5	5.3	0.2
Cheese & Chive Sauce, Smoked Fillets, Seafresh*	1 Serving/170g	201	10.4	118	14.7	1.2	6.1	0.1
Cheese Sauce, Fillets, Fresh Tastes, Asda*	½ Pack/180g	212	9.5	118	16.2	1.3	5.3	0.6
in Cheese & Leek Sauce, Fillets, SteamFresh, Birds Eye*	1 Serving/190g	165	7.0	87	11.0	2.4	3.7	0.2
Smoked Leek & Cheese Sauce, Asda*	½ Pack/200g	232	10.0	116	14.0	3.7	5.0	1.5
Tomato Herb Sauce, Fillets, BGTY, Sainsbury's*	½ Pack/165g	150	4.6	91	12.9	3.6	2.8	0.1
Watercress Sauce, GFY, Asda*	1 Pack/400g	268	6.8	67	6.0	7.0	1.7	1.4
HADDOCK WITH								
Broccoli & Cheese, Lakeland*	1 Serving/150g	280	10.5	187	10.4	20.6	7.0	0.0
Cheddar & Chive Sauce, The Saucy Fish Co.*	1 Fillet/120g	168	9.0	140	16.6	1.2	7.5	0.0
Cheese & Chive Sauce, Atlantic, Youngs*	½ Pack/180g	184	8.6	102	13.0	1.7	4.8	0.2
Creme Fraiche & Chive Sauce, Smoked, Tesco*	1 Serving/150g	154	4.6	103	16.8	2.1	3.1	0.3
Rich Cheese Crust, Smoked, Sainsbury's*	1 Serving/199g	295	18.9	148	13.0	2.5	9.5	0.9
HAGGIS								
Hall's*	1 Haggis/454g	1053	64.5	232	9.7	15.1	14.2	2.5
Neeps & Tatties, M & S*	1 Pack/300g	330	14.4	110	3.8	12.3	4.8	0.8
Traditional, Average	*1 Serving/454g*	*1119*	*66.5*	*246*	*12.3*	*17.2*	*14.6*	*1.0*
Traditional, Macsween*	1 Haggis/454g	1149	70.8	253	11.1	19.1	15.6	2.1
Vegetarian, Macsween*	1 Serving/100g	208	11.5	208	5.9	25.9	11.5	2.4
HAKE								
Fillets, Herby Mediterranean Glaze, Sensations, Youngs*	½ Pack/120g	106	2.6	88	16.8	0.4	2.2	0.0
Fillets in Breadcrumbs, Average	1oz/28g	66	3.7	234	12.9	15.9	13.3	1.0
Goujons, Average	1 Serving/150g	345	17.8	230	12.4	18.6	11.9	1.3
Raw, Average	*1oz/28g*	*29*	*0.6*	*102*	*20.4*	*0.0*	*2.2*	*0.0*
with Tomato & Basil Sauce, Vegetable Selection, Tesco*	1 Pack/450g	247	5.8	55	4.3	6.7	1.3	1.5
with Tomato & Chilli Salsa, Just Cook, Sainsbury's*	½ Pack/180g	112	1.6	62	11.4	2.2	0.9	0.0
HALIBUT								
Cooked, Average	*1oz/28g*	*38*	*1.1*	*135*	*24.6*	*0.4*	*4.0*	*0.0*
Raw	*1oz/28g*	*29*	*0.5*	*103*	*21.5*	*0.0*	*1.9*	*0.0*
with Roasted Pepper Sauce, Fillets, M & S*	1 Serving/145g	217	14.4	150	12.7	2.4	9.9	0.6
HALLOUMI								
Chargrilled with Bean & Lentil Salad, Love Life, Waitrose*	1 Pack/400g	352	12.0	88	5.1	8.5	3.0	3.3
HALVA								
Average	*1oz/28g*	*107*	*3.7*	*381*	*1.8*	*68.0*	*13.2*	*0.0*
HAM								
Applewood Smoked, Average	*1 Slice/28g*	*31*	*0.8*	*112*	*21.2*	*0.5*	*2.7*	*0.2*
Baked, Average	*1 Slice/74g*	*98*	*3.7*	*133*	*21.0*	*1.0*	*5.0*	*0.0*
Belgian, Sainsbury's*	1 Serving/100g	141	6.1	141	19.4	2.0	6.1	0.0

H

	Measure INFO/WEIGHT	per Measure KCAL	per Measure FAT	Nutrition Values per 100g / 100ml KCAL	PROT	CARB	FAT	FIBRE
HAM								
Boiled, Average	1 Pack/113g	154	6.5	136	20.6	0.6	5.7	0.0
Breaded, Average	1 Slice/37g	57	2.3	155	23.1	1.8	6.3	1.6
Breaded, Dry Cured, Average	1 Slice/33g	47	1.8	142	22.1	1.4	5.4	0.0
Brunswick, Average	1 Slice/20g	32	1.8	160	19.5	0.6	8.8	0.0
Cooked, Sliced, Average	1 Slice/17g	18	0.5	109	19.0	1.0	3.1	0.1
Cooked, Wafer Thin, Weight Watchers*	1 Serving/60g	58	1.1	97	18.2	1.8	1.8	0.1
Crumbed, Sliced, Average	1 Slice/28g	33	0.9	117	21.5	0.9	3.1	0.0
Danish, Average	1 Slice/11g	14	0.6	125	18.4	1.0	5.3	0.0
Danish, Lean, Average	1 Slice/15g	14	0.3	92	17.8	1.0	1.8	0.0
Dry Cured, Average	1 Slice/18g	26	1.0	144	22.4	1.0	5.5	0.2
Extra Lean, Average	1 Slice/11g	10	0.2	90	18.0	1.4	1.4	0.0
Gammon, Breaded, Average	1 Serving/25g	31	0.8	122	22.0	1.5	3.1	0.0
Gammon, Dry Cured, Sliced, Average	1 Slice/33g	43	1.4	131	22.9	0.4	4.2	0.0
Gammon, Honey Roast, Average	1 Serving/60g	81	2.8	134	22.4	0.4	4.7	0.0
Gammon, Mustard, Cured, Waitrose*	1 Slice/45g	54	1.8	120	21.4	0.1	4.0	0.0
Gammon, Peppered, Waitrose*	1/3 Pack/36g	51	2.3	142	20.7	0.3	6.4	0.0
Gammon, Smoked, Average	1 Slice/43g	59	2.1	137	22.3	0.7	4.9	0.2
German Black Forest, Average	½ Pack/35g	93	5.9	267	27.2	1.3	17.0	0.5
Honey & Mustard, Average	1oz/28g	39	1.2	140	20.8	4.6	4.3	0.0
Honey Roast, Average	1 Slice/20g	25	0.8	123	20.3	1.5	3.8	0.1
Honey Roast, Dry Cured, Average	1 Slice/33g	46	1.5	140	22.7	2.3	4.4	0.0
Honey Roast, Lean, Average	1 Serving/25g	28	0.8	111	18.1	2.7	3.1	0.0
Honey Roast, Wafer Thin, Average	1 Slice/10g	11	0.3	113	17.4	3.7	3.2	0.3
Honey Roast, Wafer Thin, Premium, Average	1 Slice/10g	15	0.6	149	22.0	1.6	6.0	0.0
Joint, Cured, Roasted, Average	1 Serving/100g	138	5.2	138	21.7	1.0	5.2	0.1
Lean, Average	1 Slice/18g	19	0.4	104	19.5	1.1	2.4	0.3
Oak Smoked, Average	1 Slice/20g	26	0.9	130	21.0	1.0	4.7	0.3
Parma, Average	1 Slice/10g	21	1.1	213	29.3	0.0	10.6	0.0
Parma, Premium, Average	1 Slice/14g	36	2.3	258	27.9	0.3	16.1	0.0
Peppered, Average	1 Slice/12g	13	0.3	109	18.5	2.0	2.7	0.0
Peppered, Dry Cured, Average	1 Slice/31g	43	1.5	140	23.1	1.3	4.7	0.2
Prosciutto, Average	1 Slice/12g	27	1.5	226	28.7	0.0	12.3	0.3
San Daniele, Finest, Tesco*	1 Slice/10g	24	1.3	242	30.5	0.5	13.1	0.0
Serrano, Average	1 Slice/20g	46	2.4	230	30.5	0.4	11.8	0.0
Smoked, Average	1 Slice/18g	21	0.7	117	19.7	0.9	3.7	0.0
Smoked, Dry Cured, Average	1 Slice/28g	38	1.2	137	23.0	1.4	4.4	0.1
Smoked, Wafer Thin, Average	1 Serving/40g	41	1.2	102	17.7	1.2	2.9	0.2
Thick Cut, Average	1 Slice/74g	94	2.9	127	22.4	0.6	3.9	0.1
Tinned, Average	½ Can/100g	136	8.7	136	12.2	2.0	8.7	0.0
Tinned, Lean, Average	½ Can/100g	94	2.3	94	18.1	0.2	2.3	0.4
Wafer Thin, Average	1 Slice/10g	10	0.3	101	17.9	1.4	2.6	0.1
Wiltshire, Average	1oz/28g	41	1.7	147	23.1	0.0	6.0	0.0
Wiltshire, Breaded, Average	1oz/28g	41	1.4	145	23.9	1.0	5.0	0.0
HARE								
Raw, Lean Only, Average	1oz/28g	35	1.0	125	23.5	0.2	3.5	0.0
Stewed, Lean Only, Average	1oz/28g	48	1.5	170	29.5	0.2	5.5	0.0
HARIBO*								
American Hard Gums, Haribo*	1 Pack/175g	630	3.3	360	0.3	85.5	1.9	0.2
Build a Burger, Haribo*	1oz/28g	96	0.1	344	6.6	79.0	0.2	0.3
Chamallows, Haribo*	1oz/28g	92	0.0	330	2.0	80.0	0.0	0.0
Cola Bottles, Fizzy, Haribo*	1 Pack/175g	595	0.3	340	6.3	78.3	0.2	0.3
Cola Bottles, Haribo*	1 Pack/16g	56	0.0	348	7.7	78.9	0.2	0.3
Dinosaurs, Haribo*	1oz/28g	95	0.1	340	6.3	78.3	0.2	0.5

	Measure INFO/WEIGHT	per Measure		Nutrition Values per 100g / 100ml				
		KCAL	FAT	KCAL	PROT	CARB	FAT	FIBRE
HARIBO*								
Dolly Mixtures, Haribo*	1 Pack/175g	719	8.4	411	1.8	90.2	4.8	0.2
Fantasy Mix, Haribo*	1 Pack/100g	344	0.2	344	6.6	79.0	0.2	0.3
Fried Eggs/eggstras, Haribo*	1oz/28g	96	0.1	344	6.6	79.0	0.2	0.0
Gold Bears, Haribo*	1 Pack/100g	348	0.2	348	7.7	78.9	0.2	0.3
Happy Cherries, Haribo*	1 Serving/40g	139	0.1	348	7.7	78.9	0.2	0.3
Horror Mix, Haribo*	1 Pack/100g	344	0.2	344	6.6	79.0	0.2	0.3
Jelly Babies, Haribo*	1oz/28g	97	0.1	348	4.5	82.1	0.2	0.5
Jelly Beans, Haribo*	1 Pack/100g	379	0.2	379	0.6	93.8	0.2	0.1
Kiddies Super Mix, Haribo*	1 Pack/100g	344	0.2	344	6.6	79.0	0.2	0.3
Liquorice Cream Rock, Haribo*	1oz/28g	107	1.5	382	2.3	81.2	5.3	0.3
Liquorice Favourite, Haribo*	1oz/28g	100	0.8	357	2.8	78.8	3.0	2.3
Liquorice with Stevia, Stevi-Lakritz, Haribo*	¼ Bag/25g	46	0.0	185	8.1	16.0	0.1	48.6
Magic Mix, Haribo*	1oz/28g	102	0.5	366	5.4	82.0	1.9	0.3
Maoam Stripes, Haribo*	1 Chew/7g	27	0.4	384	1.2	81.7	6.1	0.3
Mega Roulette, Haribo*	1oz/28g	97	0.1	348	7.7	78.9	0.2	0.3
Mega Roulette Sour, Haribo*	1oz/28g	95	0.1	340	6.3	78.3	0.2	0.5
Micro Mix, Haribo*	1oz/28g	106	0.7	379	4.7	84.5	2.5	0.4
Milky Mix, Haribo*	1 Pack/175g	607	0.3	347	7.1	79.6	0.2	0.4
Mint Imperials, Haribo*	1 Pack/175g	695	0.9	397	0.4	98.8	0.5	0.1
Peaches, Haribo*	1oz/28g	98	0.0	350	4.3	82.1	0.0	0.0
Pontefract Cakes, Haribo*	1 Serving/40g	118	0.1	296	5.3	68.2	0.2	0.5
Shrimps, Haribo*	1oz/28g	99	0.1	352	6.1	81.5	0.2	0.1
Snakes, Haribo*	1 Snake/8g	28	0.0	348	7.7	78.9	0.2	0.3
Starmix, Haribo*	1 Pack/100g	344	0.2	344	6.6	79.0	0.2	0.3
Tangfastics, Haribo*	1 Pack/100g	359	2.3	359	6.3	78.3	2.3	0.5
Tropifruit, Haribo*	1oz/28g	97	0.1	348	4.5	82.1	0.2	0.5
HARISSA PASTE								
Average	1 Tsp/5g	6	0.3	123	2.9	12.9	6.7	2.8
Barts*	1 Tbsp/15g	11	0.3	76	4.0	10.7	1.9	0.0
Easy, M & S*	1 Tbsp/15g	16	0.8	105	2.5	11.2	5.5	4.4
Moroccan Style, Al'fez*	1 Tsp/10g	19	1.1	190	4.0	18.2	11.2	3.4
HASH								
Barbecue Beef, COU, M & S*	1 Pack/400g	360	1.6	90	7.0	14.0	0.4	1.4
Corned Beef, Apetito*	1 Pack/380g	423	23.6	111	3.8	10.3	6.2	1.3
Corned Beef, Asda*	1 Pack/400g	416	14.4	104	6.0	12.0	3.6	1.1
Corned Beef, Chilled, Co-Op*	1 Pack/300g	345	18.0	115	9.0	5.0	6.0	1.0
Corned Beef, Frozen, Tesco*	1 Serving/400g	348	10.4	87	5.7	10.3	2.6	0.7
Corned Beef, M & S*	½ Pack/321g	385	20.2	120	8.1	7.4	6.3	1.3
Corned Beef, Tesco*	1 Serving/400g	416	10.4	104	5.3	14.8	2.6	1.7
Vegetable & Lentil, Asda*	1 Pack/289g	254	6.1	88	3.2	14.0	2.1	0.0
HASH BROWNS								
Oven Baked, Weighed Cooked, McCain*	1 Piece/38g	80	4.3	214	2.1	25.7	11.4	2.2
Oven Baked, Weighed Frozen, McCain*	1 Piece/40g	75	4.1	187	1.7	21.8	10.3	2.1
Uncooked, Average	1 Piece/45g	78	3.7	173	2.0	22.5	8.3	1.9
HAZELNUTS								
Blanched, Average	1 Serving/25g	164	15.9	656	15.3	5.8	63.5	6.5
Chopped, Average	*1 Serving/10g*	*67*	*6.4*	*665*	*16.7*	*5.6*	*64.0*	*6.5*
Whole, Average	*10 Whole/10g*	*65*	*6.3*	*655*	*15.3*	*5.8*	*63.5*	*6.5*
HEART								
Lambs, Average	*1 Heart/75g*	*91*	*4.5*	*122*	*16.0*	*1.0*	*6.0*	*0.0*
Ox, Raw	*1oz/28g*	*29*	*1.0*	*104*	*18.2*	*0.0*	*3.5*	*0.0*
Ox, Stewed	*1oz/28g*	*44*	*1.4*	*157*	*27.8*	*0.0*	*5.1*	*0.0*
Pig, Raw	*1oz/28g*	*27*	*0.9*	*97*	*17.1*	*0.0*	*3.2*	*0.0*

H

	Measure INFO/WEIGHT	per Measure KCAL	FAT	Nutrition Values per 100g / 100ml KCAL	PROT	CARB	FAT	FIBRE
HEART								
Pig, Stewed	**1oz/28g**	**45**	**1.9**	**162**	**25.1**	**0.0**	**6.8**	**0.0**
HERMESETAS								
Powdered, Hermes*	1 Tsp/0.8g	3	0.0	387	1.0	96.8	0.0	0.0
The Classic Sweetener, Hermes*	1 Tablet/0.5g	0	0.0	294	14.2	59.3	0.0	0.0
HEROES								
Dairy Milk, Whole Nut, Cadbury*	1 Sweet/11g	60	3.9	545	9.1	48.2	35.2	0.0
Fudge, Cadbury*	1 Sweet/10g	43	1.5	435	2.5	72.7	14.9	0.0
HERRING								
Canned in Tomato Sauce, Average	1oz/28g	57	4.3	204	11.9	4.1	15.5	0.1
Dried, Salted, Average	**1oz/28g**	**47**	**2.1**	**168**	**25.3**	**0.0**	**7.4**	**0.0**
Fillets, Raw, Average	**1 Herring/100g**	**185**	**12.6**	**185**	**18.4**	**0.0**	**12.6**	**0.0**
Fillets in Mustard & Dill Sauce, John West*	1 Can/190g	332	26.6	175	9.4	2.9	14.0	0.1
Fillets in Olive Oil, Succulent, Princes*	1 Serving/50g	107	7.5	215	20.0	0.0	15.0	0.0
Grilled, Average	**1oz/28g**	**51**	**3.1**	**181**	**20.1**	**0.0**	**11.2**	**0.0**
in Horseradish Sauce, John West*	1oz/28g	64	5.0	230	13.0	4.0	18.0	0.0
Pickled, Average	1oz/28g	73	5.0	262	14.2	9.6	18.0	0.0
Pickled in Mustard Sauce, Abba*	1 Serving/58g	149	10.9	260	7.0	16.0	19.0	0.0
Rollmop with Onion, Asda*	1 Rollmop/65g	89	3.1	137	13.2	10.3	4.8	0.8
Rollmops, Tesco*	1 Rollmop/65g	110	5.5	170	12.0	10.4	8.4	0.4
Smoked, Pepper in Oil, Glyngøre*	1 Can/130g	338	24.7	260	21.0	0.0	19.0	0.0
HIGH LIGHTS								
Caffe Latte, Made Up, Cadbury*	1 Serving/200g	40	1.4	20	1.0	2.5	0.7	0.0
Choc Mint, Made Up, Cadbury*	1 Mug/200ml	40	1.4	20	1.0	2.5	0.7	0.3
Chocolate, Dairy Fudge, Dry Weight, Cadbury*	1 Serving/11g	40	1.1	363	17.0	50.0	10.0	0.0
Chocolate Delights, Cadbury*	1 Bar/13g	60	2.6	480	6.4	67.0	20.5	1.2
Chocolate Orange, Made Up, Cadbury*	1 Mug/200ml	40	1.4	20	1.0	2.3	0.7	0.3
Dairy Fudge, Made Up, Cadbury*	1 Mug/200ml	40	1.0	20	1.0	2.8	0.5	0.2
Dark Chocolate, Cadbury*	1 Sachet/11g	35	0.9	315	23.1	37.3	8.1	0.0
Dark Chocolate, Made Up, Cadbury*	1 Mug/200ml	35	0.9	17	1.2	2.0	0.4	0.0
Espresso, Made Up, Cadbury*	1 Mug/200ml	35	0.9	17	1.2	1.9	0.4	0.0
Fudge, Made Up, Cadbury*	1 Mug/200ml	40	1.1	20	0.9	2.5	0.5	0.0
Hot Chocolate Drink, Instant, Dry Weight, Cadbury*	1 Sachet/11g	38	1.4	350	16.6	42.0	12.8	3.0
Hot Chocolate Drink, Instant, Made Up, Cadbury*	1 Cup/200ml	40	1.4	20	1.0	2.5	0.7	0.3
Instant Hot Chocolate, Cadbury*	1 Sachet/22g	80	2.8	364	17.3	44.5	12.7	0.0
Mint, Cadbury*	1 Mug/200ml	40	1.4	20	1.0	2.5	0.7	0.0
Toffee Flavour, Made Up, Cadbury*	1 Mug/200ml	40	1.4	20	1.0	2.6	0.7	0.0
HOKI								
Grilled	**1oz/28g**	**34**	**0.8**	**121**	**24.1**	**0.0**	**2.7**	**0.0**
in Breadcrumbs, Average	1 Piece/156g	298	13.8	191	14.5	13.9	8.9	1.2
Raw	**1oz/28g**	**24**	**0.5**	**85**	**16.9**	**0.0**	**1.9**	**0.0**
Steaks, in Batter, Crispy, Birds Eye*	1 Steak/123g	320	17.1	260	12.4	21.3	13.9	0.8
HONEY								
Acacia, Tesco*	1 Tsp/4g	12	0.0	307	0.4	76.4	0.0	0.0
Acacia Blossom, Sainsbury's*	1 Serving/24g	81	0.0	339	0.1	84.7	0.1	0.3
Australian Eucalyptus, Finest, Tesco*	1 Tsp/4g	12	0.0	307	0.4	76.4	0.0	0.0
Bio Active, New Zealand Honey Co*	1 Serving/10g	32	0.0	325	1.0	80.0	0.0	0.0
Clear, Basics, Sainsbury's*	1 Tsp/15g	46	0.0	307	0.4	76.4	0.1	0.0
Clear, Runny, Sainsbury's*	1 Serving/15g	51	0.0	339	0.1	84.7	0.1	0.3
Clear, Value, Tesco*	1 Serving/27g	86	0.0	320	1.0	78.0	0.0	0.0
Clover, Canadian, TTD, Sainsbury's*	1 Tbsp/15g	50	0.0	336	0.2	83.6	0.1	0.1
Florida Orange, Extra Special, Asda*	1 Tbsp/15g	50	0.0	334	0.5	83.0	0.0	0.0
Greek, Waitrose*	1 Tsp/6g	18	0.0	307	0.4	76.4	0.0	0.0
Pure, Clear, Average	**1 Tbsp/20g**	**63**	**0.0**	**315**	**0.5**	**78.5**	**0.0**	**0.0**

H

	Measure INFO/WEIGHT	per Measure KCAL	FAT	Nutrition Values per 100g / 100ml KCAL	PROT	CARB	FAT	FIBRE
HONEY								
Pure, Clear, Squeezy, Oak Lane*	1 Tsp/5ml	16	0.0	330	0.5	81.0	0.0	0.0
Pure, Set, Average	**1 Tbsp/20g**	**62**	**0.0**	**312**	**0.4**	**77.6**	**0.0**	**0.0**
Scottish Heather, Waitrose*	1 Serving/20g	61	0.0	307	0.4	76.4	0.0	0.0
Spanish Orange Blossom, Sainsbury's*	1 Tbsp/15g	51	0.0	339	0.1	84.7	0.0	0.3
HONEYCOMB								
Natural, Epicure*	1 Serving/100g	290	4.6	290	0.4	74.4	4.6	0.0
HOOCH*								
Vodka, Calculated Estimate, Hooch*	1 Bottle/330ml	244	0.0	74	0.3	5.1	0.0	0.0
HORLICKS								
Malted Drink, Chocolate, Extra Light, Dry Weight, Horlicks*	1 Serving/32g	95	2.5	296	9.2	47.0	7.8	17.3
Malted Drink, Extra Light, Instant, Dry Weight, Horlicks*	1 Serving/11g	35	0.7	319	8.4	57.4	6.2	10.5
Malted Drink, Light, Dry Weight, Horlicks*	1 Serving/32g	116	1.2	364	14.8	72.2	3.8	1.9
Malted Drink, Light, Made Up, Horlicks*	1 Mug/200ml	116	1.2	58	2.3	11.5	0.6	0.3
Powder, Made Up with Semi-Skimmed Milk	1 Mug/227ml	184	4.3	81	4.3	12.9	1.9	0.0
Powder, Made Up with Skimmed Milk	1 Mug/227ml	159	1.1	70	4.3	12.9	0.5	0.0
Powder, Made Up with Whole Milk	1 Mug/227ml	225	8.9	99	4.2	12.7	3.9	0.0
Snoozoo, Chocolate, Horlicks*	1 Sachet/20g	74	0.9	370	8.6	74.2	4.3	4.3
HORSE								
Meat, Raw, Average	**1 Serving/110g**	**146**	**5.1**	**133**	**21.4**	**0.0**	**4.6**	**0.0**
HORSERADISH								
Prepared, Average	**1 Tsp/5g**	**3**	**0.0**	**62**	**4.5**	**11.0**	**0.3**	**6.2**
HOT CHOCOLATE								
Balanced Lifestyle, Camelot*	1 Sachet/11g	40	1.6	363	18.5	40.6	14.1	0.5
Cadbury*	1 Serving/12g	44	0.7	370	6.3	73.3	5.9	0.0
Caramel, Whittards of Chelsea*	1 Serving/20g	71	1.5	355	7.5	64.5	7.5	13.0
Caramel Flavoured, Instant, Dry, Aldi*	1 Serving/11g	40	1.6	363	18.5	40.6	14.1	8.5
Chococino, Dulce Gusto, Nescafe*	1 Serving/34g	149	5.5	437	14.6	58.6	16.1	4.6
Chocolate Break, Dry, Tesco*	1 Serving/21g	110	6.0	524	7.9	58.9	28.5	1.7
Cocoa, Lidl*	1 Serving/20g	77	1.2	386	6.1	74.1	6.2	0.0
Dreamtime, Whittards of Chelsea*	5 Tsp/20g	72	1.0	361	6.6	72.4	5.1	8.7
Drink, Organic, Green & Black's*	1 Tsp/4g	13	0.3	374	9.1	63.5	9.3	0.1
Dry Weight, Tassimo, Suchard*	1 Cup/27g	88	2.4	325	3.2	58.0	8.9	2.6
Galaxy, Mars*	1 Sachet/28g	115	3.4	411	7.0	68.7	12.1	0.0
Horlicks*	1 Serving/32g	128	2.6	400	8.7	72.5	8.1	3.7
Impress*	1 Serving/25g	90	0.9	360	5.6	76.0	3.6	6.0
Instant, BGTY, Made Up, Sainsbury's*	1 Sachet/28g	16	0.2	56	2.1	10.6	0.6	0.3
Instant, GFY, Asda*	1 Tsp/10g	32	1.3	321	13.2	37.0	13.4	7.7
Instant, Low Fat, Solo Slim, Rosemary Conley*	1 Sachet/18g	66	0.5	368	17.0	66.7	2.8	3.8
Instant, Skinny Cow*	1 Sachet/10g	37	1.5	370	19.7	39.3	14.6	0.0
Instant, Tesco*	1 Serving/32g	155	10.3	485	10.5	38.1	32.3	5.0
Instant Break, Cadbury*	1 Sachet/28g	119	3.9	425	10.9	64.2	14.0	0.0
Light, Caramel Flavour, Kruger*	1 Sachet/10g	37	1.4	370	13.0	41.4	14.2	6.8
Light, Hazelnut Flavour, Kruger*	1 Sachet/10g	37	1.4	370	13.0	41.4	14.2	6.8
Low Calorie, Somerfield*	1 Sachet/12g	40	1.0	330	18.0	48.0	8.0	0.0
Luxury, Skinny, Whittards of Chelsea*	1 Serving/28g	92	0.8	328	12.9	67.1	2.8	13.5
Milk Drink, Low Calorie, You Count, Love Life, Waitrose*	1 Serving/11g	37	0.3	339	21.2	57.1	2.9	5.5
Orange Flavour, Solo Slim, Rosemary Conley*	1 Sachet/18g	66	0.5	368	17.1	66.7	2.8	3.9
Slim Fast*	1 Serving/59g	203	2.8	347	22.2	53.8	4.8	8.4
Value, Tesco*	1 Serving/32g	132	3.9	414	8.0	68.3	12.1	0.7
Velvet, Cadbury*	1 Serving/28g	136	6.9	487	8.6	57.8	24.6	2.0
HOT DOG								
American Style, Hunters*	1 Sausage/23g	50	3.4	220	12.5	8.7	15.0	0.1
Sausage, American Style, Average	1 Sausage/75g	180	14.3	241	11.6	6.2	19.0	0.0

H

	Measure INFO/WEIGHT	per Measure		Nutrition Values per 100g / 100ml				
		KCAL	FAT	KCAL	PROT	CARB	FAT	FIBRE
HOT DOG								
Sausage, Average	1 Sausage/23g	40	3.0	175	10.8	4.3	12.8	0.3
HOT DOG VEGETARIAN								
Meat Free, Sainsbury's*	1 Sausage/30g	71	4.5	237	18.0	7.6	15.0	1.0
Tesco*	1 Sausage/30g	66	4.5	220	18.0	2.7	15.0	2.0
HOT POT								
Beef, Apetito*	1 Pack/340g	303	10.4	89	5.1	10.3	3.1	1.3
Beef, Classic Asda*	1 Serving/400g	400	20.8	100	5.7	7.1	5.2	1.2
Beef, Healthy Options, Birds Eye*	1 Pack/350g	294	7.0	84	4.5	12.0	2.0	1.2
Beef, Minced, & Vegetable, COU, M & S*	1 Pack/400g	380	6.8	95	10.3	9.0	1.7	2.4
Beef, Minced, Bisto*	1 Pack/375g	364	13.5	97	4.1	11.3	3.6	1.4
Beef, Minced, Classic, Asda*	1 Pack/375g	397	17.2	106	6.8	8.7	4.6	1.1
Beef, Minced, Smart Price, Asda*	1 Pack/300g	199	3.9	66	3.7	10.0	1.3	0.4
Beef, Ross*	1 Pack/322g	254	11.3	79	2.5	9.4	3.5	0.4
Beef, Weight Watchers*	1 Pack/320g	231	7.7	72	3.6	8.4	2.4	1.6
Chicken, Chunky, Weight Watchers*	1 Pack/320g	275	9.0	86	4.7	10.4	2.8	0.6
Chicken, Cooked, Light Choices, Tesco*	1 Pack/361g	250	4.6	70	5.1	9.1	1.3	1.5
Chicken, Low Fat, Solo Slim, Rosemary Conley*	1 Serving/100g	81	2.9	81	6.7	7.1	2.9	2.5
Chicken, Weight Watchers*	1 Pack/320g	226	4.5	71	6.4	7.3	1.4	1.8
Chicken & Cider, Ready Meals, Waitrose*	1 Pack/400g	500	20.4	125	6.8	12.9	5.1	1.1
Chicken & Mushroom, HL, Tesco*	1 Serving/450g	369	6.7	82	6.3	11.8	1.5	0.5
Chunky Vegetable & Tomato, Big Eat, Heinz*	1 Pot/355g	213	1.4	60	2.5	11.7	0.4	4.1
Lamb, Cumbrian, Look What We Found*	1 Pack/300g	276	5.4	92	8.9	10.1	1.8	3.0
Lamb, Diet Chef Ltd*	1 Pack/300g	276	5.4	92	8.9	10.1	1.8	3.0
Lamb, Heinz*	1 Pack/340g	337	10.5	99	4.9	12.7	3.1	1.7
Lamb, Low Fat, Solo Slim, Rosemary Conley*	1 Serving/100g	92	1.8	92	8.9	10.1	1.8	3.0
Lamb, Mini, Classics, Asda*	1 Pack/300g	223	10.5	74	5.3	5.4	3.5	3.3
Lamb, Organic, Great Stuff, Asda*	1 Pack/300g	327	10.2	109	8.0	11.6	3.4	1.1
Lamb & Vegetable, Asda*	1 Pot/500g	240	2.0	48	4.0	7.0	0.4	0.0
Lamb Shank, Extra Special, Asda*	1 Pack/450g	508	20.2	113	10.2	7.8	4.5	1.3
Lancashire, M & S*	1 Pack/454g	431	15.0	95	10.1	6.7	3.3	1.0
Lancashire, Sainsbury's*	½ Pack/225g	220	8.8	98	6.1	9.5	3.9	1.0
Liver & Bacon, Tesco*	1 Pack/550g	693	31.4	126	6.4	12.3	5.7	1.5
Minced Beef, 201, Oakhouse Foods Ltd*	1 Meal/300g	330	14.1	110	6.9	10.0	4.7	1.4
Sausage, Aunt Bessie's*	¼ Pack/200g	212	9.2	106	3.6	12.6	4.6	1.9
Sausage, Smart Price, Asda*	1 Pack/300g	239	7.0	80	3.7	11.0	2.3	0.4
Sausage with Baked Beans, Heinz*	1 Can/340g	354	10.9	104	4.6	14.3	3.2	2.4
Vegetable, Gluten, Yeast & Dairy Free, Canned, GranoVita*	1 Can/420g	290	8.4	69	3.2	9.5	2.0	1.6
Vegetable, Ready Meal, Average	1 Serving/400g	261	7.4	65	1.9	10.7	1.9	1.9
Vegetable, Roast, with Gravy, Hometown Buffet*	1 Serving/113g	50	0.5	44	0.9	11.5	0.4	1.8
Vegetable, Vegetable Recipes, Ross*	1 Pack/300g	159	5.4	53	1.5	9.4	1.8	1.6
Vegetable, Weight Watchers*	1 Pack/335g	228	6.4	68	2.6	9.9	1.9	1.5
HOUMOUS								
30% Less Fat, Asda*	1oz/28g	73	5.3	259	9.0	13.0	19.0	3.8
40% Less Fat, Eat Smart, Morrisons*	½ Pack/85g	209	15.0	246	7.9	13.8	17.7	2.7
Avocado, Fresh, San Amvrosia*	1 Serving/50g	172	16.0	344	5.4	8.5	32.1	2.5
Balsamic Caramelised Red Onion, Extra Special, Asda*	½ Pack/50g	146	10.7	293	6.8	18.2	21.4	1.0
Broad Bean, Asparagus & Mint, Tesco*	¼ Pot/42g	120	9.7	285	7.1	9.7	23.0	3.7
Caramelised Onion, Tesco*	¼ Pack/50g	125	9.7	250	5.5	13.0	19.4	4.2
Carrot with Lemon & Coriander, Shapers, Boots*	1 Pack/75g	64	1.9	85	3.0	11.0	2.5	3.4
Chargrilled Red Pepper & Chilli, 30% Less Fat, Asda*	1 Serving/50g	116	8.2	233	7.5	11.5	16.4	4.9
Chilli & Red Pepper, Topped, Tesco*	½ Pack/100g	281	25.1	281	7.1	6.6	25.1	8.1
Feta, Fresh, Sainsbury's*	1 Serving/100g	292	27.4	292	8.0	3.5	27.4	6.7
Garlic & Pesto, Asda*	1 Serving/34g	107	8.8	314	8.0	12.0	26.0	0.0

HOUMOUS	Measure INFO/WEIGHT	per Measure KCAL	FAT	Nutrition Values per 100g / 100ml KCAL	PROT	CARB	FAT	FIBRE
GFY, Asda*	1 Serving/50g	136	10.0	272	9.0	14.0	20.0	3.8
Greek, Somerfield*	1 Serving/50g	152	13.4	304	7.6	8.2	26.8	5.5
Indian Spiced, Glorious!*	1 Serving/100g	78	3.9	78	5.2	14.0	3.9	3.0
Jalapeno, Asda*	1 Serving/50g	165	14.5	331	7.0	10.6	29.0	4.5
Jalapeno, Sainsbury's*	¼ Pot/50g	148	13.4	296	6.4	7.2	26.8	5.7
Jalapeno, Tesco*	½ Pot/100g	360	31.1	360	7.5	11.4	31.1	3.9
Lemon & Coriander, BGTY, Sainsbury's*	½ Tub/100g	145	9.0	145	6.3	9.7	9.0	5.9
Lemon & Coriander, GFY, Asda*	1 Serving/50g	129	9.9	259	8.3	12.0	19.8	5.1
Lemon & Coriander, Reduced Fat, Tesco*	1 Pot/60g	135	9.2	225	7.4	13.8	15.3	4.7
Lemon & Coriander, Sainsbury's*	¼ Tub/50g	145	12.5	291	7.0	9.1	25.1	6.0
Lemon & Coriander, Tesco*	1 Serving/50g	170	14.5	340	7.0	12.7	29.0	2.1
Mediterranean Deli, M & S*	¼ Pack/70g	203	17.7	290	7.8	8.0	25.3	6.5
Mixed Olive, Sainsbury's*	¼ Pot/50g	134	11.5	268	6.7	8.4	23.1	7.7
Moroccan, Tesco*	¼ Pot/50g	144	12.7	289	6.8	8.1	25.5	7.3
Moroccan Style, Sainsbury's*	¼ Pot/50g	113	9.7	227	5.5	7.3	19.5	6.6
Moroccan Style Topped, M & S*	1 Serving/100g	220	15.3	220	6.5	13.2	15.3	9.2
Moroccan with Coriander & Spices, Tesco*	¼ Pot/50g	131	9.9	262	9.4	11.6	19.8	5.2
Olive & Sundried Tomato, Tesco*	1 Serving/50g	117	9.7	235	6.5	8.0	19.5	7.4
Olive & Tomato, Mixed, Sainsbury's*	¼ Tub/50g	136	12.6	272	6.0	5.3	25.2	7.4
Organic, M & S*	¼ Pack/25g	82	7.4	330	6.9	9.1	29.7	3.3
Organic, Tesco*	¼ Tub/42g	134	11.4	320	6.5	12.3	27.2	2.4
Pesto Style Houmous, Sainsbury's*	1 Spread/25g	85	7.3	339	7.9	10.8	29.4	5.7
Red Pepper, Reduced Fat, Tesco*	¼ Pot/57g	120	7.4	205	7.7	12.5	12.6	5.3
Red Pepper Pesto, Tesco*	¼ Pot/50g	137	11.3	275	7.4	9.7	22.6	5.7
Reduced Fat, Average	1 Tbsp/30g	72	5.0	241	9.2	13.3	16.8	3.6
Reduced Fat, Mediterranean Deli, M & S*	1 Mini Pot/60g	126	9.7	210	7.5	8.3	16.2	9.3
Reduced Fat, Moroccan Style, Topped, M & S*	1 Tub/170g	374	26.0	220	6.6	13.2	15.3	9.2
Reduced Fat, Snack Pots, Mini, BGTY, Sainsbury's*	1 Mini Pot/60g	100	7.3	167	7.0	13.8	12.1	5.5
Roasted Aubergine, M & S*	½ Pot/85g	132	10.3	155	4.9	6.9	12.1	5.1
Roasted Red Pepper, 50% Less Fat, Tesco*	½ Pot/85g	156	10.5	184	7.3	10.9	12.4	9.5
Roasted Red Pepper, BGTY, Sainsbury's*	¼ Tub/50g	64	3.4	129	4.9	11.9	6.9	5.3
Roasted Red Pepper, Sainsbury's*	½ Pot/100g	317	27.2	317	6.2	9.0	27.2	5.7
Roasted Red Pepper, Somerfield*	½ Pot/85g	244	21.3	287	7.1	8.1	25.1	5.2
Roasted Red Pepper, Tesco*	1 Serving/75g	255	22.3	340	7.1	11.1	29.7	2.4
Roasted Red Pepper VLH Kitchens	1 Serving/17g	31	49.4	183	6.5	15.6	8.4	6.2
Roasted Vegetable, Fresh, Sainsbury's*	¼ Pot/50g	144	13.6	287	5.9	4.9	27.1	7.8
Sea Salt & Cracked Black Pepper, Tesco*	¼ Pot/50g	147	13.6	295	7.0	4.8	27.2	9.5
Sun Dried Tomato, Chunky, Tesco*	½ Pot/95g	322	27.0	339	6.7	14.0	28.4	3.3
Sweet Chilli, Tesco*	¼ Pot/50g	120	8.3	240	6.9	15.2	16.7	5.4
Tesco*	¼ Pot/51g	160	13.6	315	7.4	9.8	26.8	3.4
Three Bean, Reduced Fat, BGTY, Sainsbury's*	¼ Tub/50g	91	6.0	183	7.3	11.4	12.0	6.0
HULA HOOPS								
Bacon & Ketchup Flavour, KP Snacks*	1 Bag/27g	140	8.3	517	3.4	56.3	30.9	2.0
BBQ Beef, 55% Less Saturated Fat, KP Snacks*	1 Pack/34g	174	9.7	511	3.6	60.3	28.4	1.8
Cheese & Onion 55% Less Saturated Fat, KP Snacks*	1 Bag/34g	175	9.7	515	3.6	61.0	28.5	1.9
Chilli Salsa,Tortilla, KP Snacks*	1 Bag/25g	123	6.8	494	4.9	57.2	27.3	5.3
Minis, Original, KP Snacks*	1 Tub/140g	752	48.7	537	3.0	52.9	34.8	1.7
Multigrain, KP Snacks*	1 Pack/23g	113	5.9	491	5.6	60.0	25.6	4.3
Original, 55% Less Saturated Fat, KP Snacks*	1 Bag/34g	175	9.7	515	3.2	61.6	28.4	1.8
Original, KP Snacks*	1 Bag/25g	128	7.1	514	3.2	61.5	28.4	1.8
Roast Chicken, 50% Less Saturated Fat, KP Snacks*	1 Bag/34g	175	9.7	514	3.4	61.0	28.5	1.7
Salt & Vinegar, 50% Less Saturated Fat, KP Snacks*	1 Pack/25g	127	7.0	510	3.1	60.9	28.2	1.8
Sizzling Bacon, KP Snacks*	1 Bag/34g	175	9.7	514	3.4	60.9	28.5	1.7

H

ICE CREAM

INFO/WEIGHT	Measure	per Measure KCAL	FAT	Nutrition Values per 100g / 100ml KCAL	PROT	CARB	FAT	FIBRE
Aero, Bubble Ball, Nestle*	1 Ice/100ml	99	4.3	99	2.3	12.9	4.3	0.0
After Dinner, Mint, Dairy, Asda*	1 Serving/100g	182	8.0	182	3.4	24.0	8.0	0.4
After Dinner Bites, Vanilla, Magnum, Wall's Ice Cream*	1 Serving/29g	100	6.7	344	3.4	31.0	23.0	1.4
After Eight, Nestle*	1 Serving/55g	114	5.2	207	3.6	27.1	9.4	0.3
Almond Indulgence, Sainsbury's*	1 Serving/120g	286	18.8	238	2.8	21.4	15.7	0.6
Baked Alaska, Ben & Jerry's*	1 Serving/100g	260	15.0	260	4.0	29.0	15.0	0.1
Bananas Foster, Haagen-Dazs*	1 Serving/125ml	260	15.0	208	3.2	22.4	12.0	0.0
Banoffee, Haagen-Dazs*	1 Serving/120ml	274	15.6	228	4.0	23.0	13.0	0.0
Banoffee Fudge, Sainsbury's*	1/8 Pot/67g	119	4.0	178	2.8	28.7	5.9	0.2
Belgian Chocolate, Haagen-Dazs*	1oz/28g	89	5.8	318	4.6	28.4	20.7	0.0
Belgian Milk Chocolate, Tesco*	1 Lolly/85g	255	15.5	300	3.9	29.8	18.2	0.7
Billionaire Shortcake, Chokablok*	1 Scoop/100ml	225	11.4	225	2.8	27.0	11.4	0.7
Bounty, Mars*	1oz/28g	77	5.1	274	3.3	23.8	18.3	0.0
Brandy, Luxurious, M & S*	1 Serving/100g	228	13.3	228	3.8	19.1	13.3	0.2
Cappuccino, Thorntons*	1oz/28g	61	3.6	218	4.4	20.7	12.9	0.0
Caramel, Carte d'Or*	2 Boules/50g	106	4.3	212	2.6	30.8	8.7	0.0
Caramel & Cinnamon Waffle, Carte d'Or*	2 Scoops/55g	121	6.0	220	3.0	27.0	11.0	0.0
Caramel Chew Chew, Ben & Jerry's*	1 Serving/100g	270	16.0	270	3.0	29.0	16.0	0.0
Cheeky Choc, Brownie, Skinny Cow*	1 Tub/500ml	590	5.5	118	3.0	23.9	1.1	4.1
Cherry Bomb Brownie, Chokablok*	1 Scoop/87g	191	8.3	220	3.3	29.9	9.5	1.4
Cherry Garcia, Ben & Jerry's*	1 Serving/100g	250	15.0	250	3.0	26.0	15.0	0.0
Chilli Red, Purbeck*	1 Serving/50g	99	5.7	198	4.8	18.7	11.5	0.0
Choc Chip, Cookie Dough, Haagen-Dazs*	1oz/28g	74	4.7	266	3.8	24.9	16.9	0.0
Choc Chip, Haagen-Dazs*	1oz/28g	80	5.2	286	4.7	24.8	18.7	0.0
Chocolate, Haagen-Dazs*	1 Serving/120ml	269	18.0	224	4.0	19.0	15.0	0.0
Chocolate, Organic, Green & Black's*	1 Serving/125g	310	17.6	248	5.0	25.3	14.1	1.1
Chocolate, Organic, Iceland*	1oz/28g	58	2.3	208	4.9	28.6	8.2	0.0
Chocolate, Organic, M & S*	1oz/28g	71	4.5	255	5.0	24.0	16.0	1.5
Chocolate, Rich, Organic, Sainsbury's*	1 Serving/100g	213	11.7	213	4.4	22.6	11.7	1.2
Chocolate, Soft Scoop, Tesco*	1 Serving/50g	93	4.0	186	3.2	25.1	8.1	0.3
Chocolate, Swirl Pot, Skinny Cow*	1 Pot/100ml	98	0.6	98	2.9	20.2	0.6	2.7
Chocolate, Thorntons*	1oz/28g	67	3.6	238	4.6	25.1	12.9	0.0
Chocolate, Weight Watchers*	1 Serving/100ml	140	1.2	140	4.3	28.7	1.2	0.0
Chocolate & Orange, Organic, Green & Black's*	1 Serving/100g	248	14.1	248	5.0	25.3	14.1	0.1
Chocolate Brownie with Walnuts, Haagen-Dazs*	1 Cup/101g	223	16.4	221	4.4	21.0	16.2	0.0
Chocolate Chip, Baskin Robbins*	1 Serving/75g	170	10.0	227	4.0	24.0	13.3	0.0
Chocolate Flavour, Average	1 Serving/70g	149	7.9	212	4.1	23.7	11.3	0.6
Chocolate Flavour, Healthy Option, Average	1 Serving/70g	89	1.2	127	3.5	25.9	1.7	0.3
Chocolate Flavour, Soft Scoop, Sainsbury's*	1 Serving/70g	122	5.2	174	3.1	23.6	7.5	0.3
Chocolate Fudge Brownie, Ben & Jerry's*	1 Serving/50g	125	6.5	250	4.0	32.0	13.0	1.5
Chocolate Fudge Swirl, Haagen-Dazs*	1oz/28g	77	4.8	275	4.6	25.6	17.2	0.0
Chocolate Honeycomb, Co-Op*	1/4 Pot/81g	186	10.5	230	4.0	26.0	13.0	0.3
Chocolate Honeycomb, COU, M & S*	1 Serving/100ml	150	2.6	150	3.5	31.5	2.6	0.7
Chocolate Macadamia, Ben & Jerry's*	1 Serving/100g	260	18.0	260	4.0	22.0	18.0	0.8
Chocolate Midnight Cookies, Haagen-Dazs*	1oz/28g	81	4.8	289	4.9	28.7	17.2	0.0
Chocolate Orange, Deliciously Dairy, Co-Op*	1oz/28g	55	2.0	195	4.0	29.0	7.0	0.8
Chocolate Ripple, Perfectly Balanced, Waitrose*	1 Serving/125ml	205	3.1	164	4.8	30.5	2.5	4.1
Chocolate Sandwich, Skinny Cow*	1 Portion/36g	101	2.8	280	6.0	46.0	7.9	2.9
Chocolate Trio, Thorntons*	1 Bar/100g	310	20.6	310	3.3	28.0	20.6	1.8
Chocolate with Chocolate Chips, Milfina*	1oz/28g	66	3.5	235	3.8	26.7	12.5	0.8
Chunky Chocolate, Giant, M & S*	1 Lolly/90g	300	20.6	335	4.0	28.0	23.0	2.3
Chunky Monkey, Ben & Jerry's*	1 Serving/100g	290	17.0	290	4.0	27.0	17.0	1.0
Chunky Monkey, Fairtrade, Ben & Jerry's*	1 Serving/100g	290	17.0	290	4.0	27.0	17.0	1.0

ICE CREAM

	Measure INFO/WEIGHT	per Measure KCAL	FAT	Nutrition Values per 100g / 100ml KCAL	PROT	CARB	FAT	FIBRE
Clotted Cream, Cornish, Kelly's Of Cornwall*	1 Serving/125g	282	18.6	226	2.9	20.1	14.9	0.1
Coconut, Carte d'Or*	1 Serving/100ml	125	7.1	125	1.8	14.0	7.1	0.5
Coffee, Finest, Tesco*	¼ Pot/93g	236	14.9	254	4.9	22.5	16.0	0.0
Coffee, Haagen-Dazs*	1 Serving/120ml	271	18.4	226	4.1	17.9	15.3	0.0
Coffee, Waitrose*	¼ Tub/125ml	292	16.4	234	3.6	25.4	13.1	0.0
Cookie Dough, Ben & Jerry's*	1 Serving/100g	270	14.0	270	4.0	31.0	14.0	0.0
Cookie Dough Mon Star, Chokablok*	1 Serving/100g	285	17.1	285	3.3	29.5	17.1	0.6
Cookies & Cream, Haagen-Dazs*	1 Pot/100ml	226	14.7	226	4.0	19.5	14.7	0.0
Cornetto Soft, Chocolate Chip, Wall's Ice Cream*	1 Serving/80g	256	13.6	320	3.5	37.0	17.0	1.5
Cornetto Soft, Mint Chocolate Chip, Wall's Ice Cream*	1 Serving/80g	240	13.6	300	4.0	33.0	17.0	1.0
Cornetto Soft, Strawberry, Wall's Ice Cream*	1 Serving/80g	208	8.0	260	2.5	38.0	10.0	1.0
Cornetto Soft, Vanilla, Wall's Ice Cream*	1 Serving/80g	264	16.0	330	4.5	33.0	20.0	0.0
Cornish, Dairy, Tesco*	1 Serving/49g	112	6.0	228	3.2	24.7	12.3	0.1
Cornish, Dairy, Waitrose*	1 Serving/125ml	121	6.6	97	1.7	10.7	5.3	0.1
Cornish, Full Fat, Asda*	1 Serving/100g	204	11.6	204	3.5	21.4	11.6	0.1
Cornish, Strawberry, Traditional, M & S*	1oz/28g	64	3.1	229	2.3	29.7	11.2	0.2
Cornish, Vanilla, Organic, Iceland*	1oz/28g	60	3.5	214	4.1	21.4	12.4	0.0
Cornish, Vanilla, Soft Scoop, M & S*	1oz/28g	56	3.0	199	3.9	21.8	10.7	0.2
Cornish Style, Co-Op*	1oz/28g	53	2.5	190	4.0	23.0	9.0	0.1
Creamy Chocolate & Nut, Co-Op*	1oz/28g	66	3.6	235	4.0	25.0	13.0	0.5
Crema Di Mascarpone, Carte d'Or*	1 Serving/100g	207	8.9	207	2.8	29.0	8.9	0.0
Crunchie, Blast, Cadbury*	1 Lolly/100ml	225	13.2	225	2.9	23.5	13.2	0.1
Dairy, Flavoured	1oz/28g	50	2.2	179	3.5	24.7	8.0	0.0
Dairy Milk, Orange, Cadbury*	1 Serving/120ml	259	13.9	216	3.5	26.0	11.6	0.0
Dark Toffee, Organic, Green & Black's*	¼ Pot/125ml	192	9.9	154	2.8	18.1	7.9	0.1
Date & Almond Cream, Haagen-Dazs*	1 Serving/120ml	254	15.6	212	5.0	19.0	13.0	0.0
Demon Chocolate, M & S*	1 Serving/79g	208	8.8	263	3.7	37.1	11.1	0.6
Double Chocolate, Nestle*	1 Serving/78g	248	14.3	320	4.8	33.7	18.4	0.0
Dreamy Creamy Cookie, Skinny Cow*	1 Serving/100ml	117	1.1	117	2.7	24.1	1.1	3.9
Farmhouse Toffee, TTD, Sainsbury's*	¼ Pot/100g	293	18.6	293	3.2	28.3	18.6	0.6
Fig & Orange Blossom Honey, Waitrose*	1 Serving/100g	219	11.8	219	3.9	24.3	11.8	0.4
French Toast Flavour, Baskin Robbins*	1 Scoop/71g	180	9.0	254	4.2	31.0	12.7	0.0
Fruit & Fresh Tropical, Carte d'Or*	1 Serving/83g	154	7.1	185	2.5	24.5	8.5	0.0
Fun-Illa, Skinny Cow*	1 Serving/100ml	97	1.6	97	3.1	17.6	1.6	2.4
Gelato, Vanilla	1 Serving/100g	162	7.2	162	2.4	22.6	7.2	0.3
Get Fruit, Tropical, Solero*	1 Serving/125ml	162	5.5	130	1.6	20.6	4.4	0.4
Gold Digger Dynamite, Chokablok*	¼ Tub/125ml	287	14.0	230	3.2	28.2	11.2	0.9
Greek Yoghurt & Honey, Carte d'Or*	1 Serving/55g	114	4.8	207	2.7	29.0	8.8	0.0
Half Baked, Ben & Jerry's*	1 Serving/100g	270	13.0	270	5.0	32.0	13.0	1.0
Heavenly Vanilla, Cadbury*	1 Serving/250ml	355	23.2	142	2.5	12.8	9.3	0.0
Honeycomb Harvest, Mackies*	1 Serving/100g	209	10.0	209	4.0	25.0	10.0	0.0
Knickerbocker Glory	1oz/28g	31	1.4	112	1.5	16.4	5.0	0.2
Lactose Free, Hacendado*	1 Serving/100g	141	4.9	141	4.0	27.6	4.9	6.6
Lavazza, Carte d'Or*	1 Serving/55g	120	5.4	218	3.5	29.0	9.9	0.0
Lemon, Haagen-Dazs*	1 Serving/120ml	144	0.2	120	0.3	29.3	0.2	0.0
Lemon & White Chocolate, Crackpots, Iceland*	1 Serving/100g	202	8.4	202	1.7	29.9	8.4	0.3
Lemon Cream, Dairy, Sainsbury's*	1 Serving/100g	199	9.3	199	3.0	25.9	9.3	0.1
Lemon Curd Swirl, Duchy Originals*	¼ Pot/101g	247	14.2	245	3.7	25.8	14.1	0.0
Lemon Pie, Haagen-Dazs*	1oz/28g	73	4.6	261	3.9	24.5	16.3	0.0
Less Than 5% Fat, Asda*	1 Scoop/40g	56	1.8	139	2.7	22.0	4.5	0.0
Light Chocolate Ices, Co-Op*	1 Ice/62g	121	8.1	195	2.0	18.0	13.0	0.5
Log, Mint Chocolate, Sainsbury's*	1 Serving/51g	100	5.1	197	3.0	23.8	10.0	0.2
Luscious Mint Choc Chip, Morrisons*	1 Serving/50g	99	5.2	198	2.9	23.1	10.5	0.7

ICE CREAM

	Measure INFO/WEIGHT	per Measure KCAL	FAT	Nutrition Values per 100g / 100ml KCAL	PROT	CARB	FAT	FIBRE
Lychee Cream & Ginger, Haagen-Dazs*	1 Serving/120ml	258	12.7	215	3.6	26.1	10.6	0.0
Macadamia Night, Carte d'Or*	2 Scoops/56g	110	4.5	196	0.0	29.0	8.0	0.8
Macadamia Nut, Baskin Robbins*	1 Serving/113g	270	18.0	239	4.4	22.1	15.9	0.9
Madly Deeply, Skinny Cow*	1 Serving/100g	149	2.2	149	4.2	28.3	2.2	3.4
Magic Maple, M & S*	1 Ice Cream/93g	259	11.4	278	2.9	39.0	12.3	0.6
Magic Stars, Milky Way*	1 Ice Cream/53ml	67	3.3	127	2.1	15.5	6.2	0.0
Magnum, Mini, Classic, Wall's*	1 Lolly/50g	170	11.0	340	4.0	30.0	22.0	0.0
Magnum Moments, Wall's Ice Cream*	1 Serving/18ml	58	3.7	323	4.0	30.0	20.8	0.0
Mango, 98% Fat Free, Bulla*	1 Serving/70g	94	1.1	134	4.2	25.4	1.6	0.0
Maple & Walnut, American, Sainsbury's*	1/8 Pot/68g	121	4.9	179	3.1	25.6	7.2	0.2
Maple Brazil, Thorntons*	1oz/28g	66	3.8	236	4.1	24.4	13.6	0.0
Mince Pie, Finest, Tesco*	¼ Pack/188g	476	22.1	254	3.9	33.0	11.8	1.1
Mint, Majestic Luxury, Iceland*	1 Serving/80g	269	14.6	337	3.8	39.3	18.3	1.3
Mint, Thorntons*	1oz/28g	66	3.8	237	4.0	25.0	13.4	0.0
Mint & Chocolate, Sainsbury's*	1 Serving/71g	137	6.7	192	3.4	23.5	9.4	0.4
Mint & Chocolate Flavour, Average	1 Serving/70g	129	6.3	184	3.0	22.6	9.0	1.2
Mint & Chocolate Flavour, Healthy Option, Average	1 Serving/70g	101	1.8	144	4.1	29.9	2.6	4.1
Mint Chocolate Chip, Baskin Robbins*	1 Scoop/113g	270	16.0	239	4.4	24.8	14.2	0.9
Mint Crisp, Nestle*	1 Serving/75ml	232	16.4	309	2.9	25.5	21.9	0.9
Mint Crunch, Dairy Milk, Cadbury*	1 Serving/60ml	162	13.3	270	3.0	29.0	22.2	0.0
Mint Ripple, Good Choice, Iceland*	1 Scoop/50g	58	1.0	117	3.0	21.7	2.1	0.1
Mocha Coffee Indulgence, Sainsbury's*	¼ Pot/82g	178	10.6	217	3.2	22.1	12.9	0.1
Mojito, Appassionato, YSCO*	1 Serving/100g	150	2.9	150	0.3	30.2	2.9	0.2
Monster Mint, Sainsbury's*	1/8 Pot/67g	121	4.6	180	3.0	26.3	6.9	0.3
My Carte D'or, Caramel, Carte d'Or*	1 Tub/200ml	210	8.0	105	1.5	16.0	4.0	0.2
My Carte D'or, Chocolate, Carte d'Or*	1 Tub/200ml	220	11.0	110	1.7	12.5	5.5	0.4
Neapolitan, Average	1 Serving/70g	111	4.6	158	3.1	21.9	6.5	0.6
Neapolitan, Brick, Tesco*	1 Serving/50g	81	3.4	163	3.3	21.9	6.9	0.4
Neapolitan, Organic, Iceland*	1oz/28g	55	2.3	196	4.2	26.4	8.2	0.0
Neapolitan, Soft Scoop, Asda*	1 Scoop/47g	82	3.8	175	2.8	23.0	8.0	0.2
Neapolitan, Soft Scoop, M & S*	1/8 Tub/63g	100	4.6	160	2.7	21.3	7.4	0.3
Neapolitan, Soft Scoop, Sainsbury's*	1 Serving/75g	124	5.2	165	2.8	22.8	6.9	0.2
Neapolitan Brick, Co-Op*	1oz/28g	43	2.0	155	3.0	20.0	7.0	0.2
Neapolitan Easy Serve, Co-Op*	1oz/28g	42	2.0	150	3.0	20.0	7.0	0.2
Neapolitan Sandwich, Gelatelli*	1 Sandwich/106g	233	9.5	220	4.9	29.0	9.0	1.9
Neopolitan, Soft Scoop, Somerfield*	1 Serving/75g	124	5.5	166	2.8	22.6	7.3	0.3
Neopolitian, Soft Scoop, Tesco*	1 Serving/43g	70	3.0	163	3.3	21.9	6.9	0.4
Non-Dairy, Mixes	1oz/28g	51	2.2	182	4.1	25.1	7.9	0.0
Non-Dairy, Reduced Calorie	1oz/28g	33	1.7	119	3.4	13.7	6.0	0.0
Nuts About Caramel, Cadbury*	1 Ice Cream/100ml	260	13.1	260	3.4	23.8	13.1	0.0
Panna Cotta, & Raspberry Swirl, Haagen-Dazs*	1 Serving/120ml	250	14.9	208	3.2	21.0	12.4	0.0
Panna Cotta, Haagen-Dazs*	1 Serving/120ml	248	16.0	207	3.4	18.4	13.3	0.0
Peach Melba, Soft Scoop, M & S*	1oz/28g	46	2.1	165	2.8	21.4	7.6	0.3
Phish Food, Ben & Jerry's*	1 Serving/100g	260	13.0	260	3.5	35.0	13.0	0.1
Picnic, Cadbury*	1 Cone/125ml	258	11.7	207	3.4	28.9	9.4	0.3
Pistachio, Haagen-Dazs*	1 Serving/120ml	276	18.8	230	4.4	17.7	15.7	0.0
Praline, Green & Black's*	1 Sm Pot/100g	191	10.8	191	3.5	20.0	10.8	0.9
Praline & Chocolate, Thorntons*	1oz/28g	87	6.4	309	4.6	21.3	22.9	0.6
Pralines & Cream, Baskin Robbins*	1 Serving/100g	252	13.6	252	4.5	27.7	13.6	0.3
Pralines & Cream, Haagen-Dazs*	1 Serving/100g	272	16.5	272	3.9	27.2	16.5	0.0
Raspberries, Clotted Cream, Waitrose*	1 Tub/500ml	790	39.5	158	2.9	18.9	7.9	0.1
Raspberry, & Shortcake, Co-Op*	1oz/28g	64	3.9	230	3.0	23.0	14.0	0.3
Raspberry, Easy Serve, Co-Op*	1oz/28g	43	1.7	152	2.5	22.3	5.9	0.0

ICE CREAM

INFO/WEIGHT	Measure	per Measure KCAL	FAT	Nutrition Values per 100g / 100ml KCAL	PROT	CARB	FAT	FIBRE
Raspberry, Haagen-Dazs*	1 Serving/120ml	127	0.2	106	0.2	25.9	0.2	0.0
Raspberry, Swirl Pot, Skinny Cow*	1 Pot/100ml	86	0.3	86	2.5	18.4	0.3	2.2
Raspberry Ripple, Average	1 Serving/70g	93	3.3	134	1.9	20.8	4.7	0.1
Raspberry Ripple, Dairy, Waitrose*	1 Serving/186ml	195	10.0	105	1.9	12.3	5.4	0.0
Raspberry Ripple, Organic, Iceland*	1oz/28g	50	2.2	180	4.8	22.6	7.8	0.0
Raspberry Ripple, Soft Scoop, Asda*	1 Scoop/46g	78	3.2	170	2.5	24.0	7.0	0.3
Raspberry Ripple, Soft Scoop, Sainsbury's*	1 Serving/75g	127	5.2	170	2.6	24.2	7.0	0.3
Raspberry Ripple, Soft Scoop, Tesco*	1 Scoop/25g	39	1.5	157	2.5	23.0	6.1	0.2
Raspberry Ripple Brick, Tesco*	1 Serving/48g	71	2.9	148	2.6	20.8	6.0	0.2
Really Creamy After Dinner Mint, Asda*	1 Serving/100g	191	9.0	191	3.4	24.0	9.0	0.4
Really Creamy Chocolate, Asda*	1 Serving/100g	227	11.0	227	4.1	28.0	11.0	0.4
Really Creamy Lemon Meringue, Asda*	1 Serving/100ml	100	5.0	100	1.8	12.0	5.0	0.1
Really Creamy Toffee, Asda*	1 Serving/120ml	146	6.0	122	1.7	17.5	5.0	0.1
Rocky Road, M & S*	1 Tub/500g	1475	88.5	295	4.2	29.5	17.7	1.2
Rocky Road, Sainsbury's*	1/8 Pot/67g	137	4.9	205	3.8	30.9	7.3	1.0
Rolo, Nestle*	½ Tub/500ml	1180	52.5	236	3.4	31.9	10.5	0.2
Rum & Raisin, Carte d'Or*	2 Scoops/50g	100	4.0	200	2.5	24.0	8.0	1.0
Rum & Raisin, Haagen-Dazs*	1 Serving/120ml	264	17.6	220	3.4	18.6	14.7	0.0
Rum & Raisin, Organic, Iceland*	1oz/28g	55	2.0	195	4.5	28.1	7.2	0.0
Rum & Raisin, TTD, Sainsbury's*	¼ Pot/100g	220	10.4	220	3.8	27.7	10.4	1.0
Sandwich, Vanilla, Skinny Cow*	1 Portion/36g	100	3.0	277	5.4	45.1	8.2	2.1
Screwball, Asda*	1 Screwball/60g	122	6.0	203	3.3	25.0	10.0	1.5
Screwball, Co-Op*	1 Lolly/95g	190	6.6	200	2.0	31.0	7.0	0.0
Screwball, Farmfoods*	1 Lolly/72ml	127	4.4	177	3.3	27.1	6.1	0.0
Screwball, Tesco*	1 Screwball/61g	116	5.2	190	2.9	25.2	8.6	0.3
Smarties, Nestle*	1 Serving/50g	125	5.9	250	3.6	32.3	11.9	0.2
Smarties Ice Cream Pot, Nestle*	1 Pot/69g	151	5.7	218	4.4	33.6	8.2	0.0
Soft Scoop, Neapolitan, Value, Tesco*	1 Serving/100g	125	5.1	125	2.7	16.2	5.1	1.4
Soft Scoop, Vanilla, Light, Weighed in Grams, Wall's*	1 Serving/100g	140	6.0	140	3.0	19.0	6.0	2.0
Spagnola, Carte d'Or*	1 Serving/100g	187	5.7	187	2.0	32.0	5.7	0.0
Sticky Toffee, Cream O' Galloway*	1 Serving/30g	80	4.4	266	4.7	28.7	14.7	0.0
Strawberries & Cream, Deliciously Dairy, Co-Op*	1oz/28g	46	1.7	165	3.0	24.0	6.0	0.3
Strawberry, Get Fruit, Solero*	1 Serving/100ml	120	4.5	120	1.5	18.8	4.5	1.3
Strawberry, Haagen-Dazs*	1oz/28g	67	4.3	241	4.0	21.5	15.5	0.0
Strawberry, Swirl Pot, Skinny Cow*	1 Pot/100ml	89	0.3	89	2.5	19.0	0.3	2.2
Strawberry, Thorntons*	1oz/28g	52	2.6	185	3.2	22.5	9.3	0.1
Strawberry, Weight Watchers*	1 Pot/57g	81	2.2	142	2.5	23.4	3.9	0.2
Strawberry & Cream, Mivvi, Nestle*	1 Serving/60g	118	4.6	196	2.6	29.4	7.6	0.1
Strawberry & Cream, Organic, Sainsbury's*	1 Serving/100g	193	9.8	193	3.6	22.6	9.8	0.4
Strawberry & Yoghurt Delice, Carte d'Or*	1 Portion/54g	95	2.0	175	1.5	34.0	3.6	0.0
Strawberry Cheesecake, Co-Op*	1/6 Pot/86g	163	6.0	190	3.0	29.0	7.0	0.2
Tantilising Toffee, COU, M & S*	¼ Pot/125ml	125	3.5	100	0.6	18.0	2.8	0.0
Taste Sensation, Mascarpone Forest Fruits, Aldi*	1 Pot/73g	159	7.4	217	1.8	29.6	10.1	0.6
Terry's Chocolate Orange, Carte d'Or*	1 Serving/100g	182	7.1	182	2.8	27.0	7.1	0.0
The Chocolate Extremist, Chokablok*	1 Serving/100g	255	11.7	255	4.7	32.2	11.7	1.2
Tiramisu, COU, M & S*	¼ Tub/86g	120	2.5	140	2.1	26.4	2.9	3.0
Tiramisu, Haagen-Dazs*	1 Serving/120ml	303	19.6	253	3.8	22.7	16.3	0.0
Toblerone, Carte d'Or*	1 Serving/100g	211	9.1	211	3.7	29.0	9.1	0.0
Toffee, Deliciously Dairy, Co-Op*	1oz/28g	45	2.0	160	3.0	21.0	7.0	0.2
Toffee, Somerfield*	1 Serving/75g	172	6.9	229	3.4	33.2	9.2	0.9
Toffee, Swirl Pot, Skinny Cow*	1 Pot/66g	92	0.4	140	3.8	29.8	0.6	4.5
Toffee, Thorntons*	1oz/28g	61	3.2	218	4.1	24.5	11.6	0.0
Toffee & Biscuit, Weight Watchers*	1 Pot/100ml	93	2.7	93	1.5	14.9	2.7	0.1

ICE CREAM

	Measure INFO/WEIGHT	per Measure KCAL	FAT	Nutrition Values per 100g / 100ml KCAL	PROT	CARB	FAT	FIBRE
Toffee & Honeycomb Sundaes, Weight Watchers*	1 Pot/150g	222	4.6	148	2.1	32.7	3.1	1.6
Toffee & Vanilla, Sainsbury's*	1 Serving/71g	146	6.8	205	3.1	26.7	9.5	0.1
Toffee Creme, Haagen-Dazs*	1oz/28g	74	4.4	265	4.5	26.7	15.6	0.0
Toffee Fudge, Soft Scoop, Asda*	1 Serving/50g	92	3.5	185	2.6	28.0	7.0	0.0
Toffee Ripple, Tesco*	1 Serving/100g	173	7.2	173	2.7	24.4	7.2	0.1
Triple Chocolate, Brownie, Skinny Cow*	1 Ice Cream/65g	93	1.7	144	3.5	24.1	2.6	5.3
Triple Chocolate, Carte d'Or*	1 Serving/58g	122	5.7	210	3.7	27.0	9.8	0.0
Triple Chocolate, Dairy, Morrisons*	1 Serving/100g	233	10.8	233	3.8	30.0	10.8	0.4
Triple Chocolate, Dairy, Sainsbury's*	1/8 Litre/67g	123	4.4	184	3.5	27.6	6.6	1.0
Triple Chocolate Centenary, Cadbury*	1 Serving/100ml	255	15.6	255	2.5	27.1	15.6	0.0
Truffle Berry Fling, Skinny Cow*	1 Serving/100g	156	2.0	156	4.0	30.5	2.0	3.3
Truly Lovin' Toffee, Skinny Cow*	1 Tub/352g	510	3.5	145	3.5	30.5	1.0	6.6
Vanilla, Ben & Jerry's*	1 Mini Tub/116g	267	17.4	230	4.0	20.0	15.0	0.1
Vanilla, Carte d'Or*	1 Serving/50g	105	4.7	210	3.0	26.0	9.5	0.0
Vanilla, COU, M & S*	1/4 Pot/79g	111	2.2	140	1.7	25.9	2.8	0.8
Vanilla, Criminally Creamy, Co-Op*	1oz/28g	60	4.2	215	3.0	18.0	15.0	0.1
Vanilla, Dairy, Average	1 Scoop/40g	80	4.4	201	3.5	23.6	11.0	0.7
Vanilla, Dairy, Finest, Tesco*	1 Serving/92g	227	16.0	247	4.5	18.0	17.4	0.3
Vanilla, Dairy, Organic, Yeo Valley*	1 Serving/100g	206	11.2	206	4.9	21.3	11.2	0.0
Vanilla, Dairy Milk, Cadbury*	1 Serving/120g	259	13.9	216	3.5	26.0	11.6	0.1
Vanilla, Deliciously Dairy, Co-Op*	1oz/28g	49	2.2	175	3.0	23.0	8.0	0.2
Vanilla, Easy Serve, Co-Op*	1oz/28g	39	2.0	140	3.0	18.0	7.0	0.2
Vanilla, Everyday, Co-Op*	1oz/28g	41	2.0	145	3.0	18.0	7.0	0.2
Vanilla, Fairtrade, Ben & Jerry's*	1 Serving/100g	230	15.0	230	4.0	20.0	15.0	0.1
Vanilla, Haagen-Dazs*	1oz/28g	70	4.8	250	4.5	19.7	17.1	0.0
Vanilla, Light, Carte d'Or*	1 Serving/100g	136	4.4	136	2.4	22.0	4.4	4.0
Vanilla, Light Soft Scoop, 25% Less Fat, Morrisons*	1 Scoop/50g	75	2.5	150	2.9	23.2	5.0	0.2
Vanilla, Low Fat, Average	1 Scoop/50g	59	1.7	118	2.3	19.4	3.4	0.6
Vanilla, Low Fat, Weight Watchers*	1 Scoop/125ml	75	2.1	60	1.1	9.7	1.7	0.1
Vanilla, Mackies*	1 Serving/100g	193	11.0	193	4.0	18.0	11.0	0.0
Vanilla, Non-Dairy, Average	1 Serving/60g	107	5.2	178	3.2	23.1	8.7	0.0
Vanilla, Organic, Iceland*	1oz/28g	61	3.4	217	4.5	22.2	12.2	0.0
Vanilla, Organic, Sainsbury's*	1 Serving/85g	176	10.2	207	4.3	20.5	12.0	0.1
Vanilla, Organic, Tesco*	1 Serving/100g	237	17.2	237	3.7	16.8	17.2	0.0
Vanilla, Organic, Waitrose*	1 Serving/125g	177	11.2	142	2.7	12.4	9.0	0.0
Vanilla, Pecan, Haagen-Dazs*	1 Serving/120ml	316	23.5	263	4.3	17.1	19.6	0.0
Vanilla, Pizza Express*	1 Serving/100g	119	6.8	119	0.9	13.8	6.8	0.0
Vanilla, Really Creamy, Asda*	1 Serving/50g	98	5.0	196	3.5	23.0	10.0	0.1
Vanilla, Smart Price, Asda*	1 Scoop/40g	55	2.4	137	2.8	19.0	6.0	0.2
Vanilla, Soft, Non Milk Fat, Waitrose*	1 Serving/125ml	77	3.4	62	1.3	8.0	2.7	0.1
Vanilla, Soft Scoop, 25% Less Fat, Asda*	1oz/28g	42	1.4	149	2.9	23.0	5.0	0.0
Vanilla, Soft Scoop, BGTY, Sainsbury's*	1 Serving/75g	88	1.3	117	3.1	22.2	1.7	0.2
Vanilla, Soft Scoop, GFY, Asda*	1 Serving/100g	117	1.7	117	3.1	22.0	1.7	0.2
Vanilla, Soft Scoop, Light, Wall's*, Wall's Ice Cream*	1 Scoop/50ml	31	1.3	62	1.3	7.0	2.6	0.9
Vanilla, Soft Scoop, Tesco*	1oz/28g	46	2.0	164	3.1	21.8	7.1	0.1
Vanilla, Soft Scoop, Value, Tesco*	1 Scoop/42g	57	2.4	137	2.8	18.7	5.7	0.2
Vanilla, Soft Slice, Wall's Ice Cream*	1 Serving/100ml	90	4.4	90	1.4	11.2	4.4	0.1
Vanilla, Thorntons*	1oz/28g	63	3.8	225	4.9	20.5	13.6	0.0
Vanilla, Toffe Crunch, Fairtrade, Ben & Jerry's*	1 Serving/100g	280	16.0	280	4.0	29.0	16.0	0.5
Vanilla, Toffee Crunch, Ben & Jerry's*	1 Tub/407g	1099	65.1	270	4.0	29.0	16.0	0.5
Vanilla, Too Good to Be True, Wall's Ice Cream*	1 Serving/50ml	35	0.2	70	2.0	14.9	0.4	0.1
Vanilla, TTD, Sainsbury's*	1/4 Pot/100g	246	16.9	246	5.2	18.2	16.9	0.0
Vanilla, Waitrose*	1 Serving/100ml	156	10.8	156	2.6	12.0	10.8	0.0

ICE CREAM

	Measure INFO/WEIGHT	per Measure KCAL	FAT	Nutrition Values per 100g / 100ml KCAL	PROT	CARB	FAT	FIBRE
Vanilla & Cinnamon, Finest, Tesco*	1 Serving/50g	114	7.3	229	3.9	20.2	14.7	0.4
Vanilla & Strawberry, Weight Watchers*	1 Serving/100ml	81	2.2	81	1.4	13.3	2.2	0.1
Vanilla Bean, Light, Deluxe*	1 Serving/64g	110	2.5	172	4.7	26.6	3.9	0.0
Vanilla Bean, Purbeck*	1 Serving/100g	198	11.5	198	4.8	18.7	11.5	0.0
Vanilla Caramel Brownie, Haagen-Dazs*	1 Serving/150g	410	24.7	273	4.5	26.8	16.5	0.0
Vanilla Choc Fudge, Haagen-Dazs*	1oz/28g	75	4.8	267	4.3	23.5	17.2	0.0
Vanilla Chocolate, Taste Sensation, Frosty's, Aldi*	1 Pot/73g	164	7.0	224	2.1	32.4	9.6	0.7
Vanilla Flavour, Budgens*	1oz/28g	45	1.9	159	3.0	21.7	6.7	0.1
Vanilla Flavour, Soft Scoop, Sainsbury's*	1 Serving/71g	96	3.9	136	2.9	18.8	5.5	0.2
Vanilla Flavour, Soft, VLH Kitchens	1 Serving/100g	235	15.0	235	4.0	22.1	15.0	0.2
Vanilla with Strawberry Swirl, Mini Tub, Weight Watchers*	1 Mini Tub/57g	81	2.2	142	2.5	23.4	3.9	0.2
Vanilla with Vanilla Pods, Sainsbury's*	1 Serving/100g	195	10.1	195	3.5	22.5	10.1	0.1
Vanilletta, Tesco*	1 Serving/47g	82	3.8	175	4.0	21.6	8.1	0.0
Viennetta, Biscuit Caramel, Wall's Ice Cream*	1/6 Serving/58g	183	12.1	315	3.3	27.8	20.9	0.0
Viennetta, Cappuccino, Wall's Ice Cream*	1 Serving/75g	191	12.7	255	3.5	22.0	17.0	0.0
Viennetta, Chocolate, Wall's Ice Cream*	¼ Pot/80g	200	12.2	250	4.1	24.0	15.2	0.0
Viennetta, Forest Fruit, Wall's Ice Cream*	1 Serving/98g	265	15.9	270	3.4	27.2	16.2	0.0
Viennetta, Mint, Wall's Ice Cream*	1 Serving/80g	204	13.3	255	3.4	23.0	16.6	0.0
Viennetta, Selection Brownie, Wall's Ice Cream*	1 Serving/70g	194	11.3	277	4.2	28.5	16.2	0.0
Viennetta, Strawberry, Wall's Ice Cream*	1 Serving/80g	204	13.4	255	3.4	22.1	16.8	0.0
Viennetta, Vanilla, Wall's Ice Cream*	¼ Bar/80g	204	13.4	255	3.3	23.0	16.7	0.0
Voluptuous Vanilla, COU, M & S*	1 Pot/400g	520	10.4	130	4.6	22.0	2.6	0.6
Walnut & Maple, Waitrose*	1 Serving/60g	68	2.3	114	1.8	18.2	3.8	0.0

ICE CREAM BAR

Bounty, 100 Ml Bar, Mars*	1 Bar/100ml	278	18.5	278	3.4	24.7	18.5	0.7
Bournville, Cadbury*	1 Bar/120g	258	13.9	215	3.5	26.0	11.6	0.0
Choc Chip, Haagen-Dazs*	1oz/28g	90	6.0	320	4.3	27.4	21.5	0.0
Chocolate Covered	1 Bar/40g	128	9.3	320	5.0	24.0	23.3	0.0
Chunky Chocolate, Co-Op*	1 Bar/60g	204	12.0	340	5.0	35.0	20.0	1.0
Chunky Toffee, Co-Op*	1 Bar/60g	204	12.6	340	4.0	34.0	21.0	1.0
Dairy Milk, Caramel, Cadbury*	1 Bar/60ml	175	10.3	290	3.6	30.2	17.1	0.0
Dairy Milk, Fruit & Nut, Cadbury*	1 Bar/90ml	243	15.3	270	3.5	26.1	17.0	0.0
Dairy Milk, Fudge, Cadbury*	1 Bar/60g	165	10.3	275	3.0	27.6	17.2	0.0
Dream, Cadbury*	1 Bar/120ml	264	14.3	220	3.6	26.0	11.9	0.0
Dream, Cadbury*	1 Serving/118g	260	14.0	220	3.6	26.0	11.9	0.0
Dulce De Leche, Bar, Haagen-Dazs*	1 Bar/105g	370	24.0	352	3.8	32.3	22.9	0.0
Galaxy, Mars*	1 Bar/60ml	203	13.4	339	4.7	29.7	22.4	0.0
Galaxy, Mars*	1 Bar/54g	184	12.1	341	3.8	30.7	22.5	0.6
Lion, Nestle*	1 Bar/45g	166	9.9	370	4.2	39.1	21.9	1.0
Maltesers, Mars*	1 Bar/45ml	113	7.0	252	2.9	25.0	15.6	0.7
Mars, Mars*	1 Bar/65g	182	10.5	280	3.4	29.7	16.2	0.8
Peanut, Farmfoods*	1 Bar/60ml	216	12.8	360	5.3	36.6	21.4	1.2
Racer, Aldi*	1 Bar/59g	194	11.0	328	6.0	34.2	18.6	0.0
Rage, Chocolate with Caramel Sauce, Treats*	1 Bar/60g	177	10.5	295	3.3	30.9	17.5	0.0
Red Fruits, Solero*	1 Bar/80g	99	2.2	124	1.6	25.0	2.7	0.0
Snickers, Mars*	1 Bar/67g	250	15.0	373	6.0	37.3	22.4	0.0
Toffee Cream, Haagen-Dazs*	1oz/28g	97	6.2	345	4.0	31.0	22.0	0.0
Toffee Crunch, English, Weight Watchers*	1 Bar/40g	110	6.0	275	2.5	32.5	15.0	5.0
Twix, Mars*	1 Serving/43ml	130	7.8	306	4.0	30.8	18.3	1.2
Vanilla & Raspberry, Weight Watchers*	1 Serving/100g	81	0.3	81	2.0	23.0	0.3	0.0

ICE CREAM CONE

After Eight, Nestle*	1 Cone/100ml	174	8.0	174	2.4	23.0	8.0	0.9
Average	1 Cone/75g	139	6.4	186	3.5	25.5	8.5	0.0

ICE CREAM CONE

	Measure INFO/WEIGHT	per Measure KCAL	FAT	Nutrition Values per 100g / 100ml KCAL	PROT	CARB	FAT	FIBRE
Blackcurrant, GFY, Asda*	1 Cone/67g	162	6.0	241	3.0	37.0	9.0	0.1
Carousel Wafer Company*	1 Cone/5g	19	0.2	392	9.8	78.6	4.2	0.0
Choc 'n' Nut, Farmfoods*	1 Cone/120ml	334	16.8	278	5.0	33.0	14.0	1.0
Chocolate, M & S*	1oz/28g	94	6.4	335	4.0	28.0	23.0	2.3
Chocolate, Mini, Cornetto, Wall's Ice Cream*	1 Cone/19g	69	4.4	363	4.2	34.2	23.2	0.0
Chocolate, Vanilla & Hazelnut, Sainsbury's*	1 Cone/62g	190	10.5	306	4.5	33.9	16.9	0.6
Chocolate & Caramel, Skinny Cow*	1 Cone/110ml	121	2.8	110	2.5	19.3	2.5	2.7
Chocolate & Nut, Co-Op*	1 Cone/110g	307	17.0	279	3.9	31.0	15.5	0.6
Chocolate & Vanilla, Good Choice, Iceland*	1 Cone/110ml	161	7.1	146	2.7	22.9	6.5	0.8
Chocolate & Vanilla, M & S*	1oz/28g	83	4.8	295	4.2	31.8	17.0	0.7
Chocolate Flavour, Somerfield*	1 Cone/110ml	329	16.5	299	4.0	38.0	15.0	0.0
Cone, Haagen-Dazs*	1oz/28g	85	5.7	303	4.7	25.5	20.3	0.0
Cornet, Wafer Cone, Askeys*	1 Cone/4g	13	0.1	376	10.7	77.6	2.5	0.0
Cornetto, Classico, Mini, Wall's Ice Cream*	1 Cone/19g	67	4.4	353	4.2	32.6	23.2	0.0
Cornetto, Classico, Wall's Ice Cream*	1 Cone/98g	200	12.6	205	2.7	19.7	12.9	0.0
Cornetto, Flirt, Choc Chip with Hazelnut, Wall's Ice Cream*	1 Cone/70g	223	11.2	320	4.0	40.0	16.0	0.0
Cornetto, Frutti Disc, Wall's Ice Cream*	1 Cone/80g	200	8.8	250	2.5	35.0	11.0	0.0
Cornetto, GFY, Asda*	1 Cone/67g	162	6.0	241	3.0	37.0	9.0	0.1
Cornetto, Mint, Wall's Ice Cream*	1 Cone/75g	190	9.9	250	4.0	31.0	13.0	0.8
Cornetto, Wall's Ice Cream*	1 Cone/75g	195	9.7	260	3.7	34.5	12.9	0.0
Creme Egg, Cadbury*	1 Cone/115ml	270	13.3	235	2.9	29.3	11.6	0.0
Cup Cornet, Wafer Cone, Askeys*	1 Cone/4g	13	0.1	376	10.7	77.6	2.5	0.0
Extreme Raspberry, Cornetto, Nestle*	1 Cone/88g	220	8.8	250	2.5	36.0	10.0	0.2
Flake 99, Cadbury*	1 Cone/125ml	244	12.5	195	2.6	23.2	10.0	0.0
Flake 99, Strawberry, Cadbury*	1 Serving/125g	250	10.9	200	2.6	27.3	8.7	0.0
Mini, Sainsbury's*	1 Cone/18g	66	3.8	366	4.4	39.8	21.0	3.4
Mini, Tesco*	1 Cone/48g	152	9.3	316	4.1	31.5	19.3	0.8
Mint Choc Chip, Iceland*	1 Cone/72g	210	9.4	292	3.3	40.4	13.0	1.0
Raspberry & Vanilla, Refreshing, Skinny Cow*	1 Cone/110ml	122	2.8	111	1.7	20.4	2.5	1.5
Smarties, Nestle*	1 Cone/100g	177	8.1	177	2.4	23.6	8.1	0.7
Sticky Toffee, Farmfoods*	1 Cone/120ml	326	15.4	272	3.2	36.0	12.8	2.0
Strawberry, BGTY, Sainsbury's*	1 Cone/69g	151	4.5	219	2.6	37.5	6.5	1.3
Strawberry, Co-Op*	1 Cone/110g	283	13.3	257	3.5	33.6	12.1	0.5
Strawberry, M & S*	1oz/28g	74	3.9	263	3.5	31.1	14.0	0.4
Strawberry, Somerfield*	1 Cone/110g	299	12.1	272	3.0	40.0	11.0	0.0
Strawberry & Vanilla, Asda*	1 Cone/115ml	193	9.0	168	1.8	22.6	7.8	0.1
Strawberry & Vanilla, Farmfoods*	1 Cone/120ml	308	15.6	257	3.0	32.0	13.0	2.0
Strawberry & Vanilla, HL, Tesco*	1 Serving/69g	149	4.3	216	3.4	36.4	6.3	1.4
Strawberry & Vanilla, Iceland*	1 Serving/70g	182	7.6	260	3.3	37.5	10.8	0.7
Strawberry & Vanilla, M & S*	1oz/28g	81	4.6	290	4.2	30.9	16.5	0.7
Strawberry & Vanilla, Sainsbury's*	1 Cone/70g	171	6.8	243	3.4	35.6	9.7	1.0
Strawberry & Vanilla, Tesco*	1 Cone/70g	194	9.4	277	3.0	35.9	13.5	0.3
Toffee Flavoured, Somerfield*	1 Cone/110ml	320	15.4	291	4.0	39.0	14.0	0.0
Tropical, GFY, Asda*	1 Cone/100g	135	5.0	135	2.6	20.0	5.0	0.3

ICE CREAM ROLL

	Measure INFO/WEIGHT	per Measure KCAL	FAT	Nutrition Values per 100g / 100ml KCAL	PROT	CARB	FAT	FIBRE
Arctic, Average	1 Serving/70g	140	4.6	200	4.1	33.3	6.6	0.0
M & S*	1oz/28g	60	1.9	215	3.6	35.2	6.7	0.0
Mini, Cadbury*	1 Roll/45ml	99	5.9	220	3.4	24.3	13.1	0.0
Tesco*	¼ Roll/57g	131	4.9	230	3.7	34.5	8.6	0.4

ICE CREAM SANDWICH

	Measure INFO/WEIGHT	per Measure KCAL	FAT	Nutrition Values per 100g / 100ml KCAL	PROT	CARB	FAT	FIBRE
Mint, Skinny Cow*	1 Serving/71g	140	2.0	197	4.2	39.4	2.8	1.4
Vanilla, Chocolate Coated, Lidl*	1 Serving/51g	145	9.5	284	1.8	21.6	18.6	0.0
Wich, Ben & Jerry's*	1 Pack/117g	398	19.9	340	4.0	44.0	17.0	1.0

	Measure INFO/WEIGHT	per Measure KCAL	FAT	Nutrition Values per 100g / 100ml KCAL	PROT	CARB	FAT	FIBRE
ICE CREAM STICK								
Berry Blast, Smoothie, Skinny Cow*	1 Stick/110ml	71	0.1	65	0.9	15.1	0.1	1.9
Chocolate Cookies, Haagen-Dazs*	1 Stick/43g	162	10.9	376	4.9	31.8	25.4	0.0
Cookies 'n' Cream, Skinny Cow*	1 Stick/67g	89	1.0	133	4.8	25.3	1.5	3.6
Mini Chocolate Stick, Milk Chocolate, Weight Watchers*	1 Stick/32g	95	5.1	296	3.7	33.8	15.9	1.6
Mini Sticks, Milk Chocolate, Weight Watchers*	1 Mini Stick/45ml	96	5.0	213	2.7	25.8	11.1	0.7
Mint Double Chocolate, Skinny Cow*	1 Stick/110ml	94	1.8	85	2.7	15.1	1.6	2.4
Stem Ginger, with Belgian Chocolate, Waitrose*	1 Lolly/110g	255	14.4	232	2.9	25.5	13.1	1.7
Strawberries & Cream, Skinny Cow*	1 Stick/110ml	82	1.0	75	2.8	13.6	0.9	2.3
Strawberry, Majestic, Luxury, Iceland*	1 Lolly/100g	281	18.6	281	2.7	25.8	18.6	0.1
Toffee, Skinny Cow*	1 Stick/72g	87	0.4	121	3.9	25.2	0.5	4.2
Triple Chocolate, Skinny Cow*	1 Stick/68g	87	1.5	128	4.3	22.8	2.2	2.8
Tropical Moment, Asda*	1 Lolly/75g	112	3.1	150	1.7	26.1	4.2	0.4
Vanilla Macadamia, Haagen-Dazs*	1 Stick/42g	161	11.6	383	4.6	28.7	27.7	0.0
ICE LOLLY								
Assorted, De Roma*	1 Lolly/55ml	48	0.2	87	0.2	20.9	0.4	0.2
Assorted, Farmfoods*	1 Lolly/56ml	35	0.0	62	0.0	15.6	0.0	0.0
Assorted, Iceland*	1 Lolly/51g	33	0.0	65	0.0	16.2	0.0	0.0
Baby, Tesco*	1 Lolly/32g	26	0.0	80	0.1	20.0	0.0	0.1
Berry Burst, Sainsbury's*	1 Lolly/90ml	93	1.6	103	1.1	20.8	1.8	0.7
Blackcurrant, Dairy Split, Sainsbury's*	1 Lolly/73ml	88	2.6	121	1.8	20.4	3.6	0.1
Blackcurrant, Ribena*	1 Lolly/55ml	43	0.0	79	0.0	19.2	0.0	0.0
Blackcurrant Split, Iceland*	1 Lolly/75g	61	2.4	81	1.1	12.0	3.2	0.1
Bournville, Cadbury*	1 Lolly/110g	269	17.2	245	2.5	23.2	15.6	0.0
Calippo, Lemon Lime, Mini, Wall's Ice Cream*	1 Lolly/80g	68	0.0	85	0.0	21.0	0.0	0.2
Calippo, Orange, Mini, Wall's Ice Cream*	1 Lolly/78g	70	0.0	90	0.0	21.9	0.0	0.2
Calippo, Strawberry Tropical, Wall's Ice Cream*	1 Lolly/105g	89	0.1	85	0.1	21.0	0.1	0.0
Calippo Shots, Cool Lemon, Wall's Ice Cream*	1oz/28g	8	0.4	28	0.1	3.9	1.3	0.0
Calippo Shots, Twisted Berry, Wall's Ice Cream*	1oz/28g	8	0.3	28	0.1	4.2	1.2	0.0
Choc & Almond, Mini, Tesco*	1 Lolly/31g	103	7.4	331	4.4	24.8	23.8	0.9
Choc Lime Split, Morrisons*	1 Lolly/73ml	120	6.1	164	1.6	20.4	8.4	0.1
Chocolate, Mini Milk, Milk Time, Wall's Ice Cream*	1 Lolly/23g	31	0.7	135	4.3	22.0	3.1	1.0
Chocolate, Plain, Mini, Tesco*	1 Lolly/31g	94	6.6	304	3.1	24.8	21.4	1.2
Chocolate, Pooh Stick, Nestle*	1 Lolly/40g	36	1.4	89	2.1	12.9	3.6	0.0
Chocolate & Vanilla, Sainsbury's*	1 Lolly/40g	143	10.1	357	3.7	28.7	25.3	2.2
Cider Refresher, Treats*	1 Lolly/70ml	54	0.0	77	0.0	19.2	0.0	0.0
Cola Lickers, Farmfoods*	1 Lolly/56ml	38	0.0	68	0.0	17.0	0.0	0.0
Creamy Tropical Sorbet, Sticks, Waitrose*	1 Lolly/85g	100	1.8	118	1.9	22.9	2.1	0.8
Exotic Fruit, Mini, HL, Tesco*	1 Lolly/31g	41	0.6	131	1.0	26.4	2.0	1.0
Exotic Split, Bars, M & S*	1oz/28g	36	0.5	127	2.5	25.0	1.9	0.4
Fab, Nestle*	1 Lolly/57g	78	2.7	136	0.5	22.8	4.7	0.2
Fab, Orange, Nestle*	1 Lolly/58g	81	2.7	140	0.6	24.0	4.7	0.0
Feast, Chocolate, Mini, Wall's Ice Cream*	1 Lolly/52g	165	11.9	318	3.3	24.0	23.0	0.0
Feast, Ice Cream, Original, Wall's Ice Cream*	1 Lolly/92ml	294	21.6	320	3.2	23.8	23.5	0.0
Feast, Toffee, Mini, Wall's Ice Cream*	1 Lolly/52g	163	12.0	313	3.0	24.0	23.0	0.0
Feast, Wall's Ice Cream*	1 Lolly/92ml	276	20.2	300	3.2	22.0	22.0	0.0
Fruit, Assorted, Waitrose*	1 Lolly/73g	59	0.0	81	0.0	20.0	0.0	0.1
Fruit, Red, Tesco*	1 Lolly/32g	40	0.6	128	1.8	25.6	2.0	0.6
Fruit Assorted, Basics, Somerfield*	1 Lolly/56ml	32	0.0	58	0.0	15.0	0.0	0.0
Fruit Flavour, Assorted, Basics, Sainsbury's*	1 Lolly/50g	33	0.0	66	0.0	16.5	0.0	0.0
Fruit Fusion, Mini, Farmfoods*	1 Lolly/45ml	36	0.0	79	0.2	19.2	0.1	0.2
Fruit Ices, Made with Orange Juice, Del Monte*	1 Lolly/75ml	79	0.0	105	0.5	25.7	0.0	0.0
Fruit Luxury, Mini, Co-Op*	1 Lolly/45g	58	2.7	130	2.0	18.0	6.0	0.2
Fruit Pastilles, Rowntree's*	1 Lolly/65ml	61	0.0	94	0.1	23.2	0.0	0.0

ICE LOLLY

	Measure INFO/WEIGHT	per Measure KCAL	FAT	Nutrition Values per 100g / 100ml KCAL	PROT	CARB	FAT	FIBRE
Fruit Split, Asda*	1 Lolly/74g	85	2.7	115	1.7	19.0	3.6	0.0
Fruit Split, Assorted, Co-Op*	1 Lolly/73g	80	2.2	110	1.0	20.0	3.0	0.1
Fruit Split, BFY, Morrisons*	1 Lolly/73g	50	0.5	69	1.6	13.9	0.7	0.1
Fruit Split, Waitrose*	1 Lolly/73g	91	2.6	124	2.5	21.7	3.6	0.4
Fruit Splits, Assorted, Somerfield*	1 Lolly/73ml	74	2.2	102	0.0	18.0	3.0	0.0
Fruit Splits, Treats*	1 Lolly/75ml	77	3.1	103	1.4	17.6	4.1	0.0
Fruity 'n' Freezy, Asda*	1 Lolly/30ml	24	0.0	80	0.1	20.0	0.0	0.0
Funny Foot, Wall's Ice Cream*	1 Lolly/81ml	83	4.9	102	2.0	12.5	6.0	0.0
Icicles, All Flavours, Freezepops, Calypso*	1 Lolly/50ml	1	0.0	1	0.0	0.3	0.0	0.0
Kiwi Burst, Pineapple Sorbet in Kiwi Ice, Sainsbury's*	1 Lolly/90ml	76	0.1	84	0.1	20.7	0.1	0.4
Lemon & Lime, Mini Bar, M & S*	1 Lolly/50g	47	0.0	95	0.1	23.6	0.1	0.2
Lemon & Lime, Rocket Split, De Roma*	1 Lolly/60ml	65	2.6	108	1.0	16.0	4.3	0.2
Lemon & Lime, Tubes, Frozen, M & S*	1oz/28g	27	0.0	95	0.1	23.6	0.1	0.2
Lemon Sorbet, Mercadona*	1 Lolly/63g	38	0.2	61	0.5	32.4	0.3	8.0
Lemonade & Cola, Morrisons*	1 Lolly/55ml	36	0.0	65	0.0	16.2	0.0	0.0
Lemonade Sparkle, Wall's Ice Cream*	1 Lolly/55g	40	0.0	73	0.0	18.2	0.0	0.0
Mango & Lemon, BGTY, Sainsbury's*	1 Lolly/72g	84	0.2	116	0.3	28.1	0.3	0.5
Mango & Passion Fruit Bursts, Sainsbury's*	1 Lolly/89ml	75	0.1	84	0.2	20.4	0.1	0.0
Mango & Passion Fruit Smoothie, Waitrose*	1 Lolly/73g	60	0.3	82	0.7	18.9	0.4	0.7
Milk, Blue Parrot Cafe, Sainsbury's*	1 Lolly/30ml	34	1.0	113	2.7	18.0	3.3	0.3
Milk Chocolate & Crisped Wheat, Co-Op*	1 Lolly/110g	258	13.2	235	3.0	28.0	12.0	0.7
Milk Flavour, Farmfoods*	1 Lolly/50ml	91	5.0	182	2.8	20.1	10.1	0.1
Mint Chocolate, Tesco*	1 Lolly/70g	234	13.9	334	3.6	35.4	19.8	1.2
Morrisons*	1 Lolly/100g	30	0.0	30	0.0	7.4	0.0	0.0
Nobbly Bobbly, Nestle*	1 Lolly/70ml	219	11.6	312	2.9	38.1	16.5	0.6
Orange, Lidl*	1 Lolly/50g	50	0.0	100	0.5	24.4	0.0	0.0
Orange, Real Fruit Juice, Sainsbury's*	1 Lolly/73ml	49	0.1	67	0.2	16.5	0.1	0.1
Orange, Real Juice, Sainsbury's*	1 Lolly/72ml	63	0.1	88	0.7	21.0	0.1	0.1
Orange, Real Juice, Tesco*	1 Lolly/32g	25	0.0	78	0.6	18.7	0.0	0.3
Orange, Ribena*	1 Lolly/110ml	95	0.0	86	0.1	21.4	0.0	0.0
Orange, Tesco*	1 Lolly/77g	53	0.0	68	0.2	16.8	0.0	0.3
Orange, Water, Iceland*	1 Lolly/75g	73	0.0	98	0.2	24.4	0.0	0.2
Orange & Lemon Splits, Farmfoods*	1 Lolly/56ml	69	2.4	124	1.6	19.8	4.3	0.2
Orange Juice, Asda*	1 Lolly/70g	58	0.0	83	0.7	20.0	0.0	0.0
Orange Juice, Bar, M & S*	1 Lolly/75g	64	0.0	86	0.5	21.0	0.0	0.1
Orange Juice, Co-Op*	1 Lolly/73g	51	0.1	70	0.4	17.0	0.1	0.1
Orange Juice, Farmfoods*	1 Lolly/79g	74	0.0	94	0.1	23.4	0.0	0.3
Orange Juice, Freshly Squeezed, Finest, Tesco*	1 Lolly/80ml	89	0.0	111	0.7	27.0	0.0	0.0
Orange Juice, Freshly Squeezed, Waitrose*	1 Lolly/73g	88	0.1	120	0.6	29.7	0.1	0.0
Orange Juice, Milfina*	1 Lolly/79g	69	0.0	87	0.5	23.3	0.0	0.0
Orange Juice, Morrisons*	1 Lolly/55ml	46	0.0	84	0.0	20.0	0.0	0.0
Orange Juice, Tropicana*	1 Lolly/50g	42	0.0	85	0.5	20.7	0.0	0.0
Orange Maid, Nestle*	1 Lolly/73ml	66	0.0	91	0.5	21.6	0.0	0.0
Orange 'n' Cream, Tropicana*	1 Lolly/65g	83	2.9	129	1.4	20.5	4.5	0.3
Pineapple, Dairy Split, Sainsbury's*	1 Lolly/72g	84	2.6	116	1.8	19.0	3.6	0.1
Pineapple, Real Fruit Juice, Sainsbury's*	1 Lolly/73ml	55	0.1	76	0.1	19.0	0.1	0.1
Polar Snappers, Double, Farmfoods*	1 Lolly/60ml	40	0.0	66	0.0	16.5	0.0	0.0
Raspberry, Real Fruit Juice, Sainsbury's*	1 Lolly/72g	62	0.1	86	0.3	21.0	0.1	0.1
Raspberry, Smoothie, Iced, Del Monte*	1 Lolly/90ml	84	0.0	94	0.3	22.8	0.0	0.8
Raspberry & Apple, Sainsbury's*	1 Lolly/57ml	39	0.1	68	0.1	17.1	0.1	0.1
Real Fruit, Dairy Split, Sainsbury's*	1 Lolly/73ml	100	3.1	137	2.1	22.8	4.2	0.1
Real Fruit Juice, Rocket, Blue Parrot Cafe, Sainsbury's*	1 Lolly/58ml	45	0.0	77	0.2	19.1	0.0	0.1
Real Orange, Kids, Tesco*	1 Lolly/32g	25	0.0	78	0.6	18.7	0.0	0.3

	Measure INFO/WEIGHT	per Measure		Nutrition Values per 100g / 100ml				
		KCAL	FAT	KCAL	PROT	CARB	FAT	FIBRE

ICE LOLLY

Refresher, Fruit Flavour, Bassett's*	1 Lolly/45g	56	0.7	125	1.6	26.0	1.6	0.3
Rocket, Co-Op*	1 Lolly/60g	42	0.0	70	0.0	17.0	0.0	0.0
Rocket, Sainsbury's*	1 Lolly/58g	42	0.1	72	0.1	17.8	0.1	0.1
Rolo, Nestle*	1 Lolly/75ml	243	14.1	324	3.8	36.5	18.8	0.0
Scooby-Doo, Freezepops, Calypso*	1 Lolly/50ml	14	0.0	28	0.0	7.0	0.0	0.0
Seriously Fruity, Mango Sorbet, Waitrose*	1 Lolly/100ml	79	0.3	79	0.8	18.4	0.3	0.5
Skinny Dippers Minis, Caramel & Chocolate, Skinny Cow*	1 Lolly/38ml	62	1.9	162	3.4	24.3	5.0	3.3
Solero, Exotic, Wall's Ice Cream*	1 Lolly/82g	99	2.3	121	1.6	21.9	2.8	0.5
Solero, Orange Fresh, Wall's Ice Cream*	1 Lolly/96g	78	0.0	81	0.2	20.0	0.0	0.0
Solero, Red Fruits, Wall's Ice Cream*	1 Lolly/95g	99	2.1	104	1.3	21.0	2.2	0.0
Strawberries & Cream, Cadbury*	1 Lolly/100ml	225	11.7	225	2.9	27.0	11.7	0.0
Strawberries 'n' Cream, Tropicana*	1 Lolly/50g	58	0.6	117	1.6	25.0	1.2	0.0
Strawberry, Dairy Split, Sainsbury's*	1 Lolly/73ml	86	2.6	118	1.7	19.8	3.6	0.1
Strawberry, Fruit Split, Iceland*	1 Lolly/73g	77	2.4	105	0.9	17.8	3.3	0.5
Strawberry, Mini Milk, Milk Time, Wall's Ice Cream*	1 Lolly/23g	30	0.7	131	4.0	22.0	2.9	0.5
Strawberry, Orange & Pineapple, Rocket, Iceland*	1 Lolly/47g	38	0.0	81	0.0	20.2	0.0	0.1
Strawberry, So-Lo, Good Choice, Iceland*	1 Lolly/66g	85	1.2	128	2.4	25.6	1.8	0.1
Strawberry & Banana, Smoothies, Sainsbury's*	1 Lolly/60g	100	3.2	166	1.5	28.0	5.3	0.2
Strawberry & Vanilla, 99% Fat Free, So-Lo, Iceland*	1 Lolly/92g	98	0.4	107	2.3	23.5	0.4	2.2
Strawberry Fruit, Double, Del Monte*	1 Lolly/76g	84	2.0	111	1.8	20.1	2.6	0.0
Strawberry Split, Co-Op*	1 Lolly/71g	75	2.1	105	1.0	17.0	3.0	0.1
Tip Top, Calypso*	1 Lolly/20ml	6	0.0	30	0.1	7.1	0.1	0.0
Traffic Light, Co-Op*	1 Lolly/52g	55	0.4	105	0.4	25.0	0.8	0.0
Tropical, Mmmm, Tesco*	1 Lolly/73g	109	3.1	150	1.2	26.6	4.3	0.4
Tropical Fruit, Starburst, Mars*	1 Lolly/93ml	94	0.1	101	0.3	24.8	0.1	0.0
Tropical Fruit Sorbet, Waitrose*	1 Lolly/110g	90	2.2	82	1.5	14.5	2.0	0.2
Twister, Wall's Ice Cream*	1 Lolly/80ml	76	1.5	95	0.6	18.4	1.9	0.0
Vanilla, Mini Milk, Milk Time, Wall's Ice Cream*	1 Lolly/23g	29	0.7	127	3.8	21.0	2.9	0.3
Vimto Soft Drinks*	1 Lolly/73ml	84	3.0	115	1.3	18.2	4.1	0.1
Wonka Super Sour Tastic, Nestle*	1 Lolly/60ml	84	2.2	140	0.0	26.1	3.6	0.0
Zoom, Nestle*	1 Lolly/58ml	54	0.4	93	0.9	20.6	0.7	0.0

ICED DESSERT

Cafe Latte, BGTY, Sainsbury's*	1 Serving/75g	104	2.7	139	2.9	23.7	3.6	3.3
Chocolate, Honeycomb Pieces, Weight Watchers*	1 Pot/58g	92	2.5	159	3.1	26.2	4.3	0.8
Chocolate & Mallow, GFY, Asda*	1 Pot/150ml	142	1.8	95	2.0	19.0	1.2	2.3
Chocolate Mint Crisp, COU, M & S*	¼ Pot/85g	115	2.5	135	5.4	21.9	2.9	1.0
Greek Style, Yoghurt, Tesco*	1 Serving/56g	90	1.8	160	2.6	29.7	3.3	1.4
Raspberry Swirl, Weight Watchers*	1 Scoop/60g	74	1.5	124	1.7	23.4	2.5	0.3
Strawberry Swirl, Weight Watchers*	1 Pot/100ml	92	1.7	92	1.1	18.1	1.7	0.5
Summer Fruits, Yoghurt, BGTY, Sainsbury's*	¼ Pot/85g	105	0.8	124	3.3	25.6	0.9	0.5
Toffee, 3% Fat, M & S*	1oz/28g	51	0.7	183	3.1	37.2	2.4	0.5
Toffee & Walnut, Free From, Sainsbury's*	¼ Tub/81g	203	10.0	251	3.3	31.6	12.4	0.3
Toffee Flavoured, Dairy, BGTY, Sainsbury's*	1 Serving/70g	103	3.1	147	2.7	24.0	4.5	0.2
Vanilla, 3% Fat, M & S*	1oz/28g	40	0.8	143	3.5	25.9	2.8	0.7
Vanilla, Dairy, BGTY, Sainsbury's*	1 Serving/65g	78	1.0	120	3.0	23.6	1.5	0.6
Vanilla, Non Dairy, Soft, Swedish Glace*	1 Serving/100g	200	10.0	200	2.5	25.0	10.0	1.0
Vanilla & Chocolate, HL, Tesco*	1 Pot/73g	104	1.9	143	3.0	26.9	2.6	0.7

INSTANT WHIP

Chocolate Flavour, Dry, Bird's*	1oz/28g	109	1.7	390	3.8	80.5	5.9	0.7
Strawberry Flavour, Dry, Bird's*	1oz/28g	112	1.5	400	2.5	85.0	5.4	0.4

IRN BRU

Diet, Barr's*	1 Can/330ml	2	0.0	1	0.1	0.1	0.0	0.0
Original, Barr's*	1 Bottle/498ml	214	0.0	43	0.0	10.5	0.0	0.0

	Measure INFO/WEIGHT	per Measure KCAL	FAT	Nutrition Values per 100g / 100ml KCAL	PROT	CARB	FAT	FIBRE
JACKFRUIT								
Raw, Average, Flesh Only	*1 Portion/162g*	*155*	*0.5*	*95*	*1.5*	*24.4*	*0.3*	*1.6*
JALFREZI								
Chicken, & Coriander Rice, TTD, Sainsbury's*	1 Pack/473g	501	15.1	106	6.2	13.2	3.2	3.1
Chicken, & Pilau Rice, Sainsbury's*	1 Pack/500g	600	20.5	120	6.9	13.9	4.1	1.5
Chicken, & Pilau Rice, Takeaway, Asda*	1 Pack/558g	792	23.4	142	7.0	19.0	4.2	1.3
Chicken, & Rice, Serves 1, Tesco*	1 Serving/475g	589	38.0	124	7.4	5.7	8.0	1.6
Chicken, Asda*	1 Pack/340g	415	20.4	122	10.0	7.0	6.0	1.6
Chicken, Budgens*	1 Serving/200g	210	6.4	105	9.8	9.2	3.2	0.9
Chicken, Finest, Tesco*	1 Pack/350g	402	16.4	115	10.4	6.9	4.7	1.2
Chicken, GFY, Asda*	1 Pack/350g	238	3.1	68	9.0	6.0	0.9	1.8
Chicken, Hot & Spicy, Sainsbury's*	½ Pack/200g	228	11.4	114	12.8	2.9	5.7	1.0
Chicken, Indian Takeaway, Tesco*	1 Serving/350g	245	8.7	70	7.4	4.3	2.5	1.8
Chicken, Medium, GFY, Asda*	1 Pack/644g	972	27.7	151	6.0	22.0	4.3	0.9
Chicken, Somerfield*	1 Pack/350g	339	16.1	97	11.2	2.6	4.6	1.2
Chicken, with Rice, Ready Meal, Average	1 Serving/450g	557	18.9	124	6.9	14.5	4.2	1.5
Chicken, with Rice, Ready Meal, Healthy Range, Average	1 Serving/400g	363	5.7	91	7.1	12.3	1.4	1.4
Chicken Canned, Tesco*	½ Can/200g	190	6.8	95	10.8	4.1	3.4	1.4
Chicken with Basmati Rice, Weight Watchers*	1 Pack/330g	238	1.6	72	5.0	11.8	0.5	0.5
Chicken with Lemon Pilau Rice, Finest, Tesco*	1 Pack/493g	665	21.7	135	6.9	16.4	4.4	1.8
Chicken with Pilau Basmati Rice, Frozen, Patak's*	1 Pack/400g	556	18.4	139	9.8	14.7	4.6	0.9
Chicken with Pilau Rice, Asda*	1 Pack/450g	568	13.5	126	7.1	16.1	3.0	3.2
Chicken with Pilau Rice, GFY, Asda*	1 Pack/446g	495	11.1	111	8.0	14.0	2.5	1.2
Chicken with Pilau Rice, Tesco*	1 Pack/460g	506	17.5	110	5.3	13.6	3.8	0.9
Chicken with Rice, Morrisons*	1 Pack/400g	564	20.8	141	7.7	15.9	5.2	1.4
Chicken with Rice, Tesco*	1 Pack/550g	731	26.4	133	5.5	17.0	4.8	1.0
Vegetable, Co-Op*	1 Pack/400g	320	16.0	80	1.0	9.0	4.0	2.0
Vegetable, Eastern Indian, Sainsbury's*	1 Pack/400g	208	13.6	52	3.4	2.0	3.4	1.7
Vegetable, Indian, Sainsbury's*	½ Pack/200g	156	9.0	78	2.0	5.3	4.5	4.2
Vegetable, Take Away Menu for 1, BGTY, Sainsbury's*	1 Pack/148g	43	0.0	29	1.8	5.4	0.0	2.3
Vegetable, Waitrose*	1 Pack/400g	256	16.0	64	2.2	4.7	4.0	3.7
Vegetable with Rice, Birds Eye*	1 Pack/350g	353	3.9	101	2.5	20.2	1.1	1.0
JAM								
Apricot, Average	*1 Tbsp/15g*	*37*	*0.0*	*248*	*0.2*	*61.6*	*0.0*	*1.5*
Apricot, Reduced Sugar, Average	*1 Serving/20g*	*37*	*0.1*	*186*	*0.4*	*46.0*	*0.3*	*0.4*
Black Cherry, Average	*1 Tsp/5g*	*12*	*0.0*	*247*	*0.4*	*61.2*	*0.3*	*0.4*
Blackberry, Extra Special, Asda*	1 Tbsp/15g	29	0.1	190	0.9	45.0	0.7	0.0
Blackcurrant, Average	*1 Tbsp/15g*	*38*	*0.0*	*250*	*0.2*	*62.3*	*0.0*	*1.0*
Blackcurrant, Reduced Sugar, Average	*1 Tsp/6g*	*10*	*0.0*	*178*	*0.4*	*44.4*	*0.1*	*1.0*
Blueberry, Best, Hartley's*	1 Tsp/20g	49	0.0	244	0.3	60.6	0.1	0.0
Blueberry, St Dalfour*	1 Serving/20g	46	0.0	228	0.5	56.0	0.2	2.2
Blueberry & Blackberry, Baxters*	1 Tsp/15g	38	0.0	252	0.0	63.0	0.0	1.2
Blueberry & Blackcurrant, 100% Fruit, Spread, Super Jam*	1 Tsp/5g	11	0.0	222	0.3	55.0	0.1	0.0
Concorde Grape, Sugar Free, Smucker's*	1 Serving/17g	0	0.0	0	0.0	29.4	0.0	0.0
Country Berries, Luxury, Baxters*	1 Tsp/15g	38	0.0	252	0.0	63.0	0.0	1.1
Damson, Extra Fruit, Best, Hartley's*	1 Tsp/5g	12	0.0	244	0.2	60.8	0.0	0.0
Fig	1 Tsp/15g	36	0.0	242	0.5	60.0	0.0	0.0
Golden Peach, Rhapsodie De Fruit, St Dalfour*	1 Tsp/10g	23	0.0	227	0.5	56.0	0.1	1.3
Kiwi & Gooseberry, 66% Fruit, Asda*	1 Serving/30g	56	0.1	187	0.5	45.0	0.5	0.0
Mixed Fruit, Average	*1 Tbsp/15g*	*38*	*0.0*	*252*	*0.3*	*63.5*	*0.0*	*0.5*
Mixed Fruit, Value, Tesco*	1 Tsp/5g	12	0.0	250	0.1	62.1	0.0	0.8
Plum, Tesco*	1 Serving/50g	130	0.0	261	0.2	64.4	0.0	0.6
Raspberry, Average	*1 Tbsp/15g*	*36*	*0.0*	*239*	*0.6*	*58.6*	*0.1*	*0.9*
Raspberry, GFY, Asda*	1 Tbsp/19g	24	0.1	124	0.6	29.0	0.6	1.5

J

	Measure INFO/WEIGHT	per Measure KCAL	FAT	Nutrition Values per 100g / 100ml KCAL	PROT	CARB	FAT	FIBRE
JAM								
Raspberry, Grandessa, Aldi*	1 Serving/25g	45	0.1	179	1.0	41.0	0.2	1.8
Raspberry, Reduced Sugar, Average	*1 Tsp/6g*	*10*	*0.0*	*160*	*0.5*	*39.3*	*0.2*	*0.6*
Raspberry, Reduced Sugar, Baxters*	½ Tsp/5g	10	0.0	197	0.7	48.0	0.2	1.5
Raspberry, Reduced Sugar, Weight Watchers*	1 Tsp/15g	22	0.0	149	0.7	36.1	0.2	2.9
Raspberry, Seedless, Average	*1 Tsp/10g*	*26*	*0.0*	*257*	*0.4*	*63.6*	*0.0*	*0.3*
Rhubarb & Ginger, Baxters*	1 Tsp/15g	31	0.0	210	0.0	53.0	0.0	0.6
Strawberry, Average	*1 Tsp/10g*	*24*	*0.0*	*243*	*0.3*	*60.2*	*0.1*	*0.7*
Strawberry, Reduced Sugar, Average	*1 Tbsp/15g*	*28*	*0.0*	*187*	*0.4*	*45.8*	*0.3*	*0.2*
Strawberry, Reduced Sugar, Weight Watchers*	1 Serving/15g	23	0.0	154	0.5	37.5	0.2	1.2
Strawberry, Smooth, Squeezy, Hartley's*	1 Tsp/5g	10	0.0	196	0.4	48.6	0.0	0.0
Strawberry, Value, Tesco*	1 Tbsp/15g	37	0.0	246	0.3	61.2	0.0	0.5
Strawberry & Redcurrant, Reduced Sugar, Streamline*	1 Tbsp/15g	29	0.0	192	0.4	46.8	0.3	0.0
Strawberry & Vanilla, Best, Hartley's*	1 Tsp/5g	12	0.0	244	0.4	60.6	0.0	0.0
Wild Blackberry Jelly, Baxters*	1 Tsp/15g	31	0.0	210	0.0	53.0	0.0	1.2
JAMBALAYA								
American Style, Tesco*	1 Serving/275g	432	19.2	157	7.7	16.0	7.0	0.5
Cajun Chicken, Cooked, BGTY, Sainsbury's*	1 Pack/400g	392	6.5	103	6.6	14.6	1.7	1.6
Chicken, Spicy, Eat Smart, Morrisons*	1 Pack/400g	384	4.8	96	7.4	13.9	1.2	2.7
Chicken & Prawn, Love Life, Waitrose*	1 Pack/390g	417	10.9	107	5.2	14.3	2.8	1.9
COU, M & S*	1 Pack/400g	340	8.0	85	6.5	10.8	2.0	0.9
GFY, Asda*	1 Pack/450g	387	3.1	86	6.0	14.0	0.7	2.7
M & S*	1 Pack/480g	552	16.8	115	5.8	14.6	3.5	1.2
Ready Meal, Average	1 Pack/450g	569	18.2	126	6.4	15.7	4.0	1.3
Tesco*	1 Pack/550g	764	36.3	139	6.9	13.1	6.6	1.1
JELLY								
Apple & Watermelon, Low Calorie, Hartley's*	1 Serving/175g	5	0.0	3	0.0	0.3	0.0	0.3
Blackberry, Unprepared, Morrisons*	1 Serving/20g	52	0.0	261	0.3	65.0	0.0	0.0
Blackcurrant, Made Up, Rowntree's*	¼ Jelly/140ml	100	0.1	71	1.4	16.4	0.1	0.0
Blackcurrant, Made Up, Sainsbury's*	¼ Jelly/150g	97	0.0	65	1.2	15.1	0.0	0.0
Blackcurrant, Sugar Free, Unprepared, Rowntree's*	1 Pack/24g	73	0.0	305	50.0	25.0	0.0	25.0
Blackcurrant, Tesco*	1 Serving/100g	84	0.1	84	0.2	20.5	0.1	0.4
Bramble, Tesco*	1 Serving/100g	257	0.1	257	0.3	63.7	0.1	1.3
Crystals, Orange, Sugar Free, Bird's*	1 Sachet/12g	39	0.1	335	62.5	6.4	0.9	0.0
Crystals, Orange & Peach, Sugar Free, Weight Watchers*	½ Pack/204g	14	0.2	7	0.0	1.4	0.1	0.0
Crystals, Strawberry, Made Up, Tesco*	1 Serving/145g	9	0.0	6	1.3	0.3	0.0	0.0
Crystals Apple & Blackcurrant, Weight Watchers*	1 Packet/204g	14	0.2	7	0.1	1.4	0.1	0.1
Exotic Fruit, M & S*	1 Pot/175g	140	0.3	80	0.1	18.9	0.2	0.9
Fresh Fruit, M & S*	1 Pot/175g	131	0.2	75	0.2	18.4	0.1	0.3
Fruit Cocktail, M & S*	1oz/28g	31	1.3	110	0.4	16.4	4.7	0.3
Fruitini, Del Monte*	1 Serving/120g	78	0.1	65	0.3	15.3	0.1	0.5
Lemon, Unprepared, Co-Op*	1 Pack/135g	412	0.0	305	5.0	71.0	0.0	0.0
Lemon & Lime, Sugar Free, Unprepared, Rowntree's*	1oz/28g	85	0.0	305	4.5	60.7	0.0	0.0
Lime, Made Up, Rowntree's*	¼ Jelly/140ml	100	0.1	71	1.3	16.3	0.1	0.0
Lime, Unprepared, Co-Op*	1 Pack/135g	397	0.1	294	5.5	68.1	0.0	1.0
Lime Flavour, Unprepared, Waitrose*	1 Square/11g	33	0.0	296	4.5	69.5	0.0	0.0
Made Up with Water, Average	*1oz/28g*	*17*	*0.0*	*61*	*1.2*	*15.1*	*0.0*	*0.0*
Mandarin & Pineapple, Sainsbury's*	1 Pot/125g	95	0.1	76	0.2	18.9	0.1	1.2
Mixed Berry, WT5, Sainsbury's*	1 Serving/160g	112	0.3	70	0.7	16.3	0.2	1.5
Orange, Quickset, Unprepared, Rowntree's*	1oz/28g	95	0.0	340	0.0	84.0	0.0	3.0
Orange, Sugar Free, Crystals, Dry Weight, Hartley's*	1 Pack/26g	66	0.0	254	57.4	6.1	0.0	0.0
Orange, Sugar Free, Unprepared, Asda*	1 Serving/12g	36	0.0	303	63.6	12.0	0.1	0.2
Orange, Unprepared, Rowntree's*	1 Square/11g	33	0.0	296	4.4	69.6	0.0	0.0
Orange Flavour, Unprepared, Somerfield*	1 Pack/128g	379	0.0	296	5.0	69.0	0.0	0.0

J

	Measure INFO/WEIGHT	per Measure KCAL	FAT	Nutrition Values per 100g / 100ml KCAL	PROT	CARB	FAT	FIBRE
JELLY								
Peach Melba, Eat Well, M & S*	1 Pot/175g	114	0.3	65	0.2	15.9	0.2	0.2
Pineapple with Pineapple Pieces, Tesco*	1 Serving/120g	96	0.1	80	1.2	18.6	0.1	0.7
Raspberry, Crystals, Vegetarian, Just Wholefoods*	1 Packet/85g	293	0.0	345	0.5	85.7	0.0	0.0
Raspberry, Unprepared, Co-Op*	1 Pack/135g	402	0.1	298	5.5	68.9	0.0	0.0
Raspberry, Unprepared, Rowntree's*	1 Serving/135g	405	0.5	300	5.6	67.3	0.4	0.0
Raspberry, Unprepared, Somerfield*	¼ Serving/38g	111	0.0	292	6.0	66.0	0.0	0.0
Raspberry & Rose, Aroma, M & S*	1oz/28g	14	0.1	50	0.2	11.9	0.2	0.4
Raspberry Flavour, Tesco*	1 Serving/34g	22	0.0	64	1.0	15.0	0.0	0.1
Raspberry Flavoured with Raspberries, M & S*	1 Sm Pot/175g	105	0.5	60	0.2	14.0	0.3	1.5
Redcurrant, Average	***1oz/28g***	***70***	***0.0***	***250***	***0.1***	***64.4***	***0.0***	***0.0***
Strawberry, Basics, Unprepared, Somerfield*	¼ Jelly/32g	95	0.0	296	5.0	69.0	0.0	0.0
Strawberry, Goodness for Kids, Tesco*	1 Pot/75g	45	0.3	60	1.7	11.1	0.4	0.5
Strawberry, No Added Sugar, Hartley's*	1 Pot/115g	4	0.0	4	0.0	0.4	0.0	0.3
Strawberry, Sugar Free, Crystals, Dry Weight, Hartley's*	1 Sachet/26g	73	0.0	280	56.8	13.1	0.0	0.0
Strawberry, Unprepared, Co-Op*	1 Pack/135g	402	0.1	298	5.5	69.1	0.0	0.0
Strawberry, Unprepared, Somerfield*	¼ Jelly/34g	98	0.0	291	6.0	66.0	0.0	0.0
Strawberry & Raspberry, Sainsbury's*	½ Pot/280g	230	0.0	82	0.2	20.2	0.0	1.2
Strawberry Flavour, Sugar Free, Unprepared, Rowntree's*	1oz/28g	84	0.0	300	64.9	3.0	0.0	0.0
Sugar Free, Dry, Tesco*	1 Pack/13g	36	0.0	285	55.4	15.6	0.0	0.2
Tangerine, Unprepared, Rowntree's*	1 Serving/33g	99	0.1	300	5.6	67.3	0.4	0.0
Tropical Fruit, Way to Five, Sainsbury's*	1 Serving/160g	144	1.6	90	0.3	19.9	1.0	0.9
Unprepared, Hartley's*	1 Serving/31g	92	0.0	296	5.1	68.9	0.0	0.0
JELLY BABIES								
Bassett's*	1 Baby/6g	20	0.0	335	4.0	79.5	0.0	0.0
M & S*	1 Pack/125g	417	0.0	334	5.2	78.0	0.0	0.0
Mini, Waitrose*	1 Bag/125g	370	0.5	296	4.3	68.7	0.4	0.0
Somerfield*	1 Sweet/6g	21	0.0	343	4.7	80.7	0.0	0.0
JELLY BEANS								
Average	1 Serving/100g	365	0.1	365	0.1	91.2	0.1	0.1
Jelly Belly*	35 Beans/40g	140	0.0	350	0.0	90.0	0.0	0.0
No Added Sugar, Jelly Belly*	1 Serving/40g	80	0.0	200	0.0	50.0	0.0	20.0
Rowntree's*	1 Pack/35g	128	0.0	367	0.0	91.8	0.0	0.0
JELLY BEARS								
Co-Op*	1 Sweet/3g	10	0.0	325	6.0	76.0	0.1	0.0
JELLY TOTS								
Rowntree's*	1 Pack/42g	145	0.0	346	0.1	86.5	0.0	0.0
JERKY								
Beef, Peppered, Jack Link's*	1 Serving/28g	80	0.5	286	53.6	14.3	1.8	0.0
Soy, Cajun Chick'n, Vegan, Tasty Eats*	1 Pack/28g	90	3.0	321	42.9	14.3	10.7	7.1
JUICE								
100% Vegetable, V8*	1 Bottle/354ml	71	1.1	20	0.8	3.2	0.3	0.5
Apple, English with Cherry, Cawston Vale*	1 Can/250ml	117	0.2	47	0.4	11.6	0.1	0.0
Apple, Pure, Average	1 Glass/100ml	47	0.0	47	0.1	11.2	0.0	0.0
Apple, Sparkling, Apfelsaft, Thurella*	1 Bottle/500ml	225	2.5	45	0.5	11.0	0.5	0.0
Apple & Cherry, Sainsbury's*	1 Glass/200ml	96	0.0	48	0.3	10.8	0.0	0.8
Apple & Cranberry, Average	***1 Glass/250ml***	***114***	***0.0***	***45***	***0.1***	***10.1***	***0.0***	***0.0***
Apple & Elderflower, Copella*	1 Glass/250ml	107	0.2	43	0.4	10.2	0.1	0.0
Apple & Mango, Average	***1 Glass/200ml***	***108***	***0.1***	***54***	***0.3***	***12.6***	***0.0***	***0.1***
Apple & Orange, Fresh Up*	1 Glass/250ml	105	0.0	42	0.0	10.3	0.0	0.0
Apple & Pomegranate, Pommy, Sparky*	1 Glass/250ml	125	0.5	50	0.4	10.0	0.2	0.5
Apple & Raspberry, Average	***1 Glass/200ml***	***89***	***0.1***	***44***	***0.4***	***10.1***	***0.0***	***0.1***
Apple & Rhubarb, Caxton Vale*	1 Glass/250ml	115	1.0	46	0.2	9.7	0.4	0.0
Beetroot, Organic, James White*	1 Glass/250ml	105	0.2	42	0.9	9.3	0.1	0.0

J

JUICE

	Measure INFO/WEIGHT	per Measure KCAL	FAT	Nutrition Values per 100g / 100ml KCAL	PROT	CARB	FAT	FIBRE
Beetroot & Evesse Apple, Sunraysia*	1 Glass/200ml	262	0.0	131	0.4	7.3	0.0	0.0
Blackberry, Vita, Co-Op*	1 Glass/200ml	110	0.0	55	0.0	13.0	0.0	0.5
Breakfast, Ruby, Tropicana*	1 Glass/200ml	90	0.0	45	0.8	9.7	0.0	0.7
Breakfast, Sainsbury's*	1 Glass/200ml	94	0.2	47	0.7	11.3	0.1	0.3
Carrot, Average	**1 Glass/200ml**	**48**	**0.2**	**24**	**0.5**	**5.7**	**0.1**	**0.0**
Cherry, Original, Cherrygood*	1 Glass/250ml	112	0.2	45	0.0	10.5	0.1	0.0
Citrus Fruit & Veg, V8*	1 Glass/150ml	55	0.3	37	0.3	8.4	0.2	0.0
Coconut, Foco*	1 Can/520ml	182	1.1	35	0.1	8.2	0.2	0.0
Cranberry, Average	**1 Bottle/250ml**	**139**	**0.2**	**56**	**0.1**	**13.4**	**0.1**	**0.3**
Cranberry, No Added Sugar, Average	**1 Glass/200ml**	**11**	**0.1**	**5**	**0.1**	**0.8**	**0.0**	**0.0**
Exotic Fruit, Pure, Del Monte*	1 Glass/200ml	96	0.0	48	0.3	11.3	0.0	0.0
Fibre, Tropicana*	1 Glass/200ml	130	0.0	65	0.4	15.8	0.0	3.4
Go!, Tropicana*	1 Bottle/200ml	80	0.0	40	0.3	9.7	0.0	0.0
Grape, Concord, Kedem*	1 Bottle/946ml	587	0.0	62	0.0	15.4	0.0	0.0
Grape, Purple, Light, Welch's*	1 Serving/100ml	27	0.3	27	0.2	6.1	0.3	0.3
Grape, Purple, Welch's*	1 Serving/200ml	136	0.0	68	0.1	16.5	0.0	0.0
Grape, Red, Average	**1 Serving/100ml**	**62**	**0.0**	**62**	**0.1**	**15.1**	**0.0**	**0.0**
Grape, White, Average	**1 Can/160ml**	**95**	**0.1**	**59**	**0.2**	**14.3**	**0.1**	**0.1**
Grape, White, Kedem*	1 Bottle/946ml	1135	0.0	120	0.0	28.0	0.0	0.0
Grape & Peach, Don Simon*	1 Serving/200ml	94	0.0	47	0.4	11.3	0.0	0.0
Grapefruit, Pink, Average	**1 Glass/200ml**	**81**	**0.1**	**40**	**0.6**	**9.0**	**0.0**	**0.2**
Grapefruit, Pure, Average	**1 Glass/200ml**	**77**	**0.2**	**38**	**0.5**	**8.5**	**0.1**	**0.1**
Lemon, Fresh, Average	**1 Juice Lemon/35ml**	**2**	**0.0**	**7**	**0.3**	**1.6**	**0.0**	**0.1**
Lime, Fresh, Average	**1 Tsp/5ml**	**0**	**0.0**	**9**	**0.4**	**1.6**	**0.1**	**0.1**
Mandarin Orange, Tropicana*	1 Serving/200ml	94	0.0	47	0.6	10.0	0.0	0.8
Mango, Peach, Papaya, Pure, Premium, Tropicana*	1 Glass/200ml	88	0.0	44	0.5	9.8	0.0	0.1
Mango, Pure, Canned	**1 Glass/250ml**	**97**	**0.5**	**39**	**0.1**	**9.8**	**0.2**	**0.0**
Mango Veggie, Naked Juice Co*	1 Serving/240ml	150	1.0	62	1.2	15.8	0.4	2.1
Multi Vitamin, Hohes C*	1 Glass/200ml	88	0.2	44	0.1	9.4	0.1	0.5
Multivitamin, Fruit, Vitafit*	1 Glass/200ml	106	0.0	53	1.0	12.0	0.0	0.5
Orange, Apple & Mango, Calypso*	1 Carton/200ml	92	0.4	46	0.0	11.0	0.2	0.1
Orange, C, No Added Sugar, Libby's*	1 Serving/250ml	32	0.0	13	0.1	2.7	0.0	0.0
Orange, Freshly Squeezed, Average	1 Serving/200ml	66	0.0	33	0.6	8.1	0.0	1.0
Orange, No Bits, Innocent*	1 Glass/250ml	120	0.0	48	0.8	10.9	0.0	0.2
Orange, No Pulp with Calcium, Napolina*	1 Serving/240ml	110	0.0	46	0.8	10.8	0.0	0.0
Orange, Pineapple & Banana, The Feel Good Drinks Co*	1 Carton/180ml	67	0.0	37	0.3	8.5	0.0	0.0
Orange, Pulp Free, Napolina*	1 Serving/264ml	110	0.0	42	0.8	9.9	0.0	0.0
Orange, Pure, Smooth, Average	**1 Glass/200ml**	**88**	**0.1**	**44**	**0.7**	**9.8**	**0.0**	**0.2**
Orange, Pure Premium, Smooth, No Bits, Tropicana*	1 Glass/200ml	94	0.0	47	0.8	10.0	0.0	0.4
Orange, Pure with Bits, Average	**1 Glass/200ml**	**90**	**0.1**	**45**	**0.6**	**10.2**	**0.1**	**0.1**
Orange, Red, Average	**1 Glass/250ml**	**115**	**0.1**	**46**	**0.4**	**10.7**	**0.0**	**0.2**
Orange, Sparkling, 55, Britvic*	1 Bottle/275ml	135	0.3	49	0.3	11.3	0.1	0.1
Orange, Vitafit*	1 Glass/200ml	78	0.2	39	0.7	8.3	0.1	0.7
Orange & Banana, Pure, Average	**1 Glass/150ml**	**79**	**0.1**	**53**	**0.7**	**12.1**	**0.1**	**0.2**
Orange & Grapefruit, Average	**1 Glass/200ml**	**84**	**0.2**	**42**	**0.7**	**9.2**	**0.1**	**0.4**
Orange & Kiwi Fruit, Tropicana*	1 Serving/175ml	90	0.0	51	0.5	12.0	0.0	0.0
Orange & Lime, Tropicana*	1 Serving/250ml	115	0.0	46	1.1	9.4	0.0	0.6
Orange & Mango, Average	**1 Bottle/375ml**	**176**	**0.4**	**47**	**0.5**	**10.7**	**0.1**	**0.2**
Orange & Passionfruit, Tropicana*	1 Serving/200ml	94	0.0	47	0.8	10.0	0.0	0.7
Orange & Pineapple, Average	**1 Glass/120ml**	**56**	**0.6**	**46**	**0.4**	**10.5**	**0.5**	**0.5**
Orange & Raspberry, Average	**1 fl oz/30ml**	**15**	**0.0**	**50**	**0.6**	**11.4**	**0.1**	**0.2**
Orange & Raspberry, Tropicana*	1 Glass/200ml	92	0.0	46	1.2	9.0	0.0	0.9
Orange & Strawberry, Average	**1 Serving/125ml**	**64**	**0.5**	**51**	**0.6**	**10.9**	**0.4**	**0.8**

	Measure INFO/WEIGHT	per Measure KCAL	FAT	Nutrition Values per 100g / 100ml KCAL	PROT	CARB	FAT	FIBRE
JUICE								
Orange with Bits, Innocent*	1 Glass/250ml	120	0.0	48	0.8	10.9	0.0	0.3
Passion Fruit, Average	*1 Glass/200ml*	*94*	*0.2*	*47*	*0.8*	*10.7*	*0.1*	*0.0*
Peach, Mango & Passion Fruit, Sainsbury's*	1 Glass/200ml	92	0.2	46	0.3	10.3	0.1	0.5
Pear, Concentrate, Meridian Foods*	1 Serving/45ml	134	0.0	298	0.0	74.6	0.0	0.0
Pear, Pure, Heinz*	1 Serving/100ml	41	0.1	41	0.1	9.8	0.1	0.0
Pear, with a Hint of Ginger, Pressed, M & S*	1 Glass/250ml	125	0.2	50	0.3	11.7	0.1	0.0
Pineapple, Average	*1 Glass/200ml*	*100*	*0.1*	*50*	*0.3*	*11.7*	*0.1*	*0.1*
Pineapple & Coconut, Waitrose*	1 Serving/250ml	125	0.7	50	0.2	11.5	0.3	0.2
Pineapple & Guava, Tropicana*	1 Glass/200ml	106	0.0	53	0.3	12.3	0.0	1.2
Pineapple Mango Crush, Just Juice*	1 Glass/250ml	107	0.0	43	0.0	10.6	0.0	0.0
Pomegranate, Grape & Apple, Tropicana*	1 Bottle/330ml	211	0.0	64	0.2	15.5	0.0	0.6
Pomegranate, Pomegreat*	1 Glass/200ml	88	0.0	44	0.1	11.1	0.0	0.0
Pressed Apple, Strawberry & Lychee, M & S*	1 Serving/250ml	112	0.7	45	0.3	9.7	0.3	0.3
Prune, Average	*1 Serving/200ml*	*123*	*0.1*	*61*	*0.6*	*15.3*	*0.1*	*1.8*
Tomato, Average	*1 Glass/200ml*	*40*	*0.1*	*20*	*0.7*	*4.0*	*0.0*	*0.4*
Tomato, Princes*	1 Serving/100g	16	0.0	16	0.8	3.1	0.0	0.6
Tropical, Fruit & Vegetable, V8*	1 Serving/150ml	0	0.0	35	0.4	8.1	0.1	1.1
Tropical, Pure, Sainsbury's*	1 Glass/200ml	104	0.2	52	0.5	12.0	0.1	0.1
Tropical Fruit, Plenty*	1 Glass/200ml	120	0.2	60	0.5	13.7	0.1	0.0
Vegetable, Organic, Evernat*	1 Glass/200ml	36	0.2	18	0.9	3.5	0.1	0.2
Vegetable, Organic, James White*	1 Glass/100g	22	0.2	22	0.6	4.4	0.2	0.0
White Apple & Ginger, James White*	1 Glass/250ml	122	0.0	49	0.1	11.8	0.0	0.0
JUICE DRINK								
Apple, Juiceburst, Purity*	1 Bottle/500ml	220	0.0	44	0.0	11.0	0.0	0.0
Apple, Libby's*	1 Serving/100ml	43	0.0	43	0.0	10.3	0.0	0.0
Apple, Sparkling, Zing*	1 Can/250ml	92	0.0	37	0.1	8.5	0.0	0.0
Apple & Blackcurrant, Sparkling, Shapers, Boots*	1 Serving/500ml	26	0.1	5	0.0	0.9	0.0	0.0
Apple & Blueberry, The Feel Good Drinks Co*	1 Serving/375ml	163	0.4	43	0.1	10.6	0.1	0.0
Apple & Raspberry, Dr Gillian McKeith*	1 Bottle/200ml	86	0.1	43	0.1	10.6	0.1	0.0
Apple Lemonade, Cawston Press*	1 Glass/200g	106	0.2	53	0.2	11.9	0.1	0.0
Berry & Elderberry, Fusion, Oasis*	1 Bottle/375ml	11	0.0	3	0.0	0.4	0.0	0.0
Berry Blast, 5 Alive*	1 Glass/200ml	50	0.0	25	0.0	6.1	0.0	0.0
Blackcurrant, CVit*	1 Glass/200ml	4	0.0	2	0.0	0.2	0.0	0.0
Blackcurrant, Extra Light, Ribena*	1 Serving/200ml	8	0.0	4	0.0	0.5	0.0	0.0
Blackcurrant, Kids, Tesco*	1 Serving/250ml	127	0.0	51	0.0	12.4	0.0	0.0
Blackcurrant, Purity*	1 Bottle/500ml	265	0.0	53	0.0	13.2	0.0	0.0
Blackcurrant & Apple, Oasis*	1 Serving/500ml	90	0.0	18	0.0	4.1	0.0	0.0
Blackcurrant & Raspberry with Soya, Adez*	1 Glass/250ml	82	1.0	33	1.1	6.3	0.4	0.3
Citrus Burst, 5 Alive*	1 Carton/250ml	125	0.0	50	0.0	12.8	0.0	0.0
Cranberry, Classic, Ocean Spray*	1 Bottle/500ml	245	0.5	49	0.1	11.7	0.1	0.1
Cranberry, Grape & Apple, Ocean Spray*	1 Glass/200ml	108	0.0	54	0.1	12.9	0.0	0.0
Cranberry, Juice Burst, Purity*	1 Bottle/500ml	245	0.0	49	0.00	12.0	0.0	0.0
Cranberry, Light, Classic, Ocean Spray*	1 Glass/200ml	16	0.0	8	0.0	1.4	0.0	0.0
Cranberry, Original, Concentrated, Ocean Spray*	1 Serving/15ml	27	0.0	183	0.2	44.1	0.0	0.0
Cranberry, Solevita*	1 Serving/200ml	98	0.0	49	0.5	11.7	0.0	0.0
Cranberry, Tropical, Ocean Spray*	1 Glass/200ml	96	0.0	48	0.1	11.5	0.0	0.0
Cranberry & Apple, Ocean Spray*	1 Glass/200ml	92	0.0	46	0.0	11.1	0.0	0.0
Cranberry & Blackberry, Ocean Spray*	1 Glass/250ml	120	0.2	48	0.1	11.3	0.1	0.2
Cranberry & Blackcurrant, Ocean Spray*	1 Bottle/500ml	265	0.0	53	0.2	12.7	0.0	0.0
Cranberry & Blueberry, Ocean Spray*	1 Serving/100ml	48	0.0	48	0.0	11.6	0.0	0.0
Cranberry & Mango, Light, Ocean Spray*	1 Glass/250ml	22	0.0	9	0.0	2.0	0.0	0.1
Cranberry & Pomegranate, Ocean Spray*	1 Glass/250ml	120	0.0	48	0.0	11.5	0.0	0.0
Cranberry & Raspberry, Ocean Spray*	1 Glass/200ml	104	0.0	52	0.0	12.6	0.0	0.0

JUICE DRINK

	Measure INFO/WEIGHT	per Measure KCAL	FAT	Nutrition Values per 100g / 100ml KCAL	PROT	CARB	FAT	FIBRE
Cranberry Blend, Ocean Spray*	1 Glass/250ml	148	0.0	59	0.1	13.9	0.0	0.0
Exotic, Tesco*	1 Serving/250ml	127	0.0	51	0.1	12.3	0.0	0.0
Fruit Shoot, My-5, Apple & Pear, Roninson's*	1 Bottle/200ml	78	0.2	39	0.2	8.9	0.1	0.0
Grape, Apple & Raspberry, Asda*	1 Glass/200ml	90	0.0	45	0.2	11.0	0.0	0.0
Grape, Red, Sparkling, Shloer*	1 Glass/200ml	84	0.0	42	0.0	10.4	0.0	0.0
Grape, White, Sparkling, Shloer*	1 Serving/120ml	59	0.0	49	0.0	11.6	0.0	0.0
Grape & Elderflower, White, Sparkling, Shloer*	1 Glass/200ml	74	0.0	37	0.0	9.2	0.0	0.0
Grapefruit & Cranberry, M & S*	1 Serving/250ml	125	0.2	50	0.2	11.9	0.1	0.0
Grapefruit & Lime, Quest, M & S*	1 Bottle/330ml	53	0.0	16	0.0	4.0	0.0	0.0
Guava Exotic, Rubicon*	1 Carton/288ml	150	0.3	52	0.2	12.9	0.1	0.0
J20, Apple & Mango, Britvic*	1 Bottle/275ml	83	0.0	30	0.1	6.8	0.0	0.2
J20, Apple & Raspberry, Britvic*	1 Bottle/275ml	88	0.0	32	0.1	7.3	0.0	0.3
J20, Orange & Passion Fruit, Britvic*	1 Bottle/275ml	88	0.0	32	0.3	7.2	0.0	0.2
J2O, Apple & Blueberry, Britvic*	1 Bottle/275g	124	0.0	45	0.1	11.0	0.0	0.2
J2O, Glitterberry, Britvic*	1 Bottle/275ml	110	0.0	40	0.2	9.4	0.0	0.0
J2O, White Blend, White Grape & Kiwi, Britvic*	1 Bottle/275ml	91	0.0	33	0.2	7.7	0.0	0.0
Juice Burst, Pink Grapefruit, Purity*	1 Bottle/500ml	210	0.0	42	0.4	10.0	0.0	0.0
Lemon, The Feel Good Drinks Co*	1 Bottle/171ml	78	0.2	46	0.1	10.8	0.1	0.0
Lemon & Lime, Light, Oasis*	1 Bottle/250ml	6	0.0	3	0.0	0.2	0.0	0.0
Lychee, Sparkling, Rubicon*	1 Can/330g	181	0.0	55	0.0	13.6	0.0	0.0
Mango, Rubicon*	1 Serving/100ml	54	0.1	54	0.1	13.1	0.1	0.0
Mango, Sparkling, Rubicon*	1 Can/330ml	172	0.0	52	0.0	12.8	0.0	0.0
Mango & Passionfruit, Shot, Big Shotz*	1 Shot/120ml	67	0.5	56	0.0	12.1	0.4	3.4
Mango Madness, Snapple*	1 Bottle/227ml	104	0.0	46	0.0	12.0	0.0	0.0
Mega Green, Smucker's*	1 Serving/473ml	236	0.0	50	0.0	12.5	0.0	0.0
Orange, Caprisun*	1 Pouch/200ml	89	0.0	45	0.0	10.8	0.0	0.0
Orange, Carrot & Lemon, Pago*	1 Serving/200g	90	0.2	45	0.2	10.5	0.1	0.0
Orange, Juice Burst, Purity*	1 Bottle/500ml	220	0.0	44	1.0	10.2	0.0	0.0
Orange, Mango & Lime, Fruit Crush, Shapers, Boots*	1 Bottle/330ml	150	0.6	45	0.4	10.6	0.2	0.4
Passion Fruit, Exotic, Rubicon*	1 Serving/200ml	110	0.0	55	0.1	13.6	0.0	0.0
Peach, Fruit Float, Frubob*	1 Can/250ml	150	0.0	60	0.2	14.8	0.0	0.0
Peach, Passion Fruit, Extra Light, Oasis*	1 Bottle/500ml	17	0.0	3	0.0	0.6	0.0	0.0
Peach & Passionfruit Fruit, Sunmagic*	1 Serving/330ml	172	0.0	52	0.3	13.0	0.0	0.1
Pear & Plum, Shapers, Boots*	1 Bottle/500ml	10	0.0	2	0.0	0.2	0.0	0.0
Pineapple, Mango & Passionfruit, Sainsbury's*	1 Serving/200ml	74	0.0	37	0.1	8.7	0.0	0.2
Pineapple & Grapefruit, Shapers, Boots*	1 Bottle/500ml	10	0.5	2	0.1	0.2	0.1	0.0
Pink Grapefruit, Juice Burst, Purity*	1 Bottle/500ml	210	0.0	42	0.4	10.0	0.0	0.0
Pomegranate, Rubicon*	1 Can/330mll	108	0.0	54	0.0	13.5	0.0	0.0
Pomegranate & Blueberry, Weight Watchers*	1 Bottle/500ml	15	0.0	3	0.0	0.5	0.0	0.0
Pomegranate & Raspberry, Still, Shapers, Boots*	1 Bottle/500ml	45	0.0	9	0.0	2.0	0.0	0.0
Purple Grape & Mango, Welch's*	1 Glass/200ml	54	0.0	27	0.0	6.1	0.0	0.2
Raspberry, Ribena*	1 Bottle/500ml	215	0.0	43	0.0	10.4	0.0	0.0
Raspberry & Apple, No Added Sugar, Ribena*	1 Serving/200ml	8	0.0	4	0.0	0.5	0.0	0.0
Raspberry & Pear, Tesco*	1 Serving/250ml	117	0.0	47	0.0	11.3	0.0	0.0
Summer Fruits, Oasis*	1 Bottle/500ml	90	0.0	18	0.0	4.2	0.0	0.0
Tropical Hit, 5 Alive*	1 Carton/250ml	92	0.0	37	0.0	9.3	0.0	0.0
White Cranberry & Grape, Oceanspray*	1 Serving/100ml	48	0.0	48	0.0	11.6	0.0	0.0
White Cranberry & Lychee, Ocean Spray*	1 Glass/200ml	86	0.0	43	0.0	11.5	0.0	0.0
White Grape, Raspberry & Cranberry, Sparkling, Shloer*	1 Serving/250ml	117	0.0	47	0.0	11.0	0.0	0.0
White Grape & Peach, Sainsbury's*	1 Glass/250ml	95	0.2	38	0.2	9.0	0.1	0.1

JUNIPER

	Measure INFO/WEIGHT	per Measure KCAL	FAT	Nutrition Values per 100g / 100ml KCAL	PROT	CARB	FAT	FIBRE
Berries, Dried, Average	1 Tsp/2g	6	0.3	292	4.0	33.0	16.0	0.0

J

	Measure INFO/WEIGHT	per Measure		Nutrition Values per 100g / 100ml				
		KCAL	FAT	KCAL	PROT	CARB	FAT	FIBRE
KALE								
Curly, Boiled in Salted Water, Average	*1 Serving/60g*	*14*	*0.7*	*24*	*2.4*	*1.0*	*1.1*	*2.8*
Curly, Raw, Average	*1 Serving/90g*	*30*	*1.4*	*33*	*3.4*	*1.4*	*1.6*	*3.1*
KANGAROO								
Raw, Average	*1 Serving/200g*	*196*	*2.0*	*98*	*22.0*	*1.0*	*1.0*	*0.0*
Steak, Grilled, Average*	*1 Fillet/150g*	*198*	*1.8*	*132*	*30.0*	*0.0*	*1.2*	*0.0*
KEBAB								
BBQ Pork, Sainsbury's*	1 Serving/90g	65	2.2	72	11.0	1.4	2.4	0.9
Beef, & Pepper Kofta, Waitrose*	1 Kebab/138g	223	13.9	162	14.8	2.9	10.1	0.6
Beef, Hot & Spicy, Tesco*	1 Kebab/41g	111	8.4	270	15.7	4.4	20.6	1.6
Beef, Kofta, Uncooked, Tesco*	1 Kebab/73g	163	12.5	225	14.0	3.2	17.3	1.2
Beef, with Onion, Dulano, Lidl*	1 Serving/100g	224	16.0	224	18.0	2.0	16.0	0.0
Beef, with Sweet Chilli Seasoning, Sainsbury's*	1 Kebab/61g	151	8.0	248	24.1	8.5	13.1	0.8
Chicken, Barbecue, Sainsbury's*	1 Pack/200g	238	3.4	119	24.4	1.5	1.7	1.8
Chicken, Breast, Mediterranean, Sainsbury's*	1 Kebab/65g	73	2.1	113	16.5	4.6	3.2	0.6
Chicken, Breast, Salsa, Sainsbury's*	1 Kebab/80g	94	0.9	117	20.1	6.5	1.1	0.6
Chicken, Breast, Sweet, Oriental, COU, M & S*	½ Pack/200g	220	2.0	110	20.8	4.3	1.0	0.1
Chicken, Caribbean, Iceland*	1 Kebab/44g	36	0.1	82	12.0	8.0	0.2	0.5
Chicken, Chilli & Lime, Breast Fillet, Sainsbury's*	1 Kebab/77g	120	0.7	156	29.9	6.2	0.9	0.3
Chicken, Chinese, Mini, M & S*	1 Kebab/11g	24	1.4	215	19.5	5.1	12.9	0.6
Chicken, Citrus Tikka, Mini, Sainsbury's*	1 Serving/48g	72	1.1	151	30.3	2.7	2.3	0.2
Chicken, Fillet, Mini with a Tikka Marinade, Sainsbury's*	1 Kebab/25g	41	0.8	164	33.4	0.6	3.1	0.1
Chicken, Green Thai Waitrose*	1 Serving/180g	223	7.2	124	20.5	1.4	4.0	1.4
Chicken, Lemon & Ginger, Delicatezze, Waitrose*	1 Kebab/25g	50	2.8	201	24.5	0.3	11.3	2.7
Chicken, Mango & Lime, Perfectly Balanced, Waitrose*	1 Kebab/83g	103	1.3	125	26.0	1.2	1.6	1.1
Chicken, Red Pepper, Mini, Sainsbury's*	1 Kebab/52g	79	1.0	152	30.1	3.5	2.0	0.2
Chicken, Shish, Meat Only, Average	1 Kebab/250g	312	5.2	125	25.7	0.9	2.1	0.1
Chicken, Shish in Pitta Bread with Salad	1 Kebab/250g	387	10.2	155	13.5	17.2	4.1	1.0
Chicken, Sweet Chilli, Perfectly Balanced, Waitrose*	1 Kebab/83g	111	0.9	135	28.6	1.7	1.1	0.5
Chicken, Thigh, Sticky Barbecue, M & S*	1 Kebab/100g	160	7.5	160	15.6	7.4	7.5	0.8
Chicken, Thin Sliced, Heat 'n' Eat, Asda*	½ Pack/50g	92	6.0	184	15.0	3.9	12.0	1.1
Chicken, with Sweet Chilli Sauce, Finest, Tesco*	½ Pack/175g	241	1.4	138	17.9	14.7	0.8	1.2
Chicken, with Sweet Chilli Sauce, M & S*	1 Serving/165g	228	1.3	138	17.9	14.7	0.8	1.2
Chicken & Pineapple, Aldi*	1 Kebab/85g	89	2.6	105	13.9	5.3	3.1	0.0
Chicken & Pineapple, Caribbean Style, Iceland*	1 Kebab/44g	41	0.6	93	11.6	8.7	1.4	1.4
Chicken Tikka with Red Pepper & Pineapple, Tesco*	1 Kebab/80g	92	1.9	115	16.5	6.7	2.4	0.5
Chinese Chicken, Tesco*	1 Kebab/21g	37	1.6	175	19.5	5.8	7.8	0.5
Chinese Salmon, Iceland*	1 Kebab/75g	115	3.4	153	23.8	4.1	4.6	1.6
Citrus Tikka Chicken Breast, Sainsbury's*	1 Kebab/61g	79	0.3	129	25.6	5.4	0.5	0.9
Doner, Heat 'n' Eat Thin Sliced, Asda*	1 Pack/100g	196	10.6	196	16.7	8.4	10.6	1.7
Halloumi & Vegetable, Waitrose*	1 Kebab/127g	235	21.6	185	5.6	2.2	17.0	2.4
Honey & Mustard Chicken, Sainsbury's*	1 Serving/50g	65	0.9	131	24.5	4.3	1.8	0.0
Lamb, Greek Style, Lakeland*	1 Serving/100g	196	15.6	196	11.8	1.9	15.6	0.0
Lamb, Greek Style, Sainsbury's*	1 Serving/70g	196	15.3	282	16.1	4.9	22.0	1.8
Lamb, Kofta, Citrus Tikka, Sainsbury's*	1 Kebab/84g	199	11.6	235	18.1	9.8	13.7	2.6
Lamb, Shish, Sainsbury's*	1 Kebab/85g	178	11.3	210	19.7	2.8	13.3	0.7
Lamb, Shish, Waitrose*	1 Kebab/56g	114	7.1	203	15.3	6.8	12.7	1.1
Lamb, Shoulder, M & S*	½ Pack/250g	312	10.7	125	20.4	0.9	4.3	1.7
Lamb, with Halloumi Cheese & Olives, Waitrose*	1 Kebab/75g	123	6.2	164	20.0	2.4	8.3	0.2
Lamb, with Mint, Tesco*	1 Serving/80g	192	13.4	240	16.0	5.5	16.7	0.4
Lamb Kofta, Indian Style, Waitrose*	1 Kebab/125g	266	19.7	213	12.3	5.5	15.8	1.6
Lamb Shami with a Mint Raita Dip, M & S*	½ Pack/90g	189	12.1	210	12.8	9.7	13.4	3.5
Pork & Pepper, BBQ, Sainsbury's*	1 Kebab/41g	65	2.2	158	24.1	3.1	5.4	1.9
Pork & Pepper, Co-Op*	1 Kebab/74g	78	3.0	105	17.0	1.0	4.0	0.5

	Measure INFO/WEIGHT	per Measure KCAL	FAT	Nutrition Values per 100g / 100ml KCAL	PROT	CARB	FAT	FIBRE
KEBAB								
Salmon, Hot & Spicy, Tesco*	1 Kebab/75g	88	2.2	118	22.0	1.1	2.9	0.0
Shish, with Onions & Peppers	1oz/28g	59	4.5	212	12.9	3.9	16.2	1.2
Spicy Tomato Creole King Prawn, M & S*	1 Pack/240g	240	7.9	100	14.3	2.9	3.3	0.7
Sweetcorn, Tesco*	1 Kebab/130g	74	1.3	57	2.0	9.9	1.0	0.9
Tandoori, M & S*	1oz/28g	34	0.7	120	23.3	1.0	2.5	0.0
Tiger Prawn, Asda*	1oz/28g	17	0.0	59	14.6	0.0	0.1	0.0
Tikka, Mini, M & S*	1 Kebab/11g	23	1.4	205	18.4	4.0	12.7	0.6
Turkey, with Chinese Style Dressing, Sainsbury's*	1 Kebab/54g	84	2.7	157	21.4	6.4	5.1	1.7
Vegetable, Asda*	1 Kebab/40g	25	1.7	63	1.8	4.5	4.3	2.4
Vegetable, Mini, Sainsbury's*	1 Kebab/36g	22	0.8	61	2.5	7.4	2.3	2.4
Vegetable, Sainsbury's*	1 Kebab/100g	36	0.5	36	1.5	6.4	0.5	1.2
Vegetable, Tesco*	1 Kebab/120g	47	0.7	39	1.7	6.8	0.6	1.1
KEDGEREE								
Average	1oz/28g	48	2.4	171	15.9	7.8	8.7	0.1
COU, M & S*	1 Pack/370g	388	8.1	105	7.6	13.7	2.2	2.1
Smoked Haddock, Big Dish, M & S*	1 Pack/450g	585	22.5	130	8.5	13.0	5.0	1.9
KETCHUP								
Barbeque, Asda*	1 Tbsp/15g	20	0.0	136	0.9	33.0	0.0	0.0
BBQ, Heinz*	1 Serving/10g	14	0.0	137	1.3	31.3	0.3	0.3
Mild Chilli, Twisted, Heinz*	1 Tbsp/15g	16	0.0	108	1.0	24.9	0.2	0.7
Tomato, Average	**1 Tsp/5g**	**6**	**0.0**	**120**	**1.5**	**28.1**	**0.2**	**0.8**
Tomato, Reduced Salt & Sugar, HP*	1 Tbsp/17g	15	0.0	86	0.7	19.5	0.1	0.4
Tomato, Reduced Sugar, Average	**1 Tbsp/10g**	**9**	**0.1**	**87**	**2.0**	**16.9**	**1.2**	**0.9**
Tomato with Indian Spices, Heinz*	1 Tbsp/15g	17	0.1	114	1.1	24.8	0.4	0.8
KIDNEY								
Lamb, Raw, Average	**1oz/28g**	**44**	**2.2**	**156**	**21.5**	**0.0**	**7.7**	**0.0**
Ox, Raw	**1oz/28g**	**25**	**0.6**	**88**	**17.2**	**0.0**	**2.1**	**0.0**
Ox, Stewed	**1oz/28g**	**39**	**1.2**	**138**	**24.5**	**0.0**	**4.4**	**0.0**
Pig, Fried	**1oz/28g**	**57**	**2.7**	**202**	**29.2**	**0.0**	**9.5**	**0.0**
Pig, Raw	**1oz/28g**	**24**	**0.8**	**86**	**15.5**	**0.0**	**2.7**	**0.0**
Pig, Stewed	**1oz/28g**	**43**	**1.7**	**153**	**24.4**	**0.0**	**6.1**	**0.0**
Veal, Raw, Average	1 Serving/100g	99	3.1	99	15.8	0.8	3.1	0.0
KIEV								
Cheese & Herb, Mini, Bernard Matthews*	1 Kiev/23g	46	2.3	199	15.7	12.1	9.8	0.0
Chicken, Bernard Matthews*	1 Kiev/125g	374	27.9	299	10.6	13.9	22.3	2.7
Chicken, BFY, Morrisons*	1 Kiev/134g	304	17.4	227	16.1	11.5	13.0	1.0
Chicken, Breast, Hand Filled, Birds Eye*	1 Kiev/172g	330	17.2	192	15.5	9.9	10.0	2.0
Chicken, Cheesy Bean, Asda*	1 Kiev/94g	202	10.3	215	12.0	17.0	11.0	1.9
Chicken, Cooked, M Kitchen, Fresh Ideas, Morrisons*	1 Kiev/145g	359	20.8	248	17.5	12.0	14.4	0.9
Chicken, COU, M & S*	1 Kiev/150g	187	2.7	125	15.8	10.8	1.8	0.5
Chicken, Creamy Peppercorn, Sun Valley*	1 Kiev/140g	382	25.9	273	13.3	13.5	18.5	0.0
Chicken, Creamy Peppercorn, Tesco*	1 Kiev/130g	312	20.5	240	11.5	12.0	15.8	1.4
Chicken, Finest, Tesco*	1 Kiev/237g	503	26.6	212	19.5	8.2	11.2	2.6
Chicken, Garlic, 25% Less Fat, GFY, Asda*	1 Kiev/134g	296	15.7	221	17.0	11.9	11.7	0.5
Chicken, Garlic, 25% Reduced Fat, Tesco*	1 Kiev/130g	299	18.6	230	13.7	11.5	14.3	0.7
Chicken, Garlic, Fresh, Reduced Fat, Morrisons*	1 Kiev/141g	350	25.5	248	13.2	8.0	18.1	0.7
Chicken, Garlic, M & S*	1 Kiev/150g	370	24.8	247	15.6	8.2	16.5	2.9
Chicken, Garlic, Morrisons*	1 Kiev/122g	289	19.2	237	14.3	9.8	15.7	0.0
Chicken, Garlic & Herb, Reduced Fat, Sainsbury's*	1 Kiev/142g	317	18.0	223	15.1	12.1	12.7	0.6
Chicken, Garlic & Herb, Sainsbury's*	1 Kiev/134g	319	19.6	239	15.0	11.7	14.7	1.3
Chicken, Garlic & Mushroom, Sainsbury's*	1 Kiev/142g	346	19.1	243	16.2	14.5	13.4	1.4
Chicken, Garlic & Parsley, BGTY, Sainsbury's*	1 Kiev/126g	289	15.3	229	14.0	15.9	12.1	1.1
Chicken, Garlic & Parsley, Sainsbury's*	1 Kiev/120g	365	25.6	304	11.1	17.1	21.3	0.8

K

	Measure INFO/WEIGHT	per Measure KCAL	FAT	Nutrition Values per 100g / 100ml KCAL	PROT	CARB	FAT	FIBRE
KIEV								
Chicken, Garlic Butter, HL, Tesco*	1 Kiev/143g	285	16.4	200	14.3	9.9	11.5	0.6
Chicken, Garlic Butter, Somerfield*	1 Kiev/142g	425	33.9	299	12.6	8.5	23.9	1.2
Chicken, Good Choice, Iceland*	1 Kiev/120g	366	27.2	305	12.7	12.6	22.7	0.8
Chicken, Ham & Cheese, BGTY, Sainsbury's*	1 Kiev/132g	264	10.2	200	13.2	19.5	7.7	0.8
Chicken, Italian Style, Sainsbury's*	1 Kiev/135g	341	21.7	253	14.3	12.8	16.1	1.3
Chicken, Maitre Jean-Pierre*	1 Kiev/140g	385	26.7	275	13.3	12.7	19.1	0.8
Chicken, Roast Garlic & Parsley, Sainsbury's*	1 Kiev/143g	369	21.3	258	14.5	16.5	14.9	0.8
Chicken, Tomato & Mozzarella, Tesco*	1 Kiev/143g	285	17.4	200	13.4	9.0	12.2	1.4
Chicken Breast, Garlic, Frozen, Tesco*	1 Kiev/141g	430	34.7	305	13.0	6.9	24.6	1.3
Chicken Breast, Garlic Butter, Sun Valley*	1 Kiev/141g	436	32.7	309	13.2	11.8	23.2	0.9
Chicken in Crispy Breadcrumbs, Sainsbury's*	1 Kiev/117g	310	22.4	266	12.8	10.6	19.2	1.1
Garlic, Meat Free, Tesco*	1 Kiev/125g	244	11.2	195	15.0	12.5	9.0	2.6
Salmon, Fillet, Tesco*	1 Kiev/160g	376	19.5	235	13.3	18.0	12.2	2.5
Tikka Chicken, Asda*	1 Kiev/134g	274	14.8	205	12.8	13.5	11.1	0.6
Turkey, Mini, Baked, Bernard Matthews*	1 Kiev/23g	50	2.7	221	17.5	11.2	11.8	1.1
KIEV VEGETARIAN								
Aduki Bean, Cauldron Foods*	1 Kiev/110g	223	5.4	203	6.2	30.0	4.9	7.0
Cheesy Garlic, Meat Free, Sainsbury's*	1 Kiev/123g	274	15.1	223	13.8	14.3	12.3	3.5
Garlic, Meat Free, Asda*	1 Kiev/125g	239	11.2	191	15.0	12.5	9.0	2.6
Garlic Butter, Tivall*	1 Kiev/125g	366	26.2	293	15.1	10.8	21.0	2.6
Vegetable, M & S*	1 Kiev/155g	279	16.6	180	4.2	17.2	10.7	3.7
KIPPER								
Baked, Average	*1oz/28g*	*57*	*3.2*	*205*	*25.5*	*0.0*	*11.4*	*0.0*
Fillets, Raw, Average	*1 Serving/200g*	*451*	*34.3*	*226*	*17.0*	*0.0*	*17.1*	*0.0*
Fillets, Smoked with Butter, Scottish, Boil in Bag, Tesco*	1 Serving/100g	225	17.2	225	17.0	0.0	17.2	0.0
Fillets in Brine, John West*	1 Can/140g	269	16.8	192	21.0	0.0	12.0	0.0
Fillets in Sunflower Oil, John West*	1 Can/140g	321	23.8	229	19.0	0.0	17.0	0.0
Fillets with Butter, Scottish, Somerfield*	1 Serving/100g	178	12.4	178	16.5	0.0	12.4	0.0
Grilled, Average	*1oz/28g*	*71*	*5.4*	*255*	*20.1*	*0.0*	*19.4*	*0.0*
Smoked, Average	*1 Serving/150g*	*322*	*23.0*	*214*	*18.9*	*0.0*	*15.3*	*0.0*
KIT KAT								
2 Finger, Nestle*	2 Fingers/21g	107	5.4	510	6.4	62.8	25.6	2.3
4 Finger, Nestle*	4 Fingers/46g	233	11.8	512	6.3	62.6	25.9	1.1
Caramac, 4 Finger, Nestle*	4 Fingers/49g	259	14.1	532	5.9	61.9	29.0	0.6
Chunky, Caramel, Nestle*	1 Bar/48g	259	15.3	539	5.2	58.6	31.8	0.0
Chunky, Nestle*	1 Bar/48g	248	12.6	516	5.9	62.5	26.3	2.1
Chunky, Orange, Nestle*	1 Bar/48g	247	12.5	515	5.8	62.0	26.1	0.0
Chunky, Peanut, Nestle*	1 Bar/50g	268	15.7	537	8.4	54.9	31.5	0.0
Chunky, Snack Size, Nestle*	1 Bar/26g	133	7.1	513	6.6	60.4	27.2	1.1
Editions, Mango & Passionfruit, Nestle*	1 Bar/45g	225	10.5	499	4.7	69.0	23.4	0.0
Editions, Seville Orange, Nestle*	1 Bar/45g	223	10.3	496	4.6	69.3	23.0	0.8
Kubes, Nestle*	1 Pack/50g	257	13.7	515	5.9	60.9	27.5	1.0
Kubes, Orange, Nestle*	4 Kubes/13g	66	3.5	514	5.7	61.1	27.4	1.0
Lemon & Yoghurt, Nestle*	1 Pack/45g	240	13.4	533	7.3	58.0	29.8	0.4
Low Carb, 2 Finger, Nestle*	2 Fingers/21g	92	6.6	438	9.2	28.3	31.3	1.3
Low Carb, 4 Finger, Nestle*	1 Finger/11g	46	3.3	438	9.2	28.3	31.3	1.3
Mini, Nestle*	1 Bar/15g	75	3.9	502	7.5	59.4	26.0	0.0
Mint, 4 Finger, Nestle*	4 Fingers/48g	244	12.7	508	6.0	61.5	26.4	1.1
Orange, 2 Finger, Nestle*	2 Fingers/21g	107	5.6	507	5.5	61.7	26.5	0.0
Senses, Nestle*	1 Bar/31g	165	9.5	531	7.5	56.3	30.7	0.0
White, Chunky, Nestle*	1 Bar/53g	276	14.6	521	8.3	60.3	27.5	0.7
KIWI FRUIT								
Fresh, Raw, Flesh & Seeds, Average	*1 Kiwi/60g*	*29*	*0.3*	*49*	*1.1*	*10.6*	*0.5*	*1.9*

K

	Measure INFO/WEIGHT	per Measure KCAL	FAT	Nutrition Values per 100g / 100ml KCAL	PROT	CARB	FAT	FIBRE
KIWI FRUIT								
Weighed with Skin, Average	*1 Kiwi/60g*	*29*	*0.3*	*49*	*1.1*	*10.6*	*0.5*	*1.9*
KOHLRABI								
Boiled in Salted Water	*1oz/28g*	*5*	*0.1*	*18*	*1.2*	*3.1*	*0.2*	*1.9*
Raw	*1oz/28g*	*6*	*0.1*	*23*	*1.6*	*3.7*	*0.2*	*2.2*
KORMA								
Chicken, & Basmati Rice, Tesco*	1 Pot/350g	588	32.6	168	4.3	16.9	9.3	2.3
Chicken, & Pilau Rice, BGTY, Sainsbury's*	1 Pack/400g	404	5.2	101	8.0	14.3	1.3	0.6
Chicken, & Pilau Rice, GFY, Asda*	1 Pack/400g	600	24.0	150	8.0	16.0	6.0	1.3
Chicken, & Pilau Rice, Good Intentions, Somerfield*	1 Pack/400g	472	11.6	118	7.7	15.3	2.9	0.8
Chicken, & Pilau Rice, Indian, Asda*	1 Pack/456g	643	22.8	141	8.0	16.0	5.0	2.4
Chicken, & Pilau Rice, Morrisons*	1 Pack/450g	889	48.2	198	9.4	15.9	10.7	1.4
Chicken, & Pilau Rice, Saint Agur*	1 Serving/367g	367	5.5	100	6.4	14.1	1.5	2.2
Chicken, & Pilau Rice, Somerfield*	1 Pack/340g	687	37.4	202	9.0	16.0	11.0	0.0
Chicken, & Pilau Rice, Tesco*	1 Serving/460g	722	45.1	157	5.6	11.5	9.8	1.3
Chicken, & Rice, 323, Oakhouse Foods Ltd*	1 Meal/400g	552	23.6	138	7.1	14.2	5.9	0.6
Chicken, & Rice, 95% Fat Free, Birds Eye*	1 Pack/370g	444	7.0	120	6.2	19.6	1.9	1.1
Chicken, & Rice, World Flavours*	1 Pack/500g	705	23.5	141	8.7	16.0	4.7	0.0
Chicken, & White Rice, BGTY, Frozen, Sainsbury's*	1 Pack/375g	341	3.7	91	5.6	14.9	1.0	0.5
Chicken, & Yellow Pilau Rice, Chilled, Tesco*	1 Pack/550g	698	20.9	127	8.2	15.0	3.8	1.2
Chicken, Breast, Chunks, Sainsbury's*	1 Serving/227g	354	9.3	156	28.0	1.7	4.1	0.8
Chicken, Fresh, Chilled, Tesco*	1 Pack/350g	819	60.9	234	13.1	6.3	17.4	2.3
Chicken, HL, Tesco*	1 Pack/350g	371	4.2	106	7.7	15.9	1.2	0.8
Chicken, Indian, Take Away, Tesco*	½ Pack/175g	222	13.5	127	9.0	5.5	7.7	1.8
Chicken, Indian Meal for 2, Finest, Tesco*	½ Pack/200g	348	24.0	174	10.3	6.2	12.0	2.5
Chicken, Indian Takeaway, Iceland*	1 Pack/400g	656	44.0	164	11.8	4.5	11.0	1.4
Chicken, Indian Takeaway for One, Sainsbury's*	1 Serving/300g	498	30.9	166	13.0	5.3	10.3	1.6
Chicken, Less Than 3% Fat, Birds Eye*	1 Pack/358g	440	6.8	123	6.5	20.4	1.9	0.8
Chicken, Less Than 3% Fat, Frozen, GFY, Asda*	1 Pack/401g	405	6.8	101	5.3	16.2	1.7	1.2
Chicken, Morrisons*	1 Pack/350g	707	46.5	202	13.6	7.0	13.3	0.7
Chicken, Plumrose*	1 Can/392g	431	22.0	110	8.0	6.9	5.6	0.0
Chicken, Solo Slim, Rosemary Conley*	1 Pack/300g	315	12.9	105	8.7	7.9	4.3	0.8
Chicken, Tesco*	1 Pack/350g	619	41.3	177	10.8	6.8	11.8	0.6
Chicken, Tinned, Asda*	½ Can/197g	321	21.7	163	8.0	8.0	11.0	2.3
Chicken, Waitrose*	1 Pack/400g	680	46.8	170	13.7	2.4	11.7	1.9
Chicken, with Peshwari Coriander Rice, Finest, Tesco*	1 Pack/550g	907	48.4	165	7.5	13.9	8.8	0.9
Chicken, with Pilau Rice, Asda*	1 Serving/350g	735	49.0	210	12.0	9.0	14.0	2.0
Chicken, with Pilau Rice, Co-Op*	1 Pack/400g	520	20.4	130	10.3	10.7	5.1	2.6
Chicken, with Pilau Rice, Perfectly Balanced, Waitrose*	1 Pack/400g	452	6.8	113	8.9	15.4	1.7	1.3
Chicken, with Rice, Ready Meal, Average	1 Pack/350g	648	30.4	185	8.4	18.1	8.7	1.7
Chicken, with Rice, Ready Meal, Healthy Range, Average	1 Serving/400g	450	8.2	112	7.3	16.1	2.1	1.2
Vegetable, & Rice, Tesco*	1 Pack/450g	621	26.5	138	2.9	18.3	5.9	1.6
Vegetable, Ready to Cook, Fresh, Sainsbury's*	½ Pack/255g	263	17.3	103	2.8	7.7	6.8	2.1
Vegetable, Sainsbury's*	1 Serving/200g	302	25.2	151	2.7	6.6	12.6	2.2
KRISPROLLS								
Cracked Wheat, Original, Pagen*	1 Krisproll/13g	47	0.9	380	12.0	67.0	7.0	9.0
Golden, Swedish Toasts, Pagen*	1 Krisproll/12g	48	1.0	400	11.0	69.0	8.5	5.0
Organic, Bio, Pagen*	1 Krisproll/12g	46	0.8	380	12.0	67.0	7.0	8.0
Swedish Toasts, Wholegrain, Pagen*	1 Toast/13g	51	0.8	390	11.0	67.0	6.5	8.5
KULFI								
Average	*1oz/28g*	*119*	*11.2*	*424*	*5.4*	*11.8*	*39.9*	*0.6*
KUMQUATS								
Raw	*1oz/28g*	*12*	*0.1*	*43*	*0.9*	*9.3*	*0.5*	*3.8*

INFO/WEIGHT	Measure	per Measure		Nutrition Values per 100g / 100ml				
		KCAL	FAT	KCAL	PROT	CARB	FAT	FIBRE

LAGER
Alcohol Free, Becks*	1 Serving/275ml	55	0.0	20	0.7	5.0	0.0	0.0
Amstel, Heineken*	1 Pint/568ml	227	0.0	40	0.5	3.0	0.0	0.0
Average	1 Pint/568ml	233	0.0	41	0.3	3.1	0.0	0.0
Becks*	1 Can/275ml	113	0.0	41	0.0	3.0	0.0	0.0
Blanc, Kronenbourg*	½ pt/284ml	119	0.0	42	0.0	3.3	0.0	0.0
Boston, Samuel Adams*	1 Bottle/355ml	160	0.0	45	0.0	0.0	0.0	0.0
Bottled, Brahma*	1 Bottle/330ml	125	0.0	38	0.0	0.0	0.0	0.0
Budweiser, 66, Anheuser-Busch*	1 Bottle/330ml	102	0.0	31	0.0	0.0	0.0	0.0
C2, Carling*	½ Pint/284ml	80	0.0	28	0.0	3.5	0.0	0.0
Can, Carlsberg*	1 Can/440ml	141	0.0	32	0.0	2.0	0.0	0.0
Draught, Carling*	1 Pint/568ml	189	0.0	33	0.0	1.4	0.0	0.0
Edge, Carlsberg*	1 Can/300ml	126	0.0	42	0.0	4.3	0.0	0.0
Export, Carlsberg*	1 Can/440ml	185	0.0	42	0.3	2.8	0.0	0.3
Export, Foster's*	1 Pint/568ml	210	0.0	37	0.0	2.2	0.0	0.0
Foster's*	1 Pint/568ml	227	0.0	40	0.0	3.1	0.0	0.0
Gold, Foster's, Heineken*	1 Can/440ml	145	0.0	33	0.3	1.2	0.0	0.0
Grolsch*	1 Sm Can/330ml	145	0.0	44	0.0	2.2	0.0	0.0
Heineken V5, Heineken*	1 Pint/568ml	256	0.0	45	0.5	3.0	0.0	0.0
Heineken*, 5%, Heineken*	1 Bottle/250ml	110	0.0	44	0.4	3.4	0.0	0.0
Kaliber, Guinness*	1 Can/440ml	110	0.0	25	0.2	6.0	0.0	0.0
Light, Coors*	1 Pint/500ml	160	0.0	32	0.3	1.7	0.0	0.0
Light, Corona*	1 Bottle/330ml	105	0.0	32	1.5	0.0	0.0	0.0
Light, Michelob*	1 Serving/340ml	113	0.0	33	0.3	2.0	0.0	0.0
Lite, Carlsberg*	1 Bottle/330ml	89	0.0	27	0.1	0.5	0.0	0.0
Low Alcohol	1 Can/440ml	44	0.0	10	0.2	1.5	0.0	0.0
Pils, Holsten*	1 Can/440ml	167	0.0	38	0.3	2.4	0.0	0.0
Pilsner, Efes*	1 Can/500ml	226	0.0	45	0.0	7.6	0.0	0.0
Polish, Tyskie*	1 Can/550ml	236	0.0	43	0.0	0.0	0.0	0.0
Premium	1 Can/440ml	260	0.0	59	0.3	2.4	0.0	0.0
Premium, Light, Amstel*	1 Can/355ml	95	0.0	27	0.0	1.4	0.0	0.0
Tuborg Green, Carlsberg*	1 Serving/200ml	78	0.0	39	0.5	2.5	0.0	0.0
Ultra Low Carb, Michelob*	1 Bottle/275ml	88	0.0	32	0.2	0.9	0.0	0.0
Vier, Becks*	1 Bottle/275ml	110	0.0	40	0.0	3.0	0.0	0.0

LAKSA
Chicken, COU, M & S*	1 Pack/450g	360	9.9	80	7.5	7.0	2.2	1.1
Thai Noodle, with Chicken, M & S*	1 Pack/400g	460	21.6	115	7.0	9.8	5.4	1.1

LAMB
Breast, Lean, Roasted, Average	1 Serving/100g	273	18.5	273	26.7	0.0	18.5	0.0
Chops, Average	*1oz/28g*	*65*	*4.6*	*231*	*20.5*	*0.4*	*16.3*	*0.0*
Chops, Leg, De-boned, Grilled, Simply Cook, Tesco*	1 Chop/105g	330	17.7	314	39.2	0.0	16.9	0.0
Chops, Minted, Average	*1 Chop/100g*	*260*	*15.1*	*260*	*25.9*	*5.1*	*15.1*	*0.3*
Cutlets, Neck, Raw, Lean & Fat, Weighed with Bone	*1 Pack/210g*	*485*	*42.8*	*231*	*11.9*	*0.0*	*20.4*	*0.0*
Diced, From Supermarket, Healthy Range, Average	*½ Pack/200g*	*277*	*8.9*	*138*	*24.6*	*0.1*	*4.5*	*0.0*
Escalope, Asda*	1 Serving/100g	173	5.0	173	32.0	0.0	5.0	0.0
Escalope, British, HL, Tesco*	1 Piece/95g	104	3.1	110	20.1	0.0	3.3	0.0
Grill Steak, Average	*1oz/28g*	*70*	*4.7*	*250*	*20.2*	*4.4*	*16.9*	*0.4*
Grill Steak, Prime, Average	*1 Steak/63g*	*197*	*16.1*	*312*	*18.5*	*2.0*	*25.5*	*0.1*
Grill Steak, Rosemary & Mint, Tesco*	1 Steak/62g	172	10.9	277	24.4	5.6	17.6	1.8
Leg, Joint, Raw, Average	*1 Joint/510g*	*858*	*45.5*	*168*	*20.9*	*1.4*	*8.9*	*0.2*
Leg, Roasted, Lean, Average	*1oz/28g*	*58*	*2.7*	*206*	*29.9*	*0.0*	*9.6*	*0.0*
Leg, Roasted, Lean & Fat, Average	*1oz/28g*	*66*	*3.8*	*237*	*28.6*	*0.0*	*13.6*	*0.0*
Loin, Chop, Grilled, Lean & Fat, Weighed with Bone	1 Serving/100g	247	17.9	247	21.5	0.0	17.9	0.0
Loin, Chops, Raw, Lean & Fat, Weighed with Bone	1 Serving/100g	216	17.9	216	13.7	0.0	17.9	0.0

L

	Measure INFO/WEIGHT	per Measure KCAL	per Measure FAT	Nutrition Values per 100g / 100ml KCAL	PROT	CARB	FAT	FIBRE
LAMB								
Mince, Average	1oz/28g	58	4.2	207	17.6	0.5	14.8	0.0
Neck Fillet, Lean, Raw	1 Serving/100g	184	9.3	184	19.6	0.3	9.3	0.0
Rack, Raw, Lean & Fat	1oz/28g	79	6.7	283	17.3	0.0	23.8	0.0
Rack, Raw, Lean Only, Weighed with Bone	1 oz/28g	48	2.6	169	20.0	0.0	9.2	0.0
Rack, Roasted, Lean	1oz/28g	63	3.6	225	27.1	0.0	13.0	0.0
Rack, Roasted, Lean & Fat	1oz/28g	102	8.4	363	23.0	0.0	30.1	0.0
Shank, Tuscan, Somerfield*	½ Shank/200g	350	17.4	175	19.0	5.2	8.7	1.5
Shoulder, Cooked, Lean & Fat	1oz/28g	84	6.3	301	24.4	0.0	22.5	0.0
Shoulder, Fillet, Average	1oz/28g	66	5.1	235	17.6	0.0	18.3	0.0
Shoulder, Raw, Average	1oz/28g	70	5.7	248	16.7	0.0	20.2	0.0
Shoulder, Roasted, Whole, Lean	1oz/28g	61	3.4	218	27.2	0.0	12.1	0.0
Steak, Leg, Raw, Average	1 Steak/150g	169	5.5	112	20.0	0.0	3.6	0.0
Steak, Minted, Average	1 Steak/125g	212	9.0	170	22.7	3.4	7.2	0.9
Steak, Raw, Average	1 Steak/140g	190	7.6	136	21.7	0.2	5.4	0.0
Stewing, Raw, Lean & Fat	1oz/28g	57	3.5	203	22.5	0.0	12.6	0.0
Stewing, Stewed, Lean	1oz/28g	67	4.1	240	26.6	0.0	14.8	0.0
Stewing, Stewed, Lean & Fat	1oz/28g	78	5.6	279	24.4	0.0	20.1	0.0
Trimmed Fat, Raw, Average	1 Serving/100g	518	51.6	518	13.3	0.0	51.6	0.0
LAMB DINNER								
Roast, Birds Eye*	1 Dinner/340g	370	14.0	109	5.9	12.1	4.1	1.5
LAMB IN								
Garlic & Rosemary Gravy, Shank, Asda*	1 Shank/280g	451	23.2	161	19.8	1.7	8.3	0.5
Gravy, Minted, Roast, M & S*	1 Pack/200g	140	3.0	70	6.8	6.6	1.5	0.9
Gravy, Roast, Birds Eye*	1 Pack/239g	160	5.3	67	8.1	3.8	2.2	0.1
Mint Gravy, Sliced, Sainsbury's*	1 Pack/125g	134	4.7	107	15.3	2.9	3.8	0.8
Minted Gravy, Shank, Iceland*	1 Shank/350g	651	45.1	186	15.0	2.4	12.9	0.5
Rich Minted Gravy, Shank, Morrisons*	1 Pack/400g	612	26.4	153	18.8	5.2	6.6	0.0
LAMB MEDITERRANEAN								
Shanks, Finest, Tesco*	1 Serving/404g	671	35.6	166	15.0	6.6	8.8	2.0
LAMB MOROCCAN								
with Cous Cous, Perfectly Balanced, Waitrose*	1 Pack/400g	390	5.2	97	7.7	13.6	1.3	2.2
LAMB RAGU								
with Tagliatelle, Finest, Tesco*	1 Pack/400g	560	19.2	140	8.5	14.9	4.8	1.1
LAMB TAGINE								
Moroccan Style with Couscous, COU, M & S*	1 Pack/400g	340	5.6	85	8.9	8.3	1.4	1.6
LAMB WITH								
Carrot & Swede Mash, Braised, Eat Smart, Morrisons*	1 Pack/400g	304	9.2	76	5.2	8.2	2.3	1.5
Cous Cous, Moroccan Style, Tesco*	1 Pack/550g	710	14.9	129	6.6	19.6	2.7	1.3
Gravy, Joint, Tesco*	1 Serving/225g	277	13.0	123	14.9	2.8	5.8	0.0
Honey Roast Vegetables, Extra Special, Asda*	1 Pack/400g	400	14.8	100	9.9	6.7	3.7	2.5
Mango & Mint, Shoulder Chops, Waitrose*	1 Chop/250g	555	40.5	222	16.7	2.3	16.2	0.5
Mango & Mint Sauce, Boneless Joint, Asda*	1 Serving/100g	302	22.0	302	26.0	0.0	22.0	1.4
Mint, Leg Chops, Morrisons*	2 Chops/350g	857	45.1	245	29.4	2.4	12.9	0.9
Mint Butter, Leg Steaks, Waitrose*	1 Serving/155g	270	16.3	174	19.6	0.4	10.5	0.0
Mint Glaze & Redcurrant Sauce, Steaks, Leg, Asda*	½ Pack/145g	247	8.7	170	18.0	11.0	6.0	0.5
Mint Gravy, Leg Chops, Tesco*	1 Serving/175g	213	9.8	122	15.0	3.2	5.6	1.7
Mint Gravy, Shanks, Frozen, Tesco*	1 Shank/200g	420	26.4	210	20.1	1.6	13.2	0.7
Redcurrant & Rosemary Sauce, Chops, Leg, Tesco*	1 Pack/325g	604	36.1	186	17.6	4.0	11.1	0.5
Roasted Vegetables, Shank, M & S*	½ Pack/420g	660	30.6	157	14.9	8.3	7.3	0.7
Rosemary, Joint, Tesco*	1 Serving/125g	250	17.6	200	17.5	0.8	14.1	0.5
Rosemary Gravy, Shank, Sainsbury's*	1 Serving/200g	204	8.2	102	13.2	3.1	4.1	0.3
Sticky Plum & Orange Glaze, Joint, Waitrose*	1 Serving/100g	164	7.9	164	13.4	9.8	7.9	3.1
Sweet Mint & Balsamic Sauce, Chops, Asda*	½ Pack/160g	381	24.2	238	24.2	1.2	15.1	0.9

L

	Measure INFO/WEIGHT	per Measure		Nutrition Values per 100g / 100ml				
		KCAL	FAT	KCAL	PROT	CARB	FAT	FIBRE
LAMB WITH								
Sweet Mint Dressing, Joint, Tesco*	1 Serving/50g	96	5.9	193	19.9	1.8	11.8	0.6
LARD								
Average	*1oz/28g*	*249*	*27.7*	*891*	*0.0*	*0.0*	*99.0*	*0.0*
LASAGNE								
Al Forno, Beef, M & S*	1 Pack/400g	640	38.0	160	8.2	10.7	9.5	2.8
Al Forno, TTD, Sainsbury's*	1 Pack/383g	571	30.3	149	8.6	10.9	7.9	2.1
Alla Bolognese, Weight Watchers*	1 Pack/350g	416	8.7	119	8.0	16.0	2.5	0.0
Asparagus, M & S*	1 Pack/360g	432	22.0	120	4.3	11.9	6.1	1.1
Balsamic Onion & Chicken, M & S*	1 Pack/375g	562	25.1	150	9.5	12.5	6.7	1.5
Beef, BGTY, Sainsbury's*	1 Pack/390g	376	8.5	102	6.2	13.2	2.3	1.7
Beef, Frozen, Tesco*	1 Pack/450g	607	25.2	135	7.5	12.6	5.6	0.8
Beef, Frozen, Weight Watchers*	1 Pack/300g	257	7.8	86	6.1	9.3	2.6	0.4
Beef, HL, Tesco*	1 Pack/450g	450	10.3	100	6.7	12.6	2.3	1.4
Beef, Less Than 3% Fat, Frozen, GFY, Asda*	1 Pack/400g	369	10.0	92	7.3	8.9	2.5	2.5
Beef, Less Than 5% Fat, Asda*	1 Pack/400g	460	17.2	115	5.0	14.0	4.3	0.6
Beef, Little Dish*	1 Pack/200g	349	20.8	174	9.3	10.7	10.4	0.8
Beef, Ready Meal, Average	1 Serving/400g	553	24.0	138	8.2	12.7	6.0	1.4
Beef & Chunky Vegetable, HL, Tesco*	1 Pack/340g	354	9.5	104	5.9	13.8	2.8	1.2
Beef & Red Wine, & Seasoned Wedges, Weight Watchers*	1 Pack/400g	400	13.2	100	5.1	12.5	3.3	0.2
Bolognese, Co-Op*	1 Pack/500g	757	35.5	151	8.1	13.8	7.1	0.0
Bolognese, Trattorie Alfredo*	1 Serving/125g	204	11.2	163	9.0	13.0	9.0	0.0
Bolognese & Vegetable, Weight Watchers*	1 Pack/300g	279	7.8	93	5.0	12.4	2.6	0.0
Chicken, Italian, Sainsbury's*	1 Pack/450g	549	18.9	122	8.4	12.6	4.2	0.5
Chicken, Italiano, Tesco*	1 Pack/450g	490	13.5	109	8.6	12.0	3.0	0.6
Chicken, Light Choices, Tesco*	1 Pack/400g	344	6.8	86	7.1	10.5	1.7	1.8
Chilled, Somerfield*	1 Pack/300g	312	9.3	104	6.8	12.2	3.1	1.3
Classic, Deep Filled, M & S*	1 Pack/400g	760	47.6	190	10.0	11.2	11.9	0.6
Creamy Ricotta & Vegetable, HL, Tesco*	1 Pack/384g	407	10.8	106	5.5	14.6	2.8	3.6
Diet Chef Ltd*	1 Pack/270g	288	13.8	107	5.6	9.6	5.1	1.9
Family, Big Value Pack, Iceland*	¼ Pack/237g	322	14.0	136	5.0	15.9	5.9	1.4
Family, M & S*	¼ Pack/225g	281	13.9	125	10.3	6.9	6.2	1.1
Fresh, Findus*	1 Pack/350g	402	15.7	115	6.2	11.7	4.5	0.4
Frozen, You Count, Love Life, Waitrose*	1 Pack/380g	359	10.3	94	5.0	12.2	2.7	0.6
GFY, Asda*	1 Pack/410g	344	8.2	84	5.5	11.0	2.0	0.3
Italian, Tesco*	1 Pack/400g	540	28.8	135	6.3	11.1	7.2	1.5
Layered, Asda*	1 Pack/300g	444	24.0	148	5.0	14.0	8.0	0.3
Less Than 5% Fat, BFY, Morrisons*	½ Pack/350g	227	8.8	65	5.9	8.2	2.5	0.7
Light Choices, Tesco*	1 Pack/430g	396	11.2	92	5.8	11.3	2.6	1.6
Low Saturated Fat, Waitrose*	1 Pack/400g	312	6.0	78	4.7	11.4	1.5	0.4
Minced Beef, Great Stuff, Asda*	1 Pack/300g	333	13.2	111	6.2	11.7	4.4	1.3
Mushroom & Spinach, Waitrose*	1 Pack/400g	373	14.0	93	3.1	12.3	3.5	1.3
Salmon, King Prawn & Spinach, Finest, Tesco*	1 Pack/400g	600	29.6	150	10.6	9.6	7.4	0.8
Sheets, Boiled, Average	*1 Sheet/20g*	*20*	*0.1*	*100*	*3.0*	*22.0*	*0.6*	*0.9*
Sheets, Dry, Average	*1 Sheet/20g*	*70*	*0.3*	*349*	*11.9*	*72.1*	*1.5*	*2.9*
Sheets, Fresh, Dry, Average	*1 Sheet/21g*	*56*	*0.4*	*271*	*10.9*	*52.7*	*2.1*	*1.9*
Sheets, Verdi, Dry, Average	*1 Sheet/20g*	*71*	*0.4*	*355*	*12.6*	*71.1*	*2.2*	*2.7*
Sheets, Wholewheat, Cooked, Chosen By You, Asda*	1 Sheet/21g	31	0.2	148	4.8	28.3	0.9	3.7
Smoked Salmon & Asparagus, Sainsbury's*	1 Pack/350g	665	37.4	190	7.9	15.6	10.7	0.7
Spinach & Cheese, Italian, Sainsbury's*	1 Pack/450g	666	30.6	148	6.0	15.5	6.8	0.5
Spinach & Ricotta, Asda*	1 Pack/400g	488	24.0	122	4.9	12.0	6.0	1.5
Spinach & Ricotta, Finest, Tesco*	1 Pack/350g	584	37.1	167	6.1	11.7	10.6	1.2
Spinach & Ricotta, Giovanni Rana*	1 Pack/350g	728	39.6	208	7.4	19.2	11.3	0.0
Vegetable, 254, Oakhouse Foods Ltd*	1 Meal/400g	344	17.6	86	3.4	8.0	4.4	1.4

L

	Measure INFO/WEIGHT	per Measure KCAL	FAT	Nutrition Values per 100g / 100ml KCAL	PROT	CARB	FAT	FIBRE
LASAGNE								
Vegetable, Findus*	1 Pack/330g	313	8.2	95	4.0	13.0	2.5	0.0
Vegetable, Healthy Range, Average	1 Serving/400g	318	8.2	80	3.5	11.8	2.1	1.5
Vegetable, Ready Meal, Average	1 Serving/450g	459	19.8	102	4.1	12.4	4.4	1.0
Vegetable, Ross*	1 Pack/300g	270	8.4	90	2.9	13.3	2.8	1.2
Vegetable, Weight Watchers*	1 Pack/330g	251	5.6	76	3.6	11.8	1.7	0.7
LASAGNE VEGETARIAN								
Linda McCartney*	1 Pack/360g	451	20.2	125	6.3	12.4	5.6	1.4
Meat Substitute, Ready Meal, Average	1 Serving/400g	468	20.8	117	5.3	12.2	5.2	1.5
Tesco*	1 Pack/450g	630	34.6	140	6.0	11.6	7.7	1.6
LAVERBREAD								
Average	*1oz/28g*	*15*	*1.0*	*52*	*3.2*	*1.6*	*3.7*	*0.0*
LEEKS								
Boiled, Average	*1oz/28g*	*6*	*0.2*	*21*	*1.2*	*2.6*	*0.7*	*1.7*
Creamed, Frozen, Waitrose*	1 Serving/225g	115	5.4	51	1.8	5.5	2.4	0.0
Frozen, Sliced, Asda*	1 Serving/100g	27	0.5	27	1.6	2.9	0.5	2.2
Raw, Unprepared, Average	*1 Leek/166g*	*64*	*1.5*	*39*	*2.8*	*5.1*	*0.9*	*3.9*
LEMON								
Extract	¼ Tsp/1ml	5	0.0	400	0.0	0.0	0.0	0.0
Fresh, Raw, Average	1 Slice/5g	1	0.0	20	1.0	3.2	0.3	2.4
Fresh, Raw, Unwaxed, Sainsbury's*	½ Lemon/60g	12	0.2	20	1.0	3.2	0.3	0.0
Peel, Raw, Average	*1 Tbsp/6g*	*3*	*0.0*	*47*	*1.5*	*16.0*	*0.3*	*10.6*
LEMON CURD								
Average	*1 Tbsp/15g*	*44*	*0.7*	*294*	*0.7*	*62.9*	*4.7*	*0.1*
Luxury, Average	*1 Tsp/7g*	*23*	*0.6*	*326*	*2.8*	*59.7*	*8.4*	*0.1*
LEMON GRASS								
Easy, Asda*	1 Tsp/10g	5	0.1	52	0.4	7.4	1.2	5.2
Stalks, Tesco*	1 Stalk/13g	12	0.1	99	1.8	25.3	0.5	0.0
LEMON SOLE								
Fillets, Raw, Average	*1 Serving/220g*	*180*	*2.8*	*82*	*17.3*	*0.2*	*1.3*	*0.3*
Goujons, Average	1 Serving/150g	359	18.3	239	13.9	18.5	12.2	1.0
Grilled, Average	*1oz/28g*	*27*	*0.5*	*97*	*20.2*	*0.0*	*1.7*	*0.0*
in Breadcrumbs, Average	1 Fillet/142g	322	17.4	228	13.7	15.7	12.3	1.0
in White Wine & Herb Butter, Fillets, M & S*	1 Pack/220g	385	27.7	175	15.1	0.1	12.6	0.0
Steamed, Average	*1oz/28g*	*25*	*0.3*	*91*	*20.6*	*0.0*	*0.9*	*0.0*
LEMONADE								
7 Up, Light, Britvic*	1 Can/330ml	4	0.0	1	0.1	0.2	0.0	0.0
7 Up, Zero, Britvic*	1 Can/330ml	6	0.0	2	0.1	0.1	0.0	0.0
Average	1 Glass/250ml	52	0.2	21	0.1	5.0	0.1	0.1
Cloudy, Diet, Sainsbury's*	1 Can/330ml	7	0.3	2	0.1	0.2	0.1	0.3
Cloudy, Diet, Tesco*	1 Glass/200ml	6	0.0	3	0.0	0.8	0.0	0.0
Cloudy, Gastropub, M & S*	1 Bottle/500ml	25	0.0	5	0.0	0.0	0.0	0.0
Cloudy, Sainsbury's*	1 Glass/250ml	117	0.2	47	0.1	12.0	0.1	0.1
Cloudy, Shapers, Boots*	1 Bottle/500ml	15	0.0	3	0.0	0.3	0.0	0.0
Cloudy, Waitrose*	1 Glass/250ml	125	0.0	50	0.0	12.2	0.0	0.0
Diet, Amerista*	1 Glass/200ml	3	0.0	2	0.1	0.2	0.0	0.0
Diet, Average	1 Glass/250ml	4	0.1	2	0.1	0.2	0.0	0.0
Diet with Black Cherry Flavouring, Chosen By You, Asda*	1 Glass/250ml	5	0.0	2	0.0	0.0	0.0	0.0
Low Calorie, Smart Price, Asda*	1 Glass/250ml	1	0.0	0	0.0	0.1	0.0	0.0
Pink, Still, Pure Premium, Tropicana*	1 Glass/200ml	90	0.0	45	0.2	10.0	0.0	0.7
Pure Premium, Still, Tropicana *	1 Glass/200ml	86	2.0	43	0.2	9.5	1.0	0.7
R White*	1 Glass/250ml	65	0.0	26	0.1	6.2	0.0	0.0
Schweppes*	1 Glass/250ml	45	0.0	18	0.0	4.2	0.0	0.0
Sicilian, Sainsbury's*	1 Glass/200ml	98	0.2	49	0.1	11.5	0.1	0.1

L

	Measure INFO/WEIGHT	per Measure KCAL	per Measure FAT	Nutrition Values per 100g / 100ml KCAL	PROT	CARB	FAT	FIBRE
LEMONADE								
Still, Raspberry, M & S*	1 Glass/250ml	112	0.0	45	0.2	10.3	0.0	0.1
Sugar Free, Value, Tesco*	1 Glass/200ml	2	0.0	1	0.1	0.1	0.0	0.0
Traditional Style, Tesco*	1 Glass/200ml	100	0.0	50	0.0	12.3	0.0	0.0
Victorian, Fentiman's*	1 Bottle/275ml	130	0.0	47	0.0	11.3	0.0	0.0
LEMSIP								
Beechams*	1 Sachet/3g	11	0.0	387	0.0	100.0	0.0	0.0
LENTILS								
Black Beluga, Ready to Eat, Merchant Gourmet*	1 Serving/63g	92	0.7	147	10.9	20.5	1.2	5.2
Campo Largo*	1 Jar/400g	304	2.4	76	6.0	8.0	0.6	0.0
Green & Brown, Dried, Boiled in Salted Water, Average	*1 Tbsp/30g*	*31*	*0.2*	*105*	*8.8*	*16.9*	*0.7*	*3.8*
Green or Brown, Dried, Average	*1 Serving/50g*	*150*	*0.7*	*301*	*22.8*	*49.8*	*1.5*	*9.6*
Green or Brown in Water, Tinned, Average	*½ Can/132g*	*131*	*0.8*	*99*	*8.1*	*15.4*	*0.6*	*3.8*
Puy, Green, Dry, Average	1 Serving/100g	306	1.4	306	24.7	49.5	1.4	10.3
Red, Boiled in Unsalted Water, Average	*1oz/28g*	*28*	*0.1*	*101*	*7.6*	*17.5*	*0.4*	*2.6*
Red, Dried, Average	*1oz/28g*	*88*	*0.4*	*315*	*23.8*	*53.8*	*1.3*	*4.9*
Red, Split, Great Scot*	1 Serving/50g	152	0.5	304	23.8	53.2	1.0	0.0
LETTUCE								
Average, Raw	½ Cup/28g	4	0.1	14	1.1	1.8	0.3	1.2
Cos, Sweet, Baby, Somerfield*	1 Pack/600g	90	3.0	15	0.8	1.7	0.5	0.9
Curly Leaf, Sainsbury's*	1 Serving/80g	11	0.4	14	0.8	1.7	0.5	0.0
Iceberg, Average	*1 Serving/80g*	*11*	*0.3*	*13*	*0.8*	*1.8*	*0.3*	*0.5*
Iceberg, Lasting Leaf*	1 Serving/75g	12	0.2	16	0.7	1.9	0.3	1.4
Lamb's, Average	*1 Serving/80g*	*12*	*0.2*	*14*	*1.3*	*1.5*	*0.2*	*0.9*
Radicchio, Red, Raw, Average	*1 Head/220g*	*29*	*0.2*	*13*	*1.4*	*1.6*	*0.1*	*3.0*
Romaine, Average	*1 Serving/80g*	*12*	*0.4*	*15*	*0.9*	*1.7*	*0.5*	*0.7*
Romaine, Hearts, Average	*1 Serving/80g*	*12*	*0.4*	*15*	*0.9*	*1.7*	*0.5*	*1.0*
Romaine, Sweet, Average	*1 Serving/80g*	*12*	*0.4*	*15*	*0.9*	*1.6*	*0.5*	*0.8*
Round, Average	1 Serving/80g	10	0.2	13	1.3	2.2	0.2	1.1
LILT								
Fruit Crush, Coca-Cola*	1 Can/330ml	66	0.0	20	0.0	4.6	0.0	0.0
Fruit Crush, Zero, Coca-Cola*	1 Can/330ml	12	0.0	3	0.0	0.3	0.0	0.0
Z, Coca-Cola*	1 Can/330ml	10	0.0	3	0.0	0.4	0.0	0.0
LIME								
Peel, Raw	*1 Tbsp/6g*	*3*	*0.0*	*47*	*1.5*	*16.0*	*0.3*	*10.6*
Raw, Flesh Only, Average	*1 Lime/71g*	*18*	*0.1*	*25*	*0.6*	*8.8*	*0.2*	*2.3*
Raw, Weighed with Peel & Seeds, Average	*1 Lime/85g*	*25*	*0.2*	*30*	*0.7*	*10.5*	*0.2*	*2.8*
LINGUINE								
Cooked	1 Serving/100g	133	0.7	133	5.1	26.3	0.7	1.1
Crab, Rocket & Chilli, Italian, Finest, Tesco*	1 Pack/350g	717	36.4	205	6.5	20.7	10.4	1.7
Crab & Chilli, Waitrose*	1 Pack/350g	770	45.0	220	7.7	18.0	12.9	1.8
Dry, Average	*1 Serving/100g*	*352*	*2.2*	*352*	*13.1*	*70.0*	*2.2*	*2.8*
Dry, Parioli, Cucina*	1 Serving/75g	270	1.0	360	12.5	73.0	1.4	2.6
Fresh, Dry, Average	*1 Pack/250g*	*681*	*6.5*	*272*	*12.3*	*51.7*	*2.6*	*4.0*
Garlic & Basil, Asda*	1 Serving/75g	108	0.4	144	5.4	29.5	0.5	2.5
King Prawn, Asda*	1 Pack/400g	380	10.4	95	6.4	11.5	2.6	1.5
King Prawn, Meal for One, M & S*	1 Pack/400g	380	6.8	95	6.6	13.1	1.7	2.2
King Prawn, Sundried Tomato & Chilli, City Kitchen, Tesco*	1 Pack/385g	423	16.2	110	4.0	13.5	4.2	1.4
Pomodoro, M & S*	1 Pack/300g	360	10.5	120	4.1	17.6	3.5	1.2
Prawn King & Roasted Garlic, Light Choices, Tesco*	1 Pack/400g	340	5.2	85	5.6	11.9	1.3	1.5
Salmon & Prawn, Iceland*	1 Meal/450g	540	19.8	120	4.5	15.8	4.4	1.5
Smoked Salmon, Sainsbury's*	1 Serving/400g	586	28.8	146	6.2	14.2	7.2	1.2
Sun Dried Tomato & Chicken, Perfectly Balanced, Waitrose*	1 Serving/400g	316	7.6	79	7.5	8.0	1.9	3.5
Tomato & Mushroom, Perfectly Balanced, Waitrose*	1 Pack/350g	294	13.3	84	2.2	10.6	3.8	1.0

L

	Measure INFO/WEIGHT	per Measure		Nutrition Values per 100g / 100ml				
		KCAL	FAT	KCAL	PROT	CARB	FAT	FIBRE
LINGUINE								
Vegetable & Ham, BGTY, Sainsbury's*	1 Pack/450g	409	13.5	91	4.4	11.7	3.0	0.9
LINSEEDS								
Average	*1 Tsp/5g*	*23*	*1.7*	*464*	*21.7*	*18.5*	*33.5*	*26.3*
LION BAR								
Mini, Nestle*	1 Bar/16g	80	3.6	486	4.6	67.7	21.7	0.0
Nestle*	1 Bar/43g	206	9.3	478	6.5	64.6	21.6	0.0
Peanut, Nestle*	1 Bar/49g	256	14.5	522	7.1	56.9	29.6	0.0
LIQUEURS								
Amaretto, Average	*1 Shot/25ml*	*97*	*0.0*	*388*	*0.0*	*60.0*	*0.0*	*0.0*
Cointreau, Specialite De France	*1 Serving/37ml*	*80*	*0.0*	*215*	*0.0*	*0.0*	*0.0*	*0.0*
Cream, Average	*1 Shot/25ml*	*81*	*4.0*	*325*	*0.0*	*22.8*	*16.1*	*0.0*
*Grand Marnier**	*1 Shot/35ml*	*94*	*0.0*	*268*	*0.0*	*22.9*	*0.0*	*0.0*
High Strength, Average	*1 Shot/25ml*	*78*	*0.0*	*314*	*0.0*	*24.4*	*0.0*	*0.0*
Kirsch, Average	*1 Shot/25ml*	*67*	*0.0*	*267*	*0.0*	*20.0*	*0.0*	*0.0*
Marula Fruit & Cream Cocktail, Amarula*	1 fl oz/30ml	103	0.0	343	0.0	36.7	0.0	0.0
LIQUORICE								
Allsorts, Average	1 Sm Bag/56g	195	2.9	349	3.7	76.7	5.2	2.0
Allsorts, Bassett's*	1 Pack/225g	855	11.0	380	5.6	77.8	4.9	1.6
Allsorts, Fruit, Bassett's*	1 Serving/50g	160	0.2	320	1.8	76.9	0.4	0.0
Allsorts, Julian Graves*	1 Serving/30g	113	2.2	376	3.4	78.7	7.2	1.2
Assorted, Filled, Panda*	1 Sweet/4g	15	0.4	385	3.7	68.0	11.0	0.0
Bars, Panda*	1 Bar/32g	99	0.1	308	3.7	72.0	0.4	0.9
Catherine Wheels, Barratt*	1 Wheel/22g	65	0.1	290	3.8	67.2	0.3	0.7
Catherine Wheels, Sainsbury's*	1 Wheel/17g	49	0.1	286	3.8	67.2	0.3	0.7
Comfits, M & S*	1oz/28g	100	0.1	357	2.4	86.2	0.3	0.7
Organic, Laidback Liquorice*	1 Bar/28g	90	0.3	320	4.7	75.0	1.0	3.0
Panda*	1 Bar/32g	109	0.2	340	3.8	78.0	0.5	0.0
Red, Fresh, 98% Fat Free, RJ's Licorice Ltd*	1oz/28g	96	0.5	342	3.0	75.0	1.7	0.0
Shapes, Average	1oz/28g	78	0.4	278	5.5	65.0	1.4	1.9
Soft Eating, Australia, Darrell Lea*	1 Piece/20g	68	0.4	338	2.8	76.1	1.9	0.0
Sweets, Blackcurrant, Tesco*	1 Sweet/8g	32	0.3	410	0.0	92.3	3.8	0.0
Torpedos, Panda*	1 Serving/25g	91	0.0	366	1.9	88.0	0.2	1.4
Twists, Tesco*	1 Serving/63g	186	0.2	297	2.7	71.0	0.3	0.7
LIVER								
Calves, Fried	*1oz/28g*	*49*	*2.7*	*176*	*22.3*	*0.0*	*9.6*	*0.0*
Calves, Raw	*1oz/28g*	*29*	*1.0*	*104*	*18.3*	*0.0*	*3.4*	*0.0*
Chicken, Cooked, Simmered, Average	*1 Serving/100g*	*167*	*6.5*	*167*	*24.5*	*0.9*	*6.5*	*0.0*
Chicken, Fried, Average	*1oz/28g*	*47*	*2.5*	*169*	*22.1*	*0.0*	*8.9*	*0.0*
Chicken, Raw, Average	*1oz/28g*	*26*	*0.6*	*92*	*17.7*	*0.0*	*2.3*	*0.0*
Lamb's, Braised, Average	*1 Serving/100g*	*220*	*8.8*	*220*	*30.6*	*2.5*	*8.8*	*0.0*
Lamb's, Fried, Average	*1oz/28g*	*66*	*3.6*	*237*	*30.1*	*0.0*	*12.9*	*0.0*
Lamb's, Raw, Average	*1 Serving/125g*	*171*	*7.7*	*137*	*20.3*	*0.0*	*6.2*	*0.0*
Ox, Raw	*1oz/28g*	*43*	*2.2*	*155*	*21.1*	*0.0*	*7.8*	*0.0*
Ox, Stewed	*1oz/28g*	*55*	*2.7*	*198*	*24.8*	*3.6*	*9.5*	*0.0*
Pig's, Raw	*1oz/28g*	*32*	*0.9*	*113*	*21.3*	*0.0*	*3.1*	*0.0*
Pig's, Stewed	*1 Serving/70g*	*132*	*5.7*	*189*	*25.6*	*3.6*	*8.1*	*0.0*
LIVER & BACON								
Meal for One, M & S*	1 Pack/452g	430	16.7	95	7.0	8.0	3.7	1.2
with Creamy Mash, GFY, Asda*	1 Pack/386g	282	5.4	73	5.5	9.6	1.4	2.2
with Fresh Mashed Potato, Waitrose*	1 Pack/400g	416	17.2	104	7.3	9.0	4.3	1.3
with Mash, British Classics, Tesco*	1 Pack/500g	575	23.5	115	6.6	10.6	4.7	1.0
with Mash, M Kitchen, Morrisons*	1 Pack/450g	463	16.6	103	7.4	9.3	3.7	1.4

L

	Measure INFO/WEIGHT	per Measure KCAL	FAT	Nutrition Values per 100g / 100ml KCAL	PROT	CARB	FAT	FIBRE
LIVER & ONIONS								
British Classics, Tesco*	1 Pack/250g	265	12.0	106	9.7	5.9	4.8	0.5
Finest, Tesco*	½ Pack/225g	349	18.7	155	15.6	3.7	8.3	1.6
M & S*	1 Serving/200g	250	12.0	125	7.6	10.5	6.0	0.9
LIVER SAUSAGE								
Average	*1 Slice/10g*	*22*	*1.5*	*216*	*15.3*	*4.4*	*15.2*	*0.2*
LOBSTER								
Boiled, Average	*1oz/28g*	*29*	*0.4*	*103*	*22.1*	*0.0*	*1.6*	*0.0*
Dressed, John West*	1 Can/43g	45	2.1	105	13.0	2.0	5.0	0.0
Dressed, M & S*	1oz/28g	76	6.6	273	14.3	0.8	23.6	0.1
Half, M & S*	1oz/28g	66	5.5	235	12.1	2.4	19.6	0.2
Squat, Breaded, & Lemon Mayonnaise Dip, Finest, Tesco*	1 Pack/210g	380	19.1	181	6.3	18.4	9.1	0.1
Squat, Tails, Youngs*	½ Pack/125g	246	10.7	197	9.8	20.1	8.6	1.1
Thermidor, Finest, Tesco*	½ Pack/140g	381	25.2	272	15.3	12.1	18.0	1.0
Thermidor, M & S*	1 Serving/140g	287	19.2	205	10.7	9.7	13.7	0.0
LOGANBERRIES								
Raw	*1oz/28g*	*5*	*0.0*	*17*	*1.1*	*3.4*	*0.0*	*2.5*
LOLLIPOPS								
Assorted Flavours, Asda*	1 Lolly/7g	27	0.0	380	0.0	95.0	0.0	0.0
Blackcurrant, Sugar Free, Rowntree's*	1 Lolly/15g	35	0.0	233	0.1	89.4	0.0	0.0
Chocolate Lolly, M & S*	1 Lolly/45g	247	15.8	550	6.8	54.0	35.1	2.7
Chupa Chups*	1 Lolly/18g	44	0.2	247	0.0	96.5	1.3	0.0
Cremosa, Sugar Free, Chupa Chups*	1 Lolly/10g	27	0.5	275	0.2	92.5	5.4	0.0
Cuore Di Frutta, Chupa Chups*	1 Lolly/10g	25	0.1	247	0.0	96.5	1.3	0.0
No Added Sugar, Tesco*	1 Lolly/32g	26	0.0	80	0.1	20.0	0.0	0.1
Orange, Sugar Free, Rowntree's*	1 Lolly/15g	35	0.0	235	0.1	89.5	0.0	0.6
Refreshers, Bassett's*	1 Lolly/6g	25	0.0	417	0.0	108.3	0.0	0.0
Sugar Free, Simpkins*	1 Lolly/15g	51	0.0	340	0.0	88.0	0.0	0.0
Super Sour, Tesco*	1 Lolly/8g	32	0.0	385	0.1	95.6	0.2	0.5
LOQUATS								
Raw	*1oz/28g*	*8*	*0.1*	*28*	*0.7*	*6.3*	*0.2*	*0.0*
LOZENGES								
Fishermans Friend, Blackcurrant Flavour, Lofthouses*	1 Lozenge/1g	3	0.0	251	0.1	97.2	1.3	0.0
Original, Victory V*	1 Lozenge/3g	9	0.0	350	0.0	91.0	0.0	0.0
Original Extra Strong Lozenge, Fisherman's Friend*	1 Lozenge/1g	4	0.0	382	0.3	94.9	0.0	0.5
LUCOZADE								
Apple, Energy Drink, GlaxoSmithKline UK Limited*	1 Bottle/380ml	262	0.0	69	0.0	17.1	0.0	0.0
Cherry, Sport, Lite, GlaxoSmithKline UK Limited*	1 Bottle/500ml	50	0.0	10	0.0	2.0	0.0	0.0
Citrus Clear, Energy, GlaxoSmithKline UK Limited*	1 Bottle/380ml	266	0.0	70	0.1	17.0	0.0	0.0
Citrus Fruits, Hydro Active, Sport, Lucozade*	1 Bottle/500ml	50	0.0	10	0.0	2.0	0.0	0.0
Orange, Sport Lite, GlaxoSmithKline UK Limited*	1 Serving/500g	50	0.0	10	0.0	2.0	0.0	0.0
Orange Energy Drink, GlaxoSmithKline UK Limited*	1 Bottle/500ml	350	0.0	70	0.0	17.2	0.0	0.0
Original, GlaxoSmithKline UK Limited*	1 Bottle/345ml	241	0.0	70	0.0	17.2	0.0	0.0
Raspberry Sport Body Fuel, GlaxoSmithKline UK Limited*	1 Bottle/500ml	140	0.0	28	0.0	6.4	0.0	0.0
Summer Berries, Sport, Lite, GlaxoSmithKline UK Limited*	1 Serving/200ml	20	0.0	10	0.0	2.0	0.0	0.0
Tropical, GlaxoSmithKline UK Limited*	1 Bottle/380ml	266	0.0	70	0.0	17.2	0.0	0.0
LUNCHEON MEAT								
Pork, Average	*1oz/28g*	*81*	*6.8*	*288*	*13.3*	*4.0*	*24.3*	*0.0*
LYCHEES								
Fresh, Raw, Flesh Only	*1oz/28g*	*16*	*0.0*	*58*	*0.9*	*14.3*	*0.1*	*0.7*
in Juice, Amoy*	1oz/28g	13	0.0	46	0.4	10.9	0.0	0.0
in Syrup, Average	*1oz/28g*	*19*	*0.0*	*69*	*0.4*	*17.7*	*0.0*	*0.4*
Raw, Weighed with Skin & Stone	*1oz/28g*	*10*	*0.0*	*36*	*0.5*	*8.9*	*0.1*	*0.4*

L

	Measure INFO/WEIGHT	per Measure KCAL	FAT	Nutrition Values per 100g / 100ml KCAL	PROT	CARB	FAT	FIBRE
M&M'S								
Crispy, Mars*	1 Serving/36g	177	8.8	492	4.1	63.9	24.4	2.7
Mars*	1 Pack/20g	97	4.3	485	5.0	68.0	21.5	0.0
Mini, Mars*	1 Sm Pack/36g	176	8.4	489	6.3	63.6	23.2	0.0
Peanut, Mars*	1 Pack/45g	228	11.4	506	9.4	60.1	25.4	2.7
Peanut Butter, Mars*	1 Pack/42g	230	12.0	548	9.5	57.1	28.6	4.8
MACADAMIA NUTS								
Plain, Average	*1 Pack/100g*	*750*	*77.6*	*750*	*7.9*	*4.8*	*77.6*	*5.3*
Roasted, Salted, Average	*6 Nuts/10g*	*75*	*7.8*	*748*	*7.9*	*4.8*	*77.6*	*5.3*
MACARONI								
Dry, Average	*1oz/28g*	*99*	*0.5*	*354*	*11.9*	*73.5*	*1.7*	*2.6*
MACARONI CHEESE								
& Spinach, TTD, Sainsbury's*	1 Pack/500g	1025	57.5	205	6.5	18.9	11.5	1.3
Birds Eye*	1 Pack/300g	470	15.0	157	5.7	22.3	5.0	0.8
Canned	1oz/28g	39	1.8	138	4.5	16.4	6.5	0.4
Chilled, GFY, Asda*	1 Pack/443g	469	12.8	106	6.0	14.0	2.9	1.6
COU, M & S*	1 Pack/360g	360	8.6	100	5.8	13.9	2.4	1.2
Diet Chef Ltd*	1 Pouch/250g	247	7.7	99	7.3	12.7	3.1	0.4
Four Cheese, Extra Special, Asda*	1 Pack/400g	664	30.8	166	7.7	16.4	7.7	1.1
Fresh Pasta, Findus*	1 Pack/360g	360	7.2	100	5.0	16.0	2.0	0.5
HL, Tesco*	1 Serving/385g	443	4.6	115	9.3	15.9	1.2	1.0
Light Choices, Tesco*	1 Pack/385g	465	7.3	121	7.0	18.7	1.9	1.5
Ready Meal, Average	1 Serving/300g	435	19.1	145	6.0	15.8	6.4	1.0
Red Leicester, Heinz*	1 Can/400g	332	10.8	83	3.5	11.1	2.7	0.3
Ross*	1 Pack/300g	327	9.3	109	4.2	16.2	3.1	1.3
MACAROONS								
Butterscotch, Picard*	1 Macaroon/20g	85	3.6	424	9.7	55.1	18.2	0.0
Coconut, Sainsbury's*	1 Macaroon/33g	146	6.1	441	4.7	63.7	18.6	0.8
Coconut, Tesco*	1 Macaroon/33g	140	6.1	425	4.4	59.0	18.6	5.7
French, Average	1 Serving/60g	225	11.0	375	6.7	46.7	18.3	3.3
MACKEREL								
Atlantic, Raw, Average	*1 Fillet/75g*	*154*	*10.4*	*205*	*18.6*	*0.0*	*13.9*	*0.0*
Fillets, Honey Roast Smoked, Sainsbury's*	1 Serving/100g	349	27.3	349	21.5	4.5	27.3	12.4
Fillets, in a Hot Chilli Dressing, Princes*	1 Pack/125g	370	33.7	296	13.3	0.0	27.0	0.0
Fillets, in Brine, Average	*1 Can/88g*	*206*	*15.3*	*234*	*19.4*	*0.0*	*17.4*	*0.0*
Fillets, in Curry Sauce, John West*	1 Can/125g	275	20.7	220	14.2	3.5	16.6	0.2
Fillets, in Green Peppercorn Sauce, John West*	1 Can/125g	329	26.2	263	14.0	4.5	21.0	0.1
Fillets, in Mustard Sauce, Average	1 Can/125g	274	19.4	219	14.1	5.4	15.5	0.0
Fillets, in Olive Oil, Average	1 Serving/50g	149	12.2	297	18.5	1.0	24.3	0.0
Fillets, in Spicy Tomato Sauce, Average	1oz/28g	56	3.9	199	14.3	3.8	14.0	0.0
Fillets, in Sunflower Oil, Average	1 Can/94g	262	20.6	279	20.2	0.2	21.9	0.2
Fillets, in Teriyaki Sauce, Boneless & Skinless, Tesco*	1 Can/125g	320	20.3	255	12.6	13.4	16.2	2.0
Fillets, in Tomato Sauce, Average	1 Can/125g	251	18.3	200	14.3	2.7	14.7	0.0
Fillets, in White Wine & Spices, Connetable*	1 Can/120g	169	9.8	141	15.5	1.2	8.2	0.0
Fillets, Oat & Lemon Breaded, Deliciously Different, M & S*	1 Pack/300g	945	59.4	315	12.3	20.7	19.8	2.0
Fillets, Smoked, Average	*1oz/28g*	*94*	*7.9*	*335*	*19.7*	*0.5*	*28.2*	*0.3*
Fillets, with Red Pepper & Onion, Smoked, Asda*	1 Serving/90g	319	27.9	354	18.0	0.8	31.0	1.2
Fried in Blended Oil	*1oz/28g*	*76*	*5.5*	*272*	*24.0*	*0.0*	*19.5*	*0.0*
Grilled	*1oz/28g*	*67*	*4.8*	*239*	*20.8*	*0.0*	*17.3*	*0.0*
King, Raw	1 Fillet/198g	208	4.0	105	20.3	0.0	2.0	0.0
Raw with Skin, Weighed with Bone, Average	*1oz/28g*	*67*	*4.9*	*238*	*19.9*	*0.0*	*17.6*	*0.0*
Roasted, with Piri Piri, Tesco*	1 Fillet/80g	240	19.0	300	20.7	0.0	23.8	1.0
Smoked, Lemon & Parsley, Morrisons*	½ Pack/100g	282	20.0	282	20.9	4.6	20.0	1.0
Smoked, Peppered, Average	*1oz/28g*	*87*	*7.0*	*309*	*20.4*	*0.3*	*25.2*	*0.2*

	Measure INFO/WEIGHT	per Measure KCAL	FAT	Nutrition Values per 100g / 100ml KCAL	PROT	CARB	FAT	FIBRE

MADRAS

	Measure INFO/WEIGHT	KCAL	FAT	KCAL	PROT	CARB	FAT	FIBRE
Beef, Canned, BGTY, Sainsbury's*	1 Can/400g	344	14.4	86	9.5	4.0	3.6	0.9
Beef, Tesco*	1 Pack/460g	616	37.7	134	10.6	4.5	8.2	1.2
Beef, Weight Watchers*	1 Pack/320g	317	4.8	99	5.6	15.8	1.5	0.3
Chicken, Asda*	1 Serving/350g	430	31.5	123	7.0	3.6	9.0	2.3
Chicken, Frozen, GFY, Asda*	1 Pack/400g	448	5.2	112	5.6	19.4	1.3	1.2
Chicken, Indian, Tesco*	1 Pack/350g	518	31.1	148	11.3	5.6	8.9	1.9
Chicken, Indian Take Away, Tesco*	1 Serving/175g	254	17.7	145	8.2	4.8	10.1	1.7
Chicken, Sainsbury's*	1 Pack/400g	468	27.2	117	11.7	2.2	6.8	2.8
Chicken, Tesco*	1 Pack/350g	325	14.3	93	10.6	3.6	4.1	0.6
Chicken, Waitrose*	1 Pack/400g	672	42.0	168	14.6	3.7	10.5	1.8
Chicken & Pilau Rice, Asda*	1 Pack/400g	588	28.0	147	8.0	13.0	7.0	1.7
Chicken & Pilau Rice, Somerfield*	1 Pack/340g	496	23.8	146	7.0	14.0	7.0	0.0
Chicken & Rice, Hot & Spicy, Sainsbury's*	1 Pack/500g	670	25.5	134	7.1	14.9	5.1	2.2

MAGNUM

Almond, Wall's Ice Cream*	1 Bar/82g	270	17.2	330	5.0	30.0	21.0	1.5
Caramel & Almond, Temptation, Wall's Ice Cream*	1 Lolly/68g	239	15.0	351	5.4	34.0	22.0	0.0
Caramel & Nuts, Bar, Wall's Ice Cream*	1 Bar/60g	132	9.0	220	4.0	19.0	15.0	0.0
Classic, Mini, Wall's*	1 Lolly/50g	170	11.0	340	4.0	30.0	22.0	0.0
Classic, Wall's Ice Cream*	1 Lolly/86g	261	16.4	303	3.8	29.0	19.0	0.0
Double Chocolate, Wall's Ice Cream*	1 Bar/92g	346	22.0	378	4.5	36.0	24.0	0.0
Gluttony, Wall's Ice Cream*	1 Lolly/110ml	425	29.0	386	4.5	32.7	26.4	0.0
Greed, Wall's Ice Cream*	1 Bar/110ml	307	18.0	279	3.6	29.1	16.4	0.0
White, Wall's Ice Cream*	1 Lolly/87g	256	14.7	296	3.8	32.0	17.0	0.0

MAKHANI

Chicken, Sainsbury's*	½ Pack/199g	313	21.3	157	12.2	2.9	10.7	2.5
Chicken Tikka, & Pilau Rice, BGTY, Sainsbury's*	1 Pack/400g	448	4.0	112	8.3	17.5	1.0	1.9
Chicken Tikka, BGTY, Sainsbury's*	1 Pack/251g	186	4.8	74	11.3	3.0	1.9	1.7
Chicken Tikka, Waitrose*	1 Pack/400g	560	30.4	140	14.0	3.8	7.6	2.1
King Prawn, Finest, Tesco*	1 Pack/350g	514	38.8	147	6.0	6.0	11.1	1.3
Paneer, Ashoka*	½ Pouch/150g	283	23.0	189	4.7	8.0	15.3	1.0

MALT DRINK

Non-alcoholic, Supermalt*	1 Bottle/330g	210	0.0	64	0.8	15.1	0.0	0.0

MALTESERS

MaltEaster, Chocolate Bunny, Mars*	1 Bunny/29g	157	9.2	541	6.9	57.0	31.7	0.0
Mars*	1 Reg Bag/37g	187	9.2	505	8.0	61.8	25.0	0.9
Mini Bunnies, Mars*	1 Bunny/12g	64	3.6	534	8.0	53.5	30.2	0.0
White Chocolate, Mars*	1 Pack/37g	186	9.4	504	7.9	61.0	25.4	0.0

MANDARIN ORANGES

Broken, Segments in Fruit Juice, Basics, Sainsbury's*	½ Can/149g	51	0.0	34	0.7	7.7	0.0	0.3
in Juice, Average	*1oz/28g*	*11*	*0.0*	*39*	*0.7*	*9.0*	*0.0*	*0.5*
in Light Syrup, Average	*1 Can/298g*	*201*	*0.1*	*67*	*0.5*	*15.9*	*0.0*	*0.1*
in Orange Gel, Del Monte*	1 Can/128g	60	0.0	47	0.0	10.9	0.0	0.0
Weighed with Peel, Average	*1 Sm/50g*	*18*	*0.0*	*36*	*0.9*	*8.3*	*0.1*	*1.2*

MANGE TOUT

Boiled in Salted Water	*1oz/28g*	*7*	*0.0*	*26*	*3.2*	*3.3*	*0.1*	*2.2*
Raw, Average	*1 Serving/80g*	*26*	*0.2*	*32*	*3.6*	*4.2*	*0.2*	*1.1*
Stir-Fried in Blended Oil	*1oz/28g*	*20*	*1.3*	*71*	*3.8*	*3.5*	*4.8*	*2.4*

MANGO

Chunks, Fresh, Morrisons*	1 Serving/80g	53	0.2	66	0.7	14.1	0.2	2.6
Dried, Average	*1 Serving/50g*	*173*	*0.5*	*347*	*1.4*	*83.1*	*1.0*	*4.9*
Dried with Chilli, King Henry's*	1 Bag/120g	300	0.0	250	0.0	62.5	0.0	1.0
in Syrup, Average	*1oz/28g*	*22*	*0.0*	*80*	*0.3*	*20.5*	*0.0*	*0.9*
Pieces in Juice, Natures Finest*	1 Pot/220g	123	0.4	56	0.5	12.3	0.2	1.5

	Measure INFO/WEIGHT	per Measure KCAL	FAT	Nutrition Values per 100g / 100ml KCAL	PROT	CARB	FAT	FIBRE
MANGO								
Ripe, Raw, Weighed with Skin & Stone, Average	**1 Mango/225g**	**88**	**0.2**	**39**	**0.5**	**9.6**	**0.1**	**1.8**
Ripe, Raw, without Peel & Stone, Flesh Only, Average	**1 Mango/207g**	**81**	**1.0**	**39**	**0.5**	**9.6**	**0.5**	**1.8**
MANGOSTEEN								
Raw, Fresh, Average*	**1 Serving/80g**	**50**	**0.5**	**63**	**0.6**	**15.6**	**0.6**	**5.1**
MARBLE								
Cadbury*	1 Bar/46g	246	14.4	535	8.4	54.8	31.2	0.0
MARGARINE								
Average	**1 Thin Spread/7g**	**51**	**5.7**	**726**	**0.1**	**0.5**	**81.0**	**0.0**
Butter Style, Average	**1 Thin Spread/7g**	**44**	**4.8**	**627**	**0.7**	**1.1**	**68.9**	**0.0**
for Baking, Average	**1 Thin Spread/7g**	**42**	**4.7**	**607**	**0.2**	**0.4**	**67.2**	**0.0**
No Salt, Flora*	1 Thin Spread/7g	37	4.1	531	0.0	0.0	59.0	0.0
Omega 3 Plus, Flora*	1 Thin Spread/7g	24	2.7	350	0.1	3.0	38.0	0.0
Pro Activ, Extra Light, Flora*	1 Thin Spread/7g	15	1.6	218	0.1	2.9	23.0	0.2
Pro Activ, Light, Flora*	1 Thin Spread/7g	23	2.4	331	0.1	4.0	35.0	0.0
Pro Activ with Olive Oil, Flora*	1 Thin Spread/7g	23	2.4	331	0.1	4.0	35.0	0.0
Reduced Fat, Average	**1 Thin Spread/7g**	**25**	**2.7**	**356**	**0.5**	**3.0**	**38.0**	**0.0**
Soya, Granose*	1 Thin Spread/7g	52	5.7	745	0.1	0.1	82.0	0.0
Utterly Butterly*	1 Thin Spread/7g	32	3.4	452	0.3	2.5	49.0	0.0
White, Flora*	1 Thin Spread/7g	60	6.6	855	0.0	0.0	95.0	0.0
MARGARITA								
Sainsbury's*	1 Serving/100ml	53	0.1	53	0.1	12.8	0.1	0.1
MARINADE								
Barbecue, COU, M & S*	1 Serving/35g	52	0.1	150	1.2	35.5	0.2	1.0
Barbeque, Sticky, Sainsbury's*	¼ Jar/77g	112	2.8	145	0.8	26.7	3.6	1.0
BBQ, Sticky, Newman's Own*	1/3 Jar/83ml	139	0.7	167	0.9	39.0	0.8	2.5
Cajun Spice, The English Provender Co.*	1 Serving/50g	93	6.7	187	1.3	15.3	13.4	1.6
Chinese, Classic, Sharwood's*	1oz/28g	32	1.3	113	1.8	16.1	4.8	1.0
Hickory Dickory Smokey, Ainsley Harriott*	1 Pot/300ml	360	0.3	120	0.6	28.1	0.1	0.0
Lime & Coriander with Peri Peri, Nando's*	1 Tsp/5g	9	0.8	182	0.0	13.1	16.6	0.2
Peri Peri, Hot, Nando's*	1 Serving/40g	46	2.2	115	1.4	15.2	5.4	0.9
Peri Peri, Portuguese BBQ, Nando's*	1 Serving/40g	36	0.6	90	1.1	17.7	1.6	1.0
Sticky Barbecue, Tesco*	¼ Jar/70g	80	0.1	115	0.7	26.7	0.2	0.6
Sticky BBQ, Eat Well, M & S*	1 Bottle/250ml	400	1.2	160	0.7	37.8	0.5	1.0
Sun Dried Tomato & Basil with Peri-Peri, Nando's*	1 Bottle/270g	319	25.6	118	0.1	15.3	9.5	0.8
Tequila Chilli Lime, M & S*	1 Serving/75ml	116	1.2	155	0.6	34.0	1.6	0.5
MARJORAM								
Dried	**1 Tsp/1g**	**2**	**0.0**	**271**	**12.7**	**42.5**	**7.0**	**0.0**
MARLIN								
Smoked, H. Forman & Son*	1 Pack/200g	240	0.2	120	29.8	0.0	0.1	0.0
Steaks, Chargrilled, Sainsbury's*	1 Steak/240g	367	14.6	153	23.6	0.8	6.1	0.6
Steaks, Raw, Sainsbury's*	1 Steak/110g	109	0.2	99	24.3	0.0	0.2	0.0
MARMALADE								
3 Fruit, Thick Cut, Waitrose*	1 Tsp/15g	39	0.0	262	0.4	64.8	0.1	0.7
Blood Orange, Grandessa*	1 Serving/15g	36	0.0	240	0.4	59.0	0.1	0.7
Blood Orange, TTD, Sainsbury's*	1 Tbsp/15g	40	0.0	264	0.3	65.7	0.0	0.8
Christmas Orange & Whisky, M & S*	1oz/28g	67	0.1	240	0.3	59.5	0.2	1.9
Citrus Shred, Robertson*	1 Tsp/5g	13	0.0	253	0.2	63.0	0.0	0.0
Five Fruit, Tesco*	1 Serving/10g	28	0.0	278	0.2	68.2	0.1	0.9
Fresh Fruit, Three Fruits, TTD, Sainsbury's*	1 Tbsp/15g	40	0.0	268	0.3	66.7	0.0	0.8
Grapefruit, Fine Cut, Duerr's*	1 Tsp/15g	39	0.0	261	0.2	65.0	0.0	0.0
Grapefruit & Cranberry, M & S*	1 Tsp/15g	36	0.0	240	0.3	60.3	0.0	1.5
Lemon, Fine Cut, Tesco*	1 Tbsp/15g	39	0.0	257	0.2	64.0	0.0	0.5
Lemon & Lime, Average	**1 Tbsp/20g**	**53**	**0.0**	**267**	**0.1**	**66.3**	**0.1**	**0.4**

	Measure INFO/WEIGHT	per Measure		Nutrition Values per 100g / 100ml				
		KCAL	FAT	KCAL	PROT	CARB	FAT	FIBRE
MARMALADE								
Lemon Jelly, No Peel, Tesco*	1 Tsp/15g	39	0.0	263	0.1	65.0	0.0	0.4
Lemon with Shred, Average	*1 Serving/20g*	*49*	*0.0*	*247*	*0.1*	*61.6*	*0.0*	*0.6*
Lime with Shred, Average	*1 Tbsp/15g*	*39*	*0.0*	*261*	*0.1*	*65.0*	*0.1*	*0.3*
Onion, Organic, Antony Worrall Thompson's*	1 Serving/11g	20	0.1	191	1.1	44.9	0.8	1.8
Onion, Organic, Duchy Originals*	1 Serving/40g	103	1.0	257	1.0	57.8	2.4	2.6
Orange, Lemon & Grapefruit, Baxters*	1 Tsp/15g	38	0.0	252	0.0	63.0	0.0	0.1
Orange, Reduced Sugar, Average	*1 Tbsp/15g*	*26*	*0.0*	*170*	*0.4*	*42.0*	*0.1*	*0.6*
Orange, Reduced Sugar, Thin Cut, Streamline*	1 Serving/10g	18	0.0	178	0.5	43.0	0.3	0.0
Orange, Shredless, Average	*1 Tsp/10g*	*26*	*0.0*	*261*	*0.2*	*65.0*	*0.0*	*0.1*
Orange, with Drambuie, Finest, Tesco*	1 Serving/10g	33	0.0	329	0.3	82.0	0.0	0.7
Orange, with Shred, Average	*1 Tsp/5g*	*13*	*0.0*	*263*	*0.2*	*65.2*	*0.0*	*0.3*
Orange & Ginger, Average	*1 Tbsp/15g*	*40*	*0.0*	*264*	*0.2*	*65.7*	*0.1*	*0.3*
Orange & Lemon, Reduced Sugar, Zest*	1 Tsp/6g	12	0.0	195	0.3	47.1	0.2	0.0
Orange & Tangerine, Tiptree, Wilkin & Sons*	1 Tsp/15g	40	0.0	268	0.0	67.0	0.0	0.0
Pink Grapefruit, Thin Cut, Waitrose*	1 Serving/10g	26	0.0	261	0.2	65.0	0.0	0.4
Three Fruit, Diabetic, Thursday Cottage*	1 Serving/5g	8	0.0	154	0.4	38.0	0.0	1.0
Three Fruit, Finest, Tesco*	1 Serving/15g	39	0.0	262	0.5	63.6	0.2	1.6
Three Fruits, Fresh Fruit, Sainsbury's*	1 Tsp/15g	37	0.0	250	0.0	61.3	0.0	0.0
MARMITE								
XO, Marmite*	1 Serving/4g	10	0.0	250	37.5	25.0	0.2	0.2
MARMITE*								
Yeast Extract, Marmite*	1 Tsp/9g	23	0.0	252	38.7	24.1	0.1	3.4
Yeast Extract with Gold Coloured Flecks, Marmite*	1 Serving/4g	10	0.0	250	39.0	24.0	0.1	3.5
MARROW								
Boiled, Average	*1oz/28g*	*3*	*0.1*	*9*	*0.4*	*1.6*	*0.2*	*0.6*
Raw	*1oz/28g*	*3*	*0.1*	*12*	*0.5*	*2.2*	*0.2*	*0.5*
MARS								
Bar, 5 Little Ones, Mars*	1 Piece/8g	38	1.5	477	4.5	73.6	18.3	0.0
Bar, Duo, Mars*	1 Bar/42g	191	7.6	450	4.4	67.5	18.0	1.2
Bar, Funsize, Mars*	1 Bar/18g	80	3.0	446	3.5	70.1	16.8	1.1
Bar, Mars*	1 Bar/58g	260	10.2	448	4.1	68.1	17.6	1.1
Bar, Medium, 58g, Mars*	1 Bar/58g	263	10.5	453	4.6	67.9	18.1	0.0
Bar, Minis, Mars*	1 Bar/18g	80	11.6	444	3.3	0.0	64.4	1.1
Delight, Mars*	1 Bar/20g	110	6.7	552	4.5	57.8	33.6	1.3
Triple Choc, Bar, Limited Edition, Mars*	1 Bar/52g	233	9.0	448	4.5	67.7	17.3	2.0
MARSHMALLOWS								
Average	1 Mallow/5g	16	0.0	327	3.9	83.1	0.0	0.0
Chocolate Mallows, Cadbury*	1 Mallow/13g	56	2.2	435	4.7	64.7	17.4	0.8
Fat Free, Tesco*	1 Mallow/7g	24	0.0	339	3.4	80.8	0.2	0.5
Haribo*	1 Mallow/5g	16	0.0	330	3.0	80.0	0.0	0.0
No Added Sugar, Sainsbury's*	1 Mallow/2g	5	0.0	206	3.3	77.0	0.1	0.0
Pascall*	1 Mallow/5g	15	0.0	335	2.6	80.0	0.0	0.0
Princess*	1 Mallow/5g	16	0.0	314	3.4	80.0	0.0	0.0
MARZIPAN								
Bar, Chocolate, Plain, Thorntons*	1 Bar/46g	206	8.0	448	5.2	69.1	17.4	2.0
Dark Chocolate, Thorntons*	1 Serving/46g	207	8.0	451	5.2	69.4	17.4	2.1
Plain, Average	*1oz/28g*	*115*	*4.0*	*412*	*5.8*	*67.5*	*14.1*	*1.7*
MASALA								
Dal with Channa & Toor Lentils, Waitrose*	½ Pack/150g	166	6.1	111	6.6	12.0	4.1	5.0
Prawn, & Rice, Tesco*	1 Pack/475g	655	24.7	138	5.2	17.9	5.2	1.2
Prawn, King, Waitrose*	1 Pack/350g	385	25.9	110	7.1	3.8	7.4	1.8
Prawn Mango, Waitrose*	½ Pack/175g	175	11.2	100	5.8	4.3	6.4	1.3
Vegetable, Sainsbury's*	1 Pack/400g	388	30.0	97	2.1	5.2	7.5	2.5

M

MASALA	Measure INFO/WEIGHT	per Measure KCAL	FAT	Nutrition Values per 100g / 100ml KCAL	PROT	CARB	FAT	FIBRE
Vegetable, Waitrose*	1 Serving/400g	288	19.2	72	2.2	4.9	4.8	2.5
Vegetable, with Rice, Feeling Great, Findus*	1 Pack/350g	350	7.0	100	3.0	18.0	2.0	1.7
MASH								
Davidstow Cheddar, Extra Special, Asda*	1 Serving/225g	292	16.9	130	5.3	10.4	7.5	2.6
Parsnip & Parmesan, Finest, Tesco*	½ Packet/250g	245	12.2	98	1.6	11.9	4.9	2.4
Potato, Carrot, Swede, Parsnip, Cream & Butter, Asda*	½ Pack/200g	94	3.0	47	1.0	7.2	1.5	3.3
Potato, Carrot & Swede, Ready To Microwave, Waitrose*	½ Pack/225g	130	4.3	58	1.3	8.8	1.9	2.6
Root, Asda*	½ Pack/200g	142	8.0	71	0.7	8.0	4.0	3.1
Root Vegetable, Finest, Tesco*	½ Pack/250g	225	12.5	90	1.1	9.1	5.0	3.4
Vegetables, Mousline, Maggi*	1 Bag/39g	127	1.2	328	8.2	67.0	3.0	10.4
Winter Root, Sainsbury's*	1 Serving/140g	157	2.1	112	2.7	22.0	1.5	0.9
MAYONNAISE								
50% Less Fat, GFY, Asda*	1 Tbsp/10g	32	3.1	322	0.8	10.0	31.0	0.0
60% Less Fat, BGTY, Sainsbury's*	1 Tbsp/15ml	42	4.1	277	0.4	7.3	27.3	0.0
Aioli, Finest, Tesco*	1 Tsp/5g	20	2.1	408	0.8	8.5	41.2	0.0
Average	***1 Tsp/11g***	***76***	***8.3***	***690***	***0.9***	***1.6***	***75.5***	***0.0***
Deli, Caramelised Onion, Heinz*	1 Serving/20g	110	11.5	548	1.4	5.9	57.5	0.1
Deli, Moroccan, Heinz*	1 Tbsp/15g	80	8.5	532	0.9	4.6	56.5	0.1
Deli, Roasted Garlic, Heinz*	1 Tbsp/15g	81	8.5	537	1.1	5.5	56.6	0.0
Deli, Sundried Tomato, Heinz*	1 Tbsp/15g	88	9.4	589	1.3	4.9	62.5	0.0
Egg, Dairy & Gluten Free, Solesse*	1 Serving/100g	319	29.7	319	0.4	11.7	29.7	0.0
Egg & Dairy Free, Life Free From*	1 Serving/15g	76	8.0	508	0.9	5.6	53.3	0.2
Extra Light, Average	***1 Tbsp/33g***	***34***	***2.0***	***102***	***0.7***	***10.5***	***6.2***	***0.8***
Extra Light, Heinz*	1 Tbsp/12ml	9	0.4	75	0.6	11.4	3.0	0.6
Extra Light, Now Only 3% Fat, Hellmann's*	1 Serving/16g	12	0.5	73	0.6	11.0	3.0	0.6
Extra Light, Weight Watchers*	1 Serving/15g	15	0.9	97	1.1	9.6	5.9	3.2
French, Light, Sainsbury's*	1 Serving/15ml	46	4.7	307	0.4	6.1	31.1	0.2
French Style, BGTY, Sainsbury's*	1 Tbsp/15ml	55	5.5	366	0.6	7.5	36.9	0.0
Garlic, Retail, Average	1 Tsp/11g	44	4.4	403	1.2	8.6	40.3	0.0
Garlic & Herb, M & S*	1 Tsp/6g	43	4.6	712	3.4	2.4	76.9	0.9
Garlic & Herb, Reduced Calorie, Hellmann's*	1 Serving/25ml	58	4.8	233	0.7	13.1	19.3	0.4
Garlic Flavoured, Frank Cooper*	1 Tsp/6g	28	2.8	460	2.2	8.8	46.2	0.1
Heinz*	1 Tbsp/15g	99	10.8	663	0.9	3.0	71.8	0.0
Lemon, Waitrose*	1 Tsp/8ml	56	6.1	694	1.2	1.3	76.0	5.4
Light, Asda*	1 Dtsp/10g	36	3.3	364	1.0	16.1	32.8	0.0
Light, BGTY, Sainsbury's*	1 Tsp/11g	33	3.2	296	0.5	7.2	29.3	0.0
Light, Hellmann's*	1 Serving/10g	30	3.0	298	0.7	6.5	29.8	0.1
Light, Kraft*	1 Serving/25g	61	5.0	245	0.6	15.0	20.0	0.0
Light, Organic, Simply Delicious*	1 Tbsp/14g	46	4.2	328	0.8	13.0	30.3	0.4
Light, Reduced Calorie, Hellmann's*	1 Tsp/10g	30	3.0	297	0.7	6.5	29.8	0.0
Light, Reduced Fat, Heinz*	1 Tbsp/15g	42	4.0	279	1.1	7.7	26.8	0.5
Light, Squeezable, Hellmann's*	1 Tbsp/15g	44	4.4	293	0.7	6.4	29.4	0.0
Light, Squeezy, Oak Lane*	1 Serving/15ml	46	4.4	305	0.5	9.1	29.4	0.0
Light, Tesco*	1 Tbsp/15ml	41	4.0	275	0.8	7.1	26.7	0.0
Light Dijon, Benedicta*	1 Tbsp/15g	44	4.4	292	0.7	6.7	29.2	0.0
Low Fat, Belolive*	1 Serving/15ml	45	4.3	298	0.8	11.1	29.0	0.0
Made with Free Range Eggs, M & S*	1 Tbsp/15g	108	11.8	720	1.1	1.2	78.5	0.0
Mild Dijon Mustard, Frank Cooper*	1 Pot/28g	114	11.1	406	3.3	9.3	39.5	0.1
Organic, Evernat*	1 Tsp/11g	83	8.9	752	1.3	2.8	81.0	0.0
Organic, Whole Foods*	1 Tbsp/14g	100	11.0	714	0.0	7.1	78.6	0.0
Original, Egg, Dairy & Gluten Free, Tiger Tiger*	1 Tbsp/15g	66	6.8	440	1.4	5.8	45.6	0.3
Real, Best Foods*	1 Tbsp/13g	90	10.0	692	0.0	0.0	76.9	0.0
Real, Hellmann's*	1 Tsp/13g	90	10.0	692	1.1	1.3	76.9	0.0

	Measure INFO/WEIGHT	per Measure KCAL	FAT	Nutrition Values per 100g / 100ml KCAL	PROT	CARB	FAT	FIBRE
MAYONNAISE								
Real, The Big Squeeze, Hellmann's*	1 Tbsp/15ml	101	11.1	676	1.0	1.2	74.0	0.0
Reduced Calorie, Average	*1 Tsp/11g*	*33*	*3.2*	*301*	*0.7*	*8.9*	*29.0*	*0.1*
Reduced Fat, Tesco*	1 Tbsp/15ml	44	4.3	292	0.8	7.9	28.6	0.0
Squeezy, Oak Lane*	1 Tbsp/15ml	112	12.3	750	0.6	1.2	82.3	0.0
Vegetarian, Tesco*	1 Tsp/12g	89	9.7	738	1.5	0.8	81.0	0.0
with a Spark of Chilli, Hellmann's*	1 Tbsp/15ml	41	4.0	276	0.8	7.5	27.0	0.3
with a Twist of Lemon & Roast Garlic, Branston*	1 Tbsp/15ml	64	6.1	428	0.9	13.8	41.0	0.3
with a Twist of Lime & Chilli, Branston*	1 Serving/15ml	65	6.2	436	1.0	15.6	41.1	0.2
with a Twist of Pesto, Branston*	1 Tbsp/30ml	124	11.6	412	1.2	14.1	38.6	0.2
with Coarse Ground Mustard, French, Sainsbury's*	1 Serving/15ml	93	10.1	618	0.8	1.7	67.3	0.3
with Dijon Mustard, Hellmann's*	1 Tbsp/15ml	31	3.0	210	2.9	5.1	19.7	0.0
MEAL REPLACEMENT								
Bars, Chocolate, Slim Fast*	1 Bar/39g	107	3.5	274	20.6	35.3	9.0	5.5
Bars, Chocolate & Hazelnut, Tesco*	1 Bar/65g	250	7.1	385	24.2	41.0	11.0	6.3
Bars, Raspberry, Crispy, Meal, Tesco*	1 Bar/60g	216	6.7	360	22.3	42.1	11.2	7.6
Bars, Toffee Delight, Slim Fast*	1 Bar/78g	248	7.5	318	20.6	45.3	9.6	5.9
Powder, Cafe Latte, Ultra Slim, Tesco*	2 Scoops/29g	110	2.2	379	22.1	48.1	7.7	14.6
Shake, Banana Flavour, Celebrity Slim*	1 Sachet/55g	214	2.4	389	34.5	51.5	4.4	0.6
Shake, Banana Flavoured, Mealpak, All About Weight*	1 Pack/32g	120	3.3	375	37.5	30.3	10.3	8.1
Shake, Caffe Latte Flavour, Mealpak, All About Weight*	1 Pack/32g	120	3.4	375	37.5	31.3	10.6	8.1
Shake, Caramel Flavour, Celebrity Slim*	1 Pack/55g	212	2.4	385	34.2	50.9	4.4	0.6
Shake, Chocolate, Advantage, Atkins*	1 Serving/34g	121	4.2	361	49.0	8.1	12.5	15.5
Shake, Chocolate, Ready to Drink, Advantage, Atkins*	1 Carton/330ml	172	9.2	52	6.0	0.6	2.8	1.2
Shake, Chocolate Flavour, Celebrity Slim*	1 Sachet/55g	211	2.5	383	34.0	49.1	4.5	2.2
Shake, Chocolate Flavoured, Mealpak, All About Weight*	1 Pack/40g	150	4.2	375	34.9	31.5	10.6	7.2
Shake, Herbalife*	1 Serving/250ml	245	6.4	98	10.0	8.8	2.6	1.0
Shake, Neways*	1 Serving/39g	142	3.5	364	46.0	34.0	9.0	15.4
Shake, Rich Chocolate Flavour, Slim Fast*	1 Bottle/325ml	227	4.9	70	4.5	8.0	1.5	1.0
Shake, Starwberry Flavour, Meal Pack, All About Weight*	1 Pack/5g	2	0.0	40	0.0	3.5	0.0	45.0
Shake, Strawberry Flavour, Celebrity Slim*	1 Sachet/55g	214	2.4	389	34.4	51.6	4.4	0.6
Shake, Vanilla, Ready to Drink, Advantage, Atkins*	1 Carton/330ml	175	8.9	53	6.2	0.6	2.7	0.9
Shake, Vanilla Flavour, Celebrity Slim*	1 Sachet/55g	215	2.4	391	34.2	52.0	4.4	0.6
Shake, Vanilla Flavoured, Mealpak, All About Weight*	1 Shake/32g	120	3.3	375	37.5	30.6	10.3	8.1
Strawberry, High Protein, Energy Meal, Spiru-tein*	1 Serving/34g	99	0.0	291	41.2	32.3	0.0	2.9
Toffee Flavoured, Shake, Mealpak, All About Weight*	1 Sachet/36g	149	7.0	413	35.2	24.4	19.4	6.9
Ultimate Meal, The Ultimate Meal*	1/3 Cup/40g	170	4.0	425	37.5	75.0	10.0	20.0
Ultra Slim, Chocolate, Meal Bar, Tesco*	1 Bar/60g	219	6.7	365	28.5	37.3	11.1	8.2
Ultra Slim, Ready to Drink, Strawberry, Tesco*	1 Carton/330ml	231	3.0	70	4.2	10.5	0.9	1.5
Ultra Slim, Ready to Drink, Vanilla, Tesco*	1 Carton/330ml	224	3.0	68	4.2	10.5	0.9	1.5
Ultra-Slim, Ready to Drink, Chocolate, Tesco*	1 Carton/330ml	214	3.6	65	4.0	9.8	1.1	1.3
MEAT LOAF								
Beef & Pork, Co-Op*	¼ Loaf/114g	313	25.1	275	13.0	7.0	22.0	1.0
Iceland*	1 Serving/150g	331	23.5	221	10.8	9.3	15.7	0.9
in Onion Gravy, M & S*	¼ Pack/140g	203	11.9	145	11.3	6.3	8.5	1.2
Somerfield*	1 Pack/454g	867	59.0	191	10.0	8.0	13.0	0.0
Turkey & Bacon, Tesco*	1 Serving/225g	400	22.3	178	14.7	7.4	9.9	1.1
MEATBALLS								
& Mashed Potato, Tesco*	1 Pack/450g	526	29.7	117	4.0	10.4	6.6	1.0
& Pasta, Sainsbury's*	1 Serving/300g	333	9.3	111	5.3	15.5	3.1	1.9
& Pasta in Tomato Sauce, Wayfayrer*	1 Pack/300g	375	17.4	125	9.0	9.2	5.8	1.0
Aberdeen Angus, Fresh, Chilled, Waitrose*	1 Meatball/36g	92	7.1	256	18.0	1.5	19.8	0.0
Aberdeen Angus in Sauce, Perfectly Balanced, Waitrose*	½ Pack/240g	228	7.2	95	10.5	6.5	3.0	1.1
Aberdeen Angus with Tomato Sauce, Tesco*	½ Pack/250g	362	19.5	145	10.7	7.1	7.8	1.2

MEATBALLS

	Measure INFO/WEIGHT	per Measure KCAL	FAT	Nutrition Values per 100g / 100ml KCAL	PROT	CARB	FAT	FIBRE
Beef, Aberdeen Angus, 12 Pack, Waitrose*	1 Meatball/36g	93	7.1	259	18.0	2.3	19.8	0.1
Beef, British with Italian Herbs, Finest, Tesco*	1oz/28g	63	4.7	225	15.4	2.1	16.8	1.7
Beef, Diet Chef Ltd*	1 Pack/300g	408	18.6	136	11.3	8.7	6.2	2.7
Beef, Morrisons*	3 Meatballs/85g	213	13.8	251	23.1	3.1	16.2	0.9
Beef, Sainsbury's*	1 Meatball/29g	75	5.1	257	21.7	3.4	17.4	0.8
Beef, Tesco*	3 Meatballs/53g	140	11.4	265	15.0	2.9	21.5	0.9
Beef, TTD, Sainsbury's*	1 Meatball/35g	73	5.2	208	16.7	1.5	15.0	0.1
Beef in Tomato Sauce, Diet Chef Ltd*	1 Pack/300g	408	18.6	136	11.3	8.7	6.2	2.7
Chicken in Tomato Sauce, Average	1 Can/392g	580	32.9	148	7.7	10.4	8.4	0.0
Greek, M & S*	1 Serving/350g	402	18.9	115	7.7	9.1	5.4	1.5
in Bolognese Sauce, Fray Bentos*	½ Can/204g	188	5.9	92	4.8	11.6	2.9	0.7
in Bolognese Sauce, Somerfield*	1 Pack/454g	704	49.9	155	7.0	7.0	11.0	0.0
in Gravy, Campbell's*	½ Can/205g	164	5.3	80	5.6	8.6	2.6	0.0
in Gravy, Fray Bentos*	1 Meatball/21g	17	0.6	79	4.6	8.7	2.9	0.6
in Onion Gravy, Tesco*	½ Pack/200g	310	17.0	155	8.4	11.3	8.5	0.8
in Rich Gravy, Westlers*	½ Can/200g	170	6.8	85	4.1	9.5	3.4	0.4
in Sherry Sauce, Tapas, Waitrose*	1 Serving/185g	272	7.4	147	18.8	5.9	4.0	1.2
in Tomato & Basil Sauce, Go Cook, Asda*	½ Pack/270g	526	38.3	195	12.4	4.4	14.2	2.4
in Tomato Sauce, Canned, Average	1 Can/410g	387	15.1	94	5.6	9.8	3.7	0.0
in Tomato Sauce, Fray Bentos*	½ Can/206g	183	6.0	89	4.7	11.1	2.9	0.7
in Tomato Sauce, Tapas, Waitrose*	1 Pack/185g	285	16.8	154	10.8	7.2	9.1	1.3
Italian Pork, Al Forno, Sainsbury's*	1 Pack/450g	643	23.8	143	6.1	17.6	5.3	1.4
Lamb, Asda*	1 Pack/340g	928	71.4	273	16.0	5.1	21.0	0.6
Lemon Chicken with Rice, BGTY, Sainsbury's*	1 Pack/400g	388	8.4	97	6.8	12.8	2.1	1.4
Lion's Head, M & S*	1 Serving/300g	435	27.9	145	10.4	5.1	9.3	1.0
Mighty in Tomato Sauce, Westlers*	1 Can/400g	424	19.0	106	5.8	10.2	4.7	0.0
Pork, British, Simply, M & S*	½ Pack/180g	396	27.2	220	17.0	4.3	15.1	0.5
Pork, Diet Chef Ltd*	1 Pack/300g	273	5.1	91	9.4	9.4	1.7	3.2
Pork, Diet Chef Ltd*	1 Meal/300g	273	5.1	91	9.4	9.4	1.7	3.2
Pork & Beef, Swedish Style, Tesco*	1 Meatball/14g	34	2.5	245	14.3	6.5	17.7	2.0
Pork & Chorizo with Paprika Potatoes, Finest, Tesco*	½ Pack/425g	527	25.9	124	7.5	9.8	6.1	2.8
Roman-Style with Basil Mash, COU, M & S*	1 Pack/430g	344	9.5	80	3.7	10.9	2.2	1.9
Spaghetti, Tesco*	1 Pack/385g	377	16.0	98	5.4	9.8	4.2	1.2
Spiced Lamb, Feta with Paprika Potatoes, Finest, Tesco*	1 Pack/400g	460	20.0	115	6.4	7.5	5.0	6.5
Spicy, Deli Melt, Sainsbury's*	1 Pack/200g	338	21.4	169	12.7	5.5	10.7	2.9
Spicy, M & S*	1 Pack/400g	540	24.0	135	8.8	12.0	6.0	1.4
Swedish, Average	¼ Pack/88g	198	13.8	224	14.0	7.4	15.7	1.3
Turkey, GFY, Asda*	½ Pack/330g	333	12.2	101	10.0	7.0	3.7	0.0
with Paprika-Spiced Potatoes, Extra Special, Asda*	1 Pack/450g	589	23.8	131	6.5	13.4	5.3	2.0
with Spicy Potato Wedges, Bistro, TTD, Sainsbury's*	½ Pack/500g	678	8.5	136	9.4	17.3	1.7	7.1
with Spicy Tomato Sauce, Just Cook, Sainsbury's*	½ Pack/170g	246	11.9	145	14.8	5.7	7.0	0.9

MEATBALLS VEGETARIAN

Swedish Style, Sainsbury's*	1 Ball/27g	53	2.6	194	21.5	5.5	9.5	4.0
with Penne, Tesco*	1 Serving/460g	414	10.6	90	5.9	11.4	2.3	2.1

MEDLAR

Raw, Flesh Only	**1 Fruit/28g**	**11**	**0.1**	**40**	**0.5**	**10.6**	**0.4**	**10.0**

MELBA TOAST

Average	1 Serving/3g	13	0.2	396	12.0	76.0	4.9	4.6
Buitoni*	1 Serving/33g	130	1.6	395	12.1	75.5	4.9	4.6
Dutch, Light Choices, Tesco*	1 Pack/20g	75	0.5	375	13.1	75.0	2.4	4.6
Organic, Trimlyne*	2 Toasts/7g	28	0.5	407	13.7	71.6	6.8	5.3
Organic Spelt, Amisa*	2 Slices/24g	95	1.9	395	12.4	68.5	7.9	0.0
Organic Spelt, Demeter*	2 Biscuits/25g	99	2.0	395	12.4	68.5	7.9	0.0

INFO/WEIGHT	Measure	per Measure		Nutrition Values per 100g / 100ml				
		KCAL	FAT	KCAL	PROT	CARB	FAT	FIBRE
MELBA TOAST								
Original, Van Der Meulen*	1 Slice/3g	12	0.1	399	12.8	80.5	2.9	3.9
Thinly Sliced Toasted Wheat Bread, Sainsbury's*	1 Slice/3g	12	0.1	374	13.1	75.1	2.4	4.6
Tomato & Basil, Morrisons*	1 Pack/20g	77	0.6	383	13.6	75.7	2.9	2.4
Van Der Meulen*	3 Slices/39g	151	0.9	388	13.1	75.1	2.4	0.0
Wholegrain, HL, Tesco*	1 Pack/20g	74	1.0	370	16.8	63.8	4.9	8.9
with Sesame, Tesco*	1 Slice/3g	11	0.2	370	12.8	61.7	8.0	3.8
MELON								
Cantaloupe, Flesh Only, Average	*½ Melon/255g*	*87*	*0.5*	*34*	*0.8*	*8.2*	*0.2*	*0.9*
Cantaloupe, Weighed with Rind, Average	*1 Lge Wedge/100g*	*35*	*0.3*	*35*	*0.8*	*8.3*	*0.3*	*0.8*
Galia, Average	*1 Serving/240g*	*60*	*0.1*	*25*	*0.7*	*5.7*	*0.0*	*0.2*
Honeydew, Raw, Flesh Only, Average	*1oz/28g*	*8*	*0.0*	*29*	*0.7*	*6.9*	*0.1*	*0.5*
Medley, Pre Packed, Average	1 Pack/240g	66	0.3	27	0.6	6.0	0.1	0.5
MELT								
Cheese, Chilli, Fresh, Asda*	1 Melt/29g	87	4.9	301	6.0	31.0	17.0	0.0
Cheesy Fish, Youngs*	1 Pack/340g	418	22.4	123	7.6	8.3	6.6	0.9
Chilli with Spicy Potato Wedges, Asda*	1 Pack/450g	540	19.8	120	8.0	12.0	4.4	1.2
Salmon & Broccoli Wedge, From Heinz, Weight Watchers*	1 Pack/320g	298	10.6	93	5.1	10.6	3.3	1.1
Sausage & Bean, Iceland*	1 Pack/400g	588	23.2	147	6.5	17.1	5.8	1.6
Tuna, Go Large, Asda*	1 Melt/175g	509	26.2	291	12.0	27.0	15.0	0.0
Tuna, M & S*	1 Pack/218g	621	37.1	285	13.0	20.1	17.0	1.0
MENTOS								
Cola, Mentos*	1 Packet/38g	146	0.7	390	0.0	93.0	2.0	0.0
MERINGUE								
Average	*1 Meringue/8g*	*30*	*0.0*	*379*	*5.3*	*95.4*	*0.0*	*0.0*
Belgian Chocolate, Mini, Extra Special, Asda*	1 Meringue/6g	28	0.9	459	6.0	75.0	15.0	0.7
Bombe, Raspberry & Vanilla, M & S*	1 Bombe/100g	155	1.8	155	3.4	33.3	1.8	2.6
Chocolate, Waitrose*	1 Meringue/77g	341	11.3	444	2.6	75.3	14.7	0.5
Coffee Fresh Cream, Asda*	1 Meringue/28g	109	4.7	396	3.8	57.0	17.0	0.3
Cream, Fresh, Sainsbury's*	1 Meringue/35g	142	5.1	407	3.5	65.4	14.6	0.5
Cream, M & S*	1 Meringue/34g	145	7.6	425	4.1	52.6	22.2	1.4
Layered, Tesco*	1/5 Meringue/52g	146	0.8	280	3.5	63.2	1.5	1.4
Lemon, Morrisons*	1 Serving/120g	295	14.4	246	2.5	32.0	12.0	0.5
Mini, Extra Special, Asda*	1 Meringue/4g	14	0.0	394	5.0	93.0	0.2	0.5
Mini, M & S*	1 Meringue/4g	15	0.0	395	6.1	91.6	0.0	0.2
Nests, Average	1 Nest/16g	63	0.0	397	4.7	93.3	0.1	0.1
Nests, Tropical Fruit, Sainsbury's*	1 Nest/95g	234	7.4	246	2.0	42.0	7.8	2.4
Raspberry, M & S*	1 Serving/105g	215	13.8	205	1.8	20.6	13.1	3.1
Shells, Sainsbury's*	2 Shells/24g	93	0.0	387	3.9	92.8	0.0	0.0
Strawberry, COU, M & S*	1 Meringue/5g	20	0.0	385	6.4	90.0	0.1	1.4
Strawberry, Mini, Extra Special, Asda*	1 Meringue/4g	15	0.0	387	5.0	91.0	0.3	0.5
Summer Fruits, 90% Fat Free, Sara Lee*	1 Meringue/135g	308	11.5	228	2.5	35.7	8.5	2.2
Toffee, COU, M & S*	1 Mini/5g	20	0.1	395	5.0	95.3	1.7	0.7
Toffee, M & S*	1 Meringue/30g	124	6.3	415	4.1	52.2	20.9	0.8
Tropical, M & S*	1 Serving/53g	212	14.3	400	3.1	37.0	26.9	0.0
MIDGET GEMS								
M & S*	1 Bag/113g	367	0.1	325	6.3	75.1	0.1	0.0
Smart Price, Asda*	1 Pack/178g	586	0.2	329	6.0	76.0	0.1	0.0
MILK								
1% Fat, Fresh, Arla*	1 Glass/202ml	83	2.0	41	3.3	4.8	1.0	0.0
2% Low Fat, Dunkley's*	1 Cup/240ml	120	5.0	50	2.9	4.2	2.1	0.0
Alternative, Original, Good Hemp*	1 Glass/250ml	90	6.0	36	1.3	2.2	2.4	0.2
Condensed, Caramel, Carnation, Nestle*	1 Serving/50g	148	3.0	296	5.5	55.1	6.0	0.0
Condensed, Semi Skimmed, Sweetened	*1oz/28g*	*75*	*0.1*	*267*	*10.0*	*60.0*	*0.2*	*0.0*

MILK

	Measure INFO/WEIGHT	per Measure KCAL	FAT	Nutrition Values per 100g / 100ml KCAL	PROT	CARB	FAT	FIBRE
Condensed, Skimmed, Unsweetened, Average	*1oz/28g*	*30*	*1.1*	*108*	*7.5*	*10.5*	*4.0*	*0.0*
Condensed, Whole, Sweetened, Average	*1oz/28g*	*93*	*2.8*	*333*	*8.5*	*55.5*	*10.1*	*0.0*
Dried, Skimmed, Average	*1oz/28g*	*99*	*0.3*	*355*	*35.4*	*52.3*	*0.9*	*0.0*
Dried, Whole, Average	*1oz/28g*	*137*	*7.4*	*490*	*26.3*	*39.4*	*26.3*	*0.0*
Evaporated, Average	*1 Serving/85g*	*136*	*7.6*	*160*	*8.2*	*11.6*	*9.0*	*0.0*
Evaporated, Reduced Fat, Average	*1oz/28g*	*33*	*1.5*	*118*	*7.4*	*10.5*	*5.2*	*0.0*
Goats, Pasteurised	*1 fl oz/30ml*	*18*	*1.0*	*60*	*3.1*	*4.4*	*3.5*	*0.0*
Goats, Semi-Skimmed, St Helen's Farm*	1 Serving/250ml	109	4.0	44	3.0	4.3	1.6	0.0
Goats, Skimmed, St Helen's Farm*	1 Serving/125ml	37	0.1	30	3.0	4.3	0.1	0.0
Low Fat, Calcia Extra Calcium, Unigate*	1 fl oz/30ml	13	0.1	45	4.3	6.3	0.5	0.0
Semi Skimmed, Advance with Omega 3, St Ivel*	1 Glass/250ml	122	4.2	49	3.4	5.0	1.7	0.0
Semi Skimmed, Average	*1 fl oz/30ml*	*15*	*0.5*	*49*	*3.4*	*5.0*	*1.7*	*0.0*
Semi Skimmed, Lactose Free, Arla*	1 Serving/100ml	40	1.5	40	3.9	2.8	1.5	0.0
Semi Skimmed, Long Life, Average	*1 fl oz/30ml*	*15*	*0.5*	*49*	*3.4*	*5.0*	*1.7*	*0.0*
Semi Skimmed, Low Lactose, Lactofree, Arla*	1 Glass/125ml	56	1.9	45	3.4	5.0	1.5	0.0
Semi Skimmed, Low Lactose, UHT, Lactofree, Arla*	1 Serving/100ml	38	1.7	38	3.2	2.6	1.7	0.0
Semi Skimmed, Organic, Country Life*	1 fl oz/30ml	15	0.5	49	3.4	5.0	1.7	0.0
Skimmed, Albert Heijn*	1 Glass/250ml	80	0.0	32	3.0	5.0	0.0	0.0
Skimmed, Average	*1 Pint/568ml*	*194*	*0.5*	*34*	*3.3*	*5.0*	*0.1*	*0.0*
Skimmed, Uht, Average	*1 fl oz/30ml*	*10*	*0.5*	*34*	*3.3*	*5.0*	*0.1*	*0.0*
Skimmed 1% Fat, Waitrose*	1 Serving/200ml	70	0.2	35	3.4	5.0	0.1	0.0
Soya, Vitasoy*	1 Serving/250ml	130	3.7	52	3.0	5.5	1.5	2.0
Super Milk Low Fat 1%, Avonmore*	1 Litre/1000ml	420	10.0	42	3.4	5.0	1.0	0.0
Whole, Advance with Omega 3, St Ivel*	1 Serving/250ml	162	9.2	65	3.3	4.7	3.7	0.0
Whole, Average	*1 Serving/200ml*	*134*	*7.8*	*67*	*3.3*	*4.7*	*3.9*	*0.0*
Whole, Lactose Free, Lactofree, Arla*	1 Serving/200ml	116	7.0	58	3.9	2.7	3.5	0.0
Whole with Vitamin D, Oak Farms*	1 Container/236ml	150	8.0	64	3.4	4.7	3.4	0.0

MILK DRINK

Banana Flavour, Sterilised, Low Fat, Gulp*	1 Bottle/500ml	315	5.0	63	3.8	9.7	1.0	0.0
Chocolate, Break Time, Arla*	1 Bottle/500ml	290	1.5	58	3.6	10.2	0.3	0.0
Chocolate Coconut, Free From, Tesco*	1 Serving/250ml	125	5.4	49	0.4	6.8	2.1	0.7
Chocolate Flavoured, Goodness for Kids, Tesco*	1 Bottlel/330ml	247	5.9	75	3.8	10.3	1.8	0.7
Chocolate Sterilised Skimmed, Happy Shopper*	1 Bottle/500ml	295	1.5	59	3.6	10.4	0.3	0.0
Colombian Coffee Flavoured, Waitrose*	1 Serving/250ml	232	9.5	93	4.3	10.5	3.8	0.0
Family Fuel, Mars*	1 Serving/200ml	172	4.0	86	3.1	13.7	2.0	0.0
Hazelnut, Free From, Tesco*	1 Serving/250ml	85	2.5	34	0.2	5.2	1.0	1.5
Mocalatte, Cafe Met*	1 Bottle/290ml	159	3.8	55	2.9	8.0	1.3	0.0
No Added Sugar, Mars*	1 Serving/200ml	108	3.4	54	3.4	6.2	1.7	0.5
Original, Mars*	1 Serving/330g	284	6.9	86	3.1	13.7	2.1	0.0
Refuel, Mars*	1 Bottle/388ml	299	5.8	77	3.1	13.5	1.5	0.0
Semi Skimmed, Cholesterol Lowering, Pro Activ, Flora*	1 Serving/250ml	125	4.5	50	3.6	4.8	1.8	0.0
Strawberry, Probiotic, WellYou, Kaufland*	1 Bottle/125g	77	0.1	62	2.5	11.9	0.1	0.1
Strawberry Flavoured, Goodness for Kids, Tesco*	1 Bottle/330ml	247	5.6	75	4.0	9.9	1.7	0.4

MILK SHAKE

Banana, Diet Chef Ltd*	1 Drink/330ml	225	3.0	68	4.2	10.5	0.9	1.5
Banana, Yazoo, Campina*	1 Bottle/200ml	120	2.4	60	3.1	9.6	1.2	0.0
Banana Flavour, Frijj*	1 Bottle/500ml	325	4.5	65	3.7	10.5	0.9	0.0
Banana Flavour, Shapers, Boots*	1 Bottle/250ml	201	1.9	80	5.6	12.8	0.8	1.9
Cafe Latte, Diet Chef Ltd*	1 Carton/330ml	218	3.3	66	4.2	8.9	1.0	2.0
Chocolate, Asda*	1 Serving/250ml	197	9.2	79	4.4	7.0	3.7	0.4
Chocolate, Extreme, Frijj*	1 Bottle/500g	425	10.5	85	3.9	12.7	2.1	0.0
Chocolate Flavour, BGTY, Sainsbury's*	1 Bottle/500ml	290	2.5	58	5.3	8.0	0.5	0.9
Chocolate Flavour, Diet Chef Ltd*	1 Drink/330ml	210	2.3	64	4.1	8.5	0.7	1.9

	Measure INFO/WEIGHT	per Measure KCAL	per Measure FAT	Nutrition Values per 100g / 100ml KCAL	PROT	CARB	FAT	FIBRE
MILK SHAKE								
Honeycomb Choc Swirl Flavour, The Incredible, Frijj*	1 Bottle/500ml	450	12.5	90	4.0	13.0	2.5	0.2
Measure Up, Asda*	1 Glass/250ml	200	2.4	80	6.0	12.0	1.0	2.4
Mount Caramel, Frijj*	1 Bottle/500ml	360	4.5	72	3.4	12.7	0.9	0.0
Peachy Banana, Syrup, Robinson's*	1 Serving/50ml	79	0.0	158	0.0	39.0	0.0	0.0
Powder, Made Up with Semi-Skimmed Milk	1 Serving/250ml	172	4.0	69	3.2	11.3	1.6	0.0
Powder, Made Up with Whole Milk	1 Serving/250ml	217	9.2	87	3.1	11.1	3.7	0.0
Sticky Toffee Pudding Flavour, The Incredible, Frijj*	1 Bottle/500ml	445	10.0	89	4.0	13.7	2.0	0.1
Strawberry, Diet Chef Ltd*	1 Drink/330g	225	3.0	68	4.2	10.5	0.9	1.5
Strawberry, Diet Chef Ltd*	1 Carton/330ml	207	3.0	63	4.0	10.3	0.9	1.4
Strawberry, Yazoo, Campina*	1 Bottle/500ml	325	6.0	65	3.1	10.3	1.2	0.0
Strawberry & Raspberry, Syrup, Robinson's*	1 Serving/50ml	20	0.7	39	2.9	4.0	1.4	0.0
Strawberry Flavour, Thick, Low Fat, Frijj*	1 Bottle/250ml	155	2.0	62	3.4	10.1	0.8	0.0
Thick, Milky Way, Mars*	1 Bottle/440ml	282	4.8	64	3.4	10.0	1.1	0.7
Vanilla, Diet Chef Ltd*	1 Pack/330ml	225	3.0	68	4.2	10.5	0.9	1.5
Vanilla, Frijj*	1 Bottle/500ml	320	4.0	64	3.4	10.7	0.8	0.0
Vanilla Flavour, BGTY, Sainsbury's*	1 Bottle/500ml	230	0.5	46	5.3	5.9	0.1	0.4
MILKY BAR								
Buttons, Nestle*	1 Pack/30g	164	9.5	547	7.3	58.4	31.7	0.0
Choo, Nestle*	1 Bar/25g	116	4.3	464	4.2	73.1	17.2	0.0
Chunky, Nestle*	¼ Bar/38g	207	12.0	547	7.3	58.4	31.7	0.0
Crunchies, Nestle*	1 Pack/30g	168	10.4	560	7.0	54.9	34.7	0.0
Eggs, Mini, Nestle*	1 Pack/100g	500	23.3	500	4.2	68.4	23.3	0.0
Funsize, Mars*	1 Funsize Bar/17g	75	2.7	449	3.8	71.8	16.3	0.6
Munchies, Nestle*	1 Serving/70g	392	24.3	560	7.0	54.9	34.7	0.1
Nestle*	1 Sm Bar/13g	68	4.0	547	7.3	58.4	31.7	0.0
MILKY WAY								
Fun Size, Mars*	1 Bar/17g	75	2.7	447	3.8	71.6	16.2	0.0
Magic Stars, Mars*	1 Bag/33g	183	11.5	555	6.2	54.1	34.9	1.8
Mars*	1 Single Bar/22g	98	3.5	448	3.7	72.4	15.9	0.6
MINCEMEAT								
Average	**1oz/28g**	**77**	**1.2**	**274**	**0.6**	**62.1**	**4.3**	**1.3**
Traditional, Robertson*	1 Tbsp/17g	49	0.6	286	0.6	62.5	3.4	2.5
with Cherries, Almonds & Brandy, Tesco*	¼ Jar/103g	295	5.0	287	1.4	58.8	4.9	1.4
MINIS								
Cream Cheese & Chives, Ryvita*	1 Pack/30g	114	2.3	380	8.7	75.7	7.7	13.0
Salt & Vinegar, Ryvita*	1 Pack/24g	90	1.9	376	8.2	74.0	7.8	11.4
Sweet Chilli, Ryvita*	1 Pack/24g	90	1.8	376	8.5	75.9	7.4	10.3
MINSTRELS								
Galaxy, Mars*	1 Serving/100g	503	22.3	503	5.2	70.3	22.3	1.1
MINT								
Dried, Average	**1 Tsp/5g**	**14**	**0.2**	**279**	**24.8**	**34.6**	**4.6**	**0.0**
Fresh, Average	**2 Tbsp/3g**	**1**	**0.0**	**43**	**3.8**	**5.3**	**0.7**	**0.0**
MINTS								
After Dinner, Dark, Elizabeth Shaw*	1 Sweet/9g	42	2.1	469	2.8	62.5	23.1	0.0
After Dinner, Sainsbury's*	1 Mint/7g	32	1.5	456	4.1	62.1	21.2	4.1
Butter Mintoes, Tesco*	1 Sweet/7g	24	0.5	349	0.0	71.3	7.1	0.0
Clear, Co-Op*	1 Sweet/6g	24	0.0	395	0.0	98.0	0.0	0.0
Cream, Luxury, Thorntons*	1 Sweet/13g	62	3.1	477	4.2	62.3	23.8	2.3
Creams, Bassett's*	1 Sweet/11g	40	0.0	365	0.0	91.8	0.0	0.0
Curiously Strong, M & S*	1 Sweet/1g	4	0.0	390	0.4	97.5	0.0	0.0
Everton, Co-Op*	1 Sweet/6g	25	0.2	410	0.6	92.0	4.0	0.0
Extra, Peppermint Coolburst, Wrigleys^	1 Pack/22g	53	0.2	240	0.0	98.0	1.0	0.0
Extra, Spearmint, Sugar Free, Wrigleys*	1 Sweet/1g	3	0.0	244	0.0	98.5	0.8	0.0

MINTS

	Measure INFO/WEIGHT	per Measure KCAL	per Measure FAT	Nutrition Values per 100g / 100ml KCAL	PROT	CARB	FAT	FIBRE
Extra, Wrigleys*	1 Sweet/1g	3	0.0	240	0.0	64.0	1.0	0.0
Extra Strong, Peppermint, Trebor*	1 Roll/46g	180	0.1	395	0.4	98.1	0.2	0.0
Extra Strong, Spearmint, Trebor*	1 Pack/44g	174	0.0	395	0.4	98.7	0.0	0.0
Glacier, Fox's*	1 Sweet/5g	19	0.0	386	0.0	96.4	0.0	0.0
Humbugs, M & S*	1 Sweet/9g	37	0.4	407	0.6	91.1	4.4	0.0
Humbugs, Thorntons*	1 Sweet/9g	31	0.4	340	1.0	87.8	4.4	0.0
Imperials, M & S*	1 Sweet/3g	12	0.0	391	0.0	97.8	0.0	0.0
Imperials, Sainsbury's*	1 Sweet/3g	10	0.0	374	0.0	92.1	0.0	0.0
Mento, Sugar Free, Mentos*	1 Sweet/2g	5	0.1	260	1.0	87.0	5.5	0.0
Mint Assortment, M & S*	1 Sweet/7g	26	0.5	375	0.4	78.2	6.9	0.0
Mint Favourites, Bassett's*	1 Sweet/6g	22	0.4	367	0.9	77.4	5.9	0.0
Peppermints, Strong, Altoids*	1 Sweet/1g	3	0.0	385	0.5	96.0	0.0	0.0
Smooth, Weight Watchers*	1 Tube/25g	58	0.0	231	0.2	61.6	0.0	0.0
Soft, Trebor*	1 Pack/48g	182	0.0	380	0.0	94.9	0.0	0.0
Softmints, Peppermint, Trebor*	1 Pack/48g	170	0.0	355	0.0	88.9	0.0	0.0
Softmints, Spearmint, Trebor*	1 Pack/45g	170	0.0	375	0.0	94.3	0.0	0.0
Thins, Chocolate, Waitrose*	1 Thin/5g	27	1.3	509	4.2	69.6	23.8	0.2

MIRIN

Rice Wine, Sweetened, Average	*1 Tbsp/15ml*	*35*	*0.0*	*231*	*0.2*	*41.6*	*0.0*	*0.0*

MISO

Average	*1oz/28g*	*57*	*1.7*	*203*	*13.3*	*23.5*	*6.2*	*0.0*

MIXED HERBS

Average	*1 Tsp/5g*	*13*	*0.4*	*260*	*12.9*	*37.5*	*8.5*	*6.7*
Herbes De Provence, Dried, Schwartz*	1 Tsp/2g	7	0.1	364	12.9	65.0	5.8	0.0

MIXED SPICE

Rub, Moroccan, Schwartz*	1 Serving/3g	9	0.3	309	15.0	36.4	11.4	19.5
Schwartz*	1 Tsp/2g	8	0.2	390	10.4	65.8	9.5	2.0

MIXED VEGETABLES

& Mung Bean Sprouts with Asian Seasoning, Dawnfield*	1 Bag/750g	412	21.0	55	2.5	5.0	2.8	0.0
Baby, Iceland*	1 Serving/100g	20	0.0	20	1.2	3.9	0.0	2.7
Baby, Steam, Fresh, Tesco*	1 Pack/160g	72	1.3	45	2.7	6.7	0.8	3.8
Baby Corn, Mange Tout & Baby Carrots, Tesco*	1 Pack/220g	64	0.9	29	2.3	4.3	0.4	2.2
Broccoli, Sweetcorn & Peas, Rice, SteamFresh, Birds Eye*	1 Bag/160g	181	5.3	113	3.5	17.3	3.3	2.1
Broccoli & Cauliflower Florets, Baby Carrots, Asda*	1 Serving/113g	28	0.7	25	2.2	2.6	0.6	2.4
Canned, Drained, Co-Op*	½ Can/100g	45	0.1	45	2.0	9.0	0.1	2.0
Canned, Drained, Sainsbury's*	1 Can/200g	114	0.6	57	3.0	10.6	0.3	2.3
Canned, Re-Heated, Drained	1oz/28g	11	0.2	38	1.9	6.1	0.8	1.7
Carrot, Cauliflower & Broccoli, Prepared, Co-Op*	1 Pack/250g	100	1.5	40	2.4	5.0	0.6	2.7
Carrot, Swede, Leek & Onion for Casserole, M & S*	1 Serving/100g	35	0.4	35	0.8	5.6	0.4	2.6
Carrot Batons, Cauliflower & Broccoli, Steamed, Asda*	1 Bag/120g	28	0.7	23	1.8	2.6	0.6	3.1
Carrots, Broccoli & Sweetcorn, Easy Steam, Sainsbury's*	1 Pack/120g	67	1.4	56	2.6	8.7	1.2	2.0
Carrots, Broccoli & Sweetcorn, Steam Veg, Tesco*	1 Sachet/160g	80	1.8	50	2.5	7.5	1.1	3.0
Carrots, Peas, Green Beans & Sweetcorn, Frozen, Tesco*	1 Serving/80g	38	0.6	48	3.1	7.3	0.7	3.9
Casserole, Co-Op*	1 Serving/100g	40	0.3	40	1.2	7.5	0.3	2.1
Casserole, Frozen, Tesco*	1 Serving/100g	26	0.4	26	0.8	4.8	0.4	2.0
Casserole, Ready to Cook, Sainsbury's*	½ Pack/240g	74	0.7	31	0.9	6.2	0.3	1.4
Casserole, with Baby Potatoes, Fresh, M & S*	½ Pack/350g	140	1.0	40	1.2	7.8	0.3	2.1
Cauliflower, Carrots, Green Beans, SteamFresh, Birds Eye*	1 Bag/120g	40	0.6	33	2.0	5.0	0.5	2.2
Chef's Style, Ready Prepared, M & S*	1 Pack/240g	72	1.2	30	2.6	4.5	0.5	2.9
Chinese, Stir Fry, Amoy*	1 Serving/110g	27	0.3	25	1.8	3.7	0.3	0.0
Chunky, Frozen, Sainsbury's*	1 Serving/85g	31	0.6	37	2.9	4.7	0.7	3.1
Corn Baby, Fine Beans & Baby Carrots, Tesco*	1 Pack/250g	67	1.2	27	1.7	4.0	0.5	2.2
Country Selection, Budgens*	1 Serving/113g	27	0.4	24	1.6	3.6	0.4	2.9

	Measure INFO/WEIGHT	per Measure KCAL	per Measure FAT	Nutrition Values per 100g / 100ml KCAL	PROT	CARB	FAT	FIBRE
MIXED VEGETABLES								
Crunchy, Tesco*	1 Pack/210g	63	0.8	30	1.7	5.0	0.4	2.4
Farmhouse, Four Seasons*	1 Serving/100g	26	0.7	26	2.2	2.7	0.7	0.0
Farmhouse, Frozen, Four Seasons, Aldi*	1oz/28g	10	0.2	34	2.8	4.3	0.7	0.0
Farmhouse, Frozen, Waitrose*	1 Serving/90g	22	0.5	25	1.9	3.1	0.6	2.4
Fine Beans & Baby Carrots, Sweet, Tender, Waitrose*	½ Pack/125g	42	0.6	34	1.3	4.6	0.5	2.8
Freshly Frozen, Asda*	1 Serving/80g	42	0.6	52	3.2	8.0	0.8	3.0
Freshly Frozen, Iceland*	1 Serving/100g	54	0.8	54	3.3	8.3	0.8	3.7
Frozen, Boiled in Salted Water	1oz/28g	12	0.1	42	3.3	6.6	0.5	0.0
Frozen, SuperValu*	1 Serving/70g	22	0.3	31	1.7	5.1	0.4	0.0
in Salt Water, Tesco*	1/3 Can/65g	34	0.4	53	2.6	9.2	0.6	2.7
in Salted Water, Canned, Asda*	1 Serving/65g	31	0.1	48	2.6	9.0	0.2	1.7
in Salted Water, Nisa Heritage*	1 Serving/100g	39	0.8	39	1.9	6.1	0.8	1.7
Layered, Classics, M & S*	½ Pack/160g	112	6.2	70	1.2	7.3	3.9	1.2
Organic, Waitrose*	1oz/28g	19	0.4	69	4.4	10.0	1.3	2.7
Oriental, M & S*	1 Serving/250g	50	0.7	20	1.6	3.4	0.3	1.6
Peas, Carrots, & Baby Leeks, Prepared, Tesco*	½ Pack/130g	57	1.2	44	3.1	5.8	0.9	3.5
Peas & Carrots Crinkle Cut, D'Aucy*	1 Serving/265g	138	1.3	52	3.2	6.5	0.5	4.3
Potatoes, Broad Beans & Peas, M & S*	1 Pack/245g	147	3.2	60	2.9	12.9	1.3	3.4
Premium, Frozen, Somerfield*	1 Serving/100g	53	1.0	53	3.2	7.9	1.0	2.7
Ready to Roast, Asda*	½ Pack/362g	315	11.6	87	1.6	13.0	3.2	2.4
Red Peppers & Courgette, Tesco*	1 Pack/250g	67	1.2	27	1.7	3.8	0.5	2.0
Roast, Four Seasons*	1 Serving/187g	79	0.4	42	1.2	8.8	0.2	0.0
Sainsbury's*	1 Serving/230g	55	1.4	24	2.1	2.5	0.6	0.0
Seasonal Selection, Tesco*	1 Serving/100g	37	0.4	37	1.1	7.2	0.4	2.2
Special, Freshly Frozen, Morrisons*	1 Serving/100g	48	0.8	48	3.2	7.2	0.8	0.0
Special, Sainsbury's*	1 Serving/120g	68	1.2	57	3.2	8.9	1.0	2.9
Summer, Tesco*	1 Pack/167g	55	0.8	33	2.6	4.5	0.5	2.8
MOLASSES								
Average	*1 Tsp/5g*	*13*	*0.0*	*266*	*0.0*	*68.8*	*0.1*	*0.0*
MONKEY NUTS								
without Shell, Average	*1oz/28g*	*158*	*13.4*	*565*	*25.5*	*8.2*	*47.9*	*6.3*
MONKFISH								
Grilled	*1oz/28g*	*27*	*0.2*	*96*	*22.7*	*0.0*	*0.6*	*0.0*
Raw	*1oz/28g*	*18*	*0.1*	*66*	*15.7*	*0.0*	*0.4*	*0.0*
MONSTER MUNCH								
Flamin' Hot, Walkers*	1 Std Bag/22g	108	5.5	490	7.0	59.0	25.0	1.5
Pickled Onion, Walkers*	1 Std Bag/22g	108	5.5	490	6.0	60.0	25.0	1.7
Roast Beef, Walkers*	1 Std Bag/22g	108	5.5	490	7.0	59.0	25.0	1.7
Spicy, Walkers*	1 Std Bag/25g	125	7.2	500	5.0	55.0	29.0	1.3
MORNAY								
Broccoli, Somerfield*	1 Pack/400g	372	24.8	93	3.5	5.9	6.2	0.5
Cod, Fillets, Sainsbury's*	1 Serving/153g	236	14.4	154	15.2	2.2	9.4	0.9
Cod, Gratin, Cooked, Just Cook, Sainsbury's*	1 Pack/320g	518	32.2	185	13.3	6.9	11.5	0.5
Cod, Nutritionally Balanced, M & S*	1 Pack/400g	320	10.4	80	6.8	7.2	2.6	1.6
Cod, Sainsbury's*	1 Serving/180g	277	16.9	154	15.2	2.2	9.4	0.9
Cod with Mashed Potato, Carrots & Broccoli, Sainsbury's*	½ Pack/200g	144	3.4	72	6.9	7.4	1.7	1.6
Haddock, COU, M & S*	½ Pack/194g	165	3.9	85	14.5	2.6	2.0	0.6
Haddock, Perfectly Balanced, Waitrose*	1 Pack/360g	310	5.4	86	16.6	1.6	1.5	0.5
Haddock, Youngs*	½ Pack/190g	236	14.8	124	12.1	1.3	7.8	0.6
Salmon with Broccoli, Weight Watchers*	1 Pack/320g	231	9.6	72	4.5	6.5	3.0	0.5
Spinach, Waitrose*	½ Pack/125g	112	8.6	90	3.3	3.6	6.9	1.6
MOUSSAKA								
Aubergine & Lentil, Asda*	1 Pack/451g	370	17.1	82	3.9	8.1	3.8	2.9

M

MOUSSAKA

Measure INFO/WEIGHT	per Measure KCAL	FAT	Nutrition Values per 100g / 100ml KCAL	PROT	CARB	FAT	FIBRE
Beef, BGTY, Sainsbury's*	1 Pack/400g	300	10.4	75	6.1	6.8	2.6	1.2
Beef, GFY, Asda*	1 Pack/400g	300	8.4	75	7.0	7.0	2.1	0.7
Beef, HL, Tesco*	1 Pack/450g	396	12.1	88	5.0	10.9	2.7	0.8
Cafe Culture, M & S*	1 Serving/375g	619	39.4	165	9.2	7.8	10.5	0.8
COU, M & S*	1 Pack/340g	272	9.9	80	5.3	8.5	2.9	1.4
Lamb, Sainsbury's*	1 Pack/329g	497	32.3	151	8.4	7.2	9.8	1.0
Low Saturated Fat, Waitrose*	1 Pack/350g	304	10.8	87	6.3	8.4	3.1	3.1
TTD, Sainsbury's*	1 Pack/399g	546	35.9	137	8.1	5.8	9.0	0.6
Vegetable, Cooked, BGTY, Sainsbury's*	1 Pack/333g	253	6.0	76	2.6	11.5	1.8	1.6
Vegetable, COU, M & S*	1 Pack/400g	280	10.8	70	2.7	9.1	2.7	2.4
Vegetarian, Tesco*	1 Pack/300g	489	31.2	163	6.4	11.0	10.4	0.9

MOUSSE

	Measure INFO/WEIGHT	per Measure KCAL	FAT	Nutrition Values per 100g / 100ml KCAL	PROT	CARB	FAT	FIBRE
Aero Chocolate, Nestle*	1 Pot/58g	101	3.0	174	4.8	27.3	5.1	1.1
Aero Twist Cappuccino & Chocolate, Nestle*	1 Pot/75g	135	8.1	180	4.2	16.8	10.8	0.2
Apricot, Lite, Onken*	1 Pot/150g	156	2.2	104	4.6	18.0	1.5	0.3
Banoffee, COU, M & S*	1 Pot/70g	101	1.5	145	2.9	28.8	2.1	1.5
Belgian Chocolate, Finest, Tesco*	1 Pot/120g	360	22.7	300	5.1	26.6	18.9	1.1
Belgian Chocolate & Vanilla, Weight Watchers*	1 Pot/80g	106	2.2	132	4.4	22.2	2.8	0.9
Black Cherry, Lite, Onken*	1 Pot/150g	156	2.2	104	4.6	17.9	1.5	0.2
Blackcurrant, Onken*	1 Pot/150g	210	10.2	140	5.2	14.6	6.8	0.0
Cadbury's Light Chocolate, St Ivel*	1 Pot/64g	79	2.0	123	6.2	17.3	3.2	0.0
Caramel, Meringue, Cadbury*	1 Pot/65g	181	6.7	277	4.6	42.4	10.3	1.0
Caramelised Orange, COU, M & S*	1 Pot/70g	91	1.2	130	2.8	26.3	1.7	3.4
Chocolate	1 Pot/60g	83	3.2	139	4.0	19.9	5.4	0.0
Chocolate, Cadbury*	1 Pot/55g	107	4.5	195	6.1	24.6	8.2	0.0
Chocolate, COU, M & S*	1 Pot/70g	84	1.9	120	5.2	20.3	2.7	1.0
Chocolate, Finest, Tesco*	1 Pot/82g	321	26.4	391	3.7	21.7	32.2	0.0
Chocolate, GFY, Asda*	1 Pot/60g	70	1.7	117	4.8	17.9	2.9	3.5
Chocolate, Healthy Selection, Low Fat, Somerfield*	1 Pot/60g	81	2.8	135	5.3	18.2	4.6	0.0
Chocolate, Light, Cadbury*	1 Pot/55g	60	1.9	110	4.6	14.2	3.4	0.0
Chocolate, Light Choices, Light Choices, Tesco*	1 Pot/63g	80	1.3	125	5.0	20.8	2.1	1.5
Chocolate, Low Fat, Danette, Danone*	1 Pot/60g	73	1.1	121	5.1	20.8	1.9	1.5
Chocolate, Minty, Bubbly, Dessert, Aero, Nestle*	1 Pot/58g	108	5.9	186	4.6	18.9	10.2	0.3
Chocolate, White, Bubbly, Dessert, Aero, Nestle*	1 Pot/58g	108	5.8	187	4.5	19.1	10.1	0.3
Chocolate & Hazelnut, Creamy, Dr Oetker*	1 Pot/115g	158	6.9	137	3.3	17.6	6.0	0.6
Chocolate & Hazelnut, Onken*	1 Pot/125g	171	7.5	137	3.3	17.8	6.0	0.0
Chocolate & Mint, COU, M & S*	1 Pot/70g	84	1.7	120	6.2	18.7	2.5	1.0
Chocolate & Orange, COU, M & S*	1 Pot/70g	77	1.8	110	5.9	16.0	2.6	0.9
Chocolate Orange, Low Fat, Cadbury*	1 Pot/100g	110	3.0	110	5.6	15.1	3.0	0.0
Dream, Cadbury*	1 Pot/53g	100	4.2	189	6.0	22.0	8.0	0.0
Fruit Juice, Shape, Danone*	1 Pot/100g	115	2.8	115	3.5	18.5	2.8	0.0
Lemon, Classic, Onken*	1 Pot/150g	210	9.4	140	5.1	15.8	6.3	0.0
Lemon, COU, M & S*	1 Pot/70g	80	2.4	115	2.9	19.4	3.5	3.5
Lemon, Dessert, Sainsbury's*	1 Pot/63g	114	5.9	182	3.6	20.7	9.4	0.6
Lemon, GFY, Asda*	1 Pot/63g	57	1.7	92	3.6	13.0	2.8	1.7
Lemon, HL, Tesco*	1 Pot/113g	94	2.9	83	3.6	11.3	2.6	0.2
Lemon, Less Than 3% Fat, BGTY, Sainsbury's*	1 Pot/62g	70	1.7	113	4.5	17.6	2.8	0.3
Lemon, Tesco*	1 Pot/60g	67	1.6	111	3.4	18.2	2.7	0.0
Lemon Fruit Juice, Shape, Danone*	1 Pot/100g	116	2.8	116	3.5	18.6	2.8	0.0
Lemon with Meringue Style Sauce, Ski, Nestle*	1 Pot/60g	82	2.9	137	3.1	19.8	4.8	0.0
Orange, Mango & Lime, Onken*	1 Pot/150g	207	9.4	138	5.1	15.3	6.3	0.1
Peach, Onken*	1 Pot/150g	204	9.4	136	5.1	15.1	6.3	0.2
Peach, Shape, Danone*	1 Pot/100g	43	1.8	43	3.0	3.9	1.8	0.1

	Measure INFO/WEIGHT	per Measure KCAL	FAT	Nutrition Values per 100g / 100ml KCAL	PROT	CARB	FAT	FIBRE
MOUSSE								
Peach & Passion Fruit, Perfectly Balanced, Waitrose*	1 Pot/95g	118	2.7	124	3.5	21.2	2.8	0.5
Pineapple, COU, M & S*	1 Pot/70g	84	1.7	120	3.3	20.7	2.4	3.5
Raspberry, Lite, Onken*	1 Pot/150g	156	2.2	104	4.6	17.3	1.5	0.1
Raspberry & Cranberry, Luxury, Weight Watchers*	1 Pot/80g	62	1.0	78	3.8	13.0	1.2	1.0
Rhubarb, COU, M & S*	1 Pot/70g	87	1.5	125	2.9	25.7	2.1	4.2
Rhubarb, Lite, Onken*	1 Pot/150g	154	2.2	103	4.6	17.8	1.5	0.3
Rhubarb & Vanilla, Onken*	1 Pot/150g	210	9.4	140	5.0	15.8	6.3	0.2
Strawberry, Asda*	1 Pot/64g	107	5.8	167	3.5	18.0	9.0	0.2
Strawberry, HL, Tesco*	1 Pot/114g	90	3.0	79	3.8	10.2	2.6	0.8
Strawberry, Light, Muller*	1 Pot/150g	147	0.6	98	4.3	19.4	0.4	0.0
Strawberry, Lite, Onken*	1 Pot/150g	151	2.2	101	4.6	17.2	1.5	0.1
Strawberry, Morrisons*	1 Pot/63g	106	5.9	170	3.5	17.6	9.5	0.2
Strawberry, Sainsbury's*	1 Pot/63g	106	5.9	168	3.4	17.5	9.4	0.1
Strawberry, Shape, Danone*	1 Pot/100g	44	1.8	44	3.0	4.0	1.8	0.0
Strawberry & Vanilla, Weight Watchers*	1 Pot/80g	87	1.9	109	3.7	18.1	2.4	0.4
Strawberry with Strawberry Sauce, Ski, Nestle*	1 Pot/60g	79	3.1	131	3.1	18.1	5.2	0.0
Summer Fruits, Light, Muller*	1 Pot/149g	143	0.6	96	4.3	18.7	0.4	0.0
Toffee, M & S*	1 Pot/90g	180	7.2	200	4.5	27.6	8.0	0.6
Vanilla, Finesse, Aero, Rowntree's*	1 Pot/57g	127	8.3	223	3.7	18.8	14.6	0.0
White Chocolate, Finest, Tesco*	1 Pot/92g	436	34.5	474	3.9	30.2	37.5	0.0
MUFFIN								
All Butter, M & S*	1 Muffin/65g	175	4.7	270	10.3	40.8	7.3	2.1
Apple, Sultana & Cinnamon, GFY, Asda*	1 Muffin/50g	134	1.7	268	6.0	53.0	3.5	3.9
Banana & Walnut, The Handmade Flapjack Company*	1 Muffin/135g	520	30.6	385	5.3	40.5	22.7	0.0
Banana Pecan, Organic, Honeyrose Bakery*	1 Muffin/110g	300	12.6	273	4.1	38.3	11.5	4.3
Berry Burst, Asda*	1 Muffin/60g	139	1.4	232	6.2	46.7	2.3	1.7
Blueberry, & Redcurrant, BGTY, Sainsbury's*	1 Muffin/65g	159	1.6	245	5.0	50.0	2.5	3.1
Blueberry, American Style, Sainsbury's*	1 Muffin/72g	256	13.1	355	5.1	42.7	18.2	1.9
Blueberry, Asda*	1 Muffin/77g	273	13.1	353	5.0	45.0	17.0	1.3
Blueberry, Big, Asda*	1 Muffin/105g	342	11.2	326	7.5	49.8	10.7	2.3
Blueberry, GFY, Asda*	1 Muffin/59g	146	1.3	249	6.0	51.0	2.3	3.0
Blueberry, M & S*	1 Muffin/75g	255	12.6	340	4.9	41.9	16.8	1.3
Blueberry, Mini, Sainsbury's*	1 Muffin/28g	82	2.3	293	6.3	48.9	8.1	1.9
Blueberry, Mini, Tesco*	1 Muffin/28g	104	5.4	370	5.6	43.5	19.3	1.2
Blueberry, Perfectly Balanced, Waitrose*	1 Muffin/100g	225	2.2	225	4.6	46.5	2.2	1.8
Blueberry, Tesco*	1 Muffin/73g	248	12.5	340	4.7	41.0	17.1	1.9
Blueberry, The Handmade Flapjack Company*	1 Muffin/135g	479	26.6	355	4.7	39.9	19.7	0.0
Blueberry, Waitrose*	1 Muffin/65g	239	9.2	367	4.7	55.2	14.2	1.7
Blueberry, Weight Watchers*	1 Muffin/63g	156	2.0	247	4.8	46.4	3.1	7.0
Blueberry, Wild Canadian, Fabulous Bakin' Boys*	1 Muffin/40g	140	8.0	349	4.0	39.0	20.0	1.0
Blueberry Buster, McVitie's*	1 Muffin/95g	408	22.4	429	4.3	49.9	23.6	1.1
Blueberry Mega, The Handmade Flapjack Company*	1 Muffin/135g	562	30.8	416	5.1	47.8	22.8	0.0
Bran, Average	1 Muffin/57g	155	4.4	272	7.8	45.6	7.7	7.7
Bran & Sultana, Weight Watchers*	1 Muffin/60g	144	1.3	240	4.5	50.7	2.1	2.3
Cappuccino Mega, The Handmade Flapjack Company*	1 Muffin/135g	653	40.0	484	14.0	48.4	29.6	0.0
Caramel, Cadbury*	1 Muffin/116g	535	30.3	461	5.9	50.8	26.1	0.0
Carrot, Asda*	1 Muffin/59g	138	1.4	233	6.0	47.0	2.3	1.6
Carrot Cake, Entenmann's*	1 Muffin/105g	344	15.9	328	5.1	45.8	15.1	3.0
Carrot Cakelet, The Handmade Flapjack Company*	1 Muffin/135g	479	23.9	355	4.0	45.1	17.7	0.0
Cheese, Tesco*	1 Muffin/67g	150	1.9	224	13.0	36.4	2.9	3.0
Cheese & Black Pepper, TTD, Sainsbury's*	1 Muffin/67g	164	4.4	245	13.1	33.5	6.5	2.7
Cherry, The Handmade Flapjack Company*	1 Muffin/135g	499	26.6	370	4.6	43.8	19.7	0.0
Cherry Bakewell, Mr Kipling*	1 Muffin/100g	355	19.6	355	5.0	55.0	19.6	1.4

MUFFIN

MUFFIN	Measure INFO/WEIGHT	per Measure		Nutrition Values per 100g / 100ml				
		KCAL	FAT	KCAL	PROT	CARB	FAT	FIBRE
Cherry Mega, The Handmade Flapjack Company*	1 Muffin/135g	506	26.7	375	4.4	44.8	19.8	0.0
Choc Chip, Mini, Weight Watchers*	1 Muffin/15g	47	1.3	312	6.6	52.1	8.6	3.1
Chocolate, Galaxy, McVitie's*	1 Muffin/88g	319	17.1	364	5.0	44.5	19.5	0.0
Chocolate, HL, Tesco*	1 Muffin/71g	204	6.2	288	5.5	46.9	8.7	5.5
Chocolate, The Handmade Flapjack Company*	1 Muffin/135g	526	30.8	390	5.3	41.5	22.8	0.0
Chocolate Chip, American Style, Sainsbury's*	1 Muffin/72g	284	14.4	395	5.0	48.8	20.0	2.1
Chocolate Chip, BGTY, Sainsbury's*	1 Muffin/75g	282	12.3	376	5.2	51.8	16.4	1.6
Chocolate Chip, Blackfriars*	1 Muffin/50g	217	11.5	435	6.0	51.0	23.0	4.0
Chocolate Chip, Mini, Asda*	1 Muffin/22g	77	2.9	349	7.0	51.0	13.0	2.1
Chocolate Chip, Mini, BGTY, Sainsbury's*	1 Muffin/28g	91	2.4	324	6.5	55.1	8.7	1.6
Chocolate Chip, Plain, Tesco*	1 Muffin/72g	270	12.7	375	5.0	48.1	17.6	1.4
Chocolate Indulgence, McVitie's*	1 Muffin/75g	253	6.9	338	5.8	57.9	9.2	1.3
Chunky Chocolate Chip, McVitie's*	1 Muffin/94g	393	20.3	418	5.3	50.6	21.6	0.8
Cinnamon & Sultana, Morrisons*	1 Muffin/75g	183	1.0	244	8.3	48.2	1.4	2.9
Cranberry & White Chocolate, Sainsbury's*	1 Muffin/72g	253	13.3	352	5.7	40.7	18.5	1.5
Deeply Fruity, Belgian Chocolate & Forest Fruits, Waitrose*	1 Muffin/125g	451	23.0	361	5.4	43.3	18.4	0.5
Double Berry Burst, Entenmann's*	1 Muffin/59g	140	1.2	238	4.6	50.1	2.1	1.6
Double Choc Chip, Weight Watchers*	1 Muffin/65g	189	5.4	291	6.8	47.2	8.3	3.6
Double Chocolate, 95% Fat Free, Entenmann's*	1 Muffin/58g	152	2.7	262	2.6	52.3	4.7	1.8
Double Chocolate, Chocolate Chip, Mini, Tesco*	1 Muffin/28g	116	6.4	414	6.3	45.7	23.0	1.4
Double Chocolate, Free From, Tesco*	1 Muffin/70g	281	12.7	402	4.7	54.8	18.2	1.7
Double Chocolate, Mini, M & S*	1 Muffin/32g	133	6.9	416	5.4	49.8	21.7	1.1
Double Chocolate, Somerfield*	1 Muffin/70g	297	16.4	425	6.8	46.5	23.5	0.0
Double Chocolate Chip, American Style, Sainsbury's*	1 Muffin/72g	276	14.6	384	5.2	45.0	20.3	2.9
Double Chocolate Chip, Co-Op*	1 Muffin/60g	246	12.6	410	6.0	49.0	21.0	3.0
Double Chocolate Chip, Co-Op*	1 Muffin/70g	308	16.8	440	6.6	49.4	24.0	2.5
Double Chocolate Chip, Mini, Asda*	1 Muffin/19g	76	3.7	400	7.4	48.5	19.6	2.7
Double Chocolate Chip, Mini, Weight Watchers*	1 Muffin/15g	45	1.3	300	7.0	48.5	8.7	3.5
Double Chocolate Chip, Tesco*	1 Muffin/100g	360	17.9	360	6.1	44.9	17.9	5.4
English	1 Muffin/57g	120	1.0	211	7.0	43.9	1.8	1.8
English, Butter, Tesco*	1 Muffin/67g	170	3.6	253	11.2	39.8	5.4	2.0
English, Gluten, Wheat & Milk Free, Free From, Livwell*	1 Muffin/50g	160	4.9	320	4.6	52.8	9.8	3.2
English, Kingsmill*	1 Muffin/75g	167	1.4	222	9.7	40.4	1.8	2.6
English, Plain, Oakrun Bakery*	1 Muffin/57g	139	1.0	244	8.4	47.4	1.8	1.4
Family, Irwin's Bakery*	1 Muffin/40g	116	2.5	291	8.9	50.0	6.2	0.0
Finger, Double Chocolate, Bakers Delight*	1 Muffin/25g	104	4.6	416	5.8	56.9	18.4	1.7
Fruit, Spiced, TTD, Sainsbury's*	1 Muffin/70g	181	3.6	259	10.1	43.1	5.1	2.1
Lemon, Boots*	1 Muffin/110g	423	20.9	385	3.6	50.0	19.0	1.3
Lemon & Blueberry, Tesco*	1 Muffin/110g	411	23.0	374	4.0	42.4	20.9	1.1
Lemon & Poppy Seed, Entenmann's*	1 Muffin/105g	417	20.3	397	5.6	52.8	19.3	2.5
Lemon & Poppy Seed, M & S*	1 Muffin/72g	281	14.3	390	6.3	46.1	19.8	1.5
Lemon & Sultana, BGTY, Sainsbury's*	1 Muffin/75g	211	3.4	281	4.5	55.6	4.5	1.4
Lunchbox, Double Chocolate, The Fabulous Bakin' Boys*	1 Muffin/54g	218	11.8	404	5.6	46.3	21.8	1.0
Mini, Tesco*	1 Muffin/28g	120	6.3	428	6.4	50.0	22.6	1.2
Mixed Fruit, Low Fat, Abbey Bakery*	1 Muffin/35g	93	1.6	267	4.5	55.6	4.5	1.4
Morning Sunrise, Ryvita*	1 Muffin/110g	330	10.0	300	4.5	49.1	9.1	1.8
Muesli, Breakfast, Love Life, Waitrose*	1 Muffin/68g	216	6.2	318	9.1	50.0	9.1	3.4
Muesli, Sainsbury's*	1 Muffin/113g	447	25.7	396	6.3	41.5	22.7	1.4
Orange, Apricot & Almond, Organic, Honeyrose Bakery*	1 Muffin/110g	312	11.4	284	3.5	44.2	10.4	1.9
Oven Bottom, Asda*	1 Muffin/68g	173	1.0	255	10.0	50.4	1.5	2.2
Oven Bottom, Mini, Morrisons*	1 Muffin/42g	107	0.6	255	10.0	50.4	1.5	2.2
Oven Bottom, Tesco*	1 Muffin/68g	173	1.0	255	10.0	50.4	1.5	2.2
Oven Bottom, Warburton's*	1 Muffin/69g	175	2.0	253	10.9	45.8	2.9	0.0

	Measure INFO/WEIGHT	per Measure		Nutrition Values per 100g / 100ml				
		KCAL	FAT	KCAL	PROT	CARB	FAT	FIBRE
MUFFIN								
Plain, Co-Op*	1 Muffin/60g	135	1.1	225	11.2	41.3	1.9	2.4
Plain, Prepared From Recipe, Average	1 Muffin/57g	169	6.5	296	6.9	41.4	11.4	2.7
Raspberry, Perfectly Balanced, Waitrose*	1 Muffin/101g	220	2.1	219	4.7	45.4	2.1	3.7
Raspberry Cream, Sainsbury's*	1 Muffin/90g	314	19.8	349	3.9	33.8	22.0	1.3
Raspberry Injected, The Handmade Flapjack Company*	1 Muffin/135g	564	27.3	418	4.5	54.7	20.2	0.0
Rolo, Nestle*	1 Muffin/80g	289	14.4	361	5.4	44.3	18.0	0.8
Sausage, Egg & Cheese, American Style, Tesco*	1 Muffin/155g	383	20.5	247	12.2	19.9	13.2	1.0
Spiced Fruit, Co-Op*	1 Muffin/60g	159	1.2	265	11.0	52.0	2.0	3.0
Spicy Fruit, Quality Bakers*	1 Muffin/65g	146	1.0	225	9.4	38.0	1.5	3.3
Strawberry Cakelet, The Handmade Flapjack Company*	1 Muffin/135g	526	29.6	390	4.5	43.6	21.9	0.0
Sunblest*	1 Muffin/72g	166	1.3	230	9.6	43.9	1.8	2.2
Toasting, Warburton's*	1 Muffin/64g	138	1.0	216	8.9	41.4	1.6	2.9
Toffee, GFY, Asda*	1 Muffin/90g	151	2.3	168	2.1	34.0	2.6	0.0
Toffee, The Handmade Flapjack Company*	1 Muffin/135g	533	31.6	395	4.4	41.2	23.4	0.0
Toffee & Pecan, Finest, Tesco*	1 Muffin/127g	551	29.0	434	5.4	51.8	22.8	0.9
Toffee Choo Choo, Tesco*	1 Muffin/95g	402	21.3	423	6.4	49.1	22.4	1.0
Toffee Mega, The Handmade Flapjack Company*	1 Muffin/135g	567	34.7	420	4.5	43.2	25.7	0.0
Toffee Temptation, McVitie's*	1 Muffin/86g	297	8.1	347	4.7	60.8	9.5	0.8
Triple Chocolate, Triumph, Fabulous Bakin' Boys*	1 Muffin/40g	160	9.6	400	4.5	42.0	24.0	0.0
Truly Madly Chocolate, Fabulous Bakin' Boys*	1 Muffin/105g	405	23.1	386	5.0	41.0	22.0	2.0
Vanilla & Choc Chip, GFY, Asda*	1 Muffin/59g	152	1.3	260	7.0	53.0	2.2	1.6
White, All Butter, Sainsbury's*	1 Muffin/67g	173	4.2	258	10.6	39.6	6.3	3.6
White, Asda*	1 Muffin/67g	148	1.3	222	11.0	40.0	2.0	2.5
White, Finest, Tesco*	1 Muffin/70g	159	0.8	227	8.4	45.7	1.2	2.1
White, M & S*	1 Muffin/60g	135	1.1	225	11.2	43.7	1.9	2.9
White, Tesco*	1 Muffin/72g	173	2.3	240	11.3	41.6	3.2	2.8
White Chocolate & Strawberry Filled, Tesco*	1 Muffin/103g	415	20.3	405	5.2	51.3	19.8	1.3
White Chocolate Chunk Lemon, Mini, M & S*	1 Muffin/28g	130	6.7	464	6.4	55.4	23.9	2.1
Wholemeal, Tesco*	1 Muffin/65g	130	1.3	200	12.6	32.9	2.0	5.7
MULBERRIES								
Raw	*1oz/28g*	*10*	*0.0*	*36*	*1.3*	*8.1*	*0.0*	*0.0*
MULLET								
Grey, Grilled	*1oz/28g*	*42*	*1.5*	*150*	*25.7*	*0.0*	*5.2*	*0.0*
Grey, Raw	*1oz/28g*	*32*	*1.1*	*115*	*19.8*	*0.0*	*4.0*	*0.0*
Red, Grilled	*1oz/28g*	*34*	*1.2*	*121*	*20.4*	*0.0*	*4.4*	*0.0*
Red, Raw, Weighed Whole, Flesh Only	*1 Portion/100g*	*109*	*3.8*	*109*	*18.7*	*0.0*	*3.8*	*0.0*
MUNCHIES								
Mint, Nestle*	1 Pack/62g	267	10.1	432	3.8	67.5	16.4	0.0
Original, Tube, Nestle*	1 Pack/55g	272	13.3	498	4.1	65.6	24.4	0.5
MUSHROOMS								
Breaded, Average	*3 Mushrooms/51g*	*77*	*2.9*	*151*	*4.3*	*20.8*	*5.7*	*0.6*
Breaded, Garlic, Average	3 Mushrooms/50g	92	4.9	183	5.2	18.7	9.7	1.7
Buna Shimeji, Livesey Brothers*	½ Pack/75g	29	0.3	39	2.7	5.9	0.4	1.2
Button, Average	*1 Serving/50g*	*7*	*0.2*	*15*	*2.3*	*0.5*	*0.4*	*1.2*
Cheesey, Stuffed, Asda*	1 Serving/290g	322	17.4	111	4.3	10.0	6.0	0.0
Chestnut, Average	*1 Med/5g*	*1*	*0.0*	*13*	*1.8*	*0.4*	*0.5*	*0.5*
Chinese, Dried, Raw	*1oz/28g*	*80*	*0.5*	*284*	*10.0*	*59.9*	*1.8*	*0.0*
Closed Cup, Average	*1oz/28g*	*4*	*0.1*	*13*	*1.8*	*0.4*	*0.5*	*1.1*
Common, Boiled in Salted Water, Average	*1oz/28g*	*3*	*0.1*	*11*	*1.8*	*0.4*	*0.3*	*1.1*
Common, Fried, Average	*1oz/28g*	*44*	*4.5*	*157*	*2.4*	*0.3*	*16.2*	*1.5*
Common, Raw, Average	*1 Serving/80g*	*10*	*0.4*	*13*	*1.9*	*0.3*	*0.5*	*1.1*

	Measure INFO/WEIGHT	per Measure		Nutrition Values per 100g / 100ml				
		KCAL	FAT	KCAL	PROT	CARB	FAT	FIBRE
MUSHROOMS								
Creamed, Average	*1oz/28g*	*23*	*1.5*	*82*	*1.3*	*6.8*	*5.5*	*0.5*
Crispy, M & S*	1 Serving/130g	390	33.4	300	4.2	12.5	25.7	1.8
Dried	*1oz/28g*	*45*	*1.7*	*159*	*21.8*	*4.8*	*6.0*	*13.3*
Enoki, Average	*1 Serving/80g*	*34*	*0.0*	*42*	*3.0*	*7.0*	*0.0*	*3.0*
Flat, Large, Average	*1 Mushroom/52g*	*10*	*0.3*	*19*	*3.3*	*0.5*	*0.5*	*0.7*
Frozen, Cooks' Ingredients, Waitrose*	1 Portion/75g	13	0.2	18	2.1	1.8	0.3	2.5
Garlic, Average	½ Pack/150g	159	14.0	106	2.1	3.7	9.3	1.7
Hon Shimeji, Sainsbury's*	1 Serving/80g	18	0.4	22	4.0	3.9	0.5	1.1
Medley, Asda*	½ Pack/100g	89	7.8	89	3.2	1.4	7.8	2.8
Oyster, Average	*1 Serving/80g*	*12*	*0.2*	*15*	*1.6*	*1.6*	*0.2*	*1.3*
Porcini, Dried, Asda*	1 Bag/25g	65	1.2	260	30.4	24.1	4.7	17.5
Porcini, Wild, Dried, Merchant Gourmet*	1 Pack/25g	66	0.8	265	27.9	30.6	3.4	18.7
Shiitake, Cooked	*1oz/28g*	*15*	*0.1*	*55*	*1.6*	*12.3*	*0.2*	*0.0*
Shiitake, Dried, Raw	*1oz/28g*	*83*	*0.3*	*296*	*9.6*	*63.9*	*1.0*	*0.0*
Sliced, Average	*1oz/28g*	*3*	*0.1*	*12*	*1.8*	*0.4*	*0.3*	*1.1*
Sliced, Canned in Water, Drained, Value, Tesco*	½ Can/78g	8	0.2	10	1.6	0.2	0.3	2.2
Straw, Canned, Drained	*1oz/28g*	*4*	*0.1*	*15*	*2.1*	*1.2*	*0.2*	*0.0*
MUSSELS								
Boiled, Flesh Only, Average	1 Mussel/2g	2	0.1	104	16.7	3.5	2.7	0.0
Boiled, Weighed in Shell, Average	*1 Mussel/7g*	*7*	*0.2*	*104*	*16.7*	*3.5*	*2.7*	*0.0*
Cooked & Shelled, Meat, Tesco*	1 Pack/240g	216	5.0	90	13.9	3.8	2.1	0.0
Pickled, Drained, Average	*1oz/28g*	*31*	*0.6*	*112*	*20.0*	*1.5*	*2.2*	*0.0*
Raw, Weighed in Shell, Average	*1oz/28g*	*24*	*0.7*	*87*	*12.7*	*3.6*	*2.5*	*0.2*
MUSSELS IN								
Creamy Garlic Butter Sauce, Bantry Bay*	1 Serving/225g	198	7.9	88	9.0	5.2	3.5	0.6
Garlic Butter Sauce, Average	½ Pack/225g	179	11.5	79	6.3	1.9	5.1	0.1
Seasoned White Wine Sauce, Bantry Bay*	1 Serving/450g	270	9.0	60	6.3	4.1	2.0	0.1
Thai Sauce, Scottish, Waitrose*	1 Serving/250g	135	6.2	54	5.4	2.6	2.5	0.6
White Wine, Cream, Shallot & Garlic Sauce, COOK!, M & S*	1 Pack/450g	360	12.6	80	11.7	1.6	2.8	2.1
White Wine Cream Sauce, Cooked, Scottish, Morrisons*	½ Pack/250g	222	9.2	89	8.0	5.8	3.7	0.0
White Wine Sauce, Sainsbury's*	½ Pack/250g	221	9.2	88	8.0	5.8	3.7	0.0
MUSTARD								
American, Average	*1 Tsp/5g*	*5*	*0.2*	*102*	*4.4*	*10.5*	*5.0*	*2.5*
Cajun, Colman's*	1 Tsp/6g	11	0.4	187	7.0	23.0	6.5	2.7
Coarse Grain, Average	*1 Tsp/5g*	*7*	*0.4*	*141*	*7.7*	*8.4*	*8.3*	*5.9*
Dijon, Average	*1 Tsp/5g*	*8*	*0.6*	*163*	*7.4*	*7.7*	*11.3*	*1.1*
English, Average	*1 Tsp/5g*	*9*	*0.4*	*173*	*6.8*	*19.2*	*7.6*	*1.2*
English with Chillies, Sainsbury's*	1 Tsp/5g	10	0.5	204	8.3	18.1	10.9	6.4
French, Average	*1 Tsp/5g*	*5*	*0.3*	*105*	*5.4*	*8.1*	*5.6*	*1.8*
German Style, Sainsbury's*	1 Serving/10g	9	0.6	92	5.5	2.8	6.5	0.0
Honey, Colman's*	1 Tsp/6g	12	0.5	208	7.4	24.0	8.2	0.0
Powder, Average	*1 Tsp/3g*	*15*	*0.9*	*452*	*28.9*	*20.7*	*28.7*	*0.0*
Powder, Made Up, Average	*1oz/28g*	*63*	*4.0*	*226*	*14.5*	*10.4*	*14.4*	*0.0*
Smooth, Average	*1 Tsp/8g*	*11*	*0.7*	*139*	*7.1*	*9.7*	*8.2*	*0.0*
Sweet Peppers, Colman's*	1 Tsp/6g	13	0.7	218	7.9	20.0	11.0	4.9
Whole Grain, Average	*1 Tsp/8g*	*11*	*0.8*	*140*	*8.2*	*4.2*	*10.2*	*4.9*
Whole Grain with Green Peppercorns, Finest, Tesco*	1 Serving/20g	41	1.9	205	7.9	22.0	9.5	3.3
Yellow, Prepared	*1 Tbsp/15ml*	*11*	*0.6*	*73*	*4.0*	*6.0*	*4.0*	*0.0*
MUSTARD CRESS								
Raw	*1oz/28g*	*4*	*0.2*	*13*	*1.6*	*0.4*	*0.6*	*1.1*
MUTTON								
Lean, Raw, Average*	1 Serving/100g	236	13.4	236	17.9	0.1	13.4	0.0

	Measure INFO/WEIGHT	per Measure KCAL	per Measure FAT	Nutrition Values per 100g / 100ml KCAL	PROT	CARB	FAT	FIBRE
NACHOS								
American Chilli Beef, Asda*	1 Serving/200g	208	10.0	104	10.0	4.7	5.0	0.8
Cheesy with Salsa & Soured Cream, Sainsbury's*	½ Pack/170g	449	26.9	264	8.8	21.5	15.8	1.4
Chilli, Sainsbury's*	½ Pack/250g	695	32.2	278	10.9	29.5	12.9	1.3
Kit, Old El Paso*	½ Pack/260g	598	26.0	230	4.0	31.0	10.0	0.0
NASI GORENG								
Indonesian, Asda*	1 Pack/360g	778	22.7	216	7.4	32.3	6.3	1.3
NECTARINES								
Fresh, Raw, Weighed with Stone, Average	*1 Med/140g*	*53*	*0.1*	*38*	*1.3*	*8.5*	*0.1*	*1.1*
NESQUIK								
Chocolate Flavour, Powder, Dry Weight, Nesquik, Nestle*	1 Serving/15g	56	0.5	372	3.0	82.9	3.1	6.5
Strawberry Flavour, Powder, Dry Weight, Nesquik, Nestle*	1 Serving/15g	59	0.0	393	0.0	98.1	0.0	0.0
Strawberry Milk, Fresh, Nesquik, Nestle*	1 Glass/250g	175	4.0	70	3.3	10.4	1.6	0.3
NIK NAKS								
Cream 'n' Cheesy, KP Snacks*	1 Bag/34g	195	13.0	575	5.2	52.7	38.1	0.2
Nice 'n' Spicy, KP Snacks*	1 Bag/30g	171	11.5	571	4.6	51.6	38.4	1.6
Rib 'n' Saucy, Golden Wonder*	1 Bag/34g	194	12.8	571	4.5	53.7	37.6	0.5
Scampi & Lemon, KP Snacks*	1 Bag/25g	141	9.6	564	5.2	49.6	38.4	3.2
Scampi 'n' Lemon, KP Snacks*	1 Bag/34g	195	12.7	573	4.9	53.1	37.5	0.1
NOODLES								
Add to Wok Whole Wheat, Chef Kuo*	1 Serving/150g	236	0.6	157	4.6	28.6	0.4	2.6
Barbecue Beef, Instant, Asda*	1 Pack/333g	420	16.0	126	2.6	18.0	4.8	0.0
Beef, Oriental, GFY, Asda*	1 Pack/400g	372	6.8	93	7.4	12.1	1.7	1.7
Beef Flavour, Instant, Prepared, Heinz*	1 Pack/384g	257	0.4	67	2.1	14.4	0.1	0.6
Buckwheat, Cold, Famima*	1 Pack/295g	163	3.0	55	4.7	9.5	1.0	0.7
Cellophane, Glass, Dry Weight	1 Serving/100g	351	0.1	351	0.1	86.1	0.1	0.5
Char Sui, Cantonese, Sainsbury's*	1 Pack/450g	378	7.2	84	6.8	10.5	1.6	1.5
Chicken, Chinese, Asda*	1 Pot/302g	305	4.2	101	6.0	16.0	1.4	0.8
Chicken, Chinese Style, GFY, Asda*	1 Pack/393g	295	6.7	75	6.0	9.0	1.7	0.6
Chicken, Dry Weight, Heinz*	1 Pack/85g	257	0.3	302	9.5	65.3	0.4	2.7
Chicken, Instant, Less Than 1% Fat, Prepared, Heinz*	1 Pack/385g	258	0.4	67	2.1	14.4	0.1	0.6
Chicken, Instant, Weight Watchers*	1 Pack/385g	269	0.4	70	2.3	14.9	0.1	0.6
Chicken & Coconut & Lime, Simply Fuller Longer, M & S*	1 Pack/390g	448	17.5	115	8.7	10.0	4.5	1.6
Chicken & Red Thai, Easy Steam, Tesco*	1 Serving/400g	556	28.4	139	10.3	8.6	7.1	1.1
Chicken Curry Flavour, Instant, Sainsbury's*	1 Pack/85g	167	6.2	196	4.6	27.9	7.3	0.8
Chicken Flavour, 3 Minute, Dry, Blue Dragon*	1 Pack/85g	403	18.2	475	9.3	61.2	21.4	0.0
Chicken Flavour, Dry, Eldorado*	1 Pack/85g	360	12.7	423	14.0	61.0	15.0	0.0
Chicken Flavour, Dry, Princes*	1 Pack/85g	395	16.0	465	10.0	63.8	18.8	0.0
Chicken Flavour, Instant, Sainsbury's*	1 Pack/335g	549	21.4	164	4.4	22.3	6.4	1.3
Chicken Flavour, Value, Made Up, Tesco*	1 Serving/265g	450	16.7	170	4.1	23.7	6.3	1.5
Chilli Beef, Finest, Tesco*	1 Pack/450g	486	8.5	108	7.7	15.2	1.9	0.9
Chilli Chicken, GFY, Asda*	1 Pack/415g	461	3.3	111	6.0	20.0	0.8	1.0
Chilli Chicken, Tesco*	1 Pack/385g	545	15.7	142	6.4	19.5	4.1	1.4
Chinese Pork, Chosen By You, Asda*	1 Pack/400g	380	6.4	95	6.7	12.6	1.6	1.8
Chow Mein, Dry Weight, Snack in a Pot, HL, Tesco*	1 Pot/56g	202	0.8	360	13.4	72.2	1.4	5.0
Chow Mein, Instant, Made Up, Tesco*	1 Pack/168g	255	8.4	152	3.8	23.0	5.0	1.2
Chow Mein, Sainsbury's*	1 Pack/125g	136	2.2	109	3.9	19.2	1.8	0.8
Chow Mein, Snack in a Pot, Light Choices, Tesco*	1 Pot/235g	235	1.2	100	3.7	19.4	0.5	1.8
Chow Mein, Stir Fry, Tesco*	1 Serving/200g	116	2.4	58	2.1	9.7	1.2	1.0
Chow Mein Flavour, Dry, Princes*	1 Pack/85g	396	15.8	466	10.1	64.6	18.6	0.0
Crab Flavour, Dry, 3 Minute, Blue Dragon*	1 Pack/85g	393	16.3	463	9.9	62.6	19.2	0.0
Crispy, Dry, Blue Dragon*	1 Box/125g	437	0.6	350	2.4	84.0	0.5	0.0
Curry, Instant, Dry, Hoinz*	1 Serving/85g	261	0.3	307	9.5	66.4	0.4	2.7
Curry, Mealpack, All About Weight*	1 Pack/37g	152	7.5	416	35.0	22.4	20.6	5.0

NOODLES

INFO/WEIGHT	Measure	per Measure		Nutrition Values per 100g / 100ml				
		KCAL	FAT	KCAL	PROT	CARB	FAT	FIBRE
Curry Flavour, Instant, Dry, Asda*	1 Serving/65g	415	11.0	638	20.0	101.5	16.9	0.9
Curry Flavour, Instant, from Heinz, Weight Watchers*	1 Pack/385g	266	0.4	69	2.2	14.8	0.1	0.6
Curry Flavour, Instant, Sainsbury's*	1 Pack/335g	412	15.4	123	2.6	17.8	4.6	0.1
Curry Flavour, Instant, Value, Made Up, Tesco*	1 Pack/65g	83	2.4	127	3.1	20.3	3.7	0.8
Egg, Boiled	*1oz/28g*	*17*	*0.1*	*62*	*2.2*	*13.0*	*0.5*	*0.6*
Egg, Dry	*1 Block/63g*	*217*	*1.2*	*348*	*12.1*	*70.1*	*1.9*	*2.6*
Egg, Fine, Blue Dragon*	1 Serving/100g	356	1.7	356	13.8	70.0	1.7	3.4
Egg, Fine, Dry Weight, Sharwood's*	1 Block/63g	216	1.3	346	12.0	70.0	2.1	2.5
Egg, Fine, Fresh, M & S*	1 Pack/275g	330	6.0	120	4.4	20.7	2.2	1.5
Egg, Fine Thread, Dry, M & S*	1 Serving/63g	220	0.6	350	14.3	71.6	0.9	5.1
Egg, Free Range, Asda*	1 Serving/125g	205	4.9	164	5.1	27.0	3.9	1.8
Egg, Fresh, Just Stir Fry, Sainsbury's*	½ Pack/192g	314	6.5	163	5.0	28.1	3.4	1.8
Egg, Fresh, Tesco*	½ Pack/205g	287	3.9	140	4.9	25.3	1.9	2.0
Egg, Medium, Dry, Blue Dragon*	1 Serving/81g	288	1.4	356	13.8	70.0	1.7	3.4
Egg, Medium, Dry, Sharwood's*	1 Serving/63g	216	1.3	346	12.0	70.0	2.1	2.5
Egg, Medium, Sainsbury's*	1 Serving/122g	168	1.0	138	5.7	26.9	0.8	1.0
Egg, Ramen, Fresh, The Original Noodle Company*	1 Serving/63g	186	1.7	298	11.3	57.0	2.7	0.0
Egg, Raw, Medium, Waitrose*	¼ Pack/63g	221	1.6	353	15.0	67.3	2.6	3.8
Egg, Thick, Dry Weight, Sharwood's*	1 Serving/63g	214	1.1	342	10.8	71.0	1.7	2.5
Egg, Tossed in Sesame Oil, Asda*	½ Pack/150g	174	10.5	116	2.3	11.0	7.0	0.6
Egg & Bean Sprouts, Cooked, Tesco*	1 Pack/250g	237	5.2	95	4.4	14.6	2.1	1.5
Fried, Average	*1oz/28g*	*43*	*3.2*	*153*	*1.9*	*11.3*	*11.5*	*0.5*
Garlic, Chilli & Ginger, Tesco*	1 Serving/350g	507	11.2	145	4.8	24.1	3.2	2.6
Hoisin, Vegelicious, Tesco*	1 Pack/400g	440	6.8	110	4.4	18.1	1.7	1.9
Instant, Dry, Sainsbury's*	1 Pack/100g	392	14.0	392	9.4	57.0	14.0	0.2
Instant, Express, Dry, Blue Dragon*	1 Serving/75g	337	12.7	450	10.0	65.0	17.0	2.0
Instant, Value, Tesco*	1 Packet/265g	334	9.0	126	3.2	20.7	3.4	0.9
Japanese Udon, Sainsbury's*	1 Serving/150g	210	2.7	140	3.9	27.1	1.8	1.2
Meal For One, Singapore Chicken, Chosen By You, Asda*	1 Pack/400g	348	10.0	87	7.0	8.4	2.5	1.6
Medium, Egg, Dry Nests, Cooks' Ingredients, Waitrose*	1 Nest/54g	189	0.9	350	13.1	70.4	1.7	2.4
Medium, Traditional, Straight to Wok, Amoy*	1 Serving/150g	243	2.2	162	4.3	34.3	1.5	1.3
Nest, Medium, Cooked, Waitrose*	1 Nest/63g	88	0.3	139	5.0	28.6	0.5	0.6
Oriental, Chinese, Tesco*	1 Pack/200g	184	5.0	92	2.8	14.7	2.5	1.0
Oriental, Snack Pot, Dry, HL, Tesco*	1 Pot/57g	210	1.0	369	14.0	74.4	1.7	2.0
Oriental, Snack Pot, Made Up, HL, Tesco*	1 Serving/238g	221	0.7	93	3.1	19.4	0.3	0.6
Pad Thai, Ribbon, Ready to Wok, Sharwood's*	1 Serving/150g	206	1.6	137	5.0	26.3	1.1	1.0
Peking Duck, Shapers, Boots*	1 Pack/280g	395	3.9	141	7.2	25.0	1.4	1.8
Plain, Boiled	*1oz/28g*	*17*	*0.1*	*62*	*2.4*	*13.0*	*0.4*	*0.7*
Plain, Dry	*1oz/28g*	*109*	*1.7*	*388*	*11.7*	*76.1*	*6.2*	*2.9*
Ribbon, Thai Style, Ready to Wok, Sharwood's*	1 Pack/150g	205	1.6	137	5.0	26.3	1.1	1.0
Rice, Brown, 100%, Organic, King Soba*	1 Pack/83g	252	2.0	303	6.0	64.4	2.4	0.0
Rice, Cooked	1 Cup/176g	192	0.4	109	0.9	24.9	0.2	1.0
Rice, Cooked, Sharwood's*	1 Serving/200g	239	0.6	119	2.0	27.1	0.3	0.7
Rice, Dry, Blue Dragon*	1 Serving/30g	113	0.0	376	7.0	84.0	0.0	0.0
Rice, Medium, Blue Dragon*	1 Serving/63g	235	0.0	376	7.0	84.0	0.0	0.0
Rice, Oriental, Thai, Stir Fry, Dry Weight, Sharwood's*	1 Serving/63g	226	0.6	361	6.5	86.8	1.0	2.4
Rice, Stir Fry, Tesco*	½ Pack/190g	304	10.8	160	2.0	24.8	5.7	1.0
Rice, Thai, Wheat & Gluten Free, King Soba Noodles*	1 Serving/55g	193	0.8	351	8.9	75.6	1.4	0.0
Savoury Vegetable, COU, M & S*	1 Pack/450g	270	2.7	60	2.9	11.5	0.6	1.2
Shanghai Beef, COU, M & S*	1 Pack/400g	380	6.4	95	6.8	13.1	1.6	1.5
Singapore, BGTY, Sainsbury's*	1 Pack/369g	317	10.0	86	7.2	8.2	2.7	2.1
Singapore, Light Choices, Tesco*	1 Pack/450g	337	7.6	75	4.8	9.8	1.7	1.2
Singapore, Sainsbury's*	1 Pack/400g	368	6.8	92	7.5	11.6	1.7	0.9

	Measure INFO/WEIGHT	per Measure KCAL	per Measure FAT	Nutrition Values per 100g / 100ml KCAL	PROT	CARB	FAT	FIBRE
NOODLES								
Singapore, Waitrose*	1 Pack/400g	476	17.6	119	7.3	12.6	4.4	2.1
Singapore, You Count, Love Life, Waitrose*	1 Pot/260g	243	5.0	97	5.4	13.3	2.0	2.1
Singapore Style, Asda*	1 Pack/400g	688	32.0	172	7.0	18.0	8.0	1.0
Special, Chinese Takeaway, Iceland*	1 Pack/340g	422	10.9	124	6.5	17.2	3.2	0.6
Spicy, Sainsbury's*	1 Serving/180g	182	8.3	101	10.4	4.5	4.6	0.9
Spicy Thai, Instant, Heinz*	1 Pack/385g	262	0.4	68	2.1	14.6	0.1	0.6
Stir Fry, Tesco*	1 Serving/150g	202	3.6	135	5.3	23.0	2.4	1.5
Straight to Wok, Medium, Amoy*	1 Pack/150g	240	2.2	160	5.8	31.7	1.5	0.0
Straight to Wok, Rice, Amoy*	1 Pack/150g	174	0.1	116	1.6	27.4	0.1	0.0
Straight to Wok, Singapore, Amoy*	1 Serving/150g	232	4.2	155	4.8	28.4	2.8	0.0
Straight to Wok, Thread, Fine, Amoy*	1 Pack/150g	237	3.9	158	5.0	28.7	2.6	0.0
Straight to Wok, Udon, Amoy*	1 Pack/150g	211	1.9	141	4.4	28.8	1.3	0.0
Super, Bacon Flavour, Dry Weight, Batchelors*	1 Packet/100g	526	23.6	526	9.4	69.2	23.6	1.6
Super, Barbecue Beef, Made Up, Batchelors*	1 Serving/100g	156	6.7	156	3.2	20.9	6.7	1.1
Super, Barbecue Beef, to Go, 98% Fat Free, Batchelors*	1 Pack/380g	308	0.6	81	2.4	17.5	0.2	0.6
Super, Cheese & Ham, Made Up, Batchelors*	1 Serving/100g	171	7.3	171	3.4	22.9	7.3	0.6
Super, Chicken & Ham, Dry Weight, Batchelors*	1 Pack/100g	472	20.2	472	9.4	63.2	20.2	1.5
Super, Chicken & Herb, Low Fat, Dry Weight, Batchelors*	½ Pack/43g	161	0.8	379	12.2	78.3	1.9	2.3
Super, Chicken & Herb, Low Fat, Made Up, Batchelors*	1 Pack/170g	322	1.6	189	6.1	39.2	0.9	1.2
Super, Chicken Flavour, Dry Weight, Batchelors*	1 Serving/100g	449	19.2	449	8.7	60.3	19.2	2.5
Super, Chicken Flavour, Made Up, Batchelors*	1 Serving/100g	170	7.3	170	3.3	22.9	7.3	0.9
Super, Chow Mein Flavour, Made Up, Batchelors*	½ Pack/150g	262	11.8	175	3.0	23.0	7.9	0.4
Super, Mild Curry, Dry Weight, Batchelors*	½ Pack/50g	260	11.7	520	9.4	67.8	23.4	1.4
Super, Mild Curry Flavour, Made Up, Batchelors*	1 Serving/100g	157	6.7	157	3.2	20.9	6.7	1.0
Super, Mushroom Flavour, Made Up, Batchelors*	1 Serving/100g	157	6.8	157	3.2	20.9	6.8	1.0
Super, Roast Chicken, to Go, 98% Fat Free, Batchelors*	1 Serving/380g	308	0.8	81	2.6	17.2	0.2	0.5
Super, Southern Fried Chicken, Made Up, Batchelors*	1 Serving/100g	171	7.2	171	3.3	23.2	7.2	0.5
Super, Spicy Salsa, Dry Weight, Batchelors*	1 Pack/105g	474	19.5	451	7.0	63.8	18.6	1.7
Super, Sweet Thai Chilli, Dry Weight, Batchelors*	1 Pack/85g	292	1.0	343	10.6	72.5	1.2	3.0
Super, Sweet Thai Chilli Flavour, 98% Fat Free, Batchelors*	1 Pack/270g	292	1.1	108	3.3	22.8	0.4	0.9
Sweet & Sour, BGTY, Sainsbury's*	1 Serving/100g	112	3.1	112	2.3	18.6	3.1	0.0
Sweet Chilli, Sainsbury's*	½ Pack/110g	172	6.0	156	4.0	24.6	5.5	1.0
Sweet Chilli, Wok, Findus*	1 Pack/300g	300	1.5	100	3.0	20.0	0.5	0.0
Szechuan Beef Flavour, Dry, Blue Dragon*	½ Pack/100g	350	1.2	350	10.5	72.3	1.2	0.0
Thai, Spicy, Stir Fry, HL, Tesco*	½ Pack/250g	220	5.5	88	4.1	12.9	2.2	1.7
Thai, Waitrose*	1 Pack/300g	357	6.3	119	6.8	18.4	2.1	1.7
Thai Style, Asda*	1 Pot/238g	226	0.7	95	3.0	20.0	0.3	0.8
Thai Style, Sainsbury's*	1 Pack/340g	381	7.8	112	3.3	19.4	2.3	0.7
Tiger Prawn, Stir Fry, Tesco*	1 Pack/400g	596	14.8	149	6.0	23.0	3.7	2.7
Tomato & Herb in a Mug, Pot Noodle*	1 Serving/44g	28	0.1	64	2.0	13.4	0.2	0.7
Whole Wheat, Dry, Blue Dragon*	1 Serving/65g	208	1.3	320	12.5	63.0	2.0	8.0
Yaki Udan, Chicken & Prawn, M & S*	1 Pack/395g	434	14.2	110	8.1	11.9	3.6	0.8
NOUGAT								
Average	1 Sm Bar/28g	108	2.4	384	4.4	77.3	8.5	0.9
Raspberry & Orange Hazelnut, Thorntons*	1 Sweet/9g	39	1.8	433	4.8	60.0	20.0	2.2
Soft, Bar, Bassett's*	1 Bar/25g	94	1.0	375	4.0	82.0	4.0	0.0
NUT MIX								
America's, Graze*	1 Punnet/40g	263	25.3	657	16.3	6.2	63.2	6.0
Black Forest, Graze*	1 Pack/55g	258	13.8	470	6.6	54.4	25.1	0.0
Chocolate Orange Granola, Graze*	1 Punnet/41g	194	11.6	473	11.9	43.5	28.2	7.1
Cookies & Cream, Graze*	1 Punnet/38g	216	15.8	567	12.2	35.8	41.4	3.3
Fiery Almonds, Graze*	1 Punnet/35g	206	18.1	588	21.9	8.2	51.6	11.4
Honey Monster, Graze*	1 Med Pack/50g	279	20.4	559	10.8	45.2	40.8	0.0

	Measure INFO/WEIGHT	per Measure		Nutrition Values per 100g / 100ml				
		KCAL	FAT	KCAL	PROT	CARB	FAT	FIBRE
NUT MIX								
Island, Graze*	1 Pack/55g	354	33.0	643	15.1	10.5	60.0	0.0
Sweet & Sour, Graze*	1 Pack/40g	222	17.4	556	19.1	23.7	43.4	0.0
NUT ROAST								
Average	1 Serving/200g	704	51.4	352	13.3	18.3	25.7	4.2
Courgette & Spiced Tomato, Cauldron Foods*	1 Serving/100g	208	12.3	208	11.7	12.5	12.3	4.9
Leek, Cheese & Mushroom, Organic, Cauldron Foods*	½ Pack/143g	343	21.3	240	13.2	13.2	14.9	4.1
Lentil, Average	*1oz/28g*	*62*	*3.4*	*222*	*10.6*	*18.8*	*12.1*	*3.8*
NUTMEG								
Ground, Average	*1 Tsp/3g*	*16*	*1.1*	*525*	*5.8*	*45.3*	*36.3*	*0.0*
NUTS								
Almonds, Whole, Sainsbury's*	1 Serving/10g	59	4.9	588	25.8	10.2	49.3	8.5
Assortment, Eat Well, M & S*	1 Pack/70g	441	41.2	630	16.7	8.5	58.9	5.3
Bento Box, Mix, Graze*	1 Portion/30g	141	6.6	469	17.9	50.1	22.1	3.7
Fire, Graze*	1 Pack/40g	220	16.3	549	17.9	28.4	40.7	7.1
Luxury Assortment, Tesco*	1 Serving/10g	68	6.5	676	17.5	6.1	64.6	5.0
Mississippi BBQ Pistachios, Graze*	1 Punnet/30g	176	16.1	587	17.4	8.9	53.7	5.9
Mixed, Almonds, Brazil, Hazel & Walnuts, M & S*	1 Serving/25g	167	16.0	670	16.0	4.8	64.0	5.4
Mixed, Americas, Graze*	1 Punnet/40g	263	25.6	658	15.5	5.2	64.0	5.6
Mixed, Ancient Forest, Graze*	1 Pack/35g	221	21.1	632	17.6	5.9	60.3	7.0
Mixed, Average	1 Pack/40g	243	21.6	607	22.9	7.9	54.1	6.0
Mixed, Chopped, Julian Graves*	1 Serving/25g	148	12.7	591	23.2	10.0	50.9	0.0
Mixed, Chopped, Sainsbury's*	1 Serving/100g	605	50.9	605	27.1	9.6	50.9	6.0
Mixed, Chopped, Tesco*	1 Serving/25g	149	12.6	595	23.5	10.5	50.6	6.0
Mixed, Delicious, Boots*	1 Pack/50g	331	29.0	663	16.0	16.0	58.0	8.1
Mixed, Honey Roasted, Waitrose*	1 Serving/50g	291	22.5	583	17.1	27.5	45.0	5.3
Mixed, Natural, Asda*	1 Snack/30g	197	18.8	656	18.0	4.3	62.7	7.4
Mixed, Nature's Harvest*	1 Serving/25g	145	13.3	581	17.5	7.7	53.4	6.3
Mixed, Roasted, Salted, Waitrose*	1 Pack/200g	156	14.6	626	13.7	11.3	58.4	4.4
Mixed, Roasted, Waitrose*	1 Serving/25g	165	16.0	662	15.2	6.2	64.0	8.2
Mixed, Unsalted, Sainsbury's*	1 Serving/50g	311	28.8	622	18.5	7.2	57.7	8.7
Mixed, Wholesome, Love Life, Waitrose*	1 Serving/30g	205	19.6	685	14.6	5.0	65.2	5.4
Natural, Mixed, Love Life, Waitrose*	1 Serving/50g	314	25.8	628	17.4	24.9	51.6	12.1
Natural Assortment, Tesco*	1 Serving/50g	338	32.3	676	17.5	6.1	64.6	5.0
Natural Roasted Peanuts, Love Life, Waitrose*	1 Pack/250g	160	13.2	638	27.1	15.6	52.6	5.1
Oak Smoke Flavour Selection, Finest, Tesco*	1 Serving/25g	158	13.9	633	21.4	11.2	55.8	6.3
Peanuts & Cashews, Honey Roast, Tesco*	1 Serving/25g	145	10.7	579	21.6	26.6	42.9	4.2
Pecan, Wholesome, Love Life, Waitrose*	1 Serving/30g	207	21.0	691	9.2	5.8	70.1	9.6
Peri-Peri, Nando's*	1 Serving/100g	631	54.1	631	23.8	8.5	54.1	7.8
Pine, Tesco*	1 Pack/100g	699	68.6	699	16.5	4.0	68.6	1.9
Pine, Wholefoods, Tesco*	1 Serving/10g	69	6.9	690	14.0	4.0	68.6	1.9
Roasted, Salted, Assortment, Luxury, Tesco*	1 Serving/25g	161	14.5	643	21.1	9.4	57.9	8.1
Salted, Selection, Sainsbury's*	1 Serving/30g	190	17.1	634	20.6	9.7	56.9	8.2
Soya, Dry Roasted, The Food Doctor*	1 Serving/50g	203	10.7	406	37.5	15.9	21.4	16.1
Soya, Roast, Wholefoods, Tesco*	1/5 Pack/20g	80	3.8	400	38.0	19.1	19.0	13.4
Soya Beans, Roasted & Salted, Chinese Style, Tesco*	1 Serving/26g	100	5.0	385	46.1	6.9	19.2	21.8
Unsalted, Selection, Sainsbury's*	1 Serving/75g	491	48.0	655	14.7	5.0	64.0	6.7
Walnut Pieces, Morrisons*	7 Peices/6g	41	4.1	689	14.7	3.3	68.5	3.5
NUTS & RAISINS								
Mixed, Average	1 Serving/30g	144	10.2	481	14.1	31.5	34.1	4.5
Mixed, KP Snacks*	1 Serving/50g	273	20.1	546	21.4	24.4	40.3	5.2
Mixed, Nature's Harvest*	1 Serving/50g	231	16.8	463	12.4	32.9	33.7	3.4
Mixed, Tesco*	1 Serving/25g	115	6.9	450	18.6	32.6	26.8	12.5
Yoghurt Coated, Waitrose*	1 Serving/50g	263	18.3	527	10.9	38.2	36.7	3.0

	Measure INFO/WEIGHT	per Measure KCAL	FAT	Nutrition Values per 100g / 100ml KCAL	PROT	CARB	FAT	FIBRE
OAT BAKES								
Cheese, Nairn's*	1 Bag/30g	130	4.7	432	15.0	57.4	15.8	1.3
Honey & Lemon, Graze*	1 Punnet/31g	124	3.0	400	6.1	70.0	9.8	4.9
Mediterranean Tomato & Herb, Nairn's*	1 Bag/30g	129	4.7	431	8.1	64.2	15.8	8.3
Sweet Chilli, Nairn's*	1 Bag/30g	128	4.0	426	8.1	68.4	13.3	7.2
OAT CAKES								
Bran, Paterson's*	1 Cake/13g	52	2.0	416	10.0	58.5	15.8	9.5
Cheese, Nairn's*	1 Cake/9g	42	2.4	471	13.2	43.3	27.2	6.8
Fine Milled, Nairn's*	1 Cake/8g	35	1.7	449	10.5	52.6	21.8	8.6
Herb & Pumpkin Seed, Nairn's*	1 Cake/10g	43	2.1	426	12.2	46.8	21.1	13.0
Highland, Walkers*	1 Cake/12g	54	2.5	451	10.3	56.0	20.6	6.7
Oatmeal, Rough, Nairn's*	1 Cake/11g	45	2.0	421	10.6	52.8	18.6	10.5
Oatmeal, Rough, Organic, Nairn's*	1 Cake/10g	43	1.7	418	10.2	57.7	16.3	7.5
Organic, The Village Bakery*	1 Cake/13g	56	2.7	452	10.9	54.5	21.3	5.6
Orkney, Stockan's*	1 Cake/14g	63	3.2	453	11.1	50.3	23.0	6.0
Retail, Average	1 Cake/13g	57	2.4	441	10.0	63.0	18.3	0.0
Rough, Sainsbury's*	1 Cake/11g	45	1.8	426	11.7	65.2	16.9	8.6
Rough with Bran, Walkers*	1 Cake/13g	55	2.2	424	11.0	57.1	16.8	8.1
Rough with Olive Oil, Paterson's*	1 Cake/13g	54	2.1	431	10.6	58.4	17.2	8.1
Scottish, M & S*	1oz/28g	116	3.5	413	9.1	70.0	12.6	8.5
OATBRAN								
Original Pure, Mornflake*	1 Serving/30g	103	2.9	345	14.8	49.7	9.7	15.2
OATMEAL								
Raw	*1oz/28g*	*112*	*2.4*	*401*	*12.4*	*72.8*	*8.7*	*6.8*
OCTOPUS								
Chunks in Olive Oil, Palacio De Oriente*	1 Tin/111g	148	4.0	133	21.6	4.5	3.6	0.0
Raw	*1oz/28g*	*23*	*0.4*	*83*	*17.9*	*0.0*	*1.3*	*0.0*
OIL								
Avocado, Olivado*	1 Tsp/5ml	40	4.4	802	0.0	0.0	88.0	0.0
Black Truffle, Grapeseed, Cuisine Perel*	1 Tsp/5ml	43	5.0	857	0.0	7.1	100.0	0.0
Chilli, Average	*1 Tsp/5ml*	*41*	*4.6*	*823*	*0.0*	*0.0*	*91.5*	*0.0*
Coconut, Average	*1 Tsp/5ml*	*45*	*5.0*	*899*	*0.0*	*0.0*	*99.9*	*0.0*
Coconut, Virgin, Organic, Groovy Food Company*	1 Tsp/5ml	38	4.6	767	0.0	0.0	92.5	0.0
Cod Liver, Average	*1 Capsule/1g*	*9*	*1.0*	*900*	*0.0*	*0.0*	*100.0*	*0.0*
Corn, Average	*1 Tsp/5ml*	*43*	*4.8*	*864*	*0.0*	*0.0*	*95.9*	*0.0*
Cuisine, Flora*	1 Tsp/5ml	31	3.5	630	0.1	1.0	70.3	0.0
Evening Primrose, Average	*1 Serving/1g*	*9*	*1.0*	*900*	*0.0*	*0.0*	*100.0*	*0.0*
Fish, Average	*1 Serving/1g*	*9*	*1.0*	*900*	*0.0*	*0.0*	*100.0*	*0.0*
Fish, Omega 3, Capsule, Holland & Barrett*	1 Capsule/1g	10	1.0	1000	0.1	0.1	100.0	0.1
Flax Seed, Average	*1 Tbsp/15ml*	*124*	*13.9*	*829*	*0.0*	*0.0*	*92.5*	*0.0*
Fry Light, Bodyline*	1 Spray/0.25ml	1	0.1	522	0.0	0.0	55.2	0.0
Grapeseed, Average	*1 Tsp/5ml*	*43*	*4.8*	*865*	*0.0*	*0.0*	*96.1*	*0.0*
Groundnut, Average	*1 Tsp/5ml*	*41*	*4.6*	*824*	*0.0*	*0.0*	*91.8*	*0.0*
Hazelnut, Average	*1 Tsp/5ml*	*45*	*5.0*	*899*	*0.0*	*0.0*	*99.9*	*0.0*
Linseed, Organic, Biona*	1 Serving/10ml	84	9.3	837	0.0	0.0	93.0	0.0
Macadamia Nut, Oz Tukka*	1 Tsp/5ml	40	4.5	805	0.0	0.0	91.0	0.0
Olive, Average	*1 Tsp/5ml*	*43*	*4.7*	*855*	*0.0*	*0.0*	*94.9*	*0.0*
Olive, Extra Virgin, Average	*1 Tsp/5ml*	*42*	*4.7*	*848*	*0.0*	*0.0*	*94.5*	*0.0*
Olive, Extra Virgin, Only 1 Cal, Spray, Fry Light*	1 Spray/0.2ml	1	0.1	498	0.0	0.0	55.2	0.0
Olive, Garlic, Average	*1 Tbsp/15ml*	*127*	*14.1*	*848*	*0.0*	*0.0*	*94.3*	*0.0*
Olive, Mild, Average	*1 Tbsp/15mll*	*129*	*14.4*	*861*	*0.0*	*0.0*	*95.7*	*0.0*
Olive, Spray, Fry Light*	5 Sprays/1ml	5	0.5	521	0.0	0.0	54.2	0.0
Palm, Average	*1 Tsp/5ml*	*45*	*5.0*	*899*	*0.0*	*0.0*	*99.9*	*0.0*
Peanut, Average	*1 Tsp/5ml*	*45*	*5.0*	*899*	*0.0*	*0.0*	*99.9*	*0.0*

O

OIL

	Measure INFO/WEIGHT	per Measure KCAL	FAT	Nutrition Values per 100g / 100ml KCAL	PROT	CARB	FAT	FIBRE
Rapeseed, Average	*1 Tbsp/15ml*	*130*	*14.4*	*863*	*0.0*	*0.0*	*95.9*	*0.0*
Red Palm & Canola, Carotino*	1 Tsp/5ml	41	4.6	812	0.0	0.0	92.0	0.0
Rice Bran, Average	1 Tbsp/14g	120	13.6	884	0.0	0.0	100.0	0.0
Safflower, Average	*1 Tsp/5ml*	*45*	*5.0*	*899*	*0.0*	*0.0*	*99.9*	*0.0*
Sesame, Average	*1 Tsp/5ml*	*45*	*5.0*	*892*	*0.1*	*0.0*	*99.9*	*0.0*
Soya, Average	*1 Tsp/5ml*	*45*	*5.0*	*899*	*0.0*	*0.0*	*99.9*	*0.0*
Sunflower, Average	*1 Tsp/5ml*	*43*	*4.8*	*869*	*0.0*	*0.0*	*96.6*	*0.0*
Sunflower, Spray, Fry Light*	1 Spray/0.2ml	1	0.1	522	0.0	0.0	55.2	0.0
Ultimate Blend, Udo's Choice*	1 Capsule/1ml	9	1.0	900	1.3	0.0	96.8	0.0
Vegetable, Average	*1 Tbsp/15ml*	*129*	*14.3*	*858*	*0.0*	*0.0*	*95.3*	*0.0*
Walnut, Average	*1 Tsp/5ml*	*45*	*5.0*	*899*	*0.0*	*0.0*	*99.9*	*0.0*
Wheatgerm, Average	*1 Tsp/5ml*	*45*	*5.0*	*899*	*0.0*	*0.0*	*99.9*	*0.0*

OKRA

Boiled in Unsalted Water, Average	*1 Serving/80g*	*22*	*0.7*	*28*	*2.5*	*2.7*	*0.9*	*3.6*
Canned, Drained, Average	*1 Serving/80g*	*17*	*0.6*	*21*	*1.4*	*2.5*	*0.7*	*2.6*
Raw, Average	*1 Serving/80g*	*25*	*0.8*	*31*	*2.8*	*3.0*	*1.0*	*4.0*
Stir-Fried in Corn Oil, Average	*1 Serving/80g*	*215*	*20.9*	*269*	*4.3*	*4.4*	*26.1*	*6.3*

OLIVES

Black, Pitted, Average	*½ Jar/82g*	*135*	*13.3*	*164*	*1.0*	*3.5*	*16.2*	*3.1*
Black & Green with Greek Feta Cheese, Tesco*	1 Pot/100g	200	20.1	200	3.4	0.3	20.1	4.6
Green, Garlic Stuffed, Asda*	1 Olive/3g	6	0.6	174	1.8	3.5	17.0	0.0
Green, Lightly Flavoured with Lemon & Garlic, Attis*	1 Serving/50g	82	8.2	164	1.7	2.2	16.5	0.0
Green, Pitted, Average	*1 Olive/3g*	*4*	*0.4*	*129*	*1.1*	*0.9*	*13.3*	*2.5*
Green, Pitted, Stuffed with Anchovies, Sainsbury's*	1 Serving/50g	77	8.0	155	1.8	0.6	16.1	3.2
Green, Pitted & Stuffed with Minced Pimiento, Sainsbury's*	1 Olive/5g	8	0.8	147	1.2	3.9	14.1	2.0
Green, Stuffed with Almonds, Pitted, Waitrose*	1 Serving/50g	90	8.4	180	3.8	3.2	16.9	2.5
Green, Stuffed with Anchovy, Waitrose*	½ Can/40g	38	3.1	94	1.5	4.7	7.7	2.3
Green with Chilli & Garlic, Delicious, Boots*	1 Pack/60g	97	9.0	161	1.3	4.4	15.0	2.0
Green with Chilli & Garlic, Graze*	1 Punnet/44g	133	13.6	301	0.6	1.4	30.9	2.9
Kalamata, Kalamata	*1 Olive/3g*	*9*	*0.9*	*300*	*1.0*	*6.7*	*30.0*	*0.0*
Kalamata with Herbs, Graze*	1 Punnet/52g	144	15.3	277	0.6	1.7	29.4	3.1
Marinated, Mixed, M & S*	1 Serving/20g	33	3.0	165	1.6	6.5	14.9	3.0
Marinated, Selection, M & S*	4 Olives/20g	44	4.4	225	1.4	3.9	22.6	2.1
Mixed, Chilli & Garlic, Asda*	1 Serving/30g	43	4.7	144	0.9	0.0	15.6	6.1
Mixed, Marinated, Anti Pasti, Asda*	1 Serving/100g	215	22.0	215	1.8	0.7	22.0	3.1
Mixed, Marinated with Feta & Red Peppers, Asda*	1 Pot/120g	233	21.6	194	5.8	2.2	18.0	1.7
Pimento Stuffed in Brine, Tesco*	1 Serving/25g	38	4.1	153	0.8	0.1	16.4	2.1

OMELETTE

Cheese, 2 Egg, Average	1 Omelette/180g	479	40.7	266	15.9	0.0	22.6	0.0
Cheese, Findus*	1 Serving/200g	400	26.0	200	9.5	14.0	13.0	0.0
Ham & Mushroom, Farmfoods*	1 Omelette/120g	200	16.7	167	8.7	1.8	13.9	0.1
Mushroom & Cheese, Tesco*	1 Omelette/120g	248	21.5	207	9.8	1.6	17.9	0.2
Plain, 2 Egg	1 Omelette/120g	229	19.7	191	10.9	0.0	16.4	0.0
Spanish	1oz/28g	34	2.3	120	5.7	6.2	8.3	1.4
Spanish, Potato, Rapido, Unearthed*	1 Pack/175g	273	13.6	156	4.6	15.8	7.8	2.2

ONION RINGS

Battered, Asda*	1 Serving/100g	343	22.7	343	3.8	31.0	22.7	1.7
Battered, Oven Baked, Tesco*	1 Serving/50g	109	5.0	219	3.9	28.4	10.0	3.5
Battered, Sainsbury's*	1 Ring/12g	26	1.2	219	3.9	28.4	10.0	3.5
Breadcrumbs, Tesco*	1 Serving/100g	294	15.6	294	4.3	34.1	15.6	2.3
Breaded, Asda*	1 Serving/10g	29	1.5	289	4.4	34.0	15.0	2.7
Breaded, Sainsbury's*	1 Serving/100g	280	12.4	280	4.6	37.6	12.4	4.1
Oven Crisp Batter, Tesco*	1 Ring/17g	40	2.3	236	4.2	24.8	13.3	2.5

	Measure INFO/WEIGHT	per Measure KCAL	FAT	Nutrition Values per 100g / 100ml KCAL	PROT	CARB	FAT	FIBRE
ONION RINGS								
Value, Tesco*	1 Bag/14g	73	3.8	520	7.0	61.4	27.0	1.2
ONIONS								
Baked	*1oz/28g*	*29*	*0.2*	*103*	*3.5*	*22.3*	*0.6*	*3.9*
Boiled in Unsalted Water	*1oz/28g*	*5*	*0.0*	*17*	*0.6*	*3.7*	*0.1*	*0.7*
Brown, Value, Tesco*	1 Onion/100g	36	0.2	36	1.3	7.8	0.2	1.8
Dried, Raw, Average	*1oz/28g*	*88*	*0.5*	*313*	*10.2*	*68.6*	*1.7*	*12.1*
Fried, Average	*1oz/28g*	*46*	*3.1*	*164*	*2.3*	*14.1*	*11.2*	*3.1*
Pickled, Average	*1 Onion/15g*	*3*	*0.0*	*23*	*0.8*	*4.9*	*0.1*	*0.7*
Pickled, Strong, Drained, Haywards*	1 Onion/42g	10	0.0	23	0.7	4.8	0.1	0.0
Powder	1 Tsp/2g	7	0.0	341	10.4	79.1	1.0	15.2
Raw, Average	*1 Med/180g*	*69*	*0.4*	*38*	*1.2*	*7.9*	*0.2*	*1.3*
Red, Raw, Average	*1 Med/180g*	*66*	*0.4*	*37*	*1.2*	*7.9*	*0.2*	*1.5*
Spring, Raw, Average	*1 Med/15g*	*4*	*0.1*	*25*	*2.0*	*3.0*	*0.5*	*1.5*
OPTIONS								
Choca Mocha Drink, Ovaltine*	1 Sachet/11g	39	1.3	359	14.1	50.1	11.4	7.0
Chocolate Au Lait, Ovaltine*	1 Sachet/10g	35	1.0	355	11.8	54.5	10.0	7.3
Coffee, Dreamy Cappuccion, Cafe, Ovaltine*	1 Sachet/25g	64	4.2	256	12.9	58.1	16.9	0.0
Dreamy Caramel, Hot Chocolate, Ovaltine*	1 Sachet/11g	39	0.9	354	12.3	48.5	7.8	0.0
Irish Cream, Ovaltine*	1 Sachet/11g	39	1.2	357	13.9	50.0	11.3	8.1
Mint Madness, Belgian, Ovaltine*	1 Serving/11g	38	0.8	348	12.3	49.2	6.9	20.0
Outrageous Orange, Ovaltine*	1 Serving/11g	32	0.8	289	11.7	43.3	7.7	18.0
Tempting Toffee, Ovaltine*	1 Sachet/11g	43	1.0	391	13.6	66.4	9.1	0.0
Wicked White Chocolate, Ovaltine*	1 Sachet/11g	46	1.2	414	10.3	68.1	11.1	0.5
ORANGES								
Blood, Average	*1 Orange/140g*	*82*	*0.0*	*58*	*0.8*	*13.3*	*0.0*	*2.5*
Fresh, Weighed with Peel, Average	*1 Med/185g*	*115*	*0.5*	*62*	*1.0*	*15.6*	*0.3*	*3.2*
Fresh, without Peel, Average	*1 Med/145g*	*54*	*0.1*	*37*	*1.1*	*8.5*	*0.1*	*1.7*
Peel Only, Raw, Average	*1 Tbsp/6g*	*6*	*0.0*	*97*	*1.5*	*25.0*	*0.2*	*10.6*
Ruby Red, Tesco*	1 Med/130g	51	0.1	39	1.1	8.5	0.1	1.7
OREGANO								
Dried,	*1 Tsp/1g*	*3*	*0.1*	*306*	*11.0*	*49.5*	*10.3*	*0.0*
Fresh	*1 Tsp/1g*	*1*	*0.0*	*66*	*2.2*	*9.7*	*2.0*	*0.0*
OVALTINE*								
Chocolate, Light, Ovaltine*	4 Tsp/20g	76	1.2	380	8.5	70.5	6.0	4.5
Chocolate, Light, Sachet, Ovaltine*	1 Sachet/25g	96	1.5	384	7.4	73.0	5.9	4.7
Hi Malt, Light, Instant Drink, Ovaltine*	1 Sachet/20g	72	1.2	358	9.1	67.1	5.9	2.8
Powder, Made Up with Semi-Skimmed Milk, Ovaltine*	1 Mug/227ml	179	3.9	79	3.9	13.0	1.7	0.0
Powder, Made Up with Whole Milk, Ovaltine*	1 Mug/227ml	220	8.6	97	3.8	12.9	3.8	0.0
OXTAIL								
Raw	*1oz/28g*	*48*	*2.8*	*171*	*20.0*	*0.0*	*10.1*	*0.0*
Stewed, Bone Removed	*1oz/28g*	*68*	*3.8*	*243*	*30.5*	*0.0*	*13.4*	*0.0*
OYSTERS								
in Vegetable Oil, Smoked, John West*	1oz/28g	64	3.9	230	16.0	10.0	14.0	0.0
Raw, Shucked	*1 Oyster/14g*	*9*	*0.2*	*65*	*10.8*	*2.7*	*1.3*	*0.0*

O

	Measure INFO/WEIGHT	per Measure KCAL	FAT	Nutrition Values per 100g / 100ml KCAL	PROT	CARB	FAT	FIBRE
PAELLA								
Bistro, Waitrose*	1 Serving/300g	534	19.8	178	7.4	22.2	6.6	0.7
Chicken, Chorizo & King Prawn, Finest, Tesco*	½ Pack/400g	520	19.6	130	7.0	14.2	4.9	1.2
Chicken, HL, Tesco*	1 Pack/400g	432	2.0	108	6.7	19.2	0.5	1.7
Chicken, Tesco*	1 Serving/475g	575	14.2	121	7.9	15.7	3.0	1.6
Chicken & Chorizo, Asda*	1 Pack/390g	484	8.6	124	10.0	16.0	2.2	2.6
Chicken & Chorizo, Big Dish, M & S*	1 Pack/450g	630	17.5	140	7.9	18.4	3.9	1.6
Chicken & King Prawn, BGTY, Sainsbury's*	1 Pack/400g	336	5.2	84	5.4	11.8	1.3	1.9
Chicken & King Prawn, HL, Tesco*	1 Pack/385g	346	6.2	90	5.3	12.7	1.6	2.0
Chicken & Prawn, Asda*	1 Pack/400g	352	4.4	88	5.8	13.7	1.1	1.4
Chicken & Vegetable, HL, Tesco*	1 Pack/450g	441	5.8	98	9.7	11.8	1.3	1.1
Diet Chef Ltd*	1 Pack/250g	355	3.0	142	11.2	21.7	1.2	0.4
Seafood, COU, M & S*	1 Pack/400g	400	7.2	100	6.2	13.8	1.8	1.4
Seafood, Espana, M & S*	1 Bowl/380g	565	12.1	150	5.5	25.2	3.2	0.5
Seafood, M & S*	1 Pack/450g	517	17.1	115	6.4	13.7	3.8	3.2
Seafood, Sainsbury's*	1 Pack/400g	504	5.2	126	8.3	20.3	1.3	0.6
TTD, Sainsbury's*	½ Pack/374g	475	20.9	127	9.4	9.9	5.6	4.8
Vegetable, Espana, M & S*	1 Pack/375g	505	13.5	135	2.8	22.4	3.6	1.3
Vegetable, Love Life, Waitrose*	1 Pack/400g	344	12.4	86	1.6	12.9	3.1	1.7
Vegetable, Lovely Vegetables, M & S*	1 Pack/430g	387	13.8	90	2.2	13.7	3.2	1.7
Vegetable, Waitrose*	1 Serving/174g	202	3.1	116	2.2	22.7	1.8	1.5
PAIN AU CHOCOLAT								
All Butter, Tesco*	1 Serving/59g	242	11.6	410	8.2	49.4	19.7	2.3
Asda*	1 Serving/58g	244	13.9	420	8.0	43.0	24.0	3.3
Chocolate Filled, Chosen By You, Asda*	1 Pain/45g	198	11.3	441	7.1	44.9	25.2	2.9
Extra Special, Asda*	1oz/28g	113	5.9	405	8.0	46.0	21.0	3.3
M & S*	1 Pastry/60g	210	11.5	350	5.9	38.0	19.2	1.6
Mini, Asda*	1 Pastry/23g	96	5.5	420	8.0	43.0	24.0	3.3
Mini, Cafe Simple*	1 Pastry/27g	122	7.2	452	10.2	42.8	26.7	2.5
Sainsbury's*	1 Serving/58g	241	13.8	415	7.9	42.5	23.7	3.3
Small, Asda*	1 Serving/23g	106	6.0	462	8.0	49.0	26.0	0.0
TTD, Sainsbury's*	1 Pain/80g	341	18.6	426	7.5	46.9	23.2	3.0
Waitrose*	1 Pastry/53g	230	12.6	435	8.8	45.5	23.9	3.7
PAIN AU RAISIN								
Takeaway, Average	1 Pastry/100g	313	13.2	313	5.2	43.0	13.2	1.3
Twist, Extra Special, Asda*	1 Pastry/110g	421	20.9	383	7.0	46.0	19.0	2.5
PAK CHOI								
Raw, Average	*1 Leaf/14g*	*2*	*0.0*	*13*	*1.5*	*2.2*	*0.2*	*1.0*
PAKORA								
Bhaji, Onion, Fried in Vegetable Oil	1oz/28g	76	4.1	271	9.8	26.2	14.7	5.5
Bhajia, Potato Carrot & Pea, Fried in Vegetable Oil	1oz/28g	100	6.3	357	10.9	28.8	22.6	6.1
Bhajia, Vegetable, Retail	1oz/28g	66	4.1	235	6.4	21.4	14.7	3.6
Chicken, Tikka, Asda*	1 Pack/350g	696	38.5	199	16.0	9.0	11.0	1.1
Potato & Spinach, Waitrose*	1 Pakora/50g	120	8.2	240	5.5	17.3	16.5	4.7
Prawn, Indian Appetisers, Waitrose*	1 Pakora/21g	35	1.7	165	16.8	5.9	8.2	1.5
Sainsbury's*	1 Pakora/55g	166	10.1	302	7.3	26.8	18.3	1.1
Spinach, Mini, Indian Selection, Somerfield*	1 Serving/22g	61	3.5	277	6.2	26.9	16.1	4.9
Spinach, Sainsbury's*	1 Pakora/18g	35	1.9	195	5.1	19.4	10.8	3.8
Vegetable, Indian Selection, Party, Co-Op*	1 Pakora/23g	47	1.6	205	6.0	28.0	7.0	4.0
Vegetable, Indian Starter Selection, M & S*	1 Pakora/23g	61	4.2	265	6.3	19.6	18.1	2.9
Vegetable, Mini, Indian Snack Collection, Tesco*	1 Pakora/21g	36	1.9	173	6.0	16.8	9.1	4.9
Vegetable, Somerfield*	1 Pakora/15g	46	3.4	305	7.0	19.0	23.0	0.0
PANCAKE								
Apple, GFY, Asda*	1 Pancake/74g	100	1.8	135	4.2	24.0	2.5	1.0

	Measure INFO/WEIGHT	per Measure KCAL	FAT	Nutrition Values per 100g / 100ml KCAL	PROT	CARB	FAT	FIBRE
PANCAKE								
Apple & Sultana, M & S*	1 Serving/80g	160	6.3	200	2.2	30.2	7.9	1.2
Bramley Apple, Sainsbury's*	1 Pancake/85g	114	2.1	134	4.2	23.6	2.5	1.0
Cherry, GFY, Asda*	1 Serving/206g	206	3.8	100	1.9	18.9	1.8	1.8
Chinese Roll, Farmfoods*	1 Pancake/88g	125	3.8	142	4.3	21.6	4.3	1.0
Chinese Style, Cherry Valley*	1 Pancake/8g	25	0.5	310	9.2	54.7	6.0	0.0
Chocolate, M & S*	1 Pancake/80g	125	4.9	156	3.1	22.1	6.1	0.2
for Duck, Sainsbury's*	1 Pancake/10g	33	0.9	333	10.9	51.7	9.3	2.4
HL, Tesco*	1 Pancake/25g	60	0.5	240	5.8	48.8	2.0	1.9
Irish, Rankin Selection, Irwin's Bakery*	1 Pancake/40g	101	1.3	252	6.2	49.2	3.2	2.5
Lemon, M & S*	1 Pancake/38g	90	2.8	235	4.5	38.5	7.2	2.8
Lemon & Raisin, Morrisons*	1 Pancake/36g	55	0.4	153	5.3	30.4	1.2	0.9
Low Calorie, Eurodiet*	1 Serving/30g	112	2.9	373	57.5	9.2	9.8	8.4
M & S*	1 Pancake/62g	170	7.7	275	5.7	33.9	12.5	1.5
Maple & Raisin, M & S*	1 Pancake/35g	101	2.4	290	5.6	50.4	6.9	2.2
Morello Cherry, Iceland*	1 Pancake/129g	204	3.7	158	3.1	29.8	2.9	2.9
North Staffordshire Oatcakes Ltd*	1 Pancake/71g	166	4.3	234	5.0	40.9	6.1	1.0
Perfect, Kingsmill*	1 Pancake/27g	71	1.2	264	6.2	49.7	4.5	1.2
Plain, Sainsbury's*	1 Pancake/46g	102	2.4	221	6.9	36.1	5.3	1.2
Pockets, Strawberry, Kingsmill*	1 Pancake/44g	112	1.6	254	4.3	50.5	3.6	1.3
Raisin & Lemon, Asda*	1 Serving/30g	92	2.4	304	6.0	52.0	8.0	1.4
Raisin & Lemon, Co-Op*	1 Pancake/34g	92	1.9	271	8.6	45.7	5.7	0.9
Raisin & Lemon, Sainsbury's*	1 Pancake/35g	95	1.5	272	6.3	51.8	4.4	2.2
Savoury, Made with Skimmed Milk, Average	1 6"/77g	192	11.3	249	6.4	24.1	14.7	0.8
Savoury, Made with Whole Milk, Average	1 6"/77g	210	13.5	273	6.3	24.0	17.5	0.8
Scotch	1 Pancake/50g	146	5.8	292	5.8	43.6	11.7	1.4
Scotch, BGTY, Sainsbury's*	1 Pancake/30g	76	1.2	252	5.3	48.5	4.1	1.3
Scotch, Essential, Waitrose*	1 Pancake/31g	82	2.6	265	6.4	40.9	8.4	2.4
Scotch, Low Fat, Asda*	1 Pancake/32g	87	0.7	272	6.0	57.0	2.2	1.3
Scotch, M & S*	1 Pancake/34g	95	1.4	280	6.5	54.5	4.0	1.6
Sultana & Syrup, Asda*	1 Pancake/34g	89	2.4	263	5.9	43.7	7.2	1.5
Sultana & Syrup Scotch, Sainsbury's*	1 Pancake/35g	113	2.9	322	6.7	55.2	8.3	1.7
Sweet, Made with Skimmed Milk	1oz/28g	78	3.9	280	6.0	35.1	13.8	0.8
Sweet, Made with Whole Milk	1oz/28g	84	4.5	301	5.9	35.0	16.2	0.8
Sweet, Raspberry Ripple Sauce, Findus*	1 Pancake/38g	80	1.8	210	3.9	37.1	4.7	0.9
Syrup, Gluten, Wheat & Dairy Free, Free From, Livwell*	1 Pancake/40g	108	2.9	270	2.5	49.0	7.2	0.7
Syrup, Tesco*	1 Pancake/30g	79	2.5	265	4.7	42.1	8.2	1.5
Traditional, Aunt Bessie's*	1 Pancake/60g	90	1.9	150	6.1	24.6	3.1	1.1
Traditional, Tesco*	1 Pancake/62g	137	3.1	221	8.4	35.6	5.0	1.5
Vegetable Roll	1 Roll/85g	185	10.6	218	6.6	21.0	12.5	0.0
Warburton's*	1 Pancake/35g	88	2.1	252	6.4	43.0	6.0	1.8
PANCAKE MIX								
4 Grain, Wheat & Gluten Free, Organic, Hale & Hearty*	½ Pack/180g	562	2.9	312	7.8	66.6	1.6	5.7
Fresh, M & S*	1 Pancake/38g	90	5.0	235	7.5	22.4	13.1	0.5
Glutano*	1 Tbs/15g	57	0.3	378	8.9	75.6	2.2	0.0
Traditional, Asda*	1 Pack/256g	545	23.0	213	6.0	27.0	9.0	1.8
PANCETTA								
Average	***½ Pack/65g***	***212***	***18.7***	***326***	***17.0***	***0.1***	***28.7***	***0.0***
Cubes, Tesco*	1 Serving/38g	135	12.2	355	17.5	0.5	32.2	0.0
PANINI								
Bacon, British Midland*	1 Serving/150g	273	9.9	182	9.1	21.6	6.6	0.0
Chargrilled Chicken, Mozzarella & Pesto, Udo's Choice*	1 Panini/170g	389	14.6	229	16.4	21.6	8.6	2.0
Cheese, Tesco*	1 Panini/100g	249	9.1	249	10.5	31.3	9.1	3.1
Chicken Arrabiata, Ginsters*	1 Panini/200g	489	16.0	245	12.8	29.1	8.4	2.4

	Measure INFO/WEIGHT	per Measure KCAL	FAT	Nutrition Values per 100g / 100ml KCAL	PROT	CARB	FAT	FIBRE
PANINI								
Ham & Cheese, Ginsters*	1 Panini/200g	567	25.6	283	13.3	28.7	12.8	1.6
Mozzarella & Tomato, Ginsters*	1 Panini/207g	536	21.9	259	12.3	28.5	10.6	2.1
Mozzarella & Tomato, M & S*	1 Serving/176g	484	28.5	275	11.3	21.3	16.2	2.1
Tuna & Sweetcorn, Tesco*	1 Serving/250g	559	16.4	224	12.0	29.3	6.6	1.4
Tuna Melt, Ginsters*	1 Panini/210g	479	15.8	228	13.1	26.9	7.5	1.9
PANNA COTTA								
BGTY, Sainsbury's*	1 Pot/150g	150	2.8	100	2.4	18.2	1.9	1.4
Caramel, Sainsbury's*	1 Pot/120g	335	15.7	279	2.5	34.6	13.1	3.3
Sainsbury's*	1 Pot/100g	304	15.7	304	3.0	41.5	15.7	4.0
Strawberry, COU, M & S*	1 Pot/145g	145	3.8	100	2.6	15.7	2.6	0.8
PAPAYA								
Dried, Pieces, Nature's Harvest*	1 Serving/50g	177	0.0	355	0.2	85.4	0.0	2.6
Dried, Strips, Tropical Wholefoods*	1 Strip/10g	31	0.1	310	3.9	71.4	0.9	1.5
Dried, Sweetened, Tesco*	4 Pieces/25g	59	0.2	235	0.4	56.3	0.9	2.9
Raw, Flesh Only, Average	*1 Serving/140g*	*37*	*0.1*	*26*	*0.4*	*6.6*	*0.1*	*1.2*
Raw, Unripe, Flesh Only	1 Serving/100g	27	0.1	27	0.9	5.5	0.1	1.0
Raw, Weighed with Seeds & Skin	*1 Cup/140g*	*55*	*0.2*	*39*	*0.6*	*9.8*	*0.1*	*1.8*
Unripe, Raw, Weighed with Seeds & Skin	*1oz/28g*	*8*	*0.0*	*27*	*0.9*	*5.5*	*0.1*	*1.5*
PAPPARDELLE								
Basil, Fresh, Sainsbury's*	1 Serving/240g	281	3.4	117	5.0	21.2	1.4	2.0
Buitoni*	1 Serving/65g	242	3.1	373	15.0	67.5	4.8	0.0
Chilli, Fresh, Sainsbury's*	1 Serving/250g	302	4.2	121	5.7	20.7	1.7	2.0
Egg, Dry, Average	*1 Serving/100g*	*364*	*3.7*	*364*	*14.1*	*68.5*	*3.7*	*2.1*
Egg, Fresh, Waitrose*	¼ Pack/125g	350	3.4	280	12.9	51.0	2.7	1.9
Egg & Spinach, Extra Special, Asda*	½ Pack/200g	328	3.6	164	6.5	30.5	1.8	1.4
Saffron, Eat Well, M & S*	1 Serving/100g	360	2.5	360	14.0	69.0	2.5	3.2
with Salmon, COU, M & S*	1 Pack/358g	340	6.8	95	6.3	13.0	1.9	0.8
PAPRIKA								
Average	*1 Tsp/2g*	*6*	*0.3*	*289*	*14.8*	*34.9*	*13.0*	*0.0*
PARATHA								
Average	*1 Paratha/80g*	*258*	*11.4*	*322*	*8.0*	*43.2*	*14.3*	*4.0*
Lachha, Waitrose*	1 Paratha/75g	322	17.8	429	7.8	46.0	23.8	1.8
Roti, Plain, Crown Farms*	1 Slice/80g	250	10.0	312	5.0	46.2	12.5	1.2
PARCELS								
Beef Steak, Sainsbury's*	½ Pack/226g	488	35.3	216	12.2	6.6	15.6	1.0
Cheese & Ham, Sainsbury's*	1 Pack/250g	445	19.0	178	7.4	19.9	7.6	1.5
Chilli Beef, Tex Mex Feast, Asda*	1 Parcel/25g	67	3.5	270	9.0	27.0	14.0	2.1
Filo, Brie & Cranberry, Finest, Tesco*	1 Parcel/22g	73	3.7	330	9.8	33.2	17.0	1.4
Filo, Mushroom, Savoury, Creamy, Somerfield*	1oz/28g	86	5.9	308	5.0	24.0	21.0	0.0
Filo, Mushroom Leek & Gruyere, Finest, Tesco*	1 Serving/160g	440	33.6	275	6.9	20.5	21.0	1.5
Salmon, in Lemon Sauce, M & S*	1 Serving/185g	350	27.9	189	12.1	1.4	15.1	0.5
Salmon, Smoked, Sainsbury's*	1 Pack/115g	269	20.2	234	15.8	3.5	17.6	0.2
Salmon, Smoked, with Soft Cheese & Herb, Waitrose*	1 Pack/100g	246	20.2	246	14.6	1.2	20.2	0.0
Turkey Breast, with Cheddar Cheese & Chive, Asda*	1 Parcel/140g	242	9.8	173	23.0	4.6	7.0	0.9
PARSLEY								
Dried	*1 Tsp/1g*	*2*	*0.1*	*181*	*15.8*	*14.5*	*7.0*	*26.9*
Fresh, Average	*1 Tbsp/4g*	*1*	*0.0*	*34*	*3.0*	*2.7*	*1.3*	*5.0*
PARSNIP								
Boiled, Average	*1 Serving/80g*	*53*	*1.0*	*66*	*1.6*	*12.9*	*1.2*	*4.7*
Fragrant, Tesco*	1 Serving/50g	33	0.5	67	1.8	12.5	1.1	4.6
Honey Glazed, Roasting, Cooked, Betty Smith's*	1 Serving/100g	144	7.2	144	2.6	23.4	7.2	6.3
Honey Roasted, Tesco*	½ Pack/125g	165	6.6	130	1.3	16.7	5.2	5.2
Raw, Savers, Morrisons*	1 Serving/80g	61	0.9	76	1.8	12.5	1.1	4.6

	Measure INFO/WEIGHT	per Measure		Nutrition Values per 100g / 100ml				
		KCAL	FAT	KCAL	PROT	CARB	FAT	FIBRE
PARSNIP								
Raw, Unprepared, Average	*1oz/28g*	*19*	*0.3*	*66*	*1.8*	*12.5*	*1.1*	*4.6*
Roast, Honey Glazed, Baked, Aunt Bessie's*	1 Serving/125g	162	9.4	130	1.7	14.0	7.5	4.1
Roasting, Freshly Frozen, Chosen By You, Asda*	1 Serving/110g	221	8.5	201	2.5	30.4	7.7	7.8
PARTRIDGE								
Breast, Fillets, Raw, Skinned, Abel & Cole*	1 Serving/100g	145	4.7	145	25.8	0.0	4.7	0.0
Meat Only, Roasted	*1oz/28g*	*59*	*2.0*	*212*	*36.7*	*0.0*	*7.2*	*0.0*
PASANDA								
Chicken, M & S*	½ Pack/150g	240	16.3	160	11.3	3.8	10.9	1.3
Chicken, Sainsbury's*	1 Serving/200g	368	24.8	184	14.7	3.4	12.4	2.3
Chicken, Waitrose*	1oz/28g	52	3.4	185	14.8	3.8	12.3	1.1
Chicken with Pilau Rice, HL, Tesco*	1 Pack/440g	466	11.0	106	5.7	15.2	2.5	0.9
PASSATA								
Basil, Del Monte*	1 Jar/500g	160	1.0	32	1.4	5.9	0.2	0.0
Classic, Italian with Onion & Garlic, Sainsbury's*	1oz/28g	10	0.0	37	1.4	7.7	0.1	1.3
Napolina*	1 Bottle/690g	172	0.7	25	1.4	4.5	0.1	0.0
Sieved Tomato, Valfrutta*	1 Pack/500g	110	0.5	22	1.2	4.0	0.1	0.0
Smart Price, Asda*	1 Serving/100g	25	0.1	25	1.4	4.5	0.1	0.2
So Organic, Sainsbury's*	¼ Jar/175g	38	0.7	22	0.9	3.8	0.4	0.9
with Fresh Leaf Basil, Waitrose*	¼ Jar/170g	44	0.2	26	1.0	5.2	0.1	0.8
with Garlic & Herbs, Roughly Chopped, Tesco*	1 Serving/200g	56	0.0	28	1.4	5.5	0.0	1.0
with Garlic & Italian Herbs, Tesco*	1 Serving/165g	53	0.3	32	1.2	6.4	0.2	1.1
PASSION FRUIT								
Raw, Fresh, Average	*1 Fruit/30g*	*11*	*0.1*	*36*	*2.6*	*5.8*	*0.4*	*3.3*
Weighed with Skin, Average	*1 Fruit/30g*	*11*	*0.1*	*36*	*2.6*	*5.8*	*0.4*	*3.3*
PASTA								
& Chargrilled Mushrooms, Finest, Tesco*	1 Pack/200g	410	22.4	205	6.1	19.6	11.2	1.4
& Flame Grilled Chicken, M & S*	1 Pack/180g	414	25.2	230	8.2	17.5	14.0	0.8
& Roasted Vegetables, Waitrose*	1oz/28g	43	2.7	154	2.4	14.2	9.7	1.0
Angel Hair, Konjac, Slim Pasta*	1 Serving/100g	8	0.0	8	0.6	0.6	0.0	5.6
Arrabbiata Nodini, Asda*	1 Serving/150g	301	8.7	201	7.8	29.3	5.8	2.7
Arrabiata, Pasta King*	1 Serving/100g	104	1.4	104	3.5	19.5	1.4	1.8
Basilico, Pasta King*	1 Serving/100g	123	3.3	123	3.8	19.5	3.3	2.1
Bean & Tuna, BGTY, Sainsbury's*	1 Serving/200g	176	1.8	88	7.3	12.6	0.9	2.8
Boccoletti, Dried, Sainsbury's*	1 Serving/90g	321	1.5	357	12.3	73.1	1.7	2.5
Bolognese, Diet Chef Ltd*	1 Serving/300g	288	10.2	96	7.9	5.8	3.4	4.4
Bolognese, Pasta King*	1 Serving/100g	121	2.6	121	5.1	19.3	2.6	1.9
Bolognese, Vegetarian, Pasta King*	1 Serving/100g	117	2.1	117	4.9	19.7	2.1	1.9
Brown Rice, Fusilli, Gluten Free, Dove's Farm*	1 Serving/30g	101	0.4	338	7.9	70.3	1.5	4.1
Brown Rice, Penne, Gluten Free, Organic, Dove's Farm*	1 Serving/100g	338	1.5	338	7.9	70.3	1.5	4.1
Brown Rice & Maize, Ditalini, Organic, Dove's Farm*	1 Serving/100g	347	0.9	347	7.0	76.0	0.9	2.4
Cajun Chicken, GFY, Asda*	1 Serving/297g	312	8.3	105	8.0	12.0	2.8	2.1
Carbonara, Pasta King*	1 Serving/100g	122	2.9	122	5.1	19.3	2.9	1.2
Carbonara, with Cheese & Bacon, Slim Fast*	1 Serving/70g	240	4.4	343	22.7	48.9	6.3	5.7
Cheddar, Country, Bowl, Haribo*	1 Serving/269g	400	19.0	149	5.6	15.2	7.1	1.5
Cheese, Pasta King*	1 Serving/100g	117	2.3	117	5.0	19.2	2.3	1.1
Cheese & Broccoli, Tubes, Tesco*	1 Serving/202g	319	13.9	158	5.0	19.1	6.9	2.3
Chicken, Tomato & Basil, Asda*	1 Pack/400g	474	10.0	118	6.5	17.5	2.5	1.2
Chicken, Tomato & Basil, GFY, Asda*	1 Pack/400g	404	9.2	101	6.4	13.6	2.3	1.4
Chicken, Tomato & Basil, HL, Tesco*	1 Pack/400g	264	2.0	66	7.9	7.5	0.5	1.1
Chicken, Tomato & Herb, Easy Steam, Tesco*	1 Serving/400g	528	24.8	132	8.9	10.2	6.2	1.3
Chicken, Tomato & Mascarpone, Easy Steam, Tesco*	1 Pack/400g	468	16.4	117	9.7	10.3	4.1	0.9
Chicken, Tomato & Mascarpone, HL, Tesco*	1 Pack/450g	504	11.2	112	7.5	14.8	2.5	1.1
Chicken, Tomato & Mascarpone, Italiano, Tesco*	1 Pack/400g	572	24.8	143	7.4	14.3	6.2	1.3

P

PASTA

	Measure INFO/WEIGHT	per Measure KCAL	FAT	Nutrition Values per 100g / 100ml KCAL	PROT	CARB	FAT	FIBRE
Chicken & Asparagus, GFY, Asda*	1 Pack/400g	388	8.8	97	10.9	8.5	2.2	1.5
Chicken & Chorizo, Average	1 Pack/400g	174	5.7	174	10.1	20.3	5.7	1.5
Chicken & Chorizo, Quadrotti, TTD, Sainsbury's*	1 Pack/320g	675	28.8	211	11.8	20.6	9.0	2.7
Chicken & Green Pesto, HL, Tesco*	1 Serving/376g	440	4.5	117	8.3	18.5	1.2	1.4
Chicken & Ham, Easy Steam, Tesco*	1 Pack/400g	572	26.4	143	9.8	11.2	6.6	0.6
Chicken & Mushroom, Big Eat, Heinz*	1 Pot/350g	339	15.7	97	4.8	9.2	4.5	0.5
Chicken & Mushroom, Pasta & Sauce, Dry, Tesco*	1 Pack/120g	427	4.3	356	16.0	65.0	3.6	3.9
Chicken & Mushroom Flavour, Quick, Sainsbury's*	1 Pot/220g	235	6.2	107	3.3	16.1	2.8	1.9
Chicken & Pineapple, Shapers, Boots*	1 Pack/221g	210	3.3	95	5.4	15.0	1.5	0.9
Chicken & Roasted Tomato, HL, Tesco*	1 Serving/374g	426	7.1	114	7.4	16.7	1.9	1.3
Chicken & Vegetable, Mediterranean, Waitrose*	1 Serving/400g	375	9.2	94	7.5	10.5	2.3	2.2
Chicken Italiano, Pasta King*	1 Serving/100g	125	3.2	125	5.5	18.9	3.2	1.9
Chicken Penne, Weight Watchers*	1 Pot/261g	248	3.7	95	5.0	14.6	1.4	2.1
Chilli, Vegetable, Pasta King*	1 Serving/100g	121	2.1	121	5.2	20.9	2.1	2.3
Chilli Beef, Pasta King*	1 Serving/100g	125	2.6	125	5.4	20.5	2.6	2.2
Conchiglie, Dry Weight, Parioli, Cucina*	1 Serving/75g	266	1.0	355	12.5	73.0	1.4	2.6
Courgette, Green Bean & Basil Pappardelle, M & S*	1 Pack/270g	324	15.9	120	4.7	11.8	5.9	1.6
Creamy Cheese, Big Eat, Heinz*	1 Pot/350g	437	32.2	125	3.7	7.0	9.2	1.8
Creamy Garlic Mushroom, HL, Tesco*	1 Serving/100g	106	3.7	106	3.6	14.6	3.7	1.1
Creamy Mushroom, Light Choices, Tesco*	1 Pack/350g	455	4.9	130	4.3	25.0	1.4	1.3
Creamy Mushroom, Sainsbury's*	1 Serving/63g	148	9.1	237	4.5	21.7	14.6	1.2
Creamy Tomato & Chicken, Great Stuff, Asda*	1 Pack/300g	351	11.7	117	7.0	13.5	3.9	2.3
Creamy Vegetable, Meal in 5, Ainsley Harriott*	1 Pot/387g	414	10.1	107	2.8	18.1	2.6	0.8
Dischi Volanti, Tesco*	1 Serving/50g	177	0.7	355	12.5	73.0	1.4	2.6
Elicoidali, Waitrose*	1 Serving/200g	682	2.6	341	11.5	70.7	1.3	3.7
Fagottini, Wild Mushroom, Sainsbury's*	½ Pack/125g	274	9.4	219	10.2	27.7	7.5	2.7
Feta & Black Olive Girasole, Extra Special, Asda*	½ Pack/150g	360	15.4	240	8.3	28.4	10.3	0.0
Filled, Tomato & Mozzarella Caramella, Jamie Oliver*	½ Pack/165g	294	9.2	178	8.9	24.9	5.6	2.0
Fiorelli, Egg, M & S*	1 Serving/100g	355	2.8	355	13.9	68.5	2.8	3.0
Fiorelli, Mozzarella, Tomato & Basil, Waitrose*	1 Serving/125g	352	11.6	282	10.8	38.9	9.3	1.7
Fusilli, Wholewheat, Dry, Tesco*	1 Portion/75g	245	1.9	327	12.5	62.5	2.5	9.1
Fusilloni, TTD, Sainsbury's*	1 Serving/90g	321	1.5	357	12.3	73.1	1.7	2.5
Garlic Mushroom Filled, Extra Special, Asda*	1 Serving/125g	224	8.7	179	8.0	21.0	7.0	2.5
High Fibre, Uncooked, Fiber Gourmet*	1 Serving/56g	130	1.0	232	12.5	75.0	1.8	32.1
Honey & Mustard Chicken, Light Choices, Tesco*	1 Pack/375g	881	48.4	235	6.7	22.0	12.9	1.2
Honey & Mustard Chicken, Tesco*	1 Pack/375g	865	48.3	231	6.7	21.9	12.9	0.0
Hot Smoked Salmon, Tesco*	1 Pack/275g	426	17.0	155	7.1	16.6	6.2	4.1
King Prawn & Pesto, Asda*	1 Pack/400g	488	17.7	122	7.6	12.9	4.4	1.2
Linguine, Dry Weight, De Cecco*	1 Serving/100g	350	1.5	350	13.0	71.0	1.5	2.9
Lumache, Tesco*	1 Serving/100g	345	2.0	345	13.2	68.5	2.0	2.9
Lumaconi, TTD, Sainsbury's*	1 Serving/90g	321	1.5	357	12.3	73.1	1.7	2.5
Macaroni Cheese, Meal in 5, Ainsley Harriott*	1 Pot/387g	467	16.0	121	3.7	17.3	4.1	1.0
Margherite, Basil & Pinenut, TTD, Sainsbury's*	½ Pack/150g	309	10.5	206	12.6	23.2	7.0	2.7
Meat Feast, Italian, Sainsbury's*	1 Pack/450g	508	18.0	113	7.4	11.8	4.0	0.6
Medaglioni, Bolognese, Rich Red Wine, Waitrose*	½ Pack/125g	266	7.0	213	12.5	28.1	5.6	2.6
Mediterranean Vegetable, Weight Watchers*	1 Pack/400g	262	3.2	65	2.6	12.0	0.8	1.6
Mini Spirals, in Cheese Sauce, Heinz*	1 Can/154g	120	3.5	78	3.9	10.4	2.3	0.3
Organic, Gluten Free, Dove's Farm*	1 Serving/100g	338	1.5	338	7.9	70.3	1.5	4.1
Orzo, Dry, Average	1 Serving/100g	348	1.5	348	12.4	71.9	1.5	3.0
Orzo, with British Chicken, Tomato & Basil, Eat Well, M & S*	1 Pack/300g	390	11.1	130	7.9	16.5	3.7	1.9
Paccheri, Finest, Tesco*	1 Serving/100g	360	1.5	360	13.5	72.5	1.5	1.6
Parcels, Basil & Parmesan, Fresh, Sainsbury's*	1 Serving/162g	357	13.5	220	10.0	26.4	8.3	3.3
Pennoni, TTD, Sainsbury's*	1 Serving/90g	321	1.5	357	12.3	73.1	1.7	2.5

	Measure INFO/WEIGHT	per Measure KCAL	FAT	Nutrition Values per 100g / 100ml KCAL	PROT	CARB	FAT	FIBRE

PASTA

	Measure INFO/WEIGHT	KCAL	FAT	KCAL	PROT	CARB	FAT	FIBRE
Peperonata, Pasta King*	1 Serving/100g	104	1.4	104	3.5	19.4	1.4	1.8
Pepper, Zingy, Pasta King*	1 Serving/100g	106	1.5	106	3.6	19.6	1.5	1.8
Pepper & Tomato, Asda*	1 Serving/250g	340	17.5	136	3.2	15.0	7.0	2.4
Pomodoro, Pasta King*	1 Serving/100g	109	1.8	109	3.6	19.6	1.8	1.8
Pomodoro with Tomato & Herbs, Slim Fast*	1 Serving/71g	235	3.1	331	21.5	51.5	4.3	6.0
Raviolini, Gorgonzola & Walnut, M & S*	½ Pack/125g	381	16.5	305	12.6	33.6	13.2	2.0
Riccioli, Dry Weight, Buitoni*	1 Serving/75g	264	1.4	352	11.2	72.6	1.9	0.0
Roasted Vegetable Arrabbiata, Weight Watchers*	1 Pack/362g	246	1.4	68	3.4	11.4	0.4	2.8
Sausage & Tomato, Italiano, Tesco*	1 Serving/450g	679	26.5	151	5.7	18.8	5.9	1.6
Seafood, Retail	1oz/28g	31	1.3	110	8.9	7.6	4.8	0.4
Sicilian Chicken, City Kitchen, Tesco*	1 Pack/385g	500	13.5	130	9.1	14.6	3.5	0.6
Spicy Tomato, Meal in 5, Ainsley Harriott*	1 Pot/387g	369	2.1	95	2.6	19.9	0.5	1.5
Spicy Tomato & Pepperoni Sauce with Fusilli, Heinz*	1 Pack/250g	318	13.8	127	4.4	14.8	5.5	0.6
Spinach & Pine Nut, Finest, Tesco*	1 Pack/195g	546	34.9	280	6.4	23.1	17.9	1.5
Stuffed Mushroom & Emmental, Sainsbury's*	1 Pack/250g	650	23.0	260	11.3	33.5	9.2	3.7
Sundried Tomato, Sainsbury's*	1 Serving/50g	196	17.8	393	4.5	13.4	35.7	6.2
Tomato, Roasted Vegetable & Basil, Love Life, Waitrose*	1 Tub/360g	328	9.0	91	2.8	14.3	2.5	3.2
Tomato & Bacon, Value, Tesco*	1 Pack/300g	300	4.2	100	4.0	17.8	1.4	1.1
Tomato & Basil Chicken, Boots*	1 Serving/320g	621	28.8	194	9.0	19.0	9.0	1.4
Tomato & Chicken Spiralli, HL, Tesco*	1 Pack/350g	402	5.2	115	7.8	17.3	1.5	1.6
Tomato & Mascarpone, GFY, Asda*	½ Can/200g	128	4.4	64	2.1	9.0	2.2	0.0
Tomato & Mascarpone, Tesco*	1 Pack/400g	468	16.4	117	9.7	10.3	4.1	0.9
Tomato & Onion, Shells, Tesco*	1 Serving/193g	643	3.1	333	12.5	67.1	1.6	6.3
Tomato & Pepper, GFY, Asda*	1 Pack/400g	344	7.6	86	3.1	14.0	1.9	1.1
Tomato & Vegetable, Diet Chef Ltd*	1 Pack/300g	216	6.0	72	2.6	10.9	2.0	1.8
Tomato & Vegetable, Look What We Found*	1 Pouch/300g	216	6.0	72	2.6	10.9	2.0	1.8
Tomato & Vegetable, Solo Slim, Rosemary Conley*	1 Pack/300g	216	5.4	72	2.8	11.1	1.8	2.0
Tortelloni, Spinach & Ricotta, Emma Giordani*	1 Pack/250g	685	15.0	274	10.0	45.0	6.0	0.0
Tortelloni, Spinach & Ricotta, Giovanni Rana*	½ Pack/190g	376	12.3	198	7.8	27.0	6.5	3.1
Tuna Rigatoni, Diet Chef Ltd*	1 Pack/300g	336	13.2	112	5.9	12.2	4.4	1.0
Twists, Quick Cook, Morrisons*	1 Serving/75g	265	1.5	353	12.0	72.0	2.0	3.1
Twists with Tuna, Italian, Weight Watchers*	1 Can/385g	239	5.4	62	4.3	8.2	1.4	0.6
Vegetable, Creamy, BGTY, Sainsbury's*	1 Pack/400g	348	6.0	87	4.0	14.3	1.5	1.9
Vegetable, Mediterranean, Sainsbury's*	1 Pack/400g	504	11.6	126	4.0	20.9	2.9	1.8
Vegetable Rice, Dry Weight, Orgran*	1 Serving/66g	233	1.3	353	6.8	80.0	2.0	4.8
Wheat Free, Delverde*	1 Serving/63g	229	1.2	366	0.5	86.9	1.9	1.2
Whole Wheat, Bella Terra*	1 Serving/100g	375	1.7	375	12.5	78.5	1.7	10.7
Whole Wheat, Penne, Asda*	1 Serving/100g	333	2.1	333	12.1	66.3	2.1	6.9
Wholewheat, Cooked, Tesco*	1 Serving/200g	284	1.8	142	5.7	27.9	0.9	4.5

PASTA BAKE

	Measure INFO/WEIGHT	KCAL	FAT	KCAL	PROT	CARB	FAT	FIBRE
Aberdeen Angus Meatball, Waitrose*	½ Pack/350g	501	28.0	143	5.2	12.5	8.0	0.9
Bacon & Leek, Average	1 Serving/400g	633	32.3	158	6.7	14.8	8.1	1.3
Bolognese, Asda*	¼ Pack/375g	514	23.6	137	7.3	12.7	6.3	1.8
Bolognese, Finest, Tesco*	1 Serving/250g	375	15.7	150	7.3	16.1	6.3	1.1
Bolognese, GFY, Asda*	1 Pack/400g	376	8.4	94	5.8	13.1	2.1	0.9
Bolognese, Italiano, Tesco*	1/3 Pack/284g	409	14.5	144	8.7	15.7	5.1	2.3
Bolognese, Weight Watchers*	1 Pack/400g	324	8.0	81	6.1	9.6	2.0	1.3
Cheese & Bacon, Asda*	1 Serving/120g	168	14.4	140	2.9	5.2	12.0	0.3
Cheese & Bacon, Fresh Italian, Asda*	1 Serving/250g	265	20.0	106	6.0	2.6	8.0	0.5
Cheese & Tomato, Italiano, Tesco*	1 Bake/300g	354	12.6	118	3.9	16.1	4.2	1.0
Cheese & Tomato, Tesco*	1 Pack/400g	388	5.6	97	3.4	17.8	1.4	1.2
Chicken, Bacon & Mushroom, Average	1 Serving/400g	632	29.2	158	7.8	15.1	7.3	2.3
Chicken, BGTY, Sainsbury's*	1 Pack/400g	348	8.0	87	9.7	7.5	2.0	0.8

PASTA BAKE

	Measure INFO/WEIGHT	per Measure KCAL	per Measure FAT	Nutrition Values per 100g / 100ml KCAL	PROT	CARB	FAT	FIBRE
Chicken, Italiano, Tesco*	1 Serving/190g	218	7.8	115	8.4	11.2	4.1	3.1
Chicken, Morrisons*	1 Pack/402g	442	14.5	110	4.6	14.8	3.6	0.9
Chicken, Mozzarella & Tomato, Birds Eye*	1 Pack/360g	468	6.8	130	7.1	14.3	1.9	0.3
Chicken, Somerfield*	1 Pack/300g	351	18.0	117	8.0	8.0	6.0	0.0
Chicken, Tomato, & Mascarpone, Tesco*	1 Serving/400g	448	8.4	112	8.0	15.2	2.1	1.7
Chicken, Weight Watchers*	1 Pack/300g	249	2.7	83	6.0	12.1	0.9	1.1
Chicken & Bacon, Average	1 Serving/400g	627	28.7	157	9.0	13.7	7.2	1.6
Chicken & Bacon, Healthy Range, Average	1 Serving/400g	466	9.6	116	6.6	17.1	2.4	1.5
Chicken & Broccoli, Morrisons*	1 Pack/400g	452	16.0	113	6.1	13.3	4.0	0.6
Chicken & Broccoli, Pasta Presto, Findus*	1 Pack/321g	449	22.5	140	7.5	12.0	7.0	0.0
Chicken & Broccoli, Weight Watchers*	1 Bake/305g	290	4.6	95	6.0	14.2	1.5	0.9
Chicken & Courgette, Asda*	½ Pack/387g	519	23.2	134	6.0	14.0	6.0	0.6
Chicken & Leek, HL, Tesco*	1 Pack/400g	460	7.6	115	10.8	13.1	1.9	1.6
Chicken & Mushroom, Waitrose*	1 Pack/400g	532	30.8	133	6.7	9.1	7.7	0.8
Chicken & Roast Mushroom, HL, Tesco*	1 Pack/390g	413	0.4	106	8.6	17.6	0.1	1.3
Chicken & Spinach, GFY, Asda*	1 Pack/400g	374	6.0	93	5.0	15.0	1.5	1.2
Chicken & Spinach, Morrisons*	1 Serving/500g	766	36.1	153	6.6	15.5	7.2	1.4
Chicken & Spinach, Sainsbury's*	1 Pack/340g	286	9.2	84	4.9	10.0	2.7	0.6
Chilli & Cheese, American Style, Tesco*	1 Pack/425g	637	16.6	150	6.8	21.8	3.9	1.5
Creamy Mushroom, Dolmio*	½ Jar/245g	267	22.5	109	1.1	5.5	9.2	0.0
Creamy Tomato, Dolmio*	1 Serving/125g	141	9.0	113	2.3	8.4	7.2	0.0
Findus*	1 Pack/320g	448	22.4	140	7.5	12.0	7.0	0.0
Ham & Broccoli, Asda*	1 Pack/340g	309	13.9	91	3.4	10.0	4.1	0.5
Ham & Mushroom, Italiano, Tesco*	1 Pack/425g	646	20.4	152	5.8	21.3	4.8	1.7
Italian Creamy Tomato & Bacon, Asda*	1 Serving/125g	131	11.2	105	2.0	3.9	9.0	0.6
King Prawn & Salmon, GFY, Asda*	1 Pack/400g	420	11.6	105	6.9	12.7	2.9	1.2
Meat Feast, Average	1 Serving/400g	601	21.4	150	5.8	19.2	5.4	1.4
Meatball, Tesco*	1 Pack/400g	576	19.2	144	5.9	19.3	4.8	0.5
Mediterranean, Weight Watchers*	1 Pack/397g	262	3.2	66	2.6	12.0	0.8	1.6
Mediterranean Style, Tesco*	1 Pack/450g	423	1.8	94	2.9	19.6	0.4	2.0
Mix, Tuna, Colman's*	1 Sachet/45g	145	2.3	323	9.2	60.0	5.2	4.7
Mozzarella & Tomato, Asda*	1 Pack/400g	532	19.2	133	4.4	18.1	4.8	1.8
Mushroom, Creamy, Asda*	¼ Jar/118g	204	20.1	173	1.8	3.3	17.0	0.5
Penne Mozzarella, Tesco*	1 Pack/340g	408	8.5	120	4.7	19.7	2.5	0.6
Pepperoni & Ham, Tesco*	½ Pack/425g	501	2.5	118	8.9	19.3	0.6	2.5
Roasted Mediterranean Vegetables, Dolmio*	1 Serving/125g	66	2.1	53	1.3	8.1	1.7	1.2
Sausage, Average	1 Serving/400g	591	24.0	148	5.5	17.7	6.0	1.9
Spicy Tomato & Pepperoni, Asda*	1 Pack/440g	431	26.4	98	1.1	10.0	6.0	1.2
Tomato & Cheese, Light Choices, Tesco*	1 Pack/350g	385	4.5	110	3.2	20.9	1.3	1.5
Tomato & Herb, Asda*	1 Jar/436g	715	56.7	164	1.8	10.0	13.0	1.2
Tomato & Mozzarella, Average	1 Serving/400g	500	12.4	125	5.3	17.3	3.1	1.5
Tomato & Mozzarella, Light Choices, Tesco*	1 Pack/400g	368	8.0	92	3.7	14.8	2.0	1.5
Tomato & Red Pepper with Crunch Topping, Homepride*	1 Jar/535g	417	8.6	78	1.8	14.1	1.6	0.9
Tuna, Co-Op*	1 Serving/340g	306	6.8	90	7.0	12.0	2.0	1.0
Tuna, COU, M & S*	1 Pack/360g	432	15.5	120	8.0	11.9	4.3	0.8
Tuna, Good Intentions, Somerfield*	1 Serving/400g	400	8.4	100	5.9	14.5	2.1	1.2
Tuna, Lean Cuisine*	1 Pack/346g	380	8.6	110	5.0	16.0	2.5	1.5
Tuna, Light Choices, Tesco*	1 Pack/400g	380	5.2	95	10.8	10.0	1.3	2.2
Tuna, Somerfield*	1 Bake/300g	411	21.0	137	9.0	10.0	7.0	0.0
Tuna, Tesco*	1oz/28g	36	1.7	129	6.9	11.7	6.1	0.9
Tuna, Weight Watchers*	1 Pack/400g	292	3.2	73	7.0	9.4	0.8	1.4
Tuna & Sweetcorn, Average	1 Pack/400g	423	22.4	106	5.0	8.6	5.6	1.9
Tuna & Tomato, BGTY, Sainsbury's*	1 Pack/450g	553	18.9	123	8.7	12.6	4.2	0.4

	Measure INFO/WEIGHT	per Measure		Nutrition Values per 100g / 100ml				
		KCAL	FAT	KCAL	PROT	CARB	FAT	FIBRE
PASTA BAKE								
Tuna Conchiglie, M & S*	1 Pack/400g	520	17.2	130	8.6	14.3	4.3	1.1
Vegetable, Asda*	1 Serving/300g	231	10.5	77	2.4	9.0	3.5	0.8
Vegetable, Findus*	1 Pack/331g	430	21.5	130	6.0	13.0	6.5	0.0
Vegetable, M & S*	½ Pack/175g	227	9.1	130	4.9	15.5	5.2	1.6
Vegetable, Mediterranean, HL, Tesco*	1 Serving/450g	373	3.6	83	2.9	16.0	0.8	1.5
Vegetable, Mediterranean, Tesco*	1 Serving/450g	495	20.7	110	4.3	12.9	4.6	1.3
Vegetable, Ready Meals, Waitrose*	1oz/28g	44	2.4	157	5.9	14.4	8.6	1.0
Vegetable, Tesco*	1 Pack/380g	467	21.3	123	5.6	12.6	5.6	1.6
PASTA IN								
Chicken, Garlic & Wine Flavour Sauce, Dry Weight, Tesco*	1 Pack/120g	438	5.2	365	14.2	66.8	4.3	5.0
Garlic & Herb, Asda*	1 Serving/120g	487	12.0	406	10.0	69.0	10.0	2.3
Herb Sauce, Sainsbury's*	1 Pack/420g	441	0.8	105	3.5	22.4	0.2	0.8
Tomato & Mushroom Sauce, Spirals, Tesco*	1 Serving/217g	326	13.7	150	4.6	18.8	6.3	2.5
PASTA 'N' SAUCE								
Bolognese Flavour, Dry, Batchelors*	½ Pack/65g	228	1.7	353	15.1	67.2	2.6	3.9
Carbonara Flavour, Dry, Batchelors*	1 Pack/120g	463	6.0	386	14.3	71.0	5.0	3.1
Cheese, Leek & Ham, Batchelors*	1 Pack/120g	454	6.1	378	16.1	67.0	5.1	2.0
Cheese & Broccoli, Made Up, Smart Price, Asda*	1 Serving/120g	198	8.4	165	4.6	21.0	7.0	2.1
Cheese & Broccoli Sauce Mix, Made Up, Sainsbury's*	1 Pack/120g	164	6.8	137	4.2	17.2	5.7	1.1
Chicken & Mushroom, Batchelors*	½ Pack/63g	227	1.1	361	14.1	72.3	1.7	2.8
Chicken & Mushroom, Made Up, Morrisons*	1 Pack/110g	166	6.2	151	5.0	20.3	5.6	2.1
Chicken & Mushroom, Made Up, Smart Price, Asda*	1 Pack/110g	183	6.6	166	5.0	23.0	6.0	2.2
Chicken & Roasted Garlic Flavour, Dry, Batchelors*	½ Pack/60g	223	1.7	372	12.6	73.8	2.9	3.4
Creamy Tikka Masala, Dry, Batchelors*	1 Pack/122g	426	2.7	349	12.7	69.5	2.2	4.4
Creamy Tomato & Mushroom, Dry, Batchelors*	1 Pack/125g	457	4.1	366	13.0	71.0	3.3	3.2
Macaroni Cheese, Dry, Batchelors*	1 Pack/108g	402	5.1	372	17.2	65.2	4.7	2.7
Mild Cheese & Broccoli, Batchelors*	½ Pack/61g	221	2.4	363	15.0	67.0	3.9	4.0
Mushroom & Wine, Batchelors*	½ Pack/50g	242	2.8	483	18.5	89.9	5.5	4.4
Mushroom & Wine, Dry, Batchelors*	1 Pack/132g	498	6.5	377	12.0	71.3	4.9	2.5
Tomato, Onion & Herb, Made Up, Morrisons*	1 Serving/110g	141	4.9	128	3.2	18.7	4.5	2.3
Tomato, Onion & Herbs, Dry, Batchelors*	1 Pack/135g	455	1.8	337	12.8	68.5	1.3	5.8
Tomato & Bacon Flavour, Dry, Batchelors*	1 Pack/134g	476	3.5	355	13.0	70.0	2.6	3.0
Tomato & Mascarpone, BGTY, Sainsbury's*	1 Pack/380g	555	7.2	146	6.6	25.6	1.9	1.3
PASTA QUILLS								
Dry, Average	**1 Serving/75g**	**256**	**0.9**	**342**	**12.0**	**72.3**	**1.2**	**2.0**
Dry, Value, Tesco*	1 Serving/75g	261	1.1	348	12.0	71.7	1.5	3.0
Gluten Free, Salute*	1 Serving/75g	269	1.4	359	7.5	78.0	1.9	0.0
PASTA SALAD								
& Mixed Leaf, with Basil Pesto Dressing, Tesco*	1 Pack/220g	528	37.6	240	4.7	16.9	17.1	0.7
Bacon, Budgens*	1 Salad/200g	570	47.8	285	5.1	12.6	23.9	0.7
Basil & Parmesan, Tesco*	1 Serving/50g	65	1.8	130	4.3	20.2	3.6	0.6
BBQ Chicken, Positive Eating, Scottish Slimmers*	1 Serving/240g	223	4.3	93	6.4	14.0	1.8	1.3
Caesar, & Santa Tomatoes, M & S*	1 Serving/220g	495	33.7	225	5.2	15.9	15.3	0.8
Caesar, Chicken, Shapers, Boots*	1 Pack/218g	288	8.3	132	6.7	18.0	3.8	1.8
Carbonara, Waitrose*	1oz/28g	72	6.3	257	5.4	8.1	22.6	0.5
Chargrilled Chicken, & Pesto Pasta, Sainsbury's*	1 Pack/240g	454	22.1	189	7.2	19.4	9.2	0.0
Chargrilled Chicken, & Red Pepper, Tesco*	1 Pack/270g	553	24.0	205	9.8	20.3	8.9	3.1
Chargrilled Chicken, Italian Style, Fresh, Asda*	1 Pack/200g	318	14.0	159	7.0	17.0	7.0	0.4
Chargrilled Chicken, M & S*	1 Serving/190g	285	5.5	150	9.6	23.6	2.9	1.6
Chargrilled Red Pepper & Sunblush Tomato, Finest, Tesco*	1 Serving/100g	165	4.3	165	4.9	26.0	4.3	3.3
Chargrilled Vegetables, Sainsbury's*	1 Serving/178g	192	4.8	108	2.7	15.9	2.7	4.7
Chargrilled Vegetables & Tomato, Shapers, Boots*	1 Pack/175g	187	5.4	107	2.8	17.0	3.1	1.5
Cheddar Cheese, Tesco*	1 Pot/215g	546	43.9	254	5.7	12.0	20.4	0.8

PASTA SALAD

INFO/WEIGHT	Measure	per Measure		Nutrition Values per 100g / 100ml				
		KCAL	FAT	KCAL	PROT	CARB	FAT	FIBRE
Cheese, Asda*	1 Serving/40g	118	9.0	296	6.5	16.6	22.6	0.5
Cheese, Layered, Asda*	1 Pack/440g	647	40.9	147	4.5	11.4	9.3	0.0
Cheese, Morrisons*	½ Pot/125g	341	26.6	273	5.7	14.7	21.3	1.0
Cheese Layered, Asda*	1 Pack/440g	471	21.6	107	5.2	10.4	4.9	2.0
Cheese with Mayonnaise & Vinaigrette, Sainsbury's*	¼ Pot/50g	124	8.6	249	6.1	17.0	17.3	1.7
Chicken, Asda*	1 Pot/250g	322	12.2	129	5.8	15.5	4.9	1.3
Chicken & Bacon, Tesco*	½ Pack/200g	450	29.0	225	6.3	16.8	14.5	3.2
Chicken & Bacon Layered, Fresh Tastes, Asda*	1 Pack/197g	290	16.9	147	6.5	10.3	8.6	0.0
Chicken & Smoked Bacon, M & S*	1 Pack/380g	817	46.7	215	7.5	19.0	12.3	1.9
Chicken Caesar, Asda*	1 Pack/297g	683	41.3	230	9.6	16.6	13.9	2.5
Chicken Caesar, Ginsters*	1 Pack/220g	504	35.4	229	7.5	13.6	16.1	0.0
Chilli & Cheese, Sainsbury's*	1 Serving/300g	384	16.8	128	4.3	15.5	5.6	0.3
Crayfish, Rocket & Lemon, Finest, Tesco*	1 Serving/250g	727	39.7	291	8.9	28.0	15.9	4.2
Crayfish, Shapers, Boots*	1 Pack/280g	269	6.4	96	6.0	13.0	2.3	0.7
Farfalle, Prawns Tomatoes & Cucumber, Sainsbury's*	1 Serving/260g	270	12.2	104	4.5	10.9	4.7	0.7
Fire Roasted Tomato, So Good, Somerfield*	½ Pack/100g	199	10.6	199	4.4	21.6	10.6	1.5
Garlic Mushroom, Salad Bar, Asda*	1oz/28g	59	4.7	212	2.5	12.5	16.9	0.8
Goats Cheese & Mixed Pepper, Sainsbury's*	1 Pack/200g	366	18.8	183	6.4	18.2	9.4	1.5
Ham, Sainsbury's*	1 Pot/250g	610	48.2	244	4.1	13.4	19.3	0.8
Ham & Pineapple, Salad Bar, Asda*	1oz/28g	62	4.5	221	3.3	15.6	16.2	1.4
Honey & Mustard Chicken, M & S*	1 Serving/190g	304	4.7	160	8.7	26.7	2.5	1.5
Honey & Mustard Chicken, Sainsbury's*	1 Pack/190g	344	16.9	181	7.1	18.0	8.9	0.0
Honey & Mustard Chicken, Shapers, Boots*	1 Serving/252g	350	5.5	139	8.4	22.0	2.2	2.8
Hot Smoked Salmon, No Mayonnaise, Tesco*	1 Pack/275g	426	17.0	155	7.1	16.6	6.2	4.1
Italian, Bowl, Sainsbury's*	1 Serving/210g	309	15.5	147	3.1	16.9	7.4	1.9
Italian, Tesco*	½ Pack/225g	315	8.3	140	3.5	22.6	3.7	2.3
Italian Style, Iceland*	1 Serving/75g	97	4.5	129	2.6	16.2	6.0	1.6
Italian Style, Sainsbury's*	1/3 Pot/84g	129	5.3	153	3.5	20.5	6.3	1.4
Italian Style, Snack, Asda*	1 Pack/150g	141	6.0	94	3.4	11.0	4.0	4.1
Kraft*	½ Cup/68g	183	11.0	269	4.0	26.5	16.2	0.0
Lime & Coriander Chicken, M & S*	1 Serving/190g	370	23.2	195	7.6	14.4	12.2	0.6
Mediterranean, Good Intentions, Somerfield*	1 Pack/250g	290	7.0	116	2.8	19.8	2.8	1.1
Mediterranean, Tesco*	1oz/28g	24	1.3	87	2.1	9.6	4.5	1.4
Mediterranean Chicken, Waitrose*	1 Serving/200g	314	13.6	157	7.0	16.9	6.8	2.1
Mediterranean Style, Layered, Waitrose*	1 Pot/275g	190	3.6	69	2.6	11.8	1.3	1.0
Mediterranean Tuna, Shapers, Boots*	1 Serving/239g	232	3.1	97	6.2	15.0	1.3	0.9
Mediterranean Vegetable & Bean, BGTY, Sainsbury's*	1 Serving/66g	53	1.3	80	3.2	12.5	1.9	2.8
Mexican Chicken, Weight Watchers*	1 Pack/249g	284	4.2	114	7.8	16.9	1.7	3.6
Mixed Bean, Diet Chef Ltd*	1 Packet/300g	300	3.6	100	4.7	17.5	1.2	2.8
Mozzarella & Plum Tomatoes, COU, M & S*	1 Bowl/255g	204	4.1	80	4.6	11.5	1.6	1.7
Mozzarella & Sun Dried Tomato, Waitrose*	1 Serving/150g	312	18.3	208	5.8	18.8	12.2	1.3
Pepper, Side, Tesco*	1 Serving/46g	56	3.0	122	2.4	13.0	6.5	1.3
Pepper & Tomato, Fire Roasted, Finest, Tesco*	1 Pack/200g	260	8.2	130	3.7	19.4	4.1	2.5
Poached Salmon, M & S*	1 Serving/200g	340	16.8	170	7.8	16.2	8.4	1.4
Poached Salmon, Sainsbury's*	1 Serving/200g	472	30.6	236	6.7	17.9	15.3	12.0
Prawn, Layered, Asda*	½ Pack/220g	279	11.4	127	5.2	14.2	5.2	2.0
Prawn, Shapers, Boots*	1 Pot/250g	250	7.7	100	4.1	14.0	3.1	0.4
Prawn, Tesco*	½ Pack/250g	487	27.7	195	4.9	18.9	11.1	2.0
Prawn Cocktail, Shapers, Boots*	1 Pack/248g	255	6.7	103	5.0	15.0	2.7	1.6
Prawns, King & Juicy Fresh Tomatoes, COU, M & S*	1 Serving/270g	256	4.0	95	5.1	16.4	1.5	0.9
Ready to Eat, Somerfield*	½ Pack/123g	175	8.5	142	2.8	17.1	6.9	1.6
Roasted Mushroom, Spinach & Tarragon, Tesco*	1 Pot/200g	216	4.8	108	4.3	17.2	2.4	0.8
Roasted Vegetable, Waitrose*	1 Pack/190g	270	8.7	142	6.8	18.2	4.6	1.1

	Measure INFO/WEIGHT	per Measure		Nutrition Values per 100g / 100ml				
		KCAL	FAT	KCAL	PROT	CARB	FAT	FIBRE
PASTA SALAD								
Sainsbury's*	½ Pack/160g	235	9.6	147	3.2	20.0	6.0	1.5
Salmon, M & S*	1 Serving/380g	817	57.8	215	6.8	12.7	15.2	0.7
Spicy Chicken, Budgens*	1 Serving/213g	452	22.2	212	5.1	24.5	10.4	4.4
Spicy Chicken, Geo Adams*	1 Pack/230g	580	43.9	252	5.1	14.9	19.1	2.9
Spicy Chilli Pesto, Sainsbury's*	¼ Pot/63g	170	12.2	272	3.8	20.1	19.6	1.6
Sun Dried Tomato Dressing, Sainsbury's*	1 Pack/320g	442	14.1	138	3.7	20.8	4.4	3.6
Sweetcorn, Waitrose*	1oz/28g	31	0.3	112	6.4	18.9	1.2	1.1
Sweetcorn & Pepper, GFY, Asda*	1 Serving/175g	68	0.7	39	1.9	7.0	0.4	0.0
Three Cheese, Tesco*	1 Serving/300g	633	41.1	211	7.5	14.4	13.7	2.8
Tiger Prawn, Waitrose*	1 Serving/225g	544	38.5	242	5.4	16.7	17.1	0.4
Tiger Prawn & Tomato, GFY, Asda*	1 Serving/200g	250	5.8	125	4.6	20.0	2.9	2.0
Tomato, Aldi*	1 Serving/50g	58	1.8	117	3.9	18.6	3.6	0.0
Tomato, Bacon & Cheese, Ginsters*	1 Pack/220g	381	19.8	173	7.4	15.6	9.0	0.0
Tomato, Diet Chef Ltd*	1 Pack/300g	264	5.4	88	2.3	15.6	1.8	1.2
Tomato & Basil, Chicken, Waitrose*	1 Pack/205g	434	24.6	212	8.3	17.7	12.0	1.1
Tomato & Basil, M & S*	1 Pot/225g	484	35.8	215	2.9	15.0	15.9	1.2
Tomato & Basil, Perfectly Balanced, Waitrose*	1 Serving/100g	97	1.7	97	3.7	16.8	1.7	0.0
Tomato & Basil, Pot, HL, Tesco*	1 Pot/200g	242	5.4	121	2.0	22.1	2.7	2.2
Tomato & Basil, Sainsbury's*	1 Serving/62g	87	4.3	141	3.2	16.4	6.9	3.8
Tomato & Basil Chicken, M & S*	1 Serving/279g	446	22.0	160	7.0	14.8	7.9	1.8
Tomato & Basil with Red & Green Pepper, Sainsbury's*	¼ Pot/63g	89	4.3	141	3.2	16.4	6.9	3.8
Tomato & Chargrilled Vegetable, Tesco*	1 Serving/200g	248	7.8	124	3.7	18.6	3.9	1.4
Tomato & Mozzarella, Leaf, Shapers, Boots*	1 Pack/185g	356	22.3	192	5.1	16.0	12.0	2.5
Tomato & Mozzarella, Sainsbury's*	1 Pack/200g	440	22.6	220	7.5	22.2	11.3	1.3
Tomato & Mozzarella, Waitrose*	1 Pack/225g	380	27.9	169	4.3	10.0	12.4	0.6
Tomato & Pepper, HL, Tesco*	1 Serving/200g	162	3.2	81	2.6	13.9	1.6	1.4
Tomato & Tuna, Snack, Sainsbury's*	1 Serving/200g	238	2.4	119	5.3	21.7	1.2	0.0
Tuna, Arrabbiata, BGTY, Sainsbury's*	1 Serving/200g	196	2.6	98	6.8	14.7	1.3	0.0
Tuna, Mediterranean, Johnsons*	1 Serving/225g	148	6.2	66	2.8	7.5	2.8	0.9
Tuna, Perfectly Balanced, Waitrose*	1 Tub/190g	180	4.4	95	7.0	11.5	2.3	1.1
Tuna, Tesco*	1 Pot/300g	399	21.9	133	6.2	10.5	7.3	0.0
Tuna & Spinach, COU, M & S*	1 Pack/270g	256	4.9	95	6.8	14.3	1.8	3.8
Tuna & Sweetcorn, COU, M & S*	1 Pack/200g	210	1.8	105	7.1	18.3	0.9	1.2
Tuna & Sweetcorn, Sainsbury's*	1 Serving/100g	111	1.2	111	7.1	18.3	1.2	1.2
Tuna Crunch, Shapers, Boots*	1 Pack/250g	352	6.7	141	9.8	19.0	2.7	2.8
Tuna Nicoise, Waitrose*	1 Pot/190g	306	17.1	161	5.1	14.9	9.0	1.1
Vegetable, Healthy Selection, Somerfield*	1 Pot/200g	180	0.0	90	2.8	19.6	0.0	0.7
Vegetable, Somerfield*	1 Pack/200g	288	12.0	144	3.0	20.0	6.0	0.0
with Avocado & Cherry Tomatoes, M & S*	1 Pack/185g	259	14.8	140	2.9	13.9	8.0	1.2
with Italian Style Chicken, Weight Watchers*	1 Pack/185g	237	2.0	128	6.7	22.9	1.1	0.7
PASTA SAUCE								
Amatriciana, M & S*	1 Jar/340g	425	32.3	125	3.4	6.3	9.5	2.9
Amatriciana, Morrisons*	1 Tub/350g	157	5.6	45	3.7	4.6	1.6	0.5
Amatriciana, Tesco*	1 Serving/175g	108	7.2	62	2.3	4.0	4.1	0.7
Arrabbiata, Bertolli*	1 Serving/133g	120	8.8	90	1.6	5.8	6.6	1.5
Arrabbiata, Fresh, Morrisons*	1 Pot/350g	139	5.2	40	1.9	5.4	1.5	0.0
Arrabbiata, GFY, Asda*	1 Serving/350g	133	3.9	38	1.1	6.0	1.1	0.0
Arrabbiata, Italian, Waitrose*	1 Jar/320g	115	3.2	36	1.5	6.7	1.0	1.4
Arrabbiata, M & S*	1 Jar/320g	240	17.0	75	1.2	6.2	5.3	0.8
Arrabbiata, Red Pepper, Sainsbury's*	½ Pot/175g	79	5.1	45	1.4	3.3	2.9	1.6
Arrabbiata, Romano*	1 Serving/100g	69	3.4	69	2.5	7.0	3.4	0.6
Aubergine & Pepper, Sacla*	½ Pot/95g	237	23.3	250	1.8	5.6	24.5	0.0
Basil & Oregano, Ragu, Knorr*	1 Jar/500g	215	0.0	43	1.3	9.4	0.0	1.1

PASTA SAUCE

	Measure INFO/WEIGHT	per Measure KCAL	FAT	Nutrition Values per 100g / 100ml KCAL	PROT	CARB	FAT	FIBRE
Bolognese, Carb Check, Heinz*	1 Serving/150g	79	3.9	53	3.8	3.6	2.6	0.4
Bolognese, Dolmio*	1 Serving/100g	56	1.5	56	1.5	9.4	1.5	1.1
Bolognese, Finest, Tesco*	1 Serving/175g	170	10.7	97	7.0	3.8	6.1	0.5
Bolognese, Fresh, Sainsbury's*	½ Pot/150g	120	6.1	80	6.0	4.7	4.1	1.2
Bolognese, Mediterranean Vegetable, Chunky, Dolmio*	½ Jar/250g	137	4.0	55	1.3	8.8	1.6	1.1
Bolognese, Organic, Seeds of Change*	1 Jar/500g	290	6.0	58	1.3	10.4	1.2	0.8
Bolognese, Original, Asda*	1 Serving/158g	73	2.2	46	1.4	7.0	1.4	0.8
Bolognese, Original, Light, Low Fat, Dolmio*	1 Serving/125g	44	0.2	35	1.5	6.0	0.2	1.2
Bolognese, Spicy, Ragu, Knorr*	1 Jar/500g	260	1.0	52	1.9	9.7	0.2	1.4
Bolognese, Tesco*	1 Serving/175g	100	4.5	57	4.2	4.0	2.6	0.8
Bolognese, Tomato, Beef & Red Wine, Fresh, Waitrose*	1 Pot/350g	301	17.2	86	5.4	5.3	4.9	2.0
Bolognese, Traditional, Ragu, Knorr*	1 Jar/320g	157	5.4	49	1.3	7.1	1.7	1.2
Bolognese, VLH Kitchens	1 Serving/380g	316	1.1	83	6.0	4.7	4.1	1.2
Carbonara, Creamy, Dolmio Express, Dolmio*	1 Pack/150g	171	13.8	114	3.1	4.7	9.2	0.1
Carbonara, Creamy, Dolmio Express, Dolmio*	1 Pack/150g	166	13.2	111	3.3	4.7	8.8	0.1
Carbonara, Creamy, Stir in Sauce, Dolmio*	1 Serving/75g	98	8.0	130	3.3	5.2	10.6	0.2
Carbonara, Italian, Asda*	½ Pack/175g	359	29.7	205	7.0	6.0	17.0	0.1
Carbonara, Italian, Fresh, Sainsbury's*	½ Pot/176g	209	16.3	119	5.4	3.4	9.3	0.9
Carbonara, Reduced Fat, BFY, Morrisons*	½ Pot/175g	135	5.8	77	6.6	5.1	3.3	0.5
Carbonara with Pancetta, Loyd Grossman*	½ Pack/170g	209	15.5	123	2.8	7.5	9.1	0.1
Chargrilled Vegetable with Extra Virgin Olive Oil, Bertolli*	½ Jar/250g	150	4.7	60	2.1	8.7	1.9	2.4
Cheese, Fresh, Perfectly Balanced, Waitrose*	½ Pot/175g	143	5.1	82	6.1	7.9	2.9	0.5
Cherry Tomato & Basil, Sacla*	1 Serving/96g	90	7.1	94	1.2	5.3	7.4	0.0
Chilli with Jalapeno Peppers, Seeds of Change*	1 Jar/350g	322	5.2	92	3.6	16.0	1.5	2.2
Chunky Vegetable, Asda*	1 Serving/250g	122	4.2	49	1.4	7.0	1.7	1.2
Chunky Vegetable, Somerfield*	1 Jar/525g	226	5.2	43	2.0	7.0	1.0	0.0
Country Mushroom for Bolognese, Ragu, Knorr*	1 Jar/510g	347	10.7	68	2.0	9.5	2.1	1.2
Creamy Mushroom, Dolmio*	1 Pack/150g	166	15.0	111	1.3	3.7	10.0	0.0
Creamy Mushroom, Express, Dolmio*	1 Serving/150g	160	14.4	107	1.4	3.8	9.6	0.0
Creamy Tomato, Carb Check, Heinz*	1 Serving/150g	91	6.0	61	2.0	4.2	4.0	0.5
for Bolognese, Extra Mushrooms, Dolmio*	1 Jar/500g	240	6.5	48	1.6	7.6	1.3	1.1
for Bolognese, Extra Onion & Garlic, Dolmio*	1 Serving/125g	62	1.6	50	1.5	8.1	1.3	1.0
for Bolognese, Extra Spicy, Dolmio*	1 Jar/500g	260	5.5	52	1.7	8.8	1.1	0.8
for Lasagne, Tomato, Red, Ragu, Knorr*	1 Jar/500g	215	0.0	43	1.1	9.7	0.0	1.1
for Lasagne, White, Light, Ragu, Knorr*	¼ Jar/122g	88	6.1	72	0.5	6.3	5.0	0.2
for Lasagne, White, Ragu, Knorr*	1 Jar/475g	755	72.2	159	0.5	5.1	15.2	0.3
Four Cheese, Loyd Grossman*	1 Jar/350g	476	41.6	136	2.6	4.6	11.9	0.0
Four Cheese, Sainsbury's*	1 Serving/150g	295	25.5	197	6.6	4.5	17.0	0.8
Garlic, Perfectly Balanced, Waitrose*	1 Jar/440g	330	7.5	75	2.3	12.7	1.7	2.3
Garlic & Chilli, Slow Roasted, Seeds of Change*	½ Jar/175g	157	9.3	90	1.7	8.7	5.3	2.0
Garlic & Onion, Finest, Tesco*	1 Serving/126g	43	0.5	34	0.8	6.9	0.4	1.3
Grilled Vegetables, Bertolli*	1 Jar/400g	215	10.0	43	1.4	4.9	2.0	1.1
Ham & Mushroom, Creamy, Stir & Serve, Homepride*	1 Serving/92g	124	10.8	135	1.8	5.5	11.7	0.0
Hot & Spicy, Morrisons*	1 Serving/130g	81	3.1	62	1.4	8.5	2.4	1.1
Hot Mixed Peppers Bolognese, Sainsbury's*	1oz/28g	18	0.6	66	2.0	9.7	2.1	1.5
Hot Pepper & Mozzarella, Stir Through, Sacla*	½ Jar/95g	229	20.4	241	4.7	7.2	21.5	0.0
Layered Tomato & Mozzarella, Finest, Tesco*	1 Jar/160g	232	16.2	145	6.6	6.9	10.1	0.7
Light Choices, Tesco*	1oz/28g	9	0.1	33	0.7	6.9	0.3	1.2
Mediterranean, BGTY, Sainsbury's*	1oz/28g	23	1.2	82	1.9	9.0	4.3	1.4
Mediterranean, Fresh, Waitrose*	1 Pot/350g	213	13.6	61	1.4	5.0	3.9	2.4
Mediterranean Tomato, Asda*	1 Jar/500g	285	6.0	57	1.5	10.0	1.2	0.0
Mediterranean Vegetable, Organic, Pasta Reale*	1 Pack/300g	183	13.8	61	1.0	3.9	4.6	0.3
Mediterranean Vegetable, Organic, Seeds of Change*	1 Jar/350g	245	12.2	70	1.5	8.3	3.5	1.1

PASTA SAUCE	Measure INFO/WEIGHT	per Measure KCAL	FAT	Nutrition Values per 100g / 100ml KCAL	PROT	CARB	FAT	FIBRE
Mediterranean Vegetable, Rustico, Bertolli*	½ Jar/160g	141	11.5	88	1.7	4.1	7.2	0.7
Mediterranean Vegetable Pasta, Tesco*	1 Serving/166g	95	2.8	57	1.4	9.0	1.7	1.2
Mushroom, Microwaveable, Dolmio*	1 Serving/150g	160	14.4	107	1.4	3.8	9.6	0.0
Mushroom, Perfectly Balanced, Waitrose*	1 Jar/440g	330	8.4	75	2.6	11.8	1.9	2.2
Mushroom, Sainsbury's*	1 Serving/100g	66	2.1	66	2.0	9.8	2.1	1.7
Mushroom & Garlic, 98% Fat Free, Homepride*	1 Jar/450g	229	6.3	51	1.1	8.9	1.4	0.5
Mushroom & Garlic, Deliciously Good, Homepride*	1/3 Jar/147g	109	7.1	74	0.9	6.9	4.8	0.3
Mushroom & Marsala Wine, Sacla*	½ Pot/85g	165	16.0	194	2.2	3.9	18.8	0.0
Mushroom & Mascarpone, Morrisons*	½ Pot/175g	199	17.0	114	2.3	4.3	9.7	0.0
Mushroom & White Wine, Knorr*	1oz/28g	27	2.2	98	1.0	4.0	8.0	0.0
Napoletana, BGTY, Sainsbury's*	½ Pot/151g	71	3.8	47	1.2	5.0	2.5	1.3
Napoletana, Buitoni*	½ Jar/200g	146	8.2	73	1.6	7.3	4.1	2.2
Napoletana, Fresh, Waitrose*	1 Serving/175g	82	3.0	47	1.3	6.6	1.7	1.0
Napoletana, GFY, Asda*	1 Serving/175g	58	1.7	33	1.0	5.0	1.0	0.0
Olive, Barilla*	1 Serving/100g	92	5.0	92	1.5	10.3	5.0	0.0
Olive & Tomato, Sacla*	1 Serving/95g	87	7.6	92	1.3	3.6	8.0	0.0
Onion & Garlic, Co-Op*	1 Serving/125g	106	3.7	85	2.0	12.0	3.0	0.7
Onion & Garlic, Tesco*	1 Serving/125g	35	0.1	28	1.2	5.6	0.1	2.6
Onion & Roasted Garlic, Knorr*	1 Jar/500g	210	0.0	42	1.3	9.2	0.0	1.1
Original, BFY, Morrisons*	1/3 Jar/200g	100	0.2	50	1.6	10.6	0.1	1.2
Original, Tesco*	1 Jar/300g	123	4.2	41	1.0	6.1	1.4	2.3
Parmesan & Pesto, Weight Watchers*	½ Jar/175g	86	2.8	49	1.8	6.7	1.6	1.0
Pepper & Tomato, M & S*	1 Jar/320g	224	13.4	70	1.6	6.1	4.2	0.9
Pomodoro, Cirio*	1 Serving/200g	116	4.6	58	1.4	8.4	2.3	0.0
Porcini Mushroom & Pepperoni, Asda*	½ Jar/140g	158	8.4	113	3.8	11.0	6.0	0.0
Porcini Mushroom Stir in, BGTY, Sainsbury's*	½ Jar/75g	57	3.1	76	3.8	5.7	4.2	1.9
Primavera, Fresh, Morrisons*	½ Pot/175g	152	10.3	87	2.4	6.1	5.9	0.0
Primavera, Loyd Grossman*	1 Jar/350g	343	25.9	98	1.4	6.3	7.4	0.9
Puttanesca, Italian, Waitrose*	1 Jar/350g	195	9.8	56	1.5	6.1	2.8	1.3
Puttanesca, Loyd Grossman*	1 Jar/350g	315	21.7	90	1.7	6.8	6.2	0.9
Puttanesca, M & S*	1 Jar/320g	256	17.6	80	1.5	6.2	5.5	1.9
Puttanesca, Sainsbury's*	1 Serving/110g	132	9.7	120	2.0	8.1	8.8	0.0
Red Pepper & Italian Cheese, Stir Through, Asda*	½ Jar/95g	85	4.7	90	2.9	8.5	4.9	0.9
Red Pepper & Plum, Finest, Tesco*	1 Serving/63g	109	7.2	173	3.7	14.0	11.4	5.4
Red Wine, Traditional Recipe, Dolmio*	1 Serving/100g	63	0.8	63	1.5	10.3	0.8	0.0
Rich Tomato with Basil Pesto, Express, Dolmio*	1 Pack/170g	146	10.0	86	2.0	6.2	5.9	0.0
Roasted Garlic & Onion, Newman's Own*	1 Jar/680g	367	12.9	54	2.0	12.1	1.9	0.0
Roasted Garlic & Onion, Weight Watchers*	1 Jar/175g	65	0.7	37	1.3	6.4	0.4	1.2
Roasted Red Pepper & Tomato, Finest, Tesco*	1 Serving/145g	117	7.8	81	1.2	6.8	5.4	2.2
Roasted Vegetable, GFY, Asda*	½ Pot/175g	84	2.8	48	1.3	7.0	1.6	0.5
Roasted Vegetable, Microwaveable, Dolmio*	½ Pack/190g	103	3.8	54	1.4	7.6	2.0	0.0
Roasted Vegetable, Sainsbury's*	½ Pot/151g	103	5.9	68	1.6	6.7	3.9	0.4
Roasted Vegetable, Tesco*	1 Pack/175g	114	5.2	65	1.5	8.0	3.0	0.8
Roasted Vegetables & Tuna, BGTY, Sainsbury's*	½ Pot/150g	73	2.8	49	3.5	4.5	1.9	3.1
Romano*	1 Serving/235g	141	4.7	60	1.7	8.8	2.0	1.1
Rustico Mushroom, Garlic & Oregano, Bertolli*	1 Serving/100g	90	7.5	90	1.9	3.8	7.5	0.0
Rustico Sweet Chilli & Red Onion, Bertolli*	½ Jar/160g	146	11.5	91	1.7	4.9	7.2	0.7
Salsina with Onions & Garlic, Valfrutta*	1 Serving/150g	36	0.0	24	1.6	4.5	0.0	1.4
Seasonal, Bolognese, Dolmio*	1 Jar/500g	205	1.0	41	1.5	7.4	0.2	1.4
Siciliana, Sainsbury's*	1/3 Jar/113g	168	14.7	149	1.8	6.2	13.0	0.0
Sliced Mushroom, Tesco*	1 Jar/460g	161	0.9	35	1.3	7.0	0.2	0.8
Smoky Bacon, Loyd Grossman*	½ Jar/175g	142	8.4	81	3.0	6.1	4.8	0.8
Spicy Italian Chilli, Express, Dolmio*	1 Serving/170g	87	2.7	51	1.5	7.5	1.6	0.0

PASTA SAUCE

	Measure INFO/WEIGHT	per Measure		Nutrition Values per 100g / 100ml				
		KCAL	FAT	KCAL	PROT	CARB	FAT	FIBRE
Spicy Pepper, Tesco*	1 Jar/500g	245	5.0	49	1.7	8.4	1.0	1.0
Spicy Pepper & Tomato, Sacla*	½ Jar/95g	132	11.2	139	1.4	6.8	11.8	0.0
Spicy Roasted Garlic, Seeds of Change*	1 Serving/195g	123	3.9	63	1.5	9.7	2.0	1.2
Spicy Tomato, Asda*	1 Serving/155g	76	1.9	49	1.5	8.0	1.2	1.0
Spicy with Peppers, Tesco*	1 Jar/455g	177	1.4	39	1.2	7.9	0.3	1.1
Spinach & Ricotta, Asda*	½ Pot/175g	175	12.2	100	3.2	6.0	7.0	0.5
Spinach & Ricotta, BGTY, Sainsbury's*	1 Serving/150g	73	4.0	49	2.7	3.4	2.7	2.2
Spinach & Ricotta, Fresh, Perfectly Balanced, Waitrose*	½ Pot/175g	96	3.7	55	3.3	5.7	2.1	0.9
Spinach & Ricotta, Stir Through, Sacla*	½ Jar/95g	196	18.6	206	3.7	3.7	19.6	0.0
Stir & Serve, Homepride*	1 Jar/480g	187	5.8	39	1.2	6.0	1.2	0.0
Sun Dried Tomato, Asda*	½ Jar/159g	165	12.7	104	1.9	6.0	8.0	1.5
Sun Dried Tomato, Garlic & Basil, Finest, Tesco*	1 Jar/340g	493	39.1	145	1.8	7.7	11.5	2.3
Sun Dried Tomato, Stir In, Light, Dolmio*	1 Serving/75g	62	3.5	83	1.7	9.8	4.7	0.0
Sun Dried Tomato & Basil, Free From, Sainsbury's*	½ Jar/172g	124	4.8	72	2.9	8.7	2.8	1.5
Sun Dried Tomato & Garlic, Sacla*	1 Serving/95g	177	14.0	186	3.0	10.3	14.7	0.0
Sun Dried Tomato & Olive Oil, Loyd Grossman*	1oz/28g	52	4.4	187	0.8	10.3	15.8	0.3
Sun Ripened Tomato & Basil, Dolmio*	1 Serving/150g	117	6.9	78	1.3	7.9	4.6	0.0
Sun Ripened Tomato & Basil, Express, Dolmio*	1 Pouch/170g	88	2.7	52	1.5	7.9	1.6	0.0
Sun Ripened Tomato & Basil, Microwaveable, Dolmio*	½ Pack/190g	106	4.0	56	1.4	7.9	2.1	0.0
Sundried Tomato, Heinz*	½ Jar/150g	55	0.3	37	1.5	7.3	0.2	1.1
Sundried Tomato & Basil, Organic, Seeds of Change*	½ Jar/100g	155	13.1	155	1.6	7.7	13.1	0.0
Sundried Tomato & Garlic, M & S*	½ Jar/95g	147	13.0	155	2.9	4.4	13.7	0.8
Sweet Pepper, Dolmio*	1 Serving/150g	238	20.1	159	1.6	8.8	13.4	0.0
Sweet Red Pepper, Loyd Grossman*	1 Jar/350g	304	19.6	87	1.7	7.3	5.6	1.2
Three Cheeses, Co-Op*	1 Pack/300g	405	27.0	135	6.0	6.0	9.0	0.1
Tomato, Bacon & Mushroom, Asda*	½ Pot/50g	33	1.8	66	2.5	6.0	3.6	0.0
Tomato, Basil & Parmesan Stir in, BGTY, Sainsbury's*	1 Serving/75g	69	4.1	92	2.9	7.8	5.5	1.0
Tomato, Black Olive, Caper, Finest, Tesco*	1 Serving/145g	146	11.2	101	1.5	6.4	7.7	3.3
Tomato, Chilli & Onion, Bertolli*	1 Serving/100g	49	1.7	49	1.8	6.7	1.7	1.8
Tomato, Ginger & Basil, Cranks*	½ Jar/175g	129	8.2	74	1.7	6.3	4.7	1.1
Tomato, Low Price, Sainsbury's*	1 Jar/440g	220	3.1	50	0.6	10.1	0.7	0.4
Tomato, Mushroom & Roasted Garlic, Bertolli*	1 Jar/500g	235	9.5	47	1.9	5.3	1.9	0.0
Tomato, Organic, Evernat*	1oz/28g	18	0.4	64	2.8	10.2	1.3	0.0
Tomato, Pecorino Romano Cheese & Garlic, Bertolli*	1 Serving/125g	76	3.5	61	2.3	6.5	2.8	0.9
Tomato, Red Pepper & Chilli, Slow Cooked, Dress Italian*	1 Jar/350g	318	22.4	91	1.9	6.6	6.4	1.3
Tomato, Red Wine, Shallots, Bertolli*	½ Jar/250g	112	4.2	45	1.7	7.2	1.7	1.5
Tomato, Sweet Cherry, Slow Cooked, Dress Italian*	½ Jar/175g	163	11.2	93	1.8	7.2	6.4	2.1
Tomato & Basil, Bertolli*	1 Jar/500g	215	5.0	43	1.2	7.3	1.0	0.4
Tomato & Basil, Carb Check, Heinz*	1 Serving/150g	84	5.4	56	1.5	4.4	3.6	0.6
Tomato & Basil, Classic, Sacla*	1 Serving/100g	137	11.1	137	2.0	7.2	11.1	2.8
Tomato & Basil, Dolmio*	1 Serving/170g	95	3.6	56	1.4	7.9	2.1	0.0
Tomato & Basil, Loyd Grossman*	½ Jar/175g	107	5.9	61	1.5	5.8	3.4	0.8
Tomato & Basil, M & S*	1 Jar/340g	119	7.1	35	2.0	2.1	2.1	0.9
Tomato & Basil, Morrisons*	1 Serving/175g	63	1.0	36	2.0	5.6	0.6	1.0
Tomato & Basil, Organic, Pasta Reale*	1 Pack/300g	216	15.9	72	1.0	5.1	5.3	0.4
Tomato & Basil, Organic, Simply Organic*	1 Pot/300g	183	12.9	61	1.5	4.2	4.3	0.6
Tomato & Black Olive, Carb Control, Tesco*	1 Serving/110g	74	4.7	67	1.3	6.0	4.3	2.3
Tomato & Chargrilled Vegetable, Loyd Grossman*	1 Serving/150g	133	8.4	89	1.8	7.9	5.6	0.9
Tomato & Chilli, Loyd Grossman*	½ Jar/175g	101	5.9	58	1.4	5.5	3.4	0.7
Tomato & Chilli, Pour Over, M & S*	1 Jar/330g	231	12.5	70	1.3	7.6	3.8	1.8
Tomato & Chilli, Whole Cherry Tomatoes, Classic, Sacla*	½ Jar/175g	238	19.2	136	2.0	7.2	11.0	3.1
Tomato & Chilli with Pine Nuts & Raisins, Loyd Grossman*	½ Jar/175g	159	9.1	91	1.9	9.3	5.2	1.7
Tomato & Chunky Mushroom, Dolmio*	1 Pack/475g	323	17.6	68	1.2	7.6	3.7	0.0

PASTA SAUCE	Measure INFO/WEIGHT	per Measure KCAL	FAT	Nutrition Values per 100g / 100ml KCAL	PROT	CARB	FAT	FIBRE
Tomato & Creme Fraiche, Perfectly Balanced, Waitrose*	½ Pot/177g	85	2.3	48	1.8	7.1	1.3	2.0
Tomato & Garlic, Chosen By You, Asda*	½ Jar/160g	74	0.8	46	1.6	7.9	0.5	1.7
Tomato & Herb, Co-Op*	1 Serving/125g	75	2.5	60	1.0	9.0	2.0	1.0
Tomato & Herb, Iceland*	1 Serving/100g	59	2.0	59	1.4	8.9	2.0	0.7
Tomato & Herb, M & S*	1 Jar/500g	400	15.5	80	2.6	10.1	3.1	1.7
Tomato & Herb, Organic, M & S*	1 Jar/550g	302	19.8	55	1.4	4.2	3.6	2.6
Tomato & Herb, Organic, Meridian Foods*	½ Jar/220g	141	6.2	64	1.6	8.1	2.8	1.1
Tomato & Herb, Organic, Sainsbury's*	1 Serving/75g	38	1.5	51	1.2	6.6	2.0	0.5
Tomato & Herb, Perfectly Balanced, Waitrose*	½ Tub/176g	65	2.1	37	1.3	5.3	1.2	2.3
Tomato & Herb with Extra Garlic, Sainsbury's*	½ Pot/150g	61	1.6	41	1.4	6.3	1.1	1.6
Tomato & Mascarpone, BGTY, Sainsbury's*	1 Pot/300g	150	9.0	50	2.0	3.6	3.0	3.6
Tomato & Mascarpone, Finest, Tesco*	1 Serving/175g	135	8.7	77	2.7	5.4	5.0	0.8
Tomato & Mascarpone, Fresh, Budgens*	½ Pack/150g	136	10.5	91	1.9	6.0	7.0	0.8
Tomato & Mascarpone, Fresh, Sainsbury's*	1 Serving/150g	177	15.4	118	2.2	4.2	10.3	1.1
Tomato & Mascarpone, Italiano, Tesco*	½ Pot/175g	168	12.2	96	2.8	5.5	7.0	0.7
Tomato & Mascarpone, Morrisons*	½ Pot/175g	217	16.8	124	2.9	6.5	9.6	1.1
Tomato & Mascarpone, Pasta Reale*	1 Pack/300g	318	23.7	106	2.9	5.9	7.9	0.5
Tomato & Mascarpone, Sacla*	½ Jar/95g	161	14.2	169	2.2	6.2	15.0	0.0
Tomato & Mascarpone, Sainsbury's*	½ Pot/150g	137	9.9	91	2.1	5.9	6.6	1.2
Tomato & Mascarpone, So Organic, Sainsbury's*	1/3 Jar/146g	180	13.2	123	1.9	8.7	9.0	2.8
Tomato & Mascarpone, Tesco*	1 Serving/175g	194	15.2	111	2.8	5.4	8.7	0.6
Tomato & Mascarpone, Waitrose*	½ Pot/175g	184	14.7	105	1.9	5.5	8.4	1.1
Tomato & Mushroom, Chosen By You, Asda*	½ Jar/160g	70	1.0	44	2.1	7.0	0.6	1.1
Tomato & Mushroom, Organic, Sainsbury's*	1 Serving/150g	87	3.9	58	1.6	7.1	2.6	1.5
Tomato & Olives, La Doria*	1 Jar/90g	76	5.9	84	1.2	5.0	6.6	0.0
Tomato & Parmesan, Seeds of Change*	1 Serving/150g	100	4.3	67	2.5	7.8	2.9	1.1
Tomato & Pesto, Planet Cook, Heinz*	1 Jar/300g	237	17.1	79	1.7	5.2	5.7	1.0
Tomato & Ricotta, Italian, Sainsbury's*	1 Pack/390g	238	11.7	61	2.5	6.1	3.0	1.2
Tomato & Roasted Garlic, Chosen By You, Asda*	1 Pot/350g	122	2.1	35	1.5	5.0	0.6	1.7
Tomato & Roasted Garlic, Loyd Grossman*	½ Jar/175g	107	5.4	61	1.5	6.3	3.1	0.8
Tomato & Smokey Bacon, Dolmio*	1 Pot/150g	240	19.6	160	5.5	5.8	13.1	0.0
Tomato & Spicy Sausages, M & S*	1 Jar/330g	214	9.9	65	4.0	5.5	3.0	0.8
Tomato & Tuna, Loyd Grossman*	½ Jar/175g	154	7.7	88	4.4	7.5	4.4	0.8
Tomato & Wild Mushroom, Loyd Grossman*	½ Jar/175g	154	9.8	88	2.1	7.4	5.6	1.5
Tomato & Wild Mushroom, Waitrose*	1 Serving/175g	65	1.2	37	1.7	6.0	0.7	0.9
Tomato Bacon, Stir & Serve, Homepride*	1 Serving/96g	81	4.3	84	2.7	8.1	4.5	0.0
Tomato with Herbs Buon Appetito, Princes*	1 Jar/475g	214	1.9	45	0.7	9.6	0.4	0.0
Tomato with Red Wine & Herbs, Ragu, Knorr*	1 Jar/500g	215	0.5	43	1.3	9.3	0.1	1.1
Traditional, Somerfield*	1 Jar/525g	262	5.2	50	2.0	8.0	1.0	0.0
Vegetable, Chunky, Tesco*	1 Jar/455g	223	5.9	49	0.7	8.6	1.3	1.1
Vegetable & Garlic, Dolmio*	1 Serving/150g	108	6.1	72	1.3	7.4	4.1	0.0
Veneziana, M & S*	½ Jar/140g	196	15.0	140	5.7	5.5	10.7	1.6
Vine Ripened Tomato & Black Olive, Bertolli*	½ Jar/93g	145	12.3	157	2.3	7.3	13.3	0.0
Whole Cherry Tomato & Roasted Pepper, Sacla*	½ Jar/145g	93	5.9	64	1.5	5.2	4.1	0.0
Wild Mushroom & Herb, Seeds of Change*	1 Serving/190g	103	2.7	54	1.6	8.8	1.4	1.2
PASTA SHAPES								
Alphabetti, in Tomato Sauce, Heinz*	1 Can/200g	118	1.0	59	1.8	11.7	0.5	1.5
Bob The Builder, in Tomato Sauce, Heinz*	1 Can/205g	111	0.6	54	1.7	11.3	0.3	1.5
Cooked, Tesco*	1 Serving/260g	356	2.1	137	5.1	26.3	0.8	1.1
Disney Princess, in Tomato Sauce, Heinz*	1 Can/200g	114	0.6	57	1.8	11.9	0.3	1.5
Dried, Tesco*	1 Serving/100g	345	2.0	345	13.2	68.5	2.0	2.9
Durum Wheat, Dry, Basics, Sainsbury's*	1 Serving/75g	259	1.5	346	12.0	70.0	2.0	4.0
in a Cheese & Broccoli Sauce, Tesco*	1 Serving/84g	317	5.5	377	13.1	66.2	6.6	4.1

PASTA SHAPES	Measure INFO/WEIGHT	per Measure KCAL	FAT	Nutrition Values per 100g / 100ml KCAL	PROT	CARB	FAT	FIBRE
Postman Pat, HP*	1 Can/410g	279	1.6	68	1.8	14.3	0.4	0.7
Scooby Doo, HP*	1 Can/410g	279	1.6	68	1.8	14.3	0.4	0.7
Shrek, Multigrain in Tomato Sauce with Omega 3, Heinz*	1 Can/200g	120	1.0	60	1.9	12.0	0.5	1.5
Spiderman, in Tomato Sauce, Heinz*	½ Can/200g	114	1.0	57	1.7	11.4	0.5	1.5
Spiderman, with Mini Sausages in Tomato Sauce, Heinz*	1 Can/200g	178	6.2	89	3.6	11.6	3.1	0.5
Teletubbies, in Tomato Sauce, Heinz*	1 Can/400g	244	1.6	61	2.0	12.3	0.4	0.6
Thomas Tank Engine, in Tomato Sauce, Heinz*	1 Can/205g	109	0.4	53	1.7	11.0	0.2	0.5
Tweenies, in Tomato Sauce, Heinz*	1 Can/205g	121	1.0	59	1.8	11.7	0.5	1.5
PASTA SHELLS								
Dry, Average	*1 Serving/75g*	*265*	*1.5*	*353*	*11.1*	*71.8*	*2.0*	*2.0*
Egg, Fresh, Average	*1 Serving/125g*	*344*	*3.6*	*275*	*11.5*	*49.7*	*2.8*	*3.4*
Fresh, Dry, Average	*1 Serving/125g*	*216*	*2.1*	*173*	*7.4*	*32.0*	*1.6*	*1.5*
Wholewheat, Healthy Living, Co-Op*	1 Serving/75g	232	0.7	310	11.0	64.0	1.0	12.0
PASTA SNACK								
Cheese & Ham, Pot, Tesco*	1 Serving/208g	254	8.5	122	3.4	17.9	4.1	1.5
Cheese & Ham Tubes, Made Up, Tesco*	1 Serving/214g	312	11.6	146	4.9	19.5	5.4	2.6
Chicken, Morrisons*	1 Pack/250g	285	6.7	114	3.3	19.3	2.7	0.0
Chicken & Smoked Bacon, Sainsbury's*	1 Pack/190g	490	36.5	258	7.2	14.1	19.2	0.0
Chicken with Sweetcorn & Mushroom, Pot, Tesco*	1 Pot/216g	238	5.8	110	3.0	18.5	2.7	0.7
Creamy Cheese, Mug Shot, Symingtons*	1 Sachet/271g	301	6.0	111	3.7	19.1	2.2	1.0
Ham & Mushroom, Tesco*	1 Pack/300g	618	42.9	206	4.2	15.0	14.3	1.1
Roast Chicken, Mug Shot, Symingtons*	1 Sachet/258g	204	2.6	79	1.4	16.2	1.0	0.8
Tomato & Herb, in a Pot, Dry, Tesco*	1 Pot/59g	207	1.4	352	11.8	70.7	2.4	2.6
Tomato & Herb, Morrisons*	1 Pot/247g	247	2.7	100	3.1	19.5	1.1	0.9
Tomato 'n' Herb, Mug Shot*	1 Sachet/257g	265	2.1	103	2.3	21.6	0.8	1.2
PASTA SPIRALS								
Co-Op*	1 Serving/100g	350	1.0	350	12.0	73.0	1.0	3.0
Glutenfree, Glutano*	1oz/28g	100	0.3	357	4.0	83.0	1.0	0.0
PASTA TWIRLS								
Tri-Colour, Sainsbury's*	1 Serving/75g	268	1.3	357	12.3	73.1	1.7	2.5
PASTA TWISTS								
Dry, Average	*1oz/28g*	*99*	*0.4*	*354*	*12.2*	*71.8*	*1.5*	*2.2*
Wheat & Gluten Free, Glutafin*	1 Serving/75g	262	1.5	350	8.0	75.0	2.0	0.1
PASTA WITH								
Amigo Meatballs, Pasta King*	1 Serving/100g	127	3.4	127	4.7	19.5	3.4	1.8
Chargrilled Vegetables & Tomatoes, BGTY, Sainsbury's*	1 Serving/100g	96	1.6	96	2.9	17.4	1.6	0.0
Cheese & Tomato, Al Forno, Sainsbury's*	½ Pack/499g	749	29.0	150	5.5	18.9	5.8	1.8
Chicken Balti, Pasta King*	1 Serving/100g	114	2.1	114	4.7	19.4	2.1	1.8
Chicken Korma, Pasta King*	1 Serving/100g	119	2.8	119	5.3	18.5	2.8	1.2
Chicken Marrakech, Pasta King*	1 Serving/100g	118	2.2	118	5.3	19.4	2.2	1.8
Chicken Tikka, Pasta King*	1 Serving/100g	116	2.0	116	5.4	19.2	2.0	1.7
Chicken Torino, Pasta King*	1 Serving/100g	117	1.7	117	5.3	20.3	1.7	1.7
Feta Cheese & Slow Roasted Tomatoes, M & S*	1 Pack/190g	332	13.3	175	6.0	22.3	7.0	2.5
Firecracker Chicken, Pasta King*	1 Serving/100g	115	1.9	115	5.4	19.2	1.9	1.7
Firecracker Salmon, Pasta King*	1 Serving/100g	114	1.9	114	4.5	19.6	1.9	1.8
Garlic Mushrooms, Pasta King*	1 Serving/100g	113	2.3	113	4.4	18.9	2.3	0.1
Honey Mustard Chicken, COU, M & S*	1 Pack/300g	360	7.2	120	8.4	16.2	2.4	1.9
Louisiana Chicken, Pasta King*	1 Serving/100g	112	1.8	112	4.6	19.6	1.8	1.8
Maiale Meatballs, Pasta King*	1 Serving/100g	128	3.4	128	4.8	19.7	3.4	1.9
Meatballs, Sainsbury's*	1 Can/300g	339	14.7	113	6.6	10.6	4.9	1.6
Mediterranean Vegetables, Pasta King*	1 Serving/100g	121	3.2	121	3.7	19.3	3.2	2.1
Pesto, Spinach & Pine Nuts, Tesco*	1 Pack/300g	480	22.2	160	5.2	17.1	7.4	1.5
Salmon & Broccoli, Lemon Dressed, Sainsbury's*	1 Serving/300g	486	17.7	162	6.9	20.4	5.9	2.1

P

	Measure INFO/WEIGHT	per Measure KCAL	per Measure FAT	Nutrition Values per 100g / 100ml KCAL	PROT	CARB	FAT	FIBRE
PASTA WITH								
Spicy Beef, Light Choices, Tesco*	1 Pack/350g	450	4.9	129	4.8	20.6	1.4	2.2
Spicy Beef & Chipotle Chilli, HL, Tesco*	1 Pack/350g	367	7.0	105	4.8	17.0	2.0	2.7
Spicy Chicken, Sainsbury's*	1 Pot/300g	489	18.3	163	7.1	20.1	6.1	2.3
Spicy Sausage, Pasta King*	1 Serving/100g	117	2.2	117	4.8	19.7	2.2	1.7
Sweet & Sour Chicken, Pasta King*	1 Serving/100g	118	1.5	118	5.2	21.1	1.5	1.6
Sweet & Sour Vegetables, Pasta King*	1 Serving/100g	111	1.2	111	3.5	21.6	1.2	1.7
Sweet Chilli Chicken, Pasta King*	1 Serving/100g	113	1.8	113	5.3	19.2	1.8	1.7
Tomato & Basil Chicken, BGTY, Sainsbury's*	1 Pack/189g	250	2.1	132	9.2	21.2	1.1	2.7
Tuna & Roasted Peppers, M & S*	1 Serving/220g	308	8.6	140	9.1	17.7	3.9	0.9
Vegetable Balti, Pasta King*	1 Serving/100g	115	2.0	115	4.0	20.3	2.0	2.0
PASTE								
Bacon & Tomato, Tesco*	1 Serving/20g	46	3.6	232	14.0	3.4	18.0	0.1
BBQ Chicken, Princes*	1oz/28g	69	4.7	246	14.3	9.5	16.8	0.0
Beef, Asda*	1 Serving/37g	72	5.2	194	17.0	0.1	14.0	0.0
Beef, Princes*	1 Serving/18g	40	2.8	220	14.4	5.2	15.8	0.0
Beef, Sainsbury's*	1 Jar/75g	142	9.9	189	16.0	1.5	13.2	1.4
Chicken, Asda*	1 Thin Spread/7g	13	0.9	184	16.0	0.8	13.0	0.0
Chicken, Princes*	1 Thin Spread/9g	22	1.7	240	12.6	5.6	18.5	0.0
Chicken, Tesco*	1 Serving/12g	30	2.4	248	14.8	2.3	20.0	0.1
Chicken, Value, Tesco*	1 Thin Spread/9g	18	1.3	196	15.1	1.8	14.3	0.1
Chicken & Ham, Asda*	½ Jar/38g	82	6.5	217	14.0	2.1	17.0	0.0
Chicken & Ham, Princes*	1 Jar/100g	233	18.6	233	13.6	2.8	18.6	0.0
Chicken & Ham, Sainsbury's*	1 Thin Spread/9g	14	0.9	158	16.0	1.1	10.0	1.1
Chicken & Ham, Tesco*	1 Serving/19g	44	3.7	231	12.5	1.4	19.5	0.0
Chicken & Mushroom, Princes*	1 Serving/50g	93	5.5	187	17.1	5.0	11.0	0.0
Chicken & Stuffing, Asda*	½ Jar/35g	71	4.9	203	16.0	3.3	14.0	0.0
Chicken & Stuffing, Princes*	1 Jar/100g	229	17.0	229	15.7	3.3	17.0	0.0
Crab, Princes*	1 Pot/35g	36	1.2	104	13.4	4.8	3.5	0.0
Crab, Sainsbury's*	1 Thick Spread/5g	6	0.2	115	16.5	1.7	4.7	0.5
Crab, Tesco*	1 Jar/75g	116	6.3	155	14.4	4.6	8.4	0.1
Curry, Keralan, Waitrose*	¼ Jar/50g	111	8.3	223	3.2	14.9	16.7	1.9
Fruit, Golden Quince, Lowry Peaks*	1 Tsp/5g	16	0.0	321	0.8	83.6	0.2	0.0
Salmon, Asda*	1 Serving/53g	76	3.7	143	15.0	5.0	7.0	0.0
Salmon, Princes*	1 Serving/30g	58	3.8	195	13.5	6.5	12.8	0.0
Salmon, Value, Tesco*	1 Serving/10g	16	1.0	165	14.0	4.6	10.1	0.8
Salmon & Shrimp, Somerfield*	1 Thin Spread/9g	10	0.3	112	17.0	4.0	3.0	0.0
Salmon & Shrimp, Tesco*	1 Jar/75g	83	2.5	111	15.1	5.0	3.4	0.1
Sardine & Tomato, Asda*	1 Thin Spread/9g	11	0.5	123	14.0	3.3	6.0	0.0
Sardine & Tomato, Co-Op*	1 Serving/25g	34	1.5	135	16.0	3.0	6.0	2.0
Sardine & Tomato, Princes*	1 Jar/75g	130	8.1	173	13.9	3.4	10.8	3.2
Sardine & Tomato, Sainsbury's*	1 Mini Pot/35g	59	3.8	170	16.9	1.2	10.8	1.3
Sardine & Tomato, Somerfield*	1 Thin Spread/9g	13	0.6	144	15.0	5.0	7.0	0.0
Sardine & Tomato, Tesco*	1 Jar/75g	97	4.3	130	14.6	4.8	5.8	0.1
Tagine, Lemon, Spicy, Al'fez*	1 Tsp/6g	13	0.9	216	3.1	17.6	14.8	4.6
Tuna & Mayonnaise, Princes*	1 Pot/75g	86	12.3	115	16.8	3.8	16.4	0.0
Tuna & Mayonnaise, Sainsbury's*	1 Tbsp/17g	41	3.1	242	19.2	0.6	18.1	1.6
Tuna & Mayonnaise, Somerfield*	1 Thin Spread/9g	19	1.4	209	15.0	2.0	16.0	0.0
Tuna & Mayonnaise, Tesco*	1 Serving/15g	31	2.4	209	14.9	2.1	15.7	0.1
PASTILLES								
Blackcurrant, Rowntree's*	1 Tube/53g	188	0.0	353	4.4	84.0	0.0	0.0
Fruit, Average	1 Tube/33g	108	0.0	327	2.8	84.2	0.0	0.0
Fruit, Rowntree's*	1 Tube/53g	186	0.0	351	4.4	83.7	0.0	0.0
Wine, Maynards*	1 Sweet/5g	15	0.0	325	6.1	75.0	0.0	0.0

P

	Measure INFO/WEIGHT	per Measure KCAL	FAT	Nutrition Values per 100g / 100ml KCAL	PROT	CARB	FAT	FIBRE
PASTRAMI								
Beef, Average	**1 Serving/40g**	**51**	**1.4**	**128**	**23.1**	**1.1**	**3.6**	**0.2**
TTD, Sainsbury's*	1 Slice/10g	12	0.3	121	21.6	1.0	3.4	0.4
Turkey, Average	**½ Packet/35g**	**38**	**0.5**	**107**	**21.8**	**1.7**	**1.5**	**0.5**
PASTRY								
Choux, Cooked, Average	**1oz/28g**	**91**	**5.5**	**325**	**8.5**	**29.8**	**19.8**	**1.2**
Choux, Raw, Average	**1oz/28g**	**59**	**3.6**	**211**	**5.5**	**19.4**	**12.9**	**0.8**
Filo, Average	**1 Sheet/45g**	**137**	**1.2**	**304**	**9.0**	**61.4**	**2.7**	**0.9**
Filo, Frozen, Jus-Rol*	1 Sheet/45g	105	1.2	234	8.1	52.1	2.7	2.1
Flaky, Chinese, Average	**1oz/28g**	**110**	**4.6**	**392**	**5.4**	**59.3**	**16.4**	**0.0**
Flaky, Cooked, Average	**1oz/28g**	**157**	**11.4**	**560**	**5.6**	**45.9**	**40.6**	**1.8**
Flaky, Raw, Average	**1oz/28g**	**119**	**8.6**	**424**	**4.2**	**34.8**	**30.7**	**1.4**
Flan Case, Average	**1 Case/113g**	**615**	**38.0**	**544**	**7.1**	**56.7**	**33.6**	**1.8**
Greek, Average	**1oz/28g**	**90**	**4.8**	**322**	**4.7**	**40.0**	**17.0**	**0.0**
Puff, Frozen, Average	**1 Serving/47g**	**188**	**12.0**	**400**	**5.0**	**29.2**	**25.6**	**0.0**
Puff, Light, Sheet, Jus Rol*	1 Serving/50g	166	8.2	332	6.4	38.3	16.5	2.3
Shortcrust, Cooked, Average	**1oz/28g**	**146**	**9.0**	**521**	**6.6**	**54.2**	**32.3**	**2.2**
Shortcrust, Raw, Average	**1oz/28g**	**127**	**8.1**	**453**	**5.6**	**44.0**	**29.1**	**1.3**
Spring Roll Wrapper, TYJ Food Manufacturing*	1 Lge Sheet/18g	54	0.0	300	0.0	73.0	0.0	0.0
Wholemeal, Cooked, Average	**1oz/28g**	**140**	**9.2**	**499**	**8.9**	**44.6**	**32.9**	**6.3**
Wholemeal, Raw, Average	**1oz/28g**	**121**	**8.0**	**431**	**7.7**	**38.5**	**28.4**	**5.4**
PASTY								
Beef, Port Royal*	1 Pasty/130g	299	13.3	230	10.2	24.4	10.2	0.0
Cheddar & Onion, Hand Crimped, Waitrose*	1 Pasty/200g	546	42.2	273	8.8	22.5	21.1	2.2
Cheese & Onion, Aldi*	1oz/28g	80	5.2	287	7.0	22.9	18.6	1.0
Cheese & Onion, Co-Op*	1 Pasty/75g	235	14.8	313	9.2	24.5	19.8	1.7
Cheese & Onion, Farmfoods*	1 Pasty/191g	485	26.7	254	6.6	25.5	14.0	2.0
Cheese & Onion, Freshbake*	1 Pasty/135g	368	22.5	272	5.6	25.5	16.6	1.1
Cheese & Onion, Geo Adams*	1 Pasty/150g	420	23.4	280	6.9	27.9	15.6	1.1
Cheese & Onion, Sainsbury's*	1 Pasty/150g	486	32.7	324	7.4	24.5	21.8	1.3
Cheese & Onion, Somerfield*	1 Pasty/145g	419	26.1	289	7.0	24.0	18.0	0.0
Cheese & Onion, Tesco*	1 Pasty/150g	415	26.4	277	5.9	23.7	17.6	2.2
Chicken, Port Royal*	1 Pasty/130g	289	10.9	222	5.5	31.2	8.4	0.0
Chicken & Bacon, Ginsters*	1 Pasty/180g	457	29.0	254	8.0	19.3	16.1	2.8
Chicken & Vegetable, Proper Cornish Ltd*	1 Pasty/255g	671	34.7	263	7.4	30.2	13.6	2.4
Chicken Balti, Special Edition, Ginsters*	1 Pasty/180g	398	23.2	221	6.7	19.5	12.9	2.6
Corned Beef, Mega, M & S*	1oz/28g	87	5.7	310	9.5	22.3	20.2	0.9
Cornish, Asda*	1 Pasty/100g	287	19.0	287	7.0	22.0	19.0	1.2
Cornish, BGTY, Sainsbury's*	1 Pasty/135g	308	12.7	228	7.7	28.2	9.4	1.6
Cornish, Cheese & Onion, Ginsters*	1 Pasty/130g	511	33.0	393	10.4	30.7	25.4	2.3
Cornish, Chicken & Bacon, Ginsters*	1 Pasty/227g	574	34.5	253	6.9	22.2	15.2	0.8
Cornish, Co-Op*	1 Pasty/75g	200	12.3	267	6.4	23.4	16.4	1.6
Cornish, Crimped, TTD, Sainsbury's*	1 Pasty/200g	515	28.7	258	8.3	23.7	14.4	1.2
Cornish, Mega, M & S*	1oz/28g	84	6.2	300	6.0	18.7	22.1	1.2
Cornish, Mini, Iceland*	1 Pasty/70g	215	14.8	306	7.0	22.1	21.1	1.2
Cornish, Mini, M & S*	1 Pasty/75g	244	17.5	325	7.3	21.9	23.4	1.8
Cornish, Mini, Sainsbury's*	1 Pasty/70g	280	20.1	400	7.3	28.1	28.7	1.5
Cornish, Mini, Tesco*	1 Pasty/24g	66	4.2	274	5.6	23.2	17.7	0.5
Cornish, Morrisons*	1 Pasty/200g	626	37.0	313	7.5	29.1	18.5	1.0
Cornish, Multi Pack, Ginsters*	1 Pasty/130g	357	24.3	275	6.0	20.6	18.7	2.6
Cornish, Original, Ginsters*	1 Pasty/227g	549	32.2	242	5.3	23.2	14.2	3.1
Cornish, Pork Farms*	1 Pasty/250g	672	40.7	269	7.7	22.8	16.3	0.0
Cornish, Sainsbury's*	1 Pasty/150g	489	32.1	326	6.7	26.6	21.4	2.0
Cornish, Smart Price, Asda*	1 Pasty/94g	286	15.0	304	8.0	32.0	16.0	1.7

	Measure INFO/WEIGHT	per Measure KCAL	FAT	Nutrition Values per 100g / 100ml KCAL	PROT	CARB	FAT	FIBRE
PASTY								
Cornish, Snack Pack, Six, Ginsters*	1 Pasty/40g	116	8.0	289	7.2	20.3	19.9	2.8
Cornish, Tesco*	1 Pasty/150g	466	32.7	311	6.8	21.9	21.8	1.6
Cornish, Traditional Style, Geo Adams*	1 Pasty/165g	488	30.4	296	7.1	25.4	18.4	1.3
Cornish, Value, Tesco*	1 Pasty/150g	425	26.6	283	6.7	24.2	17.7	2.2
Cornish Roaster, Ginsters*	1 Pasty/130g	417	24.2	321	8.5	29.9	18.6	1.3
Lamb, Port Royal*	1 Pasty/130g	352	17.4	271	7.2	30.5	13.4	0.0
Olive & Cheese, Tapas, Waitrose*	1 Pack/130g	455	25.2	350	8.1	35.8	19.4	1.3
Salt Fish, Port Royal*	1 Pasty/130g	300	13.4	231	6.8	27.8	10.3	0.0
Tandoori & Vegetable, Holland & Barrett*	1 Pack/110g	232	9.3	211	4.3	29.4	8.5	1.8
Three Cheese & Onion, Ginsters*	1 Pasty/180g	531	36.9	295	8.0	19.7	20.5	3.1
Vegetable	1oz/28g	77	4.2	274	4.1	33.3	14.9	1.9
Vegetable, Hand Crimped, Waitrose*	1 Pasty/200g	454	22.6	227	4.5	26.8	11.3	2.2
Vegetarian, Country Slice, Linda McCartney*	1 Pasty/150g	373	20.2	249	5.6	26.5	13.5	2.9
Vegetarian, Port Royal*	1 Pasty/130g	315	13.8	242	12.5	24.1	10.6	0.0
Westcountry Cheddar & Onion, Multi Pack, Ginsters*	1 Pasty/130g	370	23.9	285	7.1	23.2	18.4	2.0
PATE								
Apricot, Asda*	1 Serving/50g	156	14.0	312	12.0	3.0	28.0	0.0
Ardennes, Asda*	1 Serving/50g	143	12.0	286	13.9	3.6	24.0	1.3
Ardennes, BGTY, Sainsbury's*	¼ Pack/50g	90	5.7	180	16.6	2.9	11.4	0.0
Ardennes, Healthy Choice, Somerfield*	1 Pack/175g	341	23.1	195	16.4	2.6	13.2	1.6
Ardennes, HL, Tesco*	½ Pack/88g	154	11.0	176	12.1	3.6	12.6	1.8
Ardennes, Iceland*	1 Serving/70g	223	19.9	318	12.0	3.4	28.5	0.5
Ardennes, Reduced Fat, Waitrose*	¼ Pack/42g	94	7.1	224	15.4	2.6	16.9	0.5
Ardennes, Tesco*	1 Tbsp/15g	53	5.0	354	13.3	0.5	33.2	1.2
Ardennes, with Bacon, Tesco*	½ Pack/85g	241	20.6	284	11.4	5.1	24.2	1.1
Bean Feast, The Redwood Co*	1 Serving/60g	161	10.2	268	7.3	21.1	17.0	3.8
Breton, Country with Apricots, Coarse, Sainsbury's*	1 Serving/21g	60	4.7	285	13.5	7.0	22.5	0.5
Brussels, 25% Less Fat, Morrisons*	¼ Pack/43g	106	8.8	249	14.2	0.7	20.6	0.0
Brussels, BGTY, 50% Less Fat, Sainsbury's*	1 Serving/100g	223	16.0	223	14.6	5.1	16.0	0.1
Brussels, Co-Op*	1 Serving/15g	51	4.6	340	11.0	4.0	31.0	2.0
Brussels, Fat Reduced, Somerfield*	1 Serving/50g	96	7.0	192	14.0	2.0	14.0	0.0
Brussels, Finest, Tesco*	½ Pack/85g	306	28.7	360	8.6	5.2	33.8	0.8
Brussels, HL, Tesco*	1 Serving/29g	66	4.4	229	14.4	8.4	15.3	1.8
Brussels, M & S*	1 Pot/170g	518	45.2	305	13.3	2.8	26.6	1.0
Brussels, Reduced Fat, Somerfield*	1 Serving/50g	138	10.5	277	14.0	8.0	21.0	0.0
Brussels, Reduced Fat, Tesco*	1 Pack/175g	420	33.2	240	11.1	5.8	19.0	1.4
Brussels, Reduced Fat, Waitrose*	1 Serving/40g	92	7.4	229	13.2	2.4	18.5	0.5
Brussels, Sainsbury's*	1 Pack/170g	663	64.9	390	10.6	1.1	38.2	0.1
Brussels, Sanpareil*	¼ Pack/37g	121	11.1	326	13.0	1.0	30.0	0.0
Brussels, Smooth, 50% Less Fat, Tesco*	1 Pack/175g	350	26.8	200	14.1	1.2	15.3	1.8
Brussels, Smooth, Reduced, Tesco*	1 Serving/40g	82	6.4	205	10.7	4.5	16.0	0.6
Brussels, Smooth, Reduced Fat, Tesco*	1 Serving/15g	30	2.3	200	14.1	1.2	15.3	1.8
Brussels, Smooth, Spreadable, Sainsbury's*	1 Serving/30g	97	8.7	323	10.7	4.7	29.0	0.0
Brussels, Tesco*	1 Serving/28g	92	8.5	330	11.0	3.0	30.5	1.1
Brussels, with Forest Mushroom, Co-Op*	1 Serving/57g	180	16.5	315	12.0	2.0	29.0	1.0
Brussels, with Garlic, Asda*	1 Serving/50g	170	15.6	340	10.7	4.0	31.3	2.5
Brussels, with Herbs, Tesco*	1 Serving/25g	87	8.1	347	8.4	6.4	32.6	1.5
Brussels & Garlic, Reduced Fat, Tesco*	1 Serving/65g	135	8.0	208	16.2	8.1	12.3	0.6
Brussels & Garlic, Tesco*	1 Serving/40g	145	13.5	363	8.7	6.0	33.8	0.0
Brussels & Mushroom, Mini, GFY, Asda*	1 Pack/40g	67	4.4	167	14.7	2.3	11.0	3.9
Brussels Style, Organic, The Redwood Co*	¼ Pack/30g	82	6.1	273	15.2	8.0	20.4	1.3
Carrot, Ginger & Spring Onion, M & S*	1 Serving/50g	72	5.5	145	1.5	9.6	11.0	0.9
Celery, Stilton & Walnut, Waitrose*	1 Pot/115g	294	26.4	256	9.0	3.2	23.0	2.2

PATE

INFO/WEIGHT	Measure	per Measure		Nutrition Values per 100g / 100ml				
		KCAL	FAT	KCAL	PROT	CARB	FAT	FIBRE
Chargrilled Vegetable, BGTY, Sainsbury's*	½ Pot/57g	43	0.7	75	4.9	10.8	1.3	2.7
Chick Pea & Black Olive, Cauldron Foods*	1 Pot/113g	193	11.9	171	7.6	11.4	10.5	6.6
Chicken, with Sauternes, TTD, Sainsbury's*	1 Serving/30g	114	11.1	381	6.5	5.3	37.1	0.6
Chicken & Brandy, Morrisons*	1 Serving/44g	133	11.8	303	10.8	4.3	26.9	0.8
Chicken Liver, Asda*	1 Serving/65g	131	10.4	202	13.0	4.0	16.0	0.8
Chicken Liver, BGTY, Sainsbury's*	1 Serving/30g	64	4.8	214	11.5	6.0	16.0	0.5
Chicken Liver, M & S*	1oz/28g	79	6.7	281	14.0	1.9	24.1	0.1
Chicken Liver, Organic, Waitrose*	½ Tub/88g	204	16.1	233	12.6	1.8	18.4	1.4
Chicken Liver, with Brandy, Tesco*	1oz/28g	82	7.2	293	11.8	3.5	25.8	1.4
Chicken Liver, with Madeira, Sainsbury's*	1 Serving/30g	84	7.3	279	13.1	1.9	24.3	0.0
Chicken Liver & Brandy, Asda*	1 Serving/50g	176	16.4	353	9.0	5.5	32.8	3.2
Chicken Liver & Garlic, Smooth, Asda*	1 Serving/31g	119	11.1	388	9.0	7.0	36.0	3.2
Chickpea, Moroccan, Organic, Cauldron Foods*	½ Pot/58g	119	7.9	207	6.8	16.3	13.7	4.9
Crab, M & S*	1oz/28g	63	4.8	225	12.1	5.9	17.3	0.0
Crab, Terrine, Orkney, Luxury, Castle MacLellan*	1 Tub/113g	250	21.4	221	7.3	5.5	18.9	0.9
Crab, Waitrose*	1 Pot/113g	218	16.7	193	12.4	2.5	14.8	0.9
De Campagne, Sainsbury's*	1 Serving/55g	129	10.0	235	16.3	1.4	18.2	0.0
Duck & Champagne, Luxury, M & S*	1oz/28g	106	9.9	380	8.3	8.3	35.2	7.8
Duck & Orange, Asda*	1 Serving/40g	94	7.2	235	16.0	2.2	18.0	0.0
Duck & Orange, Smooth, Tesco*	1 Serving/50g	188	17.7	377	10.5	4.0	35.4	0.5
Duck & Truffle, Medallions, M & S*	1 Serving/25g	91	8.7	365	9.0	4.8	35.0	1.4
Farmhouse, Coarse, Organic, Sainsbury's*	1 Serving/56g	138	11.0	246	13.3	3.7	19.7	0.8
Farmhouse, Mushroom, Asda*	1 Serving/50g	126	10.0	252	13.0	5.0	20.0	0.7
Farmhouse, with Christmas Ale, Sainsbury's*	1oz/28g	67	5.3	239	15.4	1.6	19.1	0.0
Farmhouse, with Herbes De Provence, Tesco*	1 Serving/50g	136	10.8	273	13.9	5.4	21.6	1.0
Farmhouse, with Mushrooms & Garlic, Tesco*	1 Serving/90g	256	22.8	285	13.8	0.6	25.3	1.3
Farmhouse Style, Finest, Tesco*	1 Serving/28g	83	7.3	295	11.9	3.6	25.9	1.0
Farmhouse Style, M & S*	¼ Pack/42g	90	7.1	215	14.4	1.9	16.9	1.2
Farmhouse Style, Weight Watchers*	1 Serving/37g	49	2.1	133	14.8	5.5	5.7	0.5
Forestiere, M & S*	1 Serving/20g	61	5.3	305	11.5	4.2	26.6	1.4
Kipper, Waitrose*	¼ Tub/28g	105	9.2	370	16.8	2.0	32.7	0.6
Liver, Value, Tesco*	1 Serving/50g	151	13.0	302	13.0	4.1	26.0	0.5
Liver & Bacon, Spreading, Value, Tesco*	1 Roll/150g	423	37.2	282	12.7	2.1	24.8	1.4
Liver & Bacon, Tesco*	1 Serving/10g	28	2.3	276	12.9	4.3	23.0	0.4
Liver Spreading, Somerfield*	1oz/28g	77	6.4	275	14.0	3.0	23.0	0.0
Mackerel, Smoked	1oz/28g	103	9.6	368	13.4	1.3	34.4	0.0
Mackerel, Tesco*	1 Serving/29g	102	9.5	353	14.3	0.5	32.6	0.0
Mediterranean Roast Vegetable, Tesco*	1 Serving/28g	31	2.6	112	2.4	4.3	9.4	1.2
Mousse De Canard, French, Weight Watchers*	1 Portion/50g	122	9.5	245	14.0	4.4	19.0	0.0
Mushroom, BGTY, Sainsbury's*	½ Pot/58g	29	0.3	50	4.6	6.7	0.5	3.0
Mushroom, COU, M & S*	1oz/28g	17	0.5	60	2.9	7.4	1.9	0.9
Mushroom, M & S*	1 Pot/115g	224	20.1	195	4.2	4.8	17.5	1.5
Mushroom, Organic, Cauldron Foods*	1 Pot/113g	169	15.0	150	2.9	6.2	13.3	1.5
Mushroom, Roast, Tesco*	1 Serving/25g	36	3.2	145	3.6	3.6	12.9	4.5
Mushroom, Sainsbury's*	½ Pot/58g	89	7.0	153	3.3	7.8	12.1	2.1
Mushroom, Tesco*	1oz/28g	39	2.7	138	3.3	9.8	9.5	1.0
Mushroom & Herb, Somerfield*	1oz/28g	81	7.6	289	4.0	8.0	27.0	0.0
Mushroom & Tarragon, Cauldron Foods*	1 Pot/113g	118	9.4	104	2.7	5.9	8.3	1.2
Mushroom & Tarragon, Waitrose*	1 Serving/30g	46	4.0	155	2.8	5.5	13.5	1.4
Poached Salmon & Watercress, Tesco*	1 Serving/25g	59	4.4	238	19.2	0.4	17.7	0.2
Pork & Garlic, Somerfield*	1oz/28g	83	7.0	295	14.0	3.0	25.0	0.0
Pork & Mushroom, Somerfield*	1oz/28g	95	8.7	339	11.0	3.0	31.0	0.0
Pork Liver, with Garlic, Coarse, Asda*	1 Pack/40g	130	12.0	326	13.0	1.0	30.0	0.0

P

	Measure INFO/WEIGHT	per Measure KCAL	per Measure FAT	Nutrition Values per 100g / 100ml KCAL	PROT	CARB	FAT	FIBRE
PATE								
Pork with Apple & Cider, Sainsbury's*	1 Serving/50g	151	12.6	303	12.5	6.3	25.3	1.1
Pork with Peppercorns, Tesco*	1 Serving/28g	84	7.5	300	12.9	1.4	26.8	0.7
Pork with Port & Cranberry, Tesco*	1 Serving/28g	83	7.2	296	12.1	4.3	25.6	0.6
Ricotta, Sundried Tomato & Basil, Princes*	1 Jar/110g	343	31.6	312	5.2	8.3	28.7	0.0
Roasted Carrot, Ginger & Spring Onion, M & S*	1 Serving/50g	72	5.5	145	1.5	9.6	11.0	0.9
Roasted Parsnip & Carrot, Organic, Cauldron Foods*	1 Pot/115g	132	7.7	115	3.5	10.2	6.7	4.9
Roasted Red Pepper, Oven Roasted, Castle MacLellan*	1oz/28g	46	3.8	163	3.3	8.2	13.5	0.8
Roasted Red Pepper, Princes*	1 Serving/35g	47	1.7	135	4.8	17.6	5.0	0.0
Roasted Red Pepper & Houmous, Princes*	¼ Jar/27g	32	1.6	120	4.6	12.4	5.8	0.0
Roasted Vegetable, COU, M & S*	1 Pot/115g	86	1.7	75	6.2	9.1	1.5	1.4
Salmon, John West*	1 Serving/50g	136	11.7	272	14.9	0.0	23.5	0.2
Salmon, Organic, M & S*	1oz/28g	76	6.3	270	16.9	0.0	22.5	0.0
Salmon, Smoked, Isle of Skye, TTD, Sainsbury's*	½ Pot/58g	133	9.8	231	17.5	1.8	17.1	0.2
Salmon, Smoked, M & S*	1oz/28g	74	6.2	265	16.9	0.0	22.0	0.0
Salmon Dill, Princes*	1 Serving/70g	124	7.8	177	15.4	4.0	11.1	0.5
Smoked Mackerel, M & S*	1oz/28g	104	9.7	370	13.4	0.7	34.7	0.3
Smoked Mackerel, Sainsbury's*	½ Pot/57g	215	20.1	378	14.2	0.8	35.3	0.0
Smoked Mackerel, Scottish, M & S*	½ Pot/58g	158	13.3	275	15.9	0.6	23.2	0.1
Smoked Salmon, Luxury, Morrisons*	½ Pot/57g	150	12.4	266	16.0	0.9	22.0	0.5
Smoked Salmon, Organic, Waitrose*	1oz/28g	83	7.2	296	13.9	2.4	25.6	0.0
Smoked Salmon, Scottish, Castle MacLellan*	¼ Tub/28g	62	4.5	220	13.5	5.6	16.0	0.0
Smoked Salmon, Scottish, M & S*	1 Serving/30g	81	6.7	270	17.0	0.2	22.3	0.0
Smoked Salmon, Tesco*	1 Pack/115g	282	22.0	245	15.0	3.0	19.1	1.0
Smoked Salmon, Waitrose*	½ Pot/57g	120	8.9	212	17.1	0.5	15.7	0.6
Smoked Trout, Waitrose*	½ Pot/56g	130	10.3	232	15.8	0.9	18.4	0.6
Soya & Mushroom, Cauldron Foods*	1 Pot/115g	199	10.8	173	8.8	6.4	9.4	6.5
Spiced Aubergine, Waitrose*	¼ Pack/38g	71	5.2	186	4.9	10.9	13.6	2.4
Spiced Parsnip & Carrot, Organic, Asda*	½ Pot/58g	63	3.5	109	3.7	10.0	6.0	2.6
Spicy Bean, BGTY, Sainsbury's*	½ Pot/58g	56	1.1	97	5.0	15.1	1.9	5.4
Spicy Bean, Princes*	½ Pot/55g	46	0.2	84	3.6	16.7	0.3	0.0
Spicy Bean, Weight Watchers*	1 Serving/37g	33	0.6	89	5.7	12.9	1.6	4.2
Spicy Mexican, Organic, Waitrose*	1 Serving/50g	57	3.1	115	6.2	8.6	6.2	3.5
Spinach, Cheese & Almond, Organic, Cauldron Foods*	½ Pot/58g	103	8.2	179	7.7	5.1	14.2	3.2
Sun-Dried Tomato & Basil, Cauldron Foods*	1 Pot/115g	189	11.7	164	6.9	11.1	10.2	4.6
Tofu, Spicy Mexican, Organic, GranoVita*	1 Serving/50g	108	10.0	216	6.0	3.0	20.0	0.0
Tomato, Lentil & Basil, Cauldron Foods*	1 Pot/115g	161	7.8	140	6.8	14.0	6.8	3.2
Tuna, M & S*	1oz/28g	99	8.8	355	18.0	0.0	31.3	0.0
Tuna, Tesco*	1 Pack/115g	332	26.7	289	19.8	0.3	23.2	0.2
Tuna with Butter & Lemon Juice, Sainsbury's*	½ Pot/58g	209	18.3	360	19.0	0.1	31.6	0.3
Vegetable	1oz/28g	48	3.8	173	7.5	5.9	13.4	0.0
Vegetable, Cauldron Foods*	1 Pack/113g	220	12.7	195	9.2	14.1	11.3	4.4
Vegetarian, with Mushrooms, Organic, Tartex*	¼ Tube/50g	101	8.0	203	7.7	7.0	16.0	0.0
Yeast, Garlic & Herb, Tartex*	1 Serving/30g	69	5.4	230	7.0	10.0	18.0	0.0
Yeast, Mexican Red Pepper & Wild Chilli Organic, Tartex*	1 Pot/50g	99	8.0	198	6.4	7.0	16.0	0.0
Yeast, Pateole, GranoVita*	1 Portion/30g	66	5.3	219	10.2	4.5	17.8	0.0
Yeast, Wild Mushroom, GranoVita*	1oz/28g	60	4.8	213	10.0	5.0	17.0	0.0
PAVLOVA								
Mandarin, Mini, Iceland*	1 Pavlova/22g	59	2.6	268	2.1	37.9	12.0	1.7
Raspberry, Co-Op*	1/6 Pavlova/49g	147	5.9	300	3.2	44.8	12.0	1.1
Raspberry, Individual, M & S*	1 Pavlova/65g	133	1.6	205	4.0	41.8	2.4	0.2
Raspberry, M & S*	1 Serving/84g	193	8.1	230	2.3	33.3	9.6	0.3
Raspberry, Mini, Co-Op*	1 Pavlova/19g	61	1.7	320	3.0	56.0	9.0	0.6
Raspberry, Mini, Iceland*	1 Pavlova/21g	58	2.9	273	2.3	35.1	13.7	2.6

	Measure INFO/WEIGHT	per Measure KCAL	per Measure FAT	Nutrition Values per 100g / 100ml KCAL	PROT	CARB	FAT	FIBRE
PAVLOVA								
Raspberry, Sara Lee*	1/6 Pavlova/55g	168	8.5	303	2.7	38.5	15.3	1.1
Raspberry, Tesco*	1 Serving/65g	191	8.4	294	2.7	41.8	12.9	1.1
Raspberry & Lemon, Asda*	1 Serving/43g	102	1.9	235	2.8	46.0	4.4	0.5
Sticky Toffee, Farmfoods*	1/6 Pavlova/49g	186	9.6	380	3.4	47.8	19.5	0.3
Sticky Toffee, Sainsbury's*	1/6 Pavlova/60g	249	9.8	415	3.7	63.1	16.4	0.9
Strawberry, Co-Op*	1 Serving/52g	177	7.3	340	3.0	50.0	14.0	0.4
Strawberry, COU, M & S*	1 Pot/95g	147	2.3	155	2.4	30.5	2.4	0.8
Strawberry, Farmfoods*	1/6 Pavlova/52g	152	7.8	292	2.3	36.9	15.0	2.2
Strawberry & Champagne, Mini, Co-Op*	1 Pavlova/19g	65	3.6	340	3.0	40.0	19.0	0.8
Toffee, Co-Op*	1/6 Pavlova/53g	193	8.5	365	3.0	52.0	16.0	0.6
Toffee, Mini, Iceland*	1 Pavlova/19g	68	2.9	353	3.0	51.5	15.0	1.9
Toffee Pecan, M & S*	1oz/28g	118	7.4	420	3.9	41.5	26.6	0.4
PAW-PAW								
Raw, Fresh	*1oz/28g*	*10*	*0.0*	*36*	*0.5*	*8.8*	*0.1*	*2.2*
Raw, Weighed with Skin & Pips	*1oz/28g*	*8*	*0.0*	*27*	*0.4*	*6.6*	*0.1*	*1.7*
PEACH								
Dried, Average	*1 Pack/250g*	*472*	*1.6*	*189*	*2.5*	*44.9*	*0.6*	*6.9*
in Fruit Juice, Average	*1oz/28g*	*13*	*0.0*	*47*	*0.5*	*11.2*	*0.0*	*0.7*
in Strawberry Jelly, Pieces, Fruitini, Del Monte*	1 Can/140g	91	0.1	65	0.3	15.3	0.1	0.0
in Syrup, Average	*1oz/28g*	*19*	*0.0*	*67*	*0.4*	*16.3*	*0.1*	*0.4*
Raw, Stoned, Average	1oz/28g	9	0.0	33	1.0	7.6	0.1	1.5
Raw, Weighed with Stone, Average	*1 Peach/125g*	*41*	*0.1*	*33*	*1.0*	*7.6*	*0.1*	*1.4*
Slices in Fruit Juice, Average	1 Serving/100g	49	0.0	49	0.6	11.5	0.0	0.5
Slices in Light Syrup, Value, Tesco*	4 Serving/238g	159	0.2	67	0.4	16.0	0.1	0.8
PEANUT BRITTLE								
Thorntons*	2 Pieces/32g	163	8.6	509	12.4	54.3	26.9	2.6
PEANUT BUTTER								
& Grape Jelly Stripes In Jar, Goober*	1 Tsp/15g	67	3.4	450	13.2	65.0	22.6	3.8
25% Less Fat, Tesco*	1 Tbsp/16g	85	5.6	529	22.6	30.7	35.1	6.7
Creamy, Smooth, Sun Pat*	1 Serving/15g	93	7.5	620	24.0	17.5	50.2	6.1
Crunchy, Basics, Sainsbury's*	1 Serving/10g	61	5.3	610	22.2	12.0	52.6	5.6
Crunchy, Bettabuy, Morrisons*	1 Serving/10g	61	5.2	606	22.5	17.3	52.2	5.7
Crunchy, Budgens*	1oz/28g	166	13.9	592	23.6	12.5	49.7	6.9
Crunchy, Chosen By You, Asda*	1 Serving/10g	60	4.9	603	24.5	15.5	49.2	6.6
Crunchy, Harvest Spread*	1 Serving/25g	148	12.4	592	23.6	12.5	49.7	6.9
Crunchy, No Added Sugar, Organic, Whole Earth*	1 Serving/25g	148	12.5	592	24.9	10.1	50.2	7.3
Crunchy, Organic, Evernat*	1 Tsp/10g	64	5.3	641	29.0	13.0	53.0	7.0
Crunchy, Organic, No Added Sugar, Waitrose*	1 Serving/12g	71	6.0	592	24.9	10.1	50.2	7.3
Crunchy, Organic, Tesco*	1 Serving/25g	149	12.4	595	23.6	12.5	49.7	6.9
Crunchy, Original Style, No Added Sugar, Whole Earth*	1 Serving/20g	127	10.2	637	25.7	16.8	51.1	8.7
Crunchy, Route 66*	1 Serving/10g	65	5.8	648	20.0	13.0	58.0	5.4
Crunchy, Sainsbury's*	1 Serving/10g	62	5.0	620	28.6	12.6	49.6	4.3
Crunchy, Smart Price, Asda*	1 Thin Spread/12g	73	6.0	610	23.2	16.0	50.4	6.2
Crunchy, Somerfield*	1 Tsp/10g	59	4.9	586	24.4	11.8	49.0	7.1
Crunchy, Sun Pat*	1 Serving/50g	307	24.4	615	25.3	15.1	48.9	6.8
Crunchy, Tesco*	1 Serving/20g	123	10.2	615	23.8	14.6	50.8	6.4
Crunchy, Value, Tesco*	1 Serving/10g	61	5.4	615	21.5	11.7	53.6	5.4
Crunchy, Whole Nut, Organic, Meridian Foods*	1 Serving/28g	171	13.6	612	31.2	12.2	48.7	6.5
Extra Crunch, Skippy*	2 Tbsp/40g	252	20.0	630	22.7	22.9	50.0	7.7
Extra Crunchy, Sun Pat*	1 Serving/20g	119	10.2	597	21.9	12.6	51.0	7.3
GFY, Asda*	1 Serving/15g	80	5.2	531	28.0	31.0	35.0	0.0
Organic, Rapunzel*	1 Serving/5g	31	2.6	613	29.0	4.5	53.0	0.0
Powdered, PB2, Bell Plantation*	2 Tbsp/12g	45	1.5	375	41.7	41.7	12.5	16.7

	Measure INFO/WEIGHT	per Measure KCAL	FAT	Nutrition Values per 100g / 100ml KCAL	PROT	CARB	FAT	FIBRE
PEANUT BUTTER								
Smart Price, Asda*	1 Serving/15g	87	7.5	582	23.0	10.0	50.0	6.0
Smooth, 30% Reduced Fat, Duerr's*	1 Serving/20g	107	7.0	533	22.6	31.7	35.1	6.7
Smooth, 33% Less Fat, BGTY, Sainsbury's*	1 Serving/10g	53	3.5	533	22.6	31.7	35.1	6.7
Smooth, Average	1 Serving/20g	125	10.7	623	22.6	13.1	53.7	5.4
Smooth, Chosen By You, Asda*	1 Serving/15g	91	7.4	604	24.1	15.7	49.4	6.0
Smooth, Kernel King, Duerr's*	1 Serving/15g	89	7.5	596	23.3	12.4	50.3	6.8
Smooth, Kraft*	1 Serving/20g	127	10.7	636	23.1	17.6	53.5	0.0
Smooth, Light, Kraft*	1 Serving/20g	114	7.7	571	16.3	40.1	38.6	0.0
Smooth, Morrisons*	1 Serving/15g	92	7.8	616	23.1	14.5	51.8	6.2
Smooth, No Added Sugar, Organic, Whole Earth*	1 Serving/20g	119	10.2	595	24.5	9.9	50.8	7.1
Smooth, Organic, Meridian Foods*	1 Serving/10g	61	4.9	612	31.2	12.2	48.7	6.5
Smooth, Organic, Tesco*	1 Serving/15g	90	7.5	600	23.3	12.4	50.3	6.5
Smooth, Organic, Waitrose*	1 Serving/20g	125	10.2	623	28.0	13.0	51.0	0.0
Smooth, Organic, Waitrose*	1 Serving/12g	71	6.1	595	24.6	9.9	50.8	7.1
Smooth, Somerfield*	1 Tsp/10g	59	5.0	592	24.0	11.0	50.0	0.0
Smooth, Sun Pat*	1 Serving/20g	123	9.8	614	25.0	15.2	48.9	6.7
Smooth, Tesco*	1 Serving/20g	123	10.1	614	27.8	12.0	50.5	6.5
Smooth Original, No Added Sugar, Whole Earth*	1 Serving/10g	59	5.1	595	24.6	9.9	50.8	7.1
Stripy, Sun Pat*	1 Tsp/10g	62	4.7	617	13.0	35.0	47.0	3.0
Whole Nut, Crunchy, Average	1 Tsp/10g	61	5.3	606	24.9	7.7	53.1	6.0
Wholenut, Sainsbury's*	1 Serving/15g	90	7.7	598	24.2	9.8	51.3	7.0
Wholenut, Tesco*	1 Tbsp/15g	90	7.6	590	24.9	10.1	50.0	6.3
Wholenut, Waitrose*	1 Serving/12g	70	6.0	587	24.9	9.3	50.0	6.3
PEANUTS								
Chilli, Average	½ Pack/50g	303	25.3	605	28.2	9.3	50.6	6.8
Dry Roasted, Average	1 Serving/20g	117	9.8	587	25.7	11.5	48.8	6.5
Honey Roasted, Average	1oz/28g	169	13.2	605	26.8	23.5	47.0	5.5
Hot Chilli, Holland & Barrett*	1 Pack/100g	523	31.0	523	14.0	47.0	31.0	5.5
Milk Chocolate Coated, Graze*	1 Pack/35g	187	13.1	533	14.6	34.9	37.3	0.0
Plain, Average	*10 Whole/10g*	*59*	*5.0*	*592*	*24.7*	*11.0*	*50.0*	*6.3*
Roast, Salted, Average	10 Whole/12g	74	6.3	614	27.8	7.9	52.4	4.9
Roasted, Love Life, Waitrose*	1 Serving/30g	170	13.8	567	25.6	12.5	46.1	8.0
Salted, Average	10 Whole/6g	37	3.1	609	27.0	8.3	52.0	5.4
White Chocolate Coated, Graze*	1 Pack/30g	166	11.8	553	14.7	37.8	39.3	0.0
Yoghurt Coated, Graze*	1 Pack/35g	189	12.3	540	9.9	48.1	35.1	0.0
PEARL BARLEY								
Boiled	*1oz/28g*	*34*	*0.1*	*123*	*2.3*	*28.2*	*0.4*	*3.7*
Dried, Cooked, Love Life, Waitrose*	1 Serving/80g	101	0.4	126	2.2	28.2	0.5	3.7
Raw, Average	*1oz/28g*	*99*	*0.3*	*352*	*9.9*	*77.7*	*1.2*	*15.6*
PEARS								
Abate Fetel, Average	*1 Med/133g*	*48*	*0.1*	*36*	*0.4*	*8.3*	*0.1*	*2.2*
Asian, Nashi, Raw, Average	*1 Lge/209g*	*88*	*0.5*	*42*	*0.5*	*10.6*	*0.2*	*3.6*
Blush, Morrisons*	1 Sm/148g	86	0.2	58	0.4	15.5	0.1	3.1
Cape, Quartered, Tesco*	1 Serving/100g	35	0.0	35	0.3	8.5	0.0	1.4
Comice, Raw, Weighed with Core	*1 Med/170g*	*56*	*0.0*	*33*	*0.3*	*8.5*	*0.0*	*2.0*
Conference, Average	*1 Lge/209g*	*88*	*0.2*	*42*	*0.3*	*10.1*	*0.1*	*2.0*
Dessert, Green, Sainsbury's*	1 Sm/135g	53	0.1	39	0.3	9.2	0.1	2.0
Dried, Average	*1 Pear Half/16g*	*33*	*0.1*	*204*	*1.9*	*48.4*	*0.5*	*9.7*
Dried, Williams, Love Life, Waitrose*	1 Serving/50g	110	0.2	221	1.6	52.4	0.5	8.3
Frozen, Diced, Asda*	1 Serving/50g	23	0.0	47	0.3	10.4	0.1	1.7
in Fruit Juice, Average	*1 Serving/225g*	*102*	*0.1*	*45*	*0.3*	*10.9*	*0.0*	*1.2*
in Syrup, Average	*1oz/28g*	*16*	*0.0*	*58*	*0.2*	*14.4*	*0.1*	*1.4*
Prickly, Raw, Fresh	*1oz/28g*	*14*	*0.1*	*49*	*0.7*	*11.5*	*0.3*	*0.0*

	Measure INFO/WEIGHT	per Measure		Nutrition Values per 100g / 100ml				
		KCAL	FAT	KCAL	PROT	CARB	FAT	FIBRE
PEARS								
Raw, Weighed with Core, Average	*1 Lge/209g*	*78*	*0.2*	*37*	*0.3*	*9.1*	*0.1*	*1.4*
Red, Tesco*	1 Med/180g	65	0.2	36	0.4	8.3	0.1	2.2
TTD, Sainsbury's*	1 Serving/100g	40	0.1	40	0.3	10.0	0.1	2.2
William, Raw, Average	*1 Med/170g*	*58*	*0.2*	*34*	*0.4*	*8.3*	*0.1*	*2.2*
PEAS								
Dried, Boiled in Unsalted Water, Average	*1oz/28g*	*31*	*0.2*	*109*	*6.9*	*19.9*	*0.8*	*5.5*
Dried, Raw, Average	*1oz/28g*	*85*	*0.7*	*303*	*21.6*	*52.0*	*2.4*	*13.0*
Edible Podded, Raw	*1 Cup/63g*	*26*	*0.1*	*42*	*2.8*	*7.6*	*0.2*	*2.6*
Frozen, Average	*1 Serving/85g*	*62*	*0.8*	*73*	*6.0*	*9.7*	*1.0*	*4.5*
Frozen, Boiled, Average	*1 Serving/75g*	*51*	*0.7*	*68*	*6.0*	*9.4*	*0.9*	*5.1*
Frozen, Value, Tesco*	1 Serving/75g	60	0.7	80	5.9	9.0	0.9	5.5
Garden, Canned, Drained, Sainsbury's*	1oz/28g	23	0.4	81	6.7	10.0	1.6	4.5
Garden, Canned, No Sugar Or Salt, Average	*1 Can/80g*	*36*	*0.3*	*45*	*4.4*	*6.0*	*0.4*	*2.8*
Garden, Canned with Sugar & Salt, Average	*1 Serving/90g*	*59*	*0.6*	*66*	*5.3*	*9.3*	*0.7*	*5.1*
Garden, Cooked, Value, Tesco*	3 Tbsp/80g	54	0.7	67	5.3	9.4	0.9	5.1
Garden, Frozen, Average	*1 Serving/90g*	*66*	*1.0*	*74*	*6.3*	*9.7*	*1.1*	*3.3*
Garden, Frozen, Essential, Waitrose*	1 Portion/80g	52	0.7	65	5.7	8.6	0.9	4.7
Garden, Frozen for Freshness, Chosen By You, Asda*	1 Serving/80g	72	1.3	90	6.7	10.0	1.6	4.5
Garden, Minted, Average	*1 Serving/80g*	*59*	*0.9*	*74*	*6.3*	*9.7*	*1.1*	*5.9*
Garden, TTD, Sainsbury's*	1 Serving/79g	54	0.7	68	5.9	9.0	0.9	5.5
Giant, Marrowfat, Processed, Canned, Farrows*	1 Serving/80g	70	0.6	88	6.7	13.8	0.7	5.9
Green, Muncher, Original Flavour, W L Foods*	1 Serving/70g	330	13.0	471	20.0	57.1	18.6	17.1
Gungo, Canned, Drained, Dunn's River*	½ Can/115g	137	3.3	119	7.2	16.1	2.9	4.1
Marrowfat, Average	*1 Sm Can/160g*	*140*	*0.9*	*88*	*6.4*	*14.3*	*0.6*	*3.9*
Marrowfat, Processed, Canned, Drained, Value, Tesco*	1 Can/180g	162	1.3	90	6.5	14.5	0.7	3.9
Mushy, Average	*1 Can/200g*	*173*	*1.0*	*86*	*6.2*	*14.3*	*0.5*	*2.2*
Mushy, Frozen, Cooked, Asda*	1 Serving/80g	75	0.6	94	6.3	11.8	0.8	7.2
Processed, Canned, Average	*1 Sm Can/220g*	*176*	*1.8*	*80*	*6.1*	*12.3*	*0.8*	*3.6*
Snow	*1 Serving/80g*	*24*	*0.2*	*29*	*3.3*	*3.9*	*0.2*	*2.1*
Sugar Snap, Average	*1 Serving/80g*	*27*	*0.2*	*34*	*3.3*	*4.9*	*0.2*	*1.4*
Wasabi, Average	1 Serving/28g	114	3.8	406	15.2	54.0	13.7	8.6
Wasabi, Delicious, Boots*	½ Bag/25g	98	2.4	393	19.0	51.0	9.6	15.0
Wasabi, Roasted, Savoury Snack, Humdinger*	1 Portion/20g	81	2.4	404	15.8	50.3	12.0	15.9
PEASE PUDDING								
Canned, Re-Heated, Drained	1oz/28g	26	0.2	93	6.8	16.1	0.6	1.8
PECAN NUTS								
Average	*3 Nuts/6g*	*42*	*4.2*	*692*	*10.0*	*5.6*	*70.1*	*4.7*
Honey, Golden, Graze*	1 Pack/26g	168	15.4	647	7.6	23.4	59.4	0.0
PENNE								
Arrabbiata, BGTY, Sainsbury's*	1 Pack/450g	414	7.2	92	2.9	16.5	1.6	1.9
Chicken & Red Wine, Italiana, Weight Watchers*	1 Pack/395g	249	2.8	63	3.7	10.1	0.7	0.6
Chicken & Tomato, Italian, Sainsbury's*	½ Pack/350g	472	11.2	135	7.6	19.0	3.2	1.6
Chicken & Vegetables, Tomato & Basil Sauce, Birds Eye*	1 Meal/400g	325	5.2	81	7.7	9.7	1.3	1.2
Chilli, Asda*	1 Serving/100g	148	0.7	148	5.1	30.2	0.7	2.4
Chilli & Garlic, Asda*	1 Serving/75g	259	1.1	346	12.0	71.0	1.5	3.0
Cooked, Average	*1 Serving/185g*	*244*	*1.3*	*132*	*4.7*	*26.7*	*0.7*	*1.1*
Corn, Free From, Dry Weight, Sainsbury's*	1 Serving/100g	348	2.3	348	7.6	74.2	2.3	5.2
Creamy Mushroom, Prepared, Tesco*	½ Pack/200g	288	12.8	144	4.5	17.4	6.4	3.3
Dry, Average	*1 Serving/100g*	*352*	*1.9*	*352*	*12.4*	*71.3*	*1.9*	*2.7*
Dry Weight, Parioli, Cucina*	1 Serving/76g	270	1.1	355	12.5	73.0	1.4	2.6
Egg, Fresh, Average	*1 Serving/125g*	*352*	*4.0*	*282*	*11.1*	*52.2*	*3.2*	*2.0*
Free From, Tesco*	1 Serving/100g	340	2.0	340	8.0	72.5	2.0	2.5
Fresh, Dry, Average	*1 Serving/125g*	*222*	*2.4*	*178*	*7.3*	*32.2*	*1.9*	*1.6*

	Measure INFO/WEIGHT	per Measure KCAL	FAT	Nutrition Values per 100g / 100ml KCAL	PROT	CARB	FAT	FIBRE
PENNE								
Hickory Steak, COU, M & S*	1oz/28g	22	0.3	80	5.6	11.9	1.0	1.3
Hickory Steak, M & S*	1 Pack/400g	540	12.4	135	6.9	19.3	3.1	1.3
in Tomato & Basil Sauce, Sainsbury's*	½ Pack/110g	118	0.7	107	3.6	21.8	0.6	1.1
Leek & Bacon, Al Forno, Asda*	½ Pack/300g	531	39.0	177	5.0	10.0	13.0	0.5
Mediterranean, HL, Tesco*	1 Pack/400g	296	10.8	74	2.9	9.6	2.7	1.5
Napoletana Chicken, BFY, Morrisons*	1 Pack/350g	252	5.6	72	6.4	7.2	1.6	0.2
Organic, Dry, Average	*1 Serving/100g*	*352*	*1.8*	*352*	*12.4*	*71.6*	*1.8*	*1.9*
Rigate, Dry Weight, Average	*1 Serving/90g*	*318*	*1.6*	*353*	*12.3*	*72.1*	*1.8*	*1.8*
Roasted Red Pepper, GFY, Asda*	1 Pack/400g	212	2.4	53	1.9	10.0	0.6	0.8
Tomato & Basil Sauce, Asda*	½ Pack/314g	185	11.0	59	0.8	6.0	3.5	2.0
Tomato & Roasted Vegetable, Big Eat, Heinz*	1 Pot/351g	281	10.5	80	2.5	10.7	3.0	4.6
Tuna, Tomato & Olive, Asda*	1 Pack/340g	173	6.5	51	4.2	4.2	1.9	0.6
Wholewheat, Authentic, Cooked, Italiano, Tesco*	1 Portion/75g	244	1.9	325	12.5	62.5	2.5	9.0
with Chicken & Vegetables, Eat Positive, Birds Eye*	1 Meal/396g	325	5.2	82	7.7	9.8	1.3	1.2
with Roasted Vegetables, Waitrose*	1 Pack/400g	424	15.6	106	2.8	15.0	3.9	0.8
PEPERAMI*								
Firestick, Peperami*	1 Stick/25g	127	11.0	508	24.5	3.5	44.0	1.2
Hot, Peperami*	1 Stick/25g	126	11.0	504	24.5	2.5	44.0	1.2
Mini, 30% Less Fat, Peperami*	1 Stick/10g	38	3.0	379	25.0	1.5	30.0	3.0
Mini, Peperami*	1 Sausage/10g	38	2.0	379	25.0	1.5	20.0	3.0
Original, Peperami*	1 Stick/25g	126	11.0	504	24.0	2.5	44.0	0.1
PEPPER								
Black, Freshly Ground, Average	*1 Tsp/2g*	*5*	*0.1*	*255*	*10.9*	*64.8*	*3.3*	*26.5*
Cayenne, Ground	*1 Tsp/2g*	*6*	*0.3*	*318*	*12.0*	*31.7*	*17.3*	*0.0*
Peppercorns, Black, Schwartz*	1 Tsp/2g	11	0.4	529	13.0	68.7	22.5	27.0
White	*½ Tsp/1g*	*3*	*0.0*	*296*	*10.4*	*68.6*	*2.1*	*26.2*
PEPPERS								
Chilli, Chopped, Stir Fry, Schwartz*	1 Tbsp/19g	24	1.2	130	2.2	15.6	6.5	0.0
Chilli, Crushed, Schwartz*	1 Tsp/0.5g	2	0.1	321	12.0	29.0	17.0	27.0
Chilli, Dried, Flakes, Average	1 Tsp/3g	13	0.4	425	16.0	56.0	15.0	44.0
Chilli, Dried, Whole, Red, Schwartz*	1 Tsp/0.5g	2	0.1	425	15.9	56.4	15.1	0.0
Chilli, Green, Raw, Unprepared, Average	*1 Med/13g*	*5*	*0.0*	*40*	*2.0*	*9.5*	*0.2*	*1.5*
Chilli, Green, Very Lazy, The English Provender Co.*	1 Serving/10g	11	0.4	114	4.2	15.3	4.0	0.5
Chilli, Red, Chopped, In Marinade, Chef Kuo*	1 Tbsp/15g	10	0.6	69	1.6	11.5	4.2	5.3
Chilli, Red, Raw, Unprepared, Average	*1 Sm Pepper/13g*	*5*	*0.0*	*40*	*2.0*	*9.5*	*0.2*	*1.5*
Chilli, Red, Very Lazy, The English Provender Co.*	1 Serving/15g	17	0.6	114	4.2	15.3	4.0	0.5
Flame Seared with Greek Feta, M & S*	½ Tub/85g	106	8.2	125	3.6	5.4	9.7	1.8
Greek, Roasted Red in Brine, Kunapi*	1/3 Jar/120g	31	0.2	26	1.9	3.5	0.2	1.3
Green, Boiled in Salted Water	*1oz/28g*	*5*	*0.1*	*18*	*1.0*	*2.6*	*0.5*	*1.8*
Green, Filled, Tesco*	1 Pepper/150g	117	5.2	78	2.6	9.0	3.5	0.7
Green, Raw, Unprepared, Average	*1 Med/160g*	*24*	*0.5*	*15*	*0.8*	*2.6*	*0.3*	*1.6*
Italian Style, Sainsbury's*	1 Serving/150g	160	7.5	107	3.5	14.1	5.0	2.1
Jalapeno, Crushed, Schwartz*	1 Tsp/0.5g	1	0.1	136	15.9	56.4	15.1	0.0
Jalapeno, Raw	*1 Cup, Sliced/90g*	*27*	*0.6*	*30*	*1.3*	*5.9*	*0.6*	*2.8*
Mixed, Sliced, Morrisons*	1 Pack/120g	34	0.4	28	1.0	4.5	0.3	1.6
Mixed Bag, From Supermarket, Average	*1oz/28g*	*7*	*0.1*	*25*	*1.0*	*4.4*	*0.4*	*1.7*
Orange, Sweet, Raw, Average	*1oz/28g*	*8*	*0.1*	*30*	*1.8*	*5.0*	*0.3*	*1.5*
Pickled, Hot, Turkish, Melis, Melis*	1 Serving/25g	9	0.0	35	1.0	7.9	0.0	1.0
Ramiro, Red, Sainsbury's*	1 Serving/100g	30	0.3	30	1.6	5.1	0.3	2.2
Red, Boiled in Salted Water	*1oz/28g*	*10*	*0.1*	*34*	*1.1*	*7.0*	*0.4*	*1.7*
Red, Filled, Halves, Vegetarian, M & S*	1 Pack/295g	280	10.3	95	2.9	12.3	3.5	1.1
Red, Filled with Feta, COU, M & S*	1 Pepper/154g	200	11.1	130	4.1	12.4	7.2	0.6
Red, Raw, Unprepared, Average	1oz/28g	9	0.1	32	1.0	6.4	0.4	1.6

	Measure INFO/WEIGHT	per Measure KCAL	FAT	Nutrition Values per 100g / 100ml KCAL	PROT	CARB	FAT	FIBRE
PEPPERS								
Red, Roasted, in Brine, Cooks & Co*	1 Serving/100g	23	0.3	23	1.6	4.5	0.3	0.0
Red, Roasted, Melis*	1 Serving/100g	90	1.0	90	1.1	18.8	1.0	0.2
Red, Sweet, Pointed, TTD, Sainsbury's*	1 Serving/100g	32	0.4	32	1.0	6.4	0.4	0.0
Red, Sweet Pointed, Organic, Tesco*	1 Serving/100g	33	0.4	33	1.0	6.4	0.4	1.6
Stuffed, Fresh, Asda*	1 Pepper/150g	144	7.5	96	3.8	9.0	5.0	1.2
Stuffed, Perfectly Balanced, Waitrose*	1 Pack/300g	243	7.2	81	3.0	11.8	2.4	1.3
Stuffed, Sainsbury's*	1 Serving/137g	169	9.5	123	3.3	11.8	6.9	1.0
Stuffed with Rice Based Filling, Average	1oz/28g	24	0.7	85	1.5	15.4	2.4	1.3
Stuffed with Vegetables, Cheese Topping, Average	1oz/28g	31	1.9	111	3.4	9.8	6.7	1.5
Sweet, Pointed, Extra Special, Asda*	1 Serving/100g	36	0.4	36	1.0	6.4	0.4	1.6
Sweet, Raw, Average	**1 Serving/100g**	**16**	**0.3**	**16**	**0.8**	**2.6**	**0.3**	**1.6**
Sweet, Tinned, Sainsbury's*	½ Can/125g	45	0.5	36	1.1	7.0	0.4	1.7
Yellow, Raw, Unprepared, Average	**1 Med/160g**	**42**	**0.3**	**26**	**1.2**	**5.3**	**0.2**	**1.7**
PERCH								
Raw, Atlantic	**1oz/28g**	**26**	**0.5**	**94**	**18.6**	**0.0**	**1.6**	**0.0**
PERNOD*								
19% Volume, Pernod*	**1 Shot/35ml**	**45**	**0.0**	**130**	**0.0**	**0.0**	**0.0**	**0.0**
PESTO								
Sauce, Average	1oz/28g	145	13.3	517	20.4	2.0	47.5	0.0
Sauce, Basil, M & S*	1 Serving/65g	348	30.5	535	7.5	20.7	46.9	1.4
Sauce, Dressing, Finest, Tesco*	1 Serving/30ml	108	11.1	360	3.5	2.9	37.1	0.9
Sauce, Fiery Chilli, Sacla*	½ Jar/95g	342	29.3	360	4.8	16.0	30.8	3.4
Sauce, Green, Alla Genovese, Finest, Tesco*	1 Serving/65g	188	25.7	290	5.7	1.5	39.6	2.8
Sauce, Green, Alla Genovese, TTD, Sainsbury's*	1 Serving/30g	192	19.8	640	6.2	5.4	65.9	3.1
Sauce, Green, Asda*	2 Dtsp/25g	93	9.7	374	5.0	0.8	39.0	5.0
Sauce, Green, Classic, Sacla*	1 Serving/40g	185	18.6	462	5.2	7.6	46.5	0.0
Sauce, Green, Fresh, Sainsbury's*	1 Serving/60g	328	31.7	546	9.4	8.3	52.8	0.1
Sauce, Green, Fresh, Tesco*	1oz/28g	141	13.4	505	6.5	12.2	48.0	0.1
Sauce, Green, GFY, Asda*	1 Jar/190g	338	29.6	178	5.0	4.3	15.6	3.3
Sauce, Green, Italiano, Tesco*	1 Serving/50g	251	24.5	502	9.6	5.6	49.0	1.2
Sauce, Green, Less Than 60% Fat, BGTY, Sainsbury's*	¼ Jar/48g	61	5.3	128	4.2	2.6	11.2	0.0
Sauce, Green, Morrisons*	1 Serving/50g	255	24.9	510	10.7	4.7	49.8	0.0
Sauce, Green, Sainsbury's*	1 Tsp/5g	23	2.1	451	5.9	10.1	43.0	2.0
Sauce, Green, Tesco*	¼ Jar/48g	192	20.0	405	5.6	0.6	42.2	4.4
Sauce, Green, Verde, Bertolli*	¼ Jar/46g	266	27.5	575	5.7	4.3	59.5	0.0
Sauce, Italian Style, Stir, Thru, Asda*	1 Serving/15g	55	5.2	369	4.4	9.0	35.0	0.9
Sauce, Mary Berry*	1 Serving/100g	528	49.3	528	1.1	19.4	49.3	1.1
Sauce, Red, Garlic & Chilli, Jamie Oliver*	1 Jar/190g	494	48.8	260	1.1	5.6	25.7	1.1
Sauce, Red, Italian, Tesco*	1 Serving/38g	127	11.5	340	8.2	8.2	30.6	1.2
Sauce, Red, M & S*	1oz/28g	93	9.3	331	3.6	6.9	33.2	3.5
Sauce, Red, Morrisons*	1 Tbsp/15g	47	4.3	311	5.7	6.6	29.0	5.9
Sauce, Red, Rosso, Bertolli*	1 Jar/185g	703	64.7	380	6.8	9.5	35.0	2.0
Sauce, Red, Smart Price, Asda*	1 Tsp/10g	15	0.9	147	3.8	12.1	9.3	2.4
Sauce, Red, Tesco*	¼ Jar/50g	162	15.1	325	5.6	6.3	30.3	6.0
Sauce, Ricotta & Red Pepper, Chosen By You, Asda*	1 Jar/190g	486	37.2	256	4.2	14.4	19.6	2.4
Sauce, Roasted Red Pepper, Sacla*	1 Serving/30g	72	6.8	241	4.3	4.6	22.8	5.3
Sauce, Spinach & Parmesan, Sainsbury's*	¼ Jar/46g	162	16.0	349	4.6	5.3	34.4	2.5
Sauce, Sun Dried Tomato, Sacla*	1 Serving/30g	87	8.4	289	4.2	5.2	27.9	0.0
Sauce, Verde, Traditional Italian, Sacla*	1 Serving/100g	454	45.4	454	5.3	6.0	45.4	0.0
Sauce & Balsamic Vinegar, Extra Special, Asda*	1 Tbsp/15g	33	3.0	213	0.3	8.6	19.7	0.0
PETIT POIS								
& Baby Carrots, Canned, Drained, Average	½ Can/122g	58	0.8	47	2.9	7.0	0.7	3.2
& Baby Carrots, Tesco*	½ Drained Jar/110g	47	0.5	43	3.0	4.4	0.5	4.2

	Measure INFO/WEIGHT	per Measure KCAL	FAT	Nutrition Values per 100g / 100ml KCAL	PROT	CARB	FAT	FIBRE
PETIT POIS								
Canned, Drained, Average	1 Serving/80g	50	0.4	63	4.8	8.9	0.5	2.6
Fresh, Frozen, Average	1 Serving/80g	51	0.8	63	5.4	7.1	0.9	4.7
PHEASANT								
Meat Only, Roasted	***1oz/28g***	***62***	***3.4***	***220***	***27.9***	***0.0***	***12.0***	***0.0***
Meat Only, Roasted, Weighed with Bone	***1oz/28g***	***61***	***3.3***	***219***	***27.9***	***0.0***	***11.9***	***0.0***
Stuffed, Easy Carve, Finest, Tesco*	1 Serving/200g	540	37.4	270	23.2	2.2	18.7	0.9
PHYSALIS								
Raw, without Husk, Average	***5 Fruits/30g***	***16***	***0.2***	***53***	***1.9***	***11.2***	***0.7***	***0.4***
PICCALILLI								
Dijon, Sainsbury's*	1 Dtsp/15g	14	0.1	91	1.8	19.0	0.9	0.7
Haywards*	1 Serving/28g	18	0.1	66	1.4	13.9	0.5	0.0
Heinz*	1 Serving/10g	10	0.1	99	1.0	20.5	0.6	0.6
Morrisons*	1 Serving/50g	37	0.3	75	1.6	15.0	0.7	0.6
Sainsbury's*	1 Dtsp/15g	9	0.1	60	1.8	11.9	0.6	0.7
Sandwich, Tesco*	1 Serving/20g	16	0.0	80	0.4	18.5	0.0	1.6
Spicy, Sainsbury's*	1 Serving/15g	12	0.1	80	0.7	15.3	0.5	1.0
Sweet, Asda*	1 Tbsp/15g	17	0.0	112	0.5	27.0	0.2	0.6
Sweet, Somerfield*	1 Tsp/10g	11	0.1	107	1.0	24.0	1.0	0.0
Tesco*	1 Serving/50g	51	1.8	102	0.5	17.8	3.6	2.0
Three Mustard, Finest, Tesco*	1 Serving/30g	40	0.2	134	1.3	30.7	0.7	1.0
TTD, Sainsbury's*	1 Serving/19g	13	0.2	67	0.7	13.9	0.9	1.8
PICKLE								
Beetroot, Branston*	1 Tsp/20g	25	0.1	123	1.2	28.2	0.3	1.6
Branston, Crosse & Blackwell*	1 Tsp/10g	11	0.0	109	0.8	26.1	0.2	1.1
Brinjal, Patak's*	1 Tsp/16g	59	3.9	367	2.2	34.6	24.4	0.9
Chilli, Branston*	1 Tsp/16g	21	0.1	130	0.7	30.0	0.7	1.5
Chilli, Patak's*	1 Tsp/16g	52	5.4	325	4.3	1.3	33.7	0.0
Chilli Tomato, Patak's*	1oz/28g	27	0.9	95	2.5	16.0	3.2	1.5
Cornichons, in Sweet & Sour Vinegar, Waitrose*	1 Serving/10g	3	0.0	28	0.6	6.1	0.1	0.6
Garlic, Patak's*	1 Tsp/16g	42	3.0	261	3.6	20.0	18.5	1.6
Ginger, Priya*	1 Tsp/10g	27	1.7	270	3.3	26.7	16.7	0.0
Green Chilli, Priya*	1 Tsp/10g	19	1.7	190	3.3	6.7	16.7	4.8
Hot Chilli Jam, What A Pickle*	1 Tsp/8g	14	0.0	178	0.6	44.0	0.1	1.2
Lime, Hot, Asda*	1 Dtsp/10g	12	1.0	123	2.2	6.0	10.0	1.0
Lime, Hot, Patak's*	1 Tsp/16g	31	3.0	194	2.2	4.0	18.7	0.4
Lime, M & S*	1 Tsp/16g	34	0.8	215	0.8	42.5	4.8	2.4
Lime, Sharwood's*	1 Tsp/16g	24	1.5	152	2.2	15.0	9.3	2.9
Mango, Hot, Patak's*	1 Tsp/16g	43	4.1	270	2.3	7.4	25.7	1.9
Mild Mustard, Heinz*	1 Tbsp/10g	13	0.1	129	2.2	25.7	1.3	0.9
Mixed, Drained	1 Serving/100g	14	0.2	14	1.0	1.9	0.2	1.0
Mixed, Drained, Haywards*	½ Jar/120g	22	0.4	18	1.4	2.4	0.3	0.0
Mixed, Patak's*	1 Serving/30g	78	7.7	259	2.3	4.7	25.7	0.8
Mixed, Salad Bar, Asda*	1oz/28g	11	0.0	40	0.5	9.2	0.1	0.0
Onion, Priya*	1 Tsp/10g	20	1.5	203	3.3	13.3	15.0	0.0
Red Cabbage, Asda*	1 Serving/50g	16	0.0	32	1.6	6.0	0.1	0.0
Red Chilli, Priya*	1 Tsp/10g	22	1.7	217	3.3	13.3	16.7	0.0
Sandwich, Branston*	1 Tsp/10g	14	0.0	140	0.7	34.2	0.3	1.3
Sandwich, Somerfield*	1 Tsp/10g	15	0.0	150	1.0	36.0	0.0	0.0
Sandwich, Tesco*	1 Serving/5g	7	0.0	138	1.0	33.1	0.2	1.0
Small Chunk, Branston*	1 Serving/20g	22	0.0	109	0.8	26.1	0.2	1.1
Spicy, Branston*	1 Tsp/15g	21	0.0	140	0.7	34.7	0.3	1.3
Sweet	***1 Tsp/10g***	***14***	***0.0***	***141***	***0.6***	***36.0***	***0.1***	***1.2***
Sweet, Branston*	1 Serving/30g	33	0.1	109	0.8	26.1	0.2	1.1

	Measure INFO/WEIGHT	per Measure KCAL	FAT	Nutrition Values per 100g / 100ml KCAL	PROT	CARB	FAT	FIBRE
PICKLE								
Sweet, Budgens*	1 Tsp/10g	14	0.0	141	0.8	34.0	0.2	0.0
Sweet, Country, Morrisons*	1 Tbsp/15g	19	0.0	130	0.9	31.1	0.2	0.0
Sweet, Frank Cooper*	1 Pot/20g	21	0.0	104	0.5	25.3	0.1	0.8
Sweet, Hartley's*	1 Tsp/16g	22	0.0	140	0.5	36.2	0.0	0.0
Sweet, Low Price, Sainsbury's*	1 Serving/23g	23	0.1	98	0.7	23.2	0.3	0.7
Sweet, Value, Tesco*	1 Serving/10g	10	0.0	96	0.6	23.0	0.2	0.7
Sweet Harvest, Asda*	1 Serving/25g	38	0.1	154	0.8	37.0	0.3	0.8
Tangy, Sandwich, Heinz*	1 Tsp/10g	13	0.0	134	0.7	31.4	0.2	0.9
Tomato, Priya*	1 Tsp/10g	22	1.7	217	3.3	13.3	16.7	0.0
Tomato, Tangy, Heinz*	1 Tsp/10g	10	0.0	102	2.0	22.0	0.3	1.5
PICNIC								
Cadbury*	1 Bar/48g	230	10.8	480	7.3	60.9	22.6	2.1
PIE								
2 Mini Pork, Ploughmans, Ginsters*	1 Pie/50g	190	12.6	380	8.9	29.2	25.3	2.0
Aberdeen Angus, Cottage, Bistro, M Kitchen, Morrisons*	1 Pack/700g	791	30.8	113	7.0	10.4	4.4	1.7
Admiral's, Light & Easy, Youngs*	1 Pack/360g	342	14.0	95	4.1	10.9	3.9	0.8
Admiral's, Ross*	1 Pie/340g	357	15.6	105	4.8	10.9	4.6	0.7
All Steak, Pukka Pies Ltd*	1 Pie/233g	538	32.9	231	9.9	16.2	14.1	1.6
Apple, American, Iceland*	1 Serving/92g	258	10.7	280	4.8	39.2	11.6	2.2
Apple, Asda*	¼ Pack/107g	287	11.7	269	3.6	39.0	11.0	1.7
Apple, Bramley, & Blackberry, Aunt Bessie's*	¼ Pie/138g	344	12.5	250	2.1	40.1	9.1	2.6
Apple, Bramley, & Blackberry, M & S*	¼ Pie/146g	380	14.5	260	3.4	39.8	9.9	1.3
Apple, Bramley, & Custard, Lattice Topped, Mr Kipling*	1 Pie/64g	236	9.9	369	3.8	53.7	15.4	1.1
Apple, Bramley, & Damson, M & S*	¼ Pie/142g	370	13.9	260	3.3	39.7	9.8	2.1
Apple, Bramley, Aunt Bessie's*	¼ Pie/138g	351	15.1	255	2.8	36.2	11.0	1.2
Apple, Bramley, Deep Filled, Sainsbury's*	1/6 Pie/120g	329	14.3	274	3.7	38.0	11.9	1.9
Apple, Bramley, Free From, Sainsbury's*	1 Pie/60g	220	7.6	367	1.1	61.8	12.6	1.2
Apple, Bramley, Free From, Tesco*	1 Pie/60g	225	7.5	375	1.7	63.8	12.5	0.8
Apple, Bramley, Individual, Mr Kipling*	1 Pie/66g	228	8.6	346	3.4	53.8	13.0	1.4
Apple, Bramley, Individual, Sainsbury's*	1 Pie/54g	165	5.0	307	3.6	52.2	9.3	1.3
Apple, Bramley, Individual, Tesco*	1 Pie/61g	210	7.9	344	3.4	53.1	13.0	1.5
Apple, Bramley, Large, Tesco*	1/8 Pie/87g	311	13.0	358	3.9	51.9	15.0	1.9
Apple, Bramley, Less Than 10% Fat, Sainsbury's*	1 Pie/54g	165	5.0	307	3.6	52.2	9.3	1.3
Apple, Bramley, M & S*	1 Pie/55g	184	6.4	335	2.9	57.6	11.7	1.6
Apple, Bramley, Rowan Hill Bakery*	1 Pie/64g	216	8.3	337	3.6	51.5	13.0	1.4
Apple, Bramley, Tesco*	1 Serving/106g	284	11.6	268	3.6	38.8	10.9	1.7
Apple, Bramley Somerfield*	1/6 Pie/70g	193	9.0	275	3.5	34.0	12.8	2.4
Apple, Deep Filled, Amanda Smith*	1/5 Pie/150g	420	19.8	280	2.8	37.4	13.2	1.2
Apple, Deep Filled, Farmfoods*	1oz/28g	74	3.6	266	3.6	34.3	12.7	2.2
Apple, Deep Filled, Iceland*	1 Serving/116g	332	15.3	286	2.5	39.2	13.2	1.1
Apple, Deep Filled, Sainsbury's*	¼ Pie/137g	374	17.5	273	3.8	35.6	12.8	1.6
Apple, Family, Asda*	1/6 Pie/119g	314	13.0	265	3.6	38.0	11.0	2.9
Apple, Family, Morrisons*	1/6 Pie/116g	326	14.0	281	3.1	39.9	12.1	3.1
Apple, Individual, Somerfield*	1 Pie/47g	179	8.0	379	3.5	53.2	16.9	1.3
Apple, Lattice, Tesco*	1 Serving/145g	325	13.3	224	2.2	33.2	9.2	1.4
Apple, Low Price, Sainsbury's*	¼ Pie/103g	291	15.0	283	4.4	33.5	14.6	1.3
Apple, McVitie's*	1 Serving/117g	316	12.9	270	3.0	39.0	11.0	2.0
Apple, Pastry Top & Bottom	1oz/28g	74	3.7	266	2.9	35.8	13.3	1.7
Apple, Puff Pastry, M & S*	1 Pie/135g	337	17.1	250	2.4	31.3	12.7	1.0
Apple, Ready Baked, Sara Lee*	1/6 Pie/90g	249	12.4	277	2.8	35.4	13.8	1.2
Apple, Sainsbury's*	1/6 Pie/118g	314	13.6	266	3.4	37.1	11.5	0.6
Apple, Smart Price, Asda*	1 Serving/47g	178	8.0	379	3.5	53.0	17.0	1.3
Apple, Sultana & Cinnamon, Finest, Tesco*	1 Slice/83g	193	7.3	233	2.8	35.6	8.8	5.0

PIE

INFO/WEIGHT	Measure	per Measure KCAL	FAT	Nutrition Values per 100g / 100ml KCAL	PROT	CARB	FAT	FIBRE
Apple, Tesco*	1 Pie/47g	191	8.1	406	3.3	59.4	17.2	1.5
Apple, Value, Tesco*	1 Pie/47g	127	4.7	270	2.8	41.5	9.9	1.7
Apple, VLH Kitchens	1 Serving/50g	136	22.4	272	3.7	40.0	11.2	1.7
Apple & Blackberry, Co-Op*	1 Serving/138g	338	15.2	245	3.0	33.0	11.0	2.0
Apple & Blackberry, Fruit, Finest, Tesco*	1 Pie/95g	265	11.3	279	13.7	29.3	11.9	2.8
Apple & Blackberry, Lattice Topped, BGTY, Sainsbury's*	¼ Pie/100g	256	7.5	256	2.8	44.4	7.5	3.1
Apple & Blackberry, Shortcrust, M & S*	1 Serving/142g	469	17.7	330	4.3	50.2	12.5	1.1
Apple & Blackberry, Somerfield*	¼ Pie/106g	280	12.7	264	4.0	36.0	12.0	0.0
Apple & Blackberry, Tesco*	1 Serving/106g	287	11.9	271	4.2	38.4	11.2	1.7
Apple & Blackcurrant, Mr Kipling*	1 Pie/66g	211	8.4	320	3.3	47.9	12.8	1.2
Apple Meringue, Frozen, Sara Lee*	1/6 Pie/74g	179	6.5	242	2.7	37.9	8.8	1.5
Apple with Custard	1 Serving/217g	353	18.8	163	2.4	25.2	8.7	1.1
Apricot Fruit, GFY, Asda*	1 Serving/52g	162	5.2	311	3.3	52.0	10.0	0.0
Banoffee, Individual, Sainsbury's*	1 Pie/104g	365	21.0	351	3.2	39.2	20.2	2.2
Banoffee, Mini, Waitrose*	1 Pie/26g	115	5.8	444	3.3	57.0	22.5	1.2
Banoffee, Tesco*	1/6 Pie/94g	365	19.7	390	3.9	45.8	21.1	1.5
Banoffee Cream, American Dream, Heinz*	1/6 Pie/70g	239	15.0	342	3.7	33.7	21.4	3.9
Banoffee Cream, American Dream, McVitie's*	1 Serving/70g	277	17.8	396	4.3	36.7	25.5	0.8
Beef, Lean, BGTY, Sainsbury's*	1 Serving/212g	280	12.7	132	7.3	12.2	6.0	1.5
Beef, Sainsbury's*	1 Pie/210g	535	30.0	255	10.3	21.2	14.3	2.0
Beef, Shamrock, Pieminister*	1 Pie/270g	648	30.8	240	8.8	24.5	11.4	1.8
Beef & Kidney, 208, Oakhouse Foods Ltd*	1 Meal/360g	540	24.8	150	6.5	15.1	6.9	1.8
Beef & Kidney, Farmfoods*	1oz/28g	68	3.9	242	5.6	23.9	13.8	1.1
Beef & Onion, Pukka Pies Ltd*	1 Serving/231g	529	32.6	229	7.6	17.9	14.1	3.0
Beef & Vegetable, Macdougalls, McDougalls*	¼ Pie/114g	292	19.3	256	5.3	20.6	16.9	0.3
Beef Steak, Aberdeen Angus, Top Crust, Waitrose*	½ Pie/280g	476	24.1	170	10.0	13.4	8.6	4.1
Blackberry & Apple, Sara Lee*	1 Serving/100g	272	13.9	272	2.9	34.0	13.9	0.0
Blackcurrant, Deep Filled, Sainsbury's*	1 Slice/137g	440	19.3	321	5.8	42.6	14.1	2.2
Blackcurrant, Shortcrust, M & S*	1 Pie/142g	412	14.3	290	3.9	45.6	10.1	1.3
Cheese & Onion, Hollands*	1 Pie/200g	516	24.4	258	6.3	30.9	12.2	0.0
Cheese & Onion, Oven Baked, Average	1 Serving/200g	654	40.0	327	8.2	30.4	20.0	1.2
Cheese & Potato	1oz/28g	39	2.3	139	4.8	12.6	8.1	0.7
Cheese & Potato, Aunt Bessie's*	¼ Serving/200g	288	18.8	144	4.6	11.7	9.4	1.5
Cherry, Asda*	1/6 Pie/117g	337	14.5	289	3.1	41.2	12.4	1.8
Cherry, Deep Filled, Somerfield*	1/6 Pie/90g	259	10.8	288	3.0	41.0	12.0	0.0
Cherry, Sainsbury's*	1 Serving/117g	325	13.6	278	3.9	39.6	11.6	1.7
Cherry, Tesco*	1 Serving/106g	294	12.7	277	4.0	38.3	12.0	1.8
Chicke, Leek & Sweetcorn, Love Life, Waitrose*	1 Pie/421g	358	14.3	85	5.2	8.6	3.4	1.7
Chicken, Aunt Bessie's*	¼ Pie/200g	474	24.2	237	10.6	21.4	12.1	2.1
Chicken, Bacon & Cheddar Cheese, Lattice, Birds Eye*	1 Pie/155g	454	26.8	293	13.4	21.0	17.3	1.5
Chicken, Broccoli & White Wine, Waitrose*	1 Serving/200g	605	40.5	302	12.5	17.7	20.2	2.3
Chicken, Cheese & Bacon, HL, Tesco*	1 Pack/450g	382	9.9	85	5.9	9.4	2.2	1.6
Chicken, Cheese & Broccoli Lattice, Birds Eye*	1 Pie/155g	446	25.3	288	12.6	22.7	16.3	1.1
Chicken, Cheese & Leek Lattice, Sun Valley*	1 Lattice/125g	315	21.9	252	15.2	8.6	17.5	1.0
Chicken, Cottage, Frozen, Tesco*	1 Pack/450g	292	2.2	65	2.8	11.7	0.5	1.0
Chicken, Deep Filled, Puff Pastry, Sainsbury's*	1 Pie/210g	538	31.9	256	10.0	19.9	15.2	3.1
Chicken, Finest, Tesco*	1 Pie/250g	615	32.2	246	10.7	21.9	12.9	1.2
Chicken, Ginsters*	¼ Pie/136g	374	23.7	275	10.0	19.0	17.4	1.0
Chicken, Individual, Made with 100% Breast, Birds Eye*	1 Pie/154g	455	28.1	296	7.9	25.0	18.3	1.0
Chicken, Individual Shortcrust, Asda*	1 Pie/175g	534	29.7	305	10.0	28.0	17.0	1.0
Chicken, Leek & Bacon Filo, Willow Farm, Finest, Tesco*	½ Pie/225g	574	33.1	255	11.1	18.5	14.7	1.4
Chicken, Leek & Ham, Morrisons*	1 Serving/113g	305	16.6	270	8.8	25.7	14.7	1.1
Chiokon, Nowgato*	1 Pie/142g	358	23.6	252	6.1	23.1	16.6	1.0

PIE

	Measure INFO/WEIGHT	per Measure KCAL	FAT	Nutrition Values per 100g / 100ml KCAL	PROT	CARB	FAT	FIBRE
Chicken, Puff Pastry, Tesco*	¼ Pie/114g	250	12.7	220	8.6	21.3	11.2	1.4
Chicken, Roast, & Vegetable, Pot, M & S*	1/3 Pie/183g	366	22.9	200	7.7	13.5	12.5	4.5
Chicken, Roast, COU, M & S*	1 Pack/320g	272	3.2	85	9.4	9.7	1.0	0.8
Chicken, Roast, M & S*	1/3 Pie/182g	465	24.1	255	7.8	26.4	13.2	2.2
Chicken, Roast, Puff Pastry, Deep Fill, Asda*	½ Pie/259g	739	44.1	285	10.0	23.0	17.0	0.8
Chicken, Roast, Sainsbury's*	1/3 Pie/173g	538	30.8	311	10.5	27.2	17.8	0.9
Chicken, Roast, Tesco*	1 Pack/450g	382	13.5	85	6.4	7.4	3.0	1.0
Chicken, Short Crust, M & S*	1 Pie/170g	510	29.6	300	9.7	26.2	17.4	1.7
Chicken, Tomato & Basil Lattice, Birds Eye*	1 Serving/155g	340	19.6	220	10.8	15.7	12.7	1.4
Chicken, wth Ham & Leek, Pot, Higgidy*	1 Pie/250g	710	33.5	284	13.1	19.1	13.4	1.1
Chicken & Asparagus, Lattice, Waitrose*	1 Serving/100g	295	19.6	295	7.4	22.3	19.6	1.8
Chicken & Asparagus, McDougalls*	1 Serving/170g	394	21.9	232	7.4	21.6	12.9	1.5
Chicken & Asparagus, Puff Pasty, John Bullers*	1 Pie/174g	477	29.6	274	11.0	19.0	17.0	2.0
Chicken & Asparagus, Tesco*	1 Serving/170g	467	28.7	275	8.3	22.4	16.9	0.8
Chicken & Bacon, Filo Pastry, Finest, Tesco*	1 Serving/160g	362	18.7	226	11.3	18.9	11.7	1.7
Chicken & Bacon, Puff Pastry, Deep Fill, Sainsbury's*	1/3 Pie/200g	532	34.0	266	9.1	19.1	17.0	1.3
Chicken & Bacon with Cheese Sauce, Tesco*	1 Serving/200g	540	33.6	270	12.0	17.6	16.8	0.8
Chicken & Basil, M & S*	1oz/28g	59	3.3	210	8.9	17.0	11.9	1.1
Chicken & Broccoli, BGTY, Sainsbury's*	1 Pack/450g	297	3.6	66	5.9	8.9	0.8	1.8
Chicken & Broccoli, COU, M & S*	1 Serving/320g	272	6.1	85	8.1	8.8	1.9	1.3
Chicken & Broccoli, Good Intentions, Somerfield*	1 Pack/450g	382	8.1	85	6.8	10.5	1.8	0.5
Chicken & Broccoli, Lattice, Tesco*	½ Pie/200g	496	30.8	248	8.5	18.9	15.4	2.1
Chicken & Broccoli, Light Choices, Tesco*	1 Pack/450g	382	7.2	85	7.0	10.3	1.6	0.8
Chicken & Broccoli Lattice, Sainsbury's*	½ Pie/192g	520	30.7	271	9.3	22.4	16.0	0.9
Chicken & Broccoli Potato, Top, Asda*	1 Pack/400g	319	7.0	80	5.2	10.7	1.7	0.6
Chicken & Gravy, Deep Fill, Asda*	1 Serving/130g	370	22.1	285	10.0	23.0	17.0	0.8
Chicken & Gravy, Light Choices, Tesco*	1 Pack/450g	410	10.9	90	5.9	10.6	2.4	1.4
Chicken & Gravy, Shortcrust Pastry, Large, Tesco*	½ Pie/300g	789	45.6	263	8.2	23.4	15.2	1.0
Chicken & Gravy, Shortcrust Pastry, Sainsbury's*	1 Serving/250g	637	35.2	255	8.0	24.1	14.1	1.0
Chicken & Gravy, Shortcrust Pastry, Tesco*	1 Pie/250g	617	34.5	247	6.8	23.9	13.8	1.0
Chicken & Ham, Deep Filled, Sainsbury's*	1 Pie/210g	594	37.2	283	8.0	23.0	17.7	1.0
Chicken & Ham, Deep Filled, Somerfield*	¼ Pie/138g	348	19.3	252	11.0	21.0	14.0	0.0
Chicken & Ham, Family, Farmfoods*	1oz/28g	67	3.9	241	9.9	19.4	13.8	1.2
Chicken & Ham, Morrisons*	¼ Pie/115g	267	13.7	232	8.7	22.5	11.9	0.8
Chicken & Ham, Sainsbury's*	1 Pie/128g	461	28.7	360	11.0	28.5	22.4	2.0
Chicken & Ham, Tesco*	1 Serving/113g	293	17.6	259	9.4	20.2	15.6	1.2
Chicken & Leek, Deep Filled, Puff Pastry, Sainsbury's*	1/3 Pie/451g	1109	65.4	246	10.1	18.7	14.5	1.5
Chicken & Leek, Light Choices, Tesco*	1 Pie/350g	297	5.6	85	6.6	10.3	1.6	1.3
Chicken & Leek, M & S*	1oz/28g	70	4.2	250	10.1	18.8	15.1	1.1
Chicken & Leek, Shortcrust, TTD, Sainsbury's*	½ Pie/300g	824	48.8	275	12.2	19.8	16.3	1.1
Chicken & Mushroom, & Potato, Filo, COU, M & S*	1 Pack/260g	273	7.0	105	7.5	12.1	2.7	1.5
Chicken & Mushroom, Asda*	1 Pie/150g	384	24.0	256	9.0	19.0	16.0	1.0
Chicken & Mushroom, Average	1 Serving/200g	540	31.7	270	8.0	23.8	15.9	1.0
Chicken & Mushroom, Chilled, Weight Watchers*	1 Pack/400g	304	4.8	76	5.7	9.8	1.2	1.5
Chicken & Mushroom, Chosen By You, Asda*	1 Pack/400g	329	9.2	82	6.7	8.1	2.3	1.2
Chicken & Mushroom, Co-Op*	1 Pie/150g	442	27.0	295	8.0	27.0	18.0	0.8
Chicken & Mushroom, Deep Filled, Frozen, Tesco*	¼ Pie/198g	465	22.2	235	9.0	23.8	11.2	1.2
Chicken & Mushroom, Dietary Specials*	1 Pie/140g	300	14.0	214	6.3	24.7	10.0	0.9
Chicken & Mushroom, Farmfoods*	1 Pie/110g	271	16.4	246	5.6	22.4	14.9	0.9
Chicken & Mushroom, Finest, Tesco*	1 Pie/250g	742	46.7	297	9.3	21.1	18.7	0.9
Chicken & Mushroom, Fray Bentos*	1 Pie/425g	684	40.4	161	6.7	11.5	9.5	0.0
Chicken & Mushroom, Ginsters*	1 Pie/180g	486	31.1	270	8.3	20.2	17.3	1.3
Chicken & Mushroom, Individual, Co-Op*	1 Pie/149g	465	29.7	312	8.6	24.5	19.9	1.2

P

PIE

INFO/WEIGHT	Measure	per Measure		Nutrition Values per 100g / 100ml				
		KCAL	FAT	KCAL	PROT	CARB	FAT	FIBRE
Chicken & Mushroom, Individual, Frozen, Tesco*	1 Pie/142g	347	17.9	245	8.9	23.5	12.6	1.2
Chicken & Mushroom, Morrisons*	1 Serving/100g	261	15.4	261	7.6	22.9	15.4	0.9
Chicken & Mushroom, Puff Pastry, Birds Eye*	1 Pie/152g	415	21.3	273	11.9	24.9	14.0	1.6
Chicken & Mushroom, Puff Pastry, Sainsbury's*	1 Pie/150g	450	25.0	300	7.8	29.6	16.7	0.9
Chicken & Mushroom, Pukka Pies Ltd*	1 Pie/226g	475	29.2	210	7.6	15.7	12.9	3.5
Chicken & Mushroom, Shortcrust, Somerfield*	¼ Pie/125g	410	28.4	328	6.2	24.7	22.7	1.4
Chicken & Mushroom, Weight Watchers*	1 Pie/136g	317	15.1	233	8.0	25.1	11.1	1.5
Chicken & Vegetable, Farmfoods*	1 Pie/128g	384	24.1	300	7.2	25.4	18.8	1.4
Chicken & Vegetable, Freshbake*	1 Pie/125g	319	19.6	255	6.5	21.8	15.7	2.7
Chicken & Vegetable, Individual, Somerfield*	1 Pie/142g	382	22.0	269	7.6	24.8	15.5	1.3
Chicken & Vegetable, Kids, Tesco*	1 Serving/235g	235	10.6	100	5.9	9.1	4.5	0.7
Chicken & Vegetable, Perfectly Balanced, Waitrose*	1 Serving/375g	285	5.2	76	5.1	10.8	1.4	1.3
Chicken & Vegetable, Potato Topped, Somerfield*	1 Pack/350g	270	10.5	77	3.7	8.8	3.0	2.0
Chicken & Vegetable, Value, Tesco*	1 Pie/121g	321	16.9	265	6.6	26.9	14.0	1.1
Chicken & Wiltshire Ham, Finest, Tesco*	1 Pie/250g	687	37.2	275	11.6	22.7	14.9	1.1
Chicken Balti, Ginsters*	1 Pie/180g	416	25.0	231	7.3	19.2	13.9	1.9
Chicken Curry, Iceland*	1 Pie/156g	440	23.7	282	10.2	26.2	15.2	2.0
Chicken in Gravy, Just,Fray Bentos*	½ Pie/212g	324	17.4	153	5.4	14.3	8.2	0.6
Chocolate, Mini, Waitrose*	1 Pie/24g	109	6.1	455	5.3	51.4	25.3	1.7
Cod & Prawn, M & S*	1oz/28g	43	2.5	155	10.6	8.7	8.9	0.7
Cod & Smoked Haddock, COU, M & S*	1 Pack/400g	320	9.6	80	6.1	9.0	2.4	1.2
Cottage, Aberdeen Angus, Large, Chilled, Finest, Tesco*	½ Pack/400g	420	17.2	105	7.1	8.7	4.3	1.8
Cottage, Aberdeen Angus, Waitrose*	1 Pie/350g	339	12.2	97	5.3	11.0	3.5	0.9
Cottage, Aldi*	1 Pack/440g	484	27.3	110	4.1	9.5	6.2	0.2
Cottage, Asda*	1 Pack/400g	360	9.6	90	6.5	10.6	2.4	1.0
Cottage, Aunt Bessie's*	1 Pack/350g	413	18.2	118	4.8	12.1	5.2	1.0
Cottage, Basics, Sainsbury's*	1 Pack/300g	228	9.0	76	4.4	7.9	3.0	1.5
Cottage, British Pies, Chilled, Tesco*	1 Pack/500g	450	14.0	90	4.6	10.3	2.8	1.5
Cottage, Budgens*	1 Pie/400g	404	18.0	101	5.6	9.6	4.5	1.0
Cottage, Chicken, Tesco*	1 Pack/400g	340	2.8	85	6.0	12.8	0.7	1.7
Cottage, Classic British, Sainsbury's*	1 Pack/450g	436	16.2	97	5.3	9.9	3.6	1.7
Cottage, Classics, Asda*	½ Pack/450g	531	27.0	118	7.0	9.0	6.0	1.0
Cottage, COU, M & S*	1 Pack/400g	340	8.0	85	6.0	11.0	2.0	1.5
Cottage, Diet Chef Ltd*	1 Pack/270g	235	9.7	87	3.7	9.8	3.6	1.7
Cottage, Disney, Tesco*	1 Pack/281g	250	7.0	89	4.9	11.8	2.5	1.9
Cottage, Family, Iceland*	¼ Pack/259g	262	10.6	101	4.2	11.8	4.1	0.8
Cottage, Fresh, M & S*	1 Pie/400g	460	22.4	115	6.8	9.9	5.6	0.6
Cottage, Frozen, Asda*	1 Serving/121g	146	7.3	121	4.8	12.0	6.0	0.6
Cottage, Frozen, Chosen By You, Asda*	1 Pack/400g	368	9.6	92	6.5	10.6	2.4	1.0
Cottage, Goodness, Tesco*	1 Pot/280g	238	8.4	85	5.0	9.5	3.0	2.5
Cottage, Healthy Living, Co-Op*	1 Pack/400g	320	6.4	80	5.0	11.0	1.6	2.0
Cottage, Healthy Options, Birds Eye*	1oz/28g	23	0.5	83	4.9	11.9	1.8	1.0
Cottage, Iceland*	1 Pack/400g	468	18.8	117	5.1	13.6	4.7	0.7
Cottage, Individual, Smart Price, Asda*	1 Pie/159g	149	5.9	94	3.1	12.0	3.7	0.7
Cottage, Light Choices, Tesco*	1 Pack/500g	400	8.5	80	4.5	11.4	1.7	1.7
Cottage, Luxury, M & S*	½ Pack/310g	403	21.7	130	7.9	8.3	7.0	1.8
Cottage, Meal for One, M & S*	1 Pack/445g	356	16.0	80	5.4	6.2	3.6	1.7
Cottage, Meatfree, Sainsbury's*	1 Pack/400g	364	12.0	91	4.4	11.7	3.0	0.7
Cottage, Mini, Waitrose*	1 Pack/250g	267	10.5	107	6.4	11.1	4.2	1.4
Cottage, Morrisons*	1 Pack/450g	450	18.4	100	5.2	10.7	4.1	1.2
Cottage, Ready Meals,Tesco*	1 Pack/400g	380	12.0	95	6.1	10.8	3.0	1.6
Cottage, Retail, Average	1 Pack/400g	399	15.7	100	5.5	10.5	3.9	1.3
Cottage, Ross*	1 Pack/320g	240	7.0	75	3.0	10.9	2.2	0.3

PIE

	Measure INFO/WEIGHT	per Measure KCAL	FAT	Nutrition Values per 100g / 100ml KCAL	PROT	CARB	FAT	FIBRE
Cottage, Sainsbury's*	1 Pack/300g	297	10.2	99	6.4	10.7	3.4	1.1
Cottage, Salmon, Sainsbury's*	1 Serving/299g	218	4.2	73	4.6	10.4	1.4	1.3
Cottage, The Best, Morrisons*	½ Pack/400g	424	16.4	106	7.7	9.5	4.1	1.2
Cottage, Vegetarian, Sainsbury's*	1 Pack/450g	328	9.9	73	3.0	10.2	2.2	1.8
Cottage, Waitrose*	1 Pack/400g	424	19.6	106	3.4	12.1	4.9	1.2
Cottage, Weight Watchers*	1 Pack/300g	186	3.9	62	3.6	9.0	1.3	0.3
Cottage, You Count, Love Life, Waitrose*	1 Pack/402g	338	9.1	84	4.0	11.5	2.2	1.1
Cottage with Cheddar Mash, TTD, Sainsbury's*	1 Pack/400g	582	27.7	145	9.2	11.6	6.9	2.4
Country, Vegetarian, Tesco*	1 Pie/142g	381	21.6	268	5.6	27.3	15.2	1.2
Cumberland, Asda*	1 Pack/400g	504	22.4	126	6.3	12.7	5.6	1.5
Cumberland, Beef, HL, Tesco*	1 Pack/500g	460	13.5	92	5.0	11.8	2.7	0.9
Cumberland, BGTY, Sainsbury's*	1 Pack/450g	360	9.0	80	5.3	10.1	2.0	1.6
Cumberland, Cod & Prawn, Tesco*	1 Pack/450g	427	11.2	95	7.9	9.5	2.5	1.3
Cumberland, GFY, Asda*	1 Pack/451g	469	9.9	104	11.4	11.4	2.2	2.1
Cumberland, HL, Tesco*	1 Pie/500g	430	13.5	86	4.5	10.8	2.7	1.2
Cumberland, M & S*	1 Pie/195g	312	20.3	160	6.9	10.1	10.4	1.1
Festive, McDonald's*	1 Pie/84g	310	17.6	369	4.0	42.0	21.0	1.0
Fish	1 Sm Serving/250g	262	7.5	105	8.0	12.3	3.0	0.7
Fish, BFY, Morrisons*	1 Pack/350g	301	10.1	86	5.0	10.0	2.9	0.9
Fish, Chilled, GFY, Asda*	1 Pie/450g	405	12.6	90	6.8	9.3	2.8	1.4
Fish, Creamy, Classics, Large, Finest, Tesco*	½ Pack/350g	402	19.6	115	6.4	8.6	5.6	0.9
Fish, Creamy, Classics, Small, Tesco*	1 Pack/400g	520	28.0	130	8.7	7.7	7.0	0.7
Fish, Cumberland, BGTY, Sainsbury's*	1 Serving/450g	342	8.5	76	7.3	7.3	1.9	1.8
Fish, Extra Special, Asda*	1 Pack/400g	540	30.8	135	9.8	6.5	7.7	1.1
Fish, Frozen, GFY, Asda*	1 Pack/360g	342	8.6	95	5.8	12.5	2.4	0.9
Fish, Good Intentions, Somerfield*	1 Pack/400g	300	5.2	75	5.6	10.3	1.3	0.5
Fish, Healthy Options, Birds Eye*	1 Pack/350g	238	2.8	68	3.7	11.6	0.8	0.7
Fish, HL, Tesco*	1 Pack/400g	316	8.8	79	4.0	10.8	2.2	1.7
Fish, Kids, Great Stuff, Asda*	1 Pack/300g	276	9.0	92	7.8	8.4	3.0	1.4
Fish, Kids Smart, Morrisons*	1 Pie/225g	190	4.9	93	6.3	10.8	2.4	1.7
Fish, Large (700g), Extra Special, Asda*	1 Serving/350g	525	30.8	150	9.9	7.8	8.8	0.6
Fish, Luxury, Cafe Culture, M & S*	1 Pack/660g	627	26.4	95	7.1	7.8	4.0	1.1
Fish, Luxury, M & S*	1 Pack/300g	330	16.8	110	7.3	7.6	5.6	1.5
Fish, Mariner's, Frozen, Youngs*	1 Pack/360g	382	16.2	106	5.3	11.0	4.5	1.0
Fish, Mix, Tesco*	1 Pack/320g	480	25.6	150	19.3	0.0	8.0	0.0
Fish, Pollock, Yummy, Jamie Oliver, Youngs*	1 Cooked Pie/217g	204	7.2	94	6.8	8.6	3.3	1.5
Fish, Salmon, Yummy, Jamie Oliver, Youngs*	1 Cooked Pie/207g	224	8.5	108	8.1	9.3	4.1	0.9
Fish, Salmon & Broccoli, Yummy, Jamie Oliver, Youngs*	1 Cooked Pie/220g	211	7.5	96	6.5	9.3	3.4	1.3
Fish, Seasonal, Mix, Sainsbury's*	1 Pack/320g	480	28.2	150	17.7	0.0	8.8	0.0
Fish, The Best, Morrisons*	½ Pack/225g	250	11.9	111	6.6	9.3	5.3	0.8
Fish, TTD, Sainsbury's*	½ Pack/390g	386	12.9	99	7.1	10.3	3.3	1.6
Fish, with Cheddar & Parsley Sauce, Go Cook, Asda*	½ Pack/450g	427	16.2	95	7.8	7.9	3.6	0.8
Fish, with Cheese, Ross*	1 Pack/300g	321	13.5	107	4.7	12.0	4.5	0.8
Fish, with Grated Cheddar, Asda*	¼ Pie/250g	262	12.5	105	7.0	8.0	5.0	1.0
Fish, with Vegetables, Ross*	1 Pack/300g	255	8.7	85	4.4	10.2	2.9	1.3
Fish & Prawn, Perfectly Balanced, Waitrose*	1 Serving/375g	379	13.5	101	6.8	10.4	3.6	0.7
Fisherman's, Asda*	1 Serving/300g	429	21.0	143	7.0	13.0	7.0	0.0
Fishermans, British Recipe, Waitrose*	1 Pack/400g	408	16.4	102	7.7	8.5	4.1	1.2
Fisherman's, Chilled, Co-Op*	1 Pie/300g	345	18.0	115	4.0	11.0	6.0	0.7
Fisherman's, Famous, Chilled, Youngs*	1 Pack/400g	448	22.8	112	7.6	7.6	5.7	0.9
Fisherman's, Healthy Options, Asda*	1 Pie/406g	337	10.1	83	5.0	10.0	2.5	0.9
Fisherman's, M & S*	1 Pie/248g	335	15.9	135	9.3	9.8	6.4	0.3
Fisherman's, Morrisons*	1 Serving/300g	246	9.9	82	3.8	9.5	3.3	1.0

	Measure	per Measure		Nutrition Values per 100g / 100ml				
	INFO/WEIGHT	KCAL	FAT	KCAL	PROT	CARB	FAT	FIBRE

PIE

	Measure	per Measure		Nutrition Values per 100g / 100ml				
Fisherman's, Nisa Heritage*	1 Serving/550g	588	30.8	107	5.2	9.0	5.6	0.2
Fishermans, Perfectly Balanced, Waitrose*	1 Serving/400g	436	11.2	109	8.1	12.8	2.8	0.9
Fisherman's, Sainsbury's*	1 Pack/300g	195	3.6	65	3.9	9.7	1.2	1.2
Fishermans, Smart Price, Asda*	1 Pack/300g	213	3.6	71	3.1	12.0	1.2	1.9
Fisherman's, Tesco*	1 Pie/400g	400	19.6	100	4.2	9.8	4.9	1.1
Fishermans, Value, Tesco*	1 Pie/300g	195	3.0	65	3.3	9.1	1.0	1.6
Fruit, Pastry Top & Bottom	1oz/28g	73	3.7	260	3.0	34.0	13.3	1.8
Fruit, Selection, Mr Kipling*	1 Pie/66g	232	9.0	350	3.5	53.5	13.6	1.3
Gala, Tesco*	1 Serving/70g	241	17.6	344	10.6	24.5	25.2	0.0
Haddock & Broccoli, M & S*	1 Serving/250g	262	10.0	105	8.1	9.3	4.0	0.5
Key Lime, Sainsbury's*	¼ Pie/80g	280	11.2	350	4.2	51.8	14.0	0.7
Lamb & Mint, Shortcrust Pasty, Tesco*	¼ Pack/150g	412	26.1	275	5.9	23.6	17.4	1.6
Lemon Meringue	1 Portion/120g	383	17.3	319	4.5	45.9	14.4	0.7
Lemon Meringue, 90% Fat Free, Sara Lee*	1/6 Pie/75g	204	6.7	272	2.4	46.1	8.9	0.9
Lemon Meringue, Lyons*	1 Serving/100g	310	14.4	310	0.0	45.9	14.4	0.0
Lemon Meringue, Mini, Asda*	1 Pie/26g	101	3.3	396	3.7	66.0	13.0	1.8
Lemon Meringue, Mr Kipling*	1 Pie/51g	184	6.2	360	2.9	59.9	12.1	3.0
Lemon Meringue, Sainsbury's*	¼ Pie/110g	351	9.9	319	2.3	57.3	9.0	0.5
Lemon Meringue, Sara Lee*	1oz/28g	77	2.6	276	2.6	46.6	9.2	0.9
Lemon Meringue, Tesco*	1 Pie/385g	989	28.1	257	4.0	43.7	7.3	0.5
Lemon Meringue, Weight Watchers*	1 Serving/85g	161	0.4	189	2.4	43.1	0.5	0.6
Macaroni Cheese, Countryside*	1 Serving/144g	282	10.1	196	4.9	28.3	7.0	1.2
Mariner's, Light & Easy, Youngs*	1 Pack/350g	367	14.3	105	5.0	12.0	4.1	1.1
Mariner's, Ross*	1 Pie/340g	435	20.1	128	5.0	13.9	5.9	1.0
Mashed Potato Topped Cumberland, M & S*	1/3 Pack/300g	360	17.7	120	5.8	9.6	5.9	1.0
Meat, Freshbake*	1 Pie/49g	152	10.5	313	6.6	23.2	21.6	1.0
Meat & Potato, Hollands*	1 Pie/175g	409	19.2	234	6.1	27.5	11.0	0.0
Meat & Potato, Shortcrust, Co-Op*	¼ Pie/137g	403	26.2	294	7.3	23.3	19.1	1.4
Meat & Potato, Tesco*	1 Serving/150g	414	26.8	276	5.1	23.6	17.9	1.6
Meat & Potato, Value, Tesco*	1 Pie/95g	274	17.5	288	6.9	23.8	18.4	3.5
Mince, Asda*	1 Pie/53g	204	8.0	382	3.8	58.0	15.0	1.5
Mince, Christmas, Finest, Tesco*	1 Pie/66g	257	8.8	390	4.6	62.4	13.3	2.6
Mince, Christmas, Sainsbury's*	1 Pie/37g	147	6.0	397	4.5	58.0	16.3	2.6
Mince, Deep, Morrisons*	1 Pie/65g	243	9.1	371	3.7	57.8	13.9	1.5
Mince, Deep Filled, Christmas, Tesco*	1 Pie/64g	243	8.6	380	4.2	59.8	13.5	2.9
Mince, Deep Filled, Morrisons*	1 Pie/66g	257	9.7	386	3.7	57.9	14.6	4.2
Mince, Deep Filled, Sainsbury's*	1 Pie/61g	226	8.8	365	3.7	55.7	14.2	5.7
Mince, Dusted, Mini, Finest, Tesco*	1 Pie/20g	76	2.4	379	7.3	62.9	12.2	5.0
Mince, Extra Special, Asda*	1 Pie/60g	225	8.3	378	3.9	59.0	14.0	2.2
Mince, Iced Top, Asda*	1 Pie/57g	215	7.1	378	2.8	63.7	12.4	1.1
Mince, Iced Top, Tesco*	1 Pie/55g	209	6.3	380	3.1	65.7	11.4	2.1
Mince, Iceland*	1 Pie/39g	156	6.4	405	4.4	59.6	16.6	3.8
Mince, Individual, Average	1 Pie/48g	203	9.8	423	4.3	59.0	20.4	2.1
Mince, Individual, Mr Kipling*	1 Pie/67g	250	9.2	376	3.7	59.0	13.9	1.5
Mince, Lattice, Classics, M & S*	1 Pie/53g	210	8.0	400	4.0	61.7	15.2	2.4
Mince, Luxury, Deep Filled, M & S*	1 Pie/65g	234	9.0	360	4.3	55.0	13.8	3.8
Mince, Mini, M & S*	1 Pie/28g	105	4.0	380	4.3	57.8	14.6	4.0
Mince, Mini, Waitrose*	1 Pie/30g	150	9.1	501	5.7	51.3	30.3	1.7
Mince, Organic, Sainsbury's*	1 Pie/46g	177	7.5	384	5.0	54.5	16.2	5.6
Mince, Rowan Hill Bakery*	1 Pie/55g	202	8.2	370	3.8	54.8	15.1	0.0
Mince, Shortcrust, Waitrose*	1 Pie/55g	210	8.0	385	3.6	60.0	14.6	20.9
Mince, Star Motif, Mini, Finest, Tesco*	1 Pie/17g	62	2.1	365	3.8	59.9	12.1	3.8
Mince, Topped with Nibbed Almonds, Mini, Finest, Tesco*	1 Pie/20g	77	2.8	383	4.9	59.0	14.1	3.4

P

PIE

	Measure INFO/WEIGHT	per Measure KCAL	FAT	KCAL	PROT	CARB	FAT	FIBRE
Mince, Trufree*	1 Pie/60g	238	9.8	397	2.1	58.5	16.4	3.6
Mince Puff, Tesco*	1 Pie/25g	105	4.4	420	3.3	62.0	17.6	2.0
Minced Beef, Aberdeen Angus, Shortcrust, M & S*	1 Pie/171g	435	26.6	255	9.3	19.3	15.6	3.0
Minced Beef & Onion, Birds Eye*	1 Pie/145g	419	25.1	289	7.1	26.3	17.3	0.7
Minced Beef & Onion, Denny*	1 Sm Pie/140g	288	19.7	206	6.1	17.3	14.1	0.0
Minced Beef & Onion, Farmfoods*	1 Pie/128g	378	23.9	295	7.3	24.4	18.7	1.0
Minced Beef & Onion, Tesco*	1 Pie/150g	454	28.5	303	5.7	27.4	19.0	1.7
Minced Beef & Potato, Weight Watchers*	1 Pie/200g	328	12.4	164	6.7	20.2	6.2	3.6
Minced Beef & Vegetable, Pot, M & S*	1/3 Pie/183g	366	26.5	200	7.8	9.1	14.5	7.1
Minced Steak & Onion, Puff Pastry, Individual, Sainsbury's*	1 Pie/150g	484	29.5	323	7.4	29.0	19.7	1.5
Mississippi Mud, Tesco*	1 Serving/104g	399	26.6	384	5.3	33.1	25.6	1.8
Moroccan Vegetable & Feta, Little, Higgidy*	1 Pie/180g	418	22.5	232	5.1	24.7	12.5	0.6
Mushroom & Leaf Spinach, Little, Higgidy*	1 Pie/180g	441	25.9	245	6.6	22.3	14.4	0.7
Mushroom & Parsley Potato, Waitrose*	1 Pack/350g	346	17.5	99	2.5	10.9	5.0	1.2
Ocean, Basics, Sainsbury's*	1 Serving/302g	196	3.6	65	3.9	9.7	1.2	1.2
Ocean, BGTY, Sainsbury's*	1 Pack/350g	285	4.7	81	6.3	11.1	1.3	0.8
Ocean, Frozen, BGTY, Sainsbury's*	1 Pack/350g	318	5.2	91	7.0	12.4	1.5	0.9
Ocean, M & S*	1 Pie/650g	617	22.7	95	8.2	7.6	3.5	0.9
Ocean, Original, Frozen, Youngs*	1 Pack/375g	420	21.4	112	7.6	7.6	5.7	0.9
Ocean, The Original, Light & Easy, Youngs*	1 Pack/415g	432	18.7	104	6.4	9.5	4.5	1.0
Ocean, Weight Watchers*	1 Pack/300g	196	3.3	65	4.2	9.2	1.1	0.8
Pork, Buffet, Bowyers*	1 Pie/60g	217	14.7	362	10.4	24.9	24.5	0.0
Pork, Buffet, Farmfoods*	1 Pie/65g	252	17.4	388	8.8	28.2	26.7	1.0
Pork, Buffet, Mini, Somerfield*	1 Pie/70g	292	19.9	418	10.8	29.5	28.5	0.2
Pork, Cheese & Pickle, Mini, Tesco*	1 Pie/49g	191	12.8	389	9.2	29.3	26.1	1.2
Pork, Crusty Bake, Mini, Sainsbury's*	1 Pie/43g	165	11.2	384	11.5	26.0	26.0	1.5
Pork, Crusty Bake, Sainsbury's*	1 Pie/75g	292	20.0	390	10.5	27.0	26.7	1.0
Pork, Geo Adams*	1 Pie/125g	487	34.7	390	11.8	23.1	27.8	0.9
Pork, Medium, Pork Farms*	1 Pie/200g	744	53.0	372	9.5	23.6	26.5	1.7
Pork, Melton, Mini, Pork Farms*	1 Pie/50g	199	14.6	399	8.9	26.2	29.2	0.0
Pork, Melton Mowbray, Cured, M & S*	1 Pie/290g	1044	71.0	360	10.1	25.9	24.5	1.0
Pork, Melton Mowbray, Cured, Mini, M & S*	1 Pie/50g	192	12.2	385	9.8	32.6	24.4	1.0
Pork, Melton Mowbray, Individual, Sainsbury's*	1 Pie/75g	296	20.8	395	10.2	26.1	27.7	2.4
Pork, Melton Mowbray, Large, Co-Op*	1/4 Pie/110g	418	35.2	380	11.0	12.0	32.0	5.0
Pork, Melton Mowbray, Lattice, Sainsbury's*	1 Serving/100g	342	23.6	342	10.8	21.7	23.6	1.2
Pork, Melton Mowbray, Medium, Somerfield*	1/4 Pie/70g	275	18.9	393	11.0	27.0	27.0	0.0
Pork, Melton Mowbray, Mini, Co-Op*	1 Pie/49g	189	13.2	385	11.0	24.0	27.0	2.0
Pork, Melton Mowbray, Mini, Finest, Tesco*	1 Pie/50g	179	11.3	359	12.1	26.6	22.7	0.9
Pork, Melton Mowbray, Mini, Morrisons*	1 Pie/50g	197	12.5	393	10.9	31.3	24.9	0.9
Pork, Melton Mowbray, Mini, Tesco*	1 Pie/50g	196	14.3	392	12.6	20.8	28.7	2.9
Pork, Melton Mowbray, Small, Somerfield*	1/2 Pie/64g	237	14.7	371	12.0	30.0	23.0	0.0
Pork, Melton Mowbray, Snack, Tesco*	1 Pie/75g	289	19.4	385	10.1	27.0	25.9	2.7
Pork, Melton Mowbray, Tesco*	1 Sm Pie/148g	679	49.9	459	10.0	29.0	33.7	1.3
Pork, Melton Mowbray, Uncured, Small, Tesco*	1 Pie/140g	465	29.5	332	11.2	24.4	21.1	2.4
Pork, Mini, Christmas, Tesco*	1 Pie/50g	195	13.5	390	10.6	25.7	27.0	1.4
Pork, Mini, Tesco*	1 Pie/45g	162	10.7	359	10.2	25.9	23.8	1.0
Pork, Mini, Value, Tesco*	1 Pie/70g	266	17.8	380	9.0	28.5	25.5	3.5
Pork, Somerfield*	1 Pie/110g	442	31.9	402	11.0	24.0	29.0	0.0
Pork, VLH Kitchens	1 Serving/36g	168	100.0	466	11.0	26.0	36.0	0.0
Pork & Egg, M & S*	1/4 Pie/108g	379	28.0	351	9.7	19.8	25.9	0.8
Pork & Pickle, Bowyers*	1 Pie/150g	576	40.9	384	10.0	26.3	27.3	0.0
Pork with Cheese & Pickle, Waitrose*	1 Pack/150g	568	36.9	379	10.3	29.1	24.6	2.7
Potato & Meat, Farmfoods*	1 Pie/158g	416	26.9	263	5.4	22.0	17.0	1.0

PIE

	Measure INFO/WEIGHT	per Measure KCAL	FAT	Nutrition Values per 100g / 100ml KCAL	PROT	CARB	FAT	FIBRE
Rhubarb, Sara Lee*	1 Serving/90g	224	12.4	250	2.9	28.7	13.8	1.3
Salmon, Crumble, Light & Easy, Youngs*	1 Pack/320g	282	6.4	88	5.7	11.8	2.0	1.0
Salmon, Value, Tesco*	1 Pack/300g	312	13.5	104	4.5	11.3	4.5	1.0
Salmon & Broccoli, Birds Eye*	1 Pie/351g	449	21.8	128	6.6	11.4	6.2	0.7
Salmon & Broccoli, Filo Pastry, Finest, Tesco*	1 Pie/170g	386	22.6	227	7.9	18.9	13.3	2.1
Salmon & Broccoli, Light Choices, Tesco*	1 Pack/400g	350	7.2	87	7.0	10.2	1.8	1.7
Salmon & Broccoli, Premium, Tesco*	1 Serving/170g	425	29.2	250	6.1	17.7	17.2	0.7
Salmon & Broccoli Lattice Bar, Asda*	1/3 Bar/133g	360	19.9	271	6.0	28.0	15.0	0.8
Sausage & Onion, Lattice, Puff Pastry, Tesco*	1/3 Pie/133g	480	22.5	361	9.1	20.6	16.9	4.6
Sausage & Onion, Tesco*	1 Pack/300g	333	18.3	111	2.3	11.7	6.1	0.5
Scotch, Co-Op*	1 Pie/132g	408	24.9	309	7.3	27.3	18.9	1.5
Scotch, Farmfoods*	1 Pie/151g	430	24.6	285	7.8	26.8	16.3	1.2
Shepherd's, 218, Oakhouse Foods Ltd*	1 Meal/390g	406	17.2	104	6.3	10.3	4.4	1.6
Shepherd's, Asda*	1 Pie/153g	193	9.2	126	5.0	13.0	6.0	0.8
Shepherd's, Average	1oz/28g	31	1.7	112	6.0	9.3	5.9	0.7
Shepherd's, Baked Bean Cuisine, Heinz*	1 Pie/340g	299	9.5	88	4.1	11.6	2.8	1.5
Shepherd's, British Classic, Serves 1, Sainsbury's*	1 Pack/450g	454	22.0	101	6.2	7.9	4.9	1.7
Shepherd's, British Classics, Chilled, Tesco*	1 Pack/500g	500	20.5	100	4.8	10.6	4.1	1.2
Shepherd's, Chilled, Finest, Tesco*	½ Pack/400g	460	16.4	115	6.9	8.0	4.1	1.9
Shepherd's, Chilled, Value, Tesco*	1 Pack/300g	210	4.5	70	3.0	11.0	1.5	1.0
Shepherd's, Classics, Asda*	1 Pack/455g	459	22.7	101	5.0	9.0	5.0	1.1
Shepherd's, Cooked, BGTY, Sainsbury's*	1 Pack/450g	359	8.0	85	4.2	11.8	1.9	1.3
Shepherd's, COU, M & S*	1 Pack/300g	210	3.9	70	5.2	8.6	1.3	1.6
Shepherd's, Diet Chef Ltd*	1 Serving/270g	235	10.5	87	3.2	9.8	3.9	1.9
Shepherd's, Frozen, Tesco*	1 Pack/400g	270	9.1	67	4.1	7.6	2.3	1.1
Shepherd's, GFY, Asda*	1 Pack/399g	339	10.8	85	4.0	11.1	2.7	1.4
Shepherd's, Good Intentions, Somerfield*	1oz/28g	25	0.9	90	4.1	10.9	3.2	1.6
Shepherd's, Great Value, Asda*	1 Pack/400g	376	12.0	94	4.7	12.0	3.0	0.6
Shepherd's, Iceland*	1 Serving/170g	224	9.5	132	5.4	14.7	5.6	0.8
Shepherd's, TTD, Sainsbury's*	1 Pack/397g	524	27.8	132	7.6	9.7	7.0	1.7
Shepherd's, Weight Watchers*	1 Pack/320g	217	6.3	68	3.3	8.8	2.0	1.1
Shepherd's, Welsh Hill Lamb, Gastropub, M & S*	½ Pack/330g	313	11.5	95	5.4	10.2	3.5	1.5
Squash, Butternut, Skinny, & Red Pepper, Little, Higgidy*	1 Pie/180g	367	23.6	204	4.2	17.2	13.1	1.6
Steak, Deep Fill, Frozen, Short Crust Base, Puff Lid, Tesco*	¼ Pie/200g	440	23.2	220	16.1	12.9	11.6	1.3
Steak, Deep Fill, Tesco*	¼ Pie/195g	468	25.5	240	9.7	20.0	13.1	1.5
Steak, Dietary Specials*	1 Pie/140g	328	14.4	234	9.8	25.7	10.3	0.4
Steak, in Rich Gravy, Aunt Bessie's*	¼ Pie/200g	440	20.6	220	9.6	22.0	10.3	1.5
Steak, in Rich Gravy, Shortcrust Pastry, Large, Sainsbury's*	1/3 Pie/200g	528	30.4	264	12.0	19.6	15.2	3.6
Steak, Individual, British Classics, Tesco*	1 Pie/150g	450	27.6	300	9.1	23.3	18.4	2.5
Steak, Large, Glenfell*	¼ Pie/170g	445	27.9	262	6.8	21.8	16.4	1.0
Steak, M & S*	1oz/28g	64	3.6	230	10.0	19.0	12.7	1.2
Steak, Mini, Asda*	1 Serving/67g	117	5.3	176	9.0	17.0	8.0	0.9
Steak, Mushroom & Ale, Topcrust, Waitrose*	1 Pie/250g	500	29.5	200	11.1	12.2	11.8	1.1
Steak, Puff Pastry, Deep Filled, Sainsbury's*	1 Pie/210g	535	30.0	255	10.3	21.2	14.3	2.0
Steak, Puff Pastry, Deep Filled, Somerfield*	½ Pie/275g	715	38.2	260	10.0	23.7	13.9	0.8
Steak, Scotch, Bell's Bakery*	1 Serving/150g	378	20.2	252	13.6	18.6	13.5	0.7
Steak, Short Crust, Sainsbury's*	½ Pie/118g	314	24.1	267	10.9	22.2	20.5	1.7
Steak, Shortcrust, 3½ Minute, Pukka Pies Ltd*	1 Pie/198g	586	32.5	296	9.4	28.6	16.4	2.1
Steak, Shortcrust Pastry, Finest, Tesco*	1 Pie/250g	660	37.7	264	10.9	21.2	15.1	0.8
Steak, Tesco*	1 Serving/205g	556	33.8	271	7.2	23.3	16.5	1.4
Steak, Top Crust, TTD, Sainsbury's*	½ Pie/299g	530	23.1	177	15.4	11.4	7.7	0.5
Steak, TTD, Sainsbury's*	½ Pie/300g	713	35.4	238	12.6	20.3	11.8	1.0
Steak & Ale, Average	1 Pie/200g	507	28.7	253	9.8	21.1	14.3	1.3

PIE

	Measure INFO/WEIGHT	per Measure KCAL	per Measure FAT	Nutrition Values per 100g / 100ml KCAL	PROT	CARB	FAT	FIBRE
Steak & Ale, Deep Fill, Puff Pastry, Tesco*	¼ Pie/150g	324	19.6	216	8.0	16.6	13.1	2.3
Steak & Ale, Deep Filled, Somerfield*	1 Pie/200g	550	32.0	275	12.0	22.0	16.0	0.0
Steak & Ale, Fray Bentos*	1 Pie/425g	697	38.7	164	7.6	13.0	9.1	0.0
Steak & Ale, Pub Style, Co-Op*	1 Pie/250g	537	30.0	215	9.0	17.0	12.0	2.0
Steak & Ale, Puff Pastry, Asda*	1/3 Pie/200g	520	30.2	260	10.6	20.4	15.1	1.6
Steak & Ale, TTD, Sainsbury's*	1 Pie/250g	681	35.6	272	11.6	24.4	14.2	1.4
Steak & Ale with Chips & Gravy	1 Serving/400g	825	42.2	206	7.2	20.5	10.6	0.5
Steak & Dorset Ale, Mini, Finest, Tesco*	1 Pie/30g	91	4.9	305	7.9	31.4	16.4	1.9
Steak & Guinness, Sainsbury's*	¼ Pie/137g	399	25.5	291	8.7	22.2	18.6	1.0
Steak & Kidney, Birds Eye*	1 Pie/146g	447	28.5	306	9.0	23.7	19.5	2.3
Steak & Kidney, Deep Fill, Sainsbury's*	½ Pie/125g	314	18.6	251	8.4	21.0	14.9	2.0
Steak & Kidney, Family, Co-Op*	1/6 Pie/87g	278	17.4	320	9.0	26.0	20.0	0.9
Steak & Kidney, Family, Iceland*	1/3 Pie/225g	502	29.2	223	10.2	16.3	13.0	2.1
Steak & Kidney, Individual	1 Pie/200g	646	42.4	323	9.1	25.6	21.2	0.9
Steak & Kidney, Premium, Tesco*	1 Serving/170g	428	26.3	252	9.9	18.3	15.5	1.2
Steak & Kidney, Princes*	½ Pack/212g	379	19.9	179	8.8	14.8	9.4	0.0
Steak & Kidney, Puff Pastry, Sainsbury's*	1 Pie/150g	423	23.5	282	8.2	26.9	15.7	0.9
Steak & Kidney, Pukka Pies Ltd*	1 Pie/238g	488	25.9	205	9.1	17.7	10.9	3.6
Steak & Kidney, Tesco*	1 Pie/150g	420	27.3	280	7.3	21.9	18.2	3.7
Steak & Kidney, Tinned, Fray Bentos*	½ Pie/212g	346	18.7	163	8.2	12.9	8.8	0.0
Steak & Mushroom, Asda*	1 Pie/130g	350	18.1	270	9.0	27.0	14.0	1.4
Steak & Mushroom, Deep Fill, Asda*	1/3 Pie/175g	476	28.0	272	11.0	21.0	16.0	1.1
Steak & Mushroom, Deep Fill, Puff Pastry, Tesco*	1 Slice/150g	339	20.7	226	9.1	16.3	13.8	1.9
Steak & Mushroom, Family, Iceland*	¼ Pie/164g	366	21.8	223	10.5	15.4	13.3	2.9
Steak & Mushroom, Finest, Tesco*	1 Pie/250g	640	36.5	256	9.2	21.9	14.6	1.1
Steak & Mushroom, Home Comforts, Weight Watchers*	1 Pie/136g	322	15.9	237	5.8	26.9	11.7	1.4
Steak & Mushroom, Individual, Birds Eye*	1 Pie/142g	389	24.1	274	7.5	22.7	17.0	2.0
Steak & Mushroom, McDougalls*	1 Pack/340g	779	57.8	229	9.0	10.0	17.0	0.9
Steak & Mushroom, Sainsbury's*	¼ Pie/130g	372	21.3	286	8.6	26.0	16.4	1.0
Steak & Mushroom, Tesco*	1 Pie/138g	345	19.5	250	8.3	22.2	14.1	1.8
Steak & Onion, Farmfoods*	1 Pie/127g	382	24.3	301	6.0	26.4	19.1	1.0
Steak & Onion, Ginsters*	1 Pie/180g	481	30.8	267	8.0	20.3	17.1	1.3
Steak & Onion, Minced, Aberdeen Angus, Tesco*	½ Pie/300g	897	57.6	299	9.4	22.1	19.2	0.7
Steak & Peppered Sauce, Gastro Style, McDougalls*	1 Pie/192g	495	28.8	258	8.9	21.4	15.0	0.9
Steak & Potato, Asda*	1/3 Pie/173g	442	26.0	255	6.9	23.1	15.0	0.9
Steak & Red Wine, Puff Pastry, Pub, Sainsbury's*	1 Pie/240g	497	29.5	207	7.2	16.8	12.3	2.1
Summer Fruits, Orchard Tree*	1/8 Pie/75g	242	10.3	323	3.0	46.6	13.8	1.2
Teviot, Minced Beef, Morrisons*	½ Pie/250g	382	17.2	153	8.0	14.5	6.9	1.6
Tuna & Sweetcorn, HL, Tesco*	1 Pack/450g	391	12.1	87	7.1	8.6	2.7	2.0
Turkey & Ham, Farmfoods*	1 Pie/147g	404	21.9	275	8.6	26.5	14.9	1.4
Turkey & Ham, Shortcrust, M & S*	1/3 Pie/183g	494	29.1	270	11.9	19.5	15.9	1.0
Vegetable	1oz/28g	42	2.1	151	3.0	18.9	7.6	1.5
Vegetable, Mediterranean, Cheesy, COU, M & S*	1 Pack/400g	280	8.4	70	2.1	10.6	2.1	2.1
Vegetable, Retail, Average	1 Serving/200g	348	19.0	174	3.7	18.6	9.5	1.1
Vegetable & Cheddar Cheese, Waitrose*	1 Pie/210g	475	31.5	226	4.9	17.8	15.0	1.2
Vegetable & Cheese, Asda*	1 Pie/141g	330	16.2	234	5.8	26.9	11.5	1.0
Vegetarian, Cottage, Mealpak, All About Weight*	1 Sachet/32g	120	2.8	375	28.6	36.0	8.6	10.0
Vegetarian, Deep Country, Linda McCartney*	1 Pie/166g	412	22.8	248	5.1	26.1	13.7	1.4
Vegetarian, Shepherd's, Linda McCartney*	1 Pack/340g	286	7.5	84	3.7	12.3	2.2	2.3
Vegetarian, Vegetable Cumberland, M & S*	½ Pack/211g	190	5.5	90	2.8	13.4	2.6	1.6
Welsh Lamb, Sainsbury's*	¼ Pie/120g	290	17.2	242	9.1	19.2	14.3	0.8
West Country Chicken, Sainsbury's*	1 Serving/240g	614	37.4	256	11.9	17.1	15.6	2.1

	Measure INFO/WEIGHT	per Measure KCAL	FAT	Nutrition Values per 100g / 100ml KCAL	PROT	CARB	FAT	FIBRE
PIE FILLING								
Apple, Sainsbury's*	1 Serving/75g	67	0.1	89	0.1	22.1	0.1	1.0
Black Cherry, Fruit, Sainsbury's*	1 Serving/100g	73	0.1	73	0.3	17.7	0.1	0.3
Blackcurrant, Fruit, Sainsbury's*	1 Serving/100g	82	0.1	82	0.4	20.0	0.1	1.6
Cherry	1oz/28g	23	0.0	82	0.4	21.5	0.0	0.4
Fruit	1oz/28g	22	0.0	77	0.4	20.1	0.0	1.0
Pistachio, Mix, Avidhipro*	1 Pack/25g	91	0.6	364	74.8	9.6	2.4	2.0
Summer Fruits, Fruit, Tesco*	1 Can/385g	377	0.0	98	0.4	24.1	0.0	0.9
PIGEON								
Meat Only, Roasted, Average	*1 Pigeon/115g*	*215*	*9.1*	*187*	*29.0*	*0.0*	*7.9*	*0.0*
Meat Only, Roasted, Weighed with Bone, Average	*1oz/28g*	*25*	*1.0*	*88*	*13.6*	*0.0*	*3.7*	*0.0*
PIKELETS								
Classics, M & S*	1 Pikelet/35g	70	0.5	200	7.3	39.1	1.3	1.6
Free From, Tesco*	1 Pikelet/30g	58	1.3	194	2.8	36.2	4.3	1.4
Tesco*	1 Pikelet/35g	68	0.2	193	5.8	40.9	0.7	1.7
PILAF								
Bulgar Wheat, Sainsbury's*	1 Pack/381g	347	11.1	91	3.9	12.3	2.9	6.3
Forest Mushroom & Pine Nut, Bistro, Waitrose*	1 Serving/225g	337	14.6	150	7.0	15.8	6.5	1.5
with Tomato, Average	1oz/28g	40	0.9	144	2.5	28.0	3.3	0.4
PILCHARDS								
Fillets in Tomato Sauce, Average	1 Can/120g	158	7.8	132	16.2	2.2	6.5	0.1
Fillets in Virgin Olive Oil, Glenryck*	1 Serving/92g	223	14.4	242	23.3	2.0	15.7	0.0
in Brine, Average	*½ Can/77g*	*114*	*5.6*	*148*	*20.8*	*0.0*	*7.3*	*0.0*
PIMMS*								
& Lemonade, Premixed, Canned, Pimms*	1 Can/250ml	160	0.0	64	0.0	8.4	0.0	0.0
*25% Volume, Pimms**	*1 Serving/25ml*	*40*	*0.0*	*160*	*0.0*	*5.0*	*0.0*	*0.0*
PINE NUTS								
Average	*1oz/28g*	*195*	*19.2*	*695*	*15.7*	*3.9*	*68.6*	*1.9*
Kernels, Love Life, Waitrose*	1 Serving/30g	204	20.6	680	14.0	4.0	68.6	41.4
PINEAPPLE								
Deliciously Refreshing & Sweet, Love Life, Waitrose*	8 Chunks/80g	47	0.1	59	0.5	13.1	0.1	1.4
Dried, Sweetened, Ready to Eat, Tesco*	1/5 Pack/50g	117	0.9	235	0.4	52.9	1.9	1.7
Dried, Tropical Wholefoods*	1 Slice/10g	30	0.0	305	2.9	73.9	0.2	5.2
Dried, Unsweetened, Sainsbury's*	1 Bag/75g	255	1.5	340	1.7	84.7	2.0	6.0
Fingers, Good to Go, Waitrose*	1 Pack/160g	90	0.2	56	0.5	13.1	0.1	1.4
in Juice, Average	*1 Can/106g*	*57*	*0.0*	*53*	*0.3*	*12.9*	*0.0*	*0.6*
in Own Juice, Del Monte*	1 Can/432g	298	0.4	69	0.4	15.5	0.1	0.0
in Syrup, Average	*1 Can/240g*	*158*	*0.0*	*66*	*0.3*	*16.1*	*0.0*	*0.8*
Raw, Diced, Medley, Lozzas	1 Fruit/400g	200	0.9	42	0.4	10.0	0.2	1.0
Raw, Flesh Only, Average	*1 Pineapple/472g*	*200*	*0.9*	*42*	*0.4*	*10.0*	*0.2*	*1.0*
Sliced, Snack, Shapers, Boots*	1 Pack/80g	35	0.2	44	0.4	10.0	0.2	1.2
Tidbits, Dried, Graze*	1 Pack/30g	79	0.2	263	0.6	72.0	0.6	1.0
PISTACHIO NUTS								
Black Pepper, Graze*	1 Punnet/30g	180	16.6	601	17.9	8.2	55.4	6.1
Raw, Average, without Shells	1 Serving/20g	111	8.9	557	20.6	28.0	44.4	10.3
Roasted, Graze*	1 Pack/50g	166	15.5	333	9.9	4.6	31.0	0.0
Roasted & Salted, Average	*1 Serving/25g*	*152*	*13.6*	*608*	*19.6*	*9.9*	*54.5*	*6.1*
Roasted & Salted, Love Life, Waitrose*	1 Serving/25g	144	13.0	576	18.5	8.2	52.1	6.1
Salted, Lemon, Graze*	1 Box/26g	148	12.0	568	21.4	26.8	46.0	0.0
Shelled, Kernels, Wholesome, Love Life, Waitrose*	1 Serving/30g	181	16.6	603	17.9	8.2	55.4	10.3
PIZZA								
American Hot, 12 Inch, Pizza Express*	½ Pizza/264g	562	19.8	213	10.5	25.9	7.5	2.6
American Hot, 8 Inch, Supermarket, Pizza Express*	1 Pizza/295g	652	22.4	221	11.0	27.3	7.6	3.5
American Hot, Chicago Town*	1 Pizza/170g	445	20.1	262	8.2	30.8	11.0	0.0

P

PIZZA

INFO/WEIGHT	Measure	per Measure KCAL	per Measure FAT	Nutrition Values per 100g / 100ml KCAL	PROT	CARB	FAT	FIBRE
Bacon, Mushroom & Tomato, Deep Pan, Loaded, Tesco*	½ Pizza/219g	464	12.7	212	9.3	30.6	5.8	1.5
Bacon, Mushroom & Tomato, HL, Tesco*	1 Pizza/231g	395	6.2	171	10.6	25.9	2.7	1.5
Bacon, Mushroom & Tomato, Stonebaked, Tesco*	1 Serving/173g	351	12.8	203	9.9	24.1	7.4	2.0
Bacon & Mushroom, Stone Bake, M & S*	1 Pizza/375g	750	24.0	200	9.9	27.2	6.4	1.6
Bacon & Mushroom, Stonebaked, Tesco*	1 Serving/157g	352	14.8	224	10.5	24.3	9.4	3.3
Bacon & Mushroom, Thin & Crispy, Sainsbury's*	½ Pizza/150g	396	15.9	264	12.9	29.2	10.6	1.7
Bacon & Mushroom, Thin & Crispy, Somerfield*	¼ Pizza/81g	189	8.1	233	11.0	24.0	10.0	0.0
Bacon & Mushroom, with Capers, Lozzas	1 Slice/157g	352	14.8	224	10.5	24.3	9.4	3.3
Bacon & Mushroom Pizzeria, Sainsbury's*	1 Pizza/355g	880	24.8	248	11.7	34.5	7.0	3.7
Baguette, Cheese & Tomato, Tesco*	1 Baguette/125g	275	8.5	220	11.0	28.0	6.8	2.8
Balsamic Roast Vegetable & Mozzarella, Sainsbury's*	½ Pizza/200g	444	15.6	222	8.5	29.4	7.8	2.4
BBQ Chicken, M & S*	½ Pizza/210g	430	11.8	205	11.6	27.5	5.6	1.8
BBQ Chicken, Stonebaked, Tesco*	½ Pizza/158g	285	9.5	180	10.5	20.9	6.0	3.9
BBQ Chicken, Thin & Crispy, Sainsbury's*	½ Pizza/167g	399	12.4	238	11.4	30.4	7.4	2.2
BBQ Chicken, Thin & Crispy, Tesco*	1 Serving/165g	355	7.4	215	11.9	31.6	4.5	1.2
BBQ Chicken, Weight Watchers*	1 Pizza/224g	412	7.8	184	11.5	26.5	3.5	2.7
BBQ Chicken Stuffed Crust, Asda*	½ Pizza/245g	612	24.5	250	13.0	27.0	10.0	2.7
Bianca, Bistro, Waitrose*	½ Pizza/207g	618	32.6	298	12.9	26.2	15.7	2.3
Bistro Caramelised Onion, Feta & Rosemary, Waitrose*	½ Pizza/230g	607	32.0	264	8.6	26.1	13.9	2.4
Bistro Salami & Pepperoni, Waitrose*	½ Pizza/190g	492	19.4	259	12.9	28.8	10.2	1.5
Buffalo Mozzarella, Rustic Tomato, Tuscan, Finest, Tesco*	½ Pizza/172g	354	11.4	206	6.8	29.8	6.6	1.9
Cajun Chicken, BGTY, Sainsbury's*	½ Pizza/165g	363	5.9	220	11.0	36.0	3.6	1.7
Cajun Chicken, Pizzatilla, M & S*	½ Pizza/240g	636	36.2	265	10.5	21.8	15.1	1.3
Cajun Chicken, Sainsbury's*	½ Pizza/146g	285	2.6	195	12.9	31.8	1.8	2.6
Cajun Style Chicken, Stonebaked, Tesco*	1 Pizza/561g	1318	55.0	235	11.9	24.8	9.8	1.4
Calzone Speciale, Ristorante, Dr Oetker*	½ Pizza/145g	378	23.2	261	11.5	22.1	16.0	0.0
Capricciosa, Pizza Express*	1 Serving/300g	753	29.3	251	13.6	29.0	9.8	0.0
Caprina, Pizza Express*	1 Pizza/300g	635	22.0	212	8.0	31.0	7.3	0.0
Charged Up Chilli Beef, Goodfella's*	½ Pizza/357g	857	32.8	240	12.8	26.4	9.2	1.6
Chargrilled Chicken, Iceland*	1 Pizza/381g	804	25.5	211	12.3	25.4	6.7	2.0
Chargrilled Chicken, Thin & Crispy, Asda*	1 Pizza/373g	780	18.6	209	9.0	32.0	5.0	1.6
Chargrilled Chicken & Vegetable, GFY, Asda*	½ Pizza/166g	355	3.3	214	13.0	36.0	2.0	2.0
Chargrilled Chicken & Vegetable, Low Fat, Bertorelli*	1 Pizza/180g	439	7.9	244	14.2	39.3	4.4	2.3
Chargrilled Vegetable, Frozen, BGTY, Sainsbury's*	1 Pizza/290g	548	13.3	189	10.2	26.7	4.6	3.0
Chargrilled Vegetable, Thin & Crispy, GFY, Asda*	1 Serving/188g	290	3.8	154	6.0	28.0	2.0	3.1
Cheese, Deep Pan, Tesco*	½ Pizza/455g	990	26.4	218	11.4	29.8	5.8	3.1
Cheese, Onion & Garlic, Pizzeria, Waitrose*	½ Pizza/245g	684	28.9	279	10.8	29.8	11.8	2.5
Cheese, Stuffed, Crust, Sainsbury's*	1 Pizza/525g	1428	52.5	272	14.0	31.5	10.0	2.0
Cheese, Thin & Crispy, Goodfella's*	1 Serving/275g	729	27.8	265	15.7	27.6	10.1	1.8
Cheese, Three, Slice, Microwaveable, Tesco*	1 Slice/160g	486	18.7	304	13.3	36.7	11.7	1.6
Cheese & Onion, Tesco*	1 Serving/22g	56	2.0	255	10.5	32.7	9.1	2.7
Cheese & Tomato, Average	1 Serving/300g	711	35.4	237	9.1	25.2	11.8	1.4
Cheese & Tomato, Big Value, Ross*	1 Pizza/716g	1446	33.7	202	7.8	32.2	4.7	2.7
Cheese & Tomato, Bistro, Waitrose*	½ Pizza/205g	488	19.9	238	10.0	27.6	9.7	1.2
Cheese & Tomato, Deep Pan, Co-Op*	½ Pizza/203g	476	14.2	235	12.0	32.0	7.0	1.0
Cheese & Tomato, Deep Pan, Goodfella's*	¼ Pizza/102g	259	10.8	253	11.5	29.6	10.5	3.7
Cheese & Tomato, French Bread, Co-Op*	1 Pizza/135g	270	8.1	200	9.0	27.0	6.0	2.0
Cheese & Tomato, Kids, Tesco*	1 Pizza/95g	219	5.2	231	11.5	33.9	5.5	1.9
Cheese & Tomato, Micro, McCain*	1 Pizza/122g	319	12.2	262	13.4	29.7	10.0	2.4
Cheese & Tomato, Mini, Bruschetta, Iceland*	1 Pizza/34g	63	2.3	188	8.0	23.0	7.0	2.1
Cheese & Tomato, Mini, M & S*	1 Pizza/95g	233	5.5	245	10.0	38.7	5.8	1.6
Cheese & Tomato, Piccadella, Tesco*	1 Pizza/295g	684	31.4	232	9.1	24.8	10.6	1.5
Cheese & Tomato, Retail, Frozen	1oz/28g	70	3.0	250	7.5	32.9	10.7	1.4

PIZZA

	Measure INFO/WEIGHT	per Measure KCAL	FAT	Nutrition Values per 100g / 100ml KCAL	PROT	CARB	FAT	FIBRE
Cheese & Tomato, Slices, Chosen By You, Asda*	1 Slice/14g	62	2.5	453	8.2	63.2	18.1	2.3
Cheese & Tomato, Square, Sainsbury's*	1 Square/160g	435	11.7	272	14.0	37.6	7.3	2.1
Cheese & Tomato, Stonebaked, Co-Op*	1 Pizza/325g	699	26.0	215	10.0	26.0	8.0	3.0
Cheese & Tomato, Stonebaked, Organic, Co-Op*	1 Pizza/330g	676	23.1	205	9.0	26.0	7.0	4.0
Cheese & Tomato, Stonebaked, Thin & Crispy, Tesco*	½ Pizza/161g	388	13.8	241	11.6	29.4	8.6	2.1
Cheese & Tomato, Thin & Crispy, Asda*	1 Pizza/366g	827	36.6	226	11.0	23.0	10.0	2.0
Cheese & Tomato, Thin & Crispy, Carlos*	1 Pizza/155g	405	13.0	261	11.4	35.0	8.4	1.2
Cheese & Tomato, Thin & Crispy, Organic, Tesco*	½ Pizza/147g	369	14.4	251	10.6	30.1	9.8	1.3
Cheese & Tomato, Thin & Crispy, Sainsbury's*	1 Serving/135g	344	10.0	255	14.9	32.2	7.4	5.0
Cheese & Tomato, Thin & Crispy, Stonebaked, Tesco*	1/3 Pizza/212g	509	19.5	240	10.1	29.2	9.2	1.4
Cheese & Tomato, Thin & Crispy, Waitrose*	1 Pizza/280g	658	28.3	235	12.3	23.6	10.1	2.3
Cheese & Tomato Slice, Ross*	1 Slice/77g	148	6.6	192	6.5	22.2	8.6	2.0
Cheese & Tomato Thin & Crispy, Stonebaked, Tesco*	1 Pizza/155g	355	12.1	229	11.6	28.1	7.8	1.3
Cheese Feast, Deep Pan, Asda*	½ Pizza/210g	422	18.9	201	13.0	17.0	9.0	2.3
Cheese Feast, Thin Crust, Chilled, Tesco*	½ Pizza/175g	467	22.4	267	14.7	23.4	12.8	2.5
Cheese Supreme, New Recipe, Goodfella's*	¼ Pizza/102g	269	10.2	264	12.3	31.2	10.0	2.2
Chicken & Bacon, Loaded, Tesco*	1 Serving/258g	622	25.3	241	12.8	25.4	9.8	1.9
Chicken & Bacon, Pizzeria, Italian, Sainsbury's*	½ Pizza/170g	508	24.1	300	13.6	29.4	14.2	2.7
Chicken & Bacon Carbonara, Thin Crust, Italian, Asda*	1 Pizza/492g	1156	34.4	235	12.0	31.0	7.0	3.4
Chicken & Chorizo, 12", TTD, Sainsbury's*	½ Pizza/290g	702	20.9	242	12.2	32.1	7.2	2.6
Chicken & Maple Bacon Carbonara, Asda*	½ Pizza/195g	484	15.6	248	11.0	33.0	8.0	2.2
Chicken & Pesto, Californian Style, Asda*	½ Pizza/235g	533	16.4	227	10.0	31.0	7.0	2.0
Chicken & Pesto with Red Peppers, Italian, Sainsbury's*	½ Pizza/192g	471	18.6	245	12.0	27.3	9.7	2.7
Chicken & Sweetcorn, Stonebaked, Tesco*	1 Serving/177g	354	9.6	200	11.9	26.0	5.4	2.0
Chicken & Sweetfire Red Pepper, Stonebaked, GFY, Asda*	½ Pizza/167g	363	7.7	217	10.0	34.0	4.6	1.6
Chicken & Vegetable, Chargrill, Italiano, Tesco*	½ Pizza/184g	383	14.7	208	10.6	23.3	8.0	2.4
Chicken & Vegetable, Stone Baked, GFY, Asda*	½ Pizza/161g	349	3.7	217	13.0	36.0	2.3	1.7
Chicken Alfredo, Chicago Town*	1 Pizza/265g	583	24.9	220	11.9	21.9	9.4	1.8
Chicken Arrabbiata, Italian Style, M & S*	½ Pizza/225g	495	15.7	220	12.3	26.3	7.0	2.0
Chicken Arrabiata, Sainsbury's*	½ Pizza/191g	444	12.2	232	12.1	31.4	6.4	1.7
Chicken Provencal, Goodfella's*	½ Pizza/143g	388	18.0	272	13.7	25.9	12.6	2.1
Etruscan Pepperoni, TTD, Sainsbury's*	½ Pizza/252g	676	20.9	268	13.2	35.1	8.3	2.4
Fajita Chicken, COU, M & S*	1 Pizza/255g	433	6.1	170	9.9	25.5	2.4	1.2
Fajita Chicken, Takeaway, Goodfella's*	¼ Pizza/150g	339	12.0	226	10.8	27.5	8.0	1.7
Fajita Vegetable, BGTY, Sainsbury's*	1 Pizza/214g	366	3.0	171	8.9	30.8	1.4	2.9
Fingers, Oven Baked, McCain*	1 Finger/30g	78	2.4	261	12.6	34.8	7.9	2.4
Fire Roasted Pepper, Sainsbury's*	1 Pizza/344g	605	5.2	176	5.3	35.3	1.5	1.6
Fire Roasted Peppers & Vegetables, Waitrose*	½ Pizza/235g	442	16.7	188	9.8	21.3	7.1	2.7
Five Cheese & Pepperoni, Deep & Crispy, Waitrose*	1/3 Pizza/200g	560	23.2	280	11.7	32.3	11.6	1.3
Flamed Chicken & Vegetables, BGTY, Sainsbury's*	1 Pizza/260g	660	11.4	254	14.2	39.3	4.4	2.3
Flamin' Hot, Deep Dish, Chicago Town*	1 Pizza/170g	454	20.4	267	8.6	31.1	12.0	0.0
Four Cheese, Finest, Tesco*	½ Pizza/230g	575	21.2	250	12.1	29.8	9.2	1.3
Four Cheese, Stuffed Crust, Takeaway, Chicago Town*	¼ Pizza/158g	433	17.0	275	10.8	33.0	10.8	1.9
Four Cheese, Thin & Crispy, Sainsbury's*	1 Pizza/265g	729	32.6	275	11.8	29.3	12.3	3.5
Four Cheese, Thin Crust, Tesco*	½ Pizza/142g	386	13.6	272	14.5	31.8	9.6	1.8
Four Cheese, Weight Watchers*	1 Pizza/186g	400	7.0	215	10.7	34.9	3.8	1.6
Four Cheese & Tomato, Pizzatilla, M & S*	1 Serving/69g	225	13.8	324	10.5	26.0	19.9	1.5
Four Seasons, Stonebaked, Truly Irresistible, Co-Op*	½ Pizza/245g	502	16.2	205	9.5	26.6	6.6	2.6
Four Seasons, Waitrose*	1/3 Pizza/174g	382	14.6	220	9.9	26.2	8.4	2.6
French Bread, Blue Parrot Cafe, Sainsbury's*	1 Pizza/132g	271	5.7	205	10.7	30.8	4.3	1.3
Frutti Di Mare, Express, Pizza Express*	1 Pizza/373g	500	9.5	134	9.1	20.1	2.6	0.0
Funghi, Ristorante, Dr Oetker*	1 Pizza/365g	865	43.4	237	7.9	22.5	11.9	0.0
Garlic & Mushroom, Asda*	½ Pizza/241g	698	41.0	209	10.0	24.0	17.0	1.6

P

PIZZA

INFO/WEIGHT	Measure	per Measure KCAL	FAT	Nutrition Values per 100g / 100ml KCAL	PROT	CARB	FAT	FIBRE
Garlic & Mushroom, Thin & Crispy, Sainsbury's*	1 Pizza/260g	829	43.2	319	11.1	31.2	16.6	1.7
Garlic Bread, Stonebaked, Italiono, Tesco*	1 Serving/117g	403	18.2	346	7.8	43.6	15.6	1.5
Garlic Chicken, Deep Pan, Sainsbury's*	½ Pizza/214g	464	13.9	217	11.2	28.3	6.5	3.3
Garlic Chicken, Thin & Crispy, Stonebake, Sainsbury's*	½ Pizza/160g	386	17.3	241	10.7	25.2	10.8	3.5
Garlic Mushroom, BGTY, Sainsbury's*	½ Pizza/123g	262	2.5	213	11.6	37.2	2.0	2.7
Garlic Mushroom, Ciabatta Style, Stonebake, Goodfella's*	½ Pizza/187g	474	23.0	254	10.0	27.9	12.3	2.2
Garlic Mushroom, Classico, Tesco*	½ Pizza/208g	415	13.9	200	10.0	24.9	6.7	2.6
Garlic Mushroom, Tesco*	1 Pizza/425g	829	34.0	195	9.3	21.6	8.0	5.3
Garlic Mushroom, Thin & Crispy, Chicago Town*	1 Pizza/115g	283	13.3	246	9.0	26.4	11.6	1.9
Garlic Mushroom, Thin & Crispy, Weight Watchers*	1 Pizza/240g	410	3.1	171	11.2	28.8	1.3	3.0
Garlic Mushroom, Thin Crust, Tesco*	½ Pizza/163g	340	14.6	209	11.0	21.1	9.0	3.6
Grilled Pepper, Weight Watchers*	1 Pizza/220g	392	5.1	178	10.0	29.3	2.3	1.8
Ham, Mushroom & Gruyere, Sainsbury's*	¼ Pizza/169g	404	13.7	239	10.2	31.3	8.1	3.7
Ham, Mushroom & Mascarpone, Italian Style, M & S*	1 Pizza/224g	515	21.7	230	10.0	25.5	9.7	2.9
Ham, Mushroom & Tomato, BGTY, Sainsbury's*	½ Pizza/150g	309	6.1	206	11.8	30.4	4.1	1.2
Ham, Pepperoni & Milano, M & S*	1 Pizza/290g	696	28.4	240	14.0	23.3	9.8	1.1
Ham & Cheese, Chunky, Asda*	1 Serving/90g	211	3.0	234	12.0	39.0	3.3	4.7
Ham & Cheese, Ultra Thin, Sodebo*	1 Pizza/200g	400	8.6	200	11.3	29.1	4.3	0.0
Ham & Mushroom, Average	1 Serving/250g	533	15.9	213	10.5	28.4	6.4	2.1
Ham & Mushroom, BGTY, Sainsbury's*	1 Pizza/248g	526	3.5	212	12.1	37.8	1.4	2.9
Ham & Mushroom, Calzone, Waitrose*	½ Pizza/145g	362	13.5	250	10.0	31.6	9.3	1.6
Ham & Mushroom, Deep & Crispy, Somerfield*	½ Pizza/210g	491	15.1	234	10.4	31.9	7.2	1.6
Ham & Mushroom, Deep & Crispy, Tesco*	1 Serving/210g	420	10.3	200	9.7	29.2	4.9	1.1
Ham & Mushroom, Deep Pan, Waitrose*	½ Pizza/220g	453	13.6	206	10.9	26.6	6.2	1.0
Ham & Mushroom, Finest, Tesco*	½ Pizza/240g	576	26.4	240	9.5	25.9	11.0	2.2
Ham & Mushroom, New, BGTY, Sainsbury's*	1 Pizza/248g	526	3.5	212	12.1	37.8	1.4	2.9
Ham & Mushroom, Stone Baked, Goodfella's*	½ Pizza/175g	439	19.9	251	9.6	27.6	11.4	1.2
Ham & Mushroom, Stonebaked, Stateside Foods*	¼ Pizza/101g	225	6.3	223	9.9	31.9	6.2	1.4
Ham & Mushroom, Thin & Crispy, Asda*	1 Pizza/360g	760	25.2	211	11.0	26.0	7.0	2.4
Ham & Onion, Tesco*	1 Serving/181g	452	17.4	250	11.8	29.0	9.6	2.2
Ham & Pineapple, Average	1 Serving/250g	555	16.8	222	11.0	29.2	6.7	2.1
Ham & Pineapple, Chicago Town*	1 Pizza/435g	866	19.6	199	10.0	29.7	4.5	0.0
Ham & Pineapple, Deep & Loaded, Sainsbury's*	1 Pizza/515g	1102	26.8	214	10.2	31.7	5.2	3.5
Ham & Pineapple, Deep Dish, Individual, Chicago Town*	1 Pizza/170g	410	15.1	241	9.9	30.4	8.9	1.6
Ham & Pineapple, Deep Pan, Ciabatta, Iceland*	½ Pizza/185g	440	14.4	238	11.6	30.3	7.8	0.8
Ham & Pineapple, HL, Tesco*	¼ Pizza/105g	170	2.2	162	10.0	25.9	2.1	2.4
Ham & Pineapple, Pizzerai, Simply Italian, Sainsbury's*	½ Pizza/178g	434	15.1	244	11.5	30.4	8.5	2.4
Ham & Pineapple, Stone Bake, M & S*	1 Pizza/345g	690	19.7	200	10.1	28.3	5.7	1.6
Ham & Pineapple, Stonebaked, Tesco*	1 Pizza/161g	293	9.2	182	9.2	23.5	5.7	3.5
Ham & Pineapple, Thin & Crispy, 2 Pack, Sainsbury's*	1 Pizza/163g	417	13.2	256	13.8	32.0	8.1	1.7
Ham & Pineapple, Thin & Crispy, Goodfella's*	1 Serving/163g	333	12.7	204	10.6	22.8	7.8	2.4
Ham & Pineapple, Thin & Crispy, Sainsbury's*	1 Pizza/330g	719	21.1	218	10.8	29.4	6.4	2.4
Ham & Pineapple, Thin & Crispy, Waitrose*	1 Pizza/220g	616	21.1	280	12.8	33.3	9.6	2.2
Hawaiian, San Marco*	¼ Pizza/90g	208	8.3	231	8.9	29.7	9.2	1.5
Hawaiian, Thin Crust, Tesco*	½ Pizza/192g	365	9.4	190	10.3	25.6	4.9	1.8
Hickory Steak, M & S*	1 Pizza/400g	820	26.8	205	9.9	25.7	6.7	1.4
Hot & Spicy, Deep Dish, Chicago Town*	1 Pizza/177g	434	17.5	245	8.6	30.4	9.9	0.9
Hot & Spicy, Pizzeria Style, Sainsbury's*	1 Pizza/376g	986	46.3	262	12.5	25.5	12.3	2.4
Hot & Spicy, Thin & Crispy, Morrisons*	½ Pizza/170g	393	15.8	231	10.5	26.5	9.3	3.2
Hot & Spicy Chicken, Deep Pan, Morrisons*	½ Pizza/233g	521	13.0	224	10.5	32.9	5.6	1.0
Hot & Spicy Chicken, Deep Pan, Tesco*	½ Pizza/222g	423	7.3	191	10.5	30.0	3.3	2.1
Hot Chicken, Stone Bake, M & S*	1 Pizza/380g	798	25.8	210	11.5	25.1	6.8	1.3
Italian Cheese & Ham, The Little Big Food Company*	1 Pizza/95g	236	6.2	248	10.9	36.2	6.5	1.0

PIZZA

	Measure INFO/WEIGHT	per Measure KCAL	FAT	Nutrition Values per 100g / 100ml KCAL	PROT	CARB	FAT	FIBRE
Italian Meat, Finest, Tesco*	½ Pizza/217g	449	8.5	207	13.6	29.4	3.9	1.3
Italian Meat, So Good, Somerfield*	½ Pizza/200g	468	10.8	234	14.0	32.4	5.4	2.4
Italian Meat Feast, Thin & Crispy, Waitrose*	1 Pizza/182g	477	22.9	262	10.7	26.5	12.6	1.8
Italian Mozzarella & Black Forest Ham, Asda*	¼ Pizza/110g	227	6.6	206	10.0	28.0	6.0	2.7
Italian Sausage & Roasted Peppers, Finest, Tesco*	1 Pizza/325g	650	13.6	200	7.8	31.7	4.2	1.9
Kids Smart, Morrisons*	1 Pizza/91g	203	4.0	223	8.8	36.9	4.4	3.1
Le Reine, 8 Inch, Supermarket, Pizza Express*	1 Pizza/283g	546	16.4	193	10.2	25.0	5.8	2.7
Leggera, Dr Oetker*	½ Pizza/175g	317	10.2	181	8.8	23.1	5.8	2.7
Loaded Cheese, Goodfella's*	1 Pizza/410g	1115	49.6	272	11.4	29.4	12.1	1.7
Margherita, 12 Inch, Supermarket, Pizza Express*	½ Pizza/230g	494	13.8	215	10.1	28.3	6.0	3.6
Margherita, Average	1 Slice/108g	239	8.6	239	11.0	30.5	8.6	1.2
Margherita, Cheese & Tomato, San Marco*	½ Pizza/200g	454	14.4	227	10.7	29.8	7.2	1.2
Margherita, Classico, Tesco*	1 Serving/150g	342	11.4	228	11.3	28.5	7.6	1.8
Margherita, HL, Tesco*	½ Pizza/125g	222	2.5	178	10.8	29.3	2.0	2.5
Margherita, Italian Stone Baked, Somerfield*	1 Pizza/290g	554	20.3	191	10.0	22.0	7.0	0.0
Margherita, Italian Stonebaked, Asda*	¼ Pizza/135g	323	10.8	240	11.0	31.0	8.0	1.8
Margherita, Italiano, Tesco*	½ Pizza/168g	395	12.1	235	11.7	29.9	7.2	1.2
Margherita, Light Choices, Tesco*	1 Pizza/200g	410	5.0	205	11.0	33.8	2.5	1.7
Margherita, Morrisons*	½ Pizza/163g	416	18.0	256	12.9	26.1	11.1	2.3
Margherita, Pizzeria, Italian, Sainsbury's*	½ Pizza/169g	426	17.4	253	12.2	27.9	10.3	2.5
Margherita, Primafresco, Tesco*	½ Pizza/204g	500	20.4	245	10.7	27.4	10.0	2.4
Margherita, Stone Baked, Goodfella's*	1 Slice/36g	95	4.1	263	10.9	31.9	11.4	7.6
Margherita, Stonebaked, Co-Op*	1 Pizza/350g	840	29.1	240	13.2	27.6	8.3	3.0
Margherita, Stonebaked Ciabatta, Goodfella's*	½ Pizza/150g	404	17.2	270	11.3	32.8	11.5	2.6
Margherita, The Best, Morrisons*	½ Pizza/252g	670	27.2	266	11.5	30.6	10.8	2.2
Margherita, Thin Crust, Tesco*	1 Serving/170g	354	13.4	208	10.1	24.1	7.9	3.6
Margherita, Truly Irresistible, Co-Op*	1 Pizza/465g	1023	36.7	220	8.1	27.4	7.9	3.3
Margherita, Tuscan, Finest, Tesco*	½ Pack/248g	557	22.0	225	8.2	27.7	8.9	1.3
Margherita Classico, Italiano, Tesco*	½ Pizza/191g	414	11.8	217	11.2	29.1	6.2	2.5
Massive on Meat, Deep Pan, Goodfella's*	1 Serving/106g	259	9.4	244	10.4	30.6	8.9	3.0
Meat, Mediterranean Style, Pizzeria, Waitrose*	¼ Pizza/174g	395	15.3	227	11.1	25.8	8.8	2.0
Meat Feast, Deep & Loaded, Sainsbury's*	½ Pizza/298g	818	30.0	275	13.2	32.7	10.1	2.6
Meat Feast, Deep Pan, Co-Op*	1 Pizza/450g	1102	45.0	245	11.0	28.0	10.0	2.0
Meat Feast, Hot & Spicy, Thin & Crispy, Sainsbury's*	½ Pizza/170g	462	21.6	272	13.0	26.5	12.7	3.2
Meat Feast, Large, Tesco*	1 Pizza/735g	1904	69.1	259	10.9	32.6	9.4	2.0
Meat Feast, Loaded, Deep Pan, Large, Tesco*	½ Pizza/282g	775	38.4	275	12.0	26.1	13.6	1.9
Meat Feast, Mega, Asda*	½ Pizza/428g	1044	33.8	244	9.5	33.6	7.9	3.2
Meat Feast, Stuffed Crust, Asda*	½ Pizza/238g	597	24.0	251	14.6	25.5	10.1	3.1
Meat Feast, Thin & Crispy, Asda*	½ Pizza/183g	410	14.6	224	11.0	27.0	8.0	1.4
Meat Feast, Thin Crust, Tesco*	½ Pizza/178g	430	20.2	242	13.6	21.3	11.4	2.3
Meat Mayhem, Goodfella's*	1 Pizza/437g	1100	41.9	252	10.6	30.9	9.6	2.5
Mediterranean Madness, Goodfella's*	¼ Pizza/109g	235	8.7	216	9.1	27.0	8.0	3.9
Mediterranean Vegetable, Stonebaked, Sainsbury's*	½ Pizza/260g	622	16.4	239	9.8	35.7	6.3	3.1
Mexican Style, Morrisons*	½ Pizza/180g	437	16.9	243	13.7	26.0	9.4	2.0
Mini, Party, Tesco*	1 Pizza/11g	26	1.1	248	11.4	28.6	10.5	1.9
Mozzarella, Ristorante, Dr Oetker*	1 Pizza/335g	890	13.6	266	10.5	24.2	4.1	0.5
Mozzarella & Sunblush Tomato, 12", TTD, Sainsbury's*	½ Pizza/251g	638	17.8	254	12.4	35.0	7.1	2.6
Mozzarella & Tomato, Asda*	1 Pizza/360g	824	32.4	229	12.0	25.0	9.0	2.4
Mozzarella E Provolone, La Bottega, Goodfella's*	½ Pizza/156g	372	15.0	238	10.1	27.9	9.6	2.4
Mushroom & Ham, COU, M & S*	1 Pizza/245g	355	4.4	145	8.8	24.0	1.8	2.2
Mushroom & Mascarpone, 12", TTD, Sainsbury's*	½ Pizza/255g	638	18.6	250	12.1	34.0	7.3	2.4
Mushroom & Roasted Onion, Waitrose*	½ Pizza/187g	403	12.6	215	9.8	28.9	6.7	1.3
Napoletana, Sainsbury's*	½ Pizza/186g	424	14.3	228	9.7	29.9	7.7	3.1

PIZZA

INFO/WEIGHT	Measure	per Measure KCAL	per Measure FAT	Nutrition Values per 100g / 100ml KCAL	PROT	CARB	FAT	FIBRE
Napoli, Tesco*	½ Pizza/184g	431	11.6	235	11.9	32.6	6.3	1.4
Napoli Ham & Mushroom, San Marco*	½ Pizza/219g	449	13.4	205	10.0	27.5	6.1	2.8
Oval, Ham & Pineapple, Weight Watchers*	1 Pizza/130g	220	2.3	169	11.6	26.7	1.8	3.0
Pasta, Ristorante, Dr Oetker*	½ Pizza/205g	449	18.2	219	8.0	26.6	8.9	0.0
Pepperonata, Delicata, Sainsbury's*	1 Pizza/330g	917	47.5	278	12.9	24.3	14.4	2.6
Pepperoni, American Style Deep Pan, Co-Op*	1 Pizza/395g	987	39.5	250	12.0	28.0	10.0	1.0
Pepperoni, Average	1 Serving/250g	671	28.4	269	11.8	29.6	11.4	2.1
Pepperoni, Deep Filled, Chicago Town*	1 Serving/202g	621	33.6	307	11.5	28.0	16.6	1.3
Pepperoni, Deep Pan, Goodfella's*	¼ Pizza/109g	294	12.6	270	12.7	28.9	11.6	1.6
Pepperoni, Deep Pan, Sainsbury's*	½ Pizza/191g	477	20.6	250	9.9	28.3	10.8	3.2
Pepperoni, Extra, Chicago Town*	1 Pizza/460g	994	34.0	216	9.6	27.7	7.4	0.0
Pepperoni, Feast, Deep Dish, Schwan's*	1 Pizza/435g	1188	61.8	273	9.9	26.3	14.2	0.0
Pepperoni, Goodfella's*	1 Pizza/337g	900	43.5	267	13.2	26.3	12.9	1.7
Pepperoni, Hot & Spicy, Stuffed Crust, Asda*	1 Pizza/245g	666	30.0	272	13.9	26.5	12.2	2.4
Pepperoni, Italian, Tesco*	½ Pizza/186g	484	20.6	260	11.4	28.0	11.1	1.1
Pepperoni, Italian Stonebaked, Asda*	¼ Pizza/132g	329	13.2	250	12.0	28.0	10.0	2.8
Pepperoni, Italian Style, Stonebaked, Stateside Foods*	½ Pizza/168g	436	17.9	260	11.8	29.0	10.7	2.1
Pepperoni, Sauce Stuffed Crust, Take Away, Chicago Town*	¼ Pizza/151g	427	18.4	283	12.4	31.0	12.2	2.1
Pepperoni, Speciale, Sainsbury's*	½ Pizza/179g	447	19.5	250	11.9	26.6	10.9	2.3
Pepperoni, Stone Baked, Carlos*	1 Pizza/330g	832	39.6	252	13.0	23.0	12.0	0.0
Pepperoni, Stonebake, 10", Asda*	½ Pizza/170g	435	19.0	256	12.9	25.9	11.2	2.5
Pepperoni, Stonebaked, American Hot, Sainsbury's*	½ Pizza/276g	674	30.9	244	11.6	24.1	11.2	2.9
Pepperoni, Stonebaked Ciabatta, Goodfella's*	½ Pizza/181g	503	26.1	278	11.9	27.4	14.4	2.4
Pepperoni, Thin & Crispy, Co-Op*	1 Pizza/270g	688	29.7	255	11.0	26.0	11.0	1.0
Pepperoni, Thin & Crispy, Essential, Waitrose*	½ Pizza/133g	380	18.0	286	12.3	28.8	13.5	1.0
Pepperoni, Thin & Crispy, Goodfella's*	1 Pizza/593g	1595	70.0	269	13.8	26.9	11.8	2.3
Pepperoni, Thin & Crispy, Sainsbury's*	½ Pizza/132g	405	18.9	307	13.9	30.7	14.3	2.6
Pepperoni, Weight Watchers*	1 Pizza/300g	501	9.3	167	8.0	25.4	3.1	2.8
Pepperoni, Xxx Hot, Deep & Crispy, Chilled, Tesco*	½ Pizza/262g	656	27.0	250	9.1	30.1	10.3	2.0
Pepperoni & Cheese, Asda*	½ Pizza/150g	385	13.5	257	10.0	34.0	9.0	2.7
Pepperoni & Jalapeno Chill, Asda*	1 Pizza/277g	742	22.2	268	10.0	39.0	8.0	1.8
Pepperoni & Onion, 9", Sainsbury's*	½ Pizza/207g	615	26.9	297	13.4	31.7	13.0	1.9
Pepperoni Bacon, Primo*	½ Pizza/111g	360	14.5	324	10.5	42.5	13.1	0.0
Pollo, Ristorante, Dr Oetker*	½ Pizza/178g	383	16.9	216	8.9	23.4	9.5	0.0
Pollo Ad Astra, Pizza Express*	1 Pizza/317g	602	14.9	190	11.6	25.2	4.7	2.7
Pollo Pesto, Supermarket, Pizza Express*	1 Pizza/265g	500	10.1	189	9.2	25.0	3.8	2.0
Prosciutto, Classico, Tesco*	½ Pizza/205g	461	10.0	225	11.7	33.6	4.9	2.5
Prosciutto, Italian Style, Co-Op*	½ Pizza/183g	421	12.8	230	13.0	29.0	7.0	3.0
Prosciutto, Pizzaria, Sainsbury's*	1 Pizza/325g	806	23.1	248	11.4	34.7	7.1	3.2
Prosciutto, Ristorante, Dr Oetker*	1 Pizza/330g	752	32.3	228	10.3	24.6	9.8	0.0
Quattro Formaggi, 8 Inch, Supermarket, Pizza Express*	1 Pizza/266g	646	26.1	243	12.1	26.5	9.8	2.3
Quattro Formaggi, Ristorante, Dr Oetker*	½ Pizza/175g	472	25.0	270	11.4	23.9	14.3	0.0
Quattro Formaggi Pizzeria, Sainsbury's*	½ Pizza/175g	490	21.2	280	12.8	30.8	12.1	2.5
Quattro Formaggio, Tesco*	½ Pizza/219g	583	27.4	266	13.3	25.1	12.5	1.8
Roasted Tomato & Mozzarella, BGTY, Sainsbury's*	1 Pizza/204g	526	16.4	258	17.8	28.6	8.0	6.0
Roasted Vegetable, for One, GFY, Asda*	1 Pizza/96g	190	3.6	198	9.0	32.0	3.8	1.5
Salame, Ristorante, Dr Oetker*	½ Pizza/160g	455	24.5	285	10.4	26.3	15.3	0.0
Salami, Lidl*	1 Pizza/350g	854	32.2	244	8.1	29.4	9.2	0.0
Salami & Ham, Pizzeria, Waitrose*	½ Pizza/205g	443	13.7	216	10.1	28.7	6.7	1.8
Salami & Pepperoni, Waitrose*	½ Pizza/190g	578	30.8	304	13.4	23.9	16.2	2.1
Salami Con Mozarella, Lidl*	½ Pizza/200g	534	22.4	267	9.9	31.5	11.2	0.0
Sicilian, Premium, Co-Op*	1 Pizza/600g	1320	48.0	220	9.0	27.0	8.0	2.0
Simply Cheese, Goodfella's*	¼ Pizza/82g	226	11.0	276	16.3	22.5	13.4	1.9

PIZZA

INFO/WEIGHT	Measure	per Measure KCAL	FAT	Nutrition Values per 100g / 100ml KCAL	PROT	CARB	FAT	FIBRE
Smoked Ham & Mushroom, Thin & Crispy, Co-Op*	1 Pizza/400g	792	18.0	198	9.0	30.3	4.5	1.7
Smoked Ham & Pineapple, Deep Pan, Co-Op*	1 Pizza/395g	1142	41.9	289	11.6	36.7	10.6	1.7
Smoked Ham & Pineapple, Weight Watchers*	1 Pizza/241g	429	7.0	178	10.3	27.6	2.9	1.5
Smokey New York, Takeaway, Tesco*	½ Pizza/178g	479	16.5	270	12.7	31.7	9.3	2.3
Spicy Beef, Goodfella's*	½ Pizza/148g	391	17.8	265	12.4	26.5	12.1	2.2
Spicy Chicken, Anytime, McCain*	1 Pizza/150g	382	11.7	255	15.1	32.2	7.8	2.0
Spicy Chicken, BBQ, Deep Pan, Asda*	1 Pizza/476g	1033	25.2	217	10.9	31.4	5.3	0.0
Spicy Chicken, Foccacia, Sainsbury's*	½ Pizza/245g	581	18.6	237	12.0	30.3	7.6	2.5
Spicy Chicken, Iceland*	1 Pizza/345g	797	22.8	231	13.4	29.9	6.6	1.5
Spicy Chicken, Micro, McCain*	1 Pizza/133g	388	19.9	292	12.4	26.9	15.0	0.0
Spicy Vegetable, Low Fat, Bertorelli*	1 Pizza/180g	243	4.3	135	6.0	23.4	2.4	1.9
Spinach & Bacon, Thin & Crispy, M & S*	1 Pizza/290g	739	35.1	255	10.6	26.8	12.1	1.0
Spinach & Ricotta, BGTY, Sainsbury's*	1 Pizza/265g	535	6.6	202	10.4	34.4	2.5	2.6
Spinach & Ricotta, Extra Special, Asda*	1 Pizza/400g	940	28.0	235	9.0	34.0	7.0	1.9
Spinach & Ricotta, GFY, Asda*	1 Pizza/160g	375	7.0	234	8.7	40.0	4.4	1.8
Spinach & Ricotta, Italian, Chilled, Sainsbury's*	1 Pizza/361g	859	34.7	238	9.3	28.7	9.6	2.3
Spinach & Ricotta, Italian, Somerfield*	1 Pizza/370g	918	37.0	248	10.3	29.2	10.0	2.2
Spinach & Ricotta, Perfectly Balanced, Waitrose*	½ Pizza/165g	272	2.8	165	9.7	27.7	1.7	2.6
Spinach & Ricotta, Pizzaria, Waitrose*	½ Pizza/238g	501	21.1	211	10.7	21.9	8.9	2.6
Spinach & Ricotta, Thin Crust, Italian, Tesco*	½ Pizza/190g	365	16.7	192	9.6	18.7	8.8	1.9
Spinach with Bacon & Mushroom, GFY, Asda*	1 Serving/270g	618	12.1	229	13.0	34.0	4.5	2.6
Sunblushed Tomato & Mascarpone, Pizzadella, Tesco*	1 Serving/275g	894	44.0	325	8.5	36.7	16.0	1.5
Super Supreme, Family, Chicago Town*	¼ Pizza/225g	526	24.3	234	9.6	24.5	10.8	0.0
Supreme, Deep Dish, Individual, Chicago Town*	1 Pizza/170g	456	20.4	268	9.2	30.8	12.0	1.0
Supreme, McCain*	1 Serving/125g	267	8.6	214	10.9	27.0	6.9	0.0
Supreme, Square to Share, Farmfoods*	1 Serving/93g	196	8.0	211	10.7	22.9	8.6	1.1
Sweet & Sour Chicken, Thin Crust, Tesco*	½ Pizza/186g	366	12.8	197	11.9	21.9	6.9	2.3
Sweet Chilli Chicken, BGTY, Sainsbury's*	½ Pizza/138g	276	2.3	200	13.0	33.2	1.7	2.1
The Big Cheese, Deep Pan, Goodfella's*	1/6 Pizza/118g	295	12.7	250	12.2	25.9	10.8	1.1
The Big Eat Meat X-Treme, Deep Pan, Goodfella's*	½ Pizza/352g	806	28.9	229	11.6	27.1	8.2	3.6
Three Cheese, Ultra Thin, Sodebo*	1 Pizza/180g	450	18.4	250	10.9	28.5	10.2	1.8
Three Cheese & Cherry Tomato, Weight Watchers*	1 Pizza/256g	399	4.1	156	9.8	25.6	1.6	2.3
Three Cheese Calzone, Waitrose*	1 Pizza/265g	747	31.8	282	10.4	33.0	12.0	1.4
Three Cheeses & Tomato, Stonebaked, Co-Op*	1 Pizza/415g	888	33.6	214	10.0	25.2	8.1	1.5
Three Meat, Thin & Crispy, Sainsbury's*	½ Pizza/147g	344	15.7	234	12.5	23.4	10.7	1.3
Tomato	1oz/28g	54	3.0	193	3.3	22.6	10.6	1.4
Tomato, Aubergine & Spinach, Pizzeria, Waitrose*	½ Pizza/193g	403	7.7	209	7.8	35.4	4.0	3.6
Tomato, Basil & Garlic, Weight Watchers*	1 Serving/85g	169	2.9	199	12.3	29.8	3.4	1.6
Tomato, Mushroom & Bacon, Deep Pan, Co-Op*	1 Pizza/420g	882	33.6	210	9.0	25.0	8.0	2.0
Tomato & Cheese, Stone Bake, M & S*	1 Pizza/340g	782	28.6	230	10.8	30.1	8.4	1.6
Tomato & Cheese, Thin & Crispy, M & S*	1 Pizza/300g	705	28.2	235	11.0	27.7	9.4	1.2
Tomato & Mascarpone Piccadella, Slow Roasted, Tesco*	½ Pizza/128g	280	9.7	220	8.4	29.8	7.6	1.5
Tomato & Pesto, Tesco*	1 Serving/176g	449	23.2	256	8.4	25.9	13.2	1.1
Tomato & Red Pepper, Perfectly Balanced, Waitrose*	½ Pizza/163g	313	2.4	192	6.6	38.1	1.5	1.9
Tomato & Ricotta, Waitrose*	½ Pizza/208g	444	18.5	214	7.8	25.7	8.9	2.2
Triple Cheese, Deep Dish, Chicago Town*	1 Serving/170g	418	18.2	246	9.9	27.6	10.7	0.0
Triple Cheese, Deep Pan, Morrisons*	1/6 Pizza/75g	198	9.2	265	10.4	28.2	12.3	1.9
Tuna & Caramelised Red Onion, COU, M & S*	1 Pizza/245g	429	5.6	175	9.6	26.7	2.3	1.4
Tuna Sweetcorn, BGTY, Sainsbury's*	1 Pizza/304g	602	5.8	198	13.5	31.7	1.9	2.7
Tuscan Vegetable & Mozzarella, Way to Five, Sainsbury's*	1 Pizza/317g	552	15.8	174	5.7	26.6	5.0	2.3
Tuscana, Finest, Tesco*	1 Serving/255g	643	35.7	252	13.2	18.4	14.0	5.9
Ultimato Meat Feast, Sainsbury's*	1 Pizza/465g	1302	47.9	280	13.5	35.1	10.3	1.7
Vegetable, Average	1 Serving/250g	475	13.1	190	8.2	27.5	5.2	2.4

	Measure INFO/WEIGHT	per Measure KCAL	FAT	Nutrition Values per 100g / 100ml KCAL	PROT	CARB	FAT	FIBRE
PIZZA								
Vegetable, COU, M & S*	1 Pizza/294g	397	7.1	135	6.4	23.2	2.4	1.9
Vegetable, Deep Pan, Co-Op*	1 Pizza/425g	829	29.7	195	8.0	25.0	7.0	2.0
Vegetable, Frozen, HL, Tesco*	1 Pizza/400g	604	10.8	151	8.1	23.5	2.7	4.4
Vegetable, GFY, Asda*	¼ Pizza/94g	141	2.7	150	7.0	24.0	2.9	3.7
Vegetable, HL, Tesco*	1 Serving/200g	302	5.4	151	8.1	23.5	2.7	4.4
Vegetable, Stonebake, Thin & Crispy, Sainsbury's*	½ Pizza/160g	362	14.2	225	7.4	29.0	8.8	2.8
Vegetable, Thin & Crispy, Iceland*	½ Pizza/200g	442	21.2	221	8.3	23.2	10.6	1.7
Vegetable Feast, Thin & Crispy, Iceland*	1 Slice/63g	148	6.9	237	7.8	26.5	11.1	1.8
Vegetale, Ristorante, Dr Oetker*	½ Pizza/185g	386	16.6	209	8.1	23.9	9.0	0.0
Verona, Frozen, Finest, Tesco*	1 Serving/238g	541	23.3	228	11.6	23.2	9.8	2.7
PIZZA BASE								
Deep Pan, Italian, Sainsbury's*	1 Base/220g	684	11.0	311	7.0	59.5	5.0	1.4
Deep Pan, Napolina*	1 Base/260g	757	7.8	291	7.9	58.0	3.0	0.2
Garlic Bread, Sainsbury's*	¼ Base/59g	109	4.2	186	5.1	25.4	7.1	1.8
Gluten, Wheat & Dairy Free, Free From, Livwell*	1 Base/100g	237	2.6	237	5.2	48.3	2.6	4.7
Gluten & Wheat Free, Glutafin*	1 Base/110g	309	5.5	281	3.0	56.0	5.0	6.0
Gluten Free, Glutafin*	1 Base/110g	278	5.5	253	3.0	49.0	5.0	4.5
Italian, Classic, Sainsbury's*	1 Base/150g	451	7.2	301	7.6	57.0	4.8	1.5
Italian, The Pizza Company*	1 Base/260g	624	6.8	240	7.6	46.5	2.6	0.0
Italiana, Parmalat*	1 Base/150g	450	7.3	300	9.0	55.0	4.9	0.0
Light & Crispy, Napolina*	1 Base/150g	436	4.5	291	7.9	58.0	3.0	0.2
Mini, Napolina*	1 Base/75g	218	2.2	291	7.9	58.0	3.0	0.2
Thin & Crispy, Sainsbury's*	1 Base/150g	504	7.8	336	9.9	62.3	5.2	4.3
Thin & Crispy, Tesco*	1 Serving/110g	348	8.2	316	9.2	52.9	7.5	1.5
Trufree*	1 Base/110g	345	6.6	314	3.0	63.0	6.0	4.0
Value, Tesco*	1 Base/300g	885	17.7	295	7.4	52.5	5.9	1.9
PIZZA DOUGH								
& Tomato Sauce, Uncooked, Jus-Rol*	¼ Pizza/150g	268	2.0	178	6.8	33.8	1.3	1.8
PLAICE								
Fillets, Lightly Dusted, Average	1 Fillet/113g	188	9.2	166	12.9	10.4	8.1	0.6
Fillets, Raw, Average	*1oz/28g*	*24*	*0.4*	*87*	*18.2*	*0.0*	*1.5*	*0.0*
Fillets in Breadcrumbs, Average	1 Serving/150g	331	17.9	221	12.8	15.5	11.9	0.8
Goujons, Baked	1oz/28g	85	5.1	304	8.8	27.7	18.3	0.0
Goujons, Fried in Blended Oil	1oz/28g	119	9.0	426	8.5	27.0	32.3	0.0
Grilled	*1oz/28g*	*27*	*0.5*	*96*	*20.1*	*0.0*	*1.7*	*0.0*
in Batter, Fried in Blended Oil	1oz/28g	72	4.7	257	15.2	12.0	16.8	0.5
Steamed	*1oz/28g*	*26*	*0.5*	*93*	*18.9*	*0.0*	*1.9*	*0.0*
PLAICE WITH								
Mushrooms & Prawns, Sainsbury's*	1 Serving/170g	354	18.2	208	12.0	15.9	10.7	1.7
Prawns & Garlic, Filled, Somerfield*	1 Serving/171g	366	20.3	214	12.0	14.8	11.9	0.7
Spinach & Cheddar Cheese, Fillets, Sainsbury's*	1 Serving/154g	222	13.3	144	13.6	3.1	8.6	0.8
Spinach & Ricotta Cheese, Whole, Sainsbury's*	1 Serving/159g	334	16.7	210	11.6	17.2	10.5	0.8
PLANTAIN								
Boiled in Unsalted Water	*1oz/28g*	*31*	*0.1*	*112*	*0.8*	*28.5*	*0.2*	*1.2*
Raw, Average	*1 Med/179g*	*218*	*0.7*	*122*	*1.3*	*31.9*	*0.4*	*2.3*
Ripe, Fried in Vegetable Oil	*1oz/28g*	*75*	*2.6*	*267*	*1.5*	*47.5*	*9.2*	*2.3*
PLUMS								
Average, Stewed without Sugar	*1oz/28g*	*8*	*0.0*	*30*	*0.5*	*7.3*	*0.1*	*1.3*
Fresh, Raw, Weighed without Stone, Average	1 Plum/66g	24	0.1	36	0.5	8.5	0.1	1.9
Fresh, Sweet & Juicy, Oaklands, Lidl*	1 Serving/80g	34	0.1	42	0.6	8.8	0.1	1.6
Soft Dried, Blue Parrot Cafe, Sainsbury's*	1 Pack/50g	118	0.2	237	2.6	55.6	0.5	7.1
Sunn Gold, Market, Value, Tesco*	1 Serving/80g	29	0.1	36	0.6	8.8	0.1	1.6
Weighed with Stone, Average	*1 Plum/90g*	*33*	*0.1*	*36*	*0.5*	*8.5*	*0.1*	*1.9*

	Measure INFO/WEIGHT	per Measure		Nutrition Values per 100g / 100ml				
		KCAL	FAT	KCAL	PROT	CARB	FAT	FIBRE
PLUMS								
Whole, Dried, Graze*	1 Pack/60g	143	0.3	239	2.6	56.0	0.5	0.0
Whole, Imperial, Graze*	1 Punnet/45g	124	0.0	275	2.6	56.0	0.1	7.1
Yellow, Waitrose*	1 Plum/50g	19	0.0	39	0.6	8.8	0.1	1.5
POLENTA								
Merchant Gourmet*	1 Serving/65g	232	0.9	357	7.4	78.8	1.4	1.3
Organic, Kallo*	1 Serving/150g	543	2.7	362	8.5	78.0	1.8	0.0
POLLOCK								
Breaded, Asda*	1 Serving/97g	200	9.7	206	12.0	17.0	10.0	1.0
POLO								
Citrus Sharp, Nestle*	1 Tube/34g	134	0.3	393	0.0	96.6	1.0	0.0
Fruits, Nestle*	1 Tube/37g	142	0.0	383	0.0	96.0	0.0	0.0
Mints, Clear Ice, Nestle*	1 Sweet/4g	16	0.0	390	0.0	97.5	0.0	0.0
Mints, Original, Nestle*	1 Sweet/2g	8	0.0	404	0.0	98.9	1.1	0.0
Spearmint, Nestle*	1 Tube/35g	141	0.4	402	0.0	98.2	1.1	0.0
POMEGRANATE								
Fresh, Good to Go, Waitrose*	1 Pack/110g	101	1.3	92	1.7	18.7	1.2	4.0
Raw, Fresh, Flesh Only, Average	*1 Sm Fruit/86g*	*59*	*0.3*	*68*	*0.9*	*17.2*	*0.3*	*0.6*
Raw, Weighed with Rind & Skin, Average	*1 Sm Fruit/154g*	*105*	*0.5*	*68*	*0.9*	*17.2*	*0.3*	*0.1*
POMELO								
Raw, Flesh Only, Average	1 Fruit/340g	129	0.1	38	0.8	9.6	0.0	1.0
POP TARTS								
Bustin' Berry, Kellogg's*	1 Tart/50g	200	6.0	400	4.0	69.0	12.0	2.0
Chocolate, Kellogg's*	1 Tart/50g	198	8.5	396	5.0	136.0	17.0	2.0
Chocomallow, Kellogg's*	1 Tart/50g	198	6.0	396	6.0	66.0	12.0	2.5
Cookies 'n' Creme, Kellogg's*	1 Tart/50g	197	5.0	394	4.0	72.0	10.0	1.5
Cream Cheese & Cherry Swirl, Kellogg's*	1 Tart/62g	250	11.0	403	3.2	59.7	17.7	1.0
Frosted Brown Sugar Cinnamon, Kellogg's*	1 Tart/50g	210	7.0	420	6.0	68.0	14.0	2.0
Strawberry Sensation, Kellogg's*	1 Tart/50g	197	5.5	395	4.0	70.0	11.0	2.0
POPCORN								
94% Fat Free, Orville Redenbacher's*	1 Bag/76g	220	0.0	289	13.2	65.8	0.0	0.0
Air Popped, Plain, Average	1oz/28g	110	1.3	387	12.9	77.9	4.5	14.5
Butter, 6% Fat, Orville Redenbacher's*	1 Portion/21g	86	1.2	410	11.9	77.6	5.7	14.3
Butter, Microwave, 94% Fat Free, Act II*	½ Bag/41g	130	2.5	317	9.8	68.3	6.1	12.2
Butter, Microwave, Act II*	1 Bag/90g	425	16.2	472	9.0	69.0	18.0	9.0
Butter, Microwave, Butterkist*	1 Bag/100g	395	18.5	395	8.3	49.5	18.5	8.5
Butter Flavour, Microwave, Popz*	1 Serving/100g	480	27.5	480	7.5	51.1	27.5	9.2
Butter Toffee, Asda*	1 Serving/100g	364	8.0	364	2.1	71.0	8.0	4.1
Butter Toffee, Belgian Milk Chocolate Coated, M & S*	1 Pack/100g	505	25.0	505	6.5	60.4	25.0	4.1
Butter Toffee, Snack-A-Jacks, Quaker Oats*	1 Bag/35g	149	3.1	425	3.5	86.0	9.0	4.5
Butter Toffee, Tesco*	1 Pack/350g	1417	26.9	405	2.2	81.7	7.7	4.3
Butter Toffee, Yummies*	1 Serving/50g	227	6.4	455	2.5	82.4	12.8	3.1
Choc Full Of, Cadbury*	¼ Bag/32g	160	7.6	495	4.5	64.5	23.5	2.9
Chocolate & Pecan, M & S*	1 Packet/27g	130	5.2	480	3.3	72.9	19.3	3.6
Chocolate Flavour, Toffee, Snack-A-Jacks, Quaker Oats*	1 Bag/35g	126	3.4	359	2.2	65.0	9.8	3.0
Lightly Salted, Snack-A-Jack, Quaker Oats*	1 Bag/13g	48	1.3	370	12.1	58.0	9.9	14.6
Maize, Unpopped, Love Life, Waitrose*	1 Serving/33g	200	14.1	605	6.2	48.7	42.8	12.7
Microwave, Salted, Sunsnacks*	1 Pack/100g	498	22.9	498	10.7	51.3	22.9	10.8
Organic Amaranth*	1 Serving/10g	36	0.9	365	14.6	26.8	8.8	0.0
Plain, Oil Popped, Average	1 Bag/74g	439	31.7	593	6.2	48.7	42.8	0.0
Ready Salted, Microwave, Popz*	1 Serving/20g	101	6.0	504	7.0	51.5	30.0	9.2
Salt & Vinegar, Diet Chef Ltd*	1 Serving/23g	106	3.6	461	10.4	69.8	15.8	13.0
Salt & Vinegar, Snack-A-Jacks, Quaker Oats*	1 Sm Pack/13g	47	1.3	360	12.0	55.0	9.9	14.0
Salted, Blockbuster*	1 Bowl/25g	99	2.9	397	10.6	62.2	11.7	0.6

POPCORN	Measure INFO/WEIGHT	per Measure KCAL	FAT	KCAL	PROT	CARB	FAT	FIBRE
Salted, Bop, Microwave, Zanuy*	1 Serving/25g	119	5.7	477	10.7	56.9	23.0	0.0
Salted, Diet Chef Ltd*	1 Pack/23g	107	3.8	465	10.5	68.6	16.6	14.0
Salted, Light, Microwave, Act II*	1 Pack/85g	336	6.5	395	10.6	71.0	7.6	15.8
Salted, M & S*	1 Pack/15g	82	4.7	545	9.4	56.8	31.1	6.3
Salted, Manhatten Peanuts Limited*	1 Bag/30g	135	4.3	450	10.0	70.0	14.3	13.7
Salted, Microwave, 93% Fat Free, Act II*	1 Pack/85g	345	5.9	406	10.0	76.0	7.0	13.0
Salted, Sold At Cinema, Playtime Popcorn*	1 Serving/74g	384	24.9	519	8.3	45.9	33.6	0.0
Sea Salt Flavour, Skinny, Topcorn, Metcalfe's Food Co*	1 Pack/23g	108	5.6	471	6.6	63.7	24.4	15.2
Sour Cream & Jalepeno Chilli, Tyrells*	1 Serving/20g	97	5.2	484	6.4	49.9	26.0	12.5
Super, Perri*	1 Packet/30g	139	7.0	464	8.4	55.5	23.2	8.5
Sweet, Best-In*	1 Serving/34g	161	5.8	473	7.3	72.6	17.0	0.0
Sweet, Butterkist, Butterkist*	1 Pack/120g	612	29.8	510	2.8	68.5	24.8	5.6
Sweet, Cinema Style, Butterkist*	1 Bag/120g	612	29.8	510	2.8	68.5	24.8	5.6
Sweet, Microwave, Butterkist*	½ Pack/50g	235	10.0	470	9.8	60.5	20.1	4.4
Sweet, Microwave, Cinema, Popz*	1 Bag/85g	420	21.7	494	6.0	60.0	25.5	8.2
Sweet, Vanilla & Sugar, Microwave, Act II*	1 Pack/75g	369	18.1	492	7.9	60.8	24.1	10.4
Sweet Maple, Diet Chef Ltd*	1 Pack/23g	111	3.6	483	9.7	75.2	15.7	13.0
Toffee, 90% Fat Free, Butterkist*	1 Pack/35g	142	3.3	406	2.8	77.7	9.3	0.0
Toffee, Best-In*	1 Bag/90g	356	3.2	396	5.0	85.9	3.6	0.0
Toffee, Butterkist*	1 Bag/30g	124	3.0	415	2.3	79.3	10.0	4.4
Toffee, Chicago Joes*	1 Serving/10g	31	0.5	314	3.1	84.6	4.8	0.0
Toffee, Milk Chocolate Coated, Butterkist*	1 Bag/50g	252	12.5	505	6.5	61.9	25.0	4.1
Toffee, Milk Chocolate Coated, Morrisons*	1 Serving/25g	118	5.0	474	4.9	68.8	19.9	2.8
Toffee, Milk Chocolate Coated, Sainsbury's*	¼ Bag/25g	130	6.6	520	6.5	64.1	26.4	1.3
Toffee, Sainsbury's*	1 Serving/50g	207	6.3	415	1.8	73.8	12.7	3.3
Toffee, Snack Pack, Butterkist*	1 Bag/30g	124	3.0	415	2.3	79.3	10.0	4.4
Vanilla, Cinema Sweet Microwave, Act II*	½ Pack/50g	234	8.0	468	9.0	71.0	16.0	12.0
Wasabi Flavour, Skinny, Topcorn, Metcalfe's Food Co*	1 Bag/25g	121	6.5	484	8.4	54.1	26.2	9.7
White Cheddar Cheese, Manhatten Peanuts Limited*	1 Bag/30g	132	4.1	440	10.0	70.0	13.7	13.0
Yellow, Kernel, (Unpopped), Jolly Time*	2 Tbsp/33g	110	1.0	333	12.1	78.8	3.0	21.2
POPPADOMS								
Fried in Vegetable Oil, Takeaway, Average	1 Poppadom/13g	65	5.0	501	11.5	28.3	38.8	5.8
Indian, Asda*	1 Pack/45g	232	15.7	516	14.5	36.2	34.8	7.8
Mercifully Mild, Phileas Fogg*	1 Serving/30g	150	9.8	499	14.8	36.8	32.6	6.0
Mini, Sainsbury's*	½ Pack/50g	249	16.1	498	14.9	36.9	32.3	7.6
Plain, Asda*	1 Poppadom/9g	44	2.5	484	18.0	40.0	28.0	0.0
Plain, Indian to Go, Sainsbury's*	1 Poppadom/8g	34	1.5	405	18.4	43.4	17.5	9.0
Plain, Tesco*	1 Serving/9g	41	2.0	439	17.8	44.4	21.1	4.6
Plain, Waitrose*	1 Serving/9g	37	1.7	408	21.0	39.3	18.6	9.1
Spicy, COU, M & S*	1 Pack/26g	84	0.6	325	23.5	51.9	2.4	8.1
Tesco*	1 Poppadum/9g	39	1.9	440	17.8	44.4	21.1	4.6
POPPETS*								
Chocolate Raisins, Poppets*	1 Pack/35g	140	4.7	401	4.9	65.4	13.3	0.0
Peanut, Poppets*	1 Box/100g	544	37.0	544	16.4	37.0	37.0	0.0
Toffee, Milk Chocolate, Poppets*	1 Box/100g	491	23.0	491	5.3	68.0	23.0	0.0
POPPING CORN								
Average	1 Serving/30g	112	1.3	375	10.9	73.1	4.3	12.7
PORK								
Belly, Fresh, Raw, Weighed with Skin, Average	1 Serving/100g	518	53.0	518	9.3	0.0	53.0	0.0
Belly, Roasted, Lean & Fat	1oz/28g	82	6.0	293	25.1	0.0	21.4	0.0
Belly, Slow Cooked, Waitrose*	1 Serving/225g	589	45.9	262	17.3	2.2	20.4	0.0
Chop, Lean & Fat, Boneless, Raw, Average	*1oz/28g*	*67*	*3.8*	*240*	*29.2*	*0.0*	*13.7*	*0.0*
Diced, Lean, Average	*1oz/28g*	*31*	*0.5*	*109*	*22.0*	*0.0*	*1.7*	*0.0*

	Measure INFO/WEIGHT	per Measure KCAL	FAT	Nutrition Values per 100g / 100ml KCAL	PROT	CARB	FAT	FIBRE
PORK								
Escalope, Average	*1 Escalope/75g*	*108*	*1.7*	*144*	*31.0*	*0.0*	*2.2*	*0.0*
Escalope, Lean, Healthy Range, Average	*1 Escalope/75g*	*80*	*1.5*	*106*	*22.0*	*0.0*	*2.0*	*0.0*
Haslet, Somerfield*	1oz/28g	57	3.4	205	15.0	10.0	12.0	0.0
Joint, Ready to Roast, Average	*½ Joint/254g*	*375*	*18.0*	*147*	*19.2*	*2.3*	*7.1*	*0.1*
Joint, with Crackling, Ready to Roast, Average	*1 Joint/567g*	*1283*	*80.1*	*226*	*24.2*	*0.8*	*14.1*	*0.0*
Leg, Joint, Healthy Range, Average	*1 Serving/200g*	*206*	*4.4*	*103*	*20.0*	*0.6*	*2.2*	*0.0*
Loin, Applewood Smoked, Asda*	1 Slice/15g	18	0.5	122	21.8	0.5	3.6	0.0
Loin, Chops, Boneless, Grilled, Average	*1oz/28g*	*90*	*4.4*	*320*	*29.0*	*0.0*	*15.7*	*0.0*
Loin, Chops, Grilled, Lean	*1oz/28g*	*52*	*1.8*	*184*	*31.6*	*0.0*	*6.4*	*0.0*
Loin, Joint, Roast, Lean	*1oz/28g*	*51*	*1.9*	*182*	*30.1*	*0.0*	*6.8*	*0.0*
Loin, Joint, Roasted, Lean & Fat	*1oz/28g*	*71*	*4.3*	*253*	*26.3*	*0.0*	*15.3*	*0.0*
Loin, Slices, Sweet Cure, Tesco*	1 Slice/13g	19	0.8	146	20.9	2.5	5.8	0.6
Loin, Steak, Fried, Lean	*1oz/28g*	*53*	*2.0*	*191*	*31.5*	*0.0*	*7.2*	*0.0*
Loin, Steak, Fried, Lean & Fat	*1oz/28g*	*77*	*5.2*	*276*	*27.5*	*0.0*	*18.4*	*0.0*
Loin, Steak, Lean, Raw, Average	*1 Serving/175g*	*345*	*19.6*	*197*	*22.7*	*1.8*	*11.2*	*0.4*
Loin, Stuffed, Roast, M & S*	1 Slice/12g	22	0.9	180	24.4	2.4	7.9	0.0
Medallions, Average	*1 Pack/220g*	*359*	*5.5*	*163*	*35.1*	*0.0*	*2.5*	*0.4*
Mince, Lean, Healthy Range, Average	*1 Pack/400g*	*504*	*20.2*	*126*	*19.7*	*0.4*	*5.0*	*0.3*
Mince, Raw	*1oz/28g*	*46*	*2.7*	*164*	*19.2*	*0.0*	*9.7*	*0.0*
Mince, Stewed	*1oz/28g*	*53*	*2.9*	*191*	*24.4*	*0.0*	*10.4*	*0.0*
Rashers, Streaky, British, Sainsbury's*	1 Serving/100g	320	23.4	320	27.4	0.0	23.4	0.0
Raw, Lean, Average	*1oz/28g*	*42*	*1.2*	*151*	*28.6*	*0.0*	*4.1*	*0.0*
Roast, Lean Only, Average	*1oz/28g*	*34*	*0.9*	*121*	*22.7*	*0.3*	*3.3*	*0.0*
Roast, Slices, Average	*1 Slice/30g*	*40*	*1.3*	*133*	*22.7*	*0.4*	*4.5*	*0.0*
Shoulder, Slices, Cured	*1oz/28g*	*29*	*1.0*	*103*	*16.9*	*0.9*	*3.6*	*0.0*
Shoulder, Whole, Lean & Fat, Raw, Average	*1 Serving/100g*	*236*	*18.0*	*236*	*17.2*	*0.0*	*18.0*	*0.0*
Shoulder, Whole, Lean Only, Roasted	1 Serving/150g	345	20.3	230	25.3	0.0	13.5	0.0
Shoulder Steak, Boneless, Frozen, Grilled, Tesco*	1 Steak/125g	156	4.9	125	0.0	0.0	3.9	0.0
Steak, Lean, Stewed	*1oz/28g*	*49*	*1.3*	*176*	*33.6*	*0.0*	*4.6*	*0.0*
Steak, Lean & Fat, Average	*1oz/28g*	*61*	*3.8*	*219*	*23.8*	*0.0*	*13.7*	*0.1*
Stir Fry Strips, Lean, Healthy Range, Average	*¼ Pack/113g*	*118*	*2.3*	*104*	*21.3*	*0.0*	*2.0*	*0.0*
Streaky, Boneless, Slices, British, Tesco*	1 Pack/460g	1477	106.7	321	0.0	0.0	23.2	0.0
Tenderloin, Lean, Boneless, Raw, Average	1 Serving/100g	109	2.2	109	20.9	0.0	2.2	0.0
Tenderloin, Separable Lean & Fat, Raw, Average	1 Loin/265g	318	9.4	120	20.6	0.0	3.5	0.0
PORK &								
Apricots, Aromatic, Cafe Culture, M & S*	½ Pack/420g	672	31.1	160	10.3	12.5	7.4	2.1
Chestnut Stuffing, M & S*	1oz/28g	64	4.8	230	5.3	12.6	17.1	3.7
PORK CHAR SUI								
Chinese, Tesco*	1 Pack/400g	520	17.2	130	7.2	15.7	4.3	0.6
in Cantonese Sauce, Asda*	1 Pack/360g	623	7.9	173	9.8	28.4	2.2	0.5
Oriental, Finest, Tesco*	1 Pack/350g	245	5.2	70	6.8	6.2	1.5	2.1
Takeaway, Iceland*	1 Pack/400g	412	9.6	103	7.9	12.5	2.4	1.2
with Chicken & Egg Fried Rice, Tesco*	1 Serving/450g	602	16.2	134	7.1	18.3	3.6	0.9
PORK CHINESE								
Sliced, M & S*	1 Serving/140g	224	4.3	160	26.4	6.1	3.1	0.0
Style, GFY, Asda*	1 Serving/170g	286	6.0	168	18.8	15.3	3.5	0.4
with Noodles, Tesco*	1 Serving/450g	612	25.6	136	7.0	14.2	5.7	1.1
PORK DINNER								
Roast, Birds Eye*	1 Pack/340g	410	12.0	121	7.6	14.7	3.5	1.6
PORK IN								
Light Mustard Sauce, Fillet, COU, M & S*	1 Pack/390g	312	9.4	80	10.9	3.5	2.4	0.7
Mustard & Cream, Chops	1oz/28g	73	6.0	261	14.5	2.4	21.6	0.3
Rich Sage & Onion Gravy, Steaks, Tesco*	1 Serving/160g	218	10.4	136	16.0	3.2	6.5	1.5

	Measure INFO/WEIGHT	per Measure KCAL	FAT	KCAL	PROT	CARB	FAT	FIBRE
PORK SCRATCHINGS								
Crunch, Mr Porky*	1 Pack/30g	159	9.6	531	60.4	0.5	31.9	4.6
KP Snacks*	1 Pack/20g	125	9.6	624	47.3	0.5	48.1	0.5
Tavern Snacks*	1 Pack/30g	187	14.4	624	47.3	0.5	48.1	0.5
PORK WITH								
Apricot & Orange Stuffing, Joint, Sainsbury's*	¼ Joint/200g	566	36.2	283	29.0	0.9	18.1	1.4
Bramley Apple, Medallions, M & S*	1 Serving/380g	418	12.9	110	17.7	2.5	3.4	0.5
Cheese & Pineapple, Loin Steaks, M & S*	1 Steak/141g	240	14.0	170	14.0	6.3	9.9	0.5
Herbes De Provence, Joint, Sainsbury's*	¼ Joint/200g	302	16.4	151	19.2	0.1	8.2	0.6
Honey & Mustard Sauce, Steaks, Tesco*	½ Pack/160g	258	11.8	161	16.3	8.7	7.4	1.4
Honey & Soy, Sainsbury's*	1 Serving/260g	260	7.5	100	12.3	6.2	2.9	0.3
Leek & Bacon Stuffing, Roast, Shoulder, Sainsbury's*	1 Serving/150g	237	12.4	158	18.8	2.4	8.3	0.5
Leek & Cheese Stuffing, Joint, Sainsbury's*	1 Serving/100g	231	10.5	231	31.0	3.0	10.5	1.1
Maple & BBQ Sauce, Loin Steaks, Somerfield*	½ Pack/160g	336	16.0	210	20.4	9.2	10.0	0.0
Noodles, Chinese, Tesco*	1 Serving/450g	463	13.5	103	5.3	13.7	3.0	1.4
Peppers, Marinated, Tapas, Waitrose*	1 Serving/105g	181	6.7	172	26.3	2.2	6.4	0.3
Rice & Beans, Jerk, Love Life, Waitrose*	1 Pack/380g	384	12.2	101	4.9	13.0	3.2	2.1
Roasted Rosemary Potatoes, Porchetta, Finest, Tesco*	½ Pack/370g	455	31.8	123	6.9	4.6	8.6	0.5
Sage, Onion & Lemon Stuffing, Joint, Sainsbury's*	1 Serving/260g	699	43.4	269	27.4	2.2	16.7	1.4
Sage & Onion Stuffing, Joint, BGTY, Sainsbury's*	1 Serving/150g	246	5.4	164	29.5	3.3	3.6	1.3
Sage & Onion Stuffing, Joint, Tesco*	1 Serving/200g	208	5.6	104	17.1	2.7	2.8	0.0
Spiced Apple Stuffing, Steaks, Easy Cook, Waitrose*	1 Serving/190g	237	7.8	124	19.3	2.4	4.1	0.5
Stuffing, Belly, Norfolk Outdoor Reared, Finest, Tesco*	1 Serving/180g	524	44.8	291	14.9	1.7	24.9	0.0
Thai Style Butter, Steaks, Asda*	4 Steaks/300g	810	54.0	270	26.0	1.0	18.0	0.0
Tomato & Apricot Sauce, Loin Steaks, Sainsbury's*	½ Pack/110g	216	10.6	196	24.4	3.1	9.6	0.6
PORT								
Average	**1 Serving/50ml**	**78**	**0.0**	**157**	**0.1**	**12.0**	**0.0**	**0.0**
POT NOODLE*								
Balti Curry, Made Up, Pot Noodle*	1 Pot/301g	268	1.5	89	3.1	17.8	0.5	0.5
Beef & Tomato, Made Up, Pot Noodle*	1 Pot/300g	378	14.1	126	3.1	18.1	4.7	1.1
Beef & Tomato, Mini, Pot Noodle*	1 Pot/190g	254	9.5	134	3.5	18.7	5.0	1.7
Beef & Tomato, Pot Noodle*	1 Pot/319g	424	14.7	133	3.4	19.4	4.6	1.3
Bombay Bad Boy, Made Up, Pot Noodle*	1 Pot/305g	384	14.0	126	3.1	17.9	4.6	1.1
Chicken & Mushroom, Made Up, Pot Noodle*	1 Pot/300g	384	14.1	128	3.2	18.0	4.7	1.1
Chicken & Mushroom, Mini, Made Up, Pot Noodle*	1 Pot/190g	243	8.5	128	3.8	18.2	4.5	1.4
Chicken Curry, Hot, Made Up, Pot Noodle*	1 Pot/300g	384	14.1	128	2.8	18.7	4.7	1.1
Chow Mein Flavour, Made Up, Pot Noodle*	1 Pot/320g	416	14.7	130	3.2	19.0	4.6	1.3
Hot, Made Up, Pot Noodle*	1 Pot/300g	378	15.6	126	3.0	16.9	5.2	1.1
Korma Curry, Made Up, Pot Noodle*	1 Pot/300g	273	3.3	91	2.9	17.4	1.1	0.4
Nice & Spicy, Made Up, Pot Noodle*	1 Pot/300g	381	14.1	127	2.8	18.3	4.7	1.1
Seedy Sanchez, Made Up, Pot Noodle*	1 Pot/300g	396	14.4	132	3.1	19.1	4.8	1.1
Southern Fried Chicken, Prepared, Golden Wonder*	1 Pot/318g	427	15.0	134	3.1	19.8	4.7	1.2
Spicy Chilli, Posh, Made Up, Pot Noodle*	1 Pot/301g	328	17.8	109	2.5	11.7	5.9	1.0
Spicy Curry, Made Up, Pot Noodle*	1 Pot/300g	393	14.4	131	2.9	19.1	4.8	1.1
Sweet & Sour, Dry, Pot Noodle*	1 Pot/86g	376	13.8	437	12.1	60.9	16.1	3.1
Sweet & Sour, King, Dry, Pot Noodle*	1 Pot/105g	473	20.1	450	8.8	60.0	19.1	4.8
Sweet & Sour, Oriental, Posh, Pot Noodle*	1 Pot/300g	375	13.8	125	1.7	19.2	4.6	0.5
POTATO BOMBAY								
Aloo, M & S*	½ Pack/114g	108	5.2	95	1.8	10.3	4.6	2.3
Average	1oz/28g	33	1.9	117	2.0	13.7	6.8	1.2
Canned, Tesco*	1 Can/400g	380	11.6	95	2.5	13.5	2.9	2.3
Flavours of India, Canned, Sainsbury's*	½ Can/200g	160	3.8	80	2.4	13.3	1.9	1.8
Indian Meal for Two, Sainsbury's*	½ Pack/151g	154	8.5	102	1.6	11.4	5.6	3.1
Indian Takeaway for 1, Sainsbury's*	1 Serving/200g	202	10.4	101	1.8	11.8	5.2	1.7

P

	Measure INFO/WEIGHT	per Measure KCAL	FAT	Nutrition Values per 100g / 100ml KCAL	PROT	CARB	FAT	FIBRE
POTATO BOMBAY								
Meal Solutions, Co-Op*	1 Pack/300g	210	12.0	70	1.0	8.0	4.0	2.0
POTATO CAKES								
Average	1 Cake/70g	127	1.2	180	3.8	37.5	1.7	2.4
Fried, Average	1oz/28g	66	2.5	237	4.9	35.0	9.0	0.8
POTATO FRITTERS								
Crispy, Oven Baked, Birds Eye*	1 Fritter/20g	29	1.6	145	2.0	16.3	8.0	1.2
with Sweetcorn, M & S*	1 Pack/135g	304	17.0	225	4.4	24.1	12.6	2.3
POTATO MASH								
Bacon & Cheese, Tesco*	1 Serving/200g	252	12.8	126	3.1	13.9	6.4	1.3
Bacon & Spring Onion, Finest, Tesco*	½ Pack/200g	214	10.4	107	4.3	10.8	5.2	1.6
Cabbage & Spring Onion, COU, M & S*	½ Pack/225g	157	4.0	70	1.7	11.4	1.8	2.1
Carrot & Swede, COU, M & S*	1oz/28g	20	0.6	70	1.1	12.1	2.1	2.9
Carrot & Swede, M & S*	1 Serving/225g	214	14.4	95	1.6	8.3	6.4	1.4
Carrot & Swede, Morrisons*	1 Serving/100g	71	1.6	71	1.5	12.6	1.6	2.2
Cheddar, Irish, Finest, Tesco*	½ Pack/250g	350	19.7	140	6.3	10.2	7.9	1.4
Cheese & Chive, Snack in a Pot, Tesco*	1 Pot/230g	304	21.6	132	2.2	9.6	9.4	0.9
Cheese & Onion, Eat Smart, Morrisons*	1 Pack/400g	340	6.4	85	4.4	13.2	1.6	1.3
Cheese & Onion, Tesco*	1 Serving/200g	210	9.4	105	3.2	12.6	4.7	1.0
Colcannon, Co-Op*	1 Pack/500g	325	10.0	65	2.0	10.0	2.0	2.0
Colcannon, Sainsbury's*	½ Pack/300g	192	12.0	64	0.4	6.7	4.0	1.4
Colcannon, Tesco*	1 Serving/250g	225	13.5	90	1.6	8.4	5.4	1.8
Colcannon, Waitrose*	½ Pack/225g	207	8.5	92	1.7	12.8	3.8	1.4
Creme Fraiche & Seasoning, Waitrose*	½ Pack/225g	189	6.3	84	2.0	12.7	2.8	1.4
Leek & Bacon, Tesco*	1 Serving/400g	356	14.4	89	3.0	11.1	3.6	1.9
Leek & Cheese, COU, M & S*	½ Pack/225g	180	4.7	80	3.0	12.0	2.1	1.3
Leeks, Creamy, Birds Eye*	1 Pack/300g	300	21.0	100	2.0	7.3	7.0	0.8
Mustard with Caramelised Onions, Finest, Tesco*	1 Serving/200g	232	9.2	116	2.6	16.0	4.6	1.8
Roast Onion, Snack in a Pot, Tesco*	1 Pot/218g	257	12.9	118	1.6	14.7	5.9	0.6
Spring Onion, Weight Watchers*	1 Serving/100g	77	2.2	77	1.9	10.9	2.2	1.4
Sun Dried Tomato & Basil, COU, M & S*	1 Serving/170g	127	2.5	75	1.0	14.4	1.5	1.2
with Cracked Pepper & Sea Salt, Luxury, Sainsbury's*	½ Pack/225g	389	28.3	173	1.6	13.2	12.6	1.0
with Sweetcorn & Flaked Tuna, Quick, Sainsbury's*	1 Pot/224g	240	9.2	107	2.4	15.0	4.1	2.1
with Vegetables, GFY, Asda*	1 Pack/290g	186	3.2	64	1.6	12.0	1.1	2.3
with Vegetables, Sainsbury's*	½ Pack/229g	142	2.3	62	1.8	11.4	1.0	3.1
POTATO RINGS								
Mature Cheddar & Red Onion, GFY, Asda*	1 Pack/10g	36	0.1	360	5.2	81.6	1.5	2.9
Ready Salted, M & S*	1 Serving/75g	375	21.1	500	3.5	58.9	28.1	2.6
Ready Salted, Sainsbury's*	1 Serving/50g	257	14.2	514	3.2	61.5	28.4	1.8
Salt & Vinegar, Sainsbury's*	1 Pack/25g	114	4.9	456	3.6	65.6	19.6	2.8
POTATO SKINS								
¼ Cut, Deep Fried, McCain*	1oz/28g	52	1.7	186	3.0	30.1	6.0	0.0
¼ Cut, Oven Baked, McCain*	1oz/28g	53	1.3	190	3.6	33.1	4.8	0.0
American Style, Loaded, Asda*	1 Serving/78g	294	18.0	375	15.0	27.0	23.0	2.4
American Style, Loaded, Tesco*	1 Serving/340g	388	8.2	114	6.8	16.3	2.4	3.3
Cheese & Bacon, Loaded, Asda*	½ Pack/125g	275	15.0	220	13.0	15.0	12.0	3.3
Cheese & Bacon, Loaded, Tesco*	1 Skin/59g	150	9.1	255	9.2	19.5	15.5	3.0
Cheese & Bacon, Sainsbury's*	1 Serving/140g	349	21.6	249	10.3	17.3	15.4	2.5
Cheese & Bacon, Waitrose*	1 Serving/75g	146	9.4	195	7.3	13.1	12.6	3.5
Cheese & Chive, Sainsbury's*	2 Skins/150g	286	17.8	191	7.7	13.3	11.9	2.8
Cheese & Ham, Iceland*	2 Skins/108g	155	4.9	143	6.3	19.3	4.5	2.0
Cheese & Onion, Loaded, Sour Cream & Chive Dip, Tesco*	1 Skin/60g	114	6.5	190	5.8	17.6	10.8	1.4
Soured Cream, Loaded, M & S*	½ Pack/150g	307	17.8	205	9.1	15.8	11.9	0.9
with Sour Cream	1 Serving/275g	541	34.6	197	7.2	13.8	12.6	2.1

	Measure INFO/WEIGHT	per Measure KCAL	FAT	Nutrition Values per 100g / 100ml KCAL	PROT	CARB	FAT	FIBRE
POTATO WAFFLES								
Frozen, Cooked	1oz/28g	56	2.3	200	3.2	30.3	8.2	2.3
Frozen, Grilled, Asda*	1 Waffle/57g	104	5.8	183	2.0	21.0	10.1	1.7
Mini, Farmfoods*	1oz/28g	41	1.6	145	1.9	21.6	5.7	1.7
Mini, Sainsbury's*	1 Waffle/11g	27	1.8	242	2.8	20.1	16.7	1.0
Oven Baked, Mini, McCain*	1oz/28g	62	2.4	221	3.9	32.0	8.6	0.0
Southern Fried, Asda*	1 Waffle/51g	107	5.1	209	2.8	27.0	10.0	2.1
Uncooked, Average	1 Waffle/62g	113	5.1	182	2.4	24.4	8.3	1.7
POTATO WEDGES								
Asda*	1 Wedge/40g	57	2.0	142	3.4	21.0	4.9	1.7
Baked, GFY, Asda*	1 Pack/450g	616	11.7	137	3.4	25.0	2.6	3.4
BBQ Chicken Spicy, Good Intentions, Somerfield*	1 Pack/400g	380	4.8	95	7.4	13.6	1.2	1.4
BBQ Flavour, Asda*	1 Serving/100g	185	9.0	185	2.9	23.0	9.0	1.7
BGTY, Sainsbury's*	½ Pack/190g	179	3.4	94	3.0	16.4	1.8	3.4
Bombay with Yoghurt & Mint Dip, HL, Tesco*	1 Serving/170g	139	3.6	82	1.3	14.5	2.1	0.9
Crispy, M & S*	1 Serving/200g	340	14.2	170	1.3	25.3	7.1	1.7
Four Cheese & Red Onion, Chicago Town*	1 Serving/150g	210	7.9	140	2.1	21.0	5.3	2.4
Garlic & Herb, COU, M & S*	1 Pack/300g	300	7.8	100	2.3	16.4	2.6	3.2
Garlic & Herb Crusted, Chicago Town*	1 Serving/150g	216	6.4	144	1.9	24.4	4.3	2.2
Jacket, Spicy, American Style, Frozen, Sainsbury's*	1 Serving/125g	156	5.0	125	1.9	20.3	4.0	1.1
Jumbo, Finest, Tesco*	1 Serving/126g	145	2.6	115	1.4	22.7	2.1	1.7
Mexican, Inspire, Asda*	1 Pack/500g	525	17.0	105	2.2	16.5	3.4	1.8
Micro, Tesco*	1 Pack/100g	170	6.8	170	2.6	24.5	6.8	2.3
New York Style, HL, Tesco*	1 Serving/125g	129	3.0	103	2.0	18.3	2.4	2.3
Only 5% Fat, Weighed Baked, McCain*	1 Serving/100g	173	4.3	173	3.3	30.2	4.3	2.8
Only 5% Fat, Weighed Frozen, McCain*	1 Serving/100g	123	3.0	123	2.2	21.8	3.0	1.9
Slightly Spiced, Weighed Baked, Potato Winners, McCain*	1 Serving/100g	187	5.2	187	2.7	26.9	5.2	1.8
Slightly Spiced, Weighed Frozen, Potato Winners, McCain*	1 Serving/100g	144	5.9	144	2.0	20.8	5.9	1.7
Sour Cream & Chives, McCain*	1 Serving/100g	132	4.1	132	2.4	24.0	4.1	0.0
Southern Fried, Asda*	1 Serving/100g	157	4.5	157	3.0	26.0	4.5	3.5
Southern Fried Style, Tesco*	1 Serving/155g	232	14.1	150	3.0	14.1	9.1	2.0
Spicy, Asda*	1 Serving/100g	145	5.7	145	1.8	21.8	5.7	2.1
Spicy, M & S*	½ Pack/225g	349	14.6	155	2.4	21.8	6.5	1.3
Spicy, Occasions, Sainsbury's*	1 Serving/100g	144	4.3	144	2.5	23.7	4.3	0.4
Spicy, Simple Solutions, Tesco*	1 Serving/150g	141	4.5	94	4.6	12.2	3.0	1.4
Spicy & Garlic Dip, Linda McCartney*	1 Pack/300g	366	16.8	122	2.6	15.3	5.6	3.1
POTATOES								
Alphabites, Captain Birds Eye, Birds Eye*	9 Bites/56g	75	3.0	134	2.0	19.5	5.3	1.4
Anya, Raw, TTD, Sainsbury's*	1 Serving/100g	75	0.3	75	1.5	17.8	0.3	1.1
Baby, Dressed with Garlic & Rosemary, M & S*	1 Serving/185g	129	5.2	70	2.0	9.0	2.8	2.4
Baby, Garlic & Sea Salt Roasted, Finest, Tesco*	1 Serving/200g	192	6.6	96	3.1	13.5	3.3	1.0
Baby, New with Butter, Mint & Parsley, Organic, Asda*	1 Pack/360g	414	10.4	115	1.7	20.4	2.9	2.5
Baby, Oven Bake, Aunt Bessie's*	1 Serving/120g	103	1.7	86	2.2	16.3	1.4	3.0
Baby, with Butter & Herbs, Sainsbury's*	¼ Pack/148g	103	0.9	70	1.9	14.2	0.6	2.0
Baby, with Herbs & Butter, Morrisons*	1 Serving/100g	94	2.3	94	1.9	14.6	2.3	1.9
Baby, with Paprika & Chilli Dressing, Morrisons*	1 Serving/120g	124	5.3	103	1.7	13.6	4.4	1.3
Baked, Flesh & Skin, Average	**1 Med/200g**	**218**	**0.2**	**109**	**2.3**	**25.2**	**0.1**	**2.4**
Baked, Flesh Only, Weighed with Skin, Average	**1oz/28g**	**26**	**0.0**	**93**	**2.0**	**21.6**	**0.1**	**1.5**
Baked, Jacket, Baby, Veg, COOK!, M & S*	1 Pack/675g	776	37.8	115	2.1	14.3	5.6	2.3
Baked, Jacket, Beef Chilli Filled, GFY, Asda*	1 Serving/300g	261	1.5	87	4.6	16.0	0.5	3.2
Baked, Jacket, Cheddar Cheese, COU, M & S*	1 Potato/164g	164	3.1	100	2.9	17.3	1.9	2.0
Baked, Jacket, Cheese & Beans, Somerfield*	1 Pack/340g	306	6.8	90	4.1	13.8	2.0	2.2
Baked, Jacket, Cheese Filled, Farmfoods*	2 Halves/255g	349	9.7	137	4.7	21.0	3.8	1.9
Baked, Jacket, Cheesy, GFY, Asda*	1 Serving/155g	129	1.5	83	2.6	16.0	1.0	2.1

POTATOES

	Measure INFO/WEIGHT	per Measure KCAL	FAT	Nutrition Values per 100g / 100ml KCAL	PROT	CARB	FAT	FIBRE
Baked, Jacket, Chicken Tikka, COU, M & S*	1 Serving/300g	240	4.8	80	5.4	10.9	1.6	1.3
Baked, Jacket, Chilli, BGTY, Sainsbury's*	1 Pack/350g	318	4.9	91	5.3	14.3	1.4	1.2
Baked, Jacket, Chilli Con Carne, COU, M & S*	1 Pack/300g	270	6.3	90	6.0	11.1	2.1	1.2
Baked, Jacket, Chilli Con Carne, Pro Cuisine*	1 Pack/340g	347	3.4	102	4.6	18.7	1.0	0.0
Baked, Jacket, Chilli Con Carne, Somerfield*	1 Pack/340g	319	11.6	94	5.5	10.3	3.4	1.2
Baked, Jacket, Creamy Mushroom, Asda*	1 Serving/100g	124	2.4	124	3.5	22.0	2.4	1.7
Baked, Jacket, Garlic, Mini, Asda*	1 Serving/65g	59	2.1	91	2.2	13.0	3.3	0.0
Baked, Jacket, Garlic Butter Filling, Morrisons*	1 Potato/210g	239	12.4	114	1.7	13.6	5.9	0.9
Baked, Jacket, Garlic Mushrooms, BGTY, Sainsbury's*	1 Pack/350g	262	3.1	75	2.3	14.4	0.9	1.2
Baked, Jacket, Halves, M & S*	1 Serving/250g	187	2.7	75	2.0	14.2	1.1	1.7
Baked, Jacket, Ham & Cheddar Cheese, Asda*	1 Pack/300g	435	11.1	145	7.0	21.0	3.7	1.6
Baked, Jacket, Mature Cheddar Cheese, Finest, Tesco*	1 Potato/245g	360	18.4	147	5.4	14.6	7.5	2.3
Baked, Jacket, Mature Cheddar Cheese, M & S*	½ Pack/206g	225	6.6	109	3.6	16.9	3.2	1.0
Baked, Jacket, Mature Cheddar Cheese, Morrisons*	1 Serving/400g	520	20.4	130	4.4	16.6	5.1	1.5
Baked, Jacket, Stuffed, Garlic & Herb Butter, Tesco*	1 Pack/435g	570	32.6	131	1.3	14.6	7.5	1.0
Baked, Jacket, Tuna & Sweetcorn, Average	1 Serving/300g	273	6.7	91	5.0	12.5	2.2	0.9
Baked, Jacket, Tuna & Sweetcorn, BGTY, Sainsbury's*	1 Pack/350g	360	9.5	103	6.5	13.2	2.7	1.3
Baked, Jacket, Tuna & Sweetcorn, COU, M & S*	1 Pack/300g	270	5.4	90	5.1	12.8	1.8	1.4
Baked, Jacket with Baked Bean & Sausage, Asda*	1 Pack/300g	447	9.6	149	5.0	25.0	3.2	2.7
Baked, Jacket with Baked Beans, Pro Cuisine*	1 Pack/340g	374	1.4	110	4.3	22.3	0.4	0.0
Baked, Jacket with Beef Chilli, Asda*	1 Pack/300g	381	7.8	127	5.0	21.0	2.6	2.0
Baked, Jacket with Beef Chilli, M & S*	1 Pack/360g	288	7.2	80	5.9	9.6	2.0	0.9
Baked, Jacket with Cheese, Freshly Prepared, Tesco*	½ Pack/215g	150	3.0	70	3.9	9.7	1.4	2.8
Baked, Jacket with Cheese, HL, Tesco*	1 Potato/225g	202	4.9	90	4.5	13.0	2.2	1.8
Baked, Jacket with Cheese & Bacon, Finest, Tesco*	1 Potato/245g	360	19.6	147	6.0	12.6	8.0	2.5
Baked, Jacket with Cheese & Butter, Tesco*	1 Potato/225g	263	11.2	117	3.1	14.9	5.0	2.3
Baked, Jacket with Cheese Mash, GFY, Asda*	1 Potato/200g	192	5.6	96	4.8	13.0	2.8	2.2
Baked, Jacket with Chicken Tikka, Light Choices, Tesco*	1 Potato/247g	185	2.2	75	3.4	12.6	0.9	1.3
Baked, Jacket with Smoked Bacon, Finest, Tesco*	½ Pack/200g	165	6.4	85	3.0	9.9	3.3	1.3
Baked, Jackets, Stuffed, Mini, Tesco*	1 Serving/108g	130	6.3	120	2.3	14.6	5.8	2.3
Baked, Skin Only, Average	*1oz/28g*	*55*	*0.0*	*198*	*4.3*	*46.1*	*0.1*	*7.9*
Baked, with Cheddar Cheese, Farmfoods*	1 Potato/143g	196	5.4	137	4.7	21.0	3.8	1.9
Baked, with Cheese & Chive, Light Choices, Tesco*	1 Potato/263g	250	3.7	95	3.2	16.7	1.4	1.6
Baked, with Chicken & Mushroom, Homepride*	1 Serving/105g	128	12.3	122	2.3	1.9	11.7	0.0
Baked in Microwave, Flesh & Skin, Average	*1oz/28g*	*29*	*0.0*	*105*	*2.4*	*24.1*	*0.1*	*2.3*
Baked in Microwave, Flesh Only, Average	*1oz/28g*	*28*	*0.0*	*100*	*2.1*	*23.3*	*0.1*	*1.6*
Baked in Microwave, Skin Only, Average	*1oz/28g*	*37*	*0.0*	*132*	*4.4*	*29.6*	*0.1*	*5.5*
Baking, Raw, Average	*1 Med/250g*	*197*	*0.2*	*79*	*2.1*	*18.0*	*0.1*	*1.6*
Boiled, Average	*1 Serving/120g*	*86*	*0.1*	*72*	*1.8*	*17.0*	*0.1*	*1.2*
Boiled, with Skin	*1 Potato/125g*	*97*	*0.1*	*78*	*2.9*	*17.2*	*0.1*	*3.3*
Boulangere, M & S*	½ Pack/225g	180	2.0	80	2.8	15.9	0.9	0.9
Charlotte, Average	*1 Serving/184g*	*139*	*0.5*	*76*	*1.6*	*17.4*	*0.2*	*3.3*
Dauphinoise, Average	*1 Serving/200g*	*335*	*23.9*	*167*	*2.2*	*12.7*	*11.9*	*1.5*
Dauphinoise, Cook*	1 Pack/225g	319	18.7	142	5.3	11.0	8.3	1.8
Dauphinoise, TTD, Sainsbury's*	½ Pack/174g	240	16.2	138	2.9	10.8	9.3	2.7
Desiree, Average	*1 Serving/200g*	*152*	*0.4*	*76*	*2.1*	*16.3*	*0.2*	*0.6*
Exquisa, Finest, Tesco*	¼ Pack/247g	185	0.7	75	1.7	16.1	0.3	1.1
Garlic, Tapas Selection, Sainsbury's*	1 Serving/22g	49	4.2	224	2.6	10.4	19.1	0.7
Hasselback, Average	*1 Serving/175g*	*182*	*1.6*	*104*	*1.9*	*22.0*	*0.9*	*2.9*
Italian Style & Vegetables, Waitrose*	1 Serving/126g	138	3.5	110	2.0	19.2	2.8	3.4
Jersey Royal, Canned, Average	*1 Can/186g*	*116*	*0.2*	*62*	*1.4*	*14.0*	*0.1*	*1.2*
Jersey Royal, New, Raw, Average	*1oz/28g*	*21*	*0.1*	*75*	*1.6*	*17.2*	*0.2*	*1.5*
Jersey Royal, with Mint Butter, Extra Special, Asda*	½ Pack/172g	148	5.3	86	1.6	13.0	3.1	1.5

POTATOES

	Measure INFO/WEIGHT	per Measure KCAL	FAT	Nutrition Values per 100g / 100ml KCAL	PROT	CARB	FAT	FIBRE
King Edward, Tesco*	1 Serving/100g	77	0.2	77	2.1	16.8	0.2	1.3
Maris Piper, Raw, Average	*1 Serving/200g*	*151*	*0.4*	*75*	*2.0*	*16.5*	*0.2*	*1.4*
Mashed, Fresh Mash, Light Choices, Tesco*	1 Pack/400g	280	8.8	70	2.0	9.3	2.2	1.6
Mashed, From Supermarket, Average	½ Pack/200g	197	8.1	98	1.8	13.3	4.1	1.5
Mashed, From Supermarket, Healthy Range, Average	1 Serving/200g	160	3.1	80	1.8	14.6	1.6	1.3
Mashed, From Supermarket, Premium, Average	1 Serving/225g	305	17.8	136	1.7	14.4	7.9	1.1
Mashed, Home Prepared with Whole Milk	1 Cup/210g	162	1.2	77	1.9	17.5	0.6	2.0
Mashed, Maris Piper with Cream & Butter, M & S*	½ Pack/200g	180	7.2	90	1.1	12.9	3.6	0.4
Mashed, Mash Direct*	½ Pack/200g	190	3.8	95	1.7	17.7	1.9	1.3
Mashed, Ready to Eat, Sainsbury's*	½ Pack/200g	142	3.8	71	1.4	12.1	1.9	2.0
Mashed, Vintage Cheddar Cheese, M & S*	½ Pack/225g	247	11.9	110	4.6	12.6	5.3	1.0
Mashed Maris Piper, Tesco*	½ Pack/213g	180	4.0	85	1.9	14.7	1.9	1.6
New, Average	*1 Serving/100g*	*75*	*0.3*	*75*	*1.5*	*17.8*	*0.3*	*1.1*
New, Baby, Average	*1 Serving/180g*	*135*	*0.5*	*75*	*1.7*	*17.1*	*0.3*	*1.6*
New, Baby, Canned, Average	*1 Can/120g*	*70*	*0.2*	*59*	*1.4*	*13.2*	*0.2*	*1.4*
New, Baby with Herb Dressing & Seasoned Butter, Tesco*	½ Pack/160g	112	4.2	70	1.5	10.2	2.6	2.6
New, Easy Steam with Herbs & Butter, Tesco*	1 Serving/125g	94	3.5	75	1.8	9.6	2.8	1.7
New, Garlic, Herb & Parsley Butter, Co-Op*	1 Serving/100g	115	5.0	115	1.0	15.0	5.0	2.0
New, in a Herb Marinade, Tesco*	¼ Pack/150g	151	7.3	101	1.3	13.0	4.9	1.5
New, with Butter, Chives & Mint, M & S*	¼ Pack/145g	116	2.0	80	1.1	16.2	1.4	2.3
New, with English Churned Butter, M & S*	1 Pack/180g	261	4.0	145	1.3	29.5	2.2	2.1
New, with Herbs & Butter, Asda*	½ Pack/170g	146	2.9	86	1.7	16.0	1.7	1.5
New, with Herbs & Butter, Waitrose*	1 Serving/385g	443	22.7	115	1.7	13.8	5.9	1.2
New, with Sunblush Tomato, M & S*	1 Pack/385g	346	6.9	90	1.6	17.2	1.8	1.3
Organics, Boiled, Asda*	1 Serving/200g	152	0.2	76	1.8	16.0	0.1	1.2
Pan Fried, Aldi*	1 Serving/250g	182	2.0	73	2.7	13.7	0.8	0.0
Patatas Bravas, Bistro, M Kitchen, Morrisons*	½ Pack/126g	113	4.0	90	1.1	13.6	3.2	1.3
Raw, Peeled, Flesh Only	*1 Serving/100g*	*75*	*0.2*	*75*	*2.0*	*17.3*	*0.2*	*1.4*
Red, Flesh Only, Average	*1 Serving/300g*	*217*	*0.4*	*72*	*1.9*	*16.3*	*0.1*	*1.2*
Redskin, Roasted, Frozen, Lamb Weston *	½ Packet/200g	202	4.0	101	2.4	18.0	2.0	1.9
Roast, Basted in Beef Dripping, Waitrose*	1 Serving/165g	213	8.9	129	2.2	18.0	5.4	1.9
Roast, Dry, No Oil, No Fat	1 Serving/100g	79	0.1	79	2.7	18.0	0.1	1.6
Roast, Extra Crispy, Oven Baked, Aunt Bessie's*	1 Serving/100g	223	11.8	223	2.9	26.1	11.8	3.6
Roast, Frozen, Average	1 Potato/70g	105	3.5	149	2.6	23.5	5.0	1.4
Roast, Frozen, Healthy Range, Average	1 Potato/70g	70	1.7	100	2.5	18.1	2.4	2.1
Roast, Garlic, Sainsbury's*	½ Pack/225g	358	21.8	159	3.2	14.6	9.7	1.4
Roast, New, Rosemary, Ainsley Harriott*	1 Serving/150g	133	4.0	89	2.0	16.0	2.7	1.3
Roast, Oven Baked, Aunt Bessie's*	1 Serving/165g	305	15.3	185	2.3	22.9	9.3	1.8
Roast, Seasoned, Butter Basted, Tesco*	½ Pack/225g	337	12.8	150	2.3	21.9	5.7	2.4
Roast, with Caramelised Onions, Finest, Tesco*	½ Pack/200g	500	16.4	250	5.5	38.6	8.2	2.9
Roast in Lard, Average	*1oz/28g*	*42*	*1.3*	*149*	*2.9*	*25.9*	*4.5*	*1.8*
Roast in Oil, Average	*1oz/28g*	*42*	*1.3*	*149*	*2.9*	*25.9*	*4.5*	*1.8*
Roasted with Goose Fat, TTD, Sainsbury's*	½ Pack/185g	216	4.4	117	2.7	21.1	2.4	3.0
Roasting, Average	*1 Serving/150g*	*202*	*5.2*	*135*	*2.5*	*23.3*	*3.5*	*1.6*
Rooster, Boiled, Unsalted Water, Albert Bartlett & Sons Ltd*	1 Med Potato/175g	126	0.2	72	1.8	17.0	0.1	1.2
Salad, Value, Tesco*	1 Serving/150g	111	0.4	74	1.7	16.1	0.3	1.0
Saute, Deep Fried, McCain*	1oz/28g	47	2.0	167	2.6	23.3	7.0	0.0
Saute, Oven Baked, McCain*	1oz/28g	56	1.1	199	4.4	36.9	3.8	0.0
Saute with Onion & Bacon, Country Supper, Waitrose*	¼ Pack/100g	112	4.3	112	1.9	16.4	4.3	1.3
Slices, Garlic & Herb, Heinz*	1oz/28g	23	1.1	82	1.7	10.2	3.9	0.7
Slices, in Rich Crispy Batter, Crispy, Chilled, Sainsbury's*	½ Pack/238g	591	37.0	249	2.4	24.8	15.6	2.8
Slices in Batter, Crispy, Ready To Bake, Waitrose*	1 Pack/475g	860	45.1	181	2.5	21.4	9.5	3.1
Spicy, with Chorizo, Tapas, Waitrose*	1 Serving/260g	512	35.6	197	6.7	11.8	13.7	1.1

	Measure INFO/WEIGHT	per Measure KCAL	per Measure FAT	Nutrition Values per 100g / 100ml KCAL	PROT	CARB	FAT	FIBRE
POTATOES								
Vivaldi, Boiled in Unsalted Water, Sainsbury's*	1 Serving/200g	144	0.2	72	1.8	17.0	0.1	1.2
Waves, Frozen, Lamb Weston *	1 1/100g	125	3.9	125	2.8	19.6	3.9	2.6
Wedges, Jumbo, TTD, Sainsbury's*	1 Serving/165g	279	6.8	169	2.4	30.7	4.1	3.1
White, Raw, Weighed with Skin, Flesh Only, Average	*1 Med/213g*	*160*	*0.3*	*75*	*2.0*	*16.8*	*0.2*	*1.3*
White, Vivaldi, TTD, Sainsbury's*	1 Serving/100g	76	0.1	76	1.8	17.0	0.1	1.2
with Garlic & Parsley Butter, Herb Oil Dressed, Co-Op*	1 Serving/178g	205	8.9	115	1.0	15.0	5.0	2.0
with Seafood & Seasoned Butter, Tapas, Waitrose*	1 Pack/170g	330	19.4	194	6.2	16.7	11.4	2.1
with Smoked Bacon, Oven Roasted, Extra Special, Asda*	½ Pack/200g	242	9.6	121	3.9	15.5	4.8	2.6
POTATOES INSTANT								
Mashed, Butter Flavour, Premier Foods*	1 Serving/180g	288	4.1	160	1.4	9.1	2.3	0.8
Mashed, Dry, Tesco*	1 Serving/70g	225	0.1	321	7.7	72.0	0.2	7.1
Mashed, Dry, Value, Tesco*	1/6 Pack/42g	157	0.4	373	7.0	84.0	1.0	6.9
Mashed, Made Up with Water, Average	1 Serving/180g	118	0.3	66	1.7	14.5	0.2	1.3
Mashed, Original, Dry Weight, Smash*	1 Serving/30g	107	1.4	358	10.7	68.1	4.8	3.4
Mashed with Fried Onion, Smash*	½ Pack/269g	191	3.5	71	1.6	13.4	1.3	0.7
Mashed with Smoked Bacon, Smash*	1 Serving/169g	137	3.7	81	1.7	13.6	2.2	0.6
POUSSIN								
Meat & Skin, Raw, Average	*1oz/28g*	*57*	*3.9*	*202*	*19.1*	*0.0*	*13.9*	*0.0*
Spatchcock, British, Waitrose*	½ Poussin/225g	364	20.2	162	19.0	1.2	9.0	0.0
Spatchcock with Garlic & Herbs, Finest, Tesco*	½ Poussin/235g	348	17.2	148	19.7	1.0	7.3	0.5
POWERADE								
Berry & Tropical Fruit, Coca-Cola*	1 Bottle/500ml	120	0.0	24	0.0	5.6	0.0	0.0
Citrus Charge, Coca-Cola*	1 Bottle/500ml	120	0.0	24	0.0	6.0	0.0	0.0
Gold Rush, Coca-Cola*	1 Bottle/500ml	120	0.0	24	0.0	6.0	0.0	0.0
Ice Storm, Coca-Cola*	1 Bottle/500ml	120	0.0	24	0.0	6.0	0.0	0.0
Isotonic, Sports Drink, Coca-Cola*	1 Bottle/500ml	120	0.0	24	0.0	5.6	0.0	0.0
Zero, Coca-Cola*	1 Bottle/500ml	5	0.0	1	0.0	0.0	0.0	0.0
PRAWN COCKTAIL								
& Orkney Crab, M & S*	1 Serving/90g	180	13.8	200	14.2	1.8	15.3	0.6
20% More Prawns, M & S*	½ Pack/100g	330	31.6	330	8.9	2.2	31.6	0.2
BFY, Morrisons*	1 Serving/100g	149	10.3	149	4.7	9.7	10.3	0.1
BGTY, Sainsbury's*	1 Pack/200g	330	23.4	165	10.1	4.8	11.7	0.9
Delicious, Boots*	1 Pack/250g	285	6.5	114	5.5	17.0	2.6	1.2
HL, Tesco*	1 Pack/170g	305	23.9	180	7.1	5.7	14.1	0.6
King, Sainsbury's*	1 Pack/260g	328	15.1	126	5.8	12.7	5.8	2.3
Light Choices, Tesco*	1 Pot/140g	210	16.0	150	7.5	4.3	11.4	1.3
Reduced Fat, M & S*	1 Pack/200g	260	15.0	130	11.9	3.2	7.5	0.7
Reduced Fat, Tesco*	1 Serving/200g	304	21.2	152	7.6	6.5	10.6	0.4
Sainsbury's*	1 Pot/200g	604	55.8	302	9.4	3.2	27.9	0.8
Tesco*	1 Tub/200g	834	83.0	417	7.3	3.5	41.5	0.1
TTD, Sainsbury's*	1 Serving/100g	333	30.6	333	11.5	2.9	30.6	0.5
PRAWN CRACKERS								
Asda*	1 Serving/25g	134	8.7	535	2.0	53.0	35.0	0.0
Cooked in Sunflower Oil, Sharwood's*	1 Cracker/2g	10	0.5	479	0.7	68.3	22.6	0.8
Food to Go, Sainsbury's*	1 Bag/40g	214	12.5	534	2.9	60.2	31.3	0.4
Green Thai Curry, M & S*	1 Pack/50g	250	12.9	500	3.2	62.2	25.8	1.6
M & S*	1 Bag/50g	262	15.6	525	2.8	57.4	31.3	0.8
Ready to Eat, Sharwood's*	1 Bag/60g	316	18.5	527	0.5	62.0	30.8	1.2
Red Mill*	1 Bag/50g	281	18.8	563	2.8	53.1	37.7	0.7
Uncooked, Sharwood's*	1oz/28g	136	8.3	487	0.7	52.7	29.7	1.7
Waitrose*	1 Pack/50g	266	16.0	533	2.4	58.6	32.1	1.6
PRAWN TOAST								
Dim Sum Selection, Sainsbury's*	1 Toast/8g	23	1.5	283	9.9	19.2	18.5	2.0

P

	Measure INFO/WEIGHT	per Measure KCAL	FAT	Nutrition Values per 100g / 100ml KCAL	PROT	CARB	FAT	FIBRE
PRAWN TOAST								
Mini, Oriental Selection, Party, Iceland*	1 Toast/15g	52	3.6	345	10.5	22.0	23.9	2.1
Oriental Selection, Waitrose*	1 Toast/14g	38	2.4	272	11.1	18.3	17.2	2.1
Sesame, Occasions, Sainsbury's*	1 Toast/12g	34	2.2	283	9.9	19.2	18.5	2.0
Sesame, Oriental Snack Selection, Sainsbury's*	1 Toast/12g	40	2.7	335	9.3	23.0	22.9	5.1
Sesame Prawn, Toasted Triangles, M & S*	1 Pack/220g	616	39.6	280	12.4	17.3	18.0	2.0
Waitrose*	1 Toast/21g	47	3.6	223	9.7	7.4	17.2	5.8
PRAWNS								
Atlantic, Extra Large, TTD, Sainsbury's*	¼ Pack/100g	79	1.0	79	17.4	0.1	1.0	0.5
Batter Crisp, Lyons*	1 Pack/160g	350	20.3	219	8.0	18.2	12.7	1.1
Boiled	*1 Prawn/3g*	*3*	*0.0*	*99*	*22.6*	*0.0*	*0.9*	*0.0*
Brine, John West*	½ Can/60g	58	0.6	97	21.0	1.0	1.0	0.0
Cooked & Peeled, Average	*1oz/28g*	*21*	*0.2*	*77*	*17.6*	*0.2*	*0.6*	*0.0*
Dried, Average	*1 Prawn/3g*	*8*	*0.1*	*281*	*62.4*	*0.0*	*3.5*	*0.0*
Filo Wrapped & Breaded, M & S*	1 Serving/19g	45	2.5	235	9.5	20.4	13.0	1.4
Hot & Spicy, Average	1 Serving/170g	461	26.9	271	9.4	22.8	15.8	2.1
Hot & Spicy, Whitby*	1 Portion/125g	319	16.4	255	9.3	25.0	13.1	2.2
Icelandic, Raw, Average	*1oz/28g*	*30*	*0.4*	*105*	*22.7*	*0.0*	*1.5*	*0.0*
King, Crevettes, Cooked & Peeled, Sainsbury's*	1 Pack/225g	205	1.1	91	21.8	0.1	0.5	0.3
King, Frozen, Morrisons*	½ Bag/100g	62	0.6	62	14.0	0.2	0.6	0.6
King, Jumbo, TTD, Sainsbury's*	½ Pack/90g	63	0.6	70	15.7	0.1	0.7	0.5
King, Raw, Average	*1 Bag/200g*	*145*	*1.9*	*72*	*15.8*	*0.2*	*0.9*	*0.1*
King, Raw, Peeled, Sainsbury's*	½ Pack/90g	61	0.6	68	14.3	0.8	0.7	0.5
King, Shell On, TTD, Sainsbury's*	1 Serving/100g	67	0.7	67	14.3	0.8	0.7	0.5
King, Tandoori, Average	1 Prawn/59g	33	0.6	55	5.7	5.9	1.1	0.7
King in Filo, Finest, Tesco*	1 Prawn/20g	38	0.6	189	13.0	27.8	2.9	1.6
King in Sweet Chilli Sauce with Noodles, COU, M & S*	1 Pack/400g	260	1.6	65	4.8	10.3	0.4	1.5
King with Chilli & Coriander, M & S*	1 Pack/140g	147	5.6	105	17.1	0.5	4.0	0.5
King with Garlic, Parsley & Lemon Butter, COOK!, M & S*	½ Pack/110g	160	11.3	145	12.9	0.8	10.2	0.5
King with Garlic Butter, M & S*	1 Serving/100g	165	9.0	165	12.5	9.1	9.0	0.5
King with Ginger & Spring Onion, Waitrose*	1 Pack/300g	207	5.1	69	6.4	7.1	1.7	1.9
Large, Wrapped, Party Food, M & S*	1 Wrap/26g	49	1.5	190	14.7	18.8	5.7	1.3
North Atlantic, Peeled, Cooked, Average	*1oz/28g*	*22*	*0.3*	*80*	*17.5*	*0.0*	*1.1*	*0.0*
North Atlantic, Raw, Average	*1oz/28g*	*17*	*0.1*	*61*	*14.4*	*0.0*	*0.4*	*0.0*
Peeled, TTD, Sainsbury's*	1 Serving/100g	65	0.9	65	14.1	0.1	0.9	0.5
Raw, Average	*1oz/28g*	*22*	*0.2*	*79*	*17.8*	*0.2*	*0.7*	*0.0*
Raw, Jumbo, TTD, Sainsbury's*	½ Pack/85g	115	2.4	135	25.5	2.0	2.8	0.5
Spirals, Shapers, Boots*	1 Pack/100g	468	22.0	468	3.1	64.0	22.0	2.8
Succulent King with a Sweet Chilli Sauce, Birds Eye*	1 Serving/140g	251	17.2	179	10.5	6.5	12.3	0.1
Sweet Chilli, Skewers, Tesco*	1 Skewer/22g	26	0.2	120	20.4	6.9	0.9	0.5
Tempura, Finest, Tesco*	1 Prawn/18g	31	1.6	175	11.5	11.0	9.1	4.0
Thai, M & S*	1oz/28g	29	0.9	103	5.2	13.6	3.1	1.3
Tiger, Cooked & Peeled, Average	*1 Pack/180g*	*151*	*2.0*	*84*	*18.4*	*0.1*	*1.1*	*0.0*
Tiger, Jumbo, Average	*1 Serving/50g*	*39*	*0.2*	*78*	*18.2*	*0.3*	*0.5*	*0.0*
Tiger, Raw, Average	*1 Prawn/30g*	*19*	*0.2*	*64*	*14.2*	*0.0*	*0.7*	*0.0*
Tiger, Vegetarian, Crispy, Tkc*	½ Pack/150g	225	6.0	150	12.0	17.0	4.0	5.0
Tiger, Wrapped, M & S*	1 Pack/190g	477	25.8	251	11.3	20.7	13.6	1.3
Wild Caught, Large, Canadian, Love Life, Waitrose*	1 Serving/100g	69	1.4	69	14.0	0.0	1.4	0.0
PRAWNS CHILLI								
& Coriander, King, Honduran, M & S*	½ Pack/70g	70	2.2	100	17.2	0.1	3.2	0.4
& Coriander, King, Sainsbury's*	1 Pack/140g	112	1.8	80	16.6	0.4	1.3	0.5
Battered, M & S*	1oz/28g	63	3.2	225	7.2	23.8	11.5	0.5
Sweet, Crispy, Dipping Sauce, M & S*	1 Pack/240g	515	27.8	215	7.5	19.9	11.6	2.3
Sweet, Thai, King, Sainsbury's*	1 Serving/150g	177	6.1	118	6.4	13.9	4.1	1.9

	Measure INFO/WEIGHT	per Measure KCAL	FAT	Nutrition Values per 100g / 100ml KCAL	PROT	CARB	FAT	FIBRE
PRAWNS CHILLI								
with Spicy Chilli Dip, King, Sainsbury's*	½ Pack/150g	282	10.8	188	8.6	22.2	7.2	1.0
PRAWNS CREOLE								
Spicy, BGTY, Sainsbury's*	1 Pack/350g	357	8.4	102	4.8	15.6	2.4	0.4
with Vegetable Rice, King, COU, M & S*	1 Pack/400g	300	2.4	75	4.5	13.3	0.6	0.7
PRAWNS WITH								
Chilli, Coriander & Lime, King, Waitrose*	1 Pack/140g	143	3.2	102	19.9	0.5	2.3	0.6
Creamy Lime Dip, King, Waitrose*	1 Pot/230g	517	40.7	225	15.8	0.8	17.7	0.2
Garlic & Herb Butter, King, Fresh, M & S*	1 Serving/200g	330	18.0	165	12.5	9.1	9.0	0.5
Ginger & Spring Onion, King, Budgens*	1 Pack/350g	150	4.2	43	5.9	2.1	1.2	0.7
Ginger & Spring Onion, Sainsbury's*	1 Pack/300g	198	9.3	66	4.7	4.7	3.1	0.3
Green Thai Sauce, Tiger, Waitrose*	½ Pack/117g	108	2.7	92	16.1	0.8	2.3	0.1
Lemon & Pepper, Honduran, King, M & S*	1 Pack/140g	133	3.6	95	17.4	0.4	2.6	0.7
Rice, Sweet Chilli, Tesco*	1 Pack/460g	488	10.1	106	2.4	19.2	2.2	0.5
Spicy Cajun Dip, King, Sainsbury's*	1 Pack/240g	254	4.3	106	14.8	9.1	1.8	1.4
PRETZELS								
American Style, Salted, Sainsbury's*	1 Serving/50g	201	2.2	403	10.8	79.7	4.5	1.8
Cheddar Cheese, Penn State Pretzels*	1 Sm Bag/30g	124	2.8	412	10.0	71.6	9.3	3.8
Choc Full Of, Cadbury*	½ Bag/55g	250	10.4	455	7.7	62.0	19.0	2.9
Giant, Salted, Tesco*	1 Serving/25g	99	1.1	395	12.2	75.8	4.3	3.4
Jumbo, Tesco*	1 Serving/50g	194	3.4	388	9.7	71.9	6.8	5.4
Lightly Salted, Tesco*	1 Serving/25g	99	1.8	395	9.3	73.4	7.1	5.5
Mini, 99% Fat Free, Free Natural*	1 Serving/50g	188	0.5	376	10.1	81.7	1.0	0.0
Mini, M & S*	1 Pack/45g	193	6.0	430	10.4	66.6	13.4	4.9
New York Style, Salted, Mini, Shapers, Boots*	1 Bag/25g	94	0.5	375	10.0	79.0	2.1	4.2
Salted, Average	1 Serving/30g	114	0.8	380	10.3	79.8	2.6	3.0
Salted, Mini, M & S*	1 Pack/25g	94	0.5	375	10.0	79.0	2.1	4.2
Salted, Stars, Tesco*	1oz/28g	104	1.3	371	8.2	73.7	4.8	3.1
Sea Salt & Black Pepper, Penn State Pretzels*	1 Serving/25g	94	1.0	375	10.4	73.7	4.2	4.7
Sea Salt & Black Pepper, Tesco*	1 Serving/50g	189	1.3	379	10.0	79.0	2.6	4.1
Snacks, Fabulous Bakin' Boys*	1 Pack/24g	96	1.2	401	9.0	79.5	4.9	2.5
Sour Cream & Chive, Hoops, BGTY, Sainsbury's*	1 Bag/25g	98	0.6	391	10.4	80.9	2.3	1.6
Sour Cream & Chive, Mini, HL, Tesco*	1 Pack/25g	92	0.5	369	10.9	76.3	2.2	4.6
Sour Cream & Chive, Penn State Pretzels*	1 Serving/25g	111	3.2	443	8.9	71.8	12.9	2.0
Sour Cream & Chive Flavour, Mini, Shapers, Boots*	1 Packet/25g	93	0.7	371	11.0	74.0	2.7	7.3
Sour Cream & Onion, M & S*	1 Serving/30g	136	4.3	455	11.0	70.9	14.5	0.7
Sour Cream & Onion, Tesco*	1 Serving/25g	114	4.2	457	8.4	67.7	17.0	2.3
Spicy Salsa, Penn State Pretzels*	1 Serving/25g	105	2.6	420	9.5	72.4	10.4	1.3
Sweet Thai Chilli Twists, Penn State Pretzels*	1 Serving/25g	98	2.0	393	9.8	70.1	8.2	6.8
Wheat, Gluten Free, Trufree*	1 Bag/60g	282	12.0	470	0.5	72.0	20.0	0.7
PRINGLES*								
Barbecue, Pringles*	1 Serving/50g	266	18.0	533	4.9	48.0	36.0	5.1
BBQ Spare Rib, Rice Infusions, Pringles*	1 Pack/23g	108	5.3	469	5.1	60.0	23.0	2.6
Cheese & Onion, Pringles*	1 Serving/25g	132	8.5	528	4.1	50.0	34.0	3.4
Curry, Masala, Take Aways, Pringles*	1 Serving/25g	128	8.7	514	4.3	52.0	35.0	2.6
Hot & Spicy, Pringles*	1 Serving/25g	132	8.5	530	4.6	49.0	34.0	3.7
Light, Original, Pringles*	1 Serving/25g	121	6.2	484	4.3	59.0	25.0	3.6
Light, Sour Cream & Onion, Pringles*	1 Serving/25g	122	6.2	487	4.7	57.0	25.0	3.6
Minis, Original, Pringles*	1 Pack/23g	118	6.9	514	5.1	55.0	30.0	3.7
Minis, Salt & Vinegar, Pringles*	1 Pack/23g	115	6.4	502	4.5	55.0	28.0	3.6
Minis, Sour Cream & Onion, Pringles*	1 Pack/23g	118	6.7	511	5.2	56.0	29.0	3.5
Minis, Texas BBQ Sauce, Pringles*	1 Pack/23g	116	6.4	504	5.0	56.0	28.0	3.8
Original, Pringles*	1 Serving/25g	131	8.5	526	3.9	52.0	34.0	2.6
Paprika, Pringles*	1 Serving/25g	132	8.5	529	4.9	49.0	34.0	6.5

	Measure INFO/WEIGHT	per Measure KCAL	per Measure FAT	Nutrition Values per 100g / 100ml KCAL	PROT	CARB	FAT	FIBRE
PRINGLES*								
Salt & Vinegar, Pringles*	1 Serving/25g	132	8.5	527	3.9	50.0	34.0	3.4
Sour Cream & Onion, Pringles*	1 Serving/25g	133	8.7	531	4.5	49.0	35.0	3.6
Texas BBQ Sauce, Pringles*	1 Serving/25g	132	8.5	527	4.2	50.0	34.0	3.5
PROFITEROLES								
Asda*	1 Serving/64g	218	17.2	343	5.0	20.0	27.0	0.0
Chocolate, 8 Pack, Co-Op*	¼ Pack/112g	330	17.9	295	6.0	31.0	16.0	2.0
Chocolate, Co-Op*	1 Pot/91g	260	13.7	285	6.0	33.0	15.0	3.0
Chocolate, Sainsbury's*	1/6 Pot/95g	192	8.5	202	5.4	25.1	8.9	0.8
Chocolate, Stack, Sainsbury's*	¼ Pack/76g	311	19.5	409	5.3	39.3	25.6	2.0
Chocolate, Tesco*	1 Serving/76g	293	21.8	386	5.1	26.9	28.7	0.5
Chocolate Covered, Tesco*	1 Serving/72g	295	21.2	410	5.7	29.3	29.5	2.0
Choux & Chocolate Sauce, Tesco*	1 Serving/77g	295	22.0	386	5.1	26.9	28.7	0.5
Classic French, Sainsbury's*	1 Serving/90g	284	15.5	316	6.6	33.7	17.2	0.1
Dairy Cream, Co-Op*	¼ Pack/70g	241	17.5	345	6.0	24.0	25.0	0.5
Filled with Cream, Stack, Fresh, M & S*	1 Serving/75g	281	21.4	375	5.3	23.6	28.5	1.9
Savoury, with Cheese & Chive, Chosen By You, Asda*	¼ Pack/15g	95	7.7	634	9.1	32.1	51.3	3.5
Waitrose*	4 Profiteroles/75g	269	17.9	359	4.8	31.1	23.9	0.7
PROVENCALE								
Chicken, M & S*	1 Pack/430g	365	11.6	85	13.2	2.3	2.7	0.6
King Prawn & Mushroom, M & S*	½ Pack/185g	120	4.6	65	7.2	3.9	2.5	0.9
Mushroom, Fresh, COU, M & S*	½ Pack/150g	60	2.2	40	2.6	4.1	1.5	1.8
Prawn & Mushroom with Pasta, COU, M & S*	1 Pack/400g	360	2.0	90	5.9	15.7	0.5	0.0
Ratatouille, Asda*	½ Can/195g	97	3.9	50	1.0	7.0	2.0	1.0
PRUNES								
Dried, Average	*1 Serving/50g*	*79*	*0.2*	*157*	*2.5*	*36.4*	*0.4*	*5.8*
in Apple Juice, Average	*1 Serving/90g*	*76*	*0.1*	*84*	*0.8*	*19.8*	*0.1*	*1.4*
in Fruit Juice, Average	*1oz/28g*	*25*	*0.0*	*88*	*0.9*	*21.4*	*0.2*	*3.0*
in Syrup, Average	*1oz/28g*	*26*	*0.0*	*92*	*1.0*	*22.1*	*0.2*	*2.6*
Pitted, Californian, Ready to Eat, Sweetvine, Aldi*	4 Prunes/30g	48	0.1	161	2.5	34.0	0.4	5.7
Pitted, in Juice, 825g Jar, Tesco*	1 Serving/206g	165	1.0	80	0.8	17.0	0.5	3.3
Pitted, Ready to Eat, Everyday Value, Tesco*	4 Prunes/40g	66	0.2	165	2.5	34.0	0.4	5.7
Ready to Eat, Dried, Organic, Love Life, Waitrose*	1 Serving/30g	73	0.1	243	2.2	56.8	0.4	7.3
Ready to Eat, Wholefoods, Tesco*	1 Serving/100g	230	0.3	230	1.9	54.9	0.3	6.5
Stewed with Sugar	*1oz/28g*	*29*	*0.1*	*103*	*1.3*	*25.5*	*0.2*	*3.1*
Stewed without Sugar	*1oz/28g*	*23*	*0.1*	*81*	*1.4*	*19.5*	*0.3*	*3.3*
Stoned, Ready to Eat, Asda*	6 Prunes/30g	48	0.1	161	2.5	33.9	0.4	5.7
PUDDING								
Apple & Blackberry Crumble, Custard Style, Somerfield*	1oz/28g	34	1.4	123	3.0	17.0	5.0	0.0
Apple & Custard, Sainsbury's*	1 Serving/115g	132	2.2	115	5.4	19.0	1.9	0.1
Banana Fudge Crunch, Bird's*	1oz/28g	125	3.9	445	5.4	75.0	14.0	0.8
Blackberry & Bramley Apple, M & S*	¼ Pudding/152g	365	12.5	240	3.3	38.2	8.2	2.0
Bread, Retail Average	1 Slice/120g	301	8.0	251	8.4	41.8	6.7	0.5
Butterscotch, Instant, Fat Free, Jell-O*	1 Serving/8g	25	0.1	333	1.3	78.7	1.3	0.0
Cherry Cobbler, GFY, Asda*	1 Pudding/100g	158	2.0	158	2.1	33.0	2.0	0.9
Chocolate, Gu*	1 Pack/240g	780	27.4	325	3.9	51.8	11.4	1.6
Chocolate, Low Fat, Good Intentions, Somerfield*	1 Pudding/110g	200	2.4	182	3.0	37.6	2.2	2.4
Chocolate, M & S*	¼ Pudding/76g	265	12.0	350	4.1	48.0	15.8	2.1
Chocolate, Melting Middle, M & S*	1 Pudding/155g	510	27.8	330	5.8	36.2	18.0	3.1
Chocolate, Perfectly Balanced, Waitrose*	1 Pot/105g	196	3.3	187	3.8	36.0	3.1	0.8
Chocolate, Raspberry & Chilli Puds	1 Pot/85g	212	12.8	249	3.2	25.0	15.1	1.3
Chocolate, Tesco*	1 Serving/110g	348	21.0	316	3.1	32.9	19.1	1.9
Chocolate & Vanilla Swirls, Sugar Free, Jell-O*	1 Pot/106g	60	1.5	57	0.9	12.3	1.4	0.0
Chocolate Bombe, Finest, Tesco*	¼ Pudding/100g	350	12.9	350	5.1	53.0	12.9	2.6

	Measure INFO/WEIGHT	per Measure		Nutrition Values per 100g / 100ml				
		KCAL	FAT	KCAL	PROT	CARB	FAT	FIBRE
PUDDING								
Chocolate Ganache, Mini Pot, Gu*	1 Pot/45g	199	16.6	442	3.3	26.4	36.8	2.3
Chocolate Sponge with Rich Caramel Sauce, Cadbury*	1 Pudding/110g	352	16.6	320	4.0	41.1	15.1	1.2
Christmas, Free From, Sainsbury's*	¼ Pudding/114g	346	7.8	305	1.8	58.9	6.9	4.7
Creme Aux Oeufs a la Vanille, Weight Watchers*	1 Pot/100g	116	3.2	116	4.8	17.0	3.2	0.0
Crumble, Fruit, Hot, Weight Watchers*	1 Crumble/90g	163	4.1	181	2.2	35.0	4.6	2.4
Eve's, Average	1oz/28g	67	3.7	241	3.5	28.9	13.1	1.4
Eve's, with Custard, Less Than 5% Fat, M & S*	1 Pudding/205g	318	9.4	155	3.4	24.7	4.6	0.7
Hot Chocolate, Melting Middle Puds, Gu*	1 Pud/100g	409	26.9	409	6.0	36.0	26.9	2.7
Jam, Roly Poly, Aunt Bessie's*	1 Serving/75g	290	10.3	387	3.4	62.2	13.8	0.9
Jam, Roly Poly, Sainsbury's*	¼ Pack/81g	291	11.5	359	4.4	53.3	14.2	0.5
Jam Roly Poly & Custard, Co-Op*	1 Serving/105g	262	7.3	250	3.0	44.0	7.0	0.8
Lemon, BGTY, Sainsbury's*	1 Serving/100g	151	1.9	151	2.9	31.0	1.9	0.5
Lemon, M & S*	1 Pudding/105g	328	16.0	312	4.3	39.4	15.2	2.3
Lemon, Perfectly Balanced, Waitrose*	1 Serving/105g	212	2.5	202	3.4	41.7	2.4	0.6
Luxury, Christmas X2, Tesco*	1 Serving/100g	295	8.1	295	2.6	52.1	8.1	6.0
Matured, Christmas, Finest, Tesco*	1 Serving/100g	353	13.4	353	4.6	51.4	13.4	2.0
Melting Chocolate & Pecan, Brownie Pud, Gu*	1/6 Pudding/67g	290	17.6	436	5.3	45.1	26.4	3.1
Queen of Puddings	1oz/28g	60	2.2	213	4.8	33.1	7.8	0.2
Raspberry, Jam Sponge Puddings, M & S*	1 Pot/119g	400	14.0	335	4.0	53.1	11.7	1.4
Rhubarb & Custard, BGTY, Sainsbury's*	1 Pudding/140g	137	2.8	98	2.0	18.4	2.0	1.4
Sago, Creamed, Ambrosia*	1 Serving/200g	158	3.2	79	2.5	13.6	1.6	0.2
Souffle, Hot Chocolate, Gu*	1 Pot/65g	298	23.5	458	6.0	24.1	36.2	2.5
Sponge, with Golden Syrup, Individual, Mr Kipling*	1 Pudding/85g	304	12.1	358	2.7	54.4	14.3	0.6
Sponge, with Raspberry Jam, Individual, Mr Kipling*	1 Pudding/85g	307	12.2	361	3.0	54.9	14.3	0.5
Steamed, Chocolate with a Rich Chocolate Sauce, Aunty's*	1 Pudding/110g	331	5.2	301	3.6	58.7	4.7	3.2
Sticky Toffee, & Sticky Toffee Sauce, BGTY, Sainsbury's*	1 Serving/130g	318	5.3	245	5.0	49.3	4.1	2.2
Sticky Toffee, Bistro, M Kitchen, Morrisons*	¼ Pack/100g	361	15.6	361	2.7	51.4	15.6	2.0
Sticky Toffee, Co-Op*	¼ Pudding/100g	355	20.0	355	3.0	40.0	20.0	0.7
Sticky Toffee, Extra Special, Asda*	¼ Pudding/100g	378	18.0	378	1.9	52.0	18.0	1.8
Sticky Toffee, Farmfoods*	¼ Pudding/186g	627	11.9	337	4.1	65.7	6.4	0.3
Sticky Toffee, HL, Tesco*	1 Pack/125g	245	5.6	196	4.0	34.9	4.5	0.6
Sticky Toffee, Individual, Mr Kipling*	1 Pudding/85g	266	7.2	312	2.7	56.1	8.4	0.9
Sticky Toffee, Tesco*	1 Serving/110g	287	14.7	261	3.3	31.8	13.4	0.7
Sticky Toffee, Weight Watchers*	1 Pudding/100g	172	1.1	172	3.0	27.2	1.1	20.5
Sticky Toffee, with Custard, Somerfield*	1 Pack/245g	576	19.6	235	3.0	38.0	8.0	0.0
Summer Fruits, Co-Op*	1 Pack/260g	273	0.5	105	1.0	25.0	0.2	1.0
Summer Fruits, Eat Well, M & S*	1 Pudding/135g	128	0.7	95	1.7	20.8	0.5	3.0
Summer Pudding, BGTY, Sainsbury's*	1 Pot/110g	223	5.1	203	3.2	40.9	4.6	2.4
Summer Pudding, Waitrose*	1 Pot/120g	125	0.5	104	2.0	23.1	0.4	1.4
Syrup, Individual, Co-Op*	1 Pudding/170g	603	35.7	355	3.0	38.0	21.0	1.0
Syrup, M & S*	1 Serving/105g	370	10.5	352	3.9	61.7	10.0	0.8
PUMPKIN								
Boiled in Salted Water	**1oz/28g**	**4**	**0.1**	**13**	**0.6**	**2.1**	**0.3**	**1.1**
PUPPODUMS								
Cracked Black Pepper, Ready to Eat, Sharwood's*	1 Puppodum/9g	41	2.4	461	16.7	37.2	27.3	7.3
Garlic & Coriander, Ready to Eat, Sharwood's*	1 Puppodum/9g	39	1.9	438	18.4	43.0	21.4	6.5
Plain, Cook to Eat, Sharwood's*	1 Puppodum/12g	32	0.1	273	21.9	45.7	1.0	10.1
Plain, Mini, Cook to Eat, Sharwood's*	1 Puppodum/4g	11	0.0	273	21.9	45.7	0.3	10.1
Spicy, Cook to Eat, Sharwood's*	1 Puppodum/12g	30	0.1	257	20.2	43.0	0.5	13.0

P

	Measure INFO/WEIGHT	per Measure KCAL	per Measure FAT	Nutrition Values per 100g / 100ml KCAL	PROT	CARB	FAT	FIBRE
QUAVERS								
Cheese, Walkers*	1 Bag/16g	88	4.9	534	2.7	62.5	30.1	1.1
Prawn Cocktail, Walkers*	1 Bag/16g	88	5.1	537	2.1	62.0	31.0	1.2
Salt & Vinegar, Walkers*	1 Bag/16g	86	4.9	527	1.9	62.0	30.0	1.2
QUICHE								
Asparagus & Feta, Little, Higgidy*	1 Portion/155g	369	23.4	238	8.1	17.3	15.1	1.4
Asparagus & Herby Summer Vegetable, Higgidy*	1 Quiche/400g	848	50.0	212	5.9	18.9	12.5	2.7
Asparagus & Mushroom, Tesco*	½ Quiche/200g	474	32.8	237	5.1	17.2	16.4	1.2
Baby Spinach & Gruyere, Sainsbury's*	¼ Quiche/93g	228	16.0	245	7.4	15.1	17.2	1.0
Bacon, Leek & Cheese, Weight Watchers*	1 Quiche/165g	327	15.7	198	8.2	18.0	9.5	1.8
Bacon, Leek & Mushroom, M & S*	¼ Quiche/100g	245	16.4	245	6.9	17.2	16.4	1.3
Bacon, Smoked & Mature Cheddar, Higgidy*	1 Quiche/400g	1096	74.0	274	8.4	18.6	18.5	1.5
Bacon & Cheese, Sainsbury's*	¼ Quiche/100g	237	15.0	237	7.0	18.6	15.0	0.7
Bacon & Leek, Asda*	¼ Quiche/100g	252	15.9	252	8.4	18.9	15.9	1.5
Bacon & Tomato, Asda*	1 Serving/107g	201	8.6	188	8.0	21.0	8.0	1.1
Broccoli, Budgens*	1 Serving/88g	213	15.5	243	6.3	14.8	17.7	1.0
Broccoli, Extra, Value, Tesco*	1 Serving/125g	341	24.0	273	10.0	15.1	19.2	0.8
Broccoli, Tesco*	1 Serving/100g	249	17.2	249	6.0	17.6	17.2	1.4
Broccoli, Tomato & Cheese, BGTY, Sainsbury's*	1 Quiche/390g	632	32.0	162	6.4	15.7	8.2	1.3
Broccoli, Tomato & Cheese, Deep Filled, Sainsbury's*	¼ Quiche/100g	203	12.9	203	5.2	16.9	12.9	2.3
Broccoli & Stilton with Crunchy Cheddar Crumb, Higgidy*	½ Quiche/200g	558	38.6	279	9.2	17.2	19.3	1.4
Cheese, Broccoli & Tomato, Nisa Heritage*	1 Serving/85g	234	16.6	275	7.3	17.5	19.5	1.4
Cheese, Onion & Chive, Smart Price, Asda*	¼ Quiche/83g	213	14.1	257	6.0	20.0	17.0	0.7
Cheese & Bacon, Crustless, Tesco*	1 Serving/85g	170	11.7	200	8.8	9.6	13.8	3.3
Cheese & Broccoli, Morrisons*	1/3 Quiche/134g	338	22.4	253	7.1	16.4	16.8	1.7
Cheese & Egg	1oz/28g	88	6.2	314	12.5	17.3	22.2	0.6
Cheese & Ham, Sainsbury's*	1 Serving/100g	266	19.0	266	9.3	14.4	19.0	1.2
Cheese & Ham, Somerfield*	1 Quiche/325g	835	58.5	257	7.0	18.0	18.0	0.0
Cheese & Mushroom, Budgens*	½ Quiche/170g	474	32.8	279	7.8	18.4	19.3	1.4
Cheese & Onion, 25% Reduced Fat, Asda*	½ Quiche/78g	163	7.0	209	11.0	21.0	9.0	2.4
Cheese & Onion, Asda*	½ Quiche/200g	578	39.6	289	9.0	18.6	19.8	1.5
Cheese & Onion, Crustless, Weight Watchers*	1 Quiche/160g	267	12.3	167	11.3	11.1	7.7	4.3
Cheese & Onion, Deep Filled, Sainsbury's*	¼ Quiche/100g	254	17.2	254	7.3	17.2	17.2	2.2
Cheese & Onion, Finest, Tesco*	1 Serving/130g	346	24.3	266	9.1	15.3	18.7	2.5
Cheese & Onion, Individual, Sainsbury's*	1 Quiche/180g	542	34.9	301	9.9	21.6	19.4	1.5
Cheese & Onion, M & S*	1 Slice/100g	250	17.2	250	8.2	16.1	17.2	1.5
Cheese & Onion, Reduced Fat, Eat Smart, Morrisons*	1 Quiche/400g	824	36.8	206	7.7	16.9	9.2	0.7
Cheese & Onion, Somerfield*	1 Quiche/300g	696	48.0	232	8.0	14.0	16.0	0.0
Cheese & Onion, VLH Kitchens	1 Serving/80g	133.6	7.5	167	9.6	18.1	6.0	1.8
Cheese & Onion, Weight Watchers*	1 Quiche/165g	325	15.3	197	7.0	21.2	9.3	1.6
Cheese & Tomato, Asda*	¼ Quiche/105g	274	17.8	261	8.0	19.0	17.0	0.9
Cheese & Tomato, M & S*	1 Serving/100g	230	15.6	230	7.7	15.1	15.6	1.6
Chicken, Garlic & Herb, Asda*	1/8 Quiche/52g	137	8.3	264	10.0	20.0	16.0	1.2
Chicken & Basil, Finest, Tesco*	1 Serving/134g	381	24.9	284	9.3	19.8	18.6	1.3
Crustless, Garden Vegetable, Tesco*	½ Quiche/170g	270	13.8	160	6.5	12.2	8.2	3.5
Crustless, Green Vegetable, Light Choices, Tesco*	1 Quiche/160g	200	9.3	125	6.0	11.9	5.8	4.7
Davidstow Cheddar Cheese & Caramelised Onion, Asda*	1/3 Quiche/117g	367	26.8	315	7.0	20.0	23.0	1.0
Farmhouse Cheddar & Onion, Waitrose*	¼ Quiche/100g	257	18.1	257	8.1	15.4	18.1	1.3
Gammon, Leek & Cheddar Cheese, Somerfield*	¼ Quiche/95g	251	16.2	264	7.6	19.9	17.1	0.9
Gammon, Leek & Mustard, Weight Watchers*	1 Quiche/165g	305	14.5	185	5.7	20.7	8.8	3.4
Ham, Cheese & Chive, GFY, Asda*	1 Serving/78g	173	7.8	222	9.0	24.0	10.0	1.5
Ham & Mustard, GFY, Asda*	1 Quiche/155g	327	17.0	211	9.0	19.0	11.0	3.9
Ham & Soft Cheese, Tesco*	¼ Quiche/100g	280	20.1	280	7.4	17.5	20.1	1.9
Ham & Tomato, M & S*	½ Pack/200g	440	31.0	220	8.1	12.4	15.5	2.9

INFO/WEIGHT	Measure		per Measure		Nutrition Values per 100g / 100ml				
			KCAL	FAT	KCAL	PROT	CARB	FAT	FIBRE

QUICHE

Leek, Cheese & Chive, Sainsbury's*	1/3 Quiche/125g		292	20.2	234	7.1	14.9	16.2	1.3
Leek & Sweet Potato, Waitrose*	½ Quiche/200g		440	29.0	220	5.3	17.0	14.5	2.3
Lorraine, Average	1oz/28g		109	7.9	391	16.1	19.8	28.1	0.7
Lorraine, BGTY, Sainsbury's*	1 Serving/128g		273	14.0	213	10.9	17.7	10.9	0.7
Lorraine, Crustless, Light Choices, Tesco*	1 Pack/160g		280	13.4	175	12.6	11.8	8.4	2.5
Lorraine, Crustless, You Count, Love Life, Waitrose*	1 Quiche/160g		295	15.4	185	8.9	15.2	9.6	0.9
Lorraine, Extra Special, Asda*	¼ Quiche/100g		270	18.0	270	8.0	19.0	18.0	2.3
Lorraine, Half Fat, Waitrose*	¼ Quiche/100g		189	8.9	189	8.1	19.0	8.9	1.4
Lorraine, Light Choices, Tesco*	¼ Pack/100g		170	6.4	170	12.3	15.5	6.4	3.2
Lorraine, Meat Free, Tesco*	1 Quiche/140g		335	19.3	240	9.4	19.1	13.8	2.8
Lorraine, Reduced Fat, Eat Smart, Morrisons*	¼ Quiche/100g		209	9.8	209	9.4	17.8	9.8	0.5
Lorraine, Weight Watchers*	1 Quiche/165g		292	13.2	177	8.7	17.5	8.0	3.2
Mediterranean, GFY, Asda*	1 Serving/25g		54	2.2	217	9.0	25.0	9.0	2.4
Mediterranean Style Vegetable, Classic, Sainsbury's*	1 Quiche/400g		868	50.4	217	6.2	19.8	12.6	2.2
Mediterranean Vegetable, BGTY, Sainsbury's*	½ Quiche/90g		160	7.2	178	7.3	19.2	8.0	1.7
Mediterranean Vegetable, Weight Watchers*	1 Quiche/165g		285	13.5	173	3.8	21.1	8.2	4.0
Mushroom	1oz/28g		80	5.5	284	10.0	18.3	19.5	0.9
Salmon & Broccoli, Asda*	¼ Quiche/106g		289	18.0	273	10.0	20.0	17.0	2.6
Salmon & Broccoli, Sainsbury's*	1 Serving/105g		346	22.8	260	7.9	18.5	17.1	0.8
Salmon & Broccoli, Tesco*	1 Serving/133g		311	20.1	234	7.9	16.6	15.1	0.9
Salmon & Spinach, Sainsbury's*	1/3 Quiche/125g		318	21.9	254	8.2	15.9	17.5	1.0
Sausage & Onion, Sainsbury's*	1 Serving/100g		287	20.0	287	7.1	19.7	20.0	1.2
Smoked Bacon & Cheddar, Little, Higgidy*	1 Quiche/155g		485	33.8	313	11.5	17.6	21.8	1.0
Spinach, Feta & Roasted Red Pepper, Higgidy*	1 Quiche/400g		888	53.2	222	5.8	19.9	13.3	2.2
Spinach, Ricotta & Gruyere Slice, Somerfield*	1 Serving/130g		348	26.0	268	7.0	15.0	20.0	0.0
Spinach & Gruyere, Sainsbury's*	¼ Quiche/100g		258	19.1	258	7.7	13.9	19.1	1.0
Spinach & Ricotta, Tesco*	¼ Quiche/100g		237	14.9	237	5.8	19.9	14.9	1.0
Spinach & Roast Red Pepper, Little, Higgidy*	1 Quiche/155g		397	27.3	256	9.1	15.2	17.6	1.2
Sweet Cherry Pepper & Fontal Cheese, Finest, Tesco*	¼ Quiche/100g		293	22.1	293	6.7	16.9	22.1	0.9
Sweetfire Pepper, Feta & Olive, Waitrose*	¼ Quiche/100g		238	16.9	238	5.7	15.7	16.9	1.4
Three Cheese & Onion, GFY, Asda*	1 Serving/73g		188	10.2	258	10.0	23.0	14.0	3.1
Tomato, Cheese & Courgette, Asda*	1 Quiche/100g		333	17.0	333	11.0	34.0	17.0	5.0
Tomato, GFY, Asda*	¼ Quiche/50g		94	4.0	188	8.0	21.0	8.0	0.8
Tomato, Mozzarella, & Basil, Weight Watchers*	1 Quiche/165g		300	12.2	182	6.1	22.8	7.4	1.3
Tomato, Mushroom & Bacon, Sainsbury's*	1 Serving/187g		447	30.9	239	7.5	15.2	16.5	1.1
Tomato, Pesto & Mozzarella, TTD, Sainsbury's*	1/3 Quiche/158g		370	25.6	234	5.5	16.5	16.2	2.1
Tomato & Cheese, Sainsbury's*	1/3 Quiche/133g		374	24.5	281	7.9	20.9	18.4	1.5
Tuna, Tomato & Basil, Asda*	1 Serving/125g		305	20.0	244	9.0	16.0	16.0	1.5
Vegetable, Tesco*	1 Serving/100g		257	17.7	257	6.9	17.5	17.7	1.5

QUINCE

Average	*1 Fruit/209g*		*54*	*0.2*	*26*	*0.3*	*6.3*	*0.1*	*1.9*

QUINOA

Cooked, Love Life, Waitrose*	1 Serving/180g		216	3.5	120	9.9	4.4	1.9	2.8
Dry Weight, Average	*1 Serving/70g*		*258*	*4.2*	*368*	*14.1*	*64.2*	*6.1*	*7.0*

QUORN*

Bacon Style, Rashers, Streaky, Frozen, Quorn*	¼ Pack/3 Strips		74	5.8	198	11.0	3.5	15.5	5.0
Balls, Al Forno, Quorn*	1 Serving/400g		348	7.2	87	4.7	13.1	1.8	1.8
Balls, Swedish Style, Quorn*	1 Pack/300g		354	6.0	118	17.0	8.0	2.0	2.0
Beef Style Pieces, Quorn*	½ Pack/75g		69	1.6	92	13.5	4.5	2.2	5.0
Bites, BBQ, Quorn*	1 Pack/140g		147	3.5	105	13.5	7.0	2.5	5.5
Bites, Indian, Quorn*	1 Bite/15g		34	1.5	222	6.0	27.0	10.0	3.0
Bites, Lamb Style Kofta, Quorn*	1 Bite/25g		47	2.4	186	5.0	20.0	9.5	3.0
Bites, Quorn*	½ Pack/70g		77	1.7	110	13.8	8.0	2.5	5.0

Q

QUORN*	Measure INFO/WEIGHT	per Measure KCAL	per Measure FAT	Nutrition Values per 100g / 100ml KCAL	PROT	CARB	FAT	FIBRE
Burgers, Chicken, Southern Style, Quorn*	1 Burger/63g	119	6.2	189	10.7	14.5	9.8	3.1
Burgers, Chicken Style, Quorn*	1 Burger/70g	136	6.7	194	11.0	16.0	9.6	4.6
Burgers, Minted Lamb Style, Quorn*	1 Burger/80g	86	3.2	108	12.0	6.0	4.0	4.0
Burgers, Original, Quorn*	1 Burger/50g	73	2.4	146	18.9	6.7	4.8	3.0
Burgers, Premium, Quorn*	1 Burger/82g	88	3.3	107	11.3	6.5	4.0	3.5
Burgers, Quarter Pounder, Mexican Style, Quorn*	1 Burger/113g	180	6.3	159	18.3	8.9	5.6	3.8
Burgers, Quarter Pounder, Quorn*	1 Burger/114g	158	5.1	139	18.0	6.5	4.5	4.5
Burgers, Sizzling, Quorn*	1 Burger/80g	123	4.8	154	18.0	7.0	6.0	3.0
Burgers, Southern Style, Quorn*	1 Burger/63g	119	6.2	189	10.7	14.5	9.8	3.1
Chicken Style Curry, Quorn*	1 Serving/300g	243	3.0	81	2.9	15.0	1.0	1.5
Chicken Style Dippers, Quorn*	1 Dipper/19g	32	2.0	167	11.0	7.2	10.5	4.0
Chicken Style Pieces, Frozen or Chilled, Quorn*	1 Serving/87g	93	2.3	107	16.3	4.5	2.6	0.6
Chicken Style Tikka Pieces, Quorn*	1 Pack/175g	201	5.2	115	12.5	7.0	3.0	6.0
Chilli, Vegetarian, Tesco*	1 Pack/400g	340	3.2	85	4.4	15.0	0.8	2.1
Cottage Pie, Quorn*	1 Lg Pack/500g	335	5.0	67	2.5	11.0	1.0	1.8
Crispbake, Tuna & Sweetcorn Style, Quorn*	1 Crispbake/100g	176	6.2	176	6.6	22.0	6.2	3.0
Crispbakes, Salmon Style & Dill, Quorn*	1 Crispbake/100g	182	6.6	182	7.0	22.0	6.6	3.5
Curry, Red Thai, Quorn*	1 Pack/400g	464	15.6	116	4.6	15.5	3.9	4.0
Curry & Rice, Quorn*	1 Pack/400g	412	8.0	103	3.8	17.5	2.0	1.5
Eggs, Picnic, Quorn*	1 Egg/20g	50	2.3	248	15.0	21.0	11.5	4.6
Enchiladas, Quorn*	1 Pack/401g	405	14.8	101	5.3	11.7	3.7	1.9
Escalope, Mozzarella & Pesto, Quorn*	1 Escalope/120g	260	15.6	217	10.0	15.0	13.0	4.5
Escalope, Turkey Style, Sage & Onion, Quorn*	1 Escalope/100g	195	9.1	195	9.1	19.2	9.1	3.3
Escalopes, Creamy Garlic & Mushroom, Quorn*	1 Escalope/120g	266	15.0	222	7.9	19.4	12.5	3.1
Escalopes, Creamy Peppercorn, Quorn*	1 Escalope/120g	252	15.2	210	7.8	16.0	12.7	4.0
Escalopes, Feta & Tomato, Quorn*	1 Escalope/120g	257	14.6	214	8.0	18.0	12.2	4.0
Escalopes, Garlic & Herb, Quorn*	1 Escalope/140g	293	16.5	209	8.9	16.9	11.8	3.8
Escalopes, Goats Cheese & Cranberry, Quorn*	1 Escalope/120g	281	16.8	234	10.0	17.0	14.0	4.0
Escalopes, Gruyere Cheese & Leek, Quorn*	1 Escalope/120g	244	13.2	203	9.0	17.0	11.0	5.0
Escalopes, Korma, Quorn*	1 Escalope/120g	270	15.6	225	7.0	20.0	13.0	3.0
Escalopes, Lemon & Black Pepper, Quorn*	1 Escalope/110g	256	12.9	233	9.6	20.5	11.7	2.1
Escalopes, Mature Cheddar & Broccoli, Quorn*	1 Escalope/120g	244	13.7	203	8.7	16.5	11.4	2.9
Escalopes, Spinach & Soft Cheese, Quorn*	1 Escalope/120g	236	13.2	197	8.5	16.1	11.0	2.9
Escalopes, Sweet Pepper & Mozzarella, Quorn*	1 Escalope/120g	231	12.4	193	8.7	16.1	10.4	3.8
Escalopes, Wensleydale & Blueberry, Quorn*	1 Escalope/120g	281	16.8	234	10.0	17.0	14.0	4.0
Fajita, Strips, Quorn*	½ Pack/70g	69	1.0	98	14.0	7.0	1.5	5.0
Fajita Meal Kit, Quorn*	½ Pack/214g	268	5.4	125	7.0	18.5	2.5	3.5
Fillets, Barbecue, Sliced, Quorn*	½ Packet/70g	65	0.7	93	13.0	8.0	1.0	5.0
Fillets, Cajun Spice, Quorn*	1 Serving/100g	176	8.2	176	10.9	14.7	8.2	3.4
Fillets, Chargrilled Tikka Style, Mini, Quorn*	½ Pack/85g	110	2.0	129	12.5	14.4	2.4	5.0
Fillets, Chinese Style Chargrilled, Mini, Quorn*	1 Serving/85g	115	2.3	135	12.1	15.6	2.7	4.7
Fillets, Crispy, Quorn*	1 Fillet/100g	197	9.8	197	13.0	14.2	9.8	4.0
Fillets, Garlic & Herb, Quorn*	1 Fillet/100g	208	9.8	208	13.9	16.1	9.8	4.1
Fillets, Hot & Spicy, Quorn*	1 Fillet/100g	176	8.2	176	10.9	14.7	8.2	6.4
Fillets, Lemon & Pepper, Quorn*	1 Fillet/100g	195	8.5	195	13.3	16.2	8.5	3.5
Fillets, Oriental, Sainsbury's*	1 Serving/294g	353	1.8	120	4.0	24.6	0.6	1.8
Fillets, Plain, Quorn*	1 Fillet/52g	55	0.8	106	13.0	5.0	1.5	5.0
Fillets, Provencale, Morrisons*	1 Serving/165g	94	2.3	57	5.4	5.8	1.4	1.1
Fillets, Thai, Quorn*	1 Serving/79g	96	3.6	121	11.0	9.0	4.5	4.0
Fishless Fingers, Quorn*	1 Finger/29g	66	3.0	232	10.2	22.1	10.5	4.9
Florentine, Deli, Quorn*	1 Slice/15g	21	0.9	140	15.0	5.8	6.3	3.0
Goujons, Quorn*	1 Goujon/31g	57	2.9	187	10.2	15.0	9.6	4.5
Grills, Lamb Style, Quorn*	1 Grill/89g	97	3.3	109	11.2	7.6	3.7	4.3

QUORN*

INFO/WEIGHT	Measure	per Measure KCAL	FAT	Nutrition Values per 100g / 100ml KCAL	PROT	CARB	FAT	FIBRE
Kievs, Mini, Quorn*	1 Kiev/20g	41	2.2	207	14.0	13.0	11.0	6.5
Lasagne, Frozen, Quorn*	1 Pack/300g	291	8.1	97	4.8	12.5	2.7	1.6
Light Bites, Quorn*	1 Pack/60g	86	3.0	143	16.2	5.0	5.0	6.5
Mexican Chilli, Quorn*	½ Pack/170g	143	4.3	84	6.6	6.5	2.5	4.5
Mince, Frozen & Chilled, Quorn*	1 Serving/87g	91	1.7	105	14.5	4.5	2.0	5.5
Mini Savoury Eggs, Quorn*	1 Egg/20g	50	2.3	248	15.0	21.0	11.5	4.6
Moussaka, Quorn*	1 Pack/400g	364	16.4	91	3.6	9.8	4.1	1.2
Noodles, Sweet Chilli, Quorn*	1 Pack/400g	352	9.2	88	4.2	12.7	2.3	1.5
Nuggets, Chicken Style, Quorn*	1 Nugget/20g	41	2.2	207	10.3	16.7	11.0	3.8
Nuggets, Crispy, Chicken Style, Quorn*	1 Nugget/17g	31	1.8	182	12.0	9.9	10.5	4.0
Ocean Pie, Fish Less, Quorn*	1 Pack/324g	424	24.3	131	5.8	9.0	7.5	2.0
Pasty, Cornish Style, Quorn*	1 Pasty/150g	399	24.0	266	5.5	25.0	16.0	3.0
Pate, Brussels Style, Deli, Quorn*	1/3 Pack/43g	55	2.3	128	11.3	8.5	5.4	4.0
Pate, Country Style Coarse, Quorn*	½ Pot/65g	68	2.7	104	9.2	7.3	4.2	2.7
Pie, Creamy Mushroom, Quorn*	1 Pie/142g	359	20.6	253	4.5	26.0	14.5	2.0
Pie, Creamy Mushroom, Sainsbury's*	1 Pie/134g	355	21.7	265	5.1	24.7	16.2	1.9
Pie, Mince & Onion, Quorn*	1 Pie/142g	360	19.8	254	5.0	27.0	14.0	1.5
Pie, Quorn & Mushroom, Tesco*	1 Pie/141g	378	23.7	268	5.3	23.8	16.8	1.3
Pork Style Ribsters, Quorn*	2 Ribsters/85g	105	3.3	124	15.9	6.3	3.9	2.1
Roast, Chicken Style, Quorn*	1/5 Roast/91g	96	1.8	106	15.0	4.5	2.0	4.9
Satay Skewers, Quorn*	1 Skewer/10g	19	0.7	183	16.7	14.0	6.7	4.5
Satay Sticks, Quorn*	½ Pack/90g	149	8.5	165	13.0	7.1	9.4	3.2
Sausage, Seasoned with Chopped Onion, Quorn*	1 Sausage/42g	51	1.6	120	14.9	6.7	3.7	3.3
Sausage & Mash, Quorn*	1 Pack/400g	332	9.2	83	4.6	9.5	2.3	2.7
Sausage Roll, Chilled, Quorn*	1 Roll/75g	194	9.6	258	12.0	24.0	12.7	4.0
Sausages, Bangers, BBQ, Sizzling, Quorn*	1 Banger/50g	98	5.5	195	12.0	9.5	11.0	5.0
Sausages, Bangers, Bramley Apple, Quorn*	1 Sausage/50g	59	2.3	117	11.5	7.5	4.6	3.0
Sausages, Bangers, Quorn*	1 Sausage/50g	58	2.4	116	11.7	6.6	4.8	3.0
Sausages, Cocktail, Quorn*	1 Sausage/10g	15	0.6	155	13.0	11.0	6.5	4.5
Sausages, Cumberland, Quorn*	1 Sausage/50g	86	3.5	172	13.5	12.0	7.0	3.5
Sausages, Frankfurter, Quorn*	1 Frankfurter/45g	82	5.8	183	12.5	4.0	13.0	3.0
Sausages, Leek & Pork Style, Quorn*	1 Sausage/44g	56	2.2	127	15.1	5.5	4.9	4.3
Sausages, Pork & Apple Style, Quorn*	1 Sausage/50g	58	2.3	117	11.5	7.5	4.6	3.0
Sausages, Red Leicester & Onion, Quorn*	1 Sausage/50g	72	2.9	144	13.0	10.0	5.8	3.0
Sausages, Sizzlers, BBQ, Quorn*	1 Sausage/50g	83	5.4	165	13.0	4.0	10.8	4.0
Sausages, Smoky Red Pepper Sizzlers, Quorn*	1 Sausage/50g	83	5.4	165	13.0	4.0	10.8	4.0
Sausages, Spinach & Cheese, Quorn*	1 Sausage/50g	60	2.0	120	15.1	6.0	4.0	2.8
Sausages, Sweet Chilli, Quorn*	1 Sausage/50g	63	2.3	125	14.0	7.0	4.5	3.0
Seasoned Steak, Strips, Quorn*	½ Pack/70g	76	0.9	109	14.0	7.5	1.3	5.5
Slices, Chicken Style, Deli, Quorn*	1 Slice/13g	13	0.3	107	16.3	4.5	2.6	6.0
Slices, Chicken Style, Wafer Thin, Deli, Quorn*	1/3 Pack/60g	64	1.6	107	16.3	4.5	2.6	5.9
Slices, Ham Style, Deli, Quorn*	1 Slice/13g	14	0.3	110	16.0	6.5	2.2	5.8
Slices, Ham Style, Smoky, Quorn*	½ Pack/50g	55	1.2	110	16.5	5.7	2.4	5.0
Slices, Ham Style, Wafer Thin, Deli, Quorn*	1/3 Pack/60g	66	1.3	110	16.0	6.5	2.2	5.8
Slices, Peppered Beef Style, Quorn*	½ Pack/50g	53	1.0	107	14.5	7.6	2.1	4.0
Slices, Turkey Style & Cranberry, Quorn*	½ Pack/50g	56	1.2	113	14.5	8.0	2.5	4.0
Slices, Turkey Style with Stuffing, Deli, Quorn*	½ Pack/50g	53	1.1	107	14.9	6.6	2.3	4.7
Southern Style, Fried Strips, Quorn*	1 Strip/31g	62	2.9	200	9.5	19.0	9.5	3.5
Spaghetti Bolognese, Quorn*	1 Pack/400g	240	3.6	60	3.7	9.2	0.9	1.6
Spaghetti Bolognese, Sainsbury's*	1 Pack/450g	346	4.9	77	4.9	11.9	1.1	1.8
Spaghetti Carbonara, Quorn*	1 Pack/400g	460	26.0	115	5.0	9.1	6.5	1.1
Spring Rolls, Mini, Quorn*	1 Roll/20g	41	2.1	205	4.5	23.0	10.5	2.4

Q

	Measure INFO/WEIGHT	per Measure		Nutrition Values per 100g / 100ml				
		KCAL	FAT	KCAL	PROT	CARB	FAT	FIBRE
RABBIT								
Meat Only, Raw	1oz/28g	38	1.5	137	21.9	0.0	5.5	0.0
Meat Only, Stewed	1oz/28g	32	0.9	114	21.2	0.0	3.2	0.0
Meat Only, Stewed, Weighed with Bone	1oz/28g	19	0.5	68	12.7	0.0	1.9	0.0
RADDICCIO								
Raw	1oz/28g	4	0.1	14	1.4	1.7	0.2	1.8
RADISH								
Red, Unprepared, Average	1 Radish/8g	1	0.0	12	0.7	1.9	0.2	0.9
White, Mooli, Raw	1oz/28g	4	0.0	15	0.8	2.9	0.1	0.0
RAISINS								
Seedless, Average	1 Serving/75g	215	0.4	287	2.2	68.5	0.5	3.1
White Chocolate Coated, Graze*	1 Pack/30g	135	6.6	451	4.7	59.7	21.9	0.0
RAITA								
Plain, Average	1oz/28g	16	0.6	57	4.2	5.8	2.2	0.0
RASPBERRIES								
Dried, Graze*	1 Pack/30g	85	0.8	284	3.2	62.0	2.6	0.0
Freeze Dried, Simply*	1 Serving/10g	37	0.0	370	10.0	80.0	0.0	20.0
Fresh, Raw, Average	1 Serving/80g	20	0.2	25	1.3	4.7	0.3	6.5
Frozen, Average	1 Serving/100g	27	0.3	27	1.3	4.7	0.3	5.2
in Fruit Juice, Average	1oz/28g	9	0.0	31	0.8	6.7	0.1	1.7
in Fruit Juice, Canned, John West*	1 Can/290g	93	0.6	32	0.9	6.7	0.2	1.5
in Syrup, Canned	1oz/28g	25	0.0	88	0.6	22.5	0.1	1.5
RATATOUILLE								
Average	1oz/28g	23	2.0	82	1.3	3.8	7.0	1.8
Chicken, Finest, Tesco*	1 Pack/550g	407	11.5	74	7.8	5.9	2.1	0.0
Princes*	1 Can/360g	86	1.4	24	1.0	4.2	0.4	0.0
Roasted Vegetable, Sainsbury's*	1 Pack/300g	134	3.0	45	1.4	7.5	1.0	2.3
RAVIOLI								
Asparagus, Waitrose*	1 Serving/150g	303	9.0	202	10.5	26.4	6.0	2.0
Basil & Parmesan, Organic, Sainsbury's*	½ Pack/192g	290	10.0	151	7.4	21.1	5.2	2.1
Beef	1 Serving/300g	501	13.7	167	6.4	25.0	4.6	1.4
Beef, GFY, Asda*	½ Pack/150g	288	4.8	192	7.0	33.9	3.2	1.9
Beef, in Tomato Sauce, Canned, Asda*	1 Can/400g	352	8.0	88	3.6	14.0	2.0	3.0
Beef, in Tomato Sauce, Canned, Great Stuff, Asda*	1 Can/200g	146	3.0	73	2.2	12.7	1.5	1.4
Beef, Tesco*	1 Serving/194g	175	5.0	90	4.3	12.3	2.6	1.5
Beef & Red Wine, Italiano, Tesco*	½ Pack/150g	315	9.7	210	7.3	30.0	6.5	2.3
Beef & Shiraz, Finest, Tesco*	½ Pack/200g	358	9.0	179	8.4	26.1	4.5	1.8
Cheese, Garlic & Herb, Fresh, Organic, Tesco*	1 Serving/125g	382	19.5	306	11.3	30.1	15.6	0.9
Cheese, in Tomato Sauce, Canned, Tesco*	1 Can/410g	328	8.2	80	2.5	13.0	2.0	0.5
Cheese & Asparagus, Waitrose*	1 Serving/100g	242	7.2	242	12.6	31.7	7.2	2.4
Cheese & Tomato, Fresh, Organic, Tesco*	1 Serving/125g	342	14.0	274	12.5	30.8	11.2	1.1
Cheese & Tomato, Heinz*	1 Can/400g	340	8.4	85	2.4	13.9	2.1	0.9
Cherry Tomato & Mushroom, Somerfield*	1 Pack/400g	436	24.8	109	3.5	9.8	6.2	1.2
Chicken, Tomato & Basil, Finest, Tesco*	1 Serving/200g	358	12.0	179	9.6	21.7	6.0	1.0
Chicken & Rosemary, Perfectly Balanced, Waitrose*	½ Pack/125g	266	4.4	213	14.9	30.4	3.5	2.1
Chicken & Tomato, Perfectly Balanced, Waitrose*	1 Serving/125g	265	3.4	212	13.5	33.4	2.7	2.8
Feta Cheese, M & S*	1 Serving/100g	195	8.5	195	9.1	20.5	8.5	1.3
Five Cheese, Weight Watchers*	1 Pack/330g	271	9.2	82	3.2	11.1	2.8	0.8
Florentine, Weight Watchers*	1 Serving/241g	220	5.0	91	3.7	14.1	2.1	1.2
Four Cheese, Good Intentions, Somerfield*	1 Pack/353g	367	12.4	104	4.1	14.0	3.5	1.7
Four Cheese in Tomato Sauce, COU, M & S*	1 Pack/345g	345	7.6	100	7.5	12.3	2.2	1.5
Fresh, Pasta Reale*	1 Serving/150g	459	8.8	306	13.1	53.3	5.9	0.0
Garlic & Herb, Italiano, Tesco*	1 Serving/100g	318	13.0	318	11.1	39.1	13.0	2.6
Garlic Mushroom, Finest, Tesco*	1 Serving/250g	552	18.2	221	8.9	30.0	7.3	2.0

R

	Measure INFO/WEIGHT	per Measure KCAL	FAT	Nutrition Values per 100g / 100ml KCAL	PROT	CARB	FAT	FIBRE
RAVIOLI								
Goat's Cheese & Pesto, Asda*	½ Pack/150g	204	5.4	136	6.0	20.0	3.6	0.0
Goats Cheese & Roasted Red Pepper, Finest, Tesco*	½ Pack/125g	307	9.6	246	11.4	32.8	7.7	1.8
Grana Padano & Rocket, Finest, Tesco*	½ Pack/150g	270	7.5	180	7.5	26.0	5.0	1.8
Meat, Italian, Fresh, Asda*	½ Pack/150g	261	6.3	174	8.0	26.0	4.2	0.0
Mozzarella, Tomato & Basil, Tesco*	1 Serving/125g	304	12.7	243	13.6	24.1	10.2	0.5
Mushroom, Fresh, Sainsbury's*	½ Pack/125g	196	5.1	157	7.4	22.6	4.1	1.9
Mushroom, Italiano, Tesco*	1 Serving/125g	332	16.1	266	10.4	27.0	12.9	3.0
Mushroom, Ready Meals, M & S*	1oz/28g	38	0.5	135	8.1	22.0	1.9	2.2
Mushroom, Wild, Finest, Tesco*	1 Serving/200g	472	12.2	236	10.8	34.4	6.1	1.9
Mushroomi, Tesco*	½ Pack/125g	332	16.1	266	10.4	27.0	12.9	3.0
Pancetta & Mozzarella, Finest, Tesco*	1 Serving/125g	344	13.2	275	12.2	32.8	10.6	1.8
Pork, in Tomato Sauce, Low Fat, Morrisons*	1oz/28g	23	0.3	81	2.7	15.5	0.9	1.3
Prosciuttoi, Ready Meal, M & S*	1 Pack/100g	195	8.1	195	13.3	17.0	8.1	1.0
Red Pepper, Basil & Chilli, Waitrose*	½ Pack/125g	312	10.5	250	11.6	32.0	8.4	1.7
Rich Beef & Red Wine, Morrisons*	1 Pack/300g	813	20.7	271	12.0	42.8	6.9	2.6
Roast Garlic & Herb, Tesco*	½ Pack/125g	342	13.6	274	12.8	31.1	10.9	1.1
Roasted Pepper, M & S*	1 Pack/400g	540	30.8	135	5.4	11.0	7.7	1.1
Roasted Vegetable, Asda*	½ Pack/150g	217	0.7	145	6.0	29.0	0.5	0.0
Roasted Vegetable, VLH Kitchens	½ Pack/140g	227	0.8	146	5.0	29.0	0.5	0.0
Salmon & Dill, Sainsbury's*	1 Pack/300g	615	21.3	205	8.7	26.5	7.1	3.0
Smoked Ham, Bacon & Tomato, Italiano, Tesco*	1 Can/125g	302	9.6	242	10.8	32.3	7.7	2.9
Smoked Salmon & Dill, Sainsbury's*	1 Serving/125g	256	8.9	205	8.7	26.5	7.1	0.7
Spinach & Ricotta, Waitrose*	1 Serving/125g	309	9.0	247	10.5	35.0	7.2	1.9
Sweet Pepper & Chilli, Tesco*	½ Pack/125g	324	14.0	259	12.5	27.1	11.2	2.7
Tomato, Cheese & Meat, Sainsbury's*	1 Serving/125g	314	16.1	251	12.4	21.4	12.9	2.2
Tomato, Cheese & Mortadella, Sainsbury's*	1 Serving/125g	272	13.2	218	10.3	20.3	10.6	2.4
Vegetable, Canned, Sainsbury's*	1 Can/400g	328	2.8	82	2.6	16.3	0.7	0.7
Vegetable, Tesco*	½ Can/200g	164	1.4	82	2.6	16.3	0.7	0.7
RED BULL*								
Energy Shot, Red Bull*	1 Can/60ml	27	0.0	45	0.0	10.7	0.0	0.0
Regular, Red Bull*	1 Can/250ml	112	0.0	45	0.0	11.3	0.0	0.0
REDCURRANTS								
Raw, Average	***1oz/28g***	***6***	***0.0***	***21***	***1.1***	***4.4***	***0.0***	***3.4***
Raw, Stalks Removed	1 Serving/100g	21	0.0	21	1.1	4.4	0.0	0.0
REEF*								
Orange & Passionfruit, Reef*	1 Bottle/275ml	179	0.0	65	0.0	9.5	0.0	0.0
REFRESHERS								
Bassett's*	1oz/28g	106	0.0	377	4.3	78.1	0.0	0.0
RELISH								
Barbeque, Sainsbury's*	1 Serving/50g	50	1.0	100	1.0	19.3	2.1	1.1
Burger, Juicy, Asda*	1 Tbsp/15g	17	0.1	113	1.2	25.4	0.7	0.7
Caramelised Onion & Chilli, M & S*	1 Serving/20g	47	0.2	235	1.4	55.1	1.1	1.0
Caramelised Red Onion, Tesco*	1 Serving/10g	28	0.0	280	0.6	69.1	0.1	0.7
Mango & Chilli, Levi Roots*	1 Serving/100g	110	0.2	110	0.7	25.0	0.2	1.1
Onion, Sainsbury's*	1 Serving/15g	23	0.1	151	0.9	36.0	0.4	0.7
Onion, Sweet, Heinz*	1 Tbsp/38g	38	0.1	102	1.0	23.5	0.4	0.6
Onion & Garlic, Spicy, Waitrose*	1 Tbsp/15g	35	0.2	232	0.8	54.2	1.1	1.7
Sweetcorn, American Style, Maryland, Tesco*	1 Serving/15g	15	0.0	101	1.1	23.9	0.1	0.9
Sweetcorn, Bick's*	1 Tbsp/22g	23	0.0	103	1.3	24.3	0.2	0.0
Tomato, Sweet, Heinz*	1 Serving/25g	34	0.0	136	0.9	32.6	0.2	0.9
Tomato & Chilli Texan Style, Tesco*	1 Tbsp/14g	20	0.0	140	1.7	32.0	0.1	1.1
Tomato Spicy, Bick's*	1 Serving/28g	28	0.1	99	1.3	23.2	0.2	0.0

R

	Measure INFO/WEIGHT	per Measure KCAL	FAT	Nutrition Values per 100g / 100ml KCAL	PROT	CARB	FAT	FIBRE
REVELS								
Mars*	1 Packet/35g	168	7.3	480	5.1	68.0	20.9	0.0
RHUBARB								
In Juice, Canned, Drained, Average	1 Serving/100g	46	0.0	46	0.5	10.8	0.0	0.8
Raw, Average	*1 Stalk/51g*	*11*	*0.1*	*21*	*0.9*	*4.5*	*0.2*	*1.8*
Stewed with Sugar, Average	*1oz/28g*	*32*	*0.0*	*116*	*0.4*	*31.2*	*0.0*	*2.0*
RIBENA*								
Apple Juice Drink, Ribena*	1 Carton/287ml	132	0.0	46	0.0	11.1	0.0	0.0
Blackcurrant, Diluted with Water, Ribena*	1 Serving/100ml	46	0.0	46	0.0	11.4	0.0	0.0
Blackcurrant, Original, Undiluted, Ribena*	1 Serving/20ml	46	0.0	230	0.0	57.0	0.0	0.0
Blackcurrant, Really Light, No Added Sugar, Ribena*	1 Carton/250ml	7	0.0	3	0.0	0.7	0.0	0.0
Blackcurrant & Cranberry, Ribena*	1 Bottle/500ml	205	0.0	41	0.0	9.9	0.0	0.0
Blackcurrant Juice Drink, Ready Made, Ribena*	1 Carton/200ml	86	0.0	43	0.0	10.6	0.0	0.0
Light, Ribena*	1 Carton/288ml	26	0.0	9	0.1	2.1	0.0	0.0
RIBS								
Loin, BBQ, Sainsbury's*	1 Rib/42g	104	5.5	247	24.7	7.3	13.2	0.9
Loin, Chinese, Sainsbury's*	1 Rib/42g	103	5.0	246	27.2	7.2	12.0	0.9
Loin, Chinese, Taste Summer, Sainsbury's*	1 Serving/30g	38	2.3	128	11.7	2.8	7.8	0.1
Pork, Barbecue, Average	1 Serving/100g	275	17.9	275	21.4	7.2	17.9	0.3
Pork, Chinese Style, Average	1 Serving/300g	736	44.7	245	17.9	10.0	14.9	0.7
Pork, Full Rack, Sainsbury's*	1 Serving/225g	567	38.7	252	18.0	6.5	17.2	0.9
Pork, Raw, Average	1oz/28g	47	2.8	169	18.6	1.8	9.9	0.2
Spare, Cantonese, Mini, Sainsbury's*	1 Rib/38g	97	5.0	259	17.2	17.3	13.4	1.0
Spare, Chinese Style, Meal Solutions, Co-Op*	1 Serving/165g	214	14.8	130	8.0	4.0	9.0	0.2
Spare, Chinese Style, Summer Eating, Asda*	1 Serving/116g	334	18.6	288	32.0	4.1	16.0	0.8
Spare, Sweet, Sticky, Mini, M & S*	1 Pack/300g	615	34.5	205	16.6	8.6	11.5	0.2
RICCOLI								
Egg, Fresh, Waitrose*	1oz/28g	81	1.0	289	11.4	53.1	3.4	2.1
RICE								
Arborio, Dry, Average	*1 Serving/80g*	*279*	*0.6*	*348*	*7.1*	*78.3*	*0.8*	*0.8*
Balti Style, Quick, Sainsbury's*	1 Serving/228g	192	1.1	84	4.3	15.7	0.5	2.0
Basmati, Boil in the Bag, Dry, Average	1 Serving/50g	176	0.4	352	8.4	77.8	0.8	0.4
Basmati, Brown, Dry, Average	*1 Serving/50g*	*177*	*1.5*	*353*	*9.5*	*71.8*	*3.0*	*2.2*
Basmati, Cooked, Average	*1 Serving/140g*	*189*	*1.0*	*135*	*3.1*	*29.0*	*0.7*	*0.4*
Basmati, Cooked, Tilda*	1 Serving/200g	214	0.2	107	2.4	24.0	0.1	1.2
Basmati, Dry Weight, Average	*1 Serving/60g*	*212*	*0.6*	*353*	*8.1*	*77.9*	*1.0*	*0.6*
Basmati, Indian, Dry, Average	*1 Serving/75g*	*260*	*0.7*	*346*	*8.4*	*76.1*	*0.9*	*0.1*
Basmati, Microwave, Cooked, Average	1 Serving/125g	182	2.3	145	2.7	30.0	1.8	0.0
Basmati, White, Dry, Average	*1 Serving/75g*	*262*	*0.4*	*349*	*8.1*	*77.1*	*0.6*	*2.2*
Basmati & Wild, Dry Weight, Tilda*	1 Serving/70g	244	0.3	349	9.4	77.0	0.5	1.0
Basmati with Mushroom, Dine In, Veetee*	1 Pack/280g	372	6.4	133	3.3	24.4	2.3	1.2
BBQ & Spicy, M & S*	1 Pack/250g	462	18.0	185	6.1	23.7	7.2	1.2
Beef, Savoury, Batchelors*	1 Pack/120g	431	2.8	359	8.9	75.7	2.3	2.5
Brown, Cooked, Average	*1 Serving/140g*	*173*	*1.5*	*123*	*2.6*	*26.6*	*1.1*	*0.9*
Brown, Dry, Average	*1 Serving/75g*	*266*	*2.3*	*355*	*7.5*	*76.2*	*3.0*	*1.4*
Brown, Long Grain, Dry, Average	*1 Serving/50g*	*182*	*1.4*	*363*	*7.6*	*76.8*	*2.8*	*2.0*
Brown, Short Grain, Dry, Average	*1 Serving/50g*	*175*	*1.4*	*351*	*6.8*	*77.6*	*2.8*	*0.9*
Brown, Whole Grain, Cooked, Average	*1 Serving/170g*	*223*	*1.9*	*131*	*2.6*	*27.8*	*1.1*	*1.2*
Brown, Whole Grain, Dry, Average	*1 Serving/40g*	*138*	*1.2*	*344*	*7.4*	*71.6*	*2.9*	*3.0*
Chicken, Savoury, Batchelors*	1 Pack/124g	455	1.9	367	8.9	79.4	1.5	2.6
Chilli & Coriander, TTD, Sainsbury's*	1 Pack/446g	522	12.5	117	6.5	16.5	2.8	2.2
Chinese Savoury, Batchelors*	1 Serving/50g	177	1.2	354	9.9	73.1	2.4	2.8
Coconut, M & S*	½ Pack/124g	217	5.0	175	3.1	31.8	4.0	0.3
Coconut, Thai, Sainsbury's*	½ Pack/100g	178	9.1	178	2.6	21.3	9.1	1.9

	Measure INFO/WEIGHT	per Measure KCAL	FAT	Nutrition Values per 100g / 100ml KCAL	PROT	CARB	FAT	FIBRE
RICE								
Coconut & Lime, Asda*	1 Pack/360g	695	17.6	193	4.5	32.7	4.9	0.9
Egg Fried, Average	1 Serving/300g	624	31.8	208	4.2	25.7	10.6	0.4
Express Microwave, Uncle Ben's*	1 Serving/250g	370	4.2	148	3.2	30.0	1.7	0.0
Fried, Chicken, Chinese Takeaway, Iceland*	1 Pack/340g	510	15.6	150	6.5	20.7	4.6	0.6
Fried, Duck, Chicken & Pork Celebration, Sainsbury's*	1 Pack/450g	544	16.2	121	7.9	14.2	3.6	1.5
Garlic & Butter Flavoured, Batchelors*	1 Serving/50g	175	1.4	350	8.0	79.8	2.8	5.0
Garlic & Coriander Flavoured, Patak's*	1 Serving/125g	186	2.7	149	2.6	28.9	2.2	0.0
Golden Savoury, Dry Weight, Batchelors*	1 Pack/120g	437	3.4	364	10.1	74.7	2.8	2.4
Golden Savoury, Nirvana*	1 Pack/120g	142	0.8	118	2.5	25.4	0.7	2.9
Golden Vegetable, Freshly Frozen, Asda*	1 Sachet/200g	238	2.6	119	3.2	23.6	1.3	1.3
Ground, Whitworths*	1 Serving/28g	98	0.2	349	7.7	77.7	0.8	0.7
Lemon Pepper in 5, Crosse & Blackwell*	½ Pack/163g	201	2.1	123	2.7	25.2	1.3	4.0
Lemon Pepper Speciality, Asda*	1 Serving/52g	67	0.7	129	2.0	27.0	1.4	0.1
Long Grain, & Wild, Dry, Average	*1 Serving/75g*	*254*	*1.5*	*338*	*7.6*	*72.6*	*2.0*	*1.7*
Long Grain, American, Cooked, Average	*1 Serving/160g*	*229*	*2.8*	*143*	*3.0*	*28.7*	*1.7*	*0.2*
Long Grain, American, Dry, Average	*1 Serving/50g*	*175*	*0.5*	*350*	*7.1*	*77.8*	*1.1*	*0.6*
Long Grain, Dry, Average	*1 Serving/50g*	*169*	*0.5*	*337*	*7.4*	*75.5*	*1.0*	*1.7*
Long Grain, Microwavable, Cooked, Average	1 Serving/150g	180	0.9	120	2.7	25.8	0.6	0.7
Paella, Savoury, Tesco*	1 Serving/60g	220	2.8	367	8.4	72.7	4.7	4.5
Pilau, Cooked, Average	*1 Serving/140g*	*244*	*6.2*	*174*	*3.5*	*30.3*	*4.4*	*0.8*
Pilau, Dry, Average	*1oz/28g*	*101*	*0.7*	*361*	*8.4*	*78.2*	*2.3*	*3.4*
Pudding, Dry Weight, Average	1 Serving/100g	355	1.1	355	6.9	82.0	1.1	0.3
Risotto, Dry, Average	*1 Serving/50g*	*174*	*0.6*	*348*	*7.8*	*76.2*	*1.3*	*2.4*
Saffron, Cooked, Average	*1 Serving/150g*	*208*	*4.7*	*139*	*2.5*	*25.3*	*3.1*	*0.5*
Thai, Cooked, Average	*1 Serving/100g*	*135*	*1.7*	*135*	*2.5*	*27.4*	*1.7*	*0.3*
Thai, Dry, Average	*1 Serving/50g*	*174*	*0.2*	*348*	*7.1*	*78.9*	*0.4*	*0.9*
Thai, Fragrant, Dry, Average	*1 Serving/75g*	*272*	*0.5*	*363*	*7.2*	*82.0*	*0.7*	*0.3*
Thai, Glutinous, Sticky, White, Dry, Raw	1 Serving/100g	370	0.6	370	6.8	81.7	0.6	2.8
White, Cooked, Average	*1 Serving/140g*	*182*	*1.1*	*130*	*2.6*	*28.7*	*0.8*	*0.1*
White, Cooked, Frozen, Average	*1 Serving/150g*	*168*	*0.8*	*112*	*2.9*	*23.8*	*0.5*	*1.1*
White, Flaked, Dry Weight, Average	*1oz/28g*	*97*	*0.3*	*346*	*6.6*	*77.5*	*1.2*	*0.0*
White, Fried	1oz/28g	37	0.9	131	2.2	25.0	3.2	0.6
White, Long Grain, Dry Weight, Average	*1 Serving/50g*	*181*	*1.0*	*362*	*7.1*	*79.1*	*1.9*	*0.4*
White, Microwave, Cooked, Average	1 Serving/150g	157	0.7	105	2.7	22.4	0.5	1.1
Whole, Dry Weight, Hacendado*	1 Bag/1000g	3320	29.1	332	7.2	63.3	2.9	7.8
Whole Grain, Dry, Average	*1 Serving/50g*	*171*	*1.1*	*341*	*8.2*	*72.0*	*2.3*	*4.0*
Wholegrain, Microwave, Eat Well, M & S*	½ Pack/125g	181	1.5	145	2.5	31.0	1.2	2.2
Wild, Coronation, Sainsbury's*	¼ Pot/75g	139	4.8	186	3.1	29.1	6.4	0.9
Wild, Giant Canadian, Dry Weight, Tilda*	1 Serving/75g	262	0.6	350	11.5	74.2	0.8	1.9
Yellow, Ready Cooked, Tesco*	1oz/28g	32	0.4	113	2.7	27.1	1.3	0.1
RICE CAKES								
Apple & Cinnamon Flavour, Kallo*	1 Cake/11g	41	0.2	376	6.2	83.1	2.2	3.9
Asda*	1 Cake/8g	31	0.2	386	8.7	81.1	3.0	2.8
Bacon, Asda*	1 Cake/9g	42	1.6	462	8.0	67.0	18.0	0.0
Barbecue, Sainsbury's*	1 Pack/30g	121	2.6	403	7.9	73.5	8.6	2.7
Black & White Sesame, Clearspring*	1 Cake/8g	31	0.2	385	7.4	82.2	2.9	0.0
Brink*	1 Cake/15g	55	0.3	370	8.8	78.8	2.2	0.0
Butter Popcorn, Snack-A-Jacks, Quaker Oats*	1 Cake/9g	35	0.0	389	11.1	88.9	0.0	0.0
Caramel, Jumbo, Tesco*	1 Cake/10g	34	0.3	340	7.0	74.0	3.0	5.0
Caramel, Large, Tesco*	1 Cake/10g	34	0.2	344	6.5	73.9	2.5	5.1
Caramel, Less Than 3% Fat, Sainsbury's*	1 Pack/35g	134	0.6	382	5.6	86.4	1.6	1.8
Caramel, Snack Size, Tesco*	1 Pack/35g	133	1.0	379	5.5	82.7	2.9	0.9
Caramel, Tesco*	1 Serving/2g	9	0.1	379	5.5	98.2	2.9	0.9

	Measure INFO/WEIGHT	per Measure KCAL	FAT	Nutrition Values per 100g / 100ml KCAL	PROT	CARB	FAT	FIBRE
RICE CAKES								
Caramel Flavour, Kallo*	1 Cake/10g	38	0.5	383	6.2	78.9	4.8	3.9
Cheese, Jumbo, Free From, Tesco*	1 Serving/10g	44	1.8	439	8.1	62.1	17.6	3.8
Cheese & Onion, Namchow*	1 Serving/38g	141	1.2	377	7.2	79.5	3.3	0.0
Chilli, Mini, M & S*	1 Pack/22g	88	1.7	400	6.9	74.9	7.9	3.5
Dark Chocolate, Organic, Kallo*	1 Cake/12g	57	2.9	471	6.8	57.2	24.1	7.4
Five Grain, Finncrisp*	1 Cake/10g	36	0.2	356	9.8	73.9	1.7	9.7
High Fibre, Oat & Rice, Slightly Salted, Thick Slice, Kallo*	1 Cake/8g	27	0.4	356	10.6	75.0	5.5	9.0
Honey, Kallo*	1 Cake/10g	40	0.2	388	5.4	86.6	2.2	1.6
Japanese, Miso, Clearspring*	1 Cake/7g	27	0.2	365	9.2	77.0	3.0	2.0
Lightly Salted, Perfectly Balanced, Waitrose*	1 Cake/8g	31	0.2	387	8.3	82.4	2.7	2.1
Lightly Salted, Thick Slice, Low Fat, Kallo*	1 Cake/8g	28	0.2	372	8.0	78.7	2.8	5.1
Salt & Vinegar, Jumbo, Tesco*	1 Cake/9g	31	0.2	347	8.4	72.7	2.5	6.0
Salt & Vinegar, Sainsbury's*	1 Pack/30g	121	2.5	403	8.3	73.3	8.3	2.7
Salt & Vinegar, Snack, Tesco*	1 Pack/35g	116	0.6	332	7.5	71.5	1.8	1.1
Salt & Vinegar Flavour, Morrisons*	1 Bag/30g	122	2.6	407	6.7	75.8	8.6	1.2
Savoury, Jumbo, HL, Tesco*	1 Cake/8g	31	0.2	369	11.9	75.0	2.4	3.6
Sea Salt & Balsamic Vinegar, Kallo*	1 Cake/9g	32	0.2	361	6.5	78.1	2.5	3.0
Sesame, No Added Salt, Thick Sliced, Organic, Kallo*	1 Cake/10g	37	0.3	373	8.0	78.0	3.2	5.4
Sesame, Slightly Salted, Thick Slice, Organic, Kallo*	1 Cake/8g	28	0.2	373	8.0	78.0	3.2	5.4
Sesame, Slightly Salted, Thin Slice, Organic, Kallo*	1 Cake/5g	17	0.1	373	8.0	78.0	3.2	5.4
Sesame Garlic, Clearspring*	1 Serving/8g	29	0.2	382	7.8	82.3	2.4	0.0
Sesame Teriyaki, Clearspring*	1 Cake/7g	28	0.2	377	6.5	82.8	2.2	0.0
Slightly Salted, Mrs Crimble's*	1 Slice/6g	21	0.2	380	7.6	80.4	3.1	3.2
Slightly Salted, Organic, Thin Slice, Kallo*	1 Cake/5g	17	0.1	372	8.0	78.7	2.8	5.1
Slightly Salted, Thick Slice, Organic, Kallo*	1 Cake/8g	28	0.2	372	8.0	78.7	2.8	5.1
Slightly Salted, with Cracked Pepper, Snack Size, Kallo*	1 Cake/2g	8	0.1	372	8.0	78.7	2.8	5.1
Sour Cream & Chive Flavour, Sainsbury's*	1 Pack/30g	119	2.5	396	7.9	72.0	8.5	2.9
Whole Grain, No Added Salt, Thick Slice, Organic, Kallo*	1 Cake/9g	33	0.3	365	7.6	80.0	3.1	3.4
Wholegrain, Mild Chilli, Tesco*	1 Cake/10g	38	1.4	400	7.2	59.8	14.4	5.8
Wholegrain, No Added Salt, BGTY, Sainsbury's*	1 Cake/8g	30	0.2	372	8.0	78.7	2.8	5.1
Wholegrain, Salt & Vinegar, Tesco*	1 Cake/9g	28	0.2	314	8.4	61.9	2.6	6.0
RICE CRACKERS								
Authentic Thai Chilli, Tyrrells*	½ Pack/75g	389	20.2	519	5.0	64.0	27.0	1.0
Barbecue, Sakata*	½ Pack/50g	203	1.3	407	7.3	85.2	2.6	1.6
Barbecue Flavour, Tesco*	1 Pack/25g	102	1.8	409	6.7	78.8	7.4	1.7
Black Pepperdoms & Mango Chutney, Graze*	1 Punnet/28g	106	3.2	377	3.1	65.5	11.3	1.2
Brown, Wakama*	1 Cracker/5g	19	0.0	375	8.0	84.8	0.4	0.0
Cheddar Gorge, Graze*	1 Punnet/24g	128	8.3	534	10.6	48.3	34.7	2.3
Cheese, Tesco*	1 Serving/25g	104	2.0	416	7.9	78.1	8.0	1.8
Chilli, Temptations, Tesco*	1 Serving/25g	128	7.2	512	4.4	58.0	28.8	0.0
Chilli, Whitworths*	½ Pack/50g	253	12.8	507	5.1	63.9	25.7	0.5
Cracked Pepper, Sakata*	½ Pack/50g	200	1.5	400	7.3	84.4	3.0	2.0
Crispy, Chilli & Lime, Go Ahead, McVitie's*	1 Serving/25g	101	0.9	405	7.1	83.6	3.6	2.1
Crispy, Sea Salt & Vinegar, Go Ahead, McVitie's*	1 Serving/25g	102	1.3	408	6.6	80.6	5.4	1.8
Crispy, Sour Cream & Herbs, Go Ahead, McVitie's*	1 Serving/25g	105	2.0	422	7.1	78.2	8.0	1.8
Japanese, Apollo*	1 Pack/75g	297	3.5	396	9.6	78.8	4.7	0.9
Japanese, Graze*	1 Pack/40g	159	1.9	397	9.0	79.7	4.7	0.0
Japanese, Hider*	1 Pack/70g	303	12.1	433	11.3	61.7	17.3	0.0
Japanese, Julian Graves*	1 Serving/25g	92	0.4	369	8.8	79.5	1.7	3.8
Japanese, Mini, Sunrise*	1 Serving/50g	180	0.0	360	7.0	83.0	0.0	7.0
Japanese Seaweed, Very Nori-sh, Graze*	1 Punnet/14g	64	1.8	454	5.9	78.8	12.7	1.0
Korean Chilli, Graze*	1 Pack/19g	98	5.1	519	5.0	64.0	27.0	0.5
Mix, M & S*	½ Pack/63g	225	0.1	360	6.5	82.9	0.1	1.6

R

	Measure INFO/WEIGHT	per Measure		Nutrition Values per 100g / 100ml				
		KCAL	FAT	KCAL	PROT	CARB	FAT	FIBRE
RICE CRACKERS								
Paprika Flavour, Namchow*	1 Serving/38g	141	1.2	375	7.5	78.9	3.3	0.0
Salt & Pepper, Asda*	1 Cracker/5g	19	0.0	385	7.0	87.0	1.0	2.2
Salt & Vinegar, Namchow*	1 Serving/38g	139	1.4	370	6.7	77.5	3.7	0.0
Sour Cream & Chive, Sakata*	1 Serving/25g	107	2.0	430	7.8	80.6	7.9	0.0
Spicy Mix, Asda*	1 Serving/25g	115	4.2	461	6.4	71.2	16.7	0.2
Thai, M & S*	1 Serving/55g	209	1.8	380	7.0	80.2	3.3	1.2
Thai, Sesame & Soy Sauce, M & S*	1 Pack/55g	210	2.6	385	7.6	77.8	4.8	1.4
Thai, Wakama*	1 Cracker/2g	8	0.1	400	6.9	86.9	2.7	0.5
Thai Chilli, Nature's Harvest*	1 Pack/75g	401	22.3	535	4.6	61.5	29.7	4.2
Thin, Blue Dragon*	3 Crackers/5g	20	0.2	395	6.1	84.4	3.7	0.0
Veggie Sushi Plate, Graze*	1 Punnet/24g	107	3.1	444	11.1	68.4	12.8	3.9
with Tamari, Clearspring*	1 Bag/50g	190	0.7	380	8.2	83.4	1.5	0.3
RICE MILK								
Organic, Provamel*	1 Serving/250ml	122	3.7	49	0.1	9.5	1.5	0.0
Original, Rice Dream*	1 Serving/150ml	70	1.5	47	0.1	9.4	1.0	0.1
RICE PUDDING								
50% Less Fat, Asda*	½ Can/212g	180	1.7	85	3.3	16.2	0.8	0.2
Banana, Ambrosia*	1 Pot/150g	153	3.8	102	3.2	16.6	2.5	0.0
Canned, Average	1oz/28g	25	0.7	89	3.4	14.0	2.5	0.2
Canned, GFY, Asda*	½ Can/213g	168	1.3	79	2.8	15.5	0.6	0.1
Caramel, Ambrosia*	1 Pot/150g	149	3.8	99	3.1	16.1	2.5	0.0
COU, M & S*	1 Pot/171g	145	2.9	85	2.4	15.5	1.7	0.5
Creamed, Asda*	1 Serving/215g	196	3.4	91	3.2	16.0	1.6	0.0
Creamed, Canned, Ambrosia*	1 Can/425g	382	8.1	90	3.1	15.2	1.9	0.0
Creamed, Luxury, with Added Cream, Canned, Sainsbury's*	½ Can/212.5g	272	12.1	128	3.3	15.9	5.7	0.0
Creamed, Pot, Ambrosia*	1 Pot/150g	156	3.8	104	3.3	17.0	2.5	0.1
Creamy, Ambrosia*	½ Can/212g	197	4.0	93	3.2	15.7	1.9	0.0
Creamy, Delicious, Taste of Home, Heinz*	½ Can/212g	225	4.0	106	3.4	18.6	1.9	0.2
Creamy, with Strawberry Crunch, Ambrosia*	1 Pack/205g	297	8.6	145	3.9	23.0	4.2	0.7
Creamy Rice, Shape, Danone*	1 Serving/175g	149	1.7	85	3.5	15.4	1.0	0.4
Creamy Rice with Tropical Crunch, Ambrosia*	1 Pack/210g	307	8.8	146	3.6	23.4	4.2	0.6
Light, Creamy, Delicious, Taste of Home, Heinz*	½ Can/213g	194	1.3	91	3.4	18.0	0.6	0.2
Low Fat, Budgens*	1 Can/425g	370	3.8	87	3.4	16.3	0.9	0.0
Low Fat, No Added Sugar, Canned, Weight Watchers*	½ Can/212g	155	3.2	73	3.7	11.4	1.5	0.0
Luxury Rice, Llangadog Creamery*	1 Serving/220g	310	16.9	141	3.1	15.2	7.7	0.0
Organic, Ambrosia*	1 Can/425g	455	15.7	107	3.4	15.1	3.7	0.0
Original, Mullerrice, Muller*	1 Pot/190g	196	4.9	103	3.6	16.3	2.6	0.3
Perfectly Balanced, Waitrose*	1 Serving/154g	140	2.5	91	3.4	15.7	1.6	1.2
Raspberry, BGTY, Sainsbury's*	1 Pot/135g	126	1.6	93	3.2	17.2	1.2	1.3
Raspberry, Mullerice, Muller*	1 Std Pot/200g	218	4.4	109	3.2	19.1	2.2	0.6
Rhubarb, Muller*	1 Pot/200g	226	4.4	113	3.2	20.0	2.2	0.0
Strawberry, Mullerrice, Muller*	1 Pot/200g	220	4.4	110	3.2	19.3	2.2	0.4
Strawberry Flavour, Jan Jac*	1 Pot/200g	256	6.4	128	2.4	22.4	3.2	0.2
Thick & Creamy, Co-Op*	1 Can/425g	531	25.5	125	3.0	16.0	6.0	0.0
Thick & Creamy, Nestle*	1 Can/425g	527	23.8	124	3.1	15.4	5.6	0.2
Toffee Flavour, Jan Jac*	1 Pot/200g	270	7.8	135	2.4	22.5	3.9	0.1
Vanilla Custard, Mullerrice, Muller*	1 Pot/200g	230	5.0	115	3.4	19.8	2.5	0.3
Venetian, Cafe Culture, M & S*	1 Serving/120g	300	19.7	250	3.4	21.8	16.4	0.2
RICE SALAD								
Chicken Tikka, COU, M & S*	1 Pack/390g	409	3.9	105	5.1	18.7	1.0	0.6
Hot Smoked Salmon, Deli Meal, M & S*	1 Pack/380g	570	26.2	150	6.5	15.1	6.9	0.2
Indian Style with Chickpeas & Yoghurt Dressing, M & S*	1 Pack/220g	264	7.0	120	3.7	19.3	3.2	3.4
Mexican with Beans, COU, M & S*	1 Serving/250g	250	3.5	100	6.0	15.6	1.4	1.2

R

	Measure INFO/WEIGHT	per Measure KCAL	FAT	Nutrition Values per 100g / 100ml KCAL	PROT	CARB	FAT	FIBRE
RICE SALAD								
Rainbow, M & S*	1 Serving/262g	340	8.4	130	2.5	23.3	3.2	1.5
Rainbow, Waitrose*	1/3 Pack/60g	70	1.6	117	3.2	18.1	2.7	3.6
Red with Feta, M & S*	1 Pack/244g	440	20.8	180	4.8	21.0	8.5	1.3
Spanish Style with Chicken, M & S*	1 Serving/220g	319	12.8	145	5.8	17.4	5.8	0.5
RICE WINE								
Sake, Average	**1oz/28g**	**38**	**0.0**	**134**	**0.5**	**5.0**	**0.0**	**0.0**
Shaoxing, Waitrose*	1 Tbsp/15ml	21	0.0	138	1.6	3.9	0.0	0.2
RIGATONI								
Carbonara, Tesco*	1 Serving/205g	236	11.9	115	5.2	10.6	5.8	1.2
Dry, Average	**1 Serving/80g**	**272**	**1.2**	**339**	**11.4**	**68.4**	**1.5**	**2.7**
Tomato & Cheese, Perfectly Balanced, Waitrose*	1 Pack/400g	664	9.2	166	7.6	28.6	2.3	2.3
Tuna, Diet Chef Ltd*	1 Pack/300g	336	13.2	112	5.9	12.2	4.4	1.0
RISOTTO								
Bacon & Mushroom, Solo Slim, Rosemary Conley*	1 Pack/251g	223	6.5	89	5.8	10.8	2.6	2.8
Balls, Mushroom, Occasions, Sainsbury's*	1 Ball/25g	76	3.4	304	3.8	41.2	13.8	1.7
Balls, Sun Dried Tomato, Occasions, Sainsbury's*	1 Ball/25g	71	3.7	285	6.8	30.8	15.0	2.9
Beef, Vesta*	1 Serving/100g	346	5.9	346	15.3	57.8	5.9	5.6
Beetroot & Goats Cheese, Lovely Vegetables, M & S*	1 Pack/379g	530	17.0	140	4.4	20.7	4.5	3.6
Butternut, Pearl Barely, Veg Pot, Innocent*	1 Pot/390g	285	5.1	73	2.9	12.6	1.3	3.8
Caramelised Onion & Gruyere Cheese, M & S*	1 Pack/200g	350	20.6	175	3.0	17.8	10.3	1.7
Chargrilled Chicken, Ready Meal, M & S*	1 Pack/365g	493	25.2	135	6.4	11.6	6.9	0.7
Cheese Flavour, Made Up, Ainsley Harriott*	1 Sachet/140g	565	14.6	404	7.8	69.6	10.4	9.1
Cherry Tomato, COU, M & S*	1 Pack/360g	324	8.3	90	2.0	15.4	2.3	1.8
Chicken	1 Serving/380g	494	17.4	130	7.2	15.1	4.6	1.3
Chicken, BGTY, Sainsbury's*	1 Pack/327g	356	6.2	109	7.5	15.5	1.9	1.0
Chicken, Tomato & Mozzarella, GFY, Asda*	1 Pack/400g	356	4.0	89	8.1	11.9	1.0	1.2
Chicken & Bacon, Italiano, Tesco*	1 Pack/450g	652	20.2	145	5.9	20.2	4.5	1.5
Chicken & Lemon, Weight Watchers*	1 Pack/330g	327	6.9	99	6.3	13.7	2.1	0.5
Chicken & Mushroom, Finest, Tesco*	1 Pack/400g	496	11.2	124	7.4	17.2	2.8	0.5
Chicken & Mushroom, Solo Slim, Rosemary Conley*	1 Pack/300g	270	11.4	90	6.6	7.3	3.8	2.5
Chicken & Mushroom, Waitrose*	1 Pack/350g	364	16.1	104	6.0	9.7	4.6	0.8
Chicken & Mushroom, Weight Watchers*	1 Pack/320g	323	8.0	101	5.7	13.8	2.5	0.3
Chicken & Sun Dried Tomato, Waitrose*	1 Pack/350g	385	22.0	110	6.0	7.2	6.3	0.3
Green Bean, Asparagus & Pecorino, Finest, Tesco*	1 Pack/400g	460	15.6	115	4.4	15.0	3.9	1.5
Haddock & Mushroom, COU, M & S*	1 Pack/400g	320	3.2	80	6.4	12.1	0.8	2.0
Hot Smoked Salmon & Spinach, M & S*	½ Pack/300g	420	24.0	140	6.4	11.0	8.0	0.6
Italian, Smoked Haddock, Tesco*	½ Pack/350g	400	15.1	114	4.2	14.3	4.3	0.8
Italian Red Wine with Creamed Spinach, Sainsbury's*	1 Pack/400g	596	27.6	149	2.4	19.3	6.9	0.4
King Prawn, Pea & Mint, M & S*	½ Pack/300g	405	18.6	135	3.8	15.9	6.2	0.9
King Prawn & Snow Crab, M & S*	1 Pack/365g	401	16.4	110	4.1	12.7	4.5	0.5
Lemon & Mint, Perfectly Balanced, Waitrose*	1 Pack/350g	462	12.9	132	3.9	20.7	3.7	1.0
Mushroom, BGTY, Sainsbury's*	1 Pack/400g	387	8.7	102	2.7	17.6	2.3	1.0
Mushroom, COU, M & S*	1 Pack/375g	337	5.6	90	3.0	16.1	1.5	1.5
Mushroom, Diet Chef Ltd*	1 Pack/250g	215	7.2	86	3.2	12.0	2.9	0.2
Mushroom, Italiano, Tesco*	1 Pack/340g	367	6.8	108	2.4	20.0	2.0	4.6
Mushroom, Low Saturated Fat, Waitrose*	1 Pack/400g	440	9.6	110	4.6	15.1	2.4	1.5
Mushroom, Perfectly Balanced, Waitrose*	1 Pack/400g	384	6.4	96	4.3	16.1	1.6	2.1
Mushroom & Chestnut, Waitrose*	1 Pack/400g	496	90.0	124	14.6	58.4	22.5	7.2
Pea, Broad Bean & Asparagus, Lovely Vegetables, M & S*	1 Pack/380g	418	9.9	110	4.5	15.1	2.6	2.9
Primavera, with Asparagus, Spinach & Peas, COU, M & S*	1 Pack/375g	340	7.2	90	3.6	15.0	1.9	1.0
Roasted Red Pepper & Italian Cheese, M & S*	1 Pack/400g	500	13.2	125	2.9	20.4	3.3	1.0
Roasted Vegetable, Made Up, Ainsley Harriott*	1 Sachet/140g	766	18.2	547	11.0	96.5	13.0	15.5
Roasted Vegetable & Sunblush Tomato, Finest, Tesco*	½ Pack/200g	306	18.0	153	3.7	14.5	9.0	1.4

	Measure INFO/WEIGHT	per Measure KCAL	per Measure FAT	Nutrition Values per 100g / 100ml KCAL	PROT	CARB	FAT	FIBRE
RISOTTO								
Roasted Vegetables, Stir-In, Uncle Ben's*	½ Pack/75g	86	7.3	115	1.7	5.0	9.7	0.0
Salmon & Prawn, Eat Smart, Morrisons*	1 Pack/381g	339	5.3	89	4.9	14.1	1.4	0.8
Seafood, HL, Tesco*	1 Pack/365g	328	3.6	90	5.3	14.1	1.0	0.9
Seafood, Youngs*	1 Pack/350g	423	12.9	121	4.5	17.4	3.7	0.1
Spring Vegetable, M & S*	1 Serving/330g	330	13.2	100	2.0	14.2	4.0	0.9
Tomato & Cheese, GFY, Asda*	1 Pack/400g	428	12.0	107	3.1	17.0	3.0	0.7
Tomato & Chilli, Solo Slim, Rosemary Conley*	1 Pack/300g	240	8.7	80	6.8	6.7	2.9	3.5
Tomato & Mascarpone, Cooked, Ainsley Harriott*	1 Sachet/346g	553	18.7	160	2.5	25.3	5.4	1.6
Tomato & Mascarpone, M & S*	1 Pack/360g	468	19.1	130	2.7	17.5	5.3	0.9
Vegetable, Average	1oz/28g	41	1.8	147	4.2	19.2	6.5	2.2
Vegetable, Brown Rice, Average	1oz/28g	40	1.8	143	4.1	18.6	6.4	2.4
RISSOLES								
Lentil, Fried in Vegetable Oil, Average	1oz/28g	59	2.9	211	8.9	22.0	10.5	3.6
ROCK SALMON								
Raw, Flesh Only, Average	*1oz/28g*	*43*	*2.7*	*154*	*16.6*	*0.0*	*9.7*	*0.0*
ROCKET								
Fresh, Raw, Average	*1 Serving/80g*	*12*	*0.4*	*16*	*0.8*	*1.7*	*0.5*	*1.2*
Super Hot, Steve's Leaves*	1 Bag/30g	6	0.1	20	3.4	0.6	0.4	3.1
Wild, Morrisons*	1 Serving/100g	17	0.6	17	0.9	1.7	0.6	1.4
ROE								
Cod, Average	*1 Can/100g*	*96*	*2.8*	*96*	*17.1*	*0.5*	*2.8*	*0.0*
Cod, Hard, Coated in Batter, Fried	1oz/28g	53	3.3	189	12.4	8.9	11.8	0.2
Cod, Hard, Fried in Blended Oil	1oz/28g	57	3.3	202	20.9	3.0	11.9	0.1
Herring, Soft, Fried in Blended Oil	1oz/28g	74	4.4	265	26.3	4.7	15.8	0.2
Herring, Soft, Raw	*1oz/28g*	*25*	*0.7*	*91*	*16.8*	*0.0*	*2.6*	*0.0*
ROGAN JOSH								
Chicken, & Rice, Sainsbury's*	1 Pack/500g	675	27.0	135	6.7	14.1	5.4	2.4
Chicken, with Pilau Rice, Farmfoods*	1 Pack/325g	354	6.8	109	5.3	17.1	2.1	0.4
Chicken Breast, Chunks, Hot, Sainsbury's*	½ Pack/114g	143	2.0	126	23.6	3.9	1.8	1.0
King Prawn with Rice, HL, Tesco*	1 Pack/400g	365	6.0	91	4.8	14.6	1.5	1.6
Lamb, Sainsbury's*	1 Pack/400g	660	44.4	165	11.3	4.9	11.1	1.9
Lamb, Waitrose*	½ Pack/175g	241	13.3	138	12.4	5.0	7.6	1.3
Lamb & Pilau Rice, Tesco*	1 Pack/550g	770	29.1	140	6.0	16.9	5.3	1.0
Lamb with Pilau Rice, Eastern Classics*	1 Pack/400g	604	21.6	151	5.6	19.9	5.4	1.0
Prawn, COU, M & S*	1 Pack/400g	360	2.4	90	4.9	16.2	0.6	0.8
ROLL								
All Day Breakfast, Asda*	1 Roll/220g	581	26.4	264	10.0	29.0	12.0	0.0
Beef, Weight Watchers*	1 Roll/174g	276	4.4	159	10.8	23.1	2.5	1.0
Brie & Grapes, M & S*	1 Roll/57g	174	10.4	306	11.1	24.5	18.2	1.4
Cheese, Tomato & Onion, Sainsbury's*	1 Pack/100g	518	28.1	518	18.4	47.9	28.1	0.0
Cheese & Chutney, M & S*	1 Roll/165g	256	1.2	155	13.9	23.1	0.7	1.2
Cheese & Onion, Asda*	1 Serving/67g	199	12.0	298	7.0	27.0	18.0	2.0
Cheese & Onion, M & S*	1 Roll/25g	80	5.1	320	9.6	24.7	20.5	1.3
Cheese & Onion, Sainsbury's*	1 Roll/67g	205	13.6	306	8.0	22.9	20.3	1.9
Cheese & Onion, Tesco*	1 Roll/67g	203	12.1	305	7.3	28.0	18.1	1.9
Cheese & Pickle, Sainsbury's*	1 Roll/136g	359	13.6	264	10.6	35.1	10.0	0.0
Chicken & Herb, Shapers, Boots*	1 Roll/168g	290	4.7	173	12.0	25.0	2.8	1.7
Chicken & Stuffing, Tesco*	1 Roll/323g	1043	58.8	323	10.4	29.4	18.2	1.0
Chicken & Sun Dried Tomato, Weight Watchers*	1 Pack/170g	272	3.2	160	12.9	22.7	1.9	1.2
Egg & Bacon, Sub, Shapers, Boots*	1 Serving/169g	320	7.3	189	11.0	27.0	4.3	1.3
Egg & Cress, HL, Tesco*	1 Pack/175g	322	6.8	184	9.6	27.7	3.9	1.2
Egg & Tomato, Shapers, Boots*	1 Roll/166g	301	5.3	181	8.0	30.0	3.2	2.6
Egg Mayo & Cress, Fullfillers*	1 Roll/125g	266	11.8	213	10.0	25.7	9.4	0.0

	Measure INFO/WEIGHT	per Measure KCAL	FAT	Nutrition Values per 100g / 100ml KCAL	PROT	CARB	FAT	FIBRE
ROLL								
Egg Mayonnaise & Cress, White, Soft, Somerfield*	1 Serving/211g	475	17.3	225	9.4	28.2	8.2	2.1
Ham, Darwins Deli*	1 Serving/125g	298	7.5	238	11.0	37.4	6.0	0.0
Ham & Cheese in Pastry, Pork Farms*	1 Roll/70g	216	12.5	308	8.0	28.8	17.9	0.0
Ham Salad, BGTY, Sainsbury's*	1 Roll/178g	292	3.4	164	10.8	25.9	1.9	0.0
Lincolnshire Sausage, COU, M & S*	1 Roll/175g	280	4.7	160	10.0	23.2	2.7	2.6
Mushroom & Bacon, Crusty, M & S*	1 Roll/160g	424	20.2	265	8.7	29.0	12.6	2.3
Oak Smoked Salmon, M & S*	1 Roll/55g	139	6.2	252	14.6	23.1	11.3	1.2
Ploughman's, 4 Pack, Ginsters*	1 Roll/60g	220	16.3	367	9.2	21.4	27.2	2.1
Ploughman's, Large, Ginsters*	1 Pack/140g	473	33.5	338	10.2	20.5	23.9	1.8
Roast Chicken & Mayonnaise, Big, Sainsbury's*	1 Pack/185g	479	27.4	259	9.6	21.8	14.8	0.0
Roast Chicken & Sweetcure Bacon, Boots*	1 Pack/245g	690	34.3	282	13.0	26.0	14.0	1.6
Roast Chicken Salad, Improved, Shapers, Boots*	1 Pack/188g	302	3.6	161	11.0	25.0	1.9	1.6
Roast Pork, Stuffing & Apple Sauce, Boots*	1 Roll/218g	602	26.2	276	10.0	32.0	12.0	1.8
Spicy Chicken, Crusty, M & S*	1 Roll/150g	382	16.6	255	12.8	25.8	11.1	2.0
Spicy Pork, Large, Ginsters*	1 Roll/140g	511	38.9	365	9.0	19.8	27.8	4.1
Steak & Onion, M & S*	1 Serving/150g	307	10.5	205	11.0	24.5	7.0	3.8
Tomato & Basil, Sub, COU, M & S*	1 Roll/35g	93	0.9	265	11.0	48.7	2.7	2.4
Tuna & Sweetcorn, with Mayonnaise, Shell*	1 Pack/180g	536	26.3	298	13.1	28.6	14.6	0.0
Tuna Cheese Melt, Boots*	1 Roll/199g	612	35.8	308	13.0	23.0	18.0	1.2
Tuna Mayo & Cucumber, Taste!*	1 Serving/111g	274	12.5	247	9.0	27.3	11.3	0.0
Tuna Mayonnaise with Cucumber, Yummies*	1 Serving/132g	340	18.6	257	10.4	22.5	14.0	0.0
Turkey, Stuffed, GFY, Asda*	½ Pack/225g	319	9.4	142	14.0	12.0	4.2	0.8
Turkey Salad, Northern Bites*	1 Roll/231g	323	8.3	140	8.6	19.6	3.6	3.0
White, Cheese & Onion, Shell*	1 Roll/178g	554	26.3	311	14.5	30.2	14.8	0.0
ROLO								
Chocolate, Nestle*	2 Pieces/20g	102	5.3	509	4.1	62.6	26.6	1.3
Giant, Nestle*	1 Sweet/9g	42	1.8	470	3.1	70.1	19.7	0.3
Little, Nestle*	1 Pack/40g	196	9.4	491	4.0	65.5	23.5	0.5
Nestle*	1 Sweet/5g	24	1.0	471	3.2	68.5	20.5	0.3
ROOT BEER								
Average	1 Can/330ml	135	0.0	41	0.0	10.6	0.0	0.0
Spring Water & Natural Sarsaparilla, Francis Hartridges*	1 Bottle/330ml	139	0.0	42	0.0	11.2	0.0	0.0
ROSEHIP								
Wild	1 Serving/100g	162	0.3	162	1.6	38.2	0.3	24.1
ROSEMARY								
Dried	*1 Tsp/1g*	*3*	*0.2*	*331*	*4.9*	*46.4*	*15.2*	*0.0*
Fresh	*1 Tsp/0.7g*	*1*	*0.0*	*99*	*1.4*	*13.5*	*4.4*	*0.0*
ROSTI								
Garlic & Mushroom, Finest, Tesco*	1 Serving/200g	346	19.6	173	5.7	15.4	9.8	1.7
Honey & Parsnip, Tesco*	1 Rosti/75g	79	2.4	105	1.8	17.0	3.2	3.9
Oven Baked, McCain*	1 Rosti/100g	194	9.3	194	2.6	25.0	9.3	2.3
Potato, Chicken & Sweetcorn Bake, Asda*	1 Serving/400g	440	18.8	110	7.0	10.0	4.7	0.6
Potato, McCain*	1 Rosti/95g	161	8.6	169	2.2	19.6	9.1	0.0
Potato, Mini, Party Bites, Sainsbury's*	1 Serving/100g	218	11.5	218	2.5	26.2	11.5	3.0
Potato, Onion & Gruyere, Finest, Tesco*	½ Pack/200g	206	10.6	103	3.2	10.5	5.3	2.0
Potato, Spinach & Mozzarella, Tesco*	1 Serving/140g	228	7.7	163	3.8	24.5	5.5	2.0
Potato & Leek, Sainsbury's*	½ Pack/190g	296	20.9	156	4.5	9.8	11.0	0.3
Potato & Root Vegetable, COU, M & S*	1 Rosti/100g	85	2.7	85	1.6	13.3	2.7	1.5
Potato Cakes, Baby, M & S*	1 Rosti/23g	40	1.5	175	3.5	25.1	6.7	1.6
Vegetable, Waitrose*	1 Pack/400g	248	9.2	62	1.4	8.8	2.3	1.3
Waitrose*	1 Rosti/45g	112	7.2	248	3.8	22.5	15.9	2.7
ROULADE								
Chocolate, Sainsbury's*	1 Serving/72g	264	15.7	367	5.7	36.9	21.8	1.8

R

	Measure INFO/WEIGHT	per Measure KCAL	FAT	Nutrition Values per 100g / 100ml KCAL	PROT	CARB	FAT	FIBRE
ROULADE								
Lemon, Asda*	1 Serving/100g	343	12.0	343	2.7	56.0	12.0	0.0
Mini, M & S*	1 Serving/63g	201	19.1	321	8.5	3.0	30.5	0.0
Orange & Lemon Meringue, Co-Op*	1 Serving/82g	287	9.8	350	3.0	57.0	12.0	0.3
Passion Fruit, M & S*	1oz/28g	83	2.6	295	2.8	50.0	9.2	0.2
Raspberry, M & S*	1oz/28g	88	3.1	315	3.3	50.3	11.0	0.1
Raspberry & Vanilla, Somerfield*	1oz/28g	118	5.6	420	3.0	56.0	20.0	0.0
Smoked Salmon & Asparagus, Sainsbury's*	1 Serving/60g	122	9.6	204	13.0	2.2	16.0	0.3
Smoked Salmon & Spinach, Finest, Tesco*	1 Serving/60g	91	6.1	152	11.5	3.6	10.2	0.6
Toffee Pecan, Finest, Tesco*	1 Serving/60g	218	8.9	363	3.6	53.8	14.8	0.5
RUM								
37.5% Volume	*1 Shot/35ml*	*72*	*0.0*	*207*	*0.0*	*0.0*	*0.0*	*0.0*
40% Volume	*1 Shot/35ml*	*78*	*0.0*	*222*	*0.0*	*0.0*	*0.0*	*0.0*
Captain Morgans & Cola, Premixed, Canned, Diageo*	1 Can/250ml	180	0.0	72	0.0	9.1	0.0	0.0
Malibu, 21% Volume, Pernod Ricard*	*1 Shot/35ml*	*70*	*0.0*	*200*	*0.0*	*29.0*	*0.0*	*0.0*
White	*1 Shot/35ml*	*72*	*0.0*	*207*	*0.0*	*0.0*	*0.0*	*0.0*
RUSKS								
Banana, Farleys*	1 Serving/17g	70	1.5	409	7.3	75.1	8.8	2.9
Mini, Farleys*	1 Serving/30g	121	2.2	405	7.0	77.7	7.3	2.1
Original, Farleys*	1 Rusk/17g	69	1.2	406	7.1	77.6	7.1	2.3

R

Measure INFO/WEIGHT	per Measure KCAL	FAT	Nutrition Values per 100g / 100ml KCAL	PROT	CARB	FAT	FIBRE

SAAG

	Measure INFO/WEIGHT	KCAL	FAT	KCAL	PROT	CARB	FAT	FIBRE
Aloo, Canned, Tesco*	½ Can/200g	124	3.8	62	1.8	9.3	1.9	2.0
Aloo, Fresh, Sainsbury's*	1 Pack/400g	388	13.2	97	2.0	14.7	3.3	4.8
Aloo, Jar, Sainsbury's*	½ Jar/135g	121	5.8	90	1.6	11.0	4.3	1.7
Aloo, North Indian, Sainsbury's*	1 Pack/300g	354	24.0	118	2.4	9.0	8.0	1.6
Aloo, Packet, Sainsbury's*	½ Pack/150g	184	12.4	123	2.1	9.9	8.3	2.7
Aloo, Sainsbury's*	1 Pack/300g	441	31.8	147	2.1	10.7	10.6	3.5
Aloo, Tesco*	1 Serving/200g	144	7.0	72	2.1	8.0	3.5	2.0
Aloo Gobi, M Kitchen, Morrisons*	1 Pack/225g	130	6.1	58	2.0	4.6	2.7	3.8
Aloo Gobi, Waitrose*	½ Pack/150	147	7.5	98	2.1	9.0	5.0	3.9
Chicken, Masala, M & S*	½ Pack/175g	227	12.4	130	13.3	3.1	7.1	5.2
Chicken, Masala, Waitrose*	1 Pack/400g	452	20.9	113	11.7	3.8	5.2	1.8
Gobi Aloo, M & S*	1 Pack/225g	270	19.1	120	1.9	9.3	8.5	2.4
Gobi Aloo, Tesco*	1 Serving/175g	166	8.9	95	2.1	9.5	5.1	1.9
Paneer, Sainsbury's*	1 Pack/300g	387	29.1	129	6.0	4.3	9.7	2.3

SAFFRON

	Measure INFO/WEIGHT	KCAL	FAT	KCAL	PROT	CARB	FAT	FIBRE
Average	*1 Tsp/1g*	*2*	*0.0*	*310*	*11.4*	*61.5*	*5.9*	*0.0*

SAGE

	Measure INFO/WEIGHT	KCAL	FAT	KCAL	PROT	CARB	FAT	FIBRE
Dried, Ground	*1 Tsp/1g*	*3*	*0.1*	*315*	*10.6*	*42.7*	*12.7*	*0.0*
Fresh	*1oz/28g*	*33*	*1.3*	*119*	*3.9*	*15.6*	*4.6*	*0.0*

SAGO

	Measure INFO/WEIGHT	KCAL	FAT	KCAL	PROT	CARB	FAT	FIBRE
Raw	*1oz/28g*	*99*	*0.1*	*355*	*0.2*	*94.0*	*0.2*	*0.5*

SALAD

	Measure INFO/WEIGHT	KCAL	FAT	KCAL	PROT	CARB	FAT	FIBRE
Adzuki & Edamame Bean, Waitrose*	1/3 Pack/67g	62	1.5	93	7.5	5.7	2.2	10.3
Alfresco Style, Tesco*	1 Serving/200g	40	0.6	20	0.9	3.3	0.3	2.1
American Ranch, Asda*	1 Serving/220g	253	19.8	115	2.5	6.0	9.0	2.0
American Style, Sweet & Crispy, Morrisons*	1 Serving/25g	7	0.1	28	1.2	4.2	0.3	2.0
Aromatic Herb, Waitrose*	¼ Pack/27g	4	0.1	15	0.9	1.7	0.5	1.0
Assorted, Asda*	1 Serving/100g	22	0.6	22	2.4	1.7	0.6	0.0
Avocado & Feta, Gourmet To Go, M & S*	1 Pack/320g	512	32.0	160	5.4	12.1	10.0	3.1
Baby Leaf, Asda*	1 Serving/80g	10	0.2	12	2.1	0.2	0.3	1.7
Baby Leaf, Florette*	1 Serving/40g	5	0.1	12	2.0	0.4	0.3	1.0
Baby Leaf, Sainsbury's*	1 Serving/60g	12	1.1	20	2.8	1.1	1.9	1.9
Baby Leaf, Seasonal, Sainsbury's*	¼ Bag/63g	11	0.3	17	2.8	0.5	0.5	2.7
Baby Leaf, Sweet, Seasonal, M & S*	½ Bag/60g	9	0.2	15	2.4	0.6	0.4	1.8
Baby Leaf, with Purple Basil, Finest, Tesco*	½ Pack/43g	7	0.1	17	2.9	0.9	0.2	1.8
Baby Leaf, with Watercress, Tesco*	1 Serving/30g	6	0.2	19	1.8	1.3	0.7	1.8
Baby Leaf & Beetroot, Bistro, M & S*	1 Pack/165g	41	0.0	25	2.0	3.6	0.0	2.0
Baby Leaf & Herb, Asda*	1 Serving/50g	7	0.1	14	2.3	0.7	0.2	2.4
Baby Plum & Sundried Tomato Salad, Waitrose*	1 Serving/200g	226	17.8	113	1.3	6.8	8.9	0.8
Baby Spinach, & Red Mustard, M & S*	1 Pack/170g	263	26.7	155	1.7	1.1	15.7	0.1
Baby Tomato, Tesco*	1 Pack/205g	35	0.6	17	0.8	2.8	0.3	0.9
Bag, Tesco*	1 Serving/200g	38	0.8	19	0.9	3.0	0.4	1.4
Basil, Pesto & Pine Nuts, Italian Style, Finest, Tesco*	½ Pack/90g	144	12.5	160	5.1	3.6	13.9	1.2
Bean, M & S*	1 Serving/80g	72	0.7	90	6.4	14.3	0.9	3.9
Bean, Mint & Coriander, Somerfield*	1 Pack/250g	287	2.7	115	7.0	19.4	1.1	4.7
Bean, Mixed, Vinaigrette, Tesco*	1 Can/400g	280	2.0	70	3.2	13.1	0.5	1.9
Bean, Retail	1oz/28g	41	2.6	147	4.2	12.8	9.3	3.0
Bean & Chorizo, Tapas Selection, Sainsbury's*	1 Serving/22g	29	1.4	132	8.1	10.7	6.3	1.9
Bean & Sweetcorn, Side, M & S*	1 Serving/125g	131	9.0	105	2.5	7.0	7.2	1.3
Beans, Mixed, Essential, Waitrose*	1 Serving/80g	87	1.8	109	8.7	13.6	2.2	3.1
Beetroot	1oz/28g	28	1.9	100	2.0	8.4	6.8	1.7
Beetroot, 1% Fat, M & S*	1 Serving/225g	130	6.1	58	1.1	7.7	2.7	1.7
Beetroot, Cous Cous & Quinoa, Tesco*	1 Serving/100g	70	0.6	70	2.3	12.9	0.6	2.3

SALAD

	Measure INFO/WEIGHT	per Measure KCAL	per Measure FAT	Nutrition Values per 100g / 100ml KCAL	PROT	CARB	FAT	FIBRE
Beetroot, Freshly Prepared, Tesco*	1 Pack/240g	58	0.7	24	1.9	3.3	0.3	2.7
Beetroot, GFY, Asda*	1 Pack/250g	130	1.0	52	1.1	11.0	0.4	2.3
Beetroot, Roast with Quinoa & Feta, Tesco*	1 Pack/400g	452	19.6	113	4.8	12.4	4.9	2.3
Beetroot & Carrot, Continental, Iceland*	1 Serving/100g	24	0.2	24	1.2	4.3	0.2	2.1
Beetroot & Cherry Tomato, & Lemon Dressing, M & S*	1 Pack/215g	129	8.2	60	1.3	5.2	3.8	1.5
Beetroot & Goats Cheese, Shaker, Good to Go, Waitrose*	1 Pack/240g	357	11.0	149	6.2	17.9	4.6	5.0
Beetroot & Lettuce, Asda*	1 Serving/30g	5	0.0	16	1.4	2.7	0.0	2.5
Beetroot & Spinach with Creamy Lemon Dressing, Tesco*	½ Tub/110g	80	5.9	73	1.3	3.8	5.4	1.9
Bistro, Asda*	1 Serving/180g	29	0.0	16	1.4	2.7	0.0	2.5
Bistro, Morrisons*	1 Serving/20g	5	0.0	23	1.2	4.2	0.2	2.0
Bistro, Sainsbury's*	1 Pack/150g	25	0.3	17	1.9	2.0	0.2	2.0
Bistro, Washed Ready to Eat, Tesco*	1 Pack/140g	22	0.7	16	1.1	1.7	0.5	1.0
Black Bean Salsa, Salad Bar, Waitrose*	1 Serving/100g	118	5.8	118	0.0	0.0	5.8	0.0
Black Olive, Tomato & Red Onion, Shapers, Boots*	1 Pack/80g	68	5.0	85	0.0	0.0	6.2	0.0
Caesar	1 Serving/200g	352	27.8	176	4.8	8.1	13.9	0.7
Caesar, Bacon, M & S*	1 Serving/250g	400	31.2	160	7.1	4.1	12.5	1.3
Caesar, Chicken, Asda*	1 Pack/273g	535	43.7	196	10.0	3.0	16.0	1.9
Caesar, Chicken, Bistro, M & S*	½ Pack/135g	189	14.3	140	5.0	6.5	10.6	0.6
Caesar, Chicken, Eat Well, M & S*	1 Pack/397g	595	24.6	150	9.9	18.7	6.2	2.1
Caesar, Chicken, Fresh, Sainsbury's*	1 Serving/200g	278	20.0	139	6.0	6.2	10.0	1.2
Caesar, Chicken, M & S*	½ Pack/140g	266	20.0	190	6.7	8.7	14.3	0.8
Caesar, Chicken, Shapers, Boots*	1 Pack/200g	205	5.8	102	8.2	10.0	2.9	1.0
Caesar, Chicken & Bacon, Gourmet, M & S*	1 Salad/250g	550	43.5	220	9.0	7.3	17.4	0.7
Caesar, Chicken & Bacon, Tesco*	1 Pack/200g	506	40.2	253	6.6	11.4	20.1	1.0
Caesar, Classic, Reduced Fat, M & S*	1 Serving/115g	132	5.6	115	4.8	12.7	4.9	0.5
Caesar, ClassicM & S*	½ Pack/112g	174	14.2	155	2.9	6.8	12.7	0.5
Caesar, Co-Op*	¼ Pack/50g	87	7.5	175	3.0	6.0	15.0	2.0
Caesar, Finest, Tesco*	1 Bowl/220g	374	30.6	170	4.9	5.1	13.9	1.6
Caesar, Florette*	1 Serving/100g	163	12.4	163	2.7	10.2	12.4	1.8
Caesar, GFY, Asda*	½ Pack/87g	76	2.6	87	8.0	7.0	3.0	1.5
Caesar, M & S*	1 Pack/268g	510	40.5	190	5.7	8.3	15.1	1.3
Caesar, Washed & Ready to Eat, Somerfield*	½ Bag/125g	155	10.9	124	5.0	6.5	8.7	0.8
Cajun Chicken, David Lloyd Leisure*	1 Pack/300g	429	10.0	143	11.7	17.7	3.3	1.0
Cannellini Bean & Chicken, M & S*	1 Serving/225g	250	14.7	111	5.9	7.4	6.5	3.1
Cannellini Bean & Chorizo, Sainsbury's*	1 Pack/250g	227	8.0	91	5.3	10.2	3.2	1.6
Cannellini Bean & Tuna, M & S*	1 Serving/255g	215	11.6	84	5.3	5.4	4.5	2.1
Caponata, Organic, Florentin*	1 Serving/100g	111	12.3	111	1.5	3.7	12.3	0.0
Caribbean Chicken, Shapers, Boots*	1 Pack/220g	222	5.1	101	5.8	14.0	2.3	1.2
Carrot, Courgette & Coriander, Salad Bar, Waitrose*	1 Serving/100g	92	7.9	92	0.0	0.0	7.9	0.0
Carrot, M & S*	1 Pack/215g	280	7.3	130	3.1	22.4	3.4	2.7
Carrot, Orange & Ginger, Good Intentions, Somerfield*	1 Serving/250g	275	3.5	110	2.0	22.4	1.4	1.4
Carrot, Peanut & Sultana, Asda*	1 Serving/20g	54	4.0	272	8.0	15.0	20.0	4.5
Carrot & Beetroot, Classic, Tesco*	½ Pack/83g	17	0.2	20	0.9	3.7	0.2	1.6
Carrot & Sultana, BGTY, Sainsbury's*	½ Pack/100g	55	0.3	55	0.6	12.4	0.3	0.0
Carrot & Sultana, HL, Tesco*	1 Tub/225g	142	1.3	63	1.2	13.2	0.6	2.5
Celery, Nut & Sultana, Waitrose*	1oz/28g	54	4.6	192	2.8	8.4	16.4	1.0
Celery & Apple, Salad Bar, Waitrose*	1 Serving/100g	136	12.9	136	0.0	0.0	12.9	0.0
Chargrilled Chicken, & Bacon, Tesco*	1 Pack/300g	657	37.8	219	7.8	18.7	12.6	0.9
Chargrilled Chicken, & Pesto, Sainsbury's*	1 Pack/250g	375	15.2	150	7.9	15.8	6.1	1.3
Chargrilled Chicken, & Quinoa, Shapers, Boots*	1 Pack/185g	139	1.8	75	6.2	10.0	1.0	1.8
Chargrilled Chicken, Tesco*	1 Serving/300g	384	14.4	128	6.1	15.0	4.8	2.4
Chargrilled Chicken, Weight Watchers*	1 Pack/182g	265	3.8	146	11.7	20.0	2.1	2.2
Cheese, HL, Tesco*	1 Serving/30g	32	0.9	107	18.0	2.0	3.0	0.0

SALAD

	Measure INFO/WEIGHT	per Measure KCAL	FAT	Nutrition Values per 100g / 100ml KCAL	PROT	CARB	FAT	FIBRE
Cheese, Layered, Tesco*	1 Serving/225g	437	32.0	194	5.8	10.8	14.2	0.8
Cheese, Ploughman's, Asda*	1 Bowl/300g	246	10.8	82	3.6	8.9	3.6	1.0
Cheese & Coleslaw, Tesco*	1 Serving/125g	135	10.9	108	3.4	3.4	8.7	1.1
Cheese Layered, M & S*	½ Pack/230g	300	20.5	130	4.6	9.3	8.9	1.2
Cheesy Bean Pasta, Salad Bar, Waitrose*	1 Serving/100g	143	4.3	143	0.0	0.0	4.3	0.0
Cherry Tomato, Tesco*	1 Pack/210g	136	9.4	65	0.9	4.2	4.5	1.1
Chick Pea & Cous Cous, Tesco*	1 Serving/250g	245	6.5	98	3.2	15.5	2.6	0.0
Chick Pea & Spinach, M & S*	1 Serving/260g	299	10.7	115	7.3	12.5	4.1	2.7
Chick Pea & Sweet Potato, Salad Bar, Sainsbury's*	1 Serving/100g	99	1.9	99	0.0	9.6	1.9	0.0
Chicken, Avocado & Bacon, M & S*	1 Serving/235g	235	13.6	100	8.5	2.8	5.8	2.8
Chicken, Italian Style, Snack Pot, Carb Check, Heinz*	1 Pot/218g	131	4.4	60	5.9	4.3	2.0	1.0
Chicken, Roast, & Coleslaw, Boots*	1 Serving/245g	392	34.3	160	4.5	3.9	14.0	1.3
Chicken, Roast, 93 Cals, Shapers, Boots*	1 Pack/233g	93	0.9	40	8.6	0.6	0.4	1.8
Chicken, Sweet Chilli, BGTY, Sainsbury's*	1 Serving/200g	206	0.8	103	6.0	18.7	0.4	0.0
Chicken, Tesco*	1 Serving/300g	348	22.2	116	5.3	7.0	7.4	1.0
Chicken, Tomato Chilli, & Rice, COU, M & S*	1 Pack/340g	357	5.1	105	6.8	16.0	1.5	0.9
Chicken & Bacon, Asda*	1 Pack/381g	480	22.9	126	7.0	11.0	6.0	0.0
Chicken & Bacon, Carb Control, Tesco*	1 Serving/188g	244	14.7	130	13.2	1.7	7.8	0.5
Chicken & Bacon, Layered, Asda*	1 Serving/375g	472	22.5	126	7.0	11.0	6.0	1.6
Chicken & Bacon, Layered, Waitrose*	1 Serving/200g	246	14.8	123	6.7	7.4	7.4	2.1
Chicken & Moroccan Cous Cous, Tesco*	1 Pack/210g	252	4.2	120	7.8	16.9	2.0	3.5
Chicken Fajita, Shapers, Boots*	1 Pack/258g	181	3.4	70	7.0	7.4	1.3	2.7
Chicken Noodle, Thai Style, Sainsbury's*	1 Pack/260g	283	7.5	109	6.6	14.2	2.9	1.3
Chicken Noodle & Sweet Chilli, Shapers, Boots*	1 Pack/197g	266	5.1	135	12.0	16.0	2.6	0.9
Classic, Co-Op*	½ Pack/80g	16	0.2	20	0.8	2.9	0.3	2.2
Coleslaw, Classics, M & S*	1 Pot/190g	123	4.4	65	1.9	8.8	2.3	1.3
Coleslaw Layered, Fresh, Asda*	1 Tub/197g	209	17.7	106	1.2	5.0	9.0	1.5
Complete Hot Greek, Sainsbury's*	1 Pack/299g	287	22.4	96	4.3	2.9	7.5	1.7
Continental, Co-Op*	1 Serving/80g	12	0.3	15	1.0	2.0	0.4	1.0
Continental Four Leaf, Sainsbury's*	½ Pack/100g	13	0.2	13	1.2	1.7	0.2	1.9
Coronation Rice, Tesco*	1 Serving/50g	103	7.5	207	2.0	15.9	15.1	0.8
Cosmopolitan, Fresh, Sainsbury's*	1 Bag/135g	20	0.5	15	1.2	1.6	0.4	1.9
Cous Cous, BFY, Morrisons*	½ Pot/113g	164	4.0	145	4.6	23.8	3.5	0.5
Cous Cous, BGTY, Sainsbury's*	1 Pot/200g	236	4.4	118	4.7	19.7	2.2	2.8
Cous Cous, Waitrose*	1 Pot/200g	344	10.0	172	4.9	26.9	5.0	1.4
Cous Cous & Roast Vegetable, GFY, Asda*	1 Serving/100g	120	1.6	120	3.5	23.0	1.6	2.7
Cous Cous with Chargrilled Chicken, Sainsbury's*	1 Pack/240g	446	20.9	186	7.4	19.6	8.7	0.0
Cous Cous with Mixed Peppers & Cucumber, GFY, Asda*	¼ Pot/56g	66	0.1	117	3.9	25.0	0.2	1.5
Crisp, Mix, Somerfield*	1 Pack/215g	34	0.6	16	0.9	2.4	0.3	1.6
Crisp & Crunchy, Asda*	1 Pack/250g	55	1.5	22	0.8	3.3	0.6	1.4
Crisp & Light, M & S*	1 Serving/170g	51	1.4	30	0.5	5.4	0.8	1.0
Crisp & Sweet Lettuce Leaves, Florette*	¼ Pack/70g	10	0.3	14	0.8	1.7	0.5	0.9
Crisp Mixed, Tesco*	1 Pack/200g	40	0.6	20	1.1	3.2	0.3	2.0
Crispy, Florette*	1 Portion/100g	22	0.3	22	1.5	3.4	0.3	3.0
Crispy Crunch, Lasting Leaf*	1 Serving/75g	13	0.3	18	1.1	1.5	0.4	1.9
Crispy Duck & Herb, M & S*	½ Pack/140g	378	25.6	270	20.7	3.7	18.3	1.4
Crispy Green, Sainsbury's*	1 Serving/70g	8	0.1	12	0.9	1.6	0.2	0.8
Crispy Leaf, Sainsbury's*	½ Pack/68g	9	0.3	14	1.0	1.7	0.4	1.7
Crispy Medley, Waitrose*	1 Serving/50g	7	0.2	15	0.8	1.7	0.5	0.9
Crunchy, Basics, Sainsbury's*	1 Pack/200g	50	0.4	25	1.3	3.4	0.2	2.2
Crunchy, Simple, M & S*	1 Serving/50g	7	0.2	15	1.0	1.6	0.5	1.8
Crunchy, Waitrose*	½ Pack/100g	18	0.4	18	1.0	2.6	0.4	1.5
Crunchy Layered, Tesco*	1 Serving/54g	15	0.2	27	1.1	4.9	0.3	1.7

S

SALAD

	Measure INFO/WEIGHT	per Measure KCAL	FAT	Nutrition Values per 100g / 100ml KCAL	PROT	CARB	FAT	FIBRE
Crunchy Mix, Co-Op*	1 Bag/200g	20	0.4	10	0.9	1.7	0.2	1.5
Cucumber & Cherry Tomato, Fresh Tastes, Asda*	1 Serving/100g	22	0.3	22	1.6	2.4	0.3	0.0
Edamame & Butterbean, TTD, Sainsbury's*	1/3 Pack/62g	70	2.5	113	6.6	9.9	4.1	4.9
Edamame Bean, Oriental Style, Asda*	1 Pack/220g	183	8.4	83	4.8	7.3	3.8	4.0
Edamame Beans & Peppers, Delicious, Boots*	1 Pack/87g	121	2.3	139	0.0	4.1	2.6	0.0
Egg & Baby Spinach, Waitrose*	1 Pack/215g	167	13.5	78	3.5	1.8	6.3	1.0
Egg & Coleslaw, Boots*	1 Pot/233g	405	37.3	174	3.0	4.6	16.0	1.0
Egg & Ham with Salad Cream Dressing, M & S*	1 Pack/240g	168	8.4	70	5.2	4.0	3.5	0.6
Egg & Potato, Fresh, M & S*	1 Serving/250g	150	7.2	60	3.0	4.6	2.9	0.9
Endive & Radicchio, Somerfield*	1 Pack/150g	19	0.0	13	2.0	1.0	0.0	0.0
English Garden, Tesco*	1 Serving/180g	22	0.4	12	0.7	1.8	0.2	0.7
Exotic with Mango & Chilli Dressing, Co-Op*	½ Pack/65g	25	0.4	38	0.6	7.7	0.6	0.8
Family, Florette*	1 Serving/50g	14	0.1	29	1.1	5.5	0.2	3.0
Family, Somerfield*	1 Serving/67g	12	0.3	18	0.8	2.9	0.4	1.3
Feta, & Butternut Squash, Tesco*	1 Pot/245g	404	19.1	165	6.5	14.9	7.8	3.1
Feta Cheese & Sunblushed Tomato, M & S*	1 Serving/190g	361	21.1	190	5.5	17.2	11.1	2.1
Fine Cut, Asda*	1oz/28g	7	0.1	24	1.2	4.1	0.3	2.1
Fine Noodle with Duck Breast, COU, M & S*	1 Pack/280g	294	3.1	105	5.5	18.9	1.1	1.1
Florida, Retail, Average	1oz/28g	63	5.7	224	0.9	9.7	20.5	1.0
Four Bean, Sainsbury's*	½ Pot/113g	114	2.5	101	6.7	6.2	2.2	15.0
Four Bean & Buckwheat, Waitrose*	1 Pack/220g	319	14.5	145	5.3	16.0	6.6	6.1
Four Leaf, M & S*	1 Serving/130g	19	0.4	15	0.9	2.0	0.3	1.4
French Goat's Cheese, Extra Fine, Asda*	1 Pack/185g	462	35.1	250	8.4	11.4	19.0	0.8
French Style, M & S*	1 Pack/140g	140	13.6	100	1.0	2.5	9.7	0.9
French Style, Waitrose*	½ Pack/82g	149	12.1	182	5.1	7.2	14.8	1.8
Fresh & Crispy, Tesco*	1 Serving/230g	30	0.7	13	0.7	1.9	0.3	1.3
Fruity Moroccan Cous Cous, Waitrose*	1 Pack/90g	139	3.2	154	5.0	25.6	3.6	4.6
Fruity Tabbouleh, Salad Bar, Waitrose*	1 Serving/100g	184	6.6	184	0.0	0.0	6.6	0.0
Fusion, Fully Prepared, Sainsbury's*	½ Pack/63g	15	0.5	24	3.7	0.3	0.8	3.4
Garden, Classic, Morrisons*	1 Tray/175g	33	0.5	19	0.8	3.2	0.3	2.8
Garden, Side, Asda*	1 Pack/175g	31	0.5	18	0.9	2.8	0.3	1.3
Garden, Tesco*	1 Serving/225g	34	0.7	15	1.0	2.0	0.3	0.9
Garden, Tray, Asda*	½ Pack/88g	16	0.3	18	0.7	3.1	0.3	1.6
Garden, Value, Tesco*	¼ Pack/50g	9	0.1	18	1.0	2.9	0.3	2.1
Garden, with Watercress, M & S*	1 Salad/80g	10	0.1	12	1.5	1.4	0.1	1.4
Garden, with Yoghurt & Mint Dressing, GFY, Asda*	1 Serving/195g	51	1.9	26	1.1	3.2	1.0	0.0
Goat's Cheese & Cous Cous, Waitrose*	1 Pack/300g	372	14.4	124	4.8	15.3	4.8	2.2
Greek	1oz/28g	36	3.5	130	2.7	1.9	12.5	0.8
Greek, BGTY, Sainsbury's*	1 Serving/199g	133	5.0	67	2.0	9.0	2.5	0.8
Greek, with Basil & Mint Oil Dressing, M & S*	1 Pack/200g	220	19.6	110	3.6	2.2	9.8	1.5
Greek Feta & Pepper with Cous Cous, Asda*	1 Pack/316g	262	10.4	83	3.2	10.2	3.3	0.0
Greek Style, Delphi*	1 Serving/220g	306	27.1	139	3.7	3.5	12.3	0.9
Greek Style, Fresh, Food Counter, Sainsbury's*	1 Serving/166g	247	23.2	149	1.9	2.7	14.0	0.0
Greek Style, Waitrose*	½ Pack/125g	54	2.7	43	1.9	4.0	2.2	1.2
Greek Style Feta, Tip & Mix, M & S*	1 Pack/195g	214	18.3	110	4.0	2.5	9.4	1.6
Greek Style Layered, Perfectly Balanced, Waitrose*	1 Pack/280g	134	7.8	48	2.4	3.2	2.8	0.7
Green, Average	1oz/28g	4	0.1	13	0.8	1.8	0.3	0.9
Green, Mixed, Average	1 Serving/100g	12	0.3	12	0.7	1.8	0.3	1.0
Green Lentil, Red Pepper & Spinach, Waitrose*	1 Pack/250g	485	20.0	194	8.6	22.0	8.0	2.9
Green with Honey & Mustard Dressing, M & S*	1 Pack/200g	120	9.6	60	0.9	2.7	4.8	0.8
Ham, Antony Worrall Thompson's*	1 Pack/202g	257	2.6	127	9.8	19.1	1.3	2.7
Ham & Free Range Egg, Fresh Tastes, Asda*	1 Bowl/265g	167	9.3	63	5.7	2.2	3.5	0.8
Ham Hock, Waitrose*	1 Pack/350g	245	9.5	70	6.6	4.8	2.7	2.0

SALAD

INFO/WEIGHT	Measure INFO/WEIGHT	per Measure KCAL	per Measure FAT	KCAL	PROT	CARB	FAT	FIBRE
Herb, Asda*	1 Serving/20g	2	0.1	12	1.8	0.6	0.3	2.0
Herb, M & S*	1 Pack/100g	20	0.4	20	2.9	1.4	0.4	1.9
Herb, Organic, Sainsbury's*	1 Serving/100g	17	0.5	17	1.8	1.3	0.5	1.8
Indian Spiced Chicken, Waitrose*	1 Pack/280g	328	12.0	117	7.8	8.9	4.3	5.6
Italian, Complete, Sainsbury's*	1 Pack/160g	237	14.4	148	5.4	11.4	9.0	1.6
Italian Style, Asda*	1 Serving/20g	3	0.1	15	1.1	1.6	0.5	1.2
Italian Style, Organic, Waitrose*	½ Pack/45g	7	0.2	15	0.8	1.7	0.5	0.9
Italian Style, Tesco*	1/3 Pack/40g	6	0.2	16	1.0	1.9	0.5	1.2
Italian Style with Rocket & Lambs Lettuce, M & S*	½ Bag/60g	12	0.3	20	1.3	2.3	0.5	1.3
Italian Wild Rocket & Parmesan, Sainsbury's*	1 Serving/50g	88	7.4	177	7.5	3.4	14.8	0.5
King Prawn, GFY, Asda*	1 Serving/175g	112	2.6	64	4.7	8.0	1.5	1.3
King Prawn, Thai Style, M & S*	1 Pack/295g	265	7.4	90	4.4	12.6	2.5	1.3
King Prawn & New Potato, COU, M & S*	1 Pack/300g	180	6.9	60	3.0	6.9	2.3	0.8
King Prawn & Pasta, COU, M & S*	1 Pack/270g	283	6.5	105	5.9	15.1	2.4	2.7
Leek & Pork Deli, Continental, Aldi*	¼ Tub/63g	68	3.1	108	1.9	13.9	5.0	2.3
Lemon Cous Cous & Roasted Pepper, COU, M & S*	1 Pack/340g	306	7.8	90	3.2	14.6	2.3	1.8
Lentils, Giant Cous Cous & Goats Cheese, Eat Well, M & S*	1 Pack/215g	312	10.3	145	6.9	17.4	4.8	3.3
Lovely Summer, Jamie Oliver*	½ Bag/60g	48	4.0	80	1.7	4.0	6.6	1.2
Mediterranean, Side, Sainsbury's*	1 Pack/170g	44	2.2	26	0.9	2.7	1.3	1.3
Mediterranean Style, Asda*	½ Pack/135g	22	0.0	16	1.0	3.0	0.0	0.0
Mediterranean Style, Tray, Morrisons*	1 Tray/100g	26	0.3	26	1.2	3.6	0.3	1.8
Mediterranean Style Chicken & Feta, Shapers, Boots*	1 Pack/240g	143	6.1	59	5.9	3.1	2.5	0.0
Mexican Style Bean & Cheese, M & S*	½ Pot/150g	150	5.2	100	6.1	11.2	3.5	4.8
Mix, Crisp & Sweet Lettuce Leaves, Florette*	1 Portion/67g	12	0.2	18	1.5	1.2	0.3	2.5
Mix with Cabbage, Beetroot & Carrot, Florette*	½ Pack/100g	30	0.2	30	1.3	4.4	0.2	0.0
Mixed, (Basic Mix), Albert Heijn*	1 Pack/300g	57	0.0	19	1.0	2.5	0.0	2.5
Mixed, Crisp, Mild, Tesco*	½ Pack/145g	29	0.4	20	1.2	3.0	0.3	2.1
Mixed, Florette*	1 Serving/100g	20	0.2	20	1.3	3.4	0.2	3.0
Mixed Bean, Asda*	½ Can/145g	126	3.6	87	5.0	11.0	2.5	6.0
Mixed Bean, Canned, Waitrose*	1 Can/270g	251	1.6	93	6.4	15.5	0.6	5.5
Mixed Leaf, Medley, Waitrose*	1 Serving/25g	4	0.1	15	0.8	1.7	0.5	1.4
Mixed Leaf, Tomato & Olive, Tesco*	1 Serving/170g	150	13.3	88	1.0	3.4	7.8	0.0
Mixed Leaf, with Olive Oil Dressing, Pizza Express*	1 Pack/240g	326	33.8	136	0.9	2.1	14.1	0.7
Mixed Leaves, Bondelle*	1 Serving/50g	10	0.1	21	1.4	3.3	0.2	0.0
Mixed Leaves, Tesco*	1 Serving/20g	3	0.1	14	0.9	1.6	0.4	0.9
Mixed Pepper, Asda*	½ Pack/100g	24	0.3	24	1.0	4.3	0.3	1.7
Mixed Vegetable, Aldi*	1 Serving/200g	120	4.0	60	0.6	10.0	2.0	0.0
Moroccan Style, Chicken, Shapers, Boots*	1 Pack/240g	230	4.3	96	5.6	13.0	1.8	1.6
Mozzarella & Cherry Tomato, Shapers, Boots*	1 Bowl/194g	184	14.2	95	4.1	3.3	7.3	0.9
Mozzarella & Rocket, Asda*	1 Serving/265g	435	31.8	164	7.0	7.0	12.0	1.5
Mozzarella & Sunkissed Tomato, Tesco*	1 Bag/160g	270	22.9	169	4.6	4.3	14.3	2.1
Mozzarella & Tomato, M & S*	1 Serving/310g	400	14.8	129	5.5	15.5	4.8	0.9
Mozzarella & Tomato (No Dressing)	1 Serving/105g	190	14.5	182	8.0	5.9	13.8	3.3
New Potato, Less Than 5% Fat, M & S*	1 Serving/110g	88	3.4	80	1.3	12.1	3.1	1.5
New Potato, Luxury, Morrisons*	½ Tub/125g	341	30.7	273	1.7	11.2	24.6	0.0
New Potato, M & S*	1 Serving/60g	114	9.8	190	0.9	9.9	16.3	1.3
New Potato, Tomato & Egg with Salad Cream, M & S*	1 Pack/300g	165	7.2	55	2.9	5.4	2.4	1.3
New Potato, Tuna & Egg, M & S*	1 Pack/340g	255	12.9	75	3.8	6.7	3.8	0.7
New Potato & Free Range Egg, M & S*	1 Pack/305g	213	11.6	70	2.5	7.0	3.8	0.8
New Potato & Free Range Egg, Side, Sainsbury's*	1 Pack/290g	174	12.2	60	2.5	3.1	4.2	1.4
New Potato & King Prawn, M & S*	1 Pack/210g	220	9.4	105	5.6	10.2	4.5	1.7
New Potato & Sweet Chilli Prawn, M & S*	1 Pack/210g	147	1.0	70	2.8	14.0	0.5	0.7
New Potato & Tuna Sweetcorn, Eat Well, M & S*	1 Pack/190g	133	3.4	70	5.4	8.4	1.8	1.9

SALAD

INFO/WEIGHT		per Measure KCAL	FAT	Nutrition Values per 100g / 100ml KCAL	PROT	CARB	FAT	FIBRE
Nicoise, Tesco*	1 Pack/260g	286	21.8	110	3.2	5.3	8.4	1.4
Noodle & King Prawn, Perfectly Balanced, Waitrose*	1 Pack/225g	223	2.2	99	5.0	17.4	1.0	1.0
Noodle & Sesame, Salad Bar, Waitrose*	1 Serving/100g	178	11.5	178	0.0	0.0	11.5	0.0
Noodle with Thai Style Chicken, M & S*	½ Pot/145g	159	7.1	110	5.2	11.6	4.9	1.4
Nutty Rice, Love Life, Waitrose*	1 Portion/200g	368	14.4	184	4.5	25.3	7.2	3.1
Nutty Super Wholefood, M & S*	½ Pack/115g	149	5.9	130	5.3	12.8	5.1	6.1
Pancetta, Express, Pizza Express*	1 Salad/90g	200	17.9	223	7.4	3.3	20.0	0.0
Pea & Ham, M & S*	1 Pack/335g	420	13.8	125	7.1	12.6	4.1	4.7
Pea Shoot, Baby Cos & Batavia Lettuce, Bagged, M & S*	1 Bag/120g	24	0.6	20	2.6	0.8	0.5	2.3
Pea Shoots & Baby Leaves, Steve's Leaves*	1 Pack/60g	14	0.4	24	2.7	2.0	0.6	2.0
Pepper, Sweetcorn & Cucumber, Salad Bar, Waitrose*	1 Serving/100g	71	3.1	71	0.0	0.0	3.1	0.0
Potato, 30% Less Fat, BGTY, Sainsbury's*	1 Serving/60g	64	3.7	106	1.7	11.1	6.1	1.1
Potato, Asda*	¼ Pot/57g	67	4.0	117	0.9	12.5	7.0	1.1
Potato, Chunky, Somerfield*	1oz/28g	59	6.2	212	1.0	3.0	22.0	0.0
Potato, Creamy, Asda*	½ Tub/150g	226	16.0	151	1.1	11.3	10.7	2.5
Potato, Creamy, Waitrose*	1 Serving/100g	163	11.9	163	1.3	12.7	11.9	1.1
Potato, Reduced Calorie, Pre Packed	1oz/28g	27	1.1	97	1.3	14.8	4.1	0.8
Potato, Salad Bar, Asda*	1oz/28g	52	4.3	187	0.6	11.6	15.4	1.1
Potato, Side, Waitrose*	1 Pack/250g	181	11.0	72	3.0	5.2	4.4	1.0
Potato & Cheese, Pasta & Mixed Leaf, Waitrose*	1 Serving/205g	266	17.4	130	3.2	10.1	8.5	1.1
Potato & Cheese, Sainsbury's*	1 Serving/125g	200	16.4	160	2.7	7.9	13.1	3.4
Potato & Egg, Somerfield*	½ Pack/158g	90	4.7	57	2.5	5.1	3.0	1.2
Potato & Egg with Mayonnaise, Tesco*	½ Tub/150g	115	8.5	77	2.9	3.1	5.7	1.2
Potato with Mayonnaise, Pre Packed	1oz/28g	67	5.8	239	1.6	12.2	20.8	0.9
Potato with Mayonnaise, Retail	1oz/28g	80	7.4	287	1.5	11.4	26.5	0.8
Potato with Onions & Chives, Co-Op*	1 Serving/50g	80	6.0	160	1.0	12.0	12.0	1.0
Prawn, King & Rice Noodle, M & S*	1 Pack/320g	208	2.6	65	2.9	11.6	0.8	0.9
Prawn, King with Noodles, Delicious, Boots*	1 Pack/228g	251	3.7	110	6.3	18.0	1.6	1.8
Prawn, Layered, Asda*	1 Tub/380g	403	15.6	106	5.0	11.5	4.1	0.0
Prawn, Layered, Sainsbury's*	1 Pack/275g	355	21.2	129	3.6	11.2	7.7	1.1
Prawn, Tesco*	1 Pack/280g	314	14.0	112	4.7	12.0	5.0	0.9
Prawn & Avocado, M & S*	1 Serving/220g	176	15.0	80	3.0	2.0	6.8	3.1
Prawn & Egg, Leaf, Shapers, Boots*	1 Pack/182g	193	14.4	106	6.7	2.1	7.9	1.0
Prawn Cocktail, HL, Tesco*	1 Serving/300g	279	3.0	93	5.7	15.3	1.0	2.0
Prawn Cocktail, Shapers, Boots*	1 Pack/245g	120	5.9	49	4.7	2.2	2.4	0.7
Prawn Cocktail, Tesco*	1 Pack/300g	360	18.0	120	5.7	10.9	6.0	0.8
Roast Butternut Squash & Fennel, TTD, Sainsbury's*	1 Pack/165g	214	7.6	130	3.4	15.2	4.6	6.9
Roast Chicken, Layered, HL, Tesco*	1 Salad/400g	268	4.4	67	5.8	8.4	1.1	2.1
Roast Chicken, Tesco*	1 Salad/300g	348	22.2	116	5.3	7.0	7.4	1.0
Roast Pepper Cous Cous, HL, Tesco*	1 Pot/220g	308	4.6	140	5.6	24.3	2.1	1.7
Roasted Artichoke & Pepper, M & S*	1 Serving/220g	638	53.9	290	4.1	12.8	24.5	5.1
Roasted Vegetables & Cous Cous, Sainsbury's*	1 Pot/225g	378	24.1	168	5.3	12.6	10.7	1.9
Rocket, Leafy, Asda*	1 Serving/75g	10	0.1	13	1.5	1.4	0.1	1.8
Rocket, Morrisons*	1 Serving/100g	14	0.5	14	0.8	1.7	0.5	0.0
Salad, Bistro, Somerfield*	½ Pack/50g	7	0.2	14	0.8	1.6	0.5	1.4
Salmon, Hot Smoked with Potato Salad, M & S*	1 Pack/338g	270	7.4	80	4.5	10.3	2.2	1.3
Salmon & Roquette, M & S*	1 Serving/255g	306	20.4	120	3.9	8.5	8.0	1.0
Santa Tomato, Side, M & S*	1 Pack/225g	146	12.4	65	0.8	3.3	5.5	0.9
Santini, Side, M & S*	1 Pack/195g	127	11.1	65	1.0	3.0	5.7	2.0
Sea Food, Family Mart*	1 Serving/100g	29	0.6	29	1.6	4.1	0.6	0.0
Seafood, Marinated, M & S*	1 Serving/90g	108	5.8	120	13.4	2.3	6.4	0.8
Seafood, Marinated, Waitrose*	1 Tub/160g	235	10.6	147	16.3	5.5	6.6	0.0
Seafood, Prawn & Calamari, Deli, M & S*	1 Pack/120g	132	6.1	110	14.7	1.2	5.1	0.8

SALAD

INFO/WEIGHT	Measure	per Measure KCAL	FAT	Nutrition Values per 100g / 100ml KCAL	PROT	CARB	FAT	FIBRE
Seasonal, Organic, Waitrose*	¼ Pack/25g	4	0.1	15	0.8	1.7	0.5	0.9
Seasonal Potato, Salad Bar, Waitrose*	1 Serving/100g	109	3.4	109	0.0	0.0	3.4	0.0
Selection, Fresh, M & S*	1 Pack/230g	32	0.7	14	0.7	2.1	0.3	0.9
Selection, Side, M & S*	1 Serving/255g	153	12.7	60	1.1	2.5	5.0	1.3
Shredded Beetroot, Asda*	1 Serving/140g	29	0.4	21	1.1	3.5	0.3	1.5
Skipjack Tuna, John West*	1 Can/192g	190	11.7	99	7.3	3.7	6.1	0.0
Smoked Ham, Weight Watchers*	1 Pack/181g	233	3.6	129	11.0	16.6	2.0	3.0
Spiced Potato, Salad Bar, Waitrose*	1 Serving/100g	88	2.0	88	0.0	0.0	2.0	0.0
Spicy Bean, Tesco*	1 Serving/125g	111	2.9	89	4.9	12.1	2.3	2.5
Spicy Chickpea, BGTY, Sainsbury's*	½ Pack/125g	119	2.1	95	4.7	15.3	1.7	5.5
Spicy Chickpea & Halloumi, Cranks*	1 Pack/238g	295	11.2	124	5.0	15.5	4.7	2.6
Spicy Mexican Bean, Salad Bar, Waitrose*	1 Serving/100g	119	4.7	119	0.0	0.0	4.7	0.0
Spinach, Rocket & Watercress, Asda*	1 Serving/100g	21	0.6	21	2.8	1.2	0.6	1.9
Spinach, Waitrose*	1 Pack/100g	25	0.8	25	2.8	1.6	0.8	2.1
Spring, American Style, M & S*	1 Serving/60g	9	0.1	15	1.9	1.4	0.2	1.3
Sprouted Pea & Bean, Mint Dressing, Eat Well, M & S*	1 Pot/165g	181	8.7	110	7.3	8.7	5.3	7.4
Super Wholefood Shaker, M & S*	1 Shaker/229g	389	23.6	170	5.6	13.9	10.3	5.6
Super Wholefood with Blueberries & Mango, M & S*	1 Pack/215g	260	7.7	121	4.4	17.0	3.6	8.7
Sweet, Layered, Tesco*	1 Serving/285g	80	1.1	28	1.1	5.0	0.4	1.6
Sweet, Shredded, Tesco*	1 Serving/100g	20	0.4	20	1.1	2.9	0.4	1.9
Sweet & Crispy, M & S*	1 Serving/140g	49	1.4	35	1.7	4.7	1.0	1.6
Sweet Carrot & Sultana, M & S*	1 Serving/100g	55	0.7	55	0.8	11.4	0.7	2.6
Sweet Chilli Chicken Noodle, COU, M & S*	1 Pack/340g	408	7.8	120	6.8	17.4	2.3	1.2
Sweet Green, M & S*	1 Serving/150g	22	0.4	15	1.5	1.3	0.3	2.0
Sweet Leaf, Fully Prepared, Fresh, Sainsbury's*	¼ Pack/75g	12	0.1	16	0.8	3.0	0.1	2.1
Sweet Leaf, M & S*	1 Pack/110g	38	0.9	35	1.5	5.3	0.8	2.1
Sweet Pepper, Medley, Waitrose*	½ Pack/100g	22	0.4	22	0.9	3.8	0.4	1.5
Sweet Pepper Side, Tesco*	1 Serving/54g	22	0.2	41	1.3	8.0	0.4	2.1
Sweet Pepper with Corn, Tesco*	1 Pack/270g	103	1.3	38	1.3	7.2	0.5	1.5
Tabbouleh, HL, Tesco*	1 Serving/200g	194	3.6	97	3.5	16.8	1.8	1.3
Tabbouleh, Salad Bar, Waitrose*	1 Serving/100g	94	1.7	94	0.0	0.0	1.7	0.0
Tabbouleh & Feta, Tesco*	1 Pack/225g	301	11.2	134	5.4	16.7	5.0	0.6
Tabbouleh Feta, Finest, Tesco*	1 Pack/225g	265	11.7	118	4.2	13.7	5.2	0.6
Three Bean, Pot, Tesco*	1 Pot/210g	204	9.2	97	4.1	10.2	4.4	2.3
Three Bean, Sainsbury's*	1 Serving/125g	108	6.3	86	4.2	6.0	5.0	0.0
Three Bean, Tinned, Tesco*	1 Tin/160g	176	1.6	110	7.7	17.6	1.0	5.3
Three Bean & Mint, Finest, Tesco*	½ Pack/115g	155	6.9	135	6.8	7.7	6.0	11.5
Three Bean & Pesto, Italian Style, Boots*	1 Serving/290g	374	12.5	129	8.3	14.0	4.3	1.8
Three Bean in Water, Drained, Wholefoods, Tesco*	½ Can/123g	135	1.2	110	7.7	17.6	1.0	5.3
Three Leaf Blend, Sainsbury's*	1 Pack/50g	9	0.3	19	1.7	1.8	0.6	1.2
Tomato, Avocado & Rocket, M & S*	1 Pack/350g	507	46.9	145	1.7	4.1	13.4	0.2
Tomato, Lettuce & Cucumber, Classics, M & S*	1 Serving/275g	151	11.5	55	0.9	3.3	4.2	1.6
Tomato & Cucumber, Ready To Eat, Morrisons*	¼ Pack/81g	17	0.2	21	0.9	3.7	0.3	2.0
Tomato & Mozzarella, Finest, Tesco*	1 Pack/175g	254	21.3	145	5.6	3.3	12.2	0.7
Tomato & Mozzarella, M & S*	1 Pack/220g	264	16.5	120	9.8	2.8	7.5	1.1
Tomato & Onion	1oz/28g	20	1.7	72	0.8	4.0	6.1	1.0
Tortellini & Chargrilled Vegetable, Tesco*	1 Serving/300g	492	23.1	164	5.1	18.7	7.7	1.7
Tortellini & Pepper, TTD, Sainsbury's*	1/3 Pack/74g	98	4.3	133	4.3	15.7	5.9	1.5
Tuna, Breton Style, Snack Pot, Carb Check, Heinz*	1 Pot/219g	239	13.8	109	8.4	4.6	6.3	1.5
Tuna, Layered, Tesco*	1 Serving/370g	466	29.2	126	4.4	9.4	7.9	1.0
Tuna, Pasta, Layered, Asda*	1 Serving/100g	98	2.8	98	5.4	12.7	2.8	1.9
Tuna, with Lemon Dressing, Tesco*	1 Serving/300g	282	24.0	94	4.2	1.4	8.0	1.0
Tuna & Mixed Bean	1 Serving/220g	287	14.4	131	9.5	11.2	6.6	3.7

S

	Measure INFO/WEIGHT	per Measure KCAL	FAT	Nutrition Values per 100g / 100ml KCAL	PROT	CARB	FAT	FIBRE
SALAD								
Tuna & Tomato, Boots*	1 Pack/171g	150	10.3	88	6.5	2.0	6.0	1.0
Tuna & Vegetable, Tesco*	½ Can/140g	189	10.1	135	9.0	8.5	7.2	3.3
Tuna Layer, COU, M & S*	1 Pack/340g	272	8.8	80	6.2	7.5	2.6	1.5
Tuna Layered, Waitrose*	1 Bowl/300g	636	58.8	212	4.0	4.8	19.6	1.0
Tuna Nicoise, BGTY, Sainsbury's*	1 Pack/300g	315	6.0	105	6.3	15.5	2.0	2.5
Tuna Nicoise, Finest, Tesco*	1 Serving/250g	430	23.5	172	8.5	13.3	9.4	0.8
Tuna Nicoise, No Mayonnaise, Shapers, Boots*	1 Pack/276g	133	3.6	48	4.0	5.0	1.3	0.8
Tuscan Style Bean & Sunblush Tomato, Waitrose*	1 Pot/225g	308	10.8	137	5.6	17.9	4.8	1.0
Vegetable, Canned	1oz/28g	40	2.7	143	1.6	13.0	9.8	1.2
Vegetable, Heinz*	1 Can/195g	259	16.6	133	1.5	12.6	8.5	1.3
Vegetable, Nutty Grain, Eat Well, M & S*	1 Pack/230g	299	11.7	130	5.3	12.8	5.1	6.1
Vegetable, Salad Bar, Waitrose*	1 Serving/100g	206	2.9	206	0.0	0.0	2.9	0.0
Waldorf, Average	1 Serving/100g	193	17.7	193	1.4	7.5	17.7	1.3
Watercress, Baby Spinach & Rocket, Somerfield*	1 Serving/100g	25	0.9	25	3.0	1.2	0.9	1.7
Watercress, Morrisons*	1 Bag/100g	17	0.7	17	1.7	1.2	0.7	0.0
Watercress, Mustard Leaf & Mizuna, M & S*	½ Pack/60g	9	0.2	15	2.4	0.4	0.3	3.0
Wild Rocket, Spinach & Watercress, Asda*	1 Serving/100g	21	0.6	21	2.8	1.2	0.6	1.9
Wild Rocket & Chard, Waitrose*	½ Bag/53g	8	0.3	15	0.8	1.7	0.5	1.4
Winter Roasted Vegetable, Salad Bar, Waitrose*	1 Serving/100g	139	10.3	139	0.0	0.0	10.3	0.0
Young, Whole Leaf, Tesco*	1 Pack/200g	28	1.0	14	0.8	1.6	0.5	1.4
SALAD CREAM								
Average	**1 Tsp/5g**	**17**	**1.4**	**335**	**1.7**	**18.6**	**27.8**	**0.1**
Heinz*	1 Tbsp/15g	50	4.0	332	1.4	20.0	26.8	0.0
Reduced Calorie, Average	**1 Tsp/5g**	**6**	**0.4**	**130**	**1.0**	**12.9**	**7.9**	**0.1**
Weight Watchers*	1 Serving/14g	16	0.6	115	1.5	16.2	4.4	0.0
SALAD KIT								
Caesar, Asda*	½ Pack/113g	154	9.0	136	5.0	11.0	8.0	1.4
Caesar, HL, Tesco*	½ Pack/133g	148	11.0	112	3.3	5.9	8.3	1.4
Caesar, New Improved, Tesco*	½ Pack/138g	279	25.3	202	4.7	4.5	18.3	1.3
Caesar, Tesco*	½ Pack/150g	237	19.8	158	3.2	6.7	13.2	0.7
Caesar, Waitrose*	1 Bag/250g	436	36.1	174	4.4	6.1	14.4	1.3
Ranch, HL, Tesco*	1 Serving/115g	69	2.9	60	4.4	5.0	2.5	1.8
SALAMI								
Ardennes Pepper, Waitrose*	1 Serving/7g	30	2.7	429	18.6	1.9	38.5	1.1
Average	**1 Slice/5g**	**18**	**1.3**	**360**	**28.4**	**1.8**	**26.1**	**0.0**
Danish, Average	**1 Serving/17g**	**89**	**8.8**	**524**	**13.2**	**1.3**	**51.7**	**0.0**
Emiliano, Sainsbury's*	1 Serving/70g	209	14.2	298	28.8	0.1	20.3	0.0
German, Average	**1 Serving/60g**	**200**	**16.4**	**333**	**20.3**	**1.6**	**27.3**	**0.1**
German, Peppered, Average	**3 Slices/25g**	**86**	**6.8**	**342**	**22.2**	**2.5**	**27.1**	**0.2**
Giganti, Sliced, TTD, Sainsbury's*	1 Slice/5g	21	1.8	411	25.0	0.1	34.4	0.6
Healthy Range, Average	**4 Slices/25g**	**55**	**3.6**	**220**	**22.3**	**0.6**	**14.3**	**0.0**
Milano, Average	**1 Serving/70g**	**278**	**22.6**	**397**	**25.9**	**0.9**	**32.2**	**0.0**
Napoli, Average	**1 Slice/5g**	**17**	**1.3**	**341**	**27.1**	**0.7**	**25.5**	**0.0**
Pepperoni, Italian, Morrisons*	1 Slice/6g	23	1.9	406	24.0	0.9	34.0	0.0
Spanish, Wafer Thin, Tesco*	1 Pack/80g	273	18.8	341	25.5	6.8	23.5	0.0
Ungherese, Tesco*	1 Serving/35g	136	11.2	388	24.5	0.5	32.0	0.0
SALMON								
Alaskan, Wild, TTD, Sainsbury's*	1 Fillet/115g	173	8.3	150	21.2	0.1	7.2	0.1
Alaskan Pink, Canned, Crown Prince*	¼ Cup/55g	90	4.0	164	20.0	0.0	7.3	0.0
Fillet, Dinner, Light & Easy, Youngs*	1 Pack/375g	315	10.5	84	6.7	7.9	2.8	1.6
Fillet, in Sunblush Tomato Dressing, The Saucy Fish Co.*	2 Fillets/270g	483	29.4	179	19.9	0.1	10.9	0.0
Fillet, Skin On, TTD, Sainsbury's*	1 Fillet/126g	249	14.3	197	23.5	0.2	11.3	0.0
Fillets, Cajun, Waitrose*	1 Serving/150g	214	9.7	143	20.6	0.4	6.5	0.0

S

SALMON

	Measure INFO/WEIGHT	per Measure KCAL	per Measure FAT	Nutrition Values per 100g / 100ml KCAL	PROT	CARB	FAT	FIBRE
Fillets, Chargrilled, Sainsbury's*	1 Serving/270g	270	19.5	243	20.9	0.2	17.6	0.0
Fillets, Chilli & Lemon Pink, Aldi*	1 Fillet/140g	260	10.4	186	16.9	12.9	7.4	0.7
Fillets, Fresh, Value, Tesco*	1 Slice/85g	153	9.3	180	21.6	0.0	11.0	0.0
Fillets, Honey Roast, Co-Op*	1 Fillet/100g	250	13.8	250	26.7	4.7	13.8	0.1
Fillets, Lightly Smoked, TTD, Sainsbury's*	1 Serving/100g	201	13.2	201	20.2	0.3	13.2	0.6
Fillets, Lime & Coriander, Tesco*	1 Pack/250g	282	5.2	113	18.2	5.4	2.1	0.0
Fillets, Raw, Average	**1 Fillet/79g**	**149**	**9.2**	**189**	**20.9**	**0.1**	**11.7**	**0.1**
Fillets, with Lemon & Herb Butter, Asda*	1 Fillet/125g	305	22.5	244	20.0	0.4	18.0	0.0
Fillets, with Orange & Dill Dressing, Tesco*	1 Serving/300g	540	30.9	180	17.7	4.1	10.3	0.7
Flakes, Honey Roast, Average	**1oz/28g**	**56**	**3.0**	**198**	**24.0**	**1.9**	**10.7**	**0.2**
Goujons, Average	1 Pack/150g	321	16.4	214	16.4	12.4	10.9	1.1
Gravadlax, Finest, Tesco*	1 Serving/70g	125	6.9	178	22.1	0.2	9.9	0.0
Gravadlax, M & S*	1 Serving/140g	294	16.0	210	18.4	5.3	11.4	0.5
Gravadlax, Scottish, M & S*	1 Serving/70g	147	8.0	210	18.4	5.3	11.4	0.5
Gravadlax with Mustard Sauce, Waitrose*	1 Pack/200g	382	22.2	191	21.8	1.0	11.1	0.4
Grilled	**1oz/28g**	**60**	**3.7**	**215**	**24.2**	**0.0**	**13.1**	**0.0**
Honey Roast Flakes, Sainsbury's*	½ Pack/68g	166	9.5	244	25.9	3.6	14.0	0.0
Hot Smoked, Average	**1 Serving/62g**	**103**	**4.4**	**166**	**24.0**	**0.9**	**7.2**	**0.1**
Juniper & Birch Smoked, TTD, Sainsbury's*	½ Pack/60g	132	8.4	220	23.3	0.3	14.0	0.1
Lime & Coriander, Tesco*	1 Serving/120g	176	4.4	147	21.4	7.0	3.7	0.7
Mild Oak Smoked, Average	**1 Slice/25g**	**45**	**2.5**	**182**	**22.6**	**0.1**	**10.2**	**0.0**
Mousse, Tesco*	1 Mousse/57g	100	7.0	177	13.5	2.9	12.4	0.2
Pink, Average	**1 Serving/125g**	**162**	**7.2**	**130**	**19.5**	**0.1**	**5.8**	**0.1**
Pink in Brine, Average	**1 Sm Can/105g**	**161**	**6.9**	**153**	**23.5**	**0.0**	**6.6**	**0.0**
Poached, Average	**1 Serving/90g**	**176**	**10.5**	**195**	**22.5**	**0.2**	**11.7**	**0.3**
Potted, M & S*	1 Serving/75g	184	14.5	245	17.1	0.5	19.4	1.2
Red, Average	**½ Can/90g**	**141**	**7.4**	**156**	**20.4**	**0.1**	**8.2**	**0.1**
Red in Brine, Average	**1oz/28g**	**47**	**2.5**	**169**	**22.4**	**0.0**	**8.9**	**0.0**
Rillettes, John West*	½ Can/62g	169	14.6	272	14.9	0.1	23.5	0.0
Roasted, Slices, Tesco*	1 Slice/33g	71	3.5	215	26.7	2.7	10.5	1.9
Roasties, Lemon & Pepper, Hot Smoked, Scottish, Asda*	1 Pack/100g	195	7.7	195	26.0	5.5	7.7	0.5
Smoked, Average	**1 Serving/70g**	**126**	**7.0**	**179**	**21.9**	**0.5**	**10.0**	**0.1**
Smoked, Gravadlax, Limoncello, Wild Waters*	1 Pack/150g	361	12.0	241	19.9	2.5	8.0	0.5
Smoked, Parcels, TTD, Sainsbury's*	1 Serving/58g	144	11.1	250	13.4	5.7	19.3	1.0
Smoked, Slices, Value, Tesco*	1 Serving/100g	180	9.7	180	22.9	0.1	9.7	0.0
Smoked, Sockeye, Wild, TTD, Sainsbury's*	½ Pack/60g	82	1.9	137	26.3	0.7	3.2	0.6
Smoked, Trimmings, Average	**1 Serving/55g**	**101**	**5.7**	**184**	**22.8**	**0.2**	**10.3**	**0.0**
Steaks	**1 Serving/100g**	**180**	**11.0**	**180**	**20.2**	**0.0**	**11.0**	**0.0**
Steamed	**1oz/28g**	**55**	**3.6**	**197**	**20.1**	**0.0**	**13.0**	**0.0**
Tail Joint, Lemon & Herb Butter, M & S*	1 Pack/480g	864	54.7	180	18.8	0.8	11.4	0.2
Whole, Raw, Average	1 Serving/100g	228	13.9	228	25.6	0.0	13.9	0.0
Wild Alaskan, Keta, Fillets, Sainsbury's*	1 Fillet/115g	178	6.4	155	25.9	0.2	5.6	0.3
with Basil, Lean Cuisine*	1 Pack/353g	260	7.4	74	5.3	8.8	2.1	1.7

SALMON &

Asparagus, Oakhouse Foods Ltd*	1 Meal/400g	396	17.2	99	6.1	9.0	4.3	0.7
Broccoli Potato Wedge Melt, Weight Watchers*	1 Pack/320g	298	10.6	93	5.1	10.6	3.3	1.1
Spinach, Roulade, Tesco*	1 Serving/60g	155	14.2	258	9.5	1.7	23.7	0.2
Vegetables, M & S*	1 Serving/200g	220	13.8	110	6.0	5.2	6.9	0.8

SALMON EN CROUTE

Chilled, Youngs*	1 Pastry/200g	531	37.3	265	9.6	14.8	18.6	2.3
Frozen, Tesco*	1 Serving/166g	365	18.4	220	10.1	19.1	11.1	1.1
Frozen, Youngs*	1 Pastry/185g	542	38.3	293	10.2	16.5	20.7	1.0
Iceland*	1 Serving/170g	476	31.3	280	8.5	20.1	18.4	1.0

S

	Measure INFO/WEIGHT	per Measure KCAL	per Measure FAT	Nutrition Values per 100g / 100ml KCAL	PROT	CARB	FAT	FIBRE
SALMON EN CROUTE								
M & S*	½ Pack/185g	573	40.5	310	10.4	17.3	21.9	0.6
Retail, Average	1oz/28g	81	5.3	288	11.8	18.0	19.1	0.5
Wild Alaskan, Inspired To Cook, Sainsbury's*	1 Parcel/173g	476	24.4	275	12.5	24.7	14.1	10.8
with Lemon & Dill, Easy to Cook, Waitrose*	½ Pack/185g	487	31.5	263	10.7	16.9	17.0	2.7
SALMON IN								
Chilli Lime & Ginger Dressing, The Saucy Fish Co.*	1 Fillet/140g	273	15.8	195	16.7	5.5	11.3	0.0
Creamy Horseradish Sauce, Fillets, Wonnemeyer*	1 Serving/300g	459	31.5	153	9.4	5.3	10.5	0.0
Creamy Watercress Sauce, Fillets, Scottish, Seafresh*	1 Pack/300g	528	38.7	176	13.7	1.2	12.9	0.1
Creamy White Wine Sauce, 146, Oakhouse Foods Ltd*	1 Meal/400g	448	19.6	112	5.7	11.7	4.9	1.6
Dill Sauce, Youngs*	1 Pack/435g	265	10.0	61	6.1	4.2	2.3	0.1
Lime & Coriander, Fillets, Good Choice, Iceland*	½ Pack/150g	189	4.3	126	19.8	5.1	2.9	0.8
Pancetta, Wrapped, Finest, Tesco*	1 Serving/150g	328	25.8	219	14.9	1.0	17.2	0.1
Tomato & Mascarpone Sauce, Fillets, Asda*	½ Pack/181g	279	19.9	154	13.0	0.8	11.0	0.6
Watercress Sauce, Pink, Wild Alaskan, Sainsbury's*	½ Pack/180g	194	9.7	108	13.9	0.9	5.4	0.8
Watercress Sauce, Somerfield*	1 Pack/210g	386	29.8	184	12.9	1.2	14.2	1.1
Watercress Sauce, Waitrose*	½ Pack/150g	264	19.3	176	13.7	1.2	12.9	0.1
White Wine & Cream Sauce, Tesco*	1 Serving/170g	279	19.2	164	13.5	2.0	11.3	1.2
White Wine & Parsley Dressing, Fillets, Tesco*	1 Fillet/150g	291	20.4	194	17.5	0.3	13.6	0.6
SALMON WITH								
a Cream Sauce, Scottish Fillets, M & S*	1 Serving/200g	360	26.0	180	13.8	1.0	13.0	0.1
Coriander & Lime, Pacific, Asda*	1 Serving/113g	154	3.4	137	27.0	0.5	3.0	0.0
Garlic & Herb Butter, Tesco*	1 Fillet/112g	291	23.1	260	17.6	0.0	20.6	0.0
Mozzarella & Tomato Crust, Just Cook, Sainsbury's*	½ Pack/171g	220	9.2	129	15.0	5.2	5.4	0.4
Pasta, Frozen, Youngs*	½ Bag/175g	234	7.7	134	7.4	16.3	4.4	1.2
Penne Pasta & Dill Sauce, SteamFresh, Birds Eye*	1 Pack/424g	335	6.4	79	6.4	9.9	1.5	1.1
Potatoes, Honey Roast, Light Choices, Tesco*	1 Pack/350g	332	12.2	95	6.6	8.5	3.5	2.4
Prawns & Fusilli Pasta, Frozen, Youngs*	1 Pack/375g	439	27.7	117	5.6	7.0	7.4	1.1
Rice, Oriental Style, M & S*	1 Pot/210g	252	6.9	120	5.9	16.5	3.3	3.3
Sweet Chilli, Fillets, Roasted, Tesco*	1 Fillet/100g	210	10.6	210	26.1	1.7	10.6	0.6
Sweet Chilli, Hot Smoked, Scottish, Tesco*	1 Fillet/120g	252	12.7	210	26.1	1.7	10.6	0.6
Sweet Chilli Lime & Ginger, Simply Fish, Tesco*	½ Pack/98g	235	17.1	240	17.4	3.2	17.5	0.0
Sweet Soy Sauce, Fillets, Inspired To Cook, Sainsbury's*	1 Fillet/142g	278	16.5	196	17.5	5.3	11.6	0.4
SALSA								
Bottled, M & S*	½ Jar/136g	95	3.3	70	1.2	12.0	2.4	1.5
Chunky, Sainsbury's*	½ Pot/84g	43	1.4	51	1.1	7.8	1.7	1.2
Cool, Sainsbury's*	1 Serving/100g	31	0.3	31	1.0	6.1	0.3	1.2
Fire Roasted Pepper, Somerfield*	1 Pot/120g	50	0.6	42	1.2	8.1	0.5	1.3
GFY, Asda*	½ Pot/236g	85	0.9	36	1.1	7.0	0.4	0.7
Hot, Fresh, Chilled, Tesco*	1 Tub/200g	120	4.8	60	1.4	7.5	2.4	1.2
Medium Hot, Discovery*	1 Serving/30g	17	0.1	56	1.4	11.7	0.4	0.8
Mild, Heinz*	1 Serving/20g	16	0.0	79	1.2	17.9	0.1	0.8
Mild, Original, Old El Paso*	1 Sachet/144g	60	0.7	42	1.6	9.0	0.5	0.0
Red Pepper, Sainsbury's*	1 Serving/85g	31	1.4	37	1.7	3.8	1.7	1.5
Smokey BBQ, Weight Watchers*	1 Serving/56g	20	0.1	36	1.1	7.6	0.1	2.3
Spiced Mango, Ginger & Chilli, Weight Watchers*	½ Pot/50g	42	0.1	85	1.0	19.9	0.2	2.6
Spicy, Less Than 3% Fat, M & S*	½ Pot/85g	30	0.7	35	1.3	5.6	0.8	0.8
Spicy Bean, Chosen By You, Asda*	½ Pot/100g	71	1.2	71	3.1	10.6	1.2	2.5
Spicy Mango & Lime, Morrisons*	½ Pot/85g	62	0.3	73	1.0	15.9	0.4	1.3
Spicy Red Pepper, Fresh, Waitrose*	½ Pot/85g	27	0.8	32	1.9	4.1	0.9	1.6
Sweetcorn, Fresh, Sainsbury's*	¼ Pot/51g	32	0.9	63	1.1	10.5	1.8	1.3
Tomato, Chunky, Tesco*	1 Pot/170g	68	2.2	40	1.1	5.9	1.3	1.1
Tomato, Chunky, Tex Mex, Tesco*	1 Serving/50g	26	1.2	52	1.0	6.4	2.5	1.0
Tomato, Mexican Style, Dip, Morrisons*	½ Pack/50g	25	0.9	51	1.2	7.6	1.8	0.8

S

	Measure INFO/WEIGHT	per Measure KCAL	FAT	Nutrition Values per 100g / 100ml KCAL	PROT	CARB	FAT	FIBRE
SALSA								
Tomato, Onion, Coriander & Chilli, Fresh, Waitrose*	1 Tub/170g	110	5.3	65	1.3	8.0	3.1	1.2
Tomato, Reduced Fat, Waitrose*	1 Serving/1g	0	0.0	27	1.5	4.7	0.2	1.4
Tomato, Spicy, Worldwide Sauces*	1 Serving/25g	7	0.0	30	1.2	5.9	0.2	1.2
Tomato, Sun Ripened, Tesco*	1 Serving/40g	46	1.7	115	5.0	14.2	4.2	4.6
Tomato, Vine Ripened, Tesco*	½ Tub/100g	47	1.8	47	1.0	6.7	1.8	1.1
Tomato & Avocado, Chunky, COU, M & S*	½ Pack/86g	30	1.2	35	0.8	5.4	1.4	1.4
Vine Ripened Tomato & Jalapeno, Sainsbury's*	¼ Tub/50g	34	1.7	68	1.1	8.0	3.5	1.2
SALT								
Alternative, Reduced Sodium, Losalt*	2 Tsp/10g	0	0.0	0	0.0	0.0	0.0	0.0
Rock, Average	¼ Tsp/1g	0	0.0	0	0.0	0.0	0.0	0.0
Table, Average	*1 Tsp/5g*	*0*	*0.0*	*0*	*0.0*	*0.0*	*0.0*	*0.0*
SAMOSAS								
Chicken, Mumtaz*	1 Serving/105g	177	8.3	169	19.6	4.9	7.9	0.0
Chicken Tikka, Sainsbury's*	1 Samosa/50g	119	6.4	239	8.3	22.5	12.9	3.1
Co-Op*	1oz/28g	70	2.8	250	6.0	34.0	10.0	2.0
Dim Sum Selection, Sainsbury's*	1 Samosa/12g	24	0.9	196	3.4	28.6	7.6	2.8
Indian Style Selection, Co-Op*	1 Samosa/21g	50	2.7	240	5.0	27.0	13.0	3.0
Lamb, Morrisons*	1 Samosa/50g	144	7.8	288	9.8	27.0	15.7	1.5
Vegetable, Large, Individual, Sainsbury's*	1 Samosa/110g	254	16.5	231	3.3	20.7	15.0	2.1
Vegetable, Large, Tesco*	1 Samosa/64g	148	7.9	231	4.8	25.2	12.4	3.4
Vegetable, M & S*	1 Samosa/45g	115	6.9	255	5.1	24.8	15.3	2.8
Vegetable, Mini, Asda*	1 Samosa/23g	52	2.0	233	6.0	32.0	9.0	2.6
Vegetable, Mini, Indian, Party Selection, Tesco*	1 Samosa/30g	58	1.5	195	3.6	33.9	5.0	2.2
Vegetable, Mini, Indian, Somerfield*	1 Samosa/25g	64	3.3	253	5.7	28.1	13.1	3.4
Vegetable, Mini, Indian Snack Selection, Sainsbury's*	1 Samosa/25g	70	3.9	280	4.7	29.8	15.8	3.2
Vegetable, Mini, Indian Snack Selection, Tesco*	1 Samosa/32g	76	4.2	238	4.7	25.5	13.0	3.3
Vegetable, Mini, Waitrose*	1 Samosa/29g	70	3.8	242	3.6	27.1	13.2	3.1
Vegetable, Morrisons*	1 Samosa/60g	101	3.5	169	4.9	24.1	5.8	2.0
Vegetable, Northern Indian, Sainsbury's*	1 Samosa/50g	126	5.9	252	5.8	30.6	11.8	2.6
Vegetable, Retail, Average	1 Samosa/110g	239	10.2	217	5.1	30.0	9.3	2.5
Vegetable, Somerfield*	1 Serving/50g	126	6.5	253	5.7	28.1	13.1	3.4
Vegetable, Waitrose*	1 Samosa/50g	118	7.1	236	3.7	23.1	14.3	2.7
Vegetable Lightly Spiced, Sainsbury's*	1 Samosa/50g	112	6.3	223	4.0	23.5	12.5	1.2
SAMPHIRE								
Raw, Fresh	1 Serving/80g	24	0.0	30	12.0	0.0	0.0	3.0
SANDWICH								
All Day Breakfast, BGTY, Sainsbury's*	1 Pack/188g	294	4.5	156	9.6	22.7	2.4	0.0
All Day Breakfast, Finest, Tesco*	1 Pack/275g	660	41.5	240	9.7	16.4	15.1	1.6
All Day Breakfast, Shapers, Boots*	1 Pack/207g	323	5.2	156	11.0	23.0	2.5	2.2
All Day Breakfast, Weight Watchers*	1 Pack/158g	298	4.3	189	11.0	30.2	2.7	1.9
Avocado, Mozzarella & Tomato, M & S*	1 Pack/273g	655	36.0	240	8.8	21.7	13.2	2.3
Avocado & Spinach, M & S*	1 Pack/242g	580	27.3	240	4.0	21.0	11.3	4.8
Bacon, Brie & Mango Chutney, Daily Bread*	1 Serving/213g	555	22.7	261	12.7	28.6	10.7	0.0
Bacon & Brie, Asda*	1 Pack/181g	603	38.2	333	13.3	22.9	21.1	1.3
Bacon & Brie, Finest, Tesco*	1 Pack/201g	571	33.6	284	14.1	19.4	16.7	2.1
Bacon & Brown Sauce, Ashberry*	1 Pack/419g	1207	53.6	288	12.0	31.0	12.8	0.0
Bacon & Egg, Boots*	1 Pack/179g	480	28.6	268	12.0	16.0	16.0	1.4
Bacon & Egg, Free Range, Daily Bread*	1 Serving/175g	425	22.9	243	10.1	21.5	13.1	0.0
Bacon & Egg, HL, Tesco*	1 Serving/178g	328	9.3	184	11.5	22.7	5.2	1.7
Bacon & Egg, Sainsbury's*	1 Pack/160g	384	17.8	240	13.0	22.0	11.1	1.8
Bacon & Egg, Scottish Slimmers, Tesco*	1 Pack/139g	279	6.4	201	13.6	26.3	4.6	1.2
Bacon & Tomato, COU, M & S*	1 Pack/169g	270	4.6	160	9.5	25.6	2.7	2.5
Baguette, Cheese, & Onion, Asda*	¼ Loaf/42g	154	7.4	366	12.0	39.8	17.6	1.3

S

SANDWICH

INFO/WEIGHT	Measure	per Measure		Nutrition Values per 100g / 100ml				
		KCAL	FAT	KCAL	PROT	CARB	FAT	FIBRE
Bap, Chicken, Chargrilled, Malted, Co-Op*	1 Bap/201g	492	26.1	245	9.0	23.0	13.0	2.0
Bap, Corned Beef & Onion, White, Open Choice Foods*	1 Bap/144g	331	8.8	230	12.7	30.7	6.1	0.0
Bap, Ham & Salad, Co-Op*	1 Bap/164g	295	4.9	180	8.0	30.0	3.0	2.0
Bap, Tuna & Sweetcorn, Malted, Co-Op*	1 Bap/212g	530	27.6	250	9.0	24.0	13.0	2.0
Beef, Roast, Feel Good, Shell*	1 Pack/153g	390	14.8	255	17.6	24.2	9.7	0.0
Beef, Roast, Handmade, Tesco*	1 Pack/223g	439	15.8	197	12.5	20.7	7.1	1.6
Beef, Roast, Plain, From Restaurant, Average	1 Sandwich/139g	346	13.8	249	15.5	24.1	9.9	0.0
Beef, Roast, Sainsbury's*	1 Pack/174g	426	17.4	245	9.4	29.3	10.0	0.0
Beef, Tomato & Horseradish, Asda*	1 Pack/169g	255	4.4	151	10.0	22.0	2.6	2.7
Beef & Horseradish, Deep Filled, BGTY, Sainsbury's*	1 Pack/202g	313	4.8	155	11.4	22.0	2.4	2.4
Beef & Horseradish, Sainsbury's*	1 Pack/187g	389	13.3	208	12.0	24.1	7.1	0.0
Beef & Onion, Roast, Deep Filled, Asda*	1 Pack/258g	550	27.9	213	11.3	22.6	10.8	1.1
Beef & Onion, Roast, HL, Tesco*	1 Pack/185g	278	3.5	150	13.3	20.0	1.9	2.7
Beef & Pate, M & S*	1 Pack/188g	310	7.3	165	11.2	21.6	3.9	2.4
Beef & Salad, Roast, Daily Bread*	1 Pack/202g	319	8.3	158	9.0	21.4	4.1	0.0
Bloomer, BLT, Freshly Prepared, M & S*	1 Pack/210g	430	19.5	205	8.2	21.8	9.3	1.8
Bloomer, Egg & Watercress, Freshly Prepared, M & S*	1 Pack/221g	465	26.1	210	10.2	15.3	11.8	3.0
BLT, & Chicken Salad, Co-Op*	1 Pack/230g	471	20.7	205	10.0	21.0	9.0	2.0
BLT, Bacon, Lettuce & Tomato, Light Choices, Tesco*	1 Pack/155g	310	7.9	200	9.9	26.5	5.1	2.2
BLT, BGTY, Sainsbury's*	1 Pack/196g	331	4.4	169	10.4	27.0	2.2	0.0
BLT, COU, M & S*	1 Pack/174g	278	4.7	160	9.5	25.6	2.7	2.5
BLT, Daily Bread*	1 Pack/171g	344	18.8	201	9.1	21.6	11.0	0.0
BLT, Deep Filled, Asda*	1 Pack/206g	606	35.0	294	13.3	21.8	17.0	3.0
BLT, Healthy Selection, Somerfield*	1 Pack/150g	217	3.1	145	9.4	22.2	2.1	2.5
BLT, HL, Tesco*	1 Pack/190g	287	2.7	151	10.1	24.5	1.4	1.6
BLT, Impress*	1 Pack/189g	381	13.4	202	11.5	22.8	7.1	0.0
BLT, Waitrose*	1 Pack/184g	398	16.4	216	9.5	24.5	8.9	2.3
BLT with Mayo, Seeded Malted Bread, Deep Fill, Heinz*	1 Pack/182g	444	19.8	244	10.3	26.2	10.9	3.0
Brie & Easy Calzone, Cranks*	1 Pack/160g	417	20.0	260	8.5	27.7	12.5	1.6
Brie & Grape, Finest, Tesco*	1 Pack/209g	527	31.6	252	8.5	20.6	15.1	1.5
Brie LT, Cranks*	1 Pack/192g	383	16.9	199	7.7	21.5	8.8	1.7
Brunch, St Ivel*	1 Pack/225g	580	28.3	258	10.2	26.0	12.6	0.0
Chargrilled Vegetable & Houmous, HL, Tesco*	1 Pack/167g	250	4.0	150	5.9	25.3	2.4	2.0
Cheddar, Red Leicester & Onion, Tesco*	1 Pack/182g	604	38.9	332	11.0	23.8	21.4	2.5
Cheddar & Celery, M & S*	1 Pack/200g	540	31.8	270	9.7	22.4	15.9	1.5
Cheddar & Coleslaw, Simply, Boots*	1 Pack/185g	538	33.3	291	9.2	23.0	18.0	1.8
Cheddar & Ham, M & S*	1 Pack/165g	396	18.6	240	15.1	20.0	11.3	1.7
Cheddar & Ham with Pickle, Smoked, Finest, Tesco*	1 Pack/217g	532	24.7	245	11.9	23.7	11.4	3.9
Cheddar & Pickle, Mature, Sainsbury's*	1 Pack/171g	588	27.0	344	14.3	38.7	15.8	7.0
Cheddar & Salad, Mature, Upper Crust*	1 Pack/225g	466	22.1	207	9.5	20.3	9.8	0.0
Cheddar & Tomato, Mature, Big, Sainsbury's*	1 Pack/233g	596	25.6	256	12.9	26.3	11.0	0.0
Cheddar & Tomato, Red, Tesco*	1 Pack/182g	526	31.7	289	9.2	24.0	17.4	1.1
Cheddar Gorge, Cranks*	1 Pack/190g	454	23.2	239	11.5	19.4	12.2	3.0
Cheese, Apple & Celery, Asda*	1 Pack/173g	244	4.8	141	8.0	21.0	2.8	2.7
Cheese, Apple & Grape, COU, M & S*	1 Pack/186g	270	2.2	145	8.5	24.9	1.2	2.0
Cheese, Asda*	1 Pack/262g	618	31.4	236	12.2	20.3	12.0	3.0
Cheese, Crunch, Scottish Slimmers*	1 Pack/137g	292	9.0	213	11.0	27.6	6.6	2.3
Cheese, Ham, BLT, Triple Pack, Asda*	1 Pack/260g	614	31.2	236	12.2	20.3	12.0	3.0
Cheese, Ham & Pickle, HL, Tesco*	1 Pack/201g	312	4.2	155	13.1	21.0	2.1	1.7
Cheese, Ham & Pickle, Simply, Boots*	1 Pack/225g	551	29.2	245	11.0	21.0	13.0	2.4
Cheese, Savoury, Sandwich King*	1 Pack/135g	328	11.2	243	11.6	30.2	8.3	0.0
Cheese, Three & Onion, Boots*	1 Pack/169g	566	33.8	335	11.0	28.0	20.0	1.9
Cheese, Three & Spring Onion, Shell*	1 Pack/168g	672	50.9	400	11.1	20.8	30.3	0.0

S

SANDWICH

	Measure INFO/WEIGHT	per Measure KCAL	FAT	Nutrition Values per 100g / 100ml KCAL	PROT	CARB	FAT	FIBRE
Cheese & Celery, Shapers, Boots*	1 Pack/181g	288	4.2	159	11.0	24.0	2.3	3.0
Cheese & Coleslaw, M & S*	1 Pack/186g	498	32.4	268	10.2	17.6	17.4	3.2
Cheese & Coleslaw, Shapers, Boots*	1 Pack/224g	338	4.7	151	11.0	22.0	2.1	3.2
Cheese & Ham, Baxter & Platts*	1 Pack/168g	408	21.8	243	11.3	20.5	13.0	1.7
Cheese & Marmite, No Mayonnaise, Boots*	1 Pack/156g	420	20.0	269	12.2	26.3	12.8	1.7
Cheese & Onion, Deep Fill, Tesco*	1 Pack/212g	742	51.9	350	12.3	20.2	24.5	1.3
Cheese & Onion, GFY, Asda*	1 Pack/156g	317	4.1	203	14.0	31.0	2.6	2.7
Cheese & Onion, Light Choices, Tesco*	1 Pack/144g	310	9.4	215	12.7	26.5	6.5	3.6
Cheese & Onion, Waitrose*	1 Pack/176g	579	38.7	329	12.5	20.2	22.0	2.8
Cheese & Pickle, Heinz*	1 Pack/178g	543	26.9	305	13.8	28.4	15.1	3.8
Cheese & Pickle, Shapers, Boots*	1 Pack/165g	342	8.1	207	9.8	31.0	4.9	2.3
Cheese & Pickle, Tesco*	1 Pack/140g	400	19.3	286	12.7	27.8	13.8	1.4
Cheese & Salad, COU, M & S*	1 Pack/188g	244	3.0	130	12.1	17.0	1.6	2.4
Cheese & Salad, Shapers, Boots*	1 Pack/205g	307	5.1	150	9.7	22.0	2.5	2.2
Cheese & Spring Onion, Asda*	1 Pack/160g	576	39.9	361	13.0	21.0	25.0	1.9
Cheese & Spring Onion, Mixed, Scottish Slimmers*	1 Pack/139g	298	9.1	214	12.4	26.5	6.5	2.1
Cheese & Tomato, Asda*	1 Pack/154g	388	19.7	252	11.0	23.2	12.8	3.7
Cheese & Tomato, Freshmans*	1 Pack/111g	248	18.6	223	11.0	8.0	16.8	0.0
Cheese & Tomato, Organic, M & S*	1 Pack/165g	559	35.3	339	11.8	24.8	21.4	1.9
Cheese & Tomato, Sainsbury's*	1 Pack/216g	542	26.3	251	12.9	22.8	12.2	0.0
Cheese & Tomato, Tesco*	1 Pack/182g	582	38.9	320	9.2	22.6	21.4	1.1
Chicken, & Bacon, Healthy Living, Co-Op*	1 Pack/179g	277	3.4	155	12.3	21.8	1.9	3.4
Chicken, & Bacon, HL, Tesco*	1 Pack/193g	318	6.2	165	13.5	19.5	3.2	2.7
Chicken, & Bacon, M & S*	1 Pack/185g	509	27.2	275	15.9	20.2	14.7	2.1
Chicken, & Bacon, Roast, Boots*	1 Pack/175g	413	14.0	236	15.4	26.3	8.0	2.2
Chicken, & Bacon, Shapers, Boots*	1 Pack/179g	317	8.9	177	14.0	19.0	5.0	3.1
Chicken, & Bacon, Tesco*	1 Pack/195g	486	24.2	249	14.3	20.0	12.4	2.7
Chicken, & Coleslaw, Tesco*	1 Pack/160g	305	7.1	191	12.0	25.7	4.4	2.4
Chicken, & Ham, Oak Smoked, Big, Sainsbury's*	1 Pack/244g	461	17.6	189	12.3	18.8	7.2	0.0
Chicken, & Ham, Roast, Ginsters*	1 Pack/180g	425	24.5	236	11.2	18.5	13.6	0.0
Chicken, & Ham, Roast, Tesco*	1 Pack/228g	561	31.9	246	13.3	16.6	14.0	1.2
Chicken, & Mayonnaise, Country Harvest*	1 Pack/120g	268	9.0	223	13.1	27.6	7.5	0.0
Chicken, & Pepperonata, COU, M & S*	1 Pack/171g	240	2.9	140	10.4	20.9	1.7	1.3
Chicken, & Pesto, Shapers, Boots*	1 Pack/181g	311	4.2	172	12.0	26.0	2.3	1.7
Chicken, & Pesto Salad, Bells*	1 Pack/196g	430	22.9	220	12.0	16.6	11.7	0.0
Chicken, & Roasted Peppers, Chargrilled, BHS*	1 Pack/183g	295	5.7	161	11.5	22.0	3.1	3.1
Chicken, & Salad, Bernard Matthews*	1 Pack/162g	269	8.4	166	7.0	22.7	5.2	0.0
Chicken, & Salad, Best for You, BHS*	1 Pack/315g	992	16.7	315	23.2	43.1	5.3	3.3
Chicken, & Salad, Co-Op*	1 Pack/195g	448	21.4	230	10.0	24.0	11.0	2.0
Chicken, & Salad, COU, M & S*	1 Pack/194g	262	3.7	135	9.8	19.0	1.9	1.6
Chicken, & Salad, Deep Filled, Asda*	1 Pack/247g	551	18.3	223	18.1	22.2	7.4	1.3
Chicken, & Salad, Deep Filled, Tesco*	1 Pack/238g	440	19.5	185	13.1	14.6	8.2	2.8
Chicken, & Salad, Ham & Cheese, Twin, Tesco*	1 Pack/189g	434	21.5	230	10.8	21.1	11.4	2.3
Chicken, & Salad, Healthy Living, Co-Op*	1 Pack/196g	265	3.5	135	10.4	19.1	1.8	3.9
Chicken, & Salad, Heinz*	1 Pack/166g	331	15.9	200	8.6	19.9	9.6	2.0
Chicken, & Salad, HL, Tesco*	1 Pack/207g	290	3.9	140	13.9	16.8	1.9	2.7
Chicken, & Salad, Low Fat, Heinz*	1 Pack/166g	246	2.2	148	11.8	22.3	1.3	5.3
Chicken, & Salad, Roast, COU, M & S*	1 Pack/196g	265	4.5	135	8.9	19.6	2.3	2.2
Chicken, & Salad, Roast, Feel Good, Shell*	1 Pack/191g	326	9.0	171	9.8	22.4	4.7	0.0
Chicken, & Salad, Roast, Waitrose*	1 Pack/217g	482	24.1	222	9.4	21.1	11.1	0.0
Chicken, & Salad, Sainsbury's*	1 Pack/240g	425	14.2	177	12.1	18.8	5.9	0.0
Chicken, & Salad, Scottish Slimmers*	1 Pack/169g	275	6.4	163	9.5	22.8	3.8	1.8
Chicken, & Salad, Shell*	1 Pack/201g	404	19.7	201	8.7	19.4	9.8	0.0

SANDWICH

	Measure INFO/WEIGHT	per Measure KCAL	FAT	Nutrition Values per 100g / 100ml KCAL	PROT	CARB	FAT	FIBRE
Chicken, & Salad, Tesco*	1 Pack/193g	386	17.6	200	11.9	17.6	9.1	1.5
Chicken, & Salad, Waitrose*	1 Pack/208g	406	19.8	195	10.3	17.1	9.5	2.5
Chicken, & Stuffing, Light Choices, Tesco*	1 Pack/172g	275	4.8	160	14.4	18.7	2.8	6.9
Chicken, & Stuffing, Roast, Weight Watchers*	1 Pack/159g	283	4.5	178	14.1	24.2	2.8	3.1
Chicken, & Stuffing, Tesco*	1 Pack/323g	1043	58.8	323	10.4	29.4	18.2	1.0
Chicken, & Stuffing, Waitrose*	1 Pack/183g	450	18.8	246	12.8	25.6	10.3	1.5
Chicken, & Sweetcorn, Scottish Slimmers*	1 Pack/147g	289	7.2	197	11.1	27.4	4.9	2.2
Chicken, & Sweetcorn, Shapers, Boots*	1 Pack/180g	324	6.3	180	12.0	25.0	3.5	2.0
Chicken, & Tomato Relish, Chargrilled, Shapers, Boots*	1 Pack/190g	294	5.7	155	12.0	20.0	3.0	3.1
Chicken, & Tomato Salsa, Chargrilled, BGTY, Sainsbury's*	1 Pack/225g	218	4.0	97	1.5	15.9	1.8	2.9
Chicken, & Watercress, Chargrilled, M & S*	1 Pack/173g	285	2.9	165	12.8	23.9	1.7	2.1
Chicken, & Watercress, COU, M & S*	1 Pack/164g	266	2.8	162	12.8	23.9	1.7	2.1
Chicken, Bacon, & Avocado, M & S*	1 Pack/242g	508	28.3	210	10.7	15.8	11.7	3.2
Chicken, Bacon, & Cheese, Club, M & S*	1 Pack/383g	805	37.2	210	11.9	18.5	9.7	1.9
Chicken, Bacon & Guacamole, Darwins Deli*	1 Pack/198g	340	16.4	172	3.6	15.9	8.3	1.7
Chicken, Bacon & Lettuce, No Mayo, Light Choices, Tesco*	1 Pack/186g	325	6.9	175	15.2	19.6	3.7	2.5
Chicken, Bacon & Salad, Big, Sainsbury's*	1 Pack/249g	610	31.6	245	11.1	21.7	12.7	0.0
Chicken, Bacon & Tomato, BGTY, Sainsbury's*	1 Pack/190g	270	4.4	142	11.4	19.0	2.3	0.0
Chicken, Bacon & Tomato with Paprika, Shapers, Boots*	1 Pack/184g	296	8.5	161	11.0	19.0	4.6	2.3
Chicken, Basil & Sunblush Tomato, Harry Mason*	1 Pack/164g	272	5.2	166	13.0	21.8	3.2	0.6
Chicken, Bechamel & Leek, Daily Bread*	1 Pack/210g	383	7.2	182	11.0	26.8	3.4	0.0
Chicken, BLT, Daily Bread*	1 Pack/187g	322	13.1	172	9.0	19.5	7.0	0.0
Chicken, Breast, BGTY, Sainsbury's*	1 Pack/165g	251	0.8	152	12.2	24.7	0.5	0.0
Chicken, Breast, Millers*	1 Pack/162g	343	14.4	212	13.8	19.3	8.9	0.0
Chicken, Breast, Oldfields*	1 Pack/193g	311	8.1	161	11.7	19.8	4.2	3.0
Chicken, British, & Chorizo, Finest, Tesco*	1 Pack/186g	391	12.6	210	15.7	21.2	6.8	2.7
Chicken, Caesar, & Salad, Sainsbury's*	1 Pack/186g	299	7.1	161	11.2	20.4	3.8	0.0
Chicken, Caesar, Boots*	1 Pack/226g	531	27.1	235	9.8	22.0	12.0	1.7
Chicken, Caesar, Chargrilled, Big, Sainsbury's*	1 Pack/216g	657	36.9	304	12.2	25.3	17.1	0.0
Chicken, Chargrilled, Ginsters*	1 Pack/209g	431	17.3	206	11.3	21.6	8.3	0.0
Chicken, Chargrilled, No Mayo, Rustlers*	1 Pack/150g	228	1.2	152	16.0	20.1	0.8	0.0
Chicken, Chargrilled, Pitta Pocket, M & S*	1 Pack/208g	279	7.3	134	11.2	14.5	3.5	1.6
Chicken, Chargrilled with Salad, Weight Watchers*	1 Pack/181g	264	3.8	146	11.7	20.0	2.1	2.2
Chicken, Cheese, Bacon, Big, Sainsbury's*	1 Pack/254g	734	45.5	289	11.7	18.0	17.9	0.0
Chicken, Chinese, Low Calorie, Tesco*	1 Pack/169g	270	4.2	160	11.8	22.6	2.5	2.0
Chicken, Chinese, Malted Brown Bread, Waitrose*	1 Pack/164g	333	11.2	203	13.5	21.9	6.8	3.3
Chicken, Chinese, Snack & Shop, Esso*	1 Pack/178g	409	16.0	230	13.0	22.8	9.0	4.0
Chicken, Chinese, Treat Yourself, Shell*	1 Pack/178g	409	17.1	230	13.0	22.8	9.6	0.0
Chicken, Chorizo & Chipotle Mayonaise, Tesco*	1 Pack/174g	365	13.4	210	12.1	22.7	7.7	2.3
Chicken, Coronation, Indulgence, Taste!*	1 Pack/159g	396	18.8	249	9.1	26.5	11.8	0.0
Chicken, Coronation, M & S*	1 Pack/210g	420	20.4	200	11.2	20.2	9.7	3.1
Chicken, Creole & Italian Leaves, Northern Bites*	1 Pack/190g	298	4.6	157	13.1	22.1	2.4	2.4
Chicken, Flame Grilled, Rustlers*	1 Pack/150g	346	14.2	231	16.3	20.1	9.5	0.0
Chicken, Ham, & Prawn, Triple, Weight Watchers*	1 Pack/250g	337	3.7	135	9.8	20.5	1.5	2.6
Chicken, Ham, Prawn, Triple Pack, HL, Tesco*	1 Pack/247g	350	5.2	142	10.7	20.2	2.1	2.2
Chicken, Healthier Choice, Ginsters*	1 Pack/183g	247	2.6	135	10.2	20.5	1.4	0.0
Chicken, Honey & Mustard, BGTY, Sainsbury's*	1 Pack/171g	296	4.6	173	13.1	24.0	2.7	0.0
Chicken, Jalfrezi, Naan, Ready to Go, M & S*	1 Pack/288g	576	18.1	200	9.8	26.3	6.3	2.9
Chicken, Kashmir, French Cuisiniers*	1 Pack/145g	204	2.3	141	12.9	20.3	1.6	2.9
Chicken, Lemon, & Relish, Perfectly Balanced, Waitrose*	1 Pack/151g	243	4.4	161	12.3	21.4	2.9	3.5
Chicken, No Mayo, M & S*	1 Pack/142g	248	3.3	175	16.6	20.6	2.3	3.2
Chicken, No Mayonnaise, Waitrose*	1 Pack/173g	332	9.5	192	11.6	24.0	5.5	2.1
Chicken, Pesano Pesto, Brambles*	1 Pack/417g	826	26.3	198	10.8	24.0	6.3	1.5

S

SANDWICH

	Measure INFO/WEIGHT	per Measure KCAL	FAT	KCAL	PROT	CARB	FAT	FIBRE
Chicken, Red Thai, BGTY, Sainsbury's*	1 Pack/195g	326	3.7	167	11.3	26.4	1.9	0.0
Chicken, Roast, & Salad, Shapers, Boots*	1 Pack/183g	274	4.4	150	12.0	20.0	2.4	3.4
Chicken, Roast, Breast, BGTY, Sainsbury's*	1 Pack/174g	275	4.3	158	14.8	20.9	2.5	1.8
Chicken, Roast, HL, Tesco*	1 Pack/155g	288	5.3	186	13.5	25.4	3.4	1.4
Chicken, Roast, Salad, BGTY, Sainsbury's*	1 Pack/182g	268	4.0	147	11.9	19.9	2.2	2.7
Chicken, Roast, Shapers, Boots*	1 Pack/163g	259	2.1	159	16.0	21.0	1.3	2.5
Chicken, Roast, Triple, Perfectly Balanced, Waitrose*	1 Pack/254g	356	8.1	140	8.7	19.2	3.2	2.8
Chicken, Rustlers*	1 Pack/150g	346	14.2	231	16.3	20.1	9.5	0.0
Chicken, Salad, M & S*	1 Pack/226g	350	9.3	155	10.6	18.8	4.1	3.0
Chicken, Salad on Malted Bread, BGTY, Sainsbury's*	1 Pack/216g	346	7.3	160	12.7	19.7	3.4	2.7
Chicken, Shell*	1 Pack/121g	334	15.7	276	13.9	25.9	13.0	0.0
Chicken, Smokey, BGTY, Sainsbury's*	1 Pack/178g	276	1.8	155	11.1	25.6	1.0	0.0
Chicken, Southern Spiced, M & S*	1 Pack/179g	421	23.3	235	11.2	21.7	13.0	3.1
Chicken, Spicy, Deep Filled, Co-Op*	1 Pack/216g	421	15.1	195	10.0	24.0	7.0	3.0
Chicken, Tandoori, Waitrose*	1 Pack/181g	302	5.6	167	11.6	23.0	3.1	4.1
Chicken, Tangy Lime & Ginger, Shapers, Boots*	1 Pack/168g	319	10.8	190	12.0	21.0	6.4	5.1
Chicken, Thai, BGTY, Sainsbury's*	1 Pack/196g	280	5.1	143	10.2	19.6	2.6	0.6
Chicken, Thai, Tesco*	1 Pack/244g	634	38.3	260	8.5	21.1	15.7	1.5
Chicken, Tikka, Asda*	1 Pack/186g	316	8.7	170	11.0	21.0	4.7	1.5
Chicken, Tikka, COU, M & S*	1 Pack/185g	268	3.3	145	12.1	20.5	1.8	3.2
Chicken, Tikka, M & S*	1 Pack/180g	391	19.6	217	10.4	19.5	10.9	2.0
Chicken, Tikka, Weight Watchers*	1 Pack/158g	250	2.2	158	13.1	23.2	1.4	2.9
Chicken, Tikka & Yoghurt, Taste!*	1 Pack/215g	437	21.1	203	8.2	20.4	9.8	0.0
Chicken, Tikka on Pepper Chilli Bread, Shapers, Boots*	1 Pack/172g	296	4.5	172	13.0	25.0	2.6	2.5
Chicken, Tomato & Rocket, Light Choices, Tesco*	1 Pack/184g	285	3.9	155	10.3	23.4	2.1	2.6
Chicken, Triple, GFY, Asda*	1 Pack/230g	453	11.5	197	13.0	25.0	5.0	1.6
Chicken, Working Lunch*	1 Pack/169g	298	7.7	176	14.0	19.9	4.5	1.8
Chicken & Bacon, BGTY, Sainsbury's*	1 Pack/211g	315	4.9	149	11.7	20.8	2.3	0.0
Chicken & Bacon, COU, M & S*	1 Pack/179g	250	3.6	140	13.5	15.8	2.0	3.8
Chicken & Bacon, Deep Fill, Ginsters*	1 Pack/200g	435	15.7	224	12.4	25.3	8.1	2.4
Chicken & Bacon Club, Fully Loaded, Handmade, Tesco*	1 Pack/257g	580	21.1	225	12.1	24.3	8.2	2.3
Chicken & Coriander with Lime, BGTY, Sainsbury's*	1 Pack/168g	282	5.9	168	10.6	23.5	3.5	0.0
Chicken & Lemon with Mint, Delilite*	1 Pack/179g	325	6.4	182	12.3	23.1	3.6	1.7
Chicken & Mustard Coleslaw, Good to Go, Waitrose*	1 Pack/184g	412	17.3	224	9.8	24.9	9.4	1.9
Chicken Jalfrezi, Deep Fill, Ginsters*	1 Pack/171g	389	14.6	227	8.4	29.3	8.5	1.7
Chicken Salad, Choice*	1 Pack/174g	285	5.0	164	11.5	22.9	2.9	1.7
Chicken Salad, Deep Fill, Ginsters*	1 Pack/203g	364	12.4	179	10.3	20.8	6.1	2.1
Chicken Salad, Light Choices, Tesco*	1 Pack/207g	290	3.9	140	13.9	16.8	1.9	2.7
Chicken Salad with Tomato & Basil, HL, Tesco*	1 Pack/190g	285	4.0	150	13.7	18.7	2.1	2.5
Chicken Tikka, Bellini & Blake*	1 Pack/179g	354	10.4	198	11.4	24.6	5.8	1.3
Corned Beef, Tomato & Onion, Salad Garden*	1 Pack/137g	338	14.8	247	14.2	23.0	10.8	0.0
Corned Beef on White, Simply, Brambles*	1 Pack/126g	325	10.8	258	14.2	30.8	8.6	1.4
Coronation Chicken, on Onion Bread, M & S*	1 Pack/260g	520	21.3	200	10.7	20.0	8.2	1.9
Crab, Marie Rose, Brown Bread, Royal London Hospital*	1 Pack/158g	293	11.2	185	9.7	22.0	7.1	0.0
Crayfish & Lemon Mayonnaise, Daily Bread*	1 Pack/173g	391	11.4	226	9.5	31.0	6.6	0.0
Crayfish & Rocket, Bells*	1 Pack/144g	276	11.8	192	11.2	18.4	8.2	2.0
Crayfish & Rocket, Bistro, Waitrose*	1 Pack/193g	422	19.5	219	11.5	20.4	10.1	2.4
Crayfish & Rocket, Finest, Tesco*	1 Pack/178g	365	10.5	205	9.8	27.5	5.9	2.1
Crayfish & Rocket, Shapers, Boots*	1 Pack/172g	291	3.8	169	11.0	26.0	2.2	2.5
Cream Cheese, Red Pepper & Spinach, Daily Bread*	1 Pack/156g	273	8.1	175	7.4	24.0	5.2	0.0
Cream Cheese & Ham, Tesco*	1 Pack/212g	655	36.7	309	11.0	27.2	17.3	1.2
Cream Cheese & Peppers, Taste!*	1 Pack/154g	296	10.5	192	7.3	25.5	6.8	0.0
Cream Cheese & Salad, Sandwich Box*	1 Pack/138g	250	8.0	181	5.6	26.3	5.8	0.0

S

SANDWICH

	Measure INFO/WEIGHT	per Measure KCAL	per Measure FAT	Nutrition Values per 100g / 100ml KCAL	PROT	CARB	FAT	FIBRE
Cumberland Sausage, Ginsters*	1 Pack/210g	564	29.5	268	9.3	26.0	14.0	2.4
Duck, Peking, No Mayo, Boots*	1 Pack/222g	399	10.2	180	7.7	27.0	4.6	1.7
Egg, & Bacon, & Lincolnshire Sausage, Waitrose*	1 Pack/249g	655	32.9	263	11.3	24.7	13.2	0.9
Egg, & Bacon, Weight Watchers*	1 Pack/139g	246	5.0	177	10.1	26.1	3.6	1.9
Egg, & Cress, Co-Op*	1 Pack/159g	397	23.8	250	9.0	21.0	15.0	2.0
Egg, & Cress, COU, M & S*	1 Pack/192g	240	5.2	125	9.8	15.5	2.7	2.8
Egg, & Cress, Free Range, Sainsbury's*	1 Pack/204g	404	16.9	198	10.5	20.3	8.3	3.3
Egg, & Cress, Heinz*	1 Pack/200g	610	21.6	305	14.4	37.5	10.8	4.0
Egg, & Cress, Organic, M & S*	1 Pack/185g	444	26.3	240	9.6	18.0	14.2	3.6
Egg, & Cress, Reduced Fat, Waitrose*	1 Pack/162g	262	10.4	162	9.7	16.5	6.4	6.4
Egg, & Ham, Asda*	1 Pack/262g	589	33.5	225	10.4	16.8	12.8	2.1
Egg, & Salad, Co-Op*	1 Pack/190g	285	7.6	150	7.0	22.0	4.0	4.0
Egg, & Salad, GFY, Asda*	1 Pack/157g	229	4.5	146	8.0	22.0	2.9	2.9
Egg, & Salad, Shapers, Boots*	1 Pack/184g	304	8.5	165	6.9	24.0	4.6	1.1
Egg, & Salad, Weight Watchers*	1 Pack/172g	237	4.6	138	7.1	21.3	2.7	2.2
Egg, & Tomato, Tesco*	1 Pack/172g	311	10.8	181	8.5	22.6	6.3	2.3
Egg, Co-Op*	1 Pack/190g	285	7.0	150	6.8	22.1	3.7	3.7
Egg, Tomato & Salad Cream, M & S*	1 Pack/216g	400	14.9	185	7.4	21.7	6.9	2.3
Egg & Bacon, Deep Fill, Ginsters*	1 Pack/216g	503	21.8	233	14.5	21.0	10.1	2.3
Egg & Bacon, Handmade, Tesco*	1 Pack/217g	489	20.4	225	13.4	20.8	9.4	2.0
Egg & Cress, on Wheat Germ Bread, Tesco*	1 Pack/174g	365	15.8	210	11.0	20.5	9.1	2.1
Egg & Tomato, Delicious, Boots*	1 Pack/218g	362	10.0	166	8.2	22.0	4.6	2.0
Egg Mayo, Free Range, on Oatmeal Bread, M & S*	1 Pack/180g	315	12.2	175	9.4	18.2	6.8	2.8
Egg Mayo Salad, You Count, Love Life, Waitrose*	1 Pack/205g	337	12.5	164	8.4	17.2	6.1	3.0
Egg Mayonnaise, & Cress, Go Simple, Asda*	1 Pack/169g	370	18.6	219	10.0	20.0	11.0	1.7
Egg Mayonnaise, & Cress, Millers*	1 Pack/166g	369	20.3	222	9.4	18.8	12.2	0.0
Egg Mayonnaise, & Cress, on Oatmeal Bread, Somerfield*	1 Pack/149g	346	16.6	232	9.5	23.6	11.1	2.0
Egg Mayonnaise, & Cress, Reduced Fat, Waitrose*	1 Pack/162g	300	12.8	185	10.4	18.1	7.9	3.4
Egg Mayonnaise, & Cress, Weight Watchers*	1 Pack/126g	238	4.2	189	8.8	31.1	3.3	3.3
Egg Mayonnaise, & Cress, Wheatgerm Bread, Asda*	1 Pack/158g	371	19.6	235	9.7	21.3	12.4	1.9
Egg Mayonnaise, & Gammon Ham, Strollers*	1 Pack/170g	400	19.3	236	13.0	20.5	11.4	0.0
Egg Mayonnaise, Boots*	1 Pack/184g	448	23.9	244	9.7	22.0	13.0	2.3
Egg Mayonnaise, Free Range, Finest, Tesco*	1 Pack/217g	412	19.1	190	10.9	16.8	8.8	2.3
Egg Mayonnaise, HL, Tesco*	1 Pack/162g	253	6.0	156	9.3	21.4	3.7	2.8
Egg Mayonnaise, on Hi Bran Bread, Ginsters*	1 Pack/143g	343	21.7	240	10.7	17.6	15.2	0.0
Egg Mayonnaise, Shell*	1 Pack/189g	522	29.1	276	9.8	24.7	15.4	0.0
Egg Mayonnaise, Simply, Boots*	1 Pack/181g	449	27.1	248	9.2	19.0	15.0	2.9
Feta Cheese, & Salad, Tastte*	1 Pack/178g	367	13.4	206	10.6	24.0	7.5	0.0
Feta Cheese, Bells*	1 Pack/223g	468	26.3	210	7.1	18.8	11.8	0.0
Goats Cheese, & Chargrilled Vegetables, Finest, Tesco*	1 Pack/214g	481	19.7	225	7.7	27.8	9.2	1.4
Goat's Cheese, & Cranberry, Shapers, Boots*	1 Pack/150g	323	6.3	216	8.4	36.0	4.2	2.6
Goat's Cheese, Sunblush Tomato, Deli Continental*	1 Pack/179g	480	29.4	268	9.5	20.5	16.4	0.0
Ham, & Cheese, Light Choices, Tesco*	1 Pack/158g	284	5.1	180	14.5	22.8	3.2	5.0
Ham, & Dijon Mustard, Healthy Selection, Budgens*	1 Pack/120g	190	3.0	158	9.7	21.9	2.5	2.0
Ham, & Edam, Smoked, Shapers, Boots*	1 Pack/183g	315	11.9	172	9.3	19.0	6.5	2.7
Ham, & Mustard, Heinz*	1 Pack/180g	460	20.7	255	11.8	25.6	11.5	5.0
Ham, & Mustard, Salad, BGTY, Sainsbury's*	1 Pack/183g	261	3.8	143	8.7	22.4	2.1	2.6
Ham, & Mustard, Smoked, Tesco*	1 Pack/131g	315	11.4	240	11.5	28.0	8.7	1.4
Ham, & Mustard, Somerfield*	1 Pack/144g	301	11.7	209	10.9	24.8	8.1	1.9
Ham, & Mustard, Tesco*	1 Pack/147g	437	27.9	297	10.6	20.8	19.0	1.2
Ham, & Pineapple Salsa, Maple Flavoured, Waitrose*	1 Pack/194g	329	8.9	170	8.4	23.8	4.6	3.1
Ham, & Salad, Big Fill, Somerfield*	1 Pack/222g	515	25.3	232	9.4	22.9	11.4	2.3
Ham, & Salad, British, COU, M & S*	1 Pack/204g	255	4.3	125	6.7	19.9	2.1	2.9

S

SANDWICH

	Measure INFO/WEIGHT	per Measure KCAL	FAT	Nutrition Values per 100g / 100ml KCAL	PROT	CARB	FAT	FIBRE
Ham, & Salad, Foo-Go*	1 Pack/178g	297	7.1	167	9.8	22.9	4.0	0.0
Ham, & Salad, Fullfillers*	1 Pack/180g	290	7.9	161	7.3	22.9	4.4	0.0
Ham, & Salad, Ginsters*	1 Pack/179g	287	6.2	160	8.8	23.5	3.4	0.0
Ham, & Salad, Good Intentions, Somerfield*	1 Pack/178g	287	5.5	161	9.5	23.8	3.1	1.1
Ham, & Salad, Healthy Options, Oldfields*	1 Pack/156g	229	3.0	147	8.7	24.0	1.9	0.0
Ham, & Salad, Shapers, Boots*	1 Pack/195g	269	2.7	138	9.4	22.0	1.4	1.8
Ham, & Salad, Smoked, Ainsley Harriott*	1 Pack/218g	307	6.3	141	8.9	19.9	2.9	0.0
Ham, & Salad, Snack & Shop, Esso*	1 Pack/191g	304	6.5	159	9.2	22.9	3.4	5.0
Ham, & Salad, Wild Bean Cafe*	1 Pack/212g	301	5.5	142	10.7	18.8	2.6	2.0
Ham, & Swiss Cheese, M & S*	1 Pack/159g	393	20.0	247	14.7	18.9	12.6	3.3
Ham, & Tomato, Brambles*	1 Pack/159g	288	7.3	181	11.1	24.1	4.6	3.3
Ham, & Tomato, GFY, Asda*	1 Pack/173g	254	2.9	147	10.0	23.0	1.7	1.4
Ham, & Tomato, Honey Roast, Feel Good, Shell*	1 Pack/171g	388	18.8	227	9.8	22.1	11.0	0.0
Ham, & Turkey, & Salad, Sutherland*	1 Pack/185g	303	4.8	164	9.8	25.2	2.6	0.0
Ham, & Turkey, Asda*	1 Pack/190g	393	19.4	207	12.9	15.8	10.2	2.3
Ham, & Turkey, Healthy, Felix Van Den Berghe*	1 Pack/149g	263	5.9	177	9.4	26.2	4.0	0.0
Ham, Cheese, & Pickle, Healthy Living, Co-Op*	1 Pack/185g	370	7.4	200	13.0	27.0	4.0	3.0
Ham, Cheese, & Pickle, Heinz*	1 Pack/188g	466	24.2	248	11.3	21.7	12.9	4.8
Ham, Cheese, & Pickle, Leicester, Waitrose*	1 Pack/205g	512	24.4	250	11.9	23.7	11.9	2.1
Ham, Cheese, & Pickle, Taste!*	1 Pack/174g	414	21.7	238	11.1	20.3	12.5	0.0
Ham, Cheese, Pickle & Lettuce, No Mayo, Tesco*	1 Pack/207g	435	16.2	210	12.2	23.0	7.8	2.7
Ham, Cheese & Mayo, Brown Bread, Mattessons*	1 Pack/172g	439	18.1	255	13.8	27.0	10.5	2.2
Ham, Cheese & Pickle, Deep Fill, Tesco*	1 Pack/225g	495	20.7	220	14.6	19.4	9.2	2.4
Ham, Cheese & Pickle, in a Soft Wrap, Sainsbury's*	1 Pack/195g	503	23.2	258	10.9	26.8	11.9	0.9
Ham, M & S*	1 Pack/200g	220	5.2	110	17.2	3.2	2.6	0.0
Ham, Smoked, & Mustard, on Oatmeal Bread, Sainsbury's*	1 Pack/154g	275	8.1	179	11.9	20.8	5.3	3.0
Ham, Smoked, Fresh, Taste!*	1 Pack/187g	286	9.0	153	9.1	18.4	4.8	0.0
Ham, Tomato, & Lettuce, Oldfields*	1 Pack/216g	393	17.5	182	12.3	19.0	8.1	3.5
Ham & Cheese Salad, Pick of the Pantry, On A Roll*	1 Pack/228g	431	22.6	189	10.9	13.5	9.9	2.6
Ham & Emmental, Tesco*	1 Pack/179g	305	6.8	170	10.7	22.1	3.8	1.3
Ham & Mustard, Ginsters*	1 Pack/140g	307	9.4	219	11.8	28.0	6.7	2.5
Ham & Mustard Mayo on White, Urban Eat*	1 Pack/130g	299	11.2	230	11.0	27.2	8.6	1.4
Ham & Pickle, EAT*	1 Pack/238g	371	11.9	156	7.6	20.1	5.0	1.6
Ham & Salad with Mustard, Finest, Tesco*	1 Pack/200g	466	21.0	233	15.3	19.3	10.5	1.3
Ham & Turkey with Salad, Co-Op*	1 Pack/188g	263	5.6	140	9.0	21.0	3.0	2.0
Ham Smoked, on a Roll, Cafe Life, Brambles*	1 Pack/211g	485	12.4	230	9.0	35.2	5.9	2.2
Hey Pesto, Cranks*	1 Pack/155g	427	22.5	275	10.0	24.9	14.5	2.5
Houmous, & Crunchy Salad, Oldfields*	1 Pack/180g	256	7.6	142	6.3	20.0	4.2	0.0
Houmous, & Grilled Vegetable, Deep Filled, Dd's*	1 Pack/200g	314	6.0	157	6.4	26.2	3.0	1.5
Houmous, & Olive Bread, Flora Light, Flora*	1 Pack/160g	258	9.2	161	5.0	22.4	5.7	1.9
Houmous & Carrot, Shapers, Boots*	1 Pack/204g	323	10.2	158	7.5	21.0	5.0	5.2
King Prawn, Sainsbury's*	1 Pack/204g	424	16.3	208	11.6	22.3	8.0	0.0
King Prawn & Avocado, Finest, Tesco*	1 Pack/185g	370	16.6	200	9.1	19.6	9.0	2.5
King Prawn & Harissa, Foo-Go*	1 Pack/180g	282	6.8	157	9.1	21.6	3.8	3.4
Lemon Chicken & Mangetout Salad, COU, M & S*	1 Pack/186g	260	5.0	140	10.6	19.0	2.7	3.7
Lemon Chicken with Herb Dressing, Ginsters*	1 Pack/170g	363	12.3	213	12.2	25.0	7.2	2.6
Margherita Classico Calzone, Cranks*	1 Pack/165g	359	12.4	218	8.7	27.9	7.5	1.8
Mediterranean Style, Triple, GFY, Asda*	1 Pack/211g	352	4.4	167	11.0	26.0	2.1	2.3
Mozzarella, & Pepperoni, Sainsbury's*	1 Pack/171g	380	12.2	222	10.5	29.0	7.1	0.0
Mozzarella, & Roast Vegetables, Felix Van Den Berghe*	1 Pack/158g	330	13.3	209	9.5	23.8	8.4	0.0
Mozzarella, & Tomato, Waitrose*	1 Pack/193g	359	18.1	186	9.7	15.7	9.4	2.3
Mozzarella, & Tomato Calzone, Waitrose*	1 Pack/175g	409	19.4	234	10.8	22.7	11.1	2.2
Mozzarella, Italian Style, Taste!*	1 Pack/183g	390	19.4	213	9.2	20.1	10.6	2.0

SANDWICH	Measure INFO/WEIGHT	per Measure KCAL	FAT	Nutrition Values per 100g / 100ml KCAL	PROT	CARB	FAT	FIBRE
Mozzarella, Pesto & Pine Nuts, Sainsbury's*	1 Pack/180g	423	17.5	235	10.2	26.8	9.7	2.8
Mozzarella, Tomato, & Basil, Healthy Options, Oldfields*	1 Pack/175g	285	8.4	163	8.1	22.1	4.8	3.3
New York Deli, Boots*	1 Pack/245g	397	12.5	162	10.0	19.0	5.1	1.7
New York Deli, Chosen By You, Asda*	1 Pack/200g	320	7.3	160	9.8	20.1	3.6	0.0
New York Deli, Extra Special, Asda*	1 Pack/201g	403	15.4	201	12.4	20.6	7.7	3.8
Nice & Cheesy Toastie, Cranks*	1 Pack/160g	437	18.5	272	11.5	29.8	11.5	1.5
Ploughman's, Cheddar, Heinz*	1 Pack/208g	552	27.7	265	9.3	27.1	13.3	2.4
Ploughman's, Cheddar, Mature Vintage, Sainsbury's*	1 Pack/204g	439	20.2	215	9.3	22.3	9.9	0.0
Ploughman's, Cheddar Cheese, Deep Fill, Asda*	1 Pack/229g	471	22.9	206	9.0	20.0	10.0	4.3
Ploughman's, Cheese, BGTY, Sainsbury's*	1 Pack/193g	326	8.1	169	9.8	22.8	4.2	3.6
Ploughman's, Cheese, Deep Fill, Sutherland*	1 Pack/220g	558	32.3	254	9.2	21.4	14.7	0.0
Ploughman's, Deep Fill, Ginsters*	1 Pack/232g	636	40.8	274	9.6	20.8	17.6	0.0
Ploughman's, Deep Fill, Tesco*	1 Pack/245g	551	27.4	225	10.9	20.2	11.2	1.4
Ploughman's, Deep Filled, Asda*	1 Pack/254g	650	36.8	256	10.3	21.3	14.5	2.9
Ploughmans, Light Choices, Tesco*	1 Pack/178g	320	7.5	180	12.2	22.9	4.2	3.3
Poached Salmon & Watercress, Lochmuir, M & S*	1 Pack/192g	355	11.7	185	10.3	22.3	6.1	1.6
Pork & Apple Sauce, Bells*	1 Pack/180g	341	8.1	190	11.5	26.1	4.5	0.0
Prawn, Crayfish & Rocket, Tesco*	1 Pack/193g	425	17.4	220	11.4	22.3	9.0	2.0
Prawn, Creme Fraiche, on Oatmeal Bread, Choice*	1 Pack/153g	265	5.2	173	11.7	23.8	3.4	1.9
Prawn, Egg & Chicken, Triple, Weight Watchers*	1 Pack/224g	367	6.0	164	10.2	24.8	2.7	2.9
Prawn, Marie Rose, Felix Van Den Berghe*	1 Pack/163g	372	16.3	228	12.8	21.9	10.0	0.0
Prawn, Marie Rose, Fulfilled*	1 Pack/149g	292	6.1	196	13.4	26.3	4.1	0.0
Prawn, Marie Rose, Waitrose*	1 Pack/164g	226	5.6	138	8.8	18.0	3.4	1.9
Prawn, Mayo, Tomato & Lettuce, Deep Fill, Benedicts*	1 Pack/200g	330	7.8	165	10.2	21.9	3.9	0.0
Prawn, Roast Chicken, BLT, Triple, Waitrose*	1 Pack/241g	653	42.7	271	9.2	18.8	17.7	1.6
Prawn, Salad, COU, M & S*	1 Pack/200g	230	3.6	115	8.0	16.6	1.8	3.8
Prawn, Thai Style, Ginsters*	1 Pack/183g	313	9.0	171	9.2	22.5	4.9	0.0
Prawn & Egg, Deep Filled, Asda*	1 Pack/250g	570	30.0	228	12.0	17.0	12.0	2.3
Prawn & Salmon, Waitrose*	1 Pack/154g	345	14.6	224	12.5	22.0	9.5	2.8
Prawn & Smoked Salmon, M & S*	1 Pack/445g	1135	63.6	255	11.7	19.3	14.3	1.4
Prawn & Thai Dressing, Tiger, Waitrose*	1 Pack/200g	342	8.6	171	9.6	23.6	4.3	2.2
Prawn Cocktail, Classic, Heinz*	1 Pack/193g	409	16.8	212	8.4	25.0	8.7	2.5
Prawn Cocktail, Waitrose*	1 Pack/196g	300	8.0	153	8.3	20.7	4.1	2.5
Prawn Cocktail, Weight Watchers*	1 Pack/168g	252	7.7	150	8.9	18.1	4.6	2.8
Prawn Mayo, BLT, Smoked Ham, & Cheese, Triple, Tesco*	1 Pack/265g	708	40.8	267	11.8	20.3	15.4	1.0
Prawn Mayo, Ham Salad Triple Pack, Sutherland*	1 Pack/253g	620	30.1	245	9.8	24.8	11.9	0.3
Prawn Mayonnaise, Cafe Collection*	1 Pack/165g	454	27.7	275	11.6	20.7	16.8	1.7
Prawn Mayonnaise, Co-Op*	1 Pack/154g	285	6.0	185	9.7	27.3	3.9	3.2
Prawn Mayonnaise, COU, M & S*	1 Pack/155g	240	3.6	155	10.2	22.9	2.3	2.8
Prawn Mayonnaise, Ginsters*	1 Pack/160g	397	21.1	248	9.1	23.3	13.2	2.4
Prawn Mayonnaise, Oatmeal Bread, Waitrose*	1 Pack/180g	463	27.0	257	10.2	20.4	15.0	3.2
Prawn Mayonnaise, on Oatmeal Bread, Weight Watchers*	1 Pack/148g	235	3.7	159	9.7	24.3	2.5	2.2
Prawn Mayonnaise, Sainsbury's*	1 Pack/151g	323	14.0	214	11.6	20.9	9.3	0.0
Prawn Mayonnaise, Simply, Boots*	1 Pack/261g	736	47.0	282	11.0	19.0	18.0	2.2
Prawn Mayonnaise, Triple, Asda*	1 Pack/248g	635	39.7	256	9.0	19.0	16.0	3.4
Prawn Mayonnaise, Upper Crust*	1 Pack/208g	343	10.4	165	9.2	20.9	5.0	0.0
Rib, BBQ, Pork, Rustlers*	1 Pack/170g	459	22.1	270	14.3	22.9	13.0	2.0
Roast Chicken, Bells*	1 Pack/196g	257	3.7	131	8.2	19.7	1.9	1.9
Roast Chicken, Ginsters*	1 Pack/160g	313	10.1	196	13.6	21.2	6.3	2.6
Roast Chicken & Stuffing, Light Choices, Tesco*	1 Pack/169g	304	3.4	180	14.9	24.6	2.0	1.9
Roast Chicken Salad, Light Choices, Tesco*	1 Pack/194g	300	4.3	155	11.2	22.0	2.2	1.2
Roast Chicken Salad, Pick of the Pantry, On A Roll*	1 Pack/225g	293	6.8	130	9.7	16.2	3.0	1.4
Rokafeta, Cranks*	1 Pack/185g	377	18.1	204	6.9	21.1	9.8	1.9

SANDWICH

INFO/WEIGHT	Measure	per Measure KCAL	FAT	Nutrition Values per 100g / 100ml KCAL	PROT	CARB	FAT	FIBRE
Salad, Healthy, Cambridge University Catering*	1 Pack/156g	246	4.4	158	5.9	27.4	2.8	0.0
Salad, Simply, Shapers, Boots*	1 Pack/216g	300	6.3	139	5.2	23.0	2.9	1.8
Salad & Salad Cream, Fulfilled*	1 Pack/172g	244	7.1	142	4.9	21.5	4.1	0.0
Salmon, & Black Pepper, Smoked, Fulfilled*	1 Pack/120g	293	10.3	244	13.8	29.0	8.6	0.0
Salmon, & Cucumber, Brown Bread, Waitrose*	1 Pack/150g	295	10.6	197	10.5	22.7	7.1	1.4
Salmon, & Cucumber, Light Choices, Tesco*	1 Pack/155g	262	3.9	169	12.3	24.1	2.5	2.1
Salmon, & Cucumber, M & S*	1 Pack/168g	329	13.9	196	11.0	19.5	8.3	2.6
Salmon, & Cucumber, Red, BGTY, Sainsbury's*	1 Pack/192g	278	4.4	145	9.4	21.7	2.3	2.4
Salmon, & Cucumber, Red, Healthy Choice, Asda*	1 Pack/149g	285	11.5	191	10.6	19.9	7.7	2.1
Salmon, & Cucumber, Red, Tesco*	1 Pack/144g	284	9.2	197	11.1	21.8	6.4	1.9
Salmon, & Cucumber, White Bread, Waitrose*	1 Pack/161g	305	8.6	189	9.8	25.5	5.3	1.7
Salmon, & Rocket, Poached, M & S*	1 Pack/180g	495	26.8	275	13.5	21.2	14.9	2.1
Salmon, & Soft Cheese, Feel Good, Shell*	1 Pack/174g	404	12.9	232	13.5	28.0	7.4	1.0
Salmon, & Soft Cheese, Smoked, Waitrose*	1 Pack/154g	300	10.0	195	14.8	19.2	6.5	4.2
Salmon, & Spinach, Poached, Shapers, Boots*	1 Pack/168g	284	7.6	169	9.2	23.0	4.5	3.1
Salmon, Poached, Prawn & Rocket, Waitrose*	1 Pack/166g	308	8.6	186	11.2	23.5	5.2	2.1
Salmon, Smoked, Daily Bread*	1 Pack/122g	296	10.6	243	13.5	28.0	8.7	0.0
Salmon, Smoked & Cream Cheese, M & S*	1 Pack/184g	450	22.4	245	12.7	20.8	12.2	1.8
Sausage, Caramelised Onion Chutney & Stuffing, Tesco*	1 Pack/216g	530	22.1	245	9.2	29.0	10.2	0.7
Sausage, Egg & Bacon, Boots*	1 Pack/325g	887	52.0	273	9.3	23.0	16.0	2.2
Sausage, Triple Pack, GFY, Asda*	1 Pack/215g	424	9.7	197	9.0	30.0	4.5	2.3
Seafood, Mixed, Tesco*	1 Pack/184g	502	30.9	273	7.3	23.2	16.8	0.8
Seafood Cocktail, Asda*	1 Pack/190g	486	30.0	256	6.7	21.3	15.8	1.6
Seafood Cocktail, Daily Bread*	1 Pack/147g	292	6.9	199	8.3	31.0	4.7	0.0
Seafood Cocktail, Waitrose*	1 Pack/210g	267	6.3	127	7.3	17.6	3.0	8.1
Seafood Medley, M & S*	1 Pack/227g	468	28.1	206	7.2	16.3	12.4	3.5
Spicy Falafel & Houmous Salad, Delifresh*	1 Pack/209g	429	19.7	205	6.1	24.0	9.4	2.6
Sub, Beef & Onion, M & S*	1 Pack/207g	611	31.7	295	13.3	25.6	15.3	1.5
Sub, Chicken, & Bacon, Compass Foods*	1 Pack/165g	450	20.1	273	12.2	28.7	12.2	0.0
Sub, Chicken, Caesar, Chargrilled, Sainsbury's*	1 Pack/216g	611	30.5	283	13.4	25.6	14.1	0.0
Sub, Chicken & Bacon, Sainsbury's*	1 Pack/190g	554	27.0	291	13.4	27.4	14.2	0.8
Sub, Egg Mayonnaise, Daily Bread*	1 Pack/165g	441	22.3	267	9.6	29.6	13.5	0.0
Sub, Ham, & Tomato Salad, Shapers, Boots*	1 Pack/170g	286	3.9	168	9.2	28.0	2.3	1.4
Tandoori Chicken, Handmade, Tesco*	1 Pack/178g	285	4.3	160	10.4	22.8	2.4	2.8
Three Cheese & Celery on Malted Brown, COU, M & S*	1 Pack/161g	250	4.2	155	8.0	24.7	2.6	2.1
Three Cheese & Onion, on White Bread, Weight Watchers*	1 Pack/158g	283	2.8	179	12.4	28.4	1.8	1.5
Three Cheese Salad, Shapers, Boots*	1 Pack/169g	248	2.2	147	11.0	23.0	1.3	2.7
Tuna, & Celery, Perfectly Balanced, Waitrose*	1 Pack/172g	272	5.5	158	11.7	20.5	3.2	3.9
Tuna, & Celery, Waitrose*	1 Pack/168g	254	6.1	151	10.2	19.5	3.6	3.0
Tuna, & Chargrilled Vegetables, BGTY, Sainsbury's*	1 Pack/196g	329	8.6	168	10.7	21.5	4.4	0.0
Tuna, & Cucumber, BHS*	1 Pack/210g	479	24.2	228	10.8	24.2	11.5	1.2
Tuna, & Cucumber, Healthy Living, Co-Op*	1 Pack/192g	250	3.5	130	10.9	17.9	1.8	3.0
Tuna, & Cucumber, on Malted Wheatgrain, Ginsters*	1 Pack/175g	318	7.5	182	14.1	21.8	4.3	0.0
Tuna, & Cucumber, Perfectly Balanced, Waitrose*	1 Pack/178g	240	3.6	135	11.0	18.3	2.0	3.6
Tuna, & Cucumber, Shapers, Boots*	1 Pack/167g	267	5.3	160	11.0	22.0	3.2	2.4
Tuna, & Cucumber, Shell*	1 Pack/188g	431	19.2	229	12.3	21.9	10.2	0.0
Tuna, & Cucumber, Weight Watchers*	1 Pack/173g	279	2.9	161	11.4	25.1	1.7	1.4
Tuna, & Green Pesto, BGTY, Sainsbury's*	1 Pack/211g	279	4.7	132	11.0	17.0	2.2	0.0
Tuna, & Salad, Bloomer, M & S*	1 Pack/231g	600	36.9	260	11.8	17.8	16.0	2.6
Tuna, & Salad, Classic*	1 Pack/230g	449	15.9	195	8.7	27.3	6.9	2.1
Tuna, & Salad, M & S*	1 Pack/250g	575	31.5	230	12.5	16.8	12.6	2.1
Tuna, & Salad, on White, Tesco*	1 Pack/190g	351	13.3	185	9.8	20.8	7.0	1.1
Tuna, & Sweetcorn, BGTY, Sainsbury's*	1 Pack/187g	309	5.1	165	10.8	24.7	2.7	2.8

S

	Measure INFO/WEIGHT	per Measure KCAL	FAT	Nutrition Values per 100g / 100ml KCAL	PROT	CARB	FAT	FIBRE
SANDWICH								
Tuna, & Sweetcorn, COU, M & S*	1 Pack/180g	270	4.3	150	12.6	19.0	2.4	3.8
Tuna, & Sweetcorn, Ginsters*	1 Pack/169g	348	11.4	205	9.6	26.4	6.7	2.4
Tuna, & Sweetcorn, Heinz*	1 Pack/208g	528	27.5	254	10.4	23.5	13.2	1.6
Tuna, & Sweetcorn, Light Choices, HL, Tesco*	1 Pack/168g	285	3.2	170	11.2	25.9	1.9	2.8
Tuna, & Sweetcorn, on Malt Bread, Tesco*	1 Pack/175g	350	8.2	200	11.6	27.5	4.7	2.2
Tuna, Mayonnaise & Cucumber, Finest, Tesco*	1 Pack/225g	484	19.1	215	11.6	23.1	8.5	1.7
Tuna, Mayonnaise with Cucumber, Cafe Life, Brambles*	1 Pack/176g	350	12.5	199	11.4	22.4	7.1	1.2
Tuna, Mediterranean, COU, M & S*	1 Pack/260g	364	5.7	140	10.3	19.6	2.2	1.6
Tuna, Melt, Swedish Bread, Shapers, Boots*	1 Pack/163g	254	3.6	156	14.0	20.0	2.2	2.1
Tuna, Nicoise, Taste!*	1 Pack/218g	404	14.4	185	11.3	20.1	6.6	0.0
Tuna, Simply, Ginsters*	1 Pack/167g	466	25.2	279	12.8	22.9	15.1	0.0
Tuna & Cucumber, Finest, Tesco*	1 Pack/169g	380	16.7	225	10.2	23.4	9.9	2.7
Tuna & Cucumber, You Count, Love Life, Waitrose*	1 Pack/195g	321	5.3	165	13.0	21.4	2.7	1.4
Tuna & Cucumber On Oatmeal Bread, Ginsters*	1 Pack/175g	290	7.2	166	11.7	20.7	4.1	2.4
Tuna Mayonnaise, & Cucumber, Daily Bread*	1 Pack/190g	392	16.6	206	12.1	19.8	8.7	0.0
Tuna Mayonnaise, & Cucumber, Darwins Deli*	1 Pack/155g	370	14.6	239	9.6	21.9	9.4	0.0
Tuna Mayonnaise, & Cucumber, Simply, Boots*	1 Pack/200g	498	26.0	249	12.0	21.0	13.0	2.4
Tuna Mayonnaise, & Salad, Serious About Sandwiches*	1 Pack/192g	305	9.0	159	8.6	20.5	4.7	2.9
Tuna Mayonnaise, & Sweetcorn, Whistlestop*	1 Pack/140g	378	17.7	271	13.6	25.5	12.7	0.0
Turkey, & Bacon, COU, M & S*	1 Pack/165g	256	4.0	155	12.0	21.0	2.4	1.7
Turkey, & Cranberry, COU, M & S*	1 Pack/180g	279	3.1	155	12.1	22.8	1.7	2.9
Turkey, & Lettuce & Tomato, Shapers, Boots*	1 Pack/217g	310	4.8	143	9.8	21.0	2.2	2.9
Turkey, & Sage, & Mayonnaise, Bells*	1 Pack/164g	414	22.1	253	11.6	21.2	13.5	0.0
Turkey, & Salad, Brambles*	1 Pack/170g	248	2.0	146	9.3	24.5	1.2	2.0
Turkey, Northern Bites*	1 Pack/200g	354	8.6	177	11.9	22.8	4.3	0.0
Turkey, Pork Sausage & Stuffing, Somerfield*	1 Pack/209g	475	19.5	227	11.6	24.3	9.3	2.1
Turkey, Smoked on Wholemeal, Sodhexo*	1 Pack/128g	259	6.1	202	16.1	23.8	4.8	3.6
Turkey, Stuffing & Cranberry, Boots*	1 Pack/192g	328	2.1	171	12.0	28.0	1.1	2.5
Turkey with All the Christmas Trimmings, Tesco*	1 Pack/189g	425	14.2	225	10.8	28.0	7.5	1.9
Vegetable, Roasted, Open, COU, M & S*	1 Pack/150g	260	2.2	173	8.4	31.3	1.5	4.4
Vegetable & Chilli Bean, Roasted, M & S*	1 Pack/200g	340	11.4	170	5.2	24.5	5.7	2.1
Veggie Threesome, Cranks*	1 Pack/227g	500	20.5	220	9.0	24.3	9.0	3.0
Wedge, Sausage & Egg, Tesco*	1 Pack/269g	699	38.7	260	9.1	23.6	14.4	1.1
Wedge, Tuna & Salad, Tesco*	1 Pack/205g	291	3.1	142	8.1	23.9	1.5	0.8
Wensleydale & Carmelised Carrot Chutney, Brambles*	1 Pack/181g	445	21.5	246	10.8	24.4	11.9	1.9
Wensleydale & Carrot, M & S*	1 Pack/183g	430	22.5	235	9.9	21.4	12.3	2.8
SANDWICH FILLER								
Beef & Onion, Deli, Asda*	1 Serving/50g	78	6.5	157	10.0	0.1	13.0	1.1
Big Breakfast, Asda*	1 Serving/125g	314	26.2	251	12.0	3.5	21.0	0.5
Cajun Chicken, Sainsbury's*	1 Serving/60g	109	8.1	182	13.4	1.8	13.5	1.8
Chargrilled Vegetable, Sainsbury's*	½ Pot/85g	192	19.3	226	3.4	2.2	22.7	0.6
Cheese & Bacon, Tesco*	1 Serving/50g	199	18.8	398	12.2	2.6	37.6	1.2
Cheese & Ham, Sainsbury's*	1 Serving/25g	124	12.3	497	12.4	0.8	49.3	0.3
Cheese & Onion, Deli, Asda*	1 Serving/57g	217	21.1	381	10.0	2.0	37.0	2.0
Cheese & Onion, Sainsbury's*	1 Tub/200g	632	59.6	316	8.7	3.2	29.8	2.2
Cheese & Onion, Tesco*	1 Pack/170g	721	72.4	424	10.0	0.2	42.6	1.5
Cheese & Spring Onion, M & S*	1 Serving/56g	199	18.8	355	8.5	5.0	33.6	0.2
Chicken, Bacon & Sweetcorn, BGTY, Sainsbury's*	1 Tub/300g	399	18.3	133	14.0	5.5	6.1	0.5
Chicken, Stuffing & Bacon, COU, M & S*	1 Pack/170g	170	3.7	100	13.1	6.2	2.2	1.3
Chicken, Sweetcorn & Bacon, Tesco*	1 Serving/50g	167	14.8	334	12.3	4.3	29.7	1.6
Chicken, Tomato & Sweetcure Bacon, M & S*	1 Pot/170g	501	44.9	295	11.4	2.8	26.4	0.7
Chicken & Bacon with Sweetcorn, Sainsbury's*	1 Serving/60g	123	9.4	205	12.0	4.0	15.7	0.9
Chicken & Stuffing, Sainsbury's*	½ Tub/120g	397	37.8	331	6.5	5.3	31.5	1.7

SANDWICH FILLER	Measure INFO/WEIGHT	per Measure KCAL	FAT	Nutrition Values per 100g / 100ml KCAL	PROT	CARB	FAT	FIBRE
Chicken & Sweetcorn, Sainsbury's*	1 Tub/170g	396	33.7	233	11.0	2.7	19.8	1.9
Chicken Caesar, BGTY, Sainsbury's*	½ Jar/85g	117	6.1	137	15.6	2.5	7.2	2.2
Chicken Fajita, Tesco*	1 Serving/50g	77	4.2	155	13.8	5.9	8.5	1.4
Chicken Tikka, BGTY, Sainsbury's*	½ Pot/85g	99	2.5	117	16.5	6.0	3.0	1.0
Chicken Tikka, Mild, Heinz*	1 Serving/52g	102	7.3	196	5.2	12.3	14.0	0.7
Chicken Tikka & Citrus Raita, COU, M & S*	½ Pot/85g	76	1.7	90	12.6	4.9	2.0	0.9
Chicken with Salad Vegetables, Heinz*	1 Serving/56g	114	8.5	203	5.1	11.7	15.1	0.5
Chickpea, Moroccan Style, Sainsbury's*	½ Tub/120g	160	9.4	133	4.1	11.7	7.8	4.2
Chunky Egg & Smoked Ham, Tesco*	1 Serving/100g	234	20.7	234	11.8	0.2	20.7	0.3
Chunky Seafood Cocktail, Tesco*	1 Serving/100g	308	27.8	308	6.0	8.3	27.8	2.0
Corned Beef & Onion, Deli, Asda*	1 Serving/50g	170	15.5	340	12.0	3.3	31.0	0.7
Coronation Chicken, 50 % Less Fat, Tesco*	1 Serving/50g	102	6.3	205	11.5	9.7	12.6	2.7
Coronation Chicken, BGTY, Sainsbury's*	1 Portion/50g	73	3.5	146	11.9	8.9	7.0	1.4
Coronation Chicken, Sainsbury's*	¼ Tub/60g	183	14.8	305	12.1	8.9	24.6	1.2
Coronation Tuna, BGTY, Sainsbury's*	1 Can/80g	90	2.1	112	16.5	5.7	2.6	1.0
Egg & Bacon, Fresh, Tesco*	1 Serving/45g	112	9.0	248	12.7	4.2	20.1	0.6
Egg Mayonnaise, BGTY, Sainsbury's*	1 Serving/63g	75	4.4	119	10.9	3.1	7.0	0.5
Egg Mayonnaise, Chunky Free Range, Tesco*	1 Serving/50g	104	8.9	209	11.3	0.9	17.8	1.6
Egg Mayonnaise, Free Range, Co-Op*	1 Pack/200g	260	17.6	130	10.1	2.4	8.8	0.5
Egg Mayonnaise, Morrisons*	1 Serving/50g	71	5.3	142	10.0	1.7	10.6	0.0
Egg Mayonnaise, Tesco*	1 Serving/50g	114	10.0	228	10.2	1.9	20.0	0.5
Egg Mayonnaise & Bacon, Free Range, Co-Op*	1 Pot/200g	500	44.0	250	13.0	0.9	22.0	0.6
Egg Mayonnaise 50% Less Fat, Tesco*	1 Serving/50g	65	3.8	130	10.2	3.8	7.6	0.5
Poached Salmon & Cucumber, Deli, M & S*	1 Pot/170g	348	27.7	205	14.0	1.0	16.3	0.5
Prawn Marie Rose, Sainsbury's*	1 Serving/60g	121	10.6	201	8.1	2.5	17.6	0.9
Prawn Mayonnaise, Deli, Asda*	1 Serving/50g	169	16.5	339	9.0	1.6	33.0	0.4
Prawn Mayonnaise, Waitrose*	1 Pot/170g	537	52.9	316	8.9	0.2	31.1	0.0
Roast Beef, Onion & Horseradish, Sainsbury's*	1 Serving/100g	372	36.8	372	6.4	3.7	36.8	1.2
Smoked Ham, Roasted Onion & Mustard, Sainsbury's*	1 Serving/100g	343	33.4	343	7.3	3.4	33.4	0.0
Smoked Salmon & Soft Cheese, M & S*	1 Pack/170g	450	40.6	265	11.1	4.9	23.9	0.0
Tex-Mex Chicken, Tesco*	1 Pack/250g	255	2.2	102	12.3	11.2	0.9	1.2
Tuna, Carb Check, Heinz*	1 Serving/52g	84	6.2	161	6.6	6.3	12.0	0.7
Tuna, Tomato & Black Olive, BGTY, Sainsbury's*	1 Pack/100g	88	1.6	88	12.6	5.9	1.6	1.2
Tuna & Sweetcorn, COU, M & S*	½ Pot/85g	76	1.7	90	11.6	5.7	2.0	1.3
Tuna & Sweetcorn, Deli Filler, Sainsbury's*	¼ Pack/58g	105	7.5	183	9.7	6.1	13.1	1.2
Tuna & Sweetcorn, GFY, Asda*	1/3 Pot/57g	71	2.3	125	12.0	10.0	4.1	0.8
Tuna & Sweetcorn, M & S*	1oz/28g	70	5.8	250	14.2	2.3	20.7	1.3
Tuna & Sweetcorn, Morrisons*	1 Tub/170g	382	28.4	225	15.3	7.0	16.7	3.4
Tuna & Sweetcorn with Salad Vegetables, Heinz*	1oz/28g	53	3.7	191	5.8	12.1	13.2	0.7
Tuna Mayonnaise, BGTY, Sainsbury's*	1 Serving/100g	114	3.4	114	17.6	3.5	3.4	0.1
Tuna Mayonnaise & Cucumber, Choice, Tesco*	1 Serving/200g	463	22.8	231	12.8	23.2	11.4	1.5
SANDWICH SPREAD								
Beef, Classic, Shippam*	1 Pot/75g	133	8.8	177	15.5	2.2	11.8	0.0
Chicken, Classic, Shippam*	1 Serving/35g	64	4.4	182	15.5	1.8	12.5	0.0
Chicken & Bacon, Asda*	¼ Jar/43g	153	13.2	359	18.0	2.0	31.0	1.0
Chicken Tikka, Asda*	1 Serving/50g	77	5.0	154	7.0	9.0	10.0	0.2
Crab, Classic, Shippam*	1 Jar/35g	59	3.8	170	13.1	4.6	10.9	0.0
Heinz*	1 Tbsp/10ml	22	1.3	220	1.0	24.0	13.0	1.0
Light, Heinz*	1 Tbsp/10g	16	0.9	161	1.1	18.2	9.2	0.9
Salmon, Classic, Shippam*	1 Serving/35g	70	4.9	200	14.7	4.2	14.1	0.0
Tuna & Mayonnaise, Shippam*	1 Pot/75g	189	13.9	252	18.3	3.1	18.5	0.0
SARDINES								
Boneless in Tomato Sauce, John West*	1 Can/120g	197	12.0	164	17.0	1.5	10.0	0.0

S

	Measure INFO/WEIGHT	per Measure KCAL	FAT	Nutrition Values per 100g / 100ml KCAL	PROT	CARB	FAT	FIBRE
SARDINES								
Grilled	*1oz/28g*	*55*	*2.9*	*195*	*25.3*	*0.0*	*10.4*	*0.0*
in BBQ Sauce, John West*	1 Tin/121g	177	7.7	146	16.1	6.2	6.4	0.0
in Oil, Canned, Drained	*1oz/28g*	*62*	*3.9*	*220*	*23.3*	*0.0*	*14.1*	*0.0*
in Olive Oil, Canned, Ambrosia*	1 Can/100g	320	13.7	320	22.3	0.7	13.7	0.0
in Peri Peri Sauce, John West*	1 Can/120g	181	12.3	150	12.3	2.3	10.2	0.3
in Spring Water, Portuguese, Sainsbury's*	1 Can/90g	165	9.3	183	22.4	0.0	10.3	0.0
in Tomato Sauce, Canned	1oz/28g	45	2.8	162	17.0	1.4	9.9	0.0
Raw, Whole with Head	*1oz/28g*	*46*	*2.6*	*165*	*20.6*	*0.0*	*9.2*	*0.0*
SATAY								
Chicken, Breast, Party Bites, Sainsbury's*	1 Stick/10g	16	0.1	157	34.1	2.7	0.9	0.1
Chicken, GFY, Asda*	1 Serving/168g	242	6.1	144	22.0	6.0	3.6	0.8
Chicken, Indonesian, Bighams*	1 Serving/240g	314	15.4	131	12.2	6.2	6.4	0.6
Chicken, Indonesian, Mini, Sainsbury's*	1 Stick/10g	17	0.7	171	23.0	4.0	7.0	0.7
Chicken, Kebab, Waitrose*	½ Pack/125g	246	13.5	197	18.9	6.0	10.8	0.5
Chicken, M & S*	1 Satay/43g	90	5.5	210	19.1	4.4	12.7	0.7
Chicken, Morrisons*	1 Satay/10g	17	0.7	171	23.5	3.5	7.0	0.7
Chicken, Occasions, Sainsbury's*	1 Satay/10g	15	0.6	150	22.0	2.0	6.0	0.7
Chicken, Oriental, Tesco*	1 Serving/100g	160	5.0	160	23.6	5.1	5.0	0.4
Chicken, Party, Mini, Tesco*	1 Satay/10g	13	0.3	133	23.7	3.4	2.8	1.0
Chicken, Sticks, Asda*	1 Stick/20g	43	2.8	216	18.0	4.5	14.0	0.0
Chicken, Stuffed, Asda*	½ Pack/168g	242	6.1	144	22.0	6.0	3.6	0.8
Chicken, Taste Original*	1 Stick/20g	33	1.3	164	23.0	2.5	6.5	0.7
Chicken & Turkey, Co-Op*	1 Pack/120g	264	16.8	220	20.0	4.0	14.0	0.0
Chicken & Turkey, Morrisons*	1 Stick/20g	39	2.5	197	20.3	1.0	12.4	2.3
Chicken & Turkey, Sainsbury's*	1 Stick/20g	44	2.8	222	20.0	4.0	14.0	1.9
SATSUMAS								
Fresh, Raw, Flesh Only, Average	*1 Sm/56g*	*21*	*0.0*	*37*	*0.9*	*8.6*	*0.1*	*1.3*
Weighed with Peel, Average	*1 Sm/60g*	*22*	*0.1*	*37*	*0.9*	*8.6*	*0.1*	*0.9*
SAUCE								
Apple, Baxters*	1 Tsp/15g	7	0.1	49	0.1	11.1	0.4	0.7
Apple, Bramley, M & S*	1 Tbsp/15g	21	0.0	140	0.2	32.6	0.3	0.4
Apple, Bramley, Sainsbury's*	1 Tsp/15g	17	0.0	111	0.2	27.2	0.1	1.8
Apple, Heinz*	1 Tsp/15g	8	0.0	56	0.3	13.4	0.2	1.5
Apple, Value, Tesco*	1 Serving/50g	29	0.0	58	0.1	14.4	0.0	0.5
Apple & Brandy, Asda*	1 Serving/125g	56	0.0	45	0.2	11.0	0.0	0.0
Apricot & Almond Tagine, Sainsbury's*	1/3 Jar/120g	98	1.9	82	2.0	17.9	1.6	2.5
Aromatic Cantonese, Express, Uncle Ben's*	1 Serving/170g	172	0.2	101	0.6	24.6	0.1	0.0
Arrabbiata, Don Pomodoro*	½ Pot/185g	231	20.3	125	0.5	6.0	11.0	0.0
Arrabbiata, Fresh, Waitrose*	1 Serving/100g	52	2.5	52	1.4	5.9	2.5	2.0
Arrabbiata, Lazio, Sainsbury's*	1/3 Jar/113g	154	12.3	136	2.2	7.2	10.9	0.0
Arrabbiata, Weight Watchers*	½ Pot/150g	43	0.7	29	1.1	5.0	0.5	1.7
Balti, 97% Fat Free, Homepride*	1 Serving/230g	133	4.4	58	1.1	9.1	1.9	1.8
Balti, Cooking, BGTY, Sainsbury's*	¼ Jar/129g	98	4.0	76	1.1	10.9	3.1	0.6
Balti, Cooking, Organic, Perfectly Balanced, Waitrose*	1 Jar/450g	301	5.8	67	1.6	12.1	1.3	3.1
Balti, Cooking, Organic, Sainsbury's*	1 Serving/225g	157	5.2	70	2.2	10.0	2.3	0.5
Balti, Cooking, Tesco*	1 Serving/500g	395	20.0	79	1.5	9.2	4.0	2.2
Balti, Deliciously Good, Homepride*	1/3 Jar/153g	89	2.9	58	1.1	9.1	1.9	0.6
Balti, Indian Style, Iceland*	1 Serving/220g	154	5.7	70	1.6	10.1	2.6	0.5
Balti, Ready Made, Average	1 Serving/100g	98	6.1	98	2.0	8.3	6.1	1.8
Balti, Reduced Fat, Healthy Living, Cook in, Co-Op*	½ Jar/225g	135	5.4	60	2.0	7.5	2.4	2.3
Balti, Tomato & Coriander, Canned, Patak's*	1 Can/283g	235	17.0	83	0.8	6.5	6.0	1.2
Balti, TTD, Sainsbury's*	½ Pack/175g	159	11.9	91	1.4	6.0	6.8	2.0
Balti Cooking, Chosen By You, Asda*	1 Jar/570g	473	27.9	83	1.7	6.9	4.9	2.3

SAUCE

Measure INFO/WEIGHT		per Measure		Nutrition Values per 100g / 100ml				
		KCAL	FAT	KCAL	PROT	CARB	FAT	FIBRE
Balti Curry, Tesco*	1 Serving/200g	126	9.2	63	1.7	4.3	4.6	1.7
Barbecue, Asda*	1 Serving/135g	128	0.3	95	1.2	22.0	0.2	0.6
Barbecue, Chicken Tonight, Knorr*	¼ Jar/125g	76	0.5	61	2.0	12.4	0.4	0.9
Barbeque, Cook in, Homepride*	1 Can/500g	375	7.5	75	0.7	14.6	1.5	0.6
Barbeque, Simply Sausages Ranch, Colman's*	1 Serving/130g	96	0.1	74	1.8	16.6	0.1	1.1
BBQ, Bick's*	1 Serving/100g	119	0.3	119	1.6	27.5	0.3	0.0
BBQ, Heinz*	1 Serving/20g	28	0.1	139	1.1	31.7	0.3	0.5
BBQ, HP*	1 Serving/20ml	29	0.0	143	0.8	33.1	0.2	0.0
BBQ, Spicy Mayhem, HP*	1 Serving/2g	3	0.0	156	0.9	36.7	0.1	0.0
Bearnaise, Mary Berry*	1 Serving/100g	435	39.8	435	1.7	17.3	39.8	0.4
Bearnaise, Sainsbury's*	1 Tbsp/15g	59	6.1	393	0.6	5.0	41.0	0.0
Bechamel for Lasagne, Loyd Grossman*	1 Jar/400g	396	33.2	99	0.6	5.4	8.3	0.1
Black Bean, Asda*	1 Serving/55g	55	0.8	100	2.9	19.0	1.4	0.0
Black Bean, Canton, Stir Fry, Blue Dragon*	½ Pack/60g	53	1.2	88	2.8	14.8	2.0	1.5
Black Bean, Cantonese, Sharwood's*	½ Jar/212g	131	3.0	62	1.9	10.5	1.4	1.2
Black Bean, Cooking, Tesco*	1 Tbsp/15g	13	0.3	90	2.5	14.9	2.0	0.6
Black Bean, Crushed, Stir Fry Sensations, Amoy*	1 Pouch/150g	150	4.3	100	2.4	16.9	2.9	1.0
Black Bean, Finest, Tesco*	1 Jar/350g	252	1.7	72	0.8	16.1	0.5	0.8
Black Bean, Fresh, Sainsbury's*	1 Sachet/50ml	78	1.3	156	6.7	27.5	2.6	1.7
Black Bean, Iceland*	¼ Jar/125g	131	5.2	105	1.3	15.3	4.2	0.7
Black Bean, Loyd Grossman*	1 Serving/175g	177	7.9	101	2.4	12.6	4.5	0.7
Black Bean, Ready to Stir Fry, M & S*	1 Sachet/120g	78	1.1	65	2.5	11.5	0.9	1.4
Black Bean, Stir Fry, Fresh, M & S*	1 Pot/120g	120	0.7	100	2.6	20.3	0.6	1.4
Black Bean, Stir Fry, Fresh Tastes, Asda*	1 Pack/180ml	149	5.2	83	3.7	10.4	2.9	1.4
Black Bean, Stir Fry, Morrisons*	1 Serving/50g	92	5.4	185	4.1	17.3	10.8	1.5
Black Bean, Stir Fry, Sainsbury's*	½ Pack/75ml	91	3.2	121	3.3	17.6	4.3	1.7
Black Bean, Uncle Ben's*	1 Serving/125g	89	1.6	71	2.0	12.8	1.3	0.0
Black Bean, Wing Yip*	½ Jar/61g	75	3.0	123	3.2	17.3	4.9	0.0
Black Bean & Chilli, Stir Fry, Asda*	½ Jar/97g	158	11.6	163	3.7	10.0	12.0	0.8
Black Bean & Green Pepper, Stir Fry, Sharwood's*	1 Serving/150g	82	0.4	55	2.0	11.0	0.3	0.5
Black Bean & Red Pepper, Sharwood's*	½ Jar/213g	132	3.0	62	1.9	10.5	1.4	1.2
Black Pepper, Stir Fry, Blue Dragon*	½ Sachet/60g	47	2.6	79	1.6	8.4	4.4	0.1
Bolognese, Emilia Romagna, Fresh, Sainsbury's*	½ Pot/150g	99	4.8	66	5.9	3.4	3.2	1.7
Bolognese, Loyd Grossman*	¼ Jar/106g	79	3.1	75	2.0	10.2	2.9	1.4
Bolognese, Original, Deliciously Good, Homepride*	¼ Jar/112g	39	0.2	35	1.3	7.1	0.2	0.8
Bolognese, Waitrose*	1 Serving/175g	150	8.6	86	5.4	5.3	4.9	2.0
Bolognese for Beef, Tesco*	½ Pack/175g	177	10.1	101	5.4	6.9	5.8	0.8
Bourguignon, Beef Tonight, Knorr*	¼ Jar/125g	71	3.2	57	0.6	7.6	2.6	0.4
Bread, Christmas, Tesco*	1 Serving/60g	64	3.2	107	3.3	11.8	5.3	0.5
Bread, Luxury, M & S*	1 Serving/115g	195	16.2	170	3.2	8.1	14.1	2.2
Bread, M & S*	1 Serving/85g	153	12.4	180	3.1	8.7	14.6	0.2
Bread, Made with Semi-Skimmed Milk	1 Serving/45g	42	1.4	93	4.3	12.8	3.1	0.3
Brown, Asda*	1 Serving/10g	10	0.0	97	0.7	23.0	0.2	0.4
Brown, Bottled	1 Tsp/6g	6	0.0	99	1.1	25.2	0.0	0.7
Brown, Chop, Hammonds of Yorkshire*	1 Tbsp/15g	10	0.0	66	0.3	16.1	0.1	0.3
Brown, HP*	1 Tbsp/15g	18	0.0	122	0.9	28.3	0.1	0.4
Brown, Tiptree, Wilkin & Sons*	1 Serving/100g	104	0.0	104	1.1	42.0	0.0	0.0
Brown, Value, Value, Tesco*	1 Serving/15g	13	0.0	86	0.7	18.8	0.1	0.3
Burger, Hellmann's*	1 Tbsp/15g	36	3.1	240	1.1	12.0	21.0	0.0
Butter & Tarragon, Chicken Tonight, Knorr*	¼ Jar/125g	132	13.0	106	1.0	2.1	10.4	0.7
Cantonese, Sizzling, Uncle Ben's*	½ Jar/270g	416	16.5	154	0.7	24.0	6.1	0.0
Cantonese Chow Mein Stir Fry, Sainsbury's*	½ Jar/100g	67	1.9	67	0.4	12.1	1.9	0.8
Caramelised Onion & Red Wine, M & S*	1 Serving/52g	31	1.6	60	1.9	6.7	3.1	0.6

S

SAUCE

INFO/WEIGHT	Measure	per Measure		Nutrition Values per 100g / 100ml				
		KCAL	FAT	KCAL	PROT	CARB	FAT	FIBRE
Carbonara, Less Than 5% Fat, GFY, Asda*	½ Tub/150g	121	6.7	81	5.0	5.0	4.5	0.5
Chasseur, Cook in, Homepride*	1 Can/390g	160	0.4	41	0.7	9.2	0.1	0.4
Cheddar Cheese, Colman's*	1 Serving/85ml	348	13.1	410	19.2	48.5	15.4	1.9
Cheddar Cheese, Dry, Knorr*	1 Serving/10g	47	3.2	469	7.8	38.0	31.8	0.3
Cheese, Basics, Sainsbury's*	¼ Pot/124g	71	3.1	57	2.5	6.1	2.5	0.5
Cheese, Italian, Tesco*	½ Carton/175g	238	15.6	136	5.8	8.3	8.9	0.0
Cheese, Italian Style, Finest, Tesco*	½ Pot/175g	355	20.8	203	10.1	14.0	11.9	0.0
Cheese, Italiano, Tesco*	1 Pot/350g	367	19.9	105	5.3	8.0	5.7	0.0
Cheese, Made with Semi-Skimmed Milk	1 Serving/60g	107	7.6	179	8.1	9.1	12.6	0.2
Cheese, Made with Whole Milk	1 Serving/60g	118	8.8	197	8.0	9.0	14.6	0.2
Cheese, Sainsbury's*	1 Serving/125g	140	9.4	112	5.0	6.1	7.5	1.2
Cherry Tomato, Finest, Tesco*	½ Pot/171g	120	4.4	70	1.5	9.4	2.6	1.1
Chilli, Barbeque, Encona*	1 Tbsp/15ml	19	0.0	129	1.3	30.7	0.1	0.0
Chilli, Cooking, Casa Mexico*	1 Jar/500g	275	2.5	55	1.5	10.0	0.5	2.7
Chilli, Hot, Asda*	1 Jar/570g	319	2.3	56	2.1	11.0	0.4	1.9
Chilli, Hot, Blue Dragon*	1 Tbsp/15ml	14	0.0	96	0.5	23.0	0.2	0.0
Chilli, Hot, Co-Op*	1 Jar/440g	242	2.2	55	2.0	10.0	0.5	2.0
Chilli, Hot, Heinz*	1 Portion/10g	8	0.0	80	1.4	18.0	0.0	0.0
Chilli, Hot, Mexican, Morrisons*	¼ Jar/125g	72	0.6	58	2.2	11.2	0.5	2.0
Chilli, HP*	1 Tsp/6g	8	0.0	134	1.2	32.3	0.0	0.0
Chilli, Medium, Somerfield*	¼ Jar/110g	57	0.4	52	2.4	9.6	0.4	2.1
Chilli, Mild, Healthy Eating, Asda*	½ Jar/250g	172	5.7	69	2.1	10.0	2.3	1.7
Chilli, Mild, Tesco*	1 Jar/550g	302	1.6	55	2.3	10.0	0.3	3.4
Chilli, Seeds of Change*	1 Jar/400g	408	6.0	102	4.0	18.2	1.5	2.2
Chilli, Tomato Based, Bottled, Average	*1 Tbsp/15g*	*16*	*0.0*	*104*	*2.5*	*19.8*	*0.3*	*5.9*
Chilli, Wicked, Sauce & Spice Mix, Two Step, Discovery*	1 Jar/370g	259	4.4	70	2.7	14.9	1.2	3.2
Chilli Con Carne, Asda*	1 Lge Jar/570g	370	4.0	65	2.6	12.0	0.7	0.0
Chilli Con Carne, Classic, Loyd Grossman*	1 Jar/350g	241	10.5	69	2.2	7.6	3.0	1.3
Chilli Con Carne, Sizzle & Stir, Knorr*	1 Jar/455g	505	32.3	111	2.7	9.1	7.1	2.7
Chilli Con Carne, Weight Watchers*	½ Jar/175g	84	0.3	48	1.8	9.7	0.2	2.0
Chilli Men, Spicy, Wagamama*	½ Jar/125g	137	5.9	110	2.0	14.9	4.7	0.6
Chilli Soy, Amoy*	1 Tbsp/15g	8	0.0	55	4.6	9.1	0.0	0.0
Chinese Stir Fry, Sainsbury's*	½ Sachet/75g	61	1.9	81	0.4	14.1	2.5	1.0
Chinese Style, Curry, Cooking, Chosen By You, Asda*	1 Serving/140g	89	4.3	63	1.5	7.4	3.1	3.5
Chinese Style, Stir Fry, Fresh, Asda*	½ Sachet/50ml	93	6.0	186	1.5	18.0	12.0	0.0
Chip Shop Curry, Knorr*	1 Sachet/150ml	145	6.9	97	1.7	12.4	4.6	0.7
Chop Suey, Cantonese, Sharwood's*	1 Serving/200g	146	2.8	73	0.6	14.4	1.4	0.4
Chop Suey, Stir Fry, Sharwood's*	1 Jar/160g	120	2.4	75	0.7	14.6	1.5	0.2
Chow Mein, Sainsbury's*	1 Serving/50g	35	1.2	71	1.8	10.5	2.4	0.0
Chow Mein, Stir Fry, Asda*	½ Jar/98g	97	1.0	99	1.6	21.0	1.0	0.1
Chow Mein, Stir Fry, Blue Dragon*	1 Sachet/120g	110	3.5	92	1.1	15.4	2.9	0.4
Coconut, Ginger & Lemon Grass, Stir Fry, Wagamama*	½ Jar/125g	144	7.1	115	1.2	14.7	5.7	0.4
Coconut, Lime & Coriander, Cooking, Nando's*	1 Serving/65g	88	6.5	135	1.5	12.1	10.0	1.2
Coconut, Thai Style, Stir Fry, Waitrose*	½ Pack/50ml	52	4.3	105	1.5	5.5	8.6	1.8
Coconut & Red Chilli, Noodle Sauce, Tesco*	1/3 Jar/110g	88	7.0	80	1.7	3.8	6.4	0.7
Cooking, Fiesta, Chilli, Aldi*	¼ Jar/124g	87	0.6	70	2.5	12.5	0.5	2.6
Cooking, Honey & Mustard, Light Choices, Tesco*	1 Serving/124g	93	2.0	75	1.4	13.0	1.6	1.2
Cooking, Hunters Chicken, Tesco*	1/3 Jar/163g	155	0.3	95	1.2	20.6	0.2	0.8
Cooking, Korma, Light Choices, Tesco*	¼ Jar/125g	100	4.0	80	1.6	10.2	3.2	1.6
Coronation, Heinz*	1 Tbsp/10g	33	3.1	334	0.8	13.1	31.0	0.9
Coronation Chicken, Cook in, Homepride*	1 Serving/250g	232	10.5	93	0.8	13.2	4.2	0.0
Cranberry, Tesco*	1 Tsp/15g	23	0.0	156	0.1	38.8	0.0	0.9
Cranberry, Waitrose*	1 Tbsp/20g	31	0.0	156	0.2	38.5	0.2	14.0

SAUCE

INFO/WEIGHT	Measure	per Measure		Nutrition Values per 100g / 100ml				
		KCAL	FAT	KCAL	PROT	CARB	FAT	FIBRE
Cranberry & Port, M & S*	1 Serving/75g	71	0.3	95	2.3	20.2	0.4	2.1
Cream, Graddsås, Ikea*	1 Serving/60ml	72	6.6	120	1.0	4.0	11.0	0.0
Creamy, Curry, BGTY, Sainsbury's*	¼ Jar/125g	84	4.7	67	1.4	6.8	3.8	0.5
Creamy Horseradish with Garlic, So Good, Somerfield*	1 Tsp/6g	19	1.3	317	4.1	25.0	22.3	0.0
Creamy Mushroom, Cooking, M & S*	1 Jar/510g	663	57.6	130	1.3	5.4	11.3	0.5
Creamy Mushroom, Homepride*	1 Portion/100g	76	5.6	76	1.1	5.2	5.6	0.3
Cumberland Sausage, Colman's*	¼ Jar/126g	43	0.3	34	0.7	7.4	0.2	0.8
Curry, Bettabuy, Morrisons*	1 Jar/440g	295	10.1	67	0.7	10.8	2.3	1.0
Curry, Cook in, Homepride*	½ Can/250g	140	4.7	56	1.1	8.6	1.9	0.5
Curry, Green Thai, Finest, Tesco*	1 Serving/350g	420	37.1	120	1.4	4.8	10.6	0.7
Curry, Green Thai, Sharwood's*	1 Serving/403g	431	30.6	107	1.1	8.4	7.6	0.1
Curry, Hot Madras, The Curry Sauce Company*	1 Serving/100g	162	12.5	162	2.2	10.2	12.5	1.5
Curry, Kashmiri, Bibijis*	¼ Packet/119g	51	1.7	43	2.1	7.1	1.4	1.5
Curry, Mild, Tesco*	1 Jar/500g	420	14.0	84	1.1	13.4	2.8	0.8
Curry, Red Thai, BGTY, Sainsbury's*	1 Serving/124g	77	4.8	62	0.6	6.0	3.9	1.4
Curry, Red Thai, Sharwood's*	1 Serving/138g	150	11.0	109	1.2	7.9	8.0	0.2
Curry, Red Thai, Worldwide Sauces*	1 Jar/450g	630	45.0	140	1.5	10.9	10.0	0.0
Curry, Sri Lanken, Seasoned Pioneers*	½ Pack/200g	194	16.8	97	1.8	3.4	8.4	0.8
Curry, Sweet	1 Serving/115g	105	6.4	91	1.2	9.6	5.6	1.4
Curry, Thai Coconut, Uncle Ben's*	1 Serving/125g	127	6.0	102	1.4	13.2	4.8	0.0
Curry, Value, Tesco*	1 Can/390g	355	17.5	91	1.6	11.0	4.5	1.3
Dhansak, Medium, Sharwood's*	1 Jar/420g	370	13.4	88	3.6	11.1	3.2	1.0
Dhansak, Sharwood's*	1 Jar/445g	667	34.7	150	4.7	15.2	7.8	1.4
Dill & Lemon, Delicate for Fish, Schwartz*	1 Pack/300g	387	34.2	129	1.1	5.6	11.4	0.5
Dill & Mustard for Gravadlax, Dry, Waitrose*	1 Sachet/35g	123	9.0	352	2.5	27.8	25.7	0.6
Enchilada, Medium, Old El Paso*	1 Can/270g	92	4.6	34	0.0	5.0	1.7	0.0
Exotic Curry, Heinz*	1 Serving/15ml	41	3.4	271	0.7	15.3	22.8	0.6
Fajita, Asda*	¼ Jar/125g	79	5.4	63	1.0	5.0	4.3	1.0
Four Cheese, Reduced Fat, Morrisons*	½ Tub/175g	161	9.5	92	6.1	4.8	5.4	0.5
Four Cheese for Pasta, Asda*	½ Jar/155g	242	21.7	156	3.5	3.9	14.0	0.1
Four Cheese for Pasta, Waitrose*	1 Pot/300g	392	24.8	112	6.6	5.5	7.1	0.5
Fruit Squirt, Passionfruit, Topping, Easiyo*	1 Serving/20g	34	0.0	172	1.0	38.9	0.1	6.3
Fruity, HP*	1 Tsp/6g	8	0.0	141	1.2	35.1	0.1	0.0
Garlic, Heinz*	1 Serving/10ml	32	3.0	323	1.0	12.1	29.9	1.2
Green Thai, Cooking, Perfectly Balanced, Waitrose*	½ Jar/215g	112	6.9	52	0.8	4.9	3.2	1.5
Green Thai, Loyd Grossman*	½ Jar/175g	182	11.2	104	1.6	10.0	6.4	0.8
Green Thai, Stir Fry, Sainsbury's*	½ Pack/75g	112	8.0	149	1.2	11.9	10.7	1.0
Ham & Mushroom for Pasta, Stir & Serve, Homepride*	1 Serving/100g	95	9.3	95	1.5	1.3	9.3	0.0
Hoi Sin, Chosen By You, Asda*	1 Jar/210g	309	2.3	147	0.8	31.3	1.1	1.4
Hoi Sin, M & S*	½ Pot/50ml	80	1.0	160	3.2	31.8	2.0	2.2
Hoi Sin, Rich, Stir Fry, Straight to Wok, Amoy*	½ Sachet/60g	68	1.4	114	1.8	21.4	2.3	0.7
Hoi Sin, Stir Fry, Fresh Tastes, Asda*	½ Sachet/90ml	121	0.8	135	1.8	29.7	0.9	0.0
Hoi Sin, Stir Fry, Tesco*	½ Sachet/60g	87	2.9	145	1.1	23.9	4.9	0.5
Hoi Sin & Garlic, Blue Dragon*	1 Serving/60g	80	1.6	133	1.2	26.1	2.6	0.0
Hoi Sin & Plum, Chinatown, Knorr*	¼ Jar/131g	96	0.9	73	0.8	15.8	0.7	1.2
Hoi Sin & Plum, Sweet & Fruity, Stir Fry, Sharwood's*	1 Serving/136g	128	1.8	94	0.7	19.9	1.3	0.9
Hoi Sin & Spring Onion, Stir Fry, Sharwood's*	1 Jar/165g	196	1.5	119	1.3	26.5	0.9	0.8
Hoisin, Lee Kum Kee*	1 Serving/35g	80	0.5	230	1.2	53.3	1.3	0.8
Hoisin & Plum, Dipping, Finest, Tesco*	1 Serving/50g	78	0.3	156	2.3	35.3	0.6	1.4
Hoisin & Plum, Stir Fry, HL, Tesco*	1 Serving/250g	147	3.2	59	2.1	9.7	1.3	1.3
Hollandaise, Classic, for Fish, Schwartz*	1 Sachet/300g	456	49.2	152	0.7	0.4	16.4	2.0
Hollandaise, Fresh, Average	1 Pack/150g	342	32.4	228	2.4	6.1	21.6	0.0
Hollandaise, Homemade, Average	1oz/28g	198	21.3	707	4.8	0.0	76.2	0.0

S

SAUCE

	Measure INFO/WEIGHT	per Measure KCAL	FAT	Nutrition Values per 100g / 100ml KCAL	PROT	CARB	FAT	FIBRE
Hollandaise, Sainsbury's*	1 Tbsp/15g	72	7.6	478	0.2	5.9	50.4	0.4
Honey & Coriander, Stir Fry, Blue Dragon*	1 Pack/120g	115	0.7	96	0.5	22.1	0.6	0.3
Honey & Mustard, Chicken Tonight, Knorr*	¼ Jar/131g	139	6.2	106	0.8	15.1	4.7	0.6
Honey & Mustard, COU, M & S*	½ Jar/160g	112	4.6	70	2.3	9.2	2.9	0.7
Honey & Mustard, for Cooking, Asda*	1 Serving/200g	234	14.0	117	0.6	13.0	7.0	0.0
Honey & Mustard, Low Fat, Chicken Tonight, Knorr*	¼ Jar/131g	105	3.0	80	1.0	13.8	2.3	0.8
Hong Kong Curry, Loyd Grossman*	1 Jar/350g	371	26.9	106	1.3	7.8	7.7	0.8
Horseradish, Colman's*	1 Tbsp/15ml	17	0.9	112	1.9	9.8	6.2	2.6
Horseradish, Creamed, Colman's*	1 Tsp/16g	37	2.1	229	4.3	21.4	13.3	0.0
Horseradish, Hot, Tesco*	1 Tsp/5g	9	0.5	185	2.3	19.7	10.6	2.3
Horseradish, Mustard, Sainsbury's*	1 Tsp/5g	8	0.3	163	7.9	18.2	6.6	3.5
Horseradish, Sainsbury's*	1 Dtsp/10g	14	0.7	145	1.5	17.8	6.6	2.4
Horseradish Cream, Tesco*	1 Serving/15g	29	1.8	195	2.3	18.7	11.9	2.1
Hot, Cholula Hot Sauce*	1 Tbsp/12g	3	0.1	22	1.0	2.5	1.0	0.0
Hot Chilli, Sharwood's*	1 fl oz/30ml	36	0.2	120	0.5	29.4	0.6	1.3
Hot Onion, Sainsbury's*	1 Serving/10g	17	0.0	167	0.2	41.0	0.1	0.1
Hot Pepper	1 Tsp/5g	1	0.1	26	1.6	1.7	1.5	0.0
Hot Pepper, Encona*	1 Tsp/5ml	3	0.1	52	0.5	10.5	1.2	0.0
Indian Tikka, Chicken Tonight, Knorr*	1 Serving/250g	320	23.0	128	1.3	10.0	9.2	1.2
Italian Onion & Garlic, Sainsbury's*	1 Jar/500g	375	10.0	75	2.2	12.1	2.0	1.7
Italian Tomato & Herb, for Pasta, BGTY, Sainsbury's*	½ Jar/250g	137	0.7	55	2.1	10.9	0.3	0.0
Italian Tomato & Herb, Sainsbury's*	¼ Jar/126g	88	2.5	70	2.0	11.1	2.0	1.4
Italian Tomato & Mascarpone, Sainsbury's*	½ Tub/175g	157	10.1	90	2.6	6.8	5.8	1.2
Italian Tomato & Sweet Basil, Go Organic*	1 Serving/80g	51	3.8	64	1.2	4.3	4.7	0.9
Jalfrezi, Cooking, Asda*	1 Jar/570g	519	35.9	91	1.2	7.4	6.3	1.7
Jalfrezi, Cooking, Sainsbury's*	1 Serving/250g	160	6.0	64	1.0	9.6	2.4	1.7
Jalfrezi, Sweet Pepper & Coconut, in Glass Jar, Patak's*	1 Jar/540g	626	37.8	116	1.7	11.3	7.0	1.4
Jalfrezi, TTD, Sainsbury's*	½ Jar/175g	205	16.8	117	1.3	6.4	9.6	1.5
Jamaican Jerk, Stir It Up, Chicken Tonight, Knorr*	1 Jar/80g	506	43.1	633	3.9	20.9	53.9	5.4
Jambalaya, Cajun, Seasoned Pioneers*	1 Pack/400g	248	20.4	62	0.8	3.2	5.1	1.0
Jeera & Tamarind, Daal, Indian, Seasoned Pioneers*	1 Pouch/400g	228	12.0	57	1.8	7.2	3.0	1.6
Kashmiri, Chilli & Peppers, Patak's*	½ Jar/212g	159	9.3	75	1.3	7.7	4.4	1.1
Korma, Asda*	1 Serving/225g	434	33.7	193	2.5	12.0	15.0	2.2
Korma, Authentic, VLH Kitchens	1 Serving/118g	180	11.0	153	1.9	6.7	13.0	0.8
Korma, Coconut & Coriander, Canned, Patak's*	1 Can/283g	487	37.9	172	3.4	9.2	13.4	1.7
Korma, Deliciously Good, Homepride*	1 Jar/450g	396	19.8	88	1.4	10.6	4.4	1.4
Korma, Free From, Sainsbury's*	½ Jar/175g	191	13.8	109	1.9	7.6	7.9	1.2
Korma, GFY, Asda*	1 Serving/240g	336	21.6	140	1.7	13.0	9.0	1.5
Korma, Homepride*	1 Serving/160g	110	3.2	69	1.3	11.6	2.0	0.0
Korma, Organic, Patak's*	¼ Jar/106g	148	12.7	140	1.9	5.9	12.0	0.9
Korma, Royal, TTD, Sainsbury's*	½ Pack/175g	207	12.3	118	2.4	11.4	7.0	3.9
Korma, Sizzle & Stir, Knorr*	1 Jar/455g	1092	96.5	240	1.2	11.2	21.2	2.7
Korma, Tesco*	¼ Jar/125g	192	14.6	154	2.4	9.9	11.7	1.3
Korma with Flaked Almonds, Weight Watchers*	1 Serving/175g	107	3.7	61	2.0	8.5	2.1	1.6
Lemon, Amoy*	1 Tsp/5ml	5	0.0	104	0.0	26.0	0.0	0.0
Lemon, Stir Fry, Straight to Wok, Amoy*	½ Sachet/50g	81	0.1	162	0.3	40.0	0.2	0.0
Lemon, Stir Fry, Tesco*	1 Jar/450g	369	0.9	82	0.1	19.3	0.2	0.1
Lemon & Ginger, Stir Fry, Finest, Tesco*	¼ Jar/85g	144	0.2	169	0.2	41.7	0.2	0.2
Lemon & Sesame, Stir Fry, Sharwood's*	1 Serving/100g	125	0.1	125	0.1	30.9	0.1	0.1
Lime & Coriander, Tangy for Fish, Schwartz*	1 Pack/300g	381	37.2	127	1.1	2.7	12.4	1.3
Lime Honey & Ginger, Stir Fry, Sharwood's*	1 Serving/50g	34	0.0	69	0.3	16.6	0.1	0.2
Madras, Cooking, HL, Tesco*	1 Serving/128g	55	2.6	43	1.6	4.8	2.0	2.3
Mango, Kashmiri Style, Finest, Tesco*	½ Jar/175g	285	23.8	163	2.4	7.7	13.6	0.9

SAUCE

INFO/WEIGHT	Measure	per Measure		Nutrition Values per 100g / 100ml				
		KCAL	FAT	KCAL	PROT	CARB	FAT	FIBRE
Mint, Sainsbury's*	1 Dtsp/10g	13	0.0	126	2.5	28.7	0.1	4.0
Mint, Smart Price, Asda*	1 Serving/5g	3	0.0	52	0.1	13.0	0.0	1.2
Mint, Value, Tesco*	1 Serving/10g	4	0.0	41	1.1	9.0	0.1	1.8
Mint Garden, Fresh, Tesco*	1 Tsp/5g	2	0.0	40	2.6	3.6	0.4	1.5
Moglai, Tomato & Fennel, Cooking, Patak's*	1 Jar/283g	374	25.2	132	3.1	9.7	8.9	1.8
Mornay, Cheese, Asda*	¼ Pot/71g	114	9.0	161	6.8	6.6	12.7	0.4
Mushroom, Creamy, Asda*	1 Serving/125g	76	4.6	61	0.8	6.0	3.7	0.5
Mushroom, Creamy, Chicken Tonight, Knorr*	¼ Jar/125g	101	7.9	81	0.8	5.4	6.3	0.3
Mushroom, Creamy, Low Fat, Chicken Tonight, Knorr*	¼ Jar/125g	59	3.6	47	0.8	7.3	2.9	0.4
Mushroom, Creamy, Tesco*	½ Pot/175g	142	10.1	81	1.5	5.6	5.8	0.4
Mushroom, Not Just for Pasta, Sainsbury's*	½ Pot/150g	91	6.6	61	1.7	3.6	4.4	0.9
Mushroom, Schwartz*	1 Pack/170g	207	19.2	122	1.2	3.9	11.3	0.5
Mushroom, Wild, Finest, Tesco*	½ Pack/175g	157	11.9	90	1.9	5.2	6.8	0.4
Napoletana, Fresh, Sainsbury's*	½ Pot/150g	94	4.5	63	1.7	7.3	3.0	2.3
Napoletana, Italian, Tesco*	1 Pot/350g	178	4.2	51	1.5	8.5	1.2	1.0
Napoletana, Waitrose*	1 Pot/600g	252	8.4	42	1.8	5.5	1.4	1.7
Onion, Made with Semi-Skimmed Milk	1 Serving/60g	52	3.0	86	2.9	8.4	5.0	0.4
Onion, Made with Skimmed Milk	1 Serving/60g	46	2.4	77	2.9	8.4	4.0	0.4
Oriental Sweet & Sour, Express, Uncle Ben's*	1 Serving/170g	221	3.2	130	0.8	27.5	1.9	0.0
Oyster, Blue Dragon*	1 Tsp/5ml	6	0.0	121	3.4	26.9	0.0	0.0
Oyster, Stir Fry, Sainsbury's*	1 Tbsp/15g	9	0.0	61	1.6	13.3	0.1	0.2
Oyster & Garlic, Stir Fry, Straight to Wok, Amoy*	½ Pack/50g	97	1.5	195	4.9	37.0	3.0	0.0
Paprika Chicken, Chicken Tonight, Knorr*	½ Jar/250g	240	21.7	96	0.9	3.5	8.7	1.4
Parsley, Fresh, Sainsbury's*	½ Pot/150g	117	7.6	78	2.0	5.9	5.1	0.5
Parsley, Instant, Dry, Asda*	1 Serving/23g	82	1.6	355	7.0	66.0	7.0	4.4
Parsley, Instant, Made Up, Semi Skim Milk, Sainsbury's*	¼ Sachet/51ml	34	1.1	67	3.5	8.6	2.1	0.1
Parsley, Made Up, Bisto*	1 Serving/50ml	41	2.4	82	0.6	9.2	4.8	0.0
Parsley, Tesco*	½ Pack/89g	85	5.1	95	2.8	8.1	5.7	1.1
Parsley Lemon Caper, New Covent Garden Food Co*	¼ Carton/65ml	137	12.1	211	2.5	8.7	18.6	0.8
Pasta Bake, Ham & Mushroom, Creamy, Homepride*	1 Pack/425g	489	45.5	115	1.8	2.8	10.7	0.0
Pasta Bake, Tomato & Cheese, Dolmio*	¼ Jar/125g	70	1.5	56	2.1	9.1	1.2	1.2
Pasta Bake, Tuna, Homepride*	½ Jar/250g	207	13.0	83	1.4	7.6	5.2	0.9
Peanut, Sainsbury's*	1 Sachet/70g	185	9.2	264	1.9	34.7	13.1	1.6
Peking Lemon, Stir Fry, Blue Dragon*	1 Serving/35g	47	0.2	134	0.0	31.6	0.7	0.5
Pepper, Creamy, Schwartz*	1 Pack/170g	116	9.2	68	1.5	3.4	5.4	1.0
Peppercorn, Creamy, Chicken Tonight, Knorr*	¼ Jar/125g	110	9.7	88	0.3	3.8	7.8	0.4
Peri Peri, Extra Hot, Nando's*	1 Serving/5g	4	0.2	71	0.7	8.8	3.7	1.4
Peri Peri, Garlic, Nando's*	1 Serving/15g	9	0.5	59	0.5	6.6	3.4	0.8
Peri Peri, Hot, Nando's*	1 Serving/5g	4	0.2	75	0.6	9.6	3.8	1.3
Peri Peri, Sweet, Nando's*	1 Tbsp/25g	35	0.5	142	0.5	30.7	2.1	0.0
Pesto, Green, Asda*	1 Tsp/5g	21	2.2	429	4.7	3.5	44.0	1.4
Plum & Sesame, Stir Fry, M & S*	½ Jar/115g	138	0.1	120	0.9	29.0	0.1	1.8
Prawn Cocktail, Frank Cooper*	1 Tbsp/15g	47	4.0	316	0.8	18.3	26.7	0.1
Prawn Cocktail, Morrisons*	1 Portion/15ml	81	8.5	540	1.4	5.5	56.9	1.1
Puttanesca, Fresh, Waitrose*	½ Pot/176g	118	7.7	67	1.8	6.2	4.4	1.2
Red & Yellow Pepper, Roasted, Sacla*	1 Serving/290g	232	17.1	80	1.1	5.5	5.9	0.0
Red Pepper, Fresh, Asda*	¼ Pot/82g	35	1.0	43	1.4	6.8	1.2	1.1
Red Pepper, GFY, Asda*	1 Serving/100g	43	1.1	43	1.2	7.0	1.1	0.0
Red Pepper, Sainsbury's*	1 Serving/37g	118	11.6	320	4.3	5.0	31.4	0.0
Red Thai, Cooking, Asda*	½ Jar/160g	136	9.1	85	0.9	6.8	5.7	1.5
Red Wine, Cook in, Homepride*	¼ Can/98g	47	0.6	48	0.5	10.1	0.6	0.0
Red Wine, Cooking, BGTY, Sainsbury's*	1 Serving/125g	52	0.6	42	0.5	8.8	0.5	0.8
Red Wine, Cooking, Homepride*	1 Serving/250ml	115	1.5	46	0.4	9.8	0.6	0.0

S

SAUCE

INFO/WEIGHT	per Measure KCAL	per Measure FAT	Nutrition per 100g KCAL	PROT	CARB	FAT	FIBRE
Red Wine, Cooking, Iceland*	1 Serving/100g	33	0.2	33	0.8	7.2	0.2	0.2
Red Wine & Onion, Rich, Simply Sausages, Colman's*	¼ Jar/125g	49	0.2	39	0.9	8.5	0.2	1.3
Redcurrant, Colman's*	1 Tsp/12g	44	0.0	368	0.7	90.0	0.0	0.0
Reggae Reggae, Cooking, Levi Roots*	½ Jar/175g	215	0.9	123	1.3	28.5	0.5	0.7
Reggae Reggae, Jerk BBQ, Levi Roots*	1 Jar/310g	375	0.3	121	1.1	28.8	0.1	0.5
Rendang, Indonesian, Seasoned Pioneers*	1 Pouch/400g	500	46.8	125	1.3	3.5	11.7	1.8
Rich & Fruity, Branston*	1 Serving/15g	19	0.0	130	0.0	31.5	0.0	1.6
Risotto, Mushroom & White Wine, Sacla*	1 Serving/95g	151	12.3	159	3.7	6.9	13.0	0.0
Roast Peanut Satay, Stir Fry, Straight to Wok, Amoy*	½ Pack/60g	106	6.4	176	4.0	16.3	10.6	1.3
Roast Vegetable with Basil & Tomato, M & S*	1 Serving/100g	85	4.1	85	2.0	9.5	4.1	1.2
Roasted Peanut Satay, Stir Fry Sensations, Amoy*	1 Pouch/160g	354	19.8	221	4.7	21.9	12.4	1.0
Roasted Vegetable, Finest, Tesco*	1 Serving/175g	101	4.2	58	1.4	7.8	2.4	1.0
Rogan Josh, Sharwood's*	½ Jar/210g	220	16.8	105	1.2	7.0	8.0	1.5
Rogan Josh, Tesco*	½ Can/220g	156	10.3	71	1.3	5.9	4.7	1.4
Rogan Josh, VLH Kitchens	1 Serving/460g	374	1.2	82	1.4	6.1	5.3	1.4
Romesco, with Red Peppers & Nuts, M & S*	1 Serving/25g	94	8.3	375	3.3	5.7	33.3	5.9
Royal Korma, Tilda*	1 Pack/400ml	824	73.2	206	1.9	8.4	18.3	0.7
Rum, with Lambs Navy* Rum, Finest, Tesco*	¼ Pot/125ml	377	31.4	302	2.1	13.1	25.1	1.5
Satay, Stir Fry & Dipping, Finest, Tesco*	1 Tsp/5g	22	1.7	432	9.0	20.7	34.8	2.7
Sausage Casserole, Cook in, Homepride*	½ Jar/250g	92	0.5	37	0.7	8.0	0.2	0.6
Seafood, 25% Less Fat, Tesco*	1 Tsp/5g	17	1.4	344	2.7	18.2	28.5	0.3
Seafood, Average	1 Tsp/5g	20	1.9	410	1.4	15.4	38.0	0.2
Seafood, Colman's*	1 Tbsp/15g	44	3.4	296	0.9	21.5	22.9	0.4
Seafood, GFY, Asda*	1 Dstp/10ml	31	2.7	313	0.6	17.0	27.0	0.0
Seafood, Organic, Simply Delicious*	1 Serving/35g	192	18.9	549	2.3	13.6	53.9	0.3
Soy, Average	1 Tsp/5ml	3	0.0	64	8.7	8.3	0.0	0.0
Soy, Dark, Amoy*	1 Tsp/5ml	5	0.0	106	0.9	25.6	0.0	0.0
Soy, Dark, Average	1 Tsp/5g	4	0.0	84	4.0	16.7	0.1	0.2
Soy, Light, Amoy*	1 Tsp/5ml	3	0.0	52	2.5	10.5	0.0	0.0
Soy, Light, Sharwood's*	1 Tsp/5ml	2	0.0	37	2.7	6.4	0.2	0.0
Soy, Naturally Brewed, Kikkoman*	1 Tbsp/15g	11	0.0	74	10.3	8.1	0.0	0.0
Soy, Premium, Light, Heinz*	1 Serving/15g	11	0.1	71	7.4	9.1	0.5	0.0
Soy, Reduced Salt, Amoy*	1 Tsp/5ml	3	0.0	56	4.0	10.0	0.0	0.0
Soy, Rich, Sharwood's*	1 Tsp/5ml	4	0.0	79	3.1	16.6	0.4	0.0
Soy, Wasabi & Lemon Grass, Stir Fry, Finest, Tesco*	1 Pack/125g	119	2.7	95	1.5	16.3	2.2	0.9
Soy & Garlic, Stir Fry, Fresh Tastes, Asda*	1 Pack/180g	175	6.7	97	1.7	14.1	3.7	0.5
Soy & Plum, Stir Fry Additions, M & S*	½ Sachet/60g	48	0.2	80	1.5	17.5	0.3	1.5
Soya, Japanese, Waitrose*	1 Tbsp/15ml	11	0.1	74	7.7	9.4	0.6	0.8
Spicy Pepperoni & Tomato, Stir in, Dolmio*	½ Pack/75g	115	8.7	154	3.3	9.3	11.6	0.8
Spicy Red Pepper & Roasted Vegetable, Sainsbury's*	1 Pot/302g	220	10.3	73	1.5	8.9	3.4	1.0
Spicy Sweet & Sour, Sharwood's*	1 Serving/138g	142	0.7	103	0.7	23.8	0.5	0.4
Spicy Szechuan, Safe To Eat*	1 Pouch/400g	124	2.4	31	1.0	4.8	0.6	0.3
Spicy Tomato, Italian, Somerfield*	½ Pot/149g	79	3.9	53	1.2	6.1	2.6	0.8
Spicy Tomato & Pesto, COU, M & S*	1 Serving/100g	60	2.5	60	2.2	6.8	2.5	1.3
Sticky BBQ, Spread & Bake, Heinz*	¼ Jar/78g	131	0.5	168	1.0	39.6	0.6	1.2
Sticky Plum, Stir Fry, Blue Dragon*	1 Serving/60g	145	0.2	242	0.1	35.6	0.3	0.0
Sticky Ribz, Ainsley Harriott*	1 Serving/50g	107	0.0	214	0.4	52.2	0.1	0.0
Stir Fry, Chinese, Tesco*	1 Serving/90g	85	3.1	95	1.3	14.3	3.5	0.6
Stir Fry, Chinese with Soy, Ginger & Garlic, Tesco*	1 Pack/150g	180	8.4	120	2.1	14.2	5.6	0.8
Stir Fry, Fragrant Sichuan, M & S*	1 Jar/155g	194	4.5	125	0.7	24.4	2.9	0.3
Stir Fry, Hoi Sin with Garlic & Spring Onion, Tesco*	¼ Pack/38g	46	0.4	120	2.2	25.2	1.1	0.5
Stir Fry, Laksa, Cook Asian, M & S*	½ Pack/75g	82	6.0	110	0.9	8.9	8.0	1.0
Stir Fry, Pad Thai, Amoy*	1 Pack/120g	179	5.4	149	2.5	24.7	4.5	1.3

SAUCE

	Measure INFO/WEIGHT	per Measure KCAL	FAT	Nutrition Values per 100g / 100ml KCAL	PROT	CARB	FAT	FIBRE
Stir Fry, Pad Thai, Tesco*	1 Pack/125g	112	2.9	90	1.3	15.8	2.3	0.8
Stir Fry, Sweet Chilli, Sainsbury's*	½ Pack/50ml	74	1.9	149	0.5	28.4	3.8	0.5
Stir Fry, Sweet Soy & Roasted Red Chilli, Blue Dragon*	1 Pack/120g	122	0.1	102	1.3	24.0	0.1	0.2
Stir Fry, Sweet Soy with Ginger & Garlic, Blue Dragon*	½ Pack/60g	52	0.0	87	0.8	20.6	0.0	0.1
Stir Fry, Sweet Thai Chilli, Straight to Wok, Amoy*	1 Serving/60g	68	1.1	113	0.3	23.8	1.8	0.3
Stir Fry, Wasabi Plum Shot, Blue Dragon*	1 Sachet/140g	344	1.8	246	1.7	35.3	1.3	1.7
Stroganoff, Asda*	1 Serving/285g	305	25.6	107	1.5	5.0	9.0	0.4
Stroganoff, Mushroom, Creamy, M & S*	1 Serving/75g	86	6.9	115	3.3	4.8	9.2	0.6
Stroganoff, Tesco*	1 Serving/100g	89	7.3	89	0.7	5.3	7.3	0.4
Succulent Szechuan Tomato, Stir Fry Sensations, Amoy*	1 Serving/64g	71	0.6	111	1.4	23.7	1.0	1.6
Sun Dried Tomato, Heinz*	1 Serving/10ml	7	0.1	73	1.5	14.9	0.6	0.9
Sun Dried Tomato & Basil, Free From, Sainsbury's*	1 Serving/175g	126	4.9	72	2.9	8.7	2.8	1.5
Sun Dried Tomato & Basil, Seeds of Change*	1 Serving/100g	169	13.2	169	1.8	9.3	13.2	0.0
Sundried Tomato for Pasta, Dress Italian, Siciliana *	½ Jar/175g	93	8.6	53	1.3	4.0	4.9	8.0
Supreme Garlic, A.1., Kraft*	1 Tbsp/18g	25	0.0	139	0.0	27.8	0.0	0.0
Sweet & Sour, Aromatic, Stir Fry Sensations, Amoy*	1 Pack/160g	312	0.5	195	0.4	46.8	0.3	0.8
Sweet & Sour, Cooking, Chinese, Sainsbury's*	¼ Jar/125g	155	0.1	124	0.6	30.1	0.1	0.7
Sweet & Sour, Cooking, Light Choices, Tesco*	1 Jar/510g	357	0.5	70	0.3	16.1	0.1	0.5
Sweet & Sour, Cooking, Organic, Sainsbury's*	1/3 Jar/150g	150	1.3	100	0.8	22.1	0.9	0.5
Sweet & Sour, Extra Pineapple, Uncle Ben's*	1 Serving/165g	147	0.3	89	0.3	21.2	0.2	0.7
Sweet & Sour, Fresh, Sainsbury's*	1 Sachet/50ml	102	4.3	205	0.8	31.2	8.6	0.3
Sweet & Sour, Oriental, Chicken Tonight, Knorr*	½ Jar/262g	217	2.6	83	0.4	20.8	1.0	0.5
Sweet & Sour, Original, Uncle Ben's*	1 Pack/300g	264	0.6	88	0.4	21.9	0.2	0.8
Sweet & Sour, Peking Style, Finest, Tesco*	1 Serving/175g	147	0.2	84	0.6	20.1	0.1	0.5
Sweet & Sour, Spicy, Uncle Ben's*	1 Jar/400g	364	0.4	91	0.6	22.1	0.1	0.0
Sweet & Sour, Stir Fry, Asda*	1 Serving/63g	146	3.1	232	0.8	46.0	5.0	0.0
Sweet & Sour, Stir Fry, GFY, Asda*	½ Pack/51ml	43	2.1	85	0.9	11.0	4.1	3.4
Sweet & Sour, Stir Fry, Sachet, Blue Dragon*	1 Sachet/120g	100	1.2	84	0.4	17.8	1.0	0.4
Sweet & Sour, Value, Tesco*	1 Serving/100g	83	0.2	83	0.3	20.0	0.2	1.0
Sweet & Sour, Weight Watchers*	½ Jar/125g	61	0.1	49	0.6	11.5	0.1	0.2
Sweet & Sour, with Mango, Sharwood's*	1/3 Jar/138g	134	0.1	97	0.7	23.3	0.1	1.3
Sweet Chilli, Dipping, M & S*	1 Tbsp/15g	34	0.1	225	0.9	53.2	0.7	0.6
Sweet Chilli, Dipping, Thai, Amoy*	1 Serving/10g	14	0.3	142	0.5	34.2	2.8	0.3
Sweet Chilli, Garlic, Stir Fry, Blue Dragon*	1 Pack/120g	142	0.1	118	0.2	28.8	0.1	0.3
Sweet Chilli, Heinz*	1 Serving/25g	37	0.1	150	0.3	36.5	0.4	6.4
Sweet Chilli, Lee Kum Kee*	1 Jar/215g	518	0.4	241	0.4	59.4	0.2	0.6
Sweet Chilli, Sharwood's*	1 Bottle/150ml	325	0.6	217	0.7	52.8	0.4	1.7
Sweet Chilli, Stir Fry, Additions, Tesco*	1 Serving/50g	105	3.8	211	0.3	35.2	7.6	0.6
Sweet Chilli, Stir Fry, BGTY, Sainsbury's*	1 Pack/150ml	178	2.8	119	0.6	25.0	1.9	1.1
Sweet Chilli & Coriander, Sharwood's*	1 Pack/370g	407	4.4	110	0.3	24.4	1.2	0.1
Sweet Chilli & Coriander, Sizzling, Homepride*	1 Serving/100g	51	0.2	51	0.7	11.5	0.2	0.0
Sweet Chilli & Garlic, Stir Fry & Dipping, Tesco*	½ Jar/95ml	78	0.0	82	0.3	20.1	0.0	0.1
Sweet Chilli & Lemon Grass, Stir Fry, Sharwood's*	1 Serving/155g	127	0.2	82	0.3	19.7	0.1	0.3
Sweet Chilli & Lime, Chinatown, Knorr*	1 Jar/525g	635	17.3	121	0.6	22.0	3.3	0.5
Sweet Curry, Eazy Squirt, Heinz*	1 Serving/10ml	12	0.0	124	0.7	29.0	0.3	0.5
Sweet Pepper, Stir in, Dolmio*	½ Pot/75g	103	7.7	137	1.5	9.7	10.3	0.0
Sweet Soy & Roasted Red Chilli, Stir Fry, Blue Dragon*	½ Pack/60g	49	0.0	81	0.4	19.5	0.0	0.2
Sweet Soy & Sesame, Uncle Ben's*	1 Serving/100g	110	1.7	110	0.7	23.0	1.7	0.0
Szechuan, Stir Fry, Sharwood's*	1 Jar/150g	126	1.6	84	3.0	15.5	1.1	0.4
Szechuan Style, Stir Fry, Fresh Ideas, Tesco*	1 Sachet/50g	114	4.8	228	1.9	33.4	9.7	0.1
Tabasco, Tabasco*	1 Tsp/5ml	1	0.0	12	1.3	0.8	0.8	0.6
Tagine, Cooking, Perfectly Balanced, Waitrose*	1 Jar/430g	258	8.6	60	1.0	9.6	2.0	1.5
Tamarind & Lime, Stir Fry, Sainsbury's*	1 Serving/75g	88	5.5	117	1.1	11.4	7.4	0.8

S

	Measure INFO/WEIGHT	per Measure KCAL	FAT	Nutrition Values per 100g / 100ml KCAL	PROT	CARB	FAT	FIBRE

SAUCE

	Measure/INFO/WEIGHT	KCAL	FAT	KCAL	PROT	CARB	FAT	FIBRE
Tartare	1oz/28g	84	6.9	299	1.3	17.9	24.6	0.0
Tartare, Colman's*	1 Tbsp/15g	45	3.7	290	1.5	17.0	24.0	0.6
Tartare, Rich, Colman's*	1 Tsp/5ml	14	1.1	284	1.2	17.0	23.0	0.6
Tartare with Olives, The English Provender Co.*	1 Tbsp/15g	64	6.6	425	2.2	5.7	43.7	0.7
Teriyaki, Asda*	1 Serving/98g	99	0.1	101	2.1	23.0	0.1	0.0
Teriyaki, Fresh, The Saucy Fish Co.*	1 Pack/150g	318	2.8	212	2.8	45.8	1.9	0.0
Teriyaki, Japanese Grill, Kikkoman*	1 Serving/15ml	24	0.0	158	4.5	30.8	0.0	0.0
Teriyaki, Lee Kum Kee*	1 Serving/15g	27	0.0	178	2.2	42.4	0.0	0.5
Teriyaki, Sticky, Oven Cook, Blue Dragon*	1 Jar/310g	391	0.3	126	0.7	30.4	0.1	0.0
Teriyaki, Stir Fry, Blue Dragon*	1 Sachet/120g	124	0.0	103	0.5	25.0	0.0	0.0
Teriyaki, Stir Fry, Fresh Ideas, Tesco*	1 Serving/25g	33	0.6	133	1.1	26.9	2.3	0.0
Teriyaki, Stir Fry, Sharwood's*	1 Jar/150g	144	0.4	96	0.9	22.5	0.3	0.3
Thai, Lemon Grass, Lime, & Chilli, Stir Fry, Sainsbury's*	1 Serving/50ml	145	13.2	290	4.0	10.2	26.5	3.5
Thai, Sweet Chilli, Blue Dragon*	1 Serving/15g	28	0.1	188	0.5	45.5	0.6	0.0
Thai Chilli, Dipping, Sainsbury's*	1 Tbsp/15g	30	0.0	201	0.2	49.8	0.0	5.0
Thai Curry, Yellow, Loyd Grossman*	1 Serving/100g	111	7.5	111	1.7	9.1	7.5	1.0
Thai Fish, Nuoc Mam, Amoy*	1 Tbsp/15ml	12	0.0	80	13.4	6.7	0.0	0.0
Thai Green, Barts*	½ Pack/150ml	210	18.0	140	2.0	6.0	12.0	0.0
Thai Green, Sainsbury's*	¼ Pack/125g	170	11.9	136	1.8	10.8	9.5	2.1
Thai Kaffir Lime, Chilli & Basil, Stir Fry, Sainsbury's*	½ Jar/175g	166	10.3	95	1.3	9.2	5.9	1.1
Three Pepper, Bottled, Heinz*	1 Tbsp/10g	33	3.2	329	1.5	8.7	32.0	0.0
Tikka, BFY, Morrisons*	½ Jar/238g	259	8.1	109	2.3	17.2	3.4	1.3
Tikka, Cooking, BGTY, Sainsbury's*	1 Jar/500g	370	9.5	74	1.2	12.9	1.9	0.3
Tikka Bhuna, Sizzle & Stir, Chicken Tonight, Knorr*	½ Jar/230g	267	21.6	116	1.2	6.7	9.4	1.1
Tikka Masala, Cooking, Sharwood's*	1 Tsp/2g	2	0.2	122	1.2	11.9	7.8	0.9
Tikka Masala, Deliciously Good, Homepride*	¼ Jar/149g	121	5.4	81	2.1	10.0	3.6	1.5
Tikka Masala, Light Choices, Tesco*	¼ Jar/125g	100	3.4	80	2.0	11.1	2.7	1.2
Tikka Masala, Perfectly Balanced, Waitrose*	½ Jar/175g	107	1.4	61	2.7	10.7	0.8	1.5
Tikka Masala, Shere Khan*	1 Serving/213ml	176	14.7	83	1.3	3.9	6.9	0.0
Toffee, GFY, Asda*	1 Serving/5g	15	0.1	306	2.2	68.0	2.8	0.0
Toffee, Luxury, Rowse*	1 Serving/20g	67	0.7	336	1.9	73.9	3.7	0.4
Toffee Fudge, Sainsbury's*	1 Serving/40g	134	1.5	336	1.9	73.9	3.7	0.4
Tomato, Heinz*	1 Tbsp/17g	18	0.0	103	0.9	24.1	0.1	0.7
Tomato, Indian, Sizzling, Homepride*	1 Serving/240g	82	0.5	34	0.9	7.0	0.2	0.0
Tomato, Olive & Rosemary, for Fish, Chunky, Schwartz*	1 Pack/300g	147	8.1	49	1.9	4.2	2.7	0.5
Tomato & Basil, for Meatballs, Dolmio*	¼ Jar/125g	47	0.2	38	1.5	6.9	0.2	1.3
Tomato & Basil, Fresh, Asda*	½ Tub/175g	100	3.7	57	1.5	7.9	2.1	0.5
Tomato & Basil, Fresh, Organic, Waitrose*	¼ Pot/175g	77	3.0	44	1.0	6.2	1.7	0.8
Tomato & Basil for Pasta Stir & Serve, Homepride*	1 Jar/480g	278	13.9	58	1.2	6.7	2.9	0.0
Tomato & Basil Sauce, Fresh, Tesco*	1 Pot/500g	245	9.0	49	1.5	6.8	1.8	0.8
Tomato & Chilli, Table & Dip, Heinz*	1 Tsp/10ml	8	0.0	76	1.4	16.6	0.2	0.8
Tomato & Chilli, Waitrose*	1 Pot/350g	182	9.1	52	10.0	6.2	2.6	3.2
Tomato & Marscapone, Italian, Somerfield*	½ Pot/150g	159	12.3	106	1.6	6.5	8.2	0.9
Tomato & Marscapone, Italiano, Tesco*	1 Serving/175g	194	15.2	111	2.8	5.4	8.7	0.6
Tomato & Mascarpone, Asda*	½ Tub/175g	152	10.1	87	1.8	7.0	5.8	0.5
Tomato & Mascarpone, Fresh, Tesco*	½ Pot/175g	206	15.2	118	2.8	7.1	8.7	0.6
Tomato & Mascarpone, Light Choices, Tesco*	½ Pot/175g	77	3.5	44	1.6	4.9	2.0	0.8
Tomato & Wild Mushroom, Organic, Fresh, Sainsbury's*	1 Serving/152g	102	7.4	67	1.9	3.9	4.9	1.7
Tomato & Worcester, Table, Lea & Perrins*	1 Serving/10g	10	0.0	102	0.8	23.0	0.5	0.7
Tomato Frito, Heinz*	1 Serving/16g	13	0.6	80	1.5	9.7	3.9	0.8
Vegetable, Chunky, Tesco*	1 Can/455g	155	0.9	34	1.2	7.0	0.2	1.0
Vegetables, Hoi Sin & Plum, Stir Fry, Sharwood's*	1 Pack/360g	367	4.7	102	1.1	21.4	1.3	0.2
Watercress, Fresh, The Saucy Fish Co.*	1 Pack/150g	169	14.5	113	2.2	5.8	9.7	0.0

S

	Measure INFO/WEIGHT	per Measure KCAL	FAT	Nutrition Values per 100g / 100ml KCAL	PROT	CARB	FAT	FIBRE
SAUCE								
Watercress & Creme Fraiche, COU, M & S*	½ Pack/154g	100	2.8	65	3.2	9.2	1.8	0.5
White, for Lasagne, Dolmio*	1 Jar/470g	451	34.3	96	0.6	7.0	7.3	0.0
White, Savoury, Made with Semi-Skimmed Milk	1oz/28g	36	2.2	128	4.2	11.1	7.8	0.2
White, Savoury, Made with Whole Milk	1oz/28g	42	2.9	150	4.1	10.9	10.3	0.2
White Granules, Sauce in Seconds, Dry, Asda*	1 Pack/57g	237	6.8	415	3.7	73.0	12.0	0.9
White Wine, Chardonnay, M & S*	1 Serving/160ml	184	16.0	115	1.4	4.6	10.0	0.9
White Wine, Cooking, Iceland*	1 Serving/220g	198	12.8	90	1.1	8.3	5.8	0.2
White Wine & Cream, Cook in, Classic, Homepride*	¼ Can/125g	101	5.1	81	1.0	8.0	4.1	0.4
White Wine & Mushroom, BGTY, Sainsbury's*	¼ Jar/125g	81	2.5	65	2.8	9.0	2.0	0.3
White Wine & Tarragon, French for Fish, Schwartz*	1 Pack/300g	372	33.3	124	1.1	5.0	11.1	0.8
White Wine Mushroom & Herb, 98% Fat Free, Homepride*	1 Jar/450g	180	5.4	40	0.8	7.0	1.2	0.5
Whole Cherry Tomato & Chilli, Finest, Tesco*	1 Jar/340g	255	15.6	75	1.7	6.8	4.6	2.3
Worcester, Morrisons*	1 Serving/5ml	6	0.0	120	0.0	28.0	0.0	0.0
Worcestershire, Average	***1 Tsp/5g***	***3***	***0.0***	***65***	***1.4***	***15.5***	***0.1***	***0.0***
Worcestershire, Lea & Perrins*	1 Tsp/5ml	4	0.0	88	1.1	22.0	0.0	0.0
Worcestershire, Special Edition, Lea & Perrins*	1 Serving/10ml	13	0.0	130	1.3	28.8	0.2	0.1
Yellow Bean, Stir Fry, Sainsbury's*	½ Jar/100g	126	1.3	126	1.8	26.7	1.3	0.8
Yellow Bean & Cashew, Tesco*	½ Jar/210g	170	6.1	81	1.6	11.9	2.9	0.3
Yellow Bean & Ginger, Stir Fry, Finest, Tesco*	1 Jar/350g	318	3.5	91	2.1	18.3	1.0	1.1
SAUCE MIX								
Bacon & Mushroom Tagliatelle, Schwartz*	1 Pack/33g	110	1.0	333	7.5	69.2	2.9	8.3
Beef Bourguignon, Colman's*	1 Pack/40g	123	0.6	308	4.9	68.6	1.6	2.2
Beef Stroganoff, Colman's*	1 Pack/40g	140	3.6	350	11.6	56.1	8.9	2.7
Bombay Potatoes, Schwartz*	1 Pack/33g	84	4.0	254	16.1	20.1	12.1	31.1
Bread, Colman's*	1 Pack/40g	131	0.4	327	11.4	67.9	1.1	3.2
Bread, Knorr*	½ Pint/40g	177	9.3	442	7.9	49.9	23.3	2.1
Bread, Luxury as Sold, Schwartz*	1 Pack/40g	148	1.5	369	11.5	70.3	3.8	3.7
Cajun Chicken, Schwartz*	1 Pack/38g	108	0.5	285	6.4	61.9	1.3	0.5
Chargrilled Chicken Pasta, Schwartz*	1 Pack/35g	119	3.1	341	8.6	56.8	8.8	6.1
Cheddar Cheese, Colman's*	1 Pack/40g	163	6.2	407	18.3	48.8	15.4	1.2
Cheddar Cheese, Dry Mix, Schwartz*	1 Pack/40g	144	3.0	361	18.4	55.1	7.4	2.3
Cheddar Cheese, Lidl*	1 Pack/40g	140	4.6	350	18.6	43.0	11.5	0.0
Cheese, Knorr*	1 Pack/58g	132	2.8	227	7.8	38.0	4.9	1.8
Cheese, Made Up, Crosse & Blackwell*	1 Pack/30g	26	1.0	86	5.1	9.2	3.2	0.7
Cheese, Made Up with Skimmed Milk	1 Serving/60g	47	1.4	78	5.4	9.5	2.3	0.0
Cheese & Bacon, for Pasta, Colman's*	1 Pack/50g	179	3.4	359	15.6	58.7	6.8	2.7
Chicken Chasseur, Colman's*	1 Pack/45g	128	0.7	284	8.0	59.2	1.6	3.8
Chicken Chasseur, Schwartz*	1 Pack/40g	126	1.8	316	9.6	59.1	4.6	6.8
Chicken Curry for Slow Cookers, as Sold, Schwartz*	1 Pack/33g	89	2.3	270	12.5	25.7	7.0	27.3
Chicken Korma, Colman's*	½ Pack/50g	229	15.4	459	6.6	38.8	30.8	13.2
Chicken Supreme, Colman's*	1 Pack/40g	143	3.7	358	12.1	56.7	9.2	2.4
Chilli Con Carne, Hot, Colman's*	1 Pack/40g	127	1.2	317	10.4	62.4	2.9	7.0
Chilli Con Carne, Schwartz*	1 Pack/41g	120	1.5	293	7.9	57.2	3.6	9.5
Coq Au Vin, Colman's*	1 Pack/50g	150	0.9	301	5.6	65.6	1.8	3.3
Cream, for Meatballs, Ikea*	1 Pack/40g	179	9.4	448	9.6	49.2	23.6	0.0
Creamy Pepper & Mushroom, Colman's*	1 Pack/25g	83	0.9	332	9.6	64.6	3.8	3.0
Dauphinoise Potato Bake, Schwartz*	1 Pack/40g	161	10.5	402	6.8	34.7	26.3	15.8
Four Cheese, Colman's*	1 Pack/35g	127	3.9	362	17.1	48.4	11.1	1.8
Hollandaise, Colman's*	1 Pack/28g	104	3.1	372	6.4	61.6	11.1	1.8
Hollandaise, Schwartz*	1 Pack/25g	98	3.2	394	10.6	59.2	12.8	3.7
Lamb Hotpot, Colman's*	1 Pack/40g	119	0.7	297	6.9	63.3	1.7	2.1
Lasagne, Mediterranean Vegetable, Schwartz*	1 Pack/30g	79	1.3	263	9.3	46.0	4.4	15.2
Lasagne, Schwartz*	1 Pack/36g	106	0.5	294	7.0	63.4	1.4	7.0

S

	Measure INFO/WEIGHT	per Measure KCAL	FAT	Nutrition Values per 100g / 100ml KCAL	PROT	CARB	FAT	FIBRE
SAUCE MIX								
Lemon Butter for Fish, Schwartz*	1 Pack/38g	136	3.0	357	6.1	65.3	8.0	5.8
Mexican Chilli Chicken, Schwartz*	1 Pack/35g	105	2.0	299	7.0	55.1	5.6	12.0
Mixed Herbs for Chicken, So Juicy, Maggi*	1 Pack/34g	97	1.0	285	8.3	53.8	2.8	5.5
Onion, Creamy, Schwartz*	1 Pack/25g	90	2.3	362	10.1	59.6	9.2	5.3
Onion as Sold, Colman's*	1 Pack/35g	110	0.6	313	10.7	63.9	1.7	6.7
Paprika Chicken, Creamy, Schwartz*	1 Pack/34g	116	3.3	342	9.7	53.9	9.8	9.5
Paprika For Chicken, So Juicy, Maggi*	1 Pack/34g	91	1.4	267	8.8	45.5	4.0	7.1
Parsley, Creamy, Made Up, Schwartz*	1 Serving/79g	59	2.0	75	4.2	8.7	2.5	0.3
Parsley, Dry, Colman's*	1 Pack/20g	63	0.3	313	7.2	67.9	1.4	3.8
Parsley, Knorr*	1 Sachet/48g	210	11.6	437	4.2	50.6	24.2	0.8
Parsley & Chive for Fish, Schwartz*	1 Pack/38g	132	3.2	348	9.0	58.9	8.5	7.7
Pepper, Creamy, Colman's*	1 Pack/25g	88	2.7	352	13.0	50.0	11.0	0.0
Shepherd's Pie, Schwartz*	1 Pack/38g	104	1.0	273	7.9	54.4	2.6	11.1
Spaghetti Bolognese, Colman's*	1 Pack/40g	120	0.4	300	8.9	64.1	0.9	5.2
Spaghetti Bolognese, Schwartz*	1 Pack/40g	114	0.6	285	9.2	59.0	1.6	7.0
Spaghetti Bolognese with Mushrooms, Colman's*	1 Pack/45g	138	0.4	307	7.8	66.8	0.9	4.7
Stroganoff, Mushroom, Schwartz*	1 Pack/35g	113	1.9	324	10.0	59.2	5.3	9.6
Sweet & Sour, Colman's*	1 Pack/40g	133	0.2	333	2.6	79.9	0.4	2.2
Sweet & Sour for Chicken, So Juicy, Maggi*	½ Pack/15g	42	0.3	279	7.1	55.8	2.3	3.5
Thai Green Curry, Schwartz*	1 Pack/41g	137	3.3	333	7.6	57.6	8.1	13.0
Thai Red Curry, Schwartz*	1 Pack/35g	120	2.5	342	5.9	63.5	7.1	7.6
Three Cheese for Vegetables, Schwartz*	1 Pack/40g	168	8.2	421	17.4	41.7	20.5	4.8
Tikka Masala, Creamy, Schwartz*	1 Pack/31g	100	3.5	324	11.9	43.5	11.4	18.1
Tuna & Mushroom Pasta Melt, Schwartz*	1 Pack/40g	122	2.8	304	10.2	49.7	7.1	7.7
Tuna & Pasta Bake, Colman's*	1 Pack/45g	144	2.4	319	10.4	57.1	5.4	5.2
Tuna Napolitana, Schwartz*	1 Pack/30g	107	3.9	357	10.3	49.6	13.1	0.5
Vegetable Pasta, Bake, Colmans*	1 Pack/50g	223	13.1	446	12.0	40.1	26.2	3.6
White, Instant, Made Up, Sainsbury's*	1 Serving/90ml	65	2.5	72	0.8	10.9	2.8	0.1
White, Made Up with Semi-Skimmed Milk	1oz/28g	20	0.7	73	4.0	9.6	2.4	0.0
White, Made Up with Skimmed Milk	1oz/28g	17	0.3	59	4.0	9.6	0.9	0.0
White, Savoury, Colman's*	1 Pack/25g	84	0.7	335	10.7	66.5	2.9	2.6
White, Savoury, Knorr*	½ Pack/16g	46	0.9	290	7.8	52.2	5.6	5.2
White, Savoury, Schwartz*	1 Pack/25g	108	5.7	434	11.5	45.6	22.9	5.9
White Wine with Herbs, Creamy, Schwartz*	1 Pack/26g	86	1.7	330	8.0	60.0	6.5	9.1
Wholegrain Mustard, Creamy, Schwartz*	1 Pack/25g	92	2.8	370	12.9	54.4	11.2	7.5
SAUERKRAUT								
Average	**1oz/28g**	**4**	**0.0**	**13**	**1.3**	**1.9**	**0.0**	**1.1**
SAUSAGE								
BBQ Hotdog, M & S*	1 Sausage/100g	300	25.3	300	12.1	5.4	25.3	2.0
Beef, Average	**1 Sausage/60g**	**151**	**11.1**	**252**	**14.5**	**7.0**	**18.5**	**0.6**
Beef with Onion & Red Wine, Finest, Tesco*	1 Sausage/63g	117	6.9	185	13.2	8.5	10.9	1.2
Billy Bear, Kids, Tesco*	1 Slice/20g	37	2.2	185	13.7	7.5	11.2	0.4
Bockwurst, Average	**1 Sausage/45g**	**114**	**10.3**	**253**	**10.7**	**0.7**	**23.0**	**0.0**
Bratwurst, Frozen, Lidl*	1 Sausage/80g	235	21.4	294	12.8	0.5	26.8	0.0
Cheese & Leek, Tesco*	1 Sausage/55g	135	7.9	245	6.6	21.3	14.4	3.9
Chicken, Manor Farm*	1 Sausage/65g	126	8.1	194	13.7	6.6	12.5	1.2
Chicken & Turkey, Morrisons*	1 Sausage/57g	86	4.1	152	16.0	5.8	7.2	1.1
Chilli & Coriander, TTD, Sainsbury's*	1 Sausage/44g	136	10.7	310	18.5	4.2	24.4	1.2
Chilli Beef, Boston Style, Waitrose*	1 Sausage/67g	135	9.7	203	14.7	3.4	14.6	0.9
Chipolata, Average	**1 Sausage/28g**	**81**	**6.5**	**291**	**12.1**	**8.7**	**23.1**	**0.7**
Chorizo, Average	**1 Serving/80g**	**250**	**19.4**	**313**	**21.1**	**2.6**	**24.2**	**0.2**
Chorizo, Lean, Average	**1 Sausage/67g**	**131**	**9.2**	**195**	**15.7**	**2.3**	**13.7**	**0.8**
Cocktail, Average	**1oz/28g**	**90**	**7.5**	**323**	**12.1**	**8.6**	**26.7**	**0.9**

	Measure INFO/WEIGHT	per Measure KCAL	FAT	Nutrition Values per 100g / 100ml KCAL	PROT	CARB	FAT	FIBRE
SAUSAGE								
Cumberland, Average	*1 Sausage/57g*	*167*	*13.0*	*293*	*13.8*	*8.5*	*22.7*	*0.8*
Cumberland, Healthy Range, Average	*1 Sausage/53g*	*75*	*2.1*	*142*	*17.4*	*9.0*	*4.0*	*0.9*
Garlic, Average	*1 Slice/11g*	*25*	*2.0*	*227*	*15.7*	*0.8*	*18.2*	*0.0*
German, Bierwurst, Selection, Sainsbury's*	1 Slice/4g	8	0.6	224	15.0	1.0	17.8	0.1
German, Extrawurst, Selection, Sainsbury's*	1 Slice/3g	9	0.8	279	13.1	0.5	25.0	0.1
German, Schinkenwurst, Selection, Sainsbury's*	1 Slice/3g	8	0.7	251	13.1	0.3	21.9	0.1
Irish, Average	*1 Sausage/40g*	*119*	*8.3*	*297*	*10.7*	*17.2*	*20.7*	*0.7*
Lamb, Spiced & Mint, Morrisons*	1 Sausage/34g	79	4.5	233	22.9	5.1	13.2	1.1
Lincolnshire, Average	*1 Sausage/42g*	*122*	*9.1*	*291*	*14.6*	*9.2*	*21.8*	*0.6*
Lincolnshire, Healthy Range, Average	*1 Sausage/50g*	*89*	*4.3*	*177*	*15.8*	*9.0*	*8.6*	*0.8*
Lorne, Average	*1 Sausage/25g*	*78*	*5.8*	*312*	*10.8*	*16.0*	*23.1*	*0.6*
Polish Kabanos, Sainsbury's*	1 Sausage/25g	92	7.6	366	23.0	0.1	30.4	0.1
Polony Slicing, Asda*	1oz/28g	60	3.9	214	11.0	11.0	14.0	0.0
Pork, Average	*1 Sausage/50g*	*152*	*11.9*	*305*	*12.8*	*9.8*	*23.8*	*0.7*
Pork, Bacon & Cheese, Asda*	¼ Pack/114g	329	23.9	289	18.0	7.0	21.0	0.4
Pork, Battered, Thick, Average	1oz/28g	126	10.2	448	17.3	21.7	36.3	2.0
Pork, Extra Lean, Average	*1 Sausage/54g*	*84*	*3.7*	*155*	*17.3*	*6.1*	*6.8*	*0.8*
Pork, Free From, Tesco*	1 Sausage/57g	124	8.5	218	12.1	8.5	15.0	2.2
Pork, Frozen, Fried	*1oz/28g*	*88*	*6.9*	*316*	*13.8*	*10.0*	*24.8*	*0.0*
Pork, Frozen, Grilled	*1oz/28g*	*81*	*5.9*	*289*	*14.8*	*10.5*	*21.2*	*0.0*
Pork, Garlic & Herb, Average	*1 Sausage/76g*	*203*	*16.5*	*268*	*12.0*	*5.9*	*21.8*	*1.1*
Pork, Premium, Average	*1 Sausage/74g*	*191*	*13.6*	*258*	*14.9*	*8.3*	*18.4*	*1.0*
Pork, Reduced Fat, Chilled, Grilled	*1oz/28g*	*64*	*3.9*	*230*	*16.2*	*10.8*	*13.8*	*1.5*
Pork, Reduced Fat, Chilled, Raw	*1oz/28g*	*50*	*3.0*	*180*	*13.0*	*8.7*	*10.6*	*1.2*
Pork, Reduced Fat, Healthy Range, Average	*1 Sausage/57g*	*86*	*3.4*	*151*	*15.6*	*9.0*	*6.0*	*0.9*
Pork, Skinless, Average	*1oz/28g*	*81*	*6.6*	*291*	*11.7*	*8.2*	*23.6*	*0.6*
Pork, Thick, Average	*1 Sausage/39g*	*115*	*8.7*	*296*	*13.3*	*10.0*	*22.4*	*1.0*
Pork, Thick, Reduced Fat, Healthy Range, Average	*1 Sausage/52g*	*90*	*3.8*	*172*	*14.0*	*12.3*	*7.4*	*0.8*
Pork & Apple, Average	*1 Sausage/57g*	*146*	*10.7*	*255*	*14.5*	*7.5*	*18.8*	*1.9*
Pork & Beef, Average	*1 Sausage/45g*	*133*	*10.2*	*295*	*8.7*	*13.6*	*22.7*	*0.5*
Pork & Herb, Average	*1 Sausage/75g*	*231*	*19.5*	*308*	*13.1*	*5.4*	*25.9*	*0.3*
Pork & Herb, Healthy Range, Average	*1 Sausage/59g*	*75*	*1.4*	*126*	*16.0*	*10.7*	*2.4*	*1.1*
Pork & Leek, Average	*1oz/28g*	*73*	*5.6*	*262*	*14.6*	*6.0*	*19.9*	*1.1*
Pork & Stilton, Average	*1 Sausage/57g*	*180*	*15.2*	*316*	*13.2*	*5.8*	*26.7*	*0.3*
Pork & Tomato, Grilled, Average	*1 Sausage/47g*	*127*	*9.7*	*273*	*13.9*	*7.5*	*20.8*	*0.4*
Premium, Chilled, Fried	*1oz/28g*	*77*	*5.8*	*275*	*15.8*	*6.7*	*20.7*	*0.0*
Premium, Chilled, Grilled	*1oz/28g*	*82*	*6.3*	*292*	*16.8*	*6.3*	*22.4*	*0.0*
Premium, Pork, (8 Pack), Weight Watchers*	1 Sausage/39g	60	1.6	155	20.0	7.8	4.2	1.7
Red Onion & Rosemary, Linda McCartney*	2 Sausages/100g	128	3.7	128	14.2	9.7	3.7	5.8
Smoked, Average	*1 Sausage/174g*	*588*	*52.2*	*338*	*13.0*	*4.0*	*30.0*	*0.0*
Turkey, Average	*1 Sausage/57g*	*90*	*4.6*	*157*	*15.7*	*6.3*	*8.0*	*0.0*
Turkey & Chicken, Average	*1 Sausage/57g*	*126*	*8.2*	*221*	*14.4*	*8.2*	*14.5*	*1.7*
Tuscan, M & S*	1 Sausage/66g	145	10.6	220	14.9	4.6	16.0	0.6
Venison, Grilled, Finest, Tesco*	1 Sausage/41g	86	5.5	215	16.6	6.3	13.7	0.6
Venison & Red Wine, TTD, Sainsbury's*	1 Sausage/58g	130	7.7	226	19.7	6.8	13.3	1.7
Wiejska, Polish, Sainsbury's*	1/8 Pack/50g	78	4.5	157	18.7	0.4	9.0	0.5
Wild Boar	1 Sausage/85g	220	17.0	259	16.5	1.2	20.0	0.0
SAUSAGE & MASH								
2 British Pork & Rich Onion Gravy, M & S*	1 Pack/400g	340	6.8	85	5.7	12.2	1.7	1.3
221, Oakhouse Foods Ltd*	1 Meal/400g	504	27.2	126	5.5	11.0	6.8	1.4
British Classic, Tesco*	1 Pack/450g	675	42.7	150	5.1	11.1	9.5	0.9
Everyday, Value, Tesco*	1 Pack/400g	400	16.4	100	3.6	11.5	4.1	1.2
GFY, Asda*	1 Pack/400g	330	10.0	82	4.2	10.7	2.5	1.7

	Measure INFO/WEIGHT	per Measure		Nutrition Values per 100g / 100ml				
		KCAL	FAT	KCAL	PROT	CARB	FAT	FIBRE
SAUSAGE & MASH								
Iceland*	1 Pack/440g	484	26.0	110	3.8	10.4	5.9	1.6
in Cider Gravy, with Apple & Onion, Weight Watchers*	1 Pack/400g	332	11.6	83	5.5	7.5	2.9	2.2
Light Choices, Tesco*	1 Pack/400g	360	8.8	90	4.4	11.8	2.2	1.4
Onion, M & S*	1 Pack/300g	315	17.1	105	4.1	9.0	5.7	1.5
Vegetarian, GFY, Asda*	1 Pack/400g	292	8.8	73	4.2	9.0	2.2	2.1
Vegetarian, Tesco*	1 Pack/410g	398	15.6	97	4.6	11.1	3.8	2.0
SAUSAGE MEAT								
Pork, Average	*1oz/28g*	*96*	*8.2*	*344*	*9.9*	*10.1*	*29.4*	*0.6*
SAUSAGE ROLL								
Basics, Party Size, Somerfield*	1 Roll/13g	45	2.9	343	7.0	29.0	22.0	0.0
BGTY, Sainsbury's*	1 Roll/65g	200	11.4	308	9.6	27.9	17.6	1.4
Cocktail, Average	1 Roll/15g	57	3.7	378	8.9	29.4	24.9	1.9
Large, Freshbake*	1 Roll/52g	153	9.5	294	6.6	25.9	18.3	4.6
Large, Frozen, Tesco*	1 Roll/50g	182	11.9	365	6.0	31.0	23.8	0.9
Lincolnshire, Geo Adams*	1 Roll/130g	474	31.6	365	8.3	28.2	24.3	1.1
Mini, Tesco*	1 Roll/15g	53	3.7	356	9.0	23.9	24.9	1.5
Mini, Waitrose*	1 Roll/35g	124	9.2	353	13.0	16.1	26.3	1.0
Party, Sainsbury's*	1 Roll/13g	54	4.0	422	8.7	26.7	31.1	1.2
Party Size, Tesco*	1 Roll/14g	49	3.5	350	5.9	25.0	24.9	1.1
Pork, Morrisons*	1 Roll/70g	195	9.0	278	9.6	31.2	12.8	1.5
Pork Farms*	1 Roll/54g	196	12.9	363	7.9	30.0	23.9	0.0
Puff Pastry	1 Med/60g	230	16.6	383	9.9	25.4	27.6	1.0
Reduced Fat, Sainsbury's*	1 Roll/66g	191	9.4	289	10.5	29.8	14.2	1.8
Snack, GFY, Asda*	1 Roll/34g	112	7.0	329	9.4	26.5	20.6	0.9
Snack, Sainsbury's*	1 Roll/34g	130	8.5	383	9.7	29.9	25.0	2.1
Snack Size, Tesco*	1 Roll/32g	118	8.8	369	9.1	21.7	27.4	2.3
SAUSAGE ROLL VEGETARIAN								
Linda McCartney*	1 Roll/52g	142	7.0	273	9.7	28.2	13.5	2.5
SAUSAGE VEGETARIAN								
Asda*	1 Sausage/43g	81	3.9	189	20.0	7.0	9.0	2.9
Braai Flavour, Fry's Special Vegetarian*	1 Sausage/63g	141	7.6	226	20.3	9.4	12.2	0.6
Cumberland, Cauldron Foods*	1 Sausage/46g	80	4.0	173	16.0	6.5	8.6	2.8
Glamorgan, Asda*	1 Sausage/50g	100	5.1	199	4.6	22.4	10.1	2.0
Granose*	1oz/28g	63	3.8	226	8.5	17.5	13.5	0.0
Lincolnshire, Chilled, Cauldron Foods*	1 Sausage/50g	79	4.4	159	15.5	4.0	8.8	2.6
Lincolnshire, Frozen, Tesco*	1 Sausage/50g	77	2.5	155	15.5	10.8	5.0	3.0
Linda McCartney*	1 Sausage/50g	101	4.4	202	22.6	8.2	8.8	1.6
Mushroom & Herb, Waitrose*	1 Sausage/50g	61	2.7	123	10.2	8.1	5.4	0.5
Mushroom & Tarragon, Wicken Fen*	1 Sausage/47g	82	3.5	175	10.1	17.0	7.4	2.4
Realeat*	1 Sausage/40g	66	3.9	165	17.2	2.0	9.8	8.1
SAVOURY EGGS								
Bites, Sainsbury's*	1 Egg/20g	55	3.6	277	9.6	18.8	18.2	2.1
Mini, Tesco*	1 Egg/20g	55	3.5	274	9.2	20.2	17.4	2.3
Snack, Tesco*	1 Egg/45g	133	8.9	295	9.0	19.6	19.7	1.8
SCALLOPS								
Canadian, Finest, Tesco*	½ Pack/100g	80	0.2	80	16.4	2.6	0.2	0.1
Hotbake Shells, Sainsbury's*	1 Serving/140g	241	15.7	172	9.5	8.4	11.2	0.8
Raw, Bay or Sea with Roe, Average	*1 Lge Scallop/15g*	*13*	*0.1*	*88*	*16.8*	*2.4*	*0.8*	*0.0*
Steamed, Average	1oz/28g	33	0.4	118	23.2	3.4	1.4	0.0
with Roasted Garlic Butter, Finest, Tesco*	1 Serving/100g	201	14.3	201	16.2	1.8	14.3	0.4
SCAMPI								
Breaded, Baked, Average	½ Pack/255g	565	27.4	222	10.7	20.5	10.7	1.0
Breaded, Fried in Oil, Average	1 Serving/100g	237	13.6	237	9.4	20.5	13.6	0.0

S

	Measure INFO/WEIGHT	per Measure KCAL	FAT	Nutrition Values per 100g / 100ml KCAL	PROT	CARB	FAT	FIBRE
SCAMPI & CHIPS								
Chunky, Finest, Tesco*	1 Pack/280g	420	15.4	150	5.9	18.3	5.5	1.4
with Peas	1 Serving/490g	822	43.6	168	10.1	11.3	8.9	1.2
Youngs*	1oz/28g	42	1.5	150	5.0	20.3	5.4	1.7
SCHNAPPS								
Vodkat, Intercontinental Brands Ltd*	1 Serving/25ml	31	0.0	124	0.0	0.8	0.0	0.0
SCHNITZEL VEGETARIAN								
Breaded, Tivall*	1 Schnitzel/100g	172	8.0	172	16.0	9.0	8.0	5.0
SCONE								
3% Fat, M & S*	1 Scone/65g	179	1.6	275	7.2	55.1	2.5	2.3
All Butter, Sultana, Duchy Originals*	1 Scone/78g	276	9.8	353	7.3	52.9	12.5	2.6
All Butter, Tesco*	1 Scone/41g	126	3.2	308	7.2	52.3	7.8	1.6
Cheese, Average	1 Scone/40g	145	7.1	363	10.1	43.2	17.8	1.6
Cherry, Double Butter, Genesis Crafty*	1 Scone/63g	198	4.8	314	6.8	54.5	7.6	1.4
Cherry, M & S*	1 Scone/60g	202	7.3	337	6.9	49.7	12.2	1.9
Clotted Cream, Cornish, TTD, Sainsbury's*	1 Scone/70g	269	12.7	384	8.4	46.6	18.2	2.1
Cream, Sainsbury's*	1 Scone/50g	172	8.7	345	4.6	42.5	17.4	3.1
Derby, Mother's Pride*	1 Scone/60g	208	8.4	347	5.2	49.8	14.0	1.5
Derby, Tesco*	1 Scone/60g	201	6.1	335	7.2	53.7	10.2	2.0
Devon, M & S*	1 Scone/59g	225	9.6	380	7.1	50.8	16.2	1.5
Devon, Sainsbury's*	1 Scone/54g	201	8.4	372	7.1	51.1	15.5	1.6
Double Butter, Cheese, Genesis Crafty*	1 Scone/60g	180	7.0	300	12.2	36.7	11.6	0.0
Fresh Cream, Tesco*	1 Scone/80g	242	9.9	304	15.8	32.3	12.5	0.9
Fresh Cream with Strawberry Jam, Tesco*	1 Scone/83g	290	15.6	352	4.7	40.7	18.9	1.1
Fruit, Average	1 Scone/40g	126	3.9	316	7.3	52.9	9.8	0.0
Luxury, Hovis*	1 Scone/85g	267	7.9	314	5.6	51.8	9.3	2.2
Plain, Average	1 Scone/40g	145	5.8	362	7.2	53.8	14.6	1.9
Plain, Genesis Crafty*	1 Scone/74g	227	7.4	307	6.8	49.1	10.0	0.0
Potato, Average	1 Scone/40g	118	5.7	296	5.1	39.1	14.3	1.6
Potato, Mother's Pride*	1 Scone/37g	77	0.8	207	4.7	42.0	2.2	4.3
Strawberry, Fresh Cream, BGTY, Sainsbury's*	1 Scone/50g	154	5.6	309	5.1	47.0	11.2	1.1
Strawberry, Fresh Cream, Sainsbury's*	1 Scone/60g	218	11.2	363	6.5	42.5	18.6	1.4
Sultana, BGTY, Sainsbury's*	1 Scone/63g	178	1.8	283	7.7	56.7	2.8	2.4
Sultana, Finest, Tesco*	1 Scone/70g	238	7.6	340	8.9	50.9	10.9	2.1
Sultana, GFY, Asda*	1 Scone/59g	192	2.6	324	7.0	64.0	4.4	2.0
Sultana, M & S*	1 Scone/66g	231	8.2	350	6.5	53.0	12.5	2.0
Sultana, Reduced Fat, Waitrose*	1 Scone/65g	187	3.4	287	6.6	53.2	5.3	2.6
Sultana, TTD, Sainsbury's*	1 Scone/70g	239	8.1	341	6.5	52.9	11.5	2.6
Sultana, Value, Tesco*	1 Scone/40g	134	4.0	335	6.5	53.8	10.1	2.7
Tattie, Scottish, Nick Nairn's*	1 Scone/21g	42	0.3	199	4.0	34.7	1.6	0.7
Wholemeal	1 Scone/40g	130	5.8	326	8.7	43.1	14.4	5.2
Wholemeal, Fruit	1 Scone/40g	130	5.1	324	8.1	47.2	12.8	4.9
SCONE MIX								
Fruit, Asda*	1 Scone/48g	143	2.4	301	7.0	57.0	5.0	3.7
SCOTCH EGGS								
Cumberland, Waitrose*	1 Egg/114g	243	14.3	214	13.0	12.1	12.6	1.6
Free Range, Sainsbury's*	1 Egg/113g	284	19.0	252	12.4	12.5	16.9	2.5
Ginsters*	1 Egg/95g	228	15.1	240	15.3	9.7	15.9	0.6
Retail	1 Egg/120g	301	20.5	251	12.0	13.1	17.1	0.0
Super Mini, Asda*	1 Egg/13g	38	2.6	305	10.0	19.0	21.0	2.1
SEA BASS								
Cooked, Dry Heat, Average	*1 Fillet/101g*	*125*	*2.6*	*124*	*23.6*	*0.0*	*2.6*	*0.0*
Fillet, Raw, Average	1 Fillet/113g	175	7.8	155	21.0	0.1	6.9	0.2
Raw, Average	*1oz/28g*	*32*	*1.0*	*113*	*20.3*	*0.0*	*3.5*	*0.1*

S

	Measure INFO/WEIGHT	per Measure		Nutrition Values per 100g / 100ml				
		KCAL	FAT	KCAL	PROT	CARB	FAT	FIBRE
SEA BREAM								
Fillets, Raw, Average	*1oz/28g*	**27**	**0.8**	**96**	**17.5**	**0.0**	**2.9**	**0.0**
SEAFOOD COCKTAIL								
Average	1oz/28g	24	0.4	87	15.6	2.9	1.5	0.0
Premium Quality, Lyons Seafood Co*	1 Serving/100g	76	0.9	76	13.2	3.7	0.9	1.1
SEAFOOD SELECTION								
M & S*	1 Serving/200g	170	2.0	85	17.4	1.6	1.0	0.5
Mussels, King Prawns & Squid, Frozen, Tesco*	½ Pack/200g	140	3.0	70	13.7	0.1	1.5	0.0
Sainsbury's*	½ Pack/125g	85	1.2	68	14.6	0.8	1.0	2.5
SEAFOOD STICKS								
Average	1 Stick/15g	16	0.0	106	8.0	18.4	0.2	0.2
Chilled or Frozen, Youngs*	1 Stick/14g	15	0.2	108	9.0	15.4	1.2	0.6
with Cocktail Dip, Asda*	1 Pot/95g	126	4.7	133	6.0	16.0	5.0	0.1
SEASONING MIX								
Beef Taco, Colman's*	1 Pack/30g	76	3.6	252	9.1	26.9	12.0	14.0
Cajun, Sizzle & Grill, Schwartz*	1 Tsp/4g	7	0.2	182	9.8	23.0	5.6	24.4
Chicken, Chargrilled, Grill & Sizzle, Schwartz*	1 Tsp/5g	12	0.2	232	8.2	40.8	4.0	13.1
Chicken, Simply Shake, Schwartz*	1 Serving/100g	273	8.1	273	12.3	67.9	8.1	29.1
Fajita, Chicken, Colman's*	1 Pack/40g	138	2.5	344	9.4	62.5	6.3	4.8
Fish, Schwartz*	1 Tsp/4g	9	0.1	222	6.5	55.5	2.3	11.6
Garlic & Herb Mash, Perfect Shake, Schwartz*	1 Serving/10g	29	2.2	290	7.6	43.0	21.9	20.2
Italian Herb, Schwartz*	1 Tsp/1g	3	0.0	338	11.0	64.5	4.0	0.0
Jamaican Jerk Chicken, Recipe, Schwartz*	1 Pack/27g	75	0.8	276	9.8	69.8	3.0	17.2
Lemon & Herb, Cous Cous, Asda*	1 Tbsp/15g	46	1.0	305	10.6	52.0	6.5	10.2
Mediterranean Roasted Vegetable, Schwartz*	1 Pack/30g	86	1.2	288	6.9	56.1	4.0	10.3
Potato Roasties, Rosemary & Garlic, Crispy, Schwartz*	1 Pack/33g	88	2.6	267	13.0	36.1	7.8	21.1
Potato Roasties, Southern Fried, Crispy, Schwartz*	1 Pack/35g	78	1.5	222	9.2	36.2	4.4	25.1
Potato Wedges, Cajun, Schwartz*	1 Pack/38g	112	2.9	295	9.1	47.6	7.6	14.3
Potato Wedges, Garlic & Herb, Schwartz*	1 Pack/38g	106	1.9	278	11.4	47.1	4.9	11.7
Potato Wedges, Nacho Cheese, Schwartz*	1 Pack/38g	114	3.7	299	13.6	39.3	9.7	7.7
Potato Wedges, Onion & Chive, Schwartz*	1 Pack/38g	113	0.7	297	10.9	59.4	1.8	6.5
Season-All, Schwartz*	1 Tsp/6g	4	0.1	72	2.3	11.6	1.8	0.0
Shepherd's Pie, Colman's*	1 Pack/50g	141	0.7	282	12.5	54.7	1.4	4.3
Shotz, Cajun Chicken Seasoning, Schwartz*	1 Pack/3g	8	0.2	268	9.9	45.6	5.2	0.0
Shotz, Chargrilled Chicken Seasoning, Schwartz*	1 Pack/3g	8	0.1	283	7.5	52.0	4.9	0.0
Shotz, Garlic Pepper Steak Seasoning, Schwartz*	1 Pack/3g	11	0.1	370	14.0	67.0	5.0	0.0
Shotz, Moroccan Chicken Seasoning, Schwartz*	1 Pack/3g	9	0.2	312	9.7	56.7	5.2	0.0
Shotz, Seven Pepper Steak Seasoning, Schwartz*	1 Pack/3g	7	0.1	246	8.2	47.8	2.4	0.0
SEAWEED								
Crispy, Average	*1oz/28g*	**182**	**17.3**	**651**	**7.5**	**15.6**	**61.9**	**7.0**
Irish Moss, Raw	*1oz/28g*	**2**	**0.1**	**8**	**1.5**	**0.0**	**0.2**	**12.3**
Kombu, Dried, Raw	*1oz/28g*	**12**	**0.4**	**43**	**7.1**	**0.0**	**1.6**	**58.7**
Nori, Dried, Raw	*1oz/28g*	**38**	**0.4**	**136**	**30.7**	**0.0**	**1.5**	**44.4**
Wakame, Dried, Raw	*1oz/28g*	**20**	**0.7**	**71**	**12.4**	**0.0**	**2.4**	**47.1**
SEEDS								
Chia, Black, The Chia Company*	1 Tbsp/15g	69	4.6	458	20.4	37.0	30.4	36.0
Chia, White, The Chia Company*	1 Tbsp/15g	69	5.1	458	20.4	37.0	34.0	36.0
Fenugreek, Average	*1 Tsp/4g*	**12**	**0.2**	**323**	**23.0**	**58.3**	**6.4**	**24.6**
Melon, Average	*1 Tbsp/15g*	**87**	**7.2**	**583**	**28.5**	**9.9**	**47.7**	**0.0**
Mustard, Average	*1 Tsp/3g*	**15**	**0.9**	**469**	**34.9**	**34.9**	**28.8**	**14.7**
Nigella, Average	*1 Tsp/5g*	**20**	**1.7**	**392**	**21.3**	**1.9**	**33.3**	**8.4**
Poppy, Average	*1 Tbsp/9g*	**47**	**3.9**	**533**	**18.0**	**23.7**	**44.7**	**10.0**
Pumpkin, Average	*1 Tbsp/10g*	**57**	**4.6**	**568**	**27.9**	**13.0**	**45.9**	**3.8**
Pumpkin, Whole, Roasted, Salted, Average	*1 Serving/50g*	**261**	**21.1**	**522**	**33.0**	**13.4**	**42.1**	**3.9**

S

	Measure INFO/WEIGHT	per Measure KCAL	FAT	Nutrition Values per 100g / 100ml KCAL	PROT	CARB	FAT	FIBRE
SEEDS								
Sesame, Average	*1oz/28g*	*171*	*15.8*	*610*	*22.3*	*3.6*	*56.4*	*7.7*
Sunflower, Average	*1 Tbsp/10g*	*59*	*4.9*	*585*	*23.4*	*15.0*	*48.7*	*5.7*
SEMOLINA								
Average	*1oz/28g*	*98*	*0.5*	*348*	*11.0*	*75.2*	*1.8*	*2.1*
Pudding, Creamed, Ambrosia*	1 Can/425g	344	7.2	81	3.3	13.1	1.7	0.2
SHAKES								
Assorted, Meal Replacement, The Biggest Loser*	1 Pack/55g	215	2.7	391	34.7	47.5	4.9	2.7
Cafe Latte Flavoured, Tony Ferguson*	1 Pack/55g	203	1.8	369	27.4	53.6	3.3	5.4
Caramel Flavour, Tony Ferguson*	1 Pack/55g	203	1.9	370	27.7	53.4	3.5	5.6
Chocolate & Mint Flavour, Tony Ferguson*	1 Pack/55g	205	2.4	373	27.4	52.5	4.3	5.6
Chocolate Flavour, Tony Ferguson*	1 Pack/55g	205	2.2	373	27.6	52.8	4.0	5.6
Strawberry Flavour, Tony Ferguson*	1 Pack/55g	203	1.9	370	27.6	53.8	3.4	5.5
Toffee Flavour, Tony Ferguson*	1 Pack/55g	202	2.1	368	27.2	53.6	3.8	5.5
Vanilla, Tony Ferguson*	1 Pack/55g	203	1.9	370	27.4	53.9	3.4	5.6
SHALLOTS								
Pickled in Hot & Spicy Vinegar, Tesco*	1 Onion/18g	14	0.0	77	1.0	18.0	0.1	1.9
Raw, Average	*1 Serving/80g*	*16*	*0.2*	*20*	*1.5*	*3.3*	*0.2*	*1.4*
SHANDY								
Bavaria*	1 Can/300ml	109	0.0	36	0.0	0.0	0.0	0.0
Bitter, Original, Ben Shaws*	1 Can/330ml	89	0.0	27	0.0	6.0	0.0	0.0
Canned, Morrisons*	1 Can/330ml	36	0.0	11	0.0	1.8	0.0	0.0
Homemade, Average	1 Pint/568ml	148	0.0	26	0.2	2.9	0.0	0.0
Lemonade, Schweppes*	1 Can/330ml	76	0.0	23	0.0	5.1	0.0	0.0
Lemonade, Traditional Style, Tesco*	1 Can/330ml	63	0.0	19	0.0	4.7	0.0	0.0
Traditional, Fentiman's*	1 Bottle/275ml	102	0.0	37	0.4	8.7	0.0	0.0
SHARK								
Raw	*1oz/28g*	*29*	*0.3*	*102*	*23.0*	*0.0*	*1.1*	*0.0*
SHARON FRUIT								
Average	*1oz/28g*	*20*	*0.0*	*73*	*0.8*	*18.6*	*0.0*	*1.6*
SHERBET LEMONS								
M & S*	1oz/28g	107	0.0	382	0.0	93.9	0.0	0.0
SHERRY								
Dry, Average	*1 Std Glass/120ml*	*139*	*0.0*	*116*	*0.2*	*1.4*	*0.0*	*0.0*
Medium	*1 Serving/50ml*	*58*	*0.0*	*116*	*0.1*	*5.9*	*0.0*	*0.0*
Sweet	*1 Serving/50ml*	*68*	*0.0*	*136*	*0.3*	*6.9*	*0.0*	*0.0*
SHORTBREAD								
All Butter, Assorted, Aldi*	1oz/28g	143	7.5	511	6.5	61.0	26.8	2.0
All Butter, Deans*	1 Biscuit/15g	77	3.8	511	4.9	65.7	25.4	1.2
All Butter, Fingers, Highland, Sainsbury's*	2 Biscuits/40g	208	11.5	521	4.8	59.4	28.8	2.7
All Butter, Fingers, McVitie's*	1 Finger/20g	106	5.4	530	6.5	64.7	27.2	0.0
All Butter, Fingers, Royal Edinburgh Bakery*	1 Biscuit/17g	88	4.8	519	5.8	60.3	28.3	1.8
All Butter, Fingers, Scottish, M & S*	1 Finger/18g	90	4.9	510	5.7	58.9	27.8	4.7
All Butter, Petticoat Tails, Co-Op*	1 Biscuit/13g	68	3.8	520	5.0	60.0	29.0	2.0
All Butter, Petticoat Tails, Gardiners of Scotland*	1 Biscuit/12g	64	3.4	514	5.2	62.1	27.2	0.0
All Butter, Round, Luxury, M & S*	1 Biscuit/20g	105	5.8	525	6.2	60.0	29.0	2.0
All Butter, Royal Edinburgh, Asda*	1 Biscuit/18g	93	5.1	519	5.8	60.3	28.3	1.8
All Butter, Scottish, M & S*	1 Biscuit/34g	173	9.5	510	5.7	58.9	27.8	2.3
All Butter, Thins, M & S*	1 Biscuit/10g	50	2.2	485	5.8	68.4	21.1	3.5
All Butter, Trufree*	1 Biscuit/11g	58	3.1	524	2.0	66.0	28.0	0.9
Assortment, Parkside*	1 Serving/30g	155	8.5	517	5.4	59.8	28.5	2.0
Average	1oz/28g	139	7.3	498	5.9	63.9	26.1	1.9
Belgian Chocolate Chunk, Asda*	1 Biscuit/20g	106	6.2	531	7.0	56.0	31.0	1.8
Bites, Murray*	1 Bar/21g	80	3.5	381	4.8	76.2	16.7	14.3

S

	Measure INFO/WEIGHT	per Measure		Nutrition Values per 100g / 100ml				
		KCAL	FAT	KCAL	PROT	CARB	FAT	FIBRE
SHORTBREAD								
Butter, Extra Special, Asda*	1 Serving/19g	101	5.9	531	7.0	56.0	31.0	1.8
Caramel, Millionaires, Fox's*	1 Serving/16g	75	3.9	483	6.1	57.9	25.3	0.1
Choc Chip, Fair Trade, Co-Op*	1 Biscuit/19g	100	6.0	526	5.3	57.9	31.6	2.6
Chocolate Chip, Jacob's*	1 Biscuit/17g	87	4.7	513	5.2	61.2	27.5	1.8
Chocolate Chunk, Belgian, TTD, Sainsbury's*	1 Biscuit/19g	101	5.7	521	5.1	59.1	29.4	2.0
Crawfords*	1 Biscuit/13g	67	3.4	533	6.6	65.0	27.4	2.0
Demerara, Rounds, TTD, Sainsbury's*	1 Biscuit/22g	113	5.9	508	5.1	62.2	26.5	1.8
Double Choc Chip, Petit Four, Scottish, Tesco*	1 Serving/50g	265	15.0	531	5.1	60.4	30.0	1.7
Dutch, M & S*	1 Biscuit/17g	90	5.2	530	5.7	58.2	30.6	0.9
Fingers, Asda*	1 Biscuit/18g	93	5.1	519	5.8	60.3	28.3	18.0
Fingers, Cornish Cookie*	1 Biscuit/25g	124	6.4	498	6.4	61.0	25.5	0.0
Fingers, Deans*	1 Biscuit/24g	115	5.9	488	5.1	60.1	24.8	1.4
Fingers, Highland, Organic, Sainsbury's*	1 Biscuit/16g	84	4.8	527	5.8	58.7	29.9	1.9
Fingers, Kate's Cakes Ltd*	1 Serving/100g	471	26.8	471	4.6	52.8	26.8	1.6
Fingers, Scottish, Finest, Tesco*	1 Biscuit/21g	104	5.0	498	5.1	65.5	23.9	2.0
Highland, Organic, Duchy Originals*	1 Biscuit/16g	80	4.2	515	5.2	61.8	27.4	1.7
Highland Demerara Rounds, Sainsbury's*	1 Biscuit/20g	113	5.8	565	5.5	70.5	29.0	2.0
Honey & Oatmeal, Walkers*	1 Biscuit/34g	158	7.6	465	6.7	64.1	22.4	3.8
Light & Buttery, Fingers, TTD, Sainsbury's*	1 Biscuit/20g	106	5.8	528	5.1	61.6	29.0	1.7
Mini Bites, Co-Op*	1 Biscuit/10g	53	3.0	530	7.0	59.0	30.0	2.0
Orange Marmalade & Oatflake, Deans*	1 Biscuit/20g	105	5.9	524	6.7	59.3	29.6	3.2
Organic, Waitrose*	1 Biscuit/13g	62	3.0	495	5.8	63.0	24.4	1.8
Pecan All Butter, Sainsbury's*	1 Biscuit/18g	99	6.5	548	5.3	49.9	36.3	2.5
Pure Butter, Jacob's*	1 Biscuit/20g	105	5.9	525	5.7	58.6	29.7	1.8
Raspberry & Oatmeal, Deans*	1 Biscuit/20g	103	5.7	514	4.7	63.1	28.6	1.4
Reduced Sugar, Tesco*	1 Biscuit/17g	86	4.9	519	6.7	57.1	29.4	2.1
Rings, Handbaked, Border*	1 Biscuit/17g	86	4.9	520	6.2	61.2	29.5	0.0
Royal Edinburgh*	1 Biscuit/11g	56	2.9	507	6.1	61.1	26.5	4.5
Stem Ginger, Waitrose*	1 Biscuit/15g	71	3.3	487	4.7	66.0	22.7	1.6
Wheat & Gluten Free, Free From Range, Tesco*	1 Biscuit/20g	98	5.2	490	6.0	58.0	26.0	6.0
SHRIMP								
Boiled, Average	*1 Serving/60g*	*70*	*1.4*	*117*	*23.8*	*0.0*	*2.4*	*0.0*
Dried, Average	*1oz/28g*	*69*	*0.7*	*245*	*55.8*	*0.0*	*2.4*	*0.0*
Frozen, Average	*1oz/28g*	*20*	*0.2*	*73*	*16.5*	*0.0*	*0.8*	*0.0*
in Brine, Canned, Drained, Average	*1oz/28g*	*26*	*0.3*	*94*	*20.8*	*0.0*	*1.2*	*0.0*
SILVERBEET								
Fresh, Raw	1 Serving/100g	17	0.0	17	1.6	1.1	0.0	1.9
Fresh, Steamed	1 Serving/100g	15	0.0	15	1.9	1.3	0.0	3.3
SKATE								
Grilled	*1oz/28g*	*22*	*0.1*	*79*	*18.9*	*0.0*	*0.5*	*0.0*
in Batter, Fried in Blended Oil	1oz/28g	47	2.8	168	14.7	4.9	10.1	0.2
Raw	*1oz/28g*	*18*	*0.1*	*64*	*15.1*	*0.0*	*0.4*	*0.0*
SKIPS								
Bacon, KP Snacks*	1 Bag/17g	81	3.8	474	6.5	62.1	22.2	2.3
Cheesy, KP Snacks*	1 Bag/17g	89	5.0	524	6.2	58.5	29.5	1.0
Pickled Onion, KP Snacks*	1 Bag/13g	67	4.0	512	3.4	56.4	30.3	1.4
Prawn Cocktail, KP Snacks*	1 Bag/17g	89	5.1	523	3.1	60.6	29.9	1.4
SKITTLES								
Mars*	1 Pack/55g	223	2.4	406	0.0	90.6	4.4	0.0
SLICES								
Apple & Raisin, Asda*	3 Slices/43g	173	3.3	400	6.5	74.7	7.7	2.8
Bacon & Cheese, Pastry, Tesco*	1 Slice/165g	480	32.0	291	7.4	21.7	19.4	1.0
Bacon & Cheese, Savoury, Pastry, Somerfield*	1 Slice/165g	490	33.5	297	7.4	21.2	20.3	1.5

S

	Measure INFO/WEIGHT	per Measure KCAL	FAT	Nutrition Values per 100g / 100ml KCAL	PROT	CARB	FAT	FIBRE
SLICES								
Beef, Minced, Morrisons*	1 Slice/143g	457	29.6	320	8.8	24.6	20.7	1.0
Beef, Minced Steak & Onion, Tesco*	1 Slice/150g	424	27.1	283	8.7	21.3	18.1	1.6
Beef, Minced with Onion, Sainsbury's*	1 Slice/120g	328	19.7	273	6.8	24.5	16.4	1.1
Belgian Chocolate, Weight Watchers*	1 Slice/30g	99	2.0	329	5.9	61.3	6.7	2.3
Cheddar Cheese & Onion, Ginsters*	1 Slice/180g	583	40.9	324	7.1	22.8	22.7	1.0
Cheese, Potato & Onion, Pastry, Taste!*	1 Slice/155g	501	30.4	323	8.6	28.1	19.6	0.0
Cheese & Ham, Pastry, Sainsbury's*	1 Slice/118g	352	23.2	298	7.8	22.5	19.7	1.8
Cheese & Ham, Savoury, Pastry, Somerfield*	1 Slice/150g	399	24.0	266	7.0	23.0	16.0	0.0
Cheese & Onion, Pastry, Tesco*	1 Slice/150g	502	37.0	335	8.0	20.1	24.7	1.4
Cheese & Onion, Savoury, Pastry, Somerfield*	1 Slice/165g	518	34.5	314	7.4	24.0	20.9	0.6
Chicken, Spicy, Deep Fill, Ginsters*	1 Slice/180g	499	30.6	277	9.2	21.8	17.0	1.4
Chicken & Mushroom, Asda*	1 Slice/128g	354	21.7	277	7.0	24.0	17.0	2.1
Chicken & Mushroom, Ginsters*	1 Slice/180g	439	26.8	244	8.3	19.1	14.9	1.8
Chicken & Mushroom, Sainsbury's*	1 Slice/164g	427	26.5	259	7.3	21.3	16.1	1.0
Chicken & Mushroom, Tesco*	1 Slice/165g	457	28.9	277	9.2	20.6	17.5	0.9
Chicken Fajita, Puff Pastry, Sainsbury's*	1 Pack/180g	452	23.0	251	9.1	23.6	12.8	2.5
Chicken Lattice, Ginsters*	1 Serving/200g	530	33.4	265	10.6	18.0	16.7	1.5
Custard, Pastry, Tesco*	1 Slice/108g	275	11.1	255	2.8	37.2	10.3	1.3
Fresh Cream, Tesco*	1 Slice/75g	311	21.0	414	3.5	37.4	27.9	1.0
Ham & Cheese, Ginsters*	1 Pack/180g	511	33.7	284	8.5	20.4	18.7	2.5
Ham & Cheese, Pastry, Ginsters*	1 Slice/155g	625	43.7	403	9.8	31.9	28.2	4.2
Iced Lemon, GFY, Asda*	1 Serving/30g	97	0.7	327	3.0	73.6	2.3	1.1
Meat Feast, Ginsters*	1 Slice/180g	468	32.0	260	8.0	17.2	17.8	2.2
Minced Steak & Onion, Sainsbury's*	1 Slice/165g	475	29.9	288	15.2	16.0	18.1	2.5
Mushroom, Creamy, Quorn*	1 Slice/164g	653	29.5	398	9.8	49.2	18.0	1.6
Peppered Steak, Asda*	1 Slice/164g	483	31.1	295	9.0	22.0	19.0	1.2
Pork & Egg, Gala, Tesco*	1 Slice/105g	333	24.1	317	10.3	17.2	23.0	3.4
Prawn & Avocado, Plait, Extra Special, Asda*	1 Serving/198g	331	6.7	167	11.0	23.0	3.4	1.3
Salmon & Watercress, Honey Roast, Plait, Asda*	1 Plait/166g	421	16.6	254	13.0	28.0	10.0	0.4
Sausage Meat with Onion Gravy, Lattice, Asda*	1 Serving/278g	595	38.9	214	10.0	12.0	14.0	1.7
Spicy Chicken, Ginsters*	1 Slice/180g	448	27.4	249	6.7	21.4	15.2	1.9
Spinach & Ricotta, Sainsbury's*	1 Slice/165g	500	35.3	303	6.5	21.1	21.4	2.9
Steak, Peppered, Deep Fill, Ginsters*	1 Slice/180g	513	36.2	285	9.4	16.1	20.1	3.1
Steak, Peppered, Ginsters*	1 Slice/180g	457	27.0	254	8.4	21.3	15.0	1.6
Steak & Onion, Aberdeen Angus, Tesco*	1 Slice/165g	444	27.7	269	8.7	20.7	16.8	1.3
Westcountry Cheddar & Onion, Ginsters*	1 Slice/180g	486	32.6	270	6.7	20.8	18.1	2.2
SLIMFAST*								
Cafe Latte, Ready To Drink, Slim Fast*	1 Bottle/325ml	230	6.5	71	4.5	7.0	2.0	1.0
Caramel Temptation Shake Powder, Slim Fast*	2 Scoops/60g	230	3.6	380	14.0	62.0	6.0	11.0
Meal Bar, Fruits of the Forest, Slim Fast*	1 Bar/60g	211	6.1	351	23.7	42.1	10.1	7.3
Meal Bar, Yoghurt & Muesli, Slim Fast*	1 Bar/60g	208	6.5	347	23.9	42.2	10.8	7.4
Milk Shake, Banana, Canned, Slim Fast*	1 Can/325ml	214	8.4	66	4.2	10.6	2.6	4.9
Milk Shake, Chocolate, Ready to Drink, Slim Fast*	1 Bottle/325ml	211	5.2	65	4.6	8.0	1.6	1.5
Milk Shake, Peach, Canned, Slim Fast*	1 Can/325ml	214	2.6	66	4.2	10.6	0.8	1.5
Shake, Blissful Banana, Ready To Drink, Slim Fast*	1 Bottle/325ml	230	6.6	70	4.5	7.0	2.0	1.5
Shake, Chocolate, Powder, Dry, Slim Fast*	2 Scoops/38g	136	2.8	363	13.9	59.0	7.5	10.9
Shake, Summer Strawberry, Ready to Drink, Slim Fast*	1 Bottle/325ml	230	6.6	70	4.5	7.0	2.0	1.0
Shake, Vanilla, Powder, Dry, Slim Fast*	2 Scoops/37g	131	2.4	360	13.4	60.9	6.5	11.0
Snacks, Chocolate Caramel Bar, Slim Fast*	1 Bar/26g	99	3.2	382	3.4	69.6	12.4	1.2
Snacks, Sour Cream & Chive Pretzels, Slim Fast*	1 Pack/23g	96	2.0	416	9.5	75.2	8.6	3.4
Soup, Chicken & Vegetable Pasta, Hearty's*	1 Pack/295ml	212	5.6	72	6.6	7.0	1.9	0.7
SMARTIES								
Giants, Nestle*	1 Pack/186g	882	35.9	474	4.6	70.4	19.3	0.7

S

INFO/WEIGHT	Measure	per Measure		Nutrition Values per 100g / 100ml				
		KCAL	FAT	KCAL	PROT	CARB	FAT	FIBRE
SMARTIES								
Mini Cones, Nestle*	1 Serving/44g	145	5.8	330	4.5	45.0	13.1	0.0
Mini Eggs, Nestle*	1 Lge Bag/100g	488	20.3	488	3.9	72.5	20.3	1.2
Nestle*	1 Tube/40g	184	6.6	461	4.0	73.6	16.6	0.6
Tree Decoration, Nestle*	1 Chocolate/18g	95	5.4	529	5.6	58.9	30.1	0.8
SMIRNOFF*								
Ice, Smirnoff*	1 Bottle/275ml	188	0.0	68	1.8	12.0	0.0	0.0
SMOOTHIE								
Acai Machine, Naked Juice Co*	1 Bottle/450ml	300	5.6	67	0.8	12.9	1.2	1.2
Apple, Grapes & Blackcurrant, PJ Smoothies*	1 Bottle/250ml	125	0.7	50	0.8	11.1	0.3	0.7
Apple, Kiwi & Lime, SunJuice*	1 Bottle/250ml	132	0.2	53	0.5	13.4	0.1	0.8
Banana, Dairy, Probiotic, Boots*	1 Bottle/250ml	147	1.2	59	1.6	12.0	0.5	1.0
Banana, Dairy, Tesco*	1 Bottle/250ml	165	1.0	66	1.6	14.0	0.4	0.4
Banana, M & S*	1 Bottle/500ml	400	2.0	80	1.8	16.8	0.4	1.2
Banana, Shapers, Boots*	1 Bottle/251ml	176	0.8	70	2.8	14.0	0.3	0.8
Banana & Mango, Juice, Calypso*	1 Carton/200ml	106	0.0	53	0.0	12.8	0.0	1.0
Banana Fruit with Yoghurt, Tesco*	1 Bottle/1000ml	610	7.0	61	2.1	11.3	0.7	0.4
Blackberries, Strawberries & Blackcurrants, Innocent*	1 Serving/200ml	108	0.0	54	0.6	11.9	0.0	1.5
Blackberries, Strawberries & Boysenberries, Innocent*	1 Serving/250ml	130	0.0	52	0.6	11.8	0.0	1.3
Blackcurrants & Gooseberries for Autumn, Innocent*	1 Bottle/250ml	117	0.2	47	0.5	12.5	0.1	1.0
Blueberry, Blackberry & Strawberry, COU, M & S*	1 Bottle/250ml	150	0.7	60	0.8	13.1	0.3	0.3
Blueberry, Blackcurrant & Beetroot, Love Life, Waitrose*	1 Serving/250ml	90	0.2	36	0.2	8.5	0.1	0.8
Blueberry & Pear, COU, M & S*	1 Bottle/250ml	112	0.7	45	0.3	10.4	0.3	0.3
Blueberry Hill, King Parrot Food Company*	1 Drink/450g	252	1.4	56	1.2	12.0	0.3	0.6
Cappuccino with Yoghurt, Island Oasis*	1 Carton/473ml	300	3.5	63	1.7	12.5	0.7	0.0
Cranberries, Yumberries & Blackcurrants, Innocent*	1 Bottle/250ml	130	0.2	52	0.5	14.2	0.1	1.5
Cranberries & Raspberries, Innocent*	1 Bottle/250ml	112	0.0	45	0.5	12.0	0.0	2.3
Cranberries & Strawberries, Innocent*	1 Bottle/250ml	102	0.5	41	0.5	9.5	0.2	0.0
Fruit, Cranberry & Raspberry, Juice Republic*	1 Bottle/250ml	182	1.0	73	0.5	16.0	0.4	0.0
Fruit, The Green One, Ella's Kitchen*	1 Pack/90g	52	0.0	58	0.4	13.4	0.0	1.8
Fruit, The Red One, Ella's Kitchen*	1 Pack/90g	48	0.1	53	0.6	11.6	0.1	1.9
Gold Machine, Naked Juice Co*	1 Bottle/450ml	262	0.0	58	0.8	13.3	0.0	0.0
Guavas, Mangoes & Goji Berries, Innocent*	1 Bottle/250ml	112	0.2	45	0.6	12.0	0.1	2.1
Kiwi, Apples & Limes, Innocent*	1 Bottle/250ml	125	0.2	50	0.5	11.0	0.1	1.8
Mango, Mini-me, Skinny, Boost*	1 Sm/480ml	178	1.4	37	0.5	7.7	0.3	0.4
Mango & Orange, Smoothie Smile*	1 Bottle/250ml	130	1.0	52	0.4	11.7	0.4	0.0
Mango & Orange, Sweetbird*	1 Serving/330ml	181	0.7	55	0.7	11.9	0.2	0.0
Mango & Passion Fruit, Weight Watchers*	1 Serving/90ml	90	0.1	100	0.3	23.9	0.1	0.5
Mango & West Indian Cherry, Plus, Tesco*	1 Serving/250ml	133	0.6	53	0.6	12.2	0.2	0.5
Mango Mania, King Parrot Food Company*	1 Drink/450g	248	0.5	55	1.3	12.3	0.1	0.4
Mixed Berry, Chosen By You, Asda*	1 Glass/250ml	143	0.0	57	0.6	12.6	0.0	1.6
Orange, Banana & Pineapple, Innocent*	1 Bottle/250ml	120	1.0	48	0.6	10.8	0.4	0.0
Orange, Mandarin & Guava, PJ Smoothies*	1 Bottle/250ml	122	0.0	49	0.7	10.9	0.0	1.6
Orange, Mango, Banana & Passion Fruit, Asda*	1 Serving/100ml	55	0.2	55	0.8	12.0	0.2	1.1
Oranges, Mangoes & Pineapples 1 Litre Carton, Innocent*	1 Carton/180ml	101	0.2	56	0.7	12.7	0.1	0.9
Peaches, Bananas & Passionfruit, PJ Smoothies*	1 Bottle/250g	127	0.2	51	0.4	12.1	0.1	0.0
Peaches & Passion Fruits, Innocent*	1 Bottle/250ml	120	0.2	48	0.5	10.7	0.1	1.7
Peaches & Passionfruits, Innocent For Kids*	1 Carton/180ml	95	0.0	53	0.6	14.7	0.0	0.9
Pineapple, Banana & Coconut, Chosen By You, Asda*	1 Glass/250ml	177	2.8	71	0.7	13.6	1.1	1.0
Pineapple, Banana & Pear, Asda*	1 Bottle/250ml	147	0.3	59	0.5	13.6	0.1	0.3
Pineapple, Mango & Passion Fruit, Extra Special, Asda*	½ Bottle/250ml	100	0.5	40	0.5	9.0	0.2	1.3
Pineapple, Mango & Passionfruit, 100% Fruit, Sainsbury's*	1 Bottle/250ml	162	0.2	65	0.7	15.2	0.1	1.0
Pineapple, Strawberries & Passion Fruit, PJ Smoothies*	1 Bottle/330ml	152	0.3	46	0.6	10.8	0.1	1.3
Pineapple & Passion Fruit, Sweetbird*	1 Serving/330ml	175	0.3	53	0.8	12.3	0.1	0.0

S

	Measure INFO/WEIGHT	per Measure KCAL	per Measure FAT	Nutrition Values per 100g / 100ml KCAL	PROT	CARB	FAT	FIBRE
SMOOTHIE								
Pineapples, Bananas & Coconuts, Innocent*	1 Bottle/250ml	172	2.7	69	0.7	13.6	1.1	1.0
Pomegranate, Raspberry & Cranberry, PJ Smoothies*	1 Bottle/250ml	132	0.5	53	1.1	11.6	0.2	0.0
Pomegranates, Blueberries & Acai, Special, Innocent*	1 Serving/250ml	170	0.5	68	0.6	15.6	0.2	0.8
Pomegranates & Raspberries, Innocent*	1 Bottle/250ml	150	0.2	60	0.6	15.4	0.1	2.0
Raspberry, Banana & Peach, Sainsbury's*	1 Bottle/251ml	138	0.3	55	0.8	12.8	0.1	1.5
Raspberry, M & S*	1 Bottle/250ml	137	1.5	55	1.7	12.2	0.6	1.9
Raspberry & Red Pepper, Love Life, Waitrose*	1 Bottle/250ml	90	0.2	36	0.3	8.5	0.1	0.7
Strawberries, Blackberries & Raspberries, Kids, Innocent*	1 Carton/180ml	81	0.2	45	0.5	9.9	0.1	1.3
Strawberries, Blackberries & Raspberries, Innocent*	1 Serving/180ml	81	0.2	45	0.5	9.9	0.1	0.0
Strawberries & Bananas, PJ Smoothies*	1 Bottle/250ml	117	0.2	47	0.4	11.0	0.1	0.0
Strawberries & Bananas, Pure Fruit, Innocent*	1 Bottle/250ml	132	0.2	53	0.7	13.1	0.1	1.3
Strawberry, Dairy, Finest, Tesco*	1 Bottle/250ml	162	0.2	65	2.9	13.2	0.1	0.1
Strawberry, Wild Orchard*	1 Bottle/250ml	120	0.0	48	0.6	11.8	0.0	1.4
Strawberry & Banana, Don Simon, Don Simon*	1 Carton/250ml	132	0.0	53	0.6	12.2	0.0	0.3
Strawberry & Banana, Fruit, Finest, Tesco*	1 Bottle/250ml	135	0.7	54	0.3	12.5	0.3	0.5
Strawberry & Banana, Morrisons*	1 Bottle/250ml	135	0.0	54	0.5	13.0	0.0	0.6
Strawberry & Cherry, Organic, M & S*	1 Bottle/250ml	137	0.7	55	0.8	12.3	0.3	0.4
Strawberry & Raspberry, Fruity, Sainsbury's*	1 Glass/200ml	106	0.0	53	0.6	11.9	0.0	2.4
Strawberry & White Chocolate, M & S*	1 Bottle/250ml	100	2.5	40	2.5	5.5	1.0	0.1
Summer Fruits, Tesco*	1 Bottle/250ml	140	0.0	56	0.2	13.8	0.0	0.5
Super Berry, M & S*	1 Bottle/250ml	150	1.0	60	0.9	13.0	0.4	1.2
Vanilla Bean, M & S*	1 Bottle/500ml	450	13.0	90	3.3	13.9	2.6	0.0
Vanilla Bean & Honey, Yoghurt, Serious Food Company*	1 Bottle/250ml	250	7.0	100	3.7	15.2	2.8	0.0
Yoghurt, Vanilla Bean & Honey, Thickie, Innocent*	1 Bottle/250g	242	4.5	97	4.1	16.2	1.8	0.1
SNACK-A-JACKS								
Apple Danish, Jumbo, Quaker Oats*	1 Cake/10g	39	0.2	390	5.0	87.0	2.5	1.0
Barbecue, Jumbo, Quaker Oats*	1 Cake/10g	38	0.2	380	8.0	83.0	2.0	1.7
Barbecue, Snack, Quaker Oats*	1 Bag/30g	123	1.8	410	7.5	81.0	6.0	1.0
Barbeque, Snack-A-Jacks, Quaker Oats*	1 Pack/26g	106	1.6	408	7.3	81.1	6.1	0.9
Caramel, Jumbo, Snack-A-Jacks, Quaker Oats*	1 Cake/13g	51	0.3	390	5.5	87.0	2.1	1.4
Caramel, Snack, Snack-A-Jacks, Quaker Oats*	1 Bag/30g	121	0.9	405	6.0	88.0	3.0	0.8
Cheese, Jumbo, Quaker Oats*	1 Cake/10g	38	0.2	380	8.5	81.0	2.5	1.7
Cheese, Snack, Quaker Oats*	1 Bag/26g	108	2.1	415	8.5	77.0	8.0	0.9
Cheese & Onion, Snack, Quaker Oats*	1 Bag/30g	120	2.2	400	6.7	77.0	7.5	1.5
Chocolate & Caramel, Delights, Quaker Oats*	1 Cake/15g	62	0.9	415	6.0	83.0	6.0	1.6
Chocolate & Orange, Delights, Quaker Oats*	1 Cake/15g	59	0.7	394	5.5	83.0	4.5	1.0
Chocolate Chip, Jumbo, Snack-A-Jacks, Quaker Oats*	1 Cake/15g	61	1.0	410	6.0	81.0	7.0	1.7
Hot Tomato Flavour, Snack-A-Jacks, Quaker Oats*	1 Bag/26g	105	1.9	405	7.3	77.1	7.5	1.2
Jumbo, Salt & Vinegar, Snack A Jacks*	1 Cake/10g	41	0.6	391	7.4	75.4	5.7	1.6
Mini Bagels, Cream Cheese & Chive Flavour, Quaker Oats*	1 Bag/35g	145	3.4	415	10.6	71.0	9.7	3.4
Mini Bites, Mature Cheese & Red Onion, Quaker Oats*	1 Bag/28g	116	2.5	415	7.5	76.0	9.0	2.0
Mini Bites, Smoked Ham, Quaker Oats*	1 Bag/28g	114	2.1	408	6.5	78.3	7.5	2.0
Mini Bites, Sour Cream & Sweet Chilli, Quaker Oats*	1 Bag/28g	115	2.2	410	6.5	78.0	8.0	2.0
Mini Breadsticks, Cheese & Onion, Quaker Oats*	1 Bag/35g	145	3.1	414	12.9	71.1	8.9	3.7
Prawn Cocktail, Snack, Quaker Oats*	1 Bag/30g	123	2.2	410	7.0	78.0	7.5	0.8
Prawn Cocktail, Snack-A-Jacks, Quaker Oats*	1 Bag/26g	106	1.9	408	6.9	78.3	7.5	0.9
Roast Chicken, Snack, Quaker Oats*	1 Bag/30g	124	2.4	415	7.0	77.5	8.0	1.0
Sour Cream & Chive Flavour, Snack-A-Jacks, Quaker Oats*	1 Bag/22g	91	1.7	413	7.8	78.4	7.6	1.3
Sweet Chilli Flavour, Snack-A-Jacks, Quaker Oats*	1 Packet/26g	107	1.9	412	7.3	78.9	7.5	1.1
SNAILS								
in Garlic Butter, Average	6 Snails/50g	219	20.7	438	9.7	8.0	41.5	1.0
Raw, Average	1 Snail/5g	4	0.1	90	16.1	2.0	1.4	0.0

	Measure INFO/WEIGHT	per Measure KCAL	FAT	Nutrition Values per 100g / 100ml KCAL	PROT	CARB	FAT	FIBRE
SNAPPER								
Red, Fried in Blended Oil	**1oz/28g**	**35**	**0.9**	**126**	**24.5**	**0.0**	**3.1**	**0.0**
Red, Weighed with Bone, Raw	**1oz/28g**	**25**	**0.4**	**90**	**19.6**	**0.0**	**1.3**	**0.0**
SNICKERS								
Cruncher, Mars*	1 Bar/40g	209	12.0	523	9.0	57.0	30.0	2.3
Mars*	1 Snacksize/41g	208	11.5	511	9.4	54.3	28.2	1.3
SORBET								
Blackcurrant, Iceland*	¼ Pot/100g	100	0.0	100	0.0	25.0	0.0	0.0
Elderflower, Bottle Green*	1 Serving/100g	104	0.0	104	0.1	25.6	0.0	0.0
Exotic Fruit, Sainsbury's*	1 Serving/75g	90	1.5	120	1.2	24.1	2.0	0.0
Jamaican Me Crazy, Ben & Jerry's*	1 Serving/100g	130	0.0	130	0.2	32.0	0.0	0.4
Kiwi & Papaya, World Fruit, Del Monte*	1 Lolly/90ml	61	0.3	68	0.2	16.2	0.3	0.0
Lemon	1 Scoop/60g	79	0.0	131	0.9	34.2	0.0	0.0
Mango, Del Monte*	1 Sorbet/500g	575	0.5	115	0.2	29.6	0.1	0.0
Mango, Waitrose*	1 Pot/100g	90	0.0	90	0.1	22.1	0.0	0.6
Mango Berry Swirl, Ben & Jerry's*	1 Serving/100g	100	0.0	100	0.2	25.0	0.0	1.5
Orange, Del Monte*	1 Sorbet/500g	625	0.5	125	0.2	32.1	0.1	0.0
Passion Fruit, Fat Free, M & S*	1 Sorbet/125g	129	0.0	103	0.4	25.0	0.0	0.4
Peach & Vanilla Fruit Swirl, HL, Tesco*	1 Pot/73g	93	0.6	127	1.1	28.9	0.8	0.5
Pineapple, Del Monte*	1 Sorbet/500g	600	0.5	120	0.3	30.6	0.1	0.0
Raspberry, Haagen-Dazs*	½ Cup/105g	120	0.0	114	0.0	28.6	0.0	1.9
Raspberry & Blackberry, Fat Free, M & S*	1 Sorbet/125g	140	0.0	112	0.4	27.5	0.0	0.6
Strawberry, M & S*	1oz/28g	27	0.0	95	0.3	23.4	0.1	0.5
Strawberry & Champagne, Sainsbury's*	¼ Pot/89g	95	0.0	107	0.2	25.5	0.0	0.6
Summer Berry, Swirl, Asda*	¼ Pack/89g	97	0.4	109	3.0	26.0	0.4	0.0
SOUFFLE								
Cheese	1oz/28g	71	5.4	253	11.4	9.3	19.2	0.3
Chocolate, Gu*	1 Pot/70g	307	24.9	439	6.3	24.4	35.6	2.9
Chocolate & Toffee, Gu*	1 Pot/95g	353	15.8	372	4.6	46.4	16.6	2.5
Lemon, Finest, Tesco*	1 Pot/80g	270	20.5	338	2.9	24.1	25.6	0.2
Plain	1oz/28g	56	4.1	201	7.6	10.4	14.7	0.3
Ricotta & Spinach, M & S*	1 Serving/120g	186	13.3	155	8.0	6.2	11.1	2.1
Strawberry, M & S*	1 Serving/95g	171	10.1	180	1.6	19.5	10.6	0.9
SOUP								
Apple, Carrot, Strawberry, Vie, Knorr*	1 Drink/100g	65	0.6	65	0.8	13.0	0.6	1.5
Aromatic Chicken with Thai Herbs, Deli Inspired, Baxters*	1 Can/415g	349	25.7	84	1.8	5.1	6.2	0.8
Asian Tomato Rice & Ginger, Skinny Soup, Glorious!*	½ Pot/300g	159	5.4	53	1.0	8.2	1.8	0.8
Asparagus, Fresh, Finest, Tesco*	½ Pot/300g	153	8.1	51	1.6	5.0	2.7	1.0
Asparagus, New Covent Garden Food Co*	½ Carton/300g	132	7.2	44	1.5	4.1	2.4	0.9
Asparagus, Slimline, Cup, Waitrose*	1 Sachet/204ml	51	1.4	25	0.4	4.3	0.7	0.7
Asparagus, Waitrose*	1 Serving/300g	60	3.6	20	0.9	1.5	1.2	0.9
Asparagus & Chicken, Waitrose*	1 Can/415g	166	4.6	40	2.1	5.3	1.1	0.7
Asparagus & Creme Fraiche, Morrisons*	½ Pot/300g	186	11.7	62	1.3	5.4	3.9	0.5
Asparagus in a Cup, You Count, Love Life, Waitrose*	1 Serving/200ml	57	1.6	28	0.5	4.7	0.8	0.3
Bean, Italian Style, Tesco*	1 Can/300g	153	3.6	51	2.8	7.3	1.2	1.1
Bean & Vegetable, Chunky, Chosen By You, Asda*	1 Can/400g	224	1.2	56	2.6	9.7	0.3	1.9
Beef & Mushroom, Big Soup, Heinz*	1 Can/515g	216	2.6	42	2.3	7.0	0.5	0.7
Beef & Tomato, Cup a Soup, Batchelors*	1 Serving/252g	83	1.6	33	0.6	6.3	0.6	0.4
Beef & Vegetable, Big Soup, Heinz*	1 Can/400g	212	4.0	53	3.5	7.5	1.0	0.9
Beef & Vegetable, Chunky, Canned, Sainsbury's*	1 Can/400g	188	3.2	47	3.2	6.7	0.8	1.3
Beef & Vegetable, Chunky, Meal, Tesco*	1 Can/400g	140	2.0	35	3.3	4.2	0.5	1.0
Beef & Vegetable, Ten Calorie, Gourmet Cuisine*	1 Sachet/200g	10	0.1	5	0.3	1.0	0.0	0.1
Beef Broth, Classic, Heinz*	1 Can/400g	100	2.8	45	2.2	7.2	0.7	0.8
Beef Goulash with Paprika Potatoes, Eat Live Enjoy, Tesco*	1 Pack/300g	229	3.9	76	9.1	6.7	1.3	0.7

SOUP

INFO/WEIGHT	Measure	per Measure		Nutrition Values per 100g / 100ml				
		KCAL	FAT	KCAL	PROT	CARB	FAT	FIBRE
Beef Stew & Dumplings, Taste of Home, Heinz*	1 Pot/430g	378	13.8	88	3.7	11.1	3.2	0.8
Beetroot, Tomato & Buckwheat, Stay Full, Baxters*	1 Can/400g	264	4.8	66	3.4	8.7	1.2	2.9
Beetroot, with Chopped Dill, Duchy Originals*	½ Pot/298g	152	7.4	51	1.1	5.9	2.5	0.9
Beetroot & Smokey Bacon, Daylesford Organics*	½ Carton/250ml	312	24.0	125	3.2	6.4	9.6	1.2
Blended Sweetcorn & Yellow Pepper, Heinz*	½ Can/200g	98	4.2	49	0.9	6.6	2.1	0.6
Bloody Mary, New Covent Garden Food Co*	1 Serving/300g	69	0.3	23	1.0	3.3	0.1	0.7
Boston Bean & Ham, New Covent Garden Food Co*	½ Carton/300g	171	0.6	57	2.4	7.8	0.2	1.6
Brazilian Beef & Black Bean, Glorious!*	½ Pot/300g	144	6.9	48	2.0	4.8	2.3	0.8
Broccoli, Pea & Mint, Love Life, Waitrose*	1 Pot/400g	200	9.6	50	2.7	4.3	2.4	2.1
Broccoli, Salmon & Watercress, Stay Full, Baxters*	1 Can/400g	244	8.8	61	3.3	5.8	2.2	2.4
Broccoli & Cauliflower, Cup, BFY, Morrisons*	1 Sachet/15g	56	2.1	376	4.9	57.2	14.2	4.9
Broccoli & Cauliflower, Cup-A-Soup, Made Up, Batchelors*	1 Serving/255g	107	5.1	42	0.6	5.3	2.0	1.1
Broccoli & Cheddar, Heinz*	1 Can/430g	340	24.1	79	2.6	4.4	5.6	0.6
Broccoli & Stilton, Cup Soup, Ainsley Harriott*	1 Satchet/229ml	87	1.8	38	1.0	7.0	0.8	1.3
Broccoli & Stilton, Farmers Market, Heinz*	½ Can/200g	108	7.4	54	1.5	3.2	3.7	0.9
Broccoli & Stilton, Fresh, Sainsbury's*	½ Pot/300ml	141	9.9	47	2.7	1.8	3.3	1.5
Broccoli & Stilton, New Covent Garden Food Co*	1 Carton/600ml	240	14.4	40	2.2	1.9	2.4	1.1
Broccoli & Stilton, Somerfield*	½ Pack/250g	140	9.7	56	1.6	3.5	3.9	1.5
Broccoli with Mustard, New Covent Garden Food Co*	1 Carton/568g	204	10.8	36	1.3	3.3	1.9	1.2
Broth, Chicken, Organic, Low Sodium, Pacific Foods*	1 Serving/250ml	10	0.1	4	0.4	0.4	0.0	0.0
Broth, Ten Vegetable, Morrisons*	1 Pot/600g	240	7.8	40	1.7	5.8	1.3	1.1
Broth, Wholegrain Farro & Ham Hock, Love Life, Waitrose*	1 Pot/398g	247	8.4	62	4.3	6.4	2.1	1.6
Butter Bean & Chorizo, Meal, Sainsbury's*	1 Pot/400g	257	9.6	64	3.9	5.6	2.4	2.3
Butternut Squash, Diet Chef Ltd*	1 Packet/300g	135	5.4	45	0.8	6.5	1.8	1.6
Butternut Squash, Fresh, Waitrose*	½ Pot/300g	153	8.7	51	0.5	5.8	2.9	0.8
Butternut Squash, New England, Skinny Soup, Glorious!*	½ Pot/300g	103	3.6	34	0.6	5.9	1.2	0.7
Butternut Squash & Red Pepper, Vegetarian, Baxters*	1 Can/415g	162	4.1	39	0.7	6.9	1.0	0.6
Butternut Squash & Tarragon, Waitrose*	½ Pot/300g	123	6.6	41	0.8	4.5	2.2	1.0
Cajun Black Bean & Bacon, Pret a Manger*	1 Pack/370g	250	5.4	68	3.7	8.6	1.5	2.1
Cantonese Hot & Sour Noodle, Baxters*	1 Serving/215g	133	2.8	62	1.4	11.1	1.3	0.5
Carrot, Butterbean & Coriander Soup, Chunky, Baxters*	1 Can/415g	220	2.5	53	2.1	9.9	0.6	2.2
Carrot, Coriander & Ginger, So Organic, Sainsbury's*	½ Can/197g	75	3.3	38	0.3	5.3	1.7	0.7
Carrot, Honey & Coriander, Cully And Sully*	1 Bowl/200g	56	3.2	28	0.5	3.3	1.6	1.0
Carrot, Onion & Chickpea, Healthy, Baxters*	1 Can/415ml	170	0.8	41	1.9	8.0	0.2	1.2
Carrot, Orange & Coriander, COU, M & S*	1 Pack/415g	145	2.5	35	0.6	6.9	0.6	1.2
Carrot, Orange & Ginger, Go Organic*	1 Jar/495g	119	4.0	24	0.5	3.6	0.8	1.4
Carrot, Red Lentil & Cumin, Organic, Waitrose*	1 Pack/350g	175	8.7	50	0.2	6.7	2.5	0.5
Carrot & Butterbean, Diet Chef Ltd*	1 Pack/300g	174	2.1	58	2.7	10.3	0.7	2.8
Carrot & Butterbean, Vegetarian, Baxters*	1 Can/415g	228	7.9	55	1.7	7.7	1.9	1.5
Carrot & Coriander, 'A' Meal, Feeling Great, Findus*	1 Serving/371g	130	3.7	35	1.5	5.5	1.0	1.5
Carrot & Coriander, Average	1 Serving/200g	83	4.3	42	0.6	4.8	2.2	1.0
Carrot & Coriander, Blended, Heinz*	½ Can/200g	104	5.4	52	0.7	6.2	2.7	0.6
Carrot & Coriander, Carton, Campbell's*	1 Serving/250ml	110	5.5	44	0.7	5.4	2.2	0.0
Carrot & Coriander, Fresh, New Covent Garden Food Co*	½ Carton/300g	108	4.5	36	0.6	4.2	1.5	1.4
Carrot & Coriander, Fresh, Organic, Simply Organic*	1 Pot/600g	276	18.0	46	0.5	4.5	3.0	1.3
Carrot & Coriander, Heinz*	1 Can/400g	160	6.0	40	0.5	5.8	1.5	0.9
Carrot & Coriander, Jenny Craig*	1 Packet/300g	69	1.8	23	2.2	2.1	0.6	0.9
Carrot & Coriander, Jeremy's Soups Ltd*	1 Serving/300g	96	4.8	32	0.5	4.1	1.6	0.8
Carrot & Coriander, Low Calorie, Average	1 Serving/200g	45	1.3	22	0.6	3.5	0.6	1.1
Carrot & Coriander, Low Fat, Solo Slim, Rosemary Conley*	1 Pack/300g	78	2.4	26	0.5	4.0	0.8	1.3
Carrot & Coriander, Selection, Campbell's*	1 Carton/500ml	185	5.0	37	0.6	6.4	1.0	0.6
Carrot & Coriander, Weight Watchers*	1 Pouch/300g	102	3.9	34	0.4	5.1	1.3	0.6
Carrot & Coriander with Creme Fraiche, Heinz*	1 Can/515g	232	9.3	45	0.7	6.6	1.8	0.9

S

SOUP

Measure INFO/WEIGHT	per Measure KCAL	FAT	Nutrition Values per 100g / 100ml KCAL	PROT	CARB	FAT	FIBRE
Carrot & Ginger, Fresh, Sainsbury's*	1 Pot/600g	150	5.4	25	0.4	3.9	0.9	1.0
Carrot & Ginger, Perfectly Balanced, Waitrose*	½ Pot/300g	66	2.7	22	0.4	3.1	0.9	1.0
Carrot & Lentil, Microwave, Heinz*	1 Can/303g	94	0.3	31	1.5	6.1	0.1	0.8
Carrot & Lentil, Weight Watchers*	1 Can/295g	86	0.3	29	1.3	5.5	0.1	0.7
Carrot & Orange	1oz/28g	6	0.1	20	0.4	3.7	0.5	1.0
Cassoulet, Gastropub, M & S*	½ Pot/300g	255	11.4	85	4.7	6.0	3.8	3.1
Cauliflower & Cheese, Tesco*	1oz/28g	13	0.8	47	1.9	3.0	3.0	0.9
Celeriac & Truffle, New Covent Garden Food Co*	1 Serving/300g	225	17.7	75	1.1	4.3	5.9	0.7
Chantenay Carrot & Parsnip, Fresh, Extra Special, Asda*	½ Pot/300g	114	6.3	38	0.6	4.2	2.1	0.8
Cheese, Leek & Bacon, Somerfield*	1 Carton/300g	441	36.0	147	5.0	5.0	12.0	0.0
Chicken, Coconut & Lemon Grass, Fresh, Waitrose*	½ Pot/300g	303	24.9	101	2.6	4.1	8.3	0.8
Chicken, Condensed, 99% Fat Free, Campbell's*	1 Can/295g	77	2.1	26	1.0	3.8	0.7	0.1
Chicken, Cream of, Canned, Tesco*	1 Can/400g	260	15.2	65	1.2	5.5	3.8	0.0
Chicken, Cream of, in Seconds, Dry, Knorr*	1 Pack/58g	300	21.2	518	11.2	36.0	36.6	0.3
Chicken, Cream of, Mealpak, All About Weight*	1 Pack/40g	152	3.6	380	36.1	32.1	9.0	13.3
Chicken, Cream of, Simmer & Serve, Dried, Sainsbury's*	1 Pack/500ml	181	7.5	36	0.8	4.9	1.5	0.8
Chicken, Green Thai, Sainsbury's*	1 Pot/600g	366	19.8	61	1.9	5.8	3.3	0.3
Chicken, Green Thai, Spiced, M & S*	½ Pot/300g	195	11.4	65	2.0	6.3	3.8	0.6
Chicken, Green Thai, Waitrose*	1 Pot/600g	462	30.0	77	4.4	3.5	5.0	1.6
Chicken, in a Cup, Dry, Symingtons*	1 Serving/22g	93	4.0	424	7.0	57.7	18.4	11.7
Chicken, in a Cup, Sainsbury's*	1 Serving/221ml	86	3.8	39	0.7	5.3	1.7	0.1
Chicken, Jamaican Jerk & Pumpkin, Sainsbury's*	½ Pot/300g	141	5.1	47	2.7	5.1	1.7	0.2
Chicken, Mulligatawny, Finest, Tesco*	½ Pot/300g	240	12.0	80	4.0	7.0	4.0	0.8
Chicken, Mushroom, & Potato, Big Soup, Heinz*	½ Can/200g	132	4.6	66	3.4	8.1	2.3	0.4
Chicken, Mushroom & Rice, Chilled, M & S*	½ Pot/300g	225	10.2	75	3.2	7.3	3.4	1.8
Chicken, New Covent Garden Food Co*	1 Carton/600g	510	32.4	85	3.8	5.4	5.4	0.6
Chicken, Packet, Knorr*	1 Packet/85g	423	27.5	498	7.7	44.3	32.3	0.2
Chicken, Potato, & Lentil, Weight Watchers*	1 Can/400g	136	3.6	34	1.2	5.3	0.9	0.3
Chicken, Sweetcorn & Potato, Heinz*	1 Can/400g	204	11.2	51	1.2	5.4	2.8	0.3
Chicken, Ten Calorie, Gourmet Cuisine*	1 Serving/200g	10	0.1	5	0.2	1.1	0.0	0.0
Chicken, Thai, Fresh, Finest, Tesco*	½ Tub/300g	255	16.2	85	4.1	4.2	5.4	1.1
Chicken, Thai, GFY, Asda*	1 Serving/200g	85	3.0	42	1.7	5.5	1.5	0.5
Chicken, Thai Style, Canned, Sainsbury's*	½ Can/200g	106	4.2	53	2.9	5.5	2.1	0.7
Chicken, Thai Style, Thick & Creamy, in a Mug, Tesco*	1 Sachet/28g	107	4.0	390	3.7	61.3	14.5	5.1
Chicken, Tomato & Red Pepper, Italian, Big Soup, Heinz*	½ Can/200g	78	1.8	39	1.6	6.2	0.9	0.7
Chicken, Weight Watchers*	1 Can/295g	97	2.9	33	1.6	4.4	1.0	0.0
Chicken & Broccoli, Soup-A-Slim, Asda*	1 Sachet/16g	55	1.4	341	7.0	58.0	9.0	6.0
Chicken & Country Vegetable, Farmers Market, Heinz*	1 Can/342g	229	11.3	67	3.2	6.0	3.3	0.5
Chicken & Country Vegetable, Soupfulls, Batchelors*	1 Serving/400g	164	3.6	41	5.1	3.0	0.9	1.3
Chicken & Ham, Big, Heinz*	½ Can/200g	92	2.0	46	2.3	6.9	1.0	0.7
Chicken & Ham, Chunky, Canned, Sainsbury's*	½ Can/200g	80	1.2	40	2.7	6.0	0.6	0.9
Chicken & Herb, Farmers Market, Heinz*	½ Carton/300g	183	6.9	61	2.2	7.8	2.3	0.5
Chicken & Leek, Cup a Soup, Made Up, Batchelors*	1 Serving/259g	96	4.7	37	0.5	4.7	1.8	0.7
Chicken & Leek, in a Cup, Symingtons*	1 Serving/225ml	110	5.6	49	0.5	6.0	2.5	1.2
Chicken & Leek, Soup in a Cup, Made Up, Sainsbury's*	1 Serving/200ml	82	3.3	41	0.4	6.1	1.6	0.1
Chicken & Mushroom, BFY, Dry, Morrisons*	1 Serving/14g	47	0.9	337	16.0	54.8	6.1	2.5
Chicken & Mushroom, Meal in a Mug, Tesco*	1 Sachet/40g	146	2.7	366	10.8	65.3	6.8	5.1
Chicken & Mushroom, Slim A Soup, Made Up, Batchelors*	1 Sachet/203g	63	2.0	31	0.7	4.7	1.0	0.3
Chicken & Mushroom, Soup-A-Slim, Asda*	1 Sachet/14g	51	1.4	362	10.0	58.0	10.0	4.2
Chicken & Mushroom in a Cup, Sainsbury's*	1 Sachet/223ml	107	4.2	48	0.7	7.1	1.9	0.1
Chicken & Noodle Laksa, Simply Fuller Longer, M & S*	1 Pot/385g	289	7.7	75	7.0	7.1	2.0	0.9
Chicken & Pasta Big, Heinz*	½ Can/200g	60	0.8	34	1.8	5.9	0.4	0.8
Chicken & Sweetcorn, Canned, Tesco*	1 Can/400ml	240	6.0	60	1.6	8.2	1.5	0.7

S

SOUP

	Measure INFO/WEIGHT	per Measure KCAL	FAT	Nutrition Values per 100g / 100ml KCAL	PROT	CARB	FAT	FIBRE
Chicken & Sweetcorn, Cantonese, Fresh, Sainsbury's*	½ Pot/300ml	135	1.5	45	2.1	7.9	0.5	0.5
Chicken & Sweetcorn, Fresh, Average	1 Serving/300g	145	3.1	48	2.4	7.3	1.0	0.5
Chicken & Sweetcorn, GFY, Asda*	1 Can/400g	108	2.0	27	1.5	4.2	0.5	0.2
Chicken & Sweetcorn, in a Mug, Tesco*	1 Sachet/28g	122	5.0	434	4.8	63.4	17.9	1.1
Chicken & Sweetcorn, Light Choice, Tesco*	½ Can/200g	84	0.8	42	1.7	7.9	0.4	0.2
Chicken & Sweetcorn, New Covent Garden Food Co*	1 Carton/600g	282	5.4	47	1.0	8.7	0.9	0.5
Chicken & Sweetcorn, Soupreme*	1 Serving/250g	90	0.7	36	2.7	5.6	0.3	1.7
Chicken & Tarragon, Thick & Creamy, Batchelors*	1 Sachet/281g	118	6.5	42	0.8	5.7	2.3	0.3
Chicken & Thyme, Diet Chef Ltd*	1 Pack/300g	147	9.0	49	2.2	3.4	3.0	0.7
Chicken & Vegetable, Average	1 Serving/200g	96	4.3	48	2.5	4.6	2.1	0.7
Chicken & Vegetable, Big Soup, Heinz*	½ Can/200g	104	2.8	52	3.3	6.7	1.4	0.8
Chicken & Vegetable, Classic, Heinz*	1 Can/400g	132	1.6	33	1.1	6.2	0.4	0.6
Chicken & Vegetable, Healthy, Baxters*	1 Can/415g	158	2.1	38	1.9	6.6	0.5	1.7
Chicken & Vegetable, Loyd Grossman*	1 Pack/400g	272	15.2	68	0.5	8.0	3.8	0.6
Chicken & Vegetable, Soup in a Mug, Value, Tesco*	1 Serving/19g	75	2.5	395	4.4	64.1	13.4	1.6
Chicken & Vegetable Casserole, Chunky, Chunky, Baxters*	1 Can/415g	195	2.9	47	2.4	7.8	0.7	1.1
Chicken & Vegetable Casserole, Taste of Home, Heinz*	1 Pot/430g	331	16.8	77	3.9	6.7	3.9	0.8
Chicken & Vegetable with Croutons, in a Cup, Sainsbury's*	1 Serving/24g	102	4.3	425	7.5	58.3	17.9	2.5
Chicken & Vegetable with Pasta, Select, Campbell's*	1 Can/480ml	220	1.0	46	2.9	7.9	0.2	0.8
Chicken & Vegetables, Creamy, for One, Wattie's*	1 Can/300g	115	6.3	38	0.9	3.8	2.1	0.0
Chicken & White Wine, Campbell's*	1 Serving/295g	145	9.7	49	1.0	4.0	3.3	0.0
Chicken & Wild Garlic, Fresh, Finest, Tesco*	½ Pot/300g	195	12.0	65	4.3	2.6	4.0	0.6
Chicken &Vegetable, Chunky, Love Life, Waitrose*	1 Can/400g	229	5.2	57	4.0	7.3	1.3	1.6
Chicken Arrabbiata, Meal, Fresh, Sainsbury's*	1 Pot/400g	232	6.0	58	4.1	5.3	1.5	1.5
Chicken Balti, Soupfulls, Batchelors*	1 Pack/300g	162	1.5	54	3.7	8.6	0.5	1.2
Chicken Broth, Favourites, Baxters*	1 Can/415g	129	1.7	31	1.5	5.4	0.4	0.6
Chicken Curry, Big Soup, Heinz*	1 Can/400g	196	2.8	49	2.8	7.3	0.7	1.0
Chicken Curry, Chosen By You, Asda*	½ Pot/300g	216	5.4	72	5.0	8.6	1.8	0.5
Chicken Curry, Mild, Indian, Soups of the World, Heinz*	1 Can/515g	381	21.1	74	3.6	5.9	4.1	0.3
Chicken Flavour, Tony Ferguson*	1 Pack/59g	203	1.9	344	25.6	49.8	3.2	5.1
Chicken Hotpot, Chunky, Big Soup, Heinz*	½ Can/258g	126	3.1	49	2.3	7.4	1.2	0.8
Chicken Mulligatawny, Asda*	1 Serving/300g	150	2.4	50	3.8	7.0	0.8	0.8
Chicken Mulligatawny, Chunky, Meal, Weight Watchers*	1 Pack/340g	163	4.4	48	2.2	6.8	1.3	1.5
Chicken Mulligatawny, Perfectly Balanced, Waitrose*	1 Serving/300g	138	6.0	46	1.7	5.3	2.0	0.4
Chicken Noodle, Batchelors*	1 Pack/284g	71	0.6	25	1.6	4.2	0.2	0.3
Chicken Noodle, Canned, Sainsbury's*	½ Can/217g	78	0.7	36	1.7	7.4	0.3	0.7
Chicken Noodle, Chunky, Campbell's*	½ Can/200g	86	1.2	43	2.8	6.5	0.6	0.0
Chicken Noodle, Classic, Heinz*	1 Can/400g	124	1.2	31	1.2	6.0	0.3	0.2
Chicken Noodle, Cup Soup, Made Up, Heinz*	1 Serving/218ml	48	0.4	22	0.7	4.3	0.2	0.1
Chicken Noodle, Dry, Nissin*	1 Pack/85g	364	14.1	428	9.5	62.0	16.6	3.3
Chicken Noodle, Dry, Symingtons*	½ Pack/15g	48	0.4	318	8.6	65.4	2.4	2.4
Chicken Noodle, Jeremy's Soups Ltd*	1 Serving/300g	132	5.7	44	3.5	3.3	1.9	0.7
Chicken Noodle, Simmer & Serve, Dried, Sainsbury's*	1 Pack/600ml	102	1.2	17	0.8	2.9	0.2	0.0
Chilli Bean, M & S*	½ Carton/300g	150	7.5	50	2.5	4.7	2.5	2.7
Chilli Bean, Mexican, Tesco*	1 Carton/600g	270	6.6	45	2.2	6.4	1.1	1.9
Chilli Beef, Chunky, Asda*	1 Can/400g	212	4.0	53	4.2	5.7	1.0	2.4
Chilli Beef, Mighty, Asda*	1 Can/400g	236	5.6	59	4.9	6.8	1.4	1.2
Chilli Beef with Lentils & Buckwheat, Deli Inspired, Baxters*	1 Can/415g	237	2.1	57	3.7	9.3	0.5	1.2
Chilli Con Carne, Chunky, Sainsbury's*	½ Can/200g	110	1.8	55	3.6	8.0	0.9	1.5
Chilli Pumpkin, Fresh, Sainsbury's*	½ Carton/300g	120	7.2	40	0.6	4.0	2.4	1.3
Chilli Tomato & Pasta, COU, M & S*	1 Serving/300g	150	5.7	50	1.3	7.2	1.9	0.9
Chinese Chicken & Sweetcorn, Soups of the World, Heinz*	½ Can/260g	117	3.6	45	1.9	6.2	1.4	0.3
Chinese Chicken Noodle, Dry, Knorr*	1 Pack/45g	138	2.0	307	15.1	51.8	4.4	2.9

SOUP

	Measure INFO/WEIGHT	per Measure KCAL	FAT	Nutrition Values per 100g / 100ml KCAL	PROT	CARB	FAT	FIBRE
Chinese Chicken Noodle, Slim a Soup Extra, Batchelors*	1 Sachet/246g	69	0.7	28	1.0	5.3	0.3	0.4
Chorizo & Bean, TTD, Sainsbury's*	1 Pack/298g	161	2.4	54	4.0	7.6	0.8	5.8
Chowder, Bacon & Corn, M & S*	½ Pot/300g	195	10.8	65	2.5	6.0	3.6	1.8
Chowder, Clam, New England, Select, Campbell's*	1 Cup/240ml	221	14.4	92	2.5	6.0	6.0	0.8
Chowder, Ham & Sweetcorn, Diet Chef Ltd*	1 Pack/300g	165	3.6	55	1.9	9.2	1.2	0.9
Chowder, Sweetcorn & Chicken, Heinz*	1 Serving/200g	148	5.6	74	3.3	9.1	2.8	0.6
Cock-A-Leekie, Favourites, Baxters*	1 Can/425g	93	2.1	22	1.2	2.8	0.5	0.4
Country Beef, Celebrity Slim*	1 Pack/55g	211	2.8	384	25.6	56.4	5.1	1.4
Country Garden, Vegetarian, Baxters*	1 Can/415g	116	2.1	28	0.9	4.9	0.5	0.8
Country Vegetable, Asda*	1 Serving/125g	59	3.6	47	0.6	4.5	2.9	0.8
Country Vegetable, Fresh, Sainsbury's*	½ Pot/300g	123	2.7	41	1.6	6.6	0.9	2.5
Country Vegetable, Fresh, Somerfield*	½ Pack/300g	123	6.0	41	1.1	4.6	2.0	1.2
Country Vegetable, Knorr*	1 Pack/500ml	160	3.5	32	0.9	5.5	0.7	1.2
Country Vegetable, Weight Watchers*	1 Can/295g	97	0.3	33	1.2	6.3	0.1	0.9
Country Vegetable & Herb, Farmers Market, Heinz*	½ Carton/300g	114	3.6	38	1.2	5.7	1.2	0.9
Country Vegetable Casserole, Taste of Home, Heinz*	1 Pot/430g	206	6.0	48	1.3	7.6	1.4	1.3
Courgette, Parmesan & Bacon, Somerfield*	1 Pack/500g	255	20.0	51	2.0	2.0	4.0	0.0
Courgette & Parmesan, Fresh, Sainsbury's*	1 Pack/300ml	198	16.8	66	1.5	2.5	5.6	0.4
Cumberland Sausage & Vegetable, Big Soup, Heinz*	1 Can/515g	221	4.1	43	1.9	6.7	0.8	0.8
Curry, Chunky, Big & Bold, New Covent Garden Food Co*	½ Tub/225g	133	4.3	59	2.9	7.3	1.9	0.6
Dhansak, TTD, Sainsbury's*	½ Pot/300g	180	3.9	60	3.2	9.0	1.3	1.6
English Broccoli & Stilton, Dry, Knorr*	1 Pack/65g	331	24.6	509	11.7	30.3	37.9	1.6
English Summer Garden, New Covent Garden Food Co*	½ Carton/300g	72	1.8	24	1.0	3.4	0.6	0.8
Farmhouse Chicken Leek, Dry, Knorr*	1 Pack/54g	248	15.7	459	10.3	39.3	29.0	1.5
Farmhouse Vegetable, Canned, BGTY, Sainsbury's*	½ Can/200ml	52	1.6	26	0.5	4.4	0.8	0.9
Farmhouse Vegetable, Fresh, Avonmore*	½ Carton/250g	137	5.0	55	1.9	7.4	2.0	0.8
Farmhouse Vegetable, Soup-A-Cup, GFY, Asda*	1 Sachet/219ml	59	1.1	27	0.6	4.9	0.5	0.4
Fish, Frozen, Findus*	1 Serving/85g	127	4.7	150	11.0	13.0	5.5	0.0
French Onion	1oz/28g	11	0.6	40	0.2	5.7	2.1	1.0
French Onion, Favourites, Baxters*	½ Can/208g	66	1.2	32	0.8	6.0	0.6	0.5
French Onion, Heinz*	1 Pack/400g	100	0.4	25	0.5	5.7	0.1	0.4
French Onion, Knorr*	1 Pack/40g	118	1.0	296	6.0	62.5	2.5	6.6
French Onion & Cider, Waitrose*	1 Can/425g	93	0.4	22	0.5	4.8	0.1	0.4
French Onion & Croutons, Dry, Tesco*	1 Serving/30g	106	2.3	353	7.3	63.7	7.7	2.0
French Onion & Gruyere Cheese, Fresh, Finest, Tesco*	½ Pot/300g	210	15.3	70	1.4	4.7	5.1	0.5
Fresh, Super Green, M & S*	½ Pot/300g	120	5.7	40	1.5	3.7	1.9	1.7
Fresh Minted Potato with Parsley, Yorkshire Provender*	½ Pot/300g	222	15.0	74	1.3	5.7	5.0	0.7
Garden Pea, Cream of, Jeremy's Soups Ltd*	1 Serving/300g	138	9.3	46	1.6	2.9	3.1	1.2
Garden Pea & Mint, Vegetarian, Baxters*	½ Can/200g	100	1.6	50	2.5	7.3	0.8	1.9
Garden Pea & Wiltshire Cured Ham, Finest, Tesco*	½ Pot/300g	185	8.1	62	3.4	5.9	2.7	1.6
Garden Vegetable, Dry, Slim Fast*	1 Serving/60g	224	6.2	373	23.8	45.0	10.3	7.0
Garden Vegetable, Heinz*	1 Can/400g	160	3.2	40	0.9	7.2	0.8	0.9
Garden Vegetable Flavour, Celebrity Slim*	1 Pack/55g	211	3.0	384	25.6	56.4	5.4	1.4
Garden Vegetable with Barley, Co-Op*	1 Pot/600g	240	0.6	40	2.1	7.4	0.1	0.7
Gazpacho, Canned, Average	1 Can/400g	76	0.4	19	2.9	1.8	0.1	0.2
Gazpacho, New Covent Garden Food Co*	1 Carton/600g	276	17.4	46	1.0	3.3	2.9	1.2
Goa Carnival, New Covent Garden Food Co*	½ Carton/300g	144	8.4	48	1.6	4.9	2.8	1.4
Goan Spiced Tomato & Lentil, Skinny Soup, Glorious!*	½ Pot/300g	153	3.3	51	2.1	8.1	1.1	1.2
Goats Cheese & Rocket, Fresh, Sainsbury's*	½ Carton/300g	180	13.2	60	2.0	3.2	4.4	0.3
Golden Vegetable, Asda*	1 Pack/300g	150	6.0	50	1.9	6.0	2.0	0.0
Golden Vegetable, Calorie Counter, Cup, Co-Op*	1 Sachet/12g	40	1.2	335	7.0	54.0	10.0	5.0
Golden Vegetable, Cup, GFY, Asda*	1 Sachet/217ml	52	1.1	24	0.5	4.4	0.5	0.2
Golden Vegetable, Dry, Knorr*	1 Pack/76g	299	14.4	394	10.4	45.4	19.0	3.3

S

SOUP

INFO/WEIGHT	Measure	per Measure		Nutrition Values per 100g / 100ml				
		KCAL	FAT	KCAL	PROT	CARB	FAT	FIBRE
Golden Vegetable, Slim a Soup, Batchelors*	1 Sachet/207g	58	1.7	28	0.5	4.7	0.8	0.7
Golden Vegetable, Soup-A-Slim, Asda*	1 Sachet/15g	50	1.2	336	6.0	60.0	8.0	1.9
Haddock, Smoked, Fresh, Finest, Tesco*	1 Pot/550g	302	13.7	55	2.7	5.1	2.5	0.8
Haggis Broth, Favourites, Baxters*	1 Can/415g	187	6.2	45	1.8	6.1	1.5	0.6
Harvest Vegetable, Soupfull, Batchelors*	1 Can/400g	160	0.4	40	1.4	8.4	0.1	1.6
Harvest Vegetable with Croutons in a Cup, Sainsbury's*	1 Sachet/226ml	86	2.7	38	1.0	5.9	1.2	0.9
Hearty Vegetable, 99% Fat Free, Prepared, Campbell's*	1 Can/295g	91	1.2	31	0.8	6.1	0.4	0.9
Hearty Vegetable Broth, Weight Watchers*	1 Can/295g	127	0.6	43	2.0	8.2	0.2	1.4
Hey Pesto, New Covent Garden Food Co*	1 Pack/600g	204	9.0	34	1.2	3.5	1.5	0.9
Highlander's Broth, Favourites, Baxters*	1 Can/414g	195	6.2	47	1.8	6.5	1.5	0.6
Indian Chicken, Glorious!*	½ Pot/300g	201	7.5	67	3.4	7.6	2.5	0.7
Italian, Chunky, New Covent Garden Food Co*	½ Carton/300g	111	4.2	37	1.5	4.7	1.4	0.9
Italian Bean, Fresh, Love Life, Waitrose*	½ Pot/300g	165	7.2	55	1.6	6.0	2.4	1.7
Italian Bean & Pasta, Healthy, Baxters*	1 Can/415g	224	0.8	54	2.2	9.9	0.2	1.7
Italian Meatball & Tomato, Big Soup, Heinz*	1 Can/515g	319	14.9	62	2.5	6.4	2.9	1.8
Italian Meatball Meal, Tesco*	1 Pot/379g	265	6.8	70	2.5	9.6	1.8	0.8
Italian Minestrone, Dry, Knorr*	1 Pack/62g	193	2.5	311	11.5	57.1	4.1	7.8
Italian Minestrone, M & S*	1 Can/425g	191	2.1	45	2.2	9.0	0.5	0.8
Italian Plum Tomato & Basil, Perfectly Balanced, Waitrose*	½ Pot/300g	69	1.5	23	0.9	3.8	0.5	0.9
Italian Plum Tomato & Mascarpone, Finest, Tesco*	1 Pot/600g	360	13.8	60	1.3	7.2	2.3	0.6
Lamb & Cous Cous, M & S*	½ Can/208g	100	3.7	48	2.1	6.2	1.8	0.9
Lamb & Vegetable, Big Soup, Heinz*	½ Can/200g	120	2.6	60	3.0	9.1	1.3	1.3
Lamb & Vegetable, Mega, Morrisons*	1 Pack/410g	172	4.1	42	1.9	6.3	1.0	0.8
Lamb Casserole, Chunky, Baxters*	1 Can/415g	232	3.3	56	2.4	9.0	0.8	1.6
Lancashire Lamb Hotpot, Taste of Home, Heinz*	1 Pot/430g	299	11.1	70	2.6	8.9	2.6	1.1
Leek, Cream of, Favourites, Baxters*	1 Can/415g	237	17.4	57	1.1	3.8	4.2	0.7
Leek & Chicken, Knorr*	1 Serving/300ml	82	5.2	27	0.6	2.4	1.7	0.1
Leek & Ham, Philpotts*	1 Pot/100g	87	4.4	87	1.3	9.6	4.4	1.7
Leek & Maris Piper Potato, Chilled, M & S*	1 Serving/300g	165	11.4	55	0.6	4.5	3.8	0.9
Leek & Potato, Chunky, Meal, Canned, Tesco*	½ Can/200g	60	2.6	30	1.0	3.5	1.3	1.0
Leek & Potato, Mix, Asda*	½ Pack/100g	25	0.0	25	0.6	5.7	0.0	1.5
Leek & Potato, Slim a Soup, Batchelors*	1 Serving/204g	57	1.4	28	0.4	5.0	0.7	0.2
Leek & Potato, Smooth, Vie, Knorr*	1 Pack/500ml	155	4.5	31	0.9	4.8	0.9	1.0
Leek & Potato, Solo Slim, Rosemary Conley*	1 Pack/300g	156	6.6	52	0.9	7.2	2.2	1.1
Leek & Potato, Soup in a Cup, Made Up, Waitrose*	1 Sachet/204ml	47	1.0	23	0.3	4.3	0.5	0.5
Leek & Potato, Soup in a Mug, HL, Tesco*	1 Serving/16g	54	0.9	336	4.3	67.1	5.6	7.4
Leek & Potato, Thick & Creamy, Soup in a Mug, Tesco*	1 Serving/25g	94	2.4	378	4.2	68.5	9.7	4.9
Leek & Potato, Weight Watchers*	1 Sachet/215ml	58	1.1	27	0.5	5.1	0.5	0.1
Leek & Potato in a Cup, BGTY, Sainsbury's*	1 Serving/218ml	59	1.5	27	0.3	4.9	0.7	0.2
Leek & Potato in a Mug, Light Choices, Tesco*	1 Sachet/220g	55	0.9	25	0.5	4.9	0.4	0.6
Lentil, Average	1 Carton/600g	594	22.8	99	4.4	12.7	3.8	1.1
Lentil, Bacon & Mixed Bean, Low Fat, Aldi*	1 Serving/400g	260	3.6	65	4.7	9.5	0.9	1.6
Lentil, Campbell's*	1 Can/295g	139	1.8	47	2.6	7.7	0.6	0.0
Lentil, Canned	1 Serving/220g	86	0.4	39	3.1	6.5	0.2	1.2
Lentil, Carrot & Cumin, Canned, BGTY, Sainsbury's*	1 Can/400g	204	3.6	51	2.3	8.4	0.9	0.1
Lentil, Classic, Heinz*	1 Can/400g	184	0.8	46	2.3	8.5	0.2	0.7
Lentil, Low Fat, Amy's Kitchen*	1 Can/411g	242	7.0	59	3.1	7.7	1.7	3.6
Lentil, Low Fat, Solo Slim, Rosemary Conley*	1 Pack/300g	102	0.9	34	2.0	5.8	0.3	0.3
Lentil, Redemption*	1 Pot/600g	138	1.2	23	1.6	3.2	0.2	0.0
Lentil, Spicy, Organic, Suma*	1 Can/400g	232	4.8	58	2.7	9.0	1.2	1.6
Lentil, Tomato & Vegetable, M & S*	1 Can/415g	170	3.4	41	2.0	6.3	0.8	1.4
Lentil, with Red Lentils, Carrots, Potato & Onion, Asda*	1 Can/400g	192	0.8	48	1.4	10.2	0.2	1.2
Lentil & Bacon, Canned, Tesco*	1 Serving/200g	96	1.4	48	3.2	7.2	0.7	0.5

S

SOUP

INFO/WEIGHT	Measure	per Measure KCAL	FAT	Nutrition Values per 100g / 100ml KCAL	PROT	CARB	FAT	FIBRE
Lentil & Bacon, Chunky, Canned, M & S*	1 Can/400g	180	2.4	45	3.3	5.8	0.6	2.1
Lentil & Bacon, Favourites, Baxters*	1 Can/425g	234	3.8	55	3.6	8.2	0.9	0.8
Lentil & Bean, Spicy, Canned, Organic, Asda*	1 Can/400g	212	3.2	53	2.8	8.6	0.8	3.0
Lentil & Chick Pea, Fresh, Organic, Tesco*	1 Serving/300ml	117	2.4	39	1.9	6.1	0.8	0.5
Lentil & Pancetta, Tesco*	½ Can/192g	115	2.5	60	3.1	8.0	1.3	1.6
Lentil & Parsley, Simply Organic*	1 Pot/600g	390	1.8	65	4.4	11.8	0.3	1.4
Lentil & Red Pepper, Sainsbury's*	½ Pot/300g	162	3.6	54	3.5	7.4	1.2	1.6
Lentil & Tomato, Spicy, Chunky, Fresh, Tesco*	½ Pot/300g	195	5.4	65	2.6	9.7	1.8	1.3
Lentil & Vegetable, Diet Chef Ltd*	1 Pack/300g	156	0.9	52	2.6	9.6	0.3	2.1
Lentil & Vegetable, Light Choices, Tesco*	1 Can/400g	188	0.8	47	2.5	8.8	0.2	1.1
Lentil & Vegetable Soup, Healthy, Baxters*	1 Can/415g	183	0.8	44	2.3	7.6	0.2	1.1
Lentil & Vegetable with Bacon, Organic, Baxters*	½ Can/211g	93	1.5	44	1.9	7.6	0.7	1.0
Lobster Bisque, Baxters*	1 Can/415g	187	8.7	45	3.0	3.6	2.1	0.2
Lobster Bisque, New Covent Garden Food Co*	½ Carton/300g	108	1.8	36	3.2	4.4	0.6	0.4
Lobster Bisque, Waitrose*	½ Carton/300g	201	13.8	67	0.9	5.5	4.6	0.6
Luxury Game, Baxters*	1 Can/415g	187	2.9	45	3.7	5.9	0.7	0.5
Malaysian Chicken & Sweetcorn, Dry, Knorr*	1 Pack/57g	211	6.5	370	10.6	56.3	11.4	1.8
Marvellous Meatball, Tesco*	1 Pot/400g	240	8.8	60	2.3	7.6	2.2	0.8
Mediterranean Minestrone, Campbell's*	½ Carton/250ml	95	2.7	38	0.9	6.1	1.1	0.6
Mediterranean Tomato, COU, M & S*	1 Pack/415g	104	2.1	25	0.7	4.8	0.5	0.6
Mediterranean Tomato, Dry, Slim Fast*	1 Sachet/62g	213	5.6	343	22.6	39.8	9.0	10.7
Mediterranean Tomato, Fresh, Organic, Sainsbury's*	1 Serving/250ml	77	3.5	31	1.3	3.3	1.4	1.0
Mediterranean Tomato, Instant, Weight Watchers*	1 Serving/200ml	50	0.2	25	0.7	5.2	0.1	0.1
Mediterranean Tomato, Slim a Soup, Cup, Batchelors*	1 Serving/208g	56	1.2	27	0.5	4.8	0.6	0.4
Mediterranean Tomato, Vegetarian, Baxters*	1 Can/415g	129	0.8	31	0.9	6.3	0.2	0.7
Mediterranean Tomato & Vegetable, Fresh, Tesco*	½ Pot/300g	105	2.1	35	1.0	6.2	0.7	0.7
Mediterranean Tomato & Vegetable, Soupfulls, Batchelors*	1 Pouch/400g	180	1.2	45	1.5	9.1	0.3	1.1
Mediterranean Tomato in a Cup, Waitrose*	1 Sachet/18g	52	1.5	289	8.3	45.6	8.3	10.0
Melon & Carrot, New Covent Garden Food Co*	1 Serving/300g	60	1.2	20	0.6	3.6	0.4	0.6
Mexican Bean, Safe To Eat*	1 Pouch/400g	140	1.2	35	2.4	4.7	0.3	1.8
Mexican Beef Chilli, Mighty, Asda*	1 Can/400g	192	2.8	48	3.3	7.0	0.7	0.9
Mexican Black Bean, Extra Special, Asda*	½ Pot/263g	194	10.8	74	2.3	7.0	4.1	1.7
Mexican Chilli Beef & Bean, Soups of the World, Heinz*	1 Can/515g	360	9.3	70	4.5	9.0	1.8	1.6
Mexican Chipotle Chicken, New Covent Garden Food Co*	½ Carton/300g	186	3.3	62	3.9	8.0	1.1	2.3
Mexican Mixed Pepper & Chilli, Cup Soup, Ainsley Harriott*	1 Sachet/223g	71	0.2	32	0.8	7.0	0.1	0.8
Mexican Spicy Bean, Weight Watchers*	1 Can/295g	112	1.5	38	1.2	6.8	0.5	0.9
Minestrone, Average	1 Serving/220g	139	6.6	63	1.8	7.6	3.0	0.9
Minestrone, Calorie Counter, Low Calorie Cup, Co-Op*	1 Sachet/13g	40	0.3	310	7.0	66.0	2.0	3.0
Minestrone, Canned	1oz/28g	9	0.2	32	1.4	5.1	0.8	0.6
Minestrone, Chunky, Big Soup, Heinz*	½ Can/200g	74	1.6	37	1.3	6.2	0.8	1.1
Minestrone, Chunky, Fresh, Baxters*	1 Serving/250g	95	1.7	38	1.5	6.5	0.7	1.1
Minestrone, Chunky, Love Life, Waitrose*	1 Can/400g	166	0.4	42	1.3	8.7	0.1	1.9
Minestrone, Classic, Heinz*	1 Can/400g	128	0.8	32	1.1	6.5	0.2	0.9
Minestrone, Favourites, Baxters*	1 Can/425g	153	2.1	36	1.5	6.3	0.5	1.0
Minestrone, for One, Heinz*	1 Can/300g	96	2.1	32	1.4	5.2	0.7	0.7
Minestrone, Fresh, Average	1 Carton/600g	244	4.9	41	1.7	6.8	0.8	1.1
Minestrone, Fresh, Baxters*	1 Box/568ml	233	5.7	41	1.8	6.2	1.0	0.6
Minestrone, Hearty, 99% Fat Free, Campbell's*	1 Can/295g	77	0.3	26	0.7	5.6	0.1	0.0
Minestrone, Hearty, Chilled, Farmers Market, Heinz*	½ Carton/300g	123	2.7	41	1.4	6.9	0.9	0.5
Minestrone, in a Cup, BGTY, Sainsbury's*	1 Serving/200ml	54	0.2	27	0.8	6.0	0.1	0.6
Minestrone, in a Mug, HL, Tesco*	1 Sachet/21g	72	1.3	342	3.6	67.7	6.3	3.8
Minestrone, New Covent Garden Food Co*	½ Carton/300g	102	2.1	34	1.2	5.3	0.7	1.0
Minestrone, Organic, Seeds of Change*	1 Pack/350g	227	11.5	65	1.4	7.4	3.3	0.9

SOUP

INFO/WEIGHT	Measure	per Measure		Nutrition Values per 100g / 100ml				
		KCAL	FAT	KCAL	PROT	CARB	FAT	FIBRE
Minestrone, Packet, Dry, Knorr*	1 Pack/61g	178	2.7	292	9.2	53.9	4.4	6.5
Minestrone, Soupreme*	1 Can/400g	168	2.4	42	2.1	6.4	0.6	1.1
Minestrone, Squeeze & Stir, Heinz*	1 Made Up/196g	59	1.4	30	0.8	5.0	0.7	0.4
Minestrone, Tuscan, Weight Watchers*	1 Can/295g	121	3.2	41	1.0	6.9	1.1	0.8
Minestrone, with Basil & Parmesan, Stay Full, Baxters*	1 Can/400g	276	5.2	69	3.5	9.2	1.3	2.6
Minestrone, with Borlotti Beans, Tuscan Style, Heinz*	½ Can/200g	90	1.5	45	1.4	8.0	0.7	1.1
Minestrone, with Croutons, Cup a Soup, Batchelors*	1 Serving/251g	93	1.3	37	0.7	7.3	0.5	0.3
Minestrone, with Croutons, Dry, Soupreme*	1 Serving/27g	94	1.7	349	7.6	65.3	6.4	4.4
Minestrone, with Croutons in a Mug, Tesco*	1 Sachet/23g	83	1.9	360	9.0	62.6	8.1	2.7
Minestrone, with Meatballs, Simply Fuller Longer, M & S*	1 Pack/400g	260	10.0	65	5.2	5.8	2.5	1.2
Minestrone, with Pasta, Chunky, Co-Op*	1 Pack/400g	140	2.4	35	1.0	6.0	0.6	0.7
Minestrone, with Ribbon Noodles, Extra, Dry, Aldi*	1 Serving/34g	107	0.7	315	11.0	62.8	2.2	2.0
Minestrone, with Wholemeal Pasta, Healthy, Baxters*	1 Can/400g	136	0.8	34	1.0	7.0	0.2	1.0
Minestrone Verde, New Covent Garden Food Co*	½ Carton/300g	123	2.4	41	1.8	6.1	0.8	1.2
Minted Lamb Hot Pot, Big Soup, Heinz*	1 Can/400g	228	5.2	57	2.9	8.1	1.3	1.0
Miso, Instant, Blue Dragon*	1 Sachet/18g	25	0.7	139	10.0	14.4	3.9	0.0
Miso, Instant, Dry, Sanchi*	1 Sachet/8g	27	0.6	336	18.4	48.6	7.6	0.0
Miso, Japanese, Made Up, Yutaka*	1 Serving/250ml	24	0.7	10	0.6	1.1	0.3	0.0
Miso, Naga-Negi Instant, Dry, Amano Foods*	1 Serving/7g	25	0.7	357	24.3	41.4	10.0	0.0
Miso, Organic, Instant, Sanchi*	1 Sachet/10g	27	0.3	270	14.0	47.0	3.0	0.0
Miso, Wakama*	1 Sachet/8g	27	0.6	336	18.7	48.6	7.6	0.0
Moroccan Chicken, Finest, Tesco*	½ Pot/300g	180	5.1	60	3.6	6.8	1.7	1.2
Moroccan Chicken, New Covent Garden Food Co*	1 Serving/300g	108	5.7	36	2.1	2.7	1.9	0.4
Moroccan Chicken & Vegetable, Love Life, Waitrose*	½ Pot/300g	192	5.7	64	3.7	7.9	1.9	1.9
Moroccan Lentil, Waitrose*	½ Pot/300g	153	1.5	51	3.5	8.2	0.5	3.4
Moroccan Style, Extra Special, Asda*	½ Pot/300g	183	3.9	61	2.9	9.4	1.3	1.0
Mulligatawny	1 Serving/220g	213	15.0	97	1.4	8.2	6.8	0.9
Mulligatawny, Classic, Heinz*	1 Can/400g	208	7.2	52	2.0	7.1	1.8	0.6
Mulligatawny in a Cup, Symingtons*	1 Serving/232ml	95	1.4	41	0.7	8.3	0.6	0.5
Mushroom, 98% Fat Free, Baxters*	1 Can/425g	170	6.8	40	0.9	5.6	1.6	0.3
Mushroom, Cream of, Canned	1 Serving/220g	101	6.6	46	1.1	3.9	3.0	0.1
Mushroom, Cream of, Classics, Heinz*	1 Can/400g	208	11.2	52	1.5	5.2	2.8	0.1
Mushroom, Cream of, Favourites, Baxters*	1 Can/406g	262	17.1	63	0.9	5.5	4.1	0.1
Mushroom, Cream of, Jeremy's Soups Ltd*	1 Serving/300g	135	12.6	45	0.8	1.2	4.2	0.2
Mushroom, Creamy, Farmers Market, Heinz*	1 Can/515g	237	15.4	46	1.0	3.5	3.0	0.3
Mushroom, Cully & Sully*	1 Carton/400g	192	17.6	48	0.8	1.3	4.4	1.0
Mushroom, Diet Chef Ltd*	1 Pack/300g	105	5.1	35	1.9	3.2	1.7	0.9
Mushroom, Dry, Symingtons*	1 Serving/23g	80	2.1	348	17.8	48.4	9.2	6.7
Mushroom, Farm Harvest, Green Giant*	1 Pouch/330g	122	5.9	37	0.6	5.2	1.8	1.3
Mushroom, Field, Morrisons*	1 Pack/600g	192	10.2	32	0.8	3.3	1.7	0.0
Mushroom, for One, Heinz*	1 Can/290g	148	7.8	51	1.4	5.1	2.7	0.1
Mushroom, Fresh, Average	1 Serving/300g	146	9.3	49	1.3	4.0	3.1	0.8
Mushroom, Hi Taste Low Cal, Cup Soup, Ainsley Harriott*	1 Sachet/22g	80	1.0	364	12.7	63.6	4.7	3.2
Mushroom, Simmer & Serve, Dried, Sainsbury's*	½ Pack/600ml	234	9.6	39	0.6	5.5	1.6	0.3
Mushroom, Weight Watchers*	1 Can/295g	83	2.1	28	1.1	4.5	0.7	0.1
Mushroom, Wild, New Covent Garden Food Co*	1 Carton/600g	222	7.2	37	1.5	4.1	1.2	0.9
Mushroom, with Croutons, Soup in a Mug, Tesco*	1 Pack/26g	113	4.5	435	6.1	63.3	17.5	2.9
Mushroom, with Croutons in a Cup, Waitrose*	1 Sachet/212g	102	4.2	48	0.6	6.8	2.0	0.5
Mushroom & Crouton, Cup Soup, Made Up, Heinz*	1 Cup/200ml	80	4.2	40	0.7	4.5	2.1	0.0
Mushroom & Garlic, Slimming Cup a Soup, Tesco*	1 Serving/16g	58	1.6	360	5.8	61.1	10.3	3.2
Mushroom Noodle, Mighty, Dry, Asda*	1 Serving/42g	171	4.6	407	8.0	69.0	11.0	1.9
Mushroom Potage, Baxters*	1 Can/415g	320	21.6	77	1.5	6.1	5.2	0.3
Onion, Ten Calorie, Gourmet Cuisine*	1 Serving/200g	10	0.2	5	0.3	0.8	0.1	0.1

S

SOUP

INFO/WEIGHT	Measure		per Measure		Nutrition Values per 100g / 100ml				
			KCAL	FAT	KCAL	PROT	CARB	FAT	FIBRE
Oxtail, Average	1 Serving/200g		82	2.3	41	1.9	5.8	1.1	0.4
Oxtail, Canned	1 Serving/220g		97	3.7	44	2.4	5.1	1.7	0.1
Oxtail, Classic, Heinz*	1 Can/400g		168	2.0	42	1.9	7.3	0.5	0.3
Oxtail, Condensed, Classics, Diluted, Campbell's*	1 Can/590g		236	8.8	40	1.4	5.3	1.5	0.0
Oxtail, Diet Chef Ltd*	1 Pack/300g		144	3.6	48	1.8	7.5	1.2	0.5
Oxtail, Favourites, Baxters*	1 Can/415g		199	5.0	48	1.8	7.4	1.2	0.5
Parsnip, Creamy, New Covent Garden Food Co*	½ Carton/300g		174	9.0	58	1.2	6.6	3.0	1.6
Parsnip, Fresh, Morrisons*	½ Pot/250g		100	3.7	40	0.9	5.8	1.5	1.4
Parsnip, Fresh, VLH Kitchens	1 Serving/400g		180	0.4	45	0.9	5.8	1.6	1.4
Parsnip, Honey & Ginger, COU, M & S*	1 Can/415g		124	2.5	30	0.7	5.3	0.6	0.7
Parsnip, Leek & Ginger, New Covent Garden Food Co*	1 Carton/600g		162	1.8	27	1.2	4.9	0.3	1.3
Parsnip, Mr Bean's*	1 Can/400g		208	7.6	52	1.9	6.7	1.9	0.0
Parsnip, Spicy, Average	1 Serving/400g		212	11.2	53	0.9	6.0	2.8	1.6
Parsnip & Apple, COU, M & S*	1 Can/415g		187	10.4	45	0.7	5.4	2.5	1.2
Parsnip & Butternut Squash, The Best, Morrisons*	1 Can/400g		244	8.4	61	2.4	8.1	2.1	1.6
Parsnip & Chilli, Diet Chef Ltd*	1 Serving/300g		102	4.2	34	0.8	4.6	1.4	1.3
Parsnip & Honey, Diet Chef Ltd*	1 Pack/300g		153	7.5	51	0.9	6.3	2.5	1.8
Parsnip & Honey, Fresh, Sainsbury's*	½ Carton/300g		192	12.6	64	1.1	5.4	4.2	1.5
Parsnip & Orchard Apple, Duchy Originals*	1 Pack/350g		115	3.1	33	0.7	5.4	0.9	1.0
Pasta, Tomato & Basil, Bertolli*	1 Serving/100g		47	1.1	47	1.5	7.9	1.1	1.6
Pea, Artichoke & Parmesan, The Best, Morrisons*	½ Pot/300g		171	7.8	57	2.8	5.6	2.6	1.0
Pea, in a Cup, Symingtons*	1 Sachet/31g		95	2.2	311	7.2	54.1	7.2	6.9
Pea, Organic, Suma*	1 Can/400g		272	8.8	68	2.7	9.4	2.2	0.7
Pea & Ham	1 Serving/220g		154	4.6	70	4.0	9.2	2.1	1.4
Pea & Ham, Campbell's*	1 Can/500g		310	4.5	62	4.6	7.4	0.9	2.8
Pea & Ham, Classic, Heinz*	1 Can/400g		252	3.2	63	2.8	10.1	0.8	1.1
Pea & Ham, Creamy, Chunky, Meal, Weight Watchers*	1 Pack/340g		156	3.7	46	2.3	6.8	1.1	2.0
Pea & Ham, Diet Chef Ltd*	1 Pack/300g		138	3.3	46	3.2	5.8	1.1	2.6
Pea & Ham, Extra Thick, In A Cup, Sainsbury's*	1 Sachet/224ml		85	1.8	38	1.1	6.7	0.8	0.4
Pea & Ham, Favourites, Baxters*	1 Can/425g		255	5.9	60	3.5	8.3	1.4	0.9
Pea & Ham, Very Special, Wattie's*	½ Can/265g		139	2.1	53	3.8	6.0	0.8	3.0
Pea & Mint, Baxters*	1 Serving/300g		186	9.6	62	2.3	6.1	3.2	1.5
Pea & Mint, New Covent Garden Food Co*	½ Pack/300g		168	5.7	56	2.5	7.1	1.9	1.7
Pea & Mint, Tinned, Tesco*	1 Can/400g		180	2.8	45	2.0	7.8	0.7	1.3
Pea & Smoked Ham, Farmers Market, Heinz*	½ Can/258g		103	1.0	40	3.5	5.6	0.4	0.8
Potato, Leek & Bacon, Fresh, Baxters*	½ Pot/300g		249	16.8	83	2.0	6.1	5.6	0.7
Potato, Leek & Chicken, Canned, BGTY, Sainsbury's*	½ Can/200g		62	0.8	31	1.6	5.3	0.4	0.4
Potato, Leek & Thyme, Farmers Market, Heinz*	1 Can/515g		294	15.4	57	0.9	6.7	3.0	0.6
Potato & Leek	1oz/28g		15	0.7	52	1.5	6.2	2.6	0.8
Potato & Leek, Classics, Canned, Heinz*	1 Can/400g		184	7.2	46	0.8	6.7	1.8	0.6
Potato & Leek, Favourites, Baxters*	1 Can/418g		180	3.8	43	1.0	7.7	0.9	0.9
Potato & Leek with Peppers & Chicken, Stockmeyer*	½ Can/200g		118	4.8	59	2.6	6.7	2.4	0.8
Prawn Laksa, Waitrose*	1 Pot/400g		388	25.2	97	2.5	9.7	6.3	0.6
Pumpkin, Creamy, Very Special, Heinz*	1 Sm Can/290g		188	5.5	65	1.3	9.9	1.9	1.1
Pumpkin, New Covent Garden Food Co*	½ Pint/284ml		97	3.1	34	0.4	5.5	1.1	0.6
Pumpkin, Pepper & Paprika, New Covent Garden Food Co*	1 Pack/600g		198	4.8	33	1.0	5.0	0.8	0.7
Pumpkin, Spicy, Fresh, Sainsbury's*	½ Pot/300g		87	3.0	29	0.9	4.2	1.0	1.3
Pumpkin, Sweet Potato & Red Pepper, SO, Sainsbury's*	½ Pot/300g		111	3.9	37	0.8	5.6	1.3	0.8
Pumpkin & Bramley Apple, New Covent Garden Food Co*	½ Carton/300g		99	1.8	33	1.1	5.9	0.6	0.8
Red Lentil & Tomato, Canned, Tesco*	½ Can/300g		189	3.9	63	4.0	8.9	1.3	1.1
Red Lentil & Vegetable, Favourites, Baxters*	1 Can/415g		199	2.1	48	2.6	8.3	0.5	1.2
Red Pepper, Black Olive & Tomato, Jeremy's Soups Ltd*	1 Serving/300g		105	3.0	35	1.0	5.3	1.0	1.1
Red Pepper, Tomato & Basil, M & S*	1 Can/415g		83	1.2	20	1.3	2.7	0.3	0.8

S

	Measure INFO/WEIGHT	per Measure KCAL	per Measure FAT	Nutrition Values per 100g / 100ml KCAL	PROT	CARB	FAT	FIBRE
Red Pepper & Goats Cheese, Diet Chef Ltd*	1 Pack/300g	138	6.6	46	2.2	4.4	2.2	0.9
Red Pepper & Rocket, New Covent Garden Food Co*	½ Carton/300g	129	2.7	43	1.7	6.9	0.9	1.0
Red Pepper & Tomato, Canned, Sainsbury's*	1 Can/400g	120	4.4	30	0.9	4.1	1.1	1.6
Red Pepper & Tomato, Canned, Weight Watchers*	1 Can/295g	35	0.2	12	0.4	2.4	0.1	0.4
Roast Chicken Flavour, Celebrity Slim*	1 Pack/55g	210	3.1	382	28.5	52.5	5.6	0.9
Roasted Red Pepper, Finest, Tesco*	1 Pot/600g	290	12.6	48	1.4	5.4	2.1	1.1
Roasted Red Pepper, Fresh, Waitrose*	1 Pack/600g	172	9.0	29	0.8	3.0	1.5	1.0
Root Vegetable, Medley, New Covent Garden Food Co*	1 Pot/600ml	168	4.8	28	0.7	4.9	0.8	1.1
Root Vegetable & Barley, Broth, Special, Heinz*	1 Can/400g	188	6.0	47	0.9	7.4	1.5	1.1
Root Vegetable & Butternut Squash, Deli Inspired, Baxters*	1 Can/415g	187	1.2	45	1.9	8.7	0.3	1.4
Root Vegetable & Sweet Potato, Farmers Market, Heinz*	1 Can/515g	278	9.8	54	0.9	8.5	1.9	1.1
Royal Game, Favourites, Baxters*	1 Can/415g	149	1.2	36	2.2	6.0	0.3	0.3
San Marzano Tomato & Mascarpone, M & S*	1 Serving/150g	97	6.4	65	1.4	5.7	4.3	2.0
Sausage & Bean, Spicy, Meal, Canned, Tesco*	1 Can/500g	265	7.0	53	2.8	6.4	1.4	1.2
Scotch Broth, British, Sainsbury's*	1 Can/415g	149	2.9	36	1.9	5.4	0.7	0.9
Scotch Broth, Classic, Heinz*	1 Can/400g	168	5.2	42	1.5	6.0	1.3	0.8
Scotch Broth, Favourites, Baxters*	1 Can/415g	199	4.1	48	2.0	7.8	1.0	1.3
Scotch Broth, Fresh, Baxters*	1 Serving/300g	108	2.1	36	1.6	5.9	0.7	0.6
Scotch Broth, Greenhaigh's*	1 Serving/250ml	107	2.5	43	3.3	5.1	1.0	1.0
Scotch Broth, New Covent Garden Food Co*	1 Carton/600g	300	7.2	50	2.4	7.4	1.2	1.2
Scotch Vegetable, Baxters*	1 Can/425g	183	2.5	43	1.9	7.4	0.6	1.2
Seafood Chowder, Waitrose*	1 Can/404g	226	11.3	56	2.2	5.6	2.8	0.6
Smoked Bacon & Bean, Diet Chef Ltd*	1 Pack/300g	162	3.3	54	2.8	8.2	1.1	2.1
Smoked Bacon & Three Bean, Chunky, Baxters*	1 Can/415g	241	5.0	58	2.9	8.8	1.2	1.8
Smoked Haddock Chowder, New Covent Garden Food Co*	½ Carton/300g	125	4.2	42	1.9	4.8	1.4	1.4
Smoked Salmon & Dill, Fresh, Finest, Tesco*	½ Carton/300g	240	16.5	80	2.2	5.3	5.5	0.6
Spicy, Three Bean, Tesco*	½ Carton/300g	165	4.5	55	2.8	7.3	1.5	2.1
Spicy Beef & Tomato, Diet Chef Ltd*	1 Pouch/300g	165	5.7	55	2.3	7.3	1.9	1.9
Spicy Corn Chowder, New Covent Garden Food Co*	½ Carton/300g	132	5.4	44	1.6	4.3	1.8	2.2
Spicy Lentil, Chilled, Morrisons*	1 Serving/300ml	271	8.6	90	3.9	12.3	2.9	4.0
Spicy Lentil, COU, M & S*	1 Pack/415g	187	3.7	45	2.6	6.7	0.9	1.2
Spicy Lentil, Cup, Made Up, Ainsley Harriott*	1 Sachet/226ml	86	1.1	38	1.1	7.3	0.5	0.4
Spicy Lentil, Hi Taste Low Cal, Cup Soup, Ainsley Harriott*	1 Sachet/22g	67	0.3	305	12.3	60.4	1.4	4.1
Spicy Lentil, in a Mug, Light Choices, Tesco*	1 Sachet/221ml	62	0.0	28	1.1	5.9	0.0	0.0
Spicy Lentil, Morrisons*	1 Pot/330g	198	5.6	60	2.1	9.0	1.7	0.8
Spicy Lentil, Seeds of Change*	1 Pack/422g	190	0.8	45	2.5	8.2	0.2	1.9
Spicy Lentil & Vegetable, Chilled, M & S*	½ Serving/300g	150	2.4	50	2.7	8.0	0.8	1.1
Spicy Lentil & Vegetable, Chosen By You, Asda*	1 Pot/330g	178	3.3	54	2.4	8.5	1.0	0.7
Spicy Lentil & Vegetable, Micro, Tesco*	1 Serving/330g	214	6.3	65	2.2	9.4	1.9	0.9
Spicy Mixed Bean, Big Soup, Heinz*	1 Serving/200g	78	0.6	39	2.3	6.7	0.3	2.0
Spicy Parsnip, New Covent Garden Food Co*	½ Box/297g	116	3.9	39	0.9	5.8	1.3	1.8
Spicy Parsnip, Vegetarian, Baxters*	1 Can/425g	221	10.6	52	1.2	6.1	2.5	1.5
Spicy Red Curry, Blue Dragon*	1 Serving/205g	97	5.1	47	0.4	5.8	2.5	0.3
Spicy Sweetcorn, Fresh, New Covent Garden Food Co*	½ Carton/300g	159	4.8	53	1.4	7.8	1.6	0.7
Spicy Tomato, Cup a Soup, Batchelors*	1 Sachet/23g	74	0.7	322	7.6	65.8	3.2	3.2
Spicy Tomato & Vegetable, Healthy Living, Co-Op*	1 Can/400g	180	3.2	45	2.0	8.0	0.8	2.0
Split Pea & Ham, Asda*	1 Serving/300g	129	0.6	43	3.5	6.9	0.2	0.7
Split Peas, Yellow, Simply Organic*	1 Pot/600g	354	3.0	59	4.3	10.4	0.5	2.6
Squash, Butternut, Curried, & Lentil, Seeds of Change*	1 Pack/400g	164	1.2	41	2.3	7.2	0.3	1.9
Squash, Butternut & Ginger, Waitrose*	½ Pot/300g	210	17.4	70	0.9	3.5	5.8	1.0
Steak, Potato & Ale, Chunky, Sainsbury's*	1 Can/400g	152	2.4	38	2.2	5.9	0.6	0.8
Steak & Guiness Casserole, Taste of Home, Heinz*	1 Pot/410g	260	7.0	63	3.2	8.4	1.7	0.7
Steak & Potato, Big Soup, Heinz*	½ Can/258g	129	2.1	50	3.0	7.7	0.8	0.8

SOUP

INFO/WEIGHT	Measure		per Measure		Nutrition Values per 100g / 100ml				
			KCAL	FAT	KCAL	PROT	CARB	FAT	FIBRE
Steak & Potato, with Hp Sauce, Taste of Home, Heinz*	1 Serving/410g		286	7.6	70	3.3	9.6	1.8	0.7
Stilton, Celery & Watercress, Morrisons*	1 Serving/250g		272	23.0	109	3.9	3.1	9.2	0.3
Summer Vegetable, New Covent Garden Food Co*	1 Carton/600g		336	14.4	56	1.7	6.5	2.4	0.7
Summer Vegetable with Fresh Rocket, Yorkshire Provender*	1 Pot/600g		282	15.0	47	1.6	4.0	2.5	1.1
Summer Vegetable with Pasta, Cup a Soup, Batchelors*	1 Serving/33g		16	0.4	50	1.4	8.5	1.1	1.0
Sun Dried Tomato & Basil, Heinz*	1 Serving/275ml		124	5.2	45	0.6	6.5	1.9	0.1
Sun Dried Tomato & Basil, Microwaveable Cup, Heinz*	1 Cup/275ml		118	4.9	43	0.6	6.2	1.8	0.1
Sunny Thai Chicken, Glorious!*	½ Pot/300g		201	6.6	67	3.6	8.3	2.2	1.0
Sweet Potato, Chickpea & Coriander, BGTY, Sainsbury's*	1 Can/400g		188	2.0	47	1.4	9.3	0.5	1.3
Sweet Potato & Coconut, COU, M & S*	1 Can/415g		166	5.4	40	0.7	6.7	1.3	0.8
Sweet Potato & Coconut, Dict Chef Ltd*	1 Pack/300g		147	8.7	49	0.8	4.9	2.9	0.9
Sweet Potato & Coconut, Diet Chef Ltd*	1 Pouch/300g		147	8.7	49	0.8	4.9	2.9	0.9
Sweetcorn, Cream of, Campbell's*	1 Serving/80g		41	2.2	51	0.6	6.2	2.7	0.5
Sweetcorn & Chicken, Cup, Calorie Counter, Co-Op*	1 Sachet/11g		35	1.2	315	5.0	49.0	11.0	11.0
Sweetcorn & Chilli, COU, M & S*	½ Can/275g		137	6.6	50	0.9	6.1	2.4	0.4
Sweetcorn & Chilli Chowder, Simply Organic*	½ Pot/300g		126	2.7	42	2.2	6.1	0.9	3.8
Tangy Tomato, Extra, Slim a Soup, Batchelors*	1 Pack/253g		121	2.0	48	1.2	9.0	0.8	0.4
Tangy Tomato, Slim a Soup, Batchelors*	1 Serving/230ml		81	1.0	35	1.1	6.7	0.4	0.5
Terrific Toulouse Sausage, Tesco*	1 Pot/400g		248	8.8	62	3.7	6.9	2.2	2.0
Thai, Mealpak, All About Weight*	1 Pack/40g		150	4.2	376	35.1	31.0	10.6	8.5
Thai Chicken, Cully & Sully*	1 Pack/400g		204	7.2	51	2.7	6.4	1.8	0.6
Thai Chicken, Diet Chef Ltd*	1 Pack/300g		114	4.5	38	1.0	5.1	1.5	1.0
Thai Chicken, New Covent Garden Food Co*	½ Carton/300g		174	10.5	58	2.6	4.1	3.5	0.8
Thai Chicken, Whole & Hearty, Chosen By You, Asda*	1 Pot/400g		265	8.4	66	4.3	7.1	2.1	0.9
Thai Green Curry with Chicken, Soups of the World, Heinz*	½ Can/258g		183	10.6	71	2.1	6.5	4.1	0.4
Thai Pumpkin Coconut, New Covent Garden Food Co*	1 Carton/568ml		182	7.4	32	1.3	3.5	1.3	1.1
Three Bean & Smoked Bacon, Farmers Market, Heinz*	1 Can/515g		309	9.8	60	2.7	8.1	1.9	1.9
Three Bean & Tomato, Autumn, Farmers Market, Heinz*	½ Carton/300g		132	1.5	44	2.3	7.5	0.5	0.5
Three Bean & Vegetable, Light Choices, Tesco*	½ Can/200g		110	0.6	55	2.6	9.7	0.3	1.9
Tomato, & Lentil, Mediterranean, Weight Watchers*	1 Can/400g		184	2.4	46	2.3	7.8	0.6	1.0
Tomato, 99% Fat Free, Wattie's*	1 Serving/105g		32	0.4	31	1.0	5.6	0.4	1.1
Tomato, Basil & Chilli, Microwave, Sainsbury's*	1 Pot/345g		100	2.1	29	1.0	5.0	0.6	1.2
Tomato, Canned, HL, Tesco*	½ Can/200g		110	4.0	55	0.7	7.4	2.0	0.5
Tomato, Canned, Light Choices, Tesco*	½ Can/200g		90	3.8	45	0.9	5.9	1.9	0.4
Tomato, Cannellini & Borlotti Bean, M & S*	½ Pot/300g		195	9.9	65	2.1	6.7	3.3	2.5
Tomato, Classic, Soup at Hand, Campbell's*	1 Serving/305g		427	1.5	140	3.0	30.0	0.5	0.0
Tomato, Cream of, Canned	1oz/28g		15	0.8	52	0.8	5.9	3.0	0.7
Tomato, Cream of, Classic, Heinz*	½ Can/200g		114	6.0	57	0.9	6.7	3.0	0.4
Tomato, Cream of, Condensed, Batchelors*	1 Can/295g		454	19.5	154	1.7	21.9	6.6	0.6
Tomato, Cream of, Dry, Knorr*	1 Pack/90g		391	21.2	435	4.3	51.3	23.6	3.3
Tomato, Cream of, Favourites, Baxters*	1 Can/415g		257	11.2	62	1.0	8.4	2.7	0.3
Tomato, Cream of, for One, Heinz*	1 Can/300g		189	10.8	63	0.8	6.9	3.6	0.4
Tomato, Cream of, Jeremy's Soups Ltd*	1 Serving/300g		180	10.2	60	1.2	6.3	3.4	0.7
Tomato, Cream of, Microwave, Heinz*	1 Pack/300g		204	11.4	68	0.9	7.5	3.8	0.4
Tomato, Cream of, Microwaveable Cup, Heinz*	1 Cup/275ml		169	9.4	61	0.8	6.9	3.4	0.4
Tomato, Cream of, Organic, Heinz*	1 Can/400g		220	10.4	55	1.0	7.0	2.6	0.4
Tomato, Cream of, Prepared, Campbell's*	½ Can/295g		195	9.4	66	0.8	8.5	3.2	0.0
Tomato, Cream of, Soup & Go, Heinz*	1 Cup/293ml		161	8.5	55	0.9	6.4	2.9	0.4
Tomato, Creamy, Chosen By You, Asda*	1 Pack/600g		288	12.0	48	1.2	5.5	2.0	1.4
Tomato, Creamy, Very Special, Heinz*	1 Serving/290g		148	6.4	51	0.7	6.5	2.2	0.0
Tomato, Cup a Soup, Made Up, Batchelors*	1 Sachet/256g		92	2.3	36	0.3	6.7	0.9	0.3
Tomato, Diet Chef Ltd*	1 Pack/300g		159	5.4	53	1.3	7.7	1.8	1.2
Tomato, in a Cup, Tesco*	1 Serving/23g		75	0.7	328	6.4	68.5	3.2	0.1

S

SOUP

INFO/WEIGHT	Measure	per Measure KCAL	FAT	Nutrition Values per 100g / 100ml KCAL	PROT	CARB	FAT	FIBRE
Tomato, Lighter Life*	1 Pack/36g	125	2.6	347	34.7	33.9	7.2	7.5
Tomato, Mealpak, All About Weight*	1 Pack/37g	152	7.5	416	35.0	22.4	20.6	5.0
Tomato, Mediterranean, In A Mug, Light Choices, Tesco*	1 Sachet/220ml	62	0.4	28	0.6	6.0	0.2	0.6
Tomato, Mediterranean, Rich, Fresh, Baxters*	1 Carton/600g	318	10.2	53	1.8	7.7	1.7	1.1
Tomato, Onion & Basil, GFY, Asda*	1 Can/400g	96	2.8	24	1.0	3.4	0.7	1.7
Tomato, Oriental Spiced, Skinny Soup, Glorious!*	1 Pot/600g	258	10.8	43	1.0	5.8	1.8	1.1
Tomato, Red Lentil & Pepper, Chosen By You, Asda*	½ Pot/300g	177	3.3	59	3.0	8.8	1.1	0.9
Tomato, Red Pepper & Basil, Thick & Creamy, Asda*	1 Sachet/24g	89	2.3	370	5.6	65.7	9.4	5.5
Tomato, Simmer & Serve, Dried, Sainsbury's*	1 Serving/200ml	70	2.2	35	0.3	6.0	1.1	0.4
Tomato, Smart Price, Asda*	1 Can/400g	184	7.6	46	0.6	6.5	1.9	0.9
Tomato, Spicy, & Beef, Diet Chef Ltd*	1 Pack/300ml	144	1.2	48	2.2	6.3	0.4	1.4
Tomato, Sweet Chilli, & Pasta, Classic, Heinz*	½ Can/200g	74	0.2	37	0.8	8.0	0.1	0.3
Tomato, Ten Calorie, Gourmet Cuisine*	1 Sachet/200g	10	0.1	5	0.3	1.0	0.0	0.1
Tomato, Three Bean & Bacon, Sainsbury's*	½ Can/200g	86	2.0	43	3.1	5.4	1.0	3.0
Tomato, Vegetable Garden, Campbell's*	1 Can/310g	240	2.7	77	1.6	16.1	0.9	0.0
Tomato, Vine Ripend, Green Giant*	1 Pouch/330g	129	3.0	39	0.6	7.7	0.9	1.6
Tomato, Weight Watchers*	1 Can/295g	74	1.5	25	0.7	4.5	0.5	0.3
Tomato & Basil, Campbell's*	1 Pack/500ml	205	6.5	41	0.7	6.7	1.3	1.1
Tomato & Basil, Creamy, Cully & Sully*	1 Pack/400g	216	18.5	54	0.8	2.5	4.6	0.5
Tomato & Basil, Cup, Co-Op*	1 Sachet/45g	157	1.8	350	2.0	76.0	4.0	4.0
Tomato & Basil, Cup a Soup, Made Up, GFY, Asda*	1 Serving/250ml	50	0.2	20	0.4	4.4	0.1	0.2
Tomato & Basil, Diet Chef Ltd*	1 Pack/300g	159	5.4	53	1.3	7.7	1.8	1.2
Tomato & Basil, Fresh, Finest, Tesco*	½ Pot/300g	219	14.7	73	1.0	6.3	4.9	0.6
Tomato & Basil, Fresh, Low Fat, Sainsbury's*	½ Carton/300ml	75	1.8	25	1.1	4.1	0.6	0.7
Tomato & Basil, Fresh, So Organic, Sainsbury's*	½ Carton/200g	100	4.0	50	0.5	7.5	2.0	0.2
Tomato & Basil, Fresh, The Fresh Soup Company*	½ Pot/250g	85	2.2	34	1.3	5.1	0.9	0.6
Tomato & Basil, GFY, Asda*	1 Serving/250ml	100	3.5	40	0.9	6.0	1.4	1.6
Tomato & Basil, Italian, 99% Fat Free, Baxters*	½ Can/208g	119	2.1	57	2.6	9.3	1.0	1.1
Tomato & Basil, Loyd Grossman*	½ Pack/210g	97	4.0	46	0.8	6.4	1.9	0.2
Tomato & Basil, Soup-A-Slim, Asda*	1 Sachet/16g	52	0.3	326	7.0	70.0	2.0	3.9
Tomato & Basil, Vie, Knorr*	1 Pack/500ml	145	2.0	29	0.8	5.5	0.4	0.9
Tomato & Basil, Weight Watchers*	1 Serving/295g	77	1.8	26	0.6	4.4	0.6	0.5
Tomato & Basil with Onion, Waistline, Crosse & Blackwell*	1 Serving/300g	87	1.8	29	0.9	5.1	0.6	0.3
Tomato & Brown Lentil, Healthy, Baxters*	1 Can/415g	199	0.8	48	2.6	9.0	0.2	2.7
Tomato & Brown Lentil, Healthy Choice, Heinz*	½ Can/208g	112	0.6	54	3.1	9.6	0.3	1.5
Tomato & Butterbean, Classic, Heinz*	½ Can/200g	92	1.4	46	1.3	8.1	0.7	0.8
Tomato & Butterbean, Vegetarian, Baxters*	1 Can/415g	166	5.0	40	1.2	6.1	1.2	1.0
Tomato & Chorizo, Mediterranean, Tesco*	1 Serving/200g	130	6.8	65	2.0	6.1	3.4	0.3
Tomato & Herb, Campbell's*	1 Carton/500ml	180	6.5	36	1.0	5.0	1.3	0.0
Tomato & Lentil, M & S*	½ Can/211g	95	0.4	45	2.3	8.4	0.2	1.5
Tomato & Lentil, Organic, Tideford*	1 Carton/300g	120	2.7	40	2.3	8.1	0.9	0.9
Tomato & Lentil, Spicy, Canned, Tesco*	1 Can/400g	180	0.8	45	2.1	8.7	0.2	0.8
Tomato & Red Pepper, to Go, Asda*	1 Pot/330g	102	4.3	31	0.6	4.3	1.3	0.6
Tomato & Red Pepper with Basil, Farmers Market, Heinz*	½ Carton/300g	117	4.2	39	1.3	5.2	1.4	0.5
Tomato & Roasted Red Pepper, COU, M & S*	1 Serving/415g	145	0.4	35	1.0	7.6	0.1	0.9
Tomato & Spinach, Organic, Waitrose*	1 Serving/300g	126	5.7	42	1.4	4.9	1.9	0.7
Tomato & Vegetable with Croutons, Dry, Soupreme*	1 Serving/27g	106	3.8	394	7.2	59.9	13.9	4.8
Tomato & Vegetable with Croutons in a Cup, Sainsbury's*	1 Sachet/218ml	85	2.2	39	0.5	6.8	1.0	0.2
Tomato Flavoured, Tony Ferguson*	1 Pack/58g	205	2.1	354	26.2	49.2	3.6	5.2
Traditional Vegetable, Knorr*	1 Serving/200ml	42	0.2	21	1.0	3.2	0.1	1.0
Turkey Broth, Canned, Baxters*	½ Can/208g	79	1.5	38	1.3	6.5	0.7	0.7
Turkey Broth, Favourites, Baxters*	1 Can/415g	158	2.9	38	1.3	6.5	0.7	0.7
Tuscan, Vegetable, Organic, Tideford Organics*	1 Pack/300g	195	7.8	65	2.4	8.1	2.6	0.0

SOUP

INFO/WEIGHT	Measure		per Measure		Nutrition Values per 100g / 100ml				
			KCAL	FAT	KCAL	PROT	CARB	FAT	FIBRE
Tuscan Bean, Canned, HL, Tesco*	½ Can/200ml		130	3.6	65	3.5	10.3	1.8	1.3
Tuscan Bean, New Covent Garden Food Co*	½ Carton/300g		84	2.4	28	1.6	3.7	0.8	1.0
Tuscan Bean, Organic, Fresh, Sainsbury's*	1 Pack/400g		171	3.2	43	2.6	6.3	0.8	2.0
Tuscan Bean, Perfectly Balanced, Waitrose*	½ Pot/300g		147	5.4	49	2.0	6.1	1.8	1.8
Tuscan Chicken & Orzo, Glorious!*	½ Pot/300g		120	1.2	40	2.8	6.2	0.4	0.7
Vegetable, Average	1 Serving/220g		114	8.8	52	0.9	3.2	4.0	0.9
Vegetable, Batchelors*	1 Can/400g		168	3.6	42	1.0	5.3	0.9	4.4
Vegetable, Bean & Pasta, Organic, Baxters*	1 Can/415g		212	3.3	51	2.2	8.7	0.8	1.4
Vegetable, Canned	1oz/28g		13	0.2	48	1.4	9.9	0.6	1.5
Vegetable, Chinky, Low Fat, Solo Slim, Rosemary Conley*	1 Pack/300g		114	2.4	38	1.4	6.4	0.8	1.9
Vegetable, Chunky, Diet Chef Ltd*	1 Pack/300g		114	0.9	38	1.4	7.4	0.3	1.3
Vegetable, Chunky, Diet Chef Ltd*	1 Pack/300g		105	1.8	35	1.9	5.5	0.6	3.0
Vegetable, Chunky, Fresh, Organic, Simply Organic*	½ Tub/300g		153	4.5	51	1.9	9.0	1.5	1.4
Vegetable, Chunky, Red Lentils & Pearl Barley, Waitrose*	½ Pot/298g		131	5.4	44	1.3	4.5	1.8	2.1
Vegetable, Classic, Heinz*	1 Can/400g		180	3.2	45	1.1	8.2	0.8	0.9
Vegetable, Condensed, Campbell's*	1 Can/295g		103	2.4	35	0.8	6.2	0.8	0.0
Vegetable, Condensed, Classic, Campbell's*	1 Can/295g		221	5.0	75	1.7	13.2	1.7	1.7
Vegetable, Country Garden, Green Giant*	1 Pack/330g		129	2.0	39	1.0	7.2	0.6	2.0
Vegetable, Cream of, Cup a Soup, Batchelors*	1 Sachet/33g		134	5.3	406	5.8	59.8	16.0	6.2
Vegetable, Cream of, Cup a Soup, Soupreme*	1 Pack/21g		73	2.2	356	4.9	59.5	10.7	6.3
Vegetable, Cream of, Cup Soup, Soupreme*	1 Serving/27g		95	2.8	352	4.8	59.6	10.5	6.3
Vegetable, Cream of, Fresh, Sainsbury's*	1 Pot/600g		216	12.6	36	0.5	3.8	2.1	1.2
Vegetable, Cream of, Jeremy's Soups Ltd*	1 Serving/300g		99	8.1	33	0.6	1.6	2.7	0.7
Vegetable, Cream of, Velouté De Légumes, Liebig*	1 Portion/200ml		84	4.0	42	0.7	5.3	2.0	1.0
Vegetable, Cully & Sully*	1 Pack/400g		204	14.4	51	0.6	4.2	3.6	0.9
Vegetable, Cup, Soupreme*	1 Sachet/26g		115	6.1	444	8.1	49.7	23.6	2.3
Vegetable, Cup Soup, Dry, Heinz*	1 Sachet/16g		54	1.1	348	5.8	64.5	7.1	3.2
Vegetable, Cup Soup, Eat Smart, Morrisons*	1 Pack/213ml		51	1.1	24	0.4	4.4	0.5	0.4
Vegetable, Cup Soup, Made Up, Heinz*	1 Cup/200g		50	1.0	25	0.4	4.7	0.5	0.2
Vegetable, Extra Thick, Canned, Sainsbury's*	1 Can/400g		184	2.4	46	1.5	8.6	0.6	1.4
Vegetable, for One, Heinz*	1 Can/300g		129	2.1	43	1.1	8.1	0.7	0.9
Vegetable, Fresh, Average	1 Serving/300g		118	4.1	39	1.4	5.4	1.4	1.3
Vegetable, From Heinz, Canned, Weight Watchers*	1 Can/295g		86	0.9	29	0.9	5.6	0.3	0.8
Vegetable, Golden, in a Mug, Tesco*	1 Sachet/17g		60	1.3	351	8.2	62.0	7.8	3.7
Vegetable, Hi Taste Low Cal, Cup Soup, Ainsley Harriott*	1 Sachet/22g		74	0.7	336	8.6	68.2	3.2	4.1
Vegetable, in a Cup, Weight Watchers*	1 Serving/100g		57	1.2	57	1.2	10.4	1.2	0.5
Vegetable, Mediterranean, Tesco*	½ Pot/300g		105	2.1	35	1.0	6.2	0.7	0.7
Vegetable, Provencal, M & S*	1 Serving/300g		150	7.5	50	1.0	6.0	2.5	1.1
Vegetable, Soup in a Mug, HL, Tesco*	1 Sachet/18g		66	1.4	365	7.0	66.3	8.0	2.6
Vegetable, Vie, Knorr*	1 Pack/500ml		160	3.5	32	0.9	5.5	0.7	1.2
Vegetable, Winter, Chunky, M & S*	1 Can/400g		140	0.8	35	1.2	6.3	0.2	1.5
Vegetable & Barley Broth, Canned, Organic, Sainsbury's*	½ Can/200g		48	0.8	24	1.4	3.7	0.4	0.9
Vegetable & Chilli, Chunky, Fresh, Sainsbury's*	½ Pot/300g		117	1.8	39	1.6	6.9	0.6	2.6
Vegetable & Lentil, Waitrose*	½ Pot/300g		138	4.5	46	2.9	5.2	1.5	3.5
Vegetable & Rosemary, Fresh, Sainsbury's*	½ Pack/300g		96	3.0	32	0.9	4.9	1.0	1.3
Vegetable Broth, Canned, HL, Tesco*	½ Can/200g		74	0.4	37	1.2	7.4	0.2	1.0
Vegetable Broth, M & S*	1 Pack/213g		85	3.0	40	1.0	6.3	1.4	0.8
Vegetable Chowder, New Covent Garden Food Co*	½ Carton/300g		159	5.1	53	2.9	6.6	1.7	1.1
Vegetable Curry, Chosen By You, Asda*	½ Pot/300g		240	2.1	80	4.5	13.3	0.7	1.1
Vegetable Mulligatawny, Tesco*	½ Pack/300g		210	7.5	70	1.9	9.0	2.5	1.1
Vegetable Pho Noodle, Broth, Heat to Eat, Tesco*	1 Pot/165g		43	0.3	26	1.3	4.5	0.2	0.6
Vegetable with Croutons, Soup in a Mug, Tesco*	1 Pack/23g		90	3.7	392	6.2	55.2	16.3	8.0
Vine Ripened Tomato & Basil, Fresh, Avonmore*	1 Serving/300g		141	8.1	47	1.0	4.7	2.7	0.3

S

	Measure INFO/WEIGHT	per Measure KCAL	FAT	Nutrition Values per 100g / 100ml KCAL	PROT	CARB	FAT	FIBRE
SOUP								
Vine Tomato, Harissa & Mint, The Best, Morrisons*	1 Pot/600g	294	11.4	49	1.5	6.4	1.9	1.1
Watercress, M & S*	½ Pot/300g	75	5.1	25	1.3	1.5	1.7	0.6
Watercress & Cream, Soup Chef*	1 Jar/780g	413	22.6	53	0.8	5.9	2.9	0.3
White Bean & Pancetta, Finest, Tesco*	1 Pot/600g	450	19.8	75	3.5	6.2	3.3	2.2
White Winter Vegetable, Cully Ans Sully*	1 Pot/400g	172	10.8	43	0.8	4.2	2.7	1.1
Wild Mushroom, Farmers Market, Heinz*	½ Carton/300g	93	3.3	31	0.9	4.4	1.1	0.5
Wild Mushroom, in a Cup, BGTY, Sainsbury's*	1 Serving/200ml	56	1.8	28	0.4	4.5	0.9	0.2
Wild Mushroom & Maderia, Fresh, Finest, Tesco*	½ Tub/300g	156	8.7	52	1.5	4.9	2.9	0.5
Wild Mushroom Carton, Soupreme*	1 Carton/500g	135	6.0	27	1.1	2.9	1.2	0.5
Winter Root Veg with British Beef, Yorkshire Provender*	½ Pot/300g	145	5.4	48	2.9	5.1	1.8	1.3
Winter Vegetable, Broth, Classic, Heinz*	1 Serving/200g	56	0.2	28	0.8	5.3	0.1	0.8
Winter Vegetable, Chosen By You, Asda*	1 Pot/600g	234	4.2	39	1.6	5.9	0.7	1.1
Winter Vegetable, New Covent Garden Food Co*	½ Pack/300g	117	2.1	39	2.0	5.1	0.7	2.3
Winter Vegetable, Organic, Sainsbury's*	½ Can/200g	100	2.0	50	2.3	7.9	1.0	1.3
Wonton, Blue Dragon*	1 Can/410g	102	5.3	25	1.2	2.0	1.3	0.2
SOUTHERN COMFORT								
37.5% Volume	*1 Shot/35ml*	*72*	*0.0*	*207*	*0.0*	*0.0*	*0.0*	*0.0*
SOYA								
Barbeque Chilli, Vegelicious, Tesco*	1 Portion/450g	450	15.7	100	3.1	12.9	3.5	2.7
Bolognese Style, Sainsbury's*	½ Pack/168g	113	1.2	67	3.1	13.9	0.7	2.7
Chunks, Protein, Natural, Nature's Harvest*	1 Serving/50g	172	0.5	345	50.0	38.0	1.0	4.0
Hot Pot with Sweet Potato, Vegelicious, Tesco*	1 Pack/450g	517	21.6	115	3.3	14.5	4.8	2.2
Mince, Dry Weight, Sainsbury's*	1 Serving/50g	164	0.4	328	47.2	33.2	0.8	3.6
Mince, Granules	*1oz/28g*	*74*	*1.5*	*263*	*43.2*	*11.0*	*5.4*	*0.0*
Mince, Prepared, Sainsbury's*	1 Serving/200g	164	0.4	82	11.8	8.3	0.2	0.9
Mince, Super Soya, M & S*	¼ Pack/89g	85	0.5	95	16.9	2.7	0.6	6.5
Mince with Onion, Cooked, Sainsbury's*	½ Pack/180g	122	2.9	68	5.4	8.0	1.6	1.8
SOYA MILK								
Banana Flavour, Provamel*	1 Serving/250ml	195	5.5	78	3.8	10.4	2.2	0.6
Choco Flavour, Provamel*	1 Serving/250ml	207	6.0	83	3.8	11.1	2.4	1.1
Chocolate, So Good Beverages*	1 Serving/250ml	160	2.5	64	3.6	10.8	1.0	0.0
Fat Free, Original, So Good Beverages*	1 Serving/250ml	100	0.2	40	3.6	6.4	0.1	0.0
Flavoured, Average	1 fl oz/30ml	12	0.5	40	2.8	3.6	1.7	0.0
No Added Sugar, Unsweetened, Average	*1 Serving/250ml*	*85*	*4.8*	*34*	*3.3*	*0.9*	*1.9*	*0.4*
Omega Original, (Best Taste Ever), So Good Beverages*	1 Serving/250ml	97	3.7	39	2.0	4.4	1.5	0.0
Omega Vanilla, So Good Beverages*	1 Serving/250ml	130	3.0	52	3.6	7.6	1.2	0.0
Original, No Added Sugar, So Good Beverages*	1 Serving/250ml	80	2.5	32	3.6	2.0	1.0	0.8
Strawberry, So Good Beverages*	1 Serving/250ml	160	2.5	64	3.6	10.4	1.0	0.0
Strawberry Flavour, Provamel*	1 Serving/250ml	160	5.2	64	3.6	7.7	2.1	1.2
Sweetened, Average	*1 Glass/200ml*	*93*	*4.2*	*47*	*3.4*	*3.7*	*2.1*	*0.4*
Sweetened, Calcium Enriched, Average	1 Glass/200ml	91	3.9	46	3.4	3.7	2.0	0.3
UHT, Non Dairy, Alternative to Milk, Waitrose*	1 Serving/250ml	102	4.7	41	3.3	2.7	1.9	0.2
Unsweetened, Organic, Waitrose*	1 Serving/60ml	19	1.1	31	3.3	0.2	1.9	0.0
Unsweetened, Uht, Organic, Tesco*	1 Serving/150ml	46	2.8	31	3.4	0.1	1.9	0.6
Vanilla, Fat Free, So Good Beverages*	1 Serving/250ml	140	0.2	56	3.6	10.4	0.1	0.0
Vanilla, Organic, Heinz*	1 Serving/200ml	106	3.2	53	2.6	6.9	1.6	0.2
Vanilla, So Good Beverages*	1 Serving/250ml	180	5.0	72	3.6	10.4	2.0	0.0
Vanilla Flavour, Organic, Provamel*	1 Serving/250ml	150	5.5	60	3.8	6.2	2.2	0.6
SPAGHETTI								
Brown Rice, Gluten Free, Organic, Doves Farm*	1 Serving/70g	237	1.0	338	7.9	70.3	1.5	4.1
Cooked, Average	*1oz/28g*	*33*	*0.2*	*119*	*4.1*	*24.8*	*0.6*	*1.1*
Dried, Waitrose*	1 Serving/75g	256	1.0	341	11.5	70.7	1.3	3.7
Dry, Average	*1oz/28g*	*98*	*0.4*	*350*	*12.1*	*72.1*	*1.5*	*2.4*

	Measure				Nutrition Values per 100g / 100ml				
	INFO/WEIGHT	KCAL	FAT		KCAL	PROT	CARB	FAT	FIBRE
SPAGHETTI									
Dry, Carb Check, Heinz*	1 Serving/75g	219	1.7		292	52.7	15.2	2.3	20.8
Durum Wheat, Dry, Average	*1oz/28g*	*97*	*0.1*		*347*	*12.3*	*71.7*	*0.3*	*1.4*
Egg, Fresh, Cooked, Tesco*	½ Pack/150g	480	3.7		320	9.7	62.7	2.5	3.4
Fresh, Cooked, Average	*1 Serving/125g*	*182*	*2.2*		*146*	*6.1*	*26.9*	*1.7*	*1.8*
Fresh, Dry, Average	*1 Serving/100g*	*278*	*3.0*		*278*	*10.8*	*53.0*	*3.0*	*2.2*
in Tomato & Cheese, Sainsbury's*	1 Serving/300g	345	10.2		115	4.4	16.8	3.4	1.4
In Tomato Sauce, Basics, Sainsbury's*	1 Can/410g	197	1.2		48	1.4	10.0	0.3	0.7
in Tomato Sauce, Canned	1oz/28g	18	0.1		64	1.9	14.1	0.4	0.7
in Tomato Sauce, Heinz*	½ Can/200g	120	0.6		60	1.7	12.7	0.3	2.4
in Tomato Sauce, HP*	1 Can/410g	247	0.8		60	1.5	13.1	0.2	0.4
In Tomato Sauce, Multigrain, Heinz*	½ Can/200g	120	0.6		60	1.7	12.7	0.3	2.4
in Tomato Sauce, Organic, Sainsbury's*	½ Can/205g	133	0.4		65	1.8	13.9	0.2	1.0
in Tomato Sauce, Whole Wheat, Sainsbury's*	1 Serving/205g	125	1.2		61	2.0	11.9	0.6	1.1
in Tomato Sauce with Parsley, Weight Watchers*	1 Sm Can/200g	100	0.4		50	1.8	9.9	0.2	0.6
Whole Wheat, Cooked, Average	*1oz/28g*	*32*	*0.3*		*113*	*4.7*	*23.2*	*0.9*	*3.5*
Whole Wheat, Dry, Average	*1 Serving/100g*	*324*	*2.6*		*324*	*13.5*	*62.2*	*2.6*	*8.0*
SPAGHETTI & MEATBALLS									
American, Superbowl, Asda*	1 Pack/453g	594	17.7		131	11.0	13.0	3.9	1.1
Chicken, in Tomato Sauce, Heinz*	1 Can/400g	332	9.2		83	4.2	11.3	2.3	0.5
COU, M & S*	1 Pack/400g	360	8.0		90	6.0	12.3	2.0	2.6
GFY, Asda*	1 Pack/400g	344	6.0		86	7.0	11.0	1.5	1.5
Healthy Range, Average	1 Serving/400g	375	8.3		94	5.7	12.9	2.1	1.7
Italian, Sainsbury's*	1 Pack/450g	495	21.1		110	5.0	11.9	4.7	2.7
Sainsbury's*	1 Pack/400g	497	18.4		124	6.5	14.2	4.6	2.8
Tesco*	1 Serving/475g	641	30.9		135	5.1	14.1	6.5	0.9
SPAGHETTI BOLOGNESE									
Al Forno, Sainsbury's*	1 Pack/400g	460	19.6		115	7.8	10.0	4.9	1.1
Average	1 Serving/450g	580	25.2		129	7.8	12.5	5.6	0.9
BGTY, Sainsbury's*	1 Pack/400g	416	9.2		104	6.3	14.4	2.3	1.1
Canned, Asda*	½ Can/205g	174	5.7		85	4.2	10.7	2.8	0.6
Egg Pasta in Rich Beef Sauce, Waitrose*	1 Pack/400g	404	10.4		101	7.6	11.7	2.6	1.0
Frozen, Tesco*	1 Pack/450g	472	9.0		105	5.8	15.0	2.0	1.8
GFY, Asda*	1 Pack/400g	352	6.4		88	4.9	13.4	1.6	2.2
Good Intentions, Somerfield*	1 Serving/400g	380	9.2		95	6.2	12.4	2.3	1.4
Healthy Choice, Iceland*	1 Pack/400g	428	4.0		107	6.8	17.8	1.0	1.1
Hidden Veg, Heinz*	1 Can/400g	312	6.4		78	3.4	12.6	1.6	0.9
HP*	1 Pack/410g	312	7.8		76	3.8	11.3	1.9	0.7
Lean Cuisine, Findus*	1 Pack/320g	275	7.4		86	4.5	11.5	2.3	1.1
Meat Free, Heinz*	1 Serving/200g	162	3.4		81	3.3	13.1	1.7	0.6
Perfectly Balanced, Waitrose*	1 Pack/400g	380	6.8		95	6.7	13.4	1.7	1.1
Quick Pasta, Dry, Sainsbury's*	1 Serving/63g	231	2.8		367	10.8	71.0	4.4	3.3
Ross*	1 Serving/320g	288	3.5		90	4.2	15.7	1.1	0.9
Vegetarian, Tesco*	1 Pack/340g	374	13.3		110	5.1	13.7	3.9	1.2
Weight Watchers*	1 Pack/320g	293	6.1		91	5.7	12.6	1.9	0.8
SPAGHETTI CARBONARA									
Chicken, Mushroom & Ham, Asda*	1 Pack/700g	686	14.0		98	10.0	10.0	2.0	1.5
Chicken & Asparagus, Sainsbury's*	1 Pack/450g	657	27.4		146	6.6	16.2	6.1	1.1
COU, M & S*	1 Pack/330g	346	7.2		105	6.1	15.7	2.2	0.8
Creamy, Mini Meals, Heinz*	1 Sm Can/200g	130	2.7		65	3.8	9.0	1.3	0.5
Free Range Egg with Italian Bacon, City Kitchen, Tesco*	1 Pack/385g	577	29.6		150	4.8	15.5	7.7	1.5
GFY, Asda*	1 Pack/400g	406	7.6		102	5.5	15.3	1.9	0.7
Italian, Chilled, Sainsbury's*	1 Pack/400g	492	15.6		123	5.5	16.1	3.9	1.4
Italian, Tesco*	1 Pack/450g	607	26.5		135	5.4	14.1	5.9	0.6

	Measure INFO/WEIGHT	per Measure		Nutrition Values per 100g / 100ml				
		KCAL	FAT	KCAL	PROT	CARB	FAT	FIBRE
SPAGHETTI CARBONARA								
Reduced Calorie, Chosen By You, Asda*	1 Pack/378g	363	7.2	96	5.5	13.8	1.9	0.7
SPAGHETTI HOOPS								
in Tomato Sauce, Heinz*	½ Can/200g	106	0.4	53	1.7	11.1	0.2	0.5
in Tomato Sauce, Hidden Veg, Heinz*	1 Can/400g	244	2.0	61	1.7	12.4	0.5	1.1
in Tomato Sauce, Multigrain, Snap Pot, Heinz*	1 Pot/190g	112	0.6	59	1.6	12.7	0.3	1.5
in Tomato Sauce, Snap Pot, Heinz*	1 Pot/192g	113	0.6	59	1.6	12.7	0.3	1.5
Tesco*	½ Can/205g	123	0.4	60	1.6	12.9	0.2	0.5
SPAGHETTINI								
Wholewheat, Great Stuff, Asda*	1 Serving/100g	99	0.7	99	3.4	19.7	0.7	2.4
SPAM*								
Pork & Ham, Chopped, Spam*	1 Serving/100g	296	24.2	296	14.5	3.2	24.2	0.0
SPELT								
Organic, Easy Grain, Food Doctor*	1 Pack/225g	326	4.0	145	5.2	26.6	1.8	5.9
Pearled, Sharpham Park*	1 Portion/100g	314	1.8	314	12.0	68.4	1.8	6.0
SPINACH								
Baby, Average	*1 Serving/90g*	*22*	*0.7*	*25*	*2.8*	*1.6*	*0.8*	*2.1*
Boiled Or Steamed, Average	*1 Serving/80g*	*17*	*0.6*	*21*	*2.6*	*0.9*	*0.8*	*2.1*
Canned, Average	*1 Serving/80g*	*18*	*0.4*	*22*	*3.0*	*1.4*	*0.5*	*2.9*
Chopped, Frozen, Waitrose*	1 Serving/80g	20	0.6	25	2.8	1.6	0.8	2.7
Creamed, Frozen, Weight Watchers*	1 Portion/112g	48	1.1	43	2.5	5.0	1.0	1.5
Raw, Average	*1 Serving/80g*	*19*	*0.6*	*24*	*2.9*	*1.4*	*0.7*	*2.2*
SPIRALI								
Dry, Average	*1 Serving/50g*	*176*	*0.8*	*351*	*12.1*	*72.5*	*1.6*	*2.7*
SPIRITS								
37.5% Volume	*1 Shot/35ml*	*72*	*0.0*	*207*	*0.0*	*0.0*	*0.0*	*0.0*
40% Volume	*1 Shot/35ml*	*78*	*0.0*	*222*	*0.0*	*0.0*	*0.0*	*0.0*
SPLENDIPS								
Cheesecake, Philadelphia, Kraft*	1 Pack/85g	200	7.1	235	6.1	34.0	8.3	2.9
Chives, Philadelphia, Kraft*	1 Pack/85g	159	4.4	187	7.5	27.0	5.2	1.7
Nachos, Philadelphia, Kraft*	1 Pack/85g	150	6.5	177	6.4	20.0	7.6	1.0
Poppadoms & Mango Chutney, Light, Philadelphia, Kraft*	1 Pack/76g	131	3.6	172	5.1	26.5	4.7	1.9
SPLIT PEAS								
Dried, Average	*1oz/28g*	*89*	*0.5*	*319*	*22.1*	*57.4*	*1.7*	*3.1*
Green, Dried, Boiled, Average	*1 Tbsp/35g*	*40*	*0.2*	*115*	*8.3*	*19.8*	*0.6*	*3.9*
Yellow, Morrisons*	1 Serving/120g	338	1.4	282	21.3	62.2	1.2	15.6
Yellow, Wholefoods, Tesco*	1 Serving/15g	52	0.4	345	22.1	58.2	2.4	6.3
SPONGE FINGERS								
Boudoir, Sainsbury's*	1 Finger/5g	20	0.2	396	8.1	82.8	3.6	0.4
Tesco*	1 Finger/5g	19	0.2	386	7.6	80.6	3.7	1.0
SPONGE PUDDING								
Average	1 Portion/170g	578	27.7	340	5.8	45.3	16.3	1.1
Banoffee, Heinz*	¼ Can/78g	239	9.5	307	2.8	46.6	12.2	0.6
Blackcurrant, BGTY, Sainsbury's*	1 Serving/110g	155	1.0	141	2.5	30.7	0.9	3.2
Blackcurrant, Low Fat, Iceland*	1 Pudding/90g	159	1.0	177	2.2	39.5	1.1	1.6
Canned, Average	1 Serving/75g	214	8.5	285	3.1	45.4	11.4	0.8
Cherry & Almond Flavour, Sainsbury's*	¼ Pudding/110g	334	15.7	304	3.5	40.3	14.3	0.7
Chocolate, BGTY, Sainsbury's*	1 Pudding/105g	137	2.5	131	4.4	23.1	2.4	2.7
Chocolate, Cadbury*	1 Pack/370g	1276	73.3	345	4.9	36.7	19.8	0.0
Chocolate, Free From, Sainsbury's*	1 Pudding/110g	388	10.2	353	5.2	62.0	9.3	0.3
Chocolate, GFY, Asda*	1 Pudding/105g	187	4.4	178	3.0	32.0	4.2	2.6
Chocolate, Heinz*	¼ Pudding/77g	229	8.9	298	4.6	44.0	11.5	1.2
Chocolate, HL, Tesco*	1 Serving/125g	239	4.7	191	4.4	34.7	3.8	0.9
Chocolate, Less Than 3% Fat, BGTY, Sainsbury's*	1 Pudding/105g	180	2.0	171	4.5	34.0	1.9	0.9

	Measure INFO/WEIGHT	per Measure KCAL	FAT	Nutrition Values per 100g / 100ml KCAL	PROT	CARB	FAT	FIBRE
SPONGE PUDDING								
Chocolate, M & S*	¼ Pudding/131g	524	32.2	400	6.1	38.6	24.6	1.8
Chocolate, Sainsbury's*	¼ Pudding/110g	464	28.3	422	5.4	42.3	25.7	0.8
Chocolate, Somerfield*	¼ Pudding/100g	369	23.0	369	5.0	35.0	23.0	0.0
Chocolate, Tesco*	1 Pudding/115g	195	4.7	170	4.7	28.3	4.1	2.8
Chocolate, Trufree*	1 Serving/115g	374	17.2	325	2.5	44.0	15.0	2.0
Chocolate, Waitrose*	1 Pudding/110g	400	22.5	363	3.6	41.4	20.4	1.7
Circus, & Custard, Weight Watchers*	1 Serving/140g	239	4.1	171	4.2	32.1	2.9	0.9
Fruit, Co-Op*	1 Can/300g	1110	48.0	370	3.0	53.0	16.0	2.0
Fruited with Brandy Sauce, Sainsbury's*	1 Pudding/125g	261	8.4	209	3.6	33.6	6.7	0.8
Fruits of the Forest, Asda*	1 Pudding/115g	323	4.4	281	2.8	59.0	3.8	1.3
Golden Syrup, Co-Op*	1 Can/300g	945	39.0	315	2.0	47.0	13.0	0.6
Lemon, COU, M & S*	1 Pudding/100g	157	2.3	157	2.0	32.1	2.3	1.9
Lemon, M & S*	1 Pudding/105g	325	16.0	310	4.3	39.4	15.2	2.3
Lemon, Waitrose*	1 Serving/105g	212	2.5	202	3.4	41.7	2.4	1.4
Lemon Curd, Heinz*	¼ Can/78g	236	9.1	302	2.6	46.7	11.7	0.6
Pear & Ginger, COU, M & S*	1 Pudding/100g	175	0.7	175	1.9	39.8	0.7	1.1
Raspberry Jam, Asda*	½ Pudding/147g	481	16.2	327	3.1	54.0	11.0	4.1
St Clements, GFY, Asda*	1 Pudding/116g	332	4.5	286	2.6	60.0	3.9	1.2
Sticky Toffee, COU, M & S*	1 Pack/150g	277	2.5	185	2.5	39.3	1.7	1.8
Sticky Toffee, Microwavable, Heinz*	1 Serving/75g	233	9.0	311	3.3	47.4	12.0	0.7
Sticky Toffee, Mini, Somerfield*	1 Pudding/110g	384	14.3	349	3.0	54.0	13.0	0.0
Strawberry, Co-Op*	1 Can/300g	960	39.0	320	2.0	48.0	13.0	0.8
Strawberry Jam, Heinz*	¼ Can/82g	230	6.2	281	2.6	50.4	7.6	0.6
Sultana with Toffee Sauce, HL, Tesco*	1 Serving/80g	280	2.2	350	3.2	60.2	2.7	1.0
Summer Fruits, BGTY, Sainsbury's*	1 Serving/110g	243	4.7	221	2.7	42.9	4.3	1.0
Syrup, & Custard, Iceland*	1 Pudding/130g	409	21.1	315	3.6	38.8	16.2	0.4
Syrup, BGTY, Sainsbury's*	1 Pudding/110g	338	4.5	307	2.8	64.6	4.1	0.4
Syrup, Finest, Tesco*	1 Pudding/115g	330	9.0	287	3.1	51.2	7.8	0.6
Syrup, GFY, Asda*	1 Sponge/105g	207	4.3	197	2.0	38.0	4.1	2.6
Syrup, Individual, Tesco*	1 Pudding/110g	390	14.5	355	3.1	55.6	13.2	0.5
Syrup, Morrisons*	1 Pot/110g	404	13.7	367	3.4	59.7	12.5	0.8
Treacle, Heinz*	1 Serving/160g	445	13.0	278	2.5	48.9	8.1	0.6
Treacle, Super Sticky, Heinz*	1 Pudding/110g	318	12.2	289	1.9	45.3	11.1	1.6
Treacle, Waitrose*	1 Pudding/105g	385	13.8	367	2.8	59.5	13.1	0.5
with Custard	1 Serving/200g	521	24.9	261	4.8	34.1	12.4	0.9
with Dried Fruit	1oz/28g	93	4.0	331	5.4	48.1	14.3	1.2
with Jam or Treacle	1oz/28g	93	4.0	333	5.1	48.7	14.4	1.0
with Lyles Golden Syrup, Heinz*	½ Pudding/95g	368	14.4	386	3.1	53.3	15.1	0.5
SPOTTED DICK								
Average	1 Serving/105g	343	17.5	327	4.2	42.7	16.7	1.0
with Custard	1 Serving/210g	438	15.6	209	3.4	31.5	7.4	1.3
SPRATS								
Fried	*1oz/28g*	*116*	*9.8*	*415*	*24.9*	*0.0*	*35.0*	*0.0*
Raw	*1oz/28g*	*48*	*3.1*	*172*	*18.3*	*0.0*	*11.0*	*0.0*
SPREAD								
British Butterspread, Asda*	1 Serving/10g	70	7.7	699	0.4	0.5	77.3	0.0
Butter Me Up, Light, Tesco*	1 Thin Spread/7g	24	2.7	350	0.3	0.5	38.0	0.0
Butter Me Up, Tesco*	1 Thin Spread/7g	38	4.1	540	0.8	1.2	59.0	0.0
Butterlicious, Vegetable, Sainsbury's*	1 Thin Spread/7g	44	4.8	628	0.6	1.1	69.0	0.0
Buttersoft, Light, Reduced Fat, Sainsbury's*	1 Thin Spread/7g	38	4.2	544	0.4	0.5	60.0	0.0
Buttery Gold, Somerfield*	1 Thin Spread/7g	44	4.8	627	0.5	1.0	69.0	0.0
Buttery Taste, Benecol*	1 Thin Spread/7g	40	4.4	575	0.0	0.8	63.3	0.0
Dairy Free, Organic, Pure Spreads*	1 Thin Spread/7g	37	4.1	533	0.5	0.0	59.0	0.0

S

	Measure INFO/WEIGHT	per Measure KCAL	FAT	Nutrition Values per 100g / 100ml KCAL	PROT	CARB	FAT	FIBRE
SPREAD								
Diet, Delight*	1 Thin Spread/7g	16	1.6	228	3.6	1.6	23.0	0.0
Enriched Olive, Tesco*	1 Thin Spread/7g	38	4.1	540	0.2	1.2	59.0	0.0
From Soya, Kallo*	1 Thin Spread/7g	27	2.6	380	7.0	6.0	37.0	0.0
Gold, Low Fat, Omega 3, St Ivel*	1 Thin Spread/7g	25	2.7	360	0.5	3.1	38.0	0.0
Gold, Low Fat, St Ivel*	1 Thin Spread/7g	23	2.4	330	0.5	3.1	35.0	0.0
Gold, Lowest Fat with Omega 3, St Ivel*	1 Thin Spread/7g	13	1.3	192	0.8	4.3	19.0	1.3
Heart, Cholesterol Reducing, Dairygold	1 Thin Spread/7g	24	2.5	338	0.7	2.8	36.0	0.0
Irish, Dairy, Original, Low Low*	1 Thin Spread/7g	24	2.7	346	0.4	0.5	38.0	0.0
Light, Benecol*	1 Thin Spread/7g	23	2.4	333	2.5	0.0	35.0	0.0
Low Fat, Average	1 Thin Spread/7g	27	2.8	390	5.8	0.5	40.5	0.0
Olive, Reduced Fat, Asda*	1 Thin Spread/7g	38	4.1	536	0.2	1.1	59.0	0.0
Olive, Reduced Fat, M & S*	1 Thin Spread/7g	38	4.1	536	0.2	1.1	59.0	0.0
Olive, Reduced Fat, Morrisons*	1 Thin Spread/7g	38	4.2	537	0.9	0.0	59.3	0.3
Olive, Reduced Fat, So Organic, Sainsbury's*	1 Thin Spread/7g	38	4.2	537	0.1	0.4	59.5	0.0
Olive, Waitrose*	1 Thin Spread/7g	37	4.1	534	0.2	0.5	59.0	0.0
Olive Gold, Reduced Fat, Co-Op*	1 Thin Spread/7g	37	4.1	535	0.2	1.0	59.0	0.0
Olive Light, GFY, Asda*	1 Thin Spread/7g	24	2.7	345	0.8	0.0	38.0	0.0
Olive Light, Sainsbury's*	1 Thin Spread/7g	24	2.7	348	1.5	0.0	38.0	0.0
Olive Oil, 55% Reduced Fat, Benecol*	1 Thin Spread/7g	35	3.8	498	0.3	0.5	55.0	0.0
Olive Oil, Bertolli*	1 Thin Spread/7g	38	4.1	536	0.2	1.0	59.0	0.0
Olivite, Low Fat, Weight Watchers*	1 Thin Spread/7g	25	2.7	351	0.0	0.2	38.9	0.0
Organic, Dairy Free, M & S*	1 Thin Spread/7g	37	4.1	531	0.0	0.0	59.0	0.0
Pure Gold, Light, 65% Less Fat, Asda*	1 Thin Spread/7g	17	1.7	239	2.5	1.0	25.0	0.0
Soft, Reduced Fat, Basics, Sainsbury's*	1 Thin Spread/7g	30	3.4	425	0.0	0.0	48.1	0.0
Soft, Sainsbury's*	1 Thin Spread/7g	44	4.9	630	0.1	0.1	70.0	0.0
Sunflower, Average	1 Thin Spread/7g	42	4.6	595	0.1	0.3	65.9	0.4
Sunflower, Enriched, Light, HL, Tesco*	1 Thin Spread/7g	24	2.7	350	0.3	1.0	38.0	0.0
Sunflower, Enriched, Tesco*	1 Thin Spread/7g	37	4.1	535	0.1	0.2	59.0	0.0
Sunflower, Light, BFY, Morrisons*	1 Thin Spread/7g	24	2.7	342	0.0	0.0	38.0	0.0
Sunflower, Light, BGTY, Sainsbury's*	1 Thin Spread/7g	19	2.0	265	0.1	0.8	29.0	0.0
Sunflower, Light, Reduced Fat, Asda*	1 Thin Spread/7g	24	2.7	347	0.3	1.0	38.0	0.1
Sunflower, Low Fat, M & S*	1 Thin Spread/7g	24	2.7	342	0.0	0.0	38.0	1.0
Sunflower, Low Fat, Somerfield*	1 Thin Spread/7g	24	2.7	342	0.0	0.0	38.0	1.0
Vegetable, Dairy Free, Free From, Sainsbury's*	1 Thin Spread/7g	44	4.9	630	0.0	0.0	70.0	3.0
Vegetable, Soft, Tesco*	1 Thin Spread/7g	46	5.1	661	0.1	1.0	73.0	0.0
Vitalite, St Ivel*	1 Thin Spread/7g	35	3.9	503	0.0	0.0	56.0	0.8
with Soya, Dairy Free, Pure Spreads*	1 Thin Spread/7g	37	4.1	532	0.0	0.0	59.0	0.0
with Sunflower, Dairy Free, Organic, Pure Spreads*	1 Thin Spread/7g	42	4.7	603	0.0	0.0	67.0	0.0
SPRING ROLLS								
Chicken, & Chilli, Cantonese, Sainsbury's*	1 Roll/51g	85	2.8	166	9.7	19.4	5.5	0.6
Chicken, & Chilli, Sainsbury's*	1 Roll/50g	92	4.6	185	9.6	15.6	9.3	2.8
Chicken, Asda*	1 Roll/58g	115	5.2	199	4.6	25.0	9.0	3.4
Chicken, Finest, Tesco*	1 Roll/60g	118	5.0	196	10.1	20.1	8.3	1.0
Chicken, Tesco*	1 Roll/50g	115	5.6	231	8.1	24.5	11.2	1.5
Dim Sum, Sainsbury's*	1 Roll/12g	26	1.2	216	4.1	28.2	9.6	2.9
Duck, M & S*	1 Roll/30g	75	3.4	250	9.8	27.7	11.2	1.5
Duck, Mini, Asda*	1 Roll/18g	47	1.9	259	8.7	32.8	10.3	1.9
Duck, Morrisons*	1 Roll/65g	147	6.7	226	6.2	27.2	10.3	1.2
Mini, Sainsbury's*	1 Roll/12g	27	1.2	221	4.2	28.7	9.9	1.6
Mini Vegetable, Co-Op*	1 Roll/18g	40	1.6	220	4.1	30.9	9.1	2.7
Prawn, Cantonese, Sainsbury's*	1 Roll/28g	46	1.7	162	6.8	20.3	6.0	2.5
Prawn, Crispy, M & S*	1 Roll/34g	75	3.4	220	10.0	22.2	9.9	1.3
Prawn, Tesco*	1 Roll/33g	70	3.1	211	8.7	22.8	9.4	1.4

	Measure INFO/WEIGHT	per Measure KCAL	per Measure FAT	Nutrition Values per 100g / 100ml KCAL	PROT	CARB	FAT	FIBRE
SPRING ROLLS								
Thai, Sainsbury's*	1 Roll/30g	69	3.4	229	2.9	28.8	11.3	3.5
Thai Prawn, Waitrose*	1 Roll/50g	109	4.7	219	8.0	25.4	9.5	2.4
Vegetable, Cantonese, Sainsbury's*	1 Roll/36g	84	4.2	233	3.6	28.1	11.7	1.4
Vegetable, Chilled, Tesco*	1 Roll/68g	149	7.6	221	4.0	25.9	11.3	1.6
Vegetable, Chinese, Sainsbury's*	1 Roll/26g	50	2.0	193	4.1	26.9	7.7	1.4
Vegetable, Frozen, Tesco*	1 Roll/60g	123	6.4	205	3.5	23.0	10.6	1.3
Vegetable, M & S*	1 Roll/37g	80	3.6	215	4.3	27.8	9.6	2.0
Vegetable, Mini, Tesco*	1 Roll/18g	36	1.5	205	4.4	26.4	8.6	1.5
Vegetable, Oriental, Sainsbury's*	1 Roll/61g	137	7.2	224	3.8	24.3	11.8	2.9
Vegetable, Waitrose*	1 Roll/57g	107	5.3	187	3.7	22.1	9.3	3.4
Vegetable & Chicken, Tesco*	1 Roll/60g	110	4.6	183	6.1	22.2	7.7	2.5
Waitrose*	1 Roll/33g	61	2.8	184	3.6	23.1	8.6	2.5
SPRITE*								
Sprite*	1 Bottle/500ml	215	0.0	43	0.0	10.5	0.0	0.0
Zero, Lemon & Lime, Sprite*	1 Bottle/500ml	6	0.0	1	0.0	0.0	0.0	0.0
Zero, Sprite*	1 Can/330ml	3	0.0	1	0.0	0.0	0.0	0.0
SPRITZER								
Red Grape, Non-Alcoholic, Extra Special, Asda*	1 Bottle/750ml	330	0.0	44	0.0	11.0	0.0	0.0
Rose & Grape, Non Alcoholic, Extra Special, Asda*	1 Bottle/750ml	90	0.0	12	0.0	3.0	0.0	0.0
White Wine, Echo Falls*	1 Serving/125ml	78	0.0	39	0.0	0.0	0.0	0.0
with White Zinfadel, Echo Falls*	1 Serving/200ml	216	0.0	108	0.0	0.0	0.0	0.0
SQUASH								
Apple, Blackcurrant, Low Sugar, Diluted, Sainsbury's*	1 Glass/250ml	5	0.2	2	0.1	0.2	0.1	0.1
Apple, Cherry & Raspberry, High Juice, Robinson's*	1 Serving/25ml	49	0.0	196	0.2	47.6	0.1	0.0
Apple, Hi Juice, Tesco*	1 fl oz/30ml	52	0.0	173	0.0	42.5	0.0	0.0
Apple, No Added Sugar, Morrisons*	1 Serving/40ml	8	0.0	21	0.1	4.1	0.0	0.0
Apple & Blackcurrant, Fruit, Robinson's*	1 Glass/50ml	18	0.0	36	0.1	8.0	0.0	0.0
Apple & Blackcurrant, No Added Sugar, Tesco*	1 Serving/30ml	4	0.0	15	0.2	2.0	0.0	0.0
Apple & Blackcurrant, Special R, Diluted, Robinson's*	1 fl oz/30ml	2	0.0	8	0.1	1.1	0.1	0.0
Blackcurrant, High Juice, Tesco*	1 Serving/75ml	215	0.0	287	0.3	70.0	0.0	0.0
Cherries & Berries, Sugar Free, Diluted, Tesco*	1 Glass/250ml	5	0.0	2	0.0	0.3	0.0	0.0
Cherries & Berries, Tesco*	1 Serving/25ml	5	0.0	21	0.2	3.2	0.0	0.0
Cranberry, Light, Classic, Undiluted, Ocean Spray*	1 Serving/50ml	31	0.0	63	0.2	14.1	0.0	0.0
Dandelion & Burdock, Morrisons*	1 Serving/50ml	1	0.0	3	0.0	0.0	0.0	0.0
Forest Fruits, High Juice, Undiluted, Robinson's*	1 Serving/25ml	51	0.0	206	0.2	50.0	0.1	0.0
Fruit & Barley, No Added Sugar, Robinson's*	1 fl oz/30ml	4	0.0	14	0.3	2.0	0.0	0.0
Fruit & Barley, Tropical, No Added Sugar, Robinson's*	1 Serving/60ml	7	0.0	12	0.2	1.6	0.0	0.0
Fruit & Barley Orange, Diluted, Robinson's*	1 Serving/50ml	6	0.0	12	0.2	1.7	0.0	0.1
Grape & Passion Fruit, High Juice, Diluted, Sainsbury's*	1 Serving/250ml	100	0.2	40	0.1	9.8	0.1	0.1
Grapefruit, High Juice, No Added Sugar, Sainsbury's*	1 Serving/25ml	1	0.0	6	0.1	1.1	0.0	0.0
Lemon, High Juice, Diluted, Sainsbury's*	1 Glass/250ml	97	0.2	39	0.1	9.1	0.1	0.1
Lemon, High Juice, Tesco*	1 Serving/80ml	141	0.1	176	0.3	43.6	0.1	0.0
Lemon, No Added Sugar, Double Concentrate, Tesco*	1 Serving/25ml	4	0.0	16	0.3	0.7	0.0	0.0
Lemon, No Sugar, Asda*	1 Serving/200ml	5	0.2	2	0.1	0.3	0.1	0.1
Lemon & Lime, Double Strength, No Added Sugar, Asda*	1 Glass/200ml	4	0.0	2	0.0	0.0	0.0	0.0
Mixed Fruit, Diluted, Kia Ora*	1 Serving/250ml	5	0.0	2	0.0	0.3	0.0	0.0
Mixed Fruit, Low Sugar, Sainsbury's*	1 Glass/250ml	5	0.2	2	0.1	0.2	0.1	0.1
Orange, Double Concentrate, Made Up, Smart Price, Asda*	1 Serving/250ml	2	0.0	1	0.0	0.1	0.0	0.0
Orange, Fruit & Barley, Chosen By You, Asda*	1 Serving/100ml	2	0.0	2	0.0	0.2	0.0	0.0
Orange, Hi Juice, Tesco*	1 Serving/75ml	140	0.1	187	0.3	45.0	0.1	0.0
Orange, High Juice, Undiluted, Robinson's*	1 Serving/200ml	364	0.2	182	0.3	44.0	0.1	0.0
Orange, No Added Sugar, High Juice, Sainsbury's*	1 Serving/100ml	6	0.1	6	0.1	1.1	0.1	0.1
Orange, Sainsbury's*	1 Glass/250ml	7	0.2	3	0.1	0.5	0.1	0.1

S

	Measure INFO/WEIGHT	per Measure KCAL	FAT	Nutrition Values per 100g / 100ml KCAL	PROT	CARB	FAT	FIBRE
SQUASH								
Orange, Special R, Diluted, Robinson's*	1 fl oz/30ml	2	0.0	8	0.2	0.7	0.1	0.0
Orange & Mandarin, Fruit Spring, Robinson's*	1 Serving/440ml	26	0.0	6	0.1	0.8	0.0	0.0
Orange & Mango, Low Sugar, Sainsbury's*	1 Serving/250ml	5	0.2	2	0.1	0.2	0.1	0.1
Orange & Mango, No Added Sugar, Robinson's*	1 Serving/25ml	2	0.0	8	0.2	0.9	0.0	0.0
Orange & Pineapple, Original, Undiluted, Robinson's*	1 Serving/250ml	137	0.0	55	1.0	13.0	0.0	0.0
Peach, High Juice, Undiluted, Robinson's*	1 fl oz/30ml	54	0.0	181	0.5	43.0	0.1	0.0
Pink Grapefruit, High Juice, Diluted, Sainsbury's*	1 Serving/250ml	85	0.0	34	0.0	8.1	0.0	0.0
Pink Grapefruit, High Juice, Low Sugar, Tesco*	1 Serving/75ml	12	0.1	16	0.2	3.7	0.1	0.0
Pink Grapefruit, High Juice, Tesco*	1 Serving/75ml	135	0.1	180	0.2	44.6	0.1	0.0
Pink Grapefruit, High Juice, Undiluted, Robinson's*	1 Glass/250ml	455	0.2	182	0.2	43.3	0.1	0.0
Summer Fruit, No Added Sugar, Sainsbury's*	1 Serving/250ml	5	0.2	2	0.1	0.2	0.1	0.1
Summer Fruits, High Juice, Undiluted, Robinson's*	1 fl oz/30ml	61	0.0	203	0.1	49.0	0.1	0.0
Summer Fruits, High Juice, Waitrose*	1 Serving/250ml	102	0.0	41	0.0	10.0	0.0	0.0
Summer Fruits, Robinson's*	1 Measure/25ml	14	0.0	56	0.1	13.0	0.0	0.0
Summer Fruits & Barley, no Added Sugar, Tesco*	1 Serving/50ml	5	0.0	11	0.2	1.7	0.0	0.0
Summerfruits, High Juice, Tesco*	1 Serving/50ml	11	0.0	23	0.2	4.5	0.0	0.0
Tropical, High Juice, Tesco*	1 Glass/75ml	141	0.1	188	0.2	46.6	0.1	0.1
Tropical, No Added Sugar, Diluted, Tesco*	1 Glass/200ml	18	0.0	9	0.2	0.9	0.0	0.0
Tropical Fruits, Sainsbury's*	1 Serving/250ml	95	0.2	38	0.1	9.3	0.1	0.1
Winter, Acorn, Baked, Average	*1oz/28g*	*16*	*0.0*	*56*	*1.1*	*12.6*	*0.1*	*3.2*
Winter, Acorn, Raw, Average	*1oz/28g*	*11*	*0.0*	*40*	*0.8*	*9.0*	*0.1*	*2.3*
Winter, All Varieties, Flesh Only, Raw, Average	*1oz/28g*	*10*	*0.0*	*34*	*0.9*	*8.6*	*0.1*	*1.5*
Winter, Butternut, Baked, Average	*1oz/28g*	*9*	*0.0*	*32*	*0.9*	*7.4*	*0.1*	*1.4*
Winter, Butternut, Raw, Prepared, Average	1 Serving/80g	29	0.1	36	1.1	8.3	0.1	1.6
Winter, Butternut, Raw, Unprepared, Average	*1 Serving/80g*	*29*	*0.1*	*36*	*1.1*	*8.3*	*0.1*	*1.6*
Winter, Spaghetti, Baked	*1oz/28g*	*6*	*0.1*	*23*	*0.7*	*4.3*	*0.3*	*2.1*
Winter, Spaghetti, Including Pips & Rind, Raw	*1oz/28g*	*7*	*0.2*	*26*	*0.6*	*4.6*	*0.6*	*2.3*
SQUID								
Calamari, Battered with Tartar Sauce Dip, Tesco*	1 Pack/210g	573	40.9	273	8.9	15.4	19.5	0.6
Dried, Average	*1oz/28g*	*88*	*1.3*	*313*	*63.3*	*4.8*	*4.6*	*0.0*
in Batter, Fried in Blended Oil, Average	1oz/28g	55	2.8	195	11.5	15.7	10.0	0.5
Pieces in Squid Ink, Palacio De Oriente*	1 Can/120g	274	21.6	228	13.0	3.6	18.0	0.0
Raw, Average	*1oz/28g*	*23*	*0.5*	*81*	*15.4*	*1.2*	*1.7*	*0.0*
STAR FRUIT								
Average, Tesco	*1oz/28g*	*9*	*0.1*	*32*	*0.5*	*7.3*	*0.3*	*1.3*
STARBAR								
Cadbury*	1 Bar/53g	260	14.8	491	10.7	49.0	27.9	0.0
STARBURST								
Fruit Chews, Tropical, Mars*	1 Tube/45g	168	3.3	373	0.0	76.9	7.3	0.0
Joosters, Mars*	1 Pack/45g	160	0.0	356	0.0	88.8	0.1	0.0
Juicy Gums, Mars*	1 Pack/45g	139	1.8	309	5.9	71.0	4.1	0.0
Mars*	1 Pack/45g	185	3.4	411	0.3	85.3	7.6	0.0
STEAK & KIDNEY PUDDING								
Fray Bentos*	1 Tin/213g	477	26.8	224	7.8	19.8	12.6	0.0
M & S*	1 Pudding/121g	260	13.4	215	9.2	19.4	11.1	3.2
Sainsbury's*	1 Pudding/435g	1135	62.6	261	10.5	22.3	14.4	0.8
Waitrose*	1 Pudding/223g	497	26.1	223	8.9	20.4	11.7	1.2
STEAMED PUDDING								
Apple & Sultana, BGTY, Sainsbury's*	1 Pudding/110g	294	3.2	267	2.9	57.4	2.9	0.8
Apple with Wild Berry Sauce, BGTY, Sainsbury's*	1 Pudding/110g	308	3.7	280	2.6	59.7	3.4	1.4
Chocolate Fudge, Less Than 5% Fat, Aunty's*	1 Pudding/110g	329	5.3	299	3.0	58.2	4.8	1.6
Golden Syrup, Aunty's*	1 Pudding/110g	324	4.5	295	2.9	58.6	4.1	0.7
Lemon, BGTY, Sainsbury's*	1 Pudding/110g	307	3.2	279	3.0	60.2	2.9	0.7

S

	Measure INFO/WEIGHT	per Measure KCAL	FAT	Nutrition Values per 100g / 100ml KCAL	PROT	CARB	FAT	FIBRE
STEAMED PUDDING								
Sticky Toffee, Aunty's*	1 Pudding/110g	331	5.3	301	2.6	58.4	4.8	1.2
Toffee & Date, Aunty's*	1 Pudding/110g	320	5.1	291	2.6	59.1	4.6	1.1
STEW								
Beef, & Dumplings, Frozen, Tesco*	1 Serving/400g	380	12.8	95	5.7	10.5	3.2	1.5
Beef, Asda*	½ Can/196g	178	4.9	91	10.0	7.0	2.5	1.5
Beef, Meal for One, M & S*	1 Pack/440g	350	8.4	80	7.0	8.7	1.9	2.0
Beef, Value, Tesco*	1 Serving/200g	170	9.8	85	4.0	6.2	4.9	1.0
Beef, with Dumplings, Classic British, Sainsbury's*	1 Pack/450g	531	23.4	118	7.7	10.2	5.2	0.5
Beef, with Dumplings, COU, M & S*	1 Pack/454g	431	11.8	95	8.9	9.1	2.6	0.8
Beef, with Dumplings, Sainsbury's*	1 Pack/450g	603	27.4	134	9.3	10.5	6.1	0.7
Beef & Dumplings	1 Serving/652g	766	32.7	117	7.4	10.7	5.0	0.8
Beef & Dumplings, Birds Eye*	1 Pack/400g	308	8.4	77	4.4	10.0	2.1	0.9
Beef & Dumplings, Countryside*	1 Pack/300g	246	6.9	82	8.1	7.3	2.3	0.5
Beef & Dumplings, Plumrose*	½ Can/196g	143	3.9	73	6.1	9.0	2.0	0.0
Beef & Dumplings, Weight Watchers*	1 Pack/327g	262	6.9	80	5.2	10.0	2.1	0.8
Chicken, & Dumplings, Birds Eye*	1 Pack/320g	282	8.6	88	7.0	8.9	2.7	0.5
Chicken, & Dumplings, Tesco*	1 Serving/450g	567	29.7	126	7.6	9.1	6.6	0.7
Irish, Diet Chef Ltd*	1 Pack/300g	252	8.1	84	8.7	6.3	2.7	1.7
Irish, Morrisons*	1 Can/392g	243	4.7	62	3.8	8.9	1.2	0.0
Irish, Plumrose*	1 Can/392g	318	9.8	81	7.5	7.2	2.5	0.0
Irish, Sainsbury's*	1 Pack/450g	274	9.4	61	5.7	4.8	2.1	0.5
Lentil & Vegetable, Organic, Simply Organic*	1 Pack/400g	284	6.0	71	3.5	11.0	1.5	1.3
Lentil & Winter Vegetable, Organic, Pure & Pronto*	1 Pack/400g	364	9.6	91	3.6	14.0	2.4	4.0
Mixed Vegetable Topped with Herb Dumplings, Tesco*	1 Pack/420g	508	26.0	121	1.9	14.5	6.2	1.3
Pearl Barley Gumbo, Chosen By You, Asda*	1 Pack/350g	336	6.6	96	3.0	14.5	1.9	4.4
Tuscan Bean, Tasty Veg Pot, Innocent*	1 Pot/400g	320	7.6	80	3.1	12.5	1.9	3.6
STIR FRY								
Baby Leaf, Ready Prepared, M & S*	1 Serving/125g	25	0.1	20	1.7	4.9	0.1	2.5
Baby Leaf, Waitrose*	1 Pack/265g	50	0.3	19	1.7	2.9	0.1	2.0
Baby Leaf & Baby Corn, Morrisons*	½ Pack/127g	33	0.5	26	1.3	4.3	0.4	1.4
Baby Vegetable & Pak Choi, Two Step, Tesco*	½ Pack/95g	29	0.8	31	2.1	4.0	0.8	2.3
Bean Sprout, Chinese, Sainsbury's*	1 Pack/300g	144	8.4	48	1.9	5.1	2.8	1.5
Bean Sprout, Ready to Eat, Washed, Sainsbury's*	1 Serving/150g	82	5.8	55	1.5	3.3	3.9	1.8
Bean Sprouts & Vegetables, Asda*	½ Pack/173g	107	6.9	62	2.0	4.5	4.0	1.8
Beef, BGTY, Sainsbury's*	½ Pack/125g	156	5.1	125	22.0	0.1	4.1	0.0
Beef, Less Than 10% Fat, Asda*	1 Pack/227g	275	6.4	121	24.0	0.0	2.8	0.8
Beef, Less Than 3% Fat, BGTY, Sainsbury's*	½ Pack/125g	134	2.6	107	22.1	0.0	2.1	0.0
Chicken Chow Mein, Orient Express, Oriental Express*	1 Pack/400g	384	10.8	96	7.3	10.7	2.7	2.2
Chicken Noodle, GFY, Asda*	1 Pack/330g	403	10.9	122	7.0	16.0	3.3	2.4
Chinese, Eastern Inspirations*	½ Pack/170g	49	0.8	29	2.7	3.5	0.5	1.8
Chinese, Family, Sainsbury's*	1 Serving/150g	60	3.0	40	2.3	3.3	2.0	3.6
Chinese Bean Sprout, Sainsbury's*	½ Pack/313g	150	8.8	48	1.9	5.1	2.8	1.5
Chinese Chicken, Sizzling, Oriental Express*	1 Pack/400g	400	8.0	100	6.6	13.8	2.0	1.7
Chinese Exotic Vegetable, Sainsbury's*	1 Pack/350g	133	7.7	38	1.7	2.8	2.2	1.8
Chinese Prawn, Iceland*	1 Pack/340g	235	4.4	69	3.1	11.1	1.3	2.1
Chinese Style, Co-Op*	1 Pack/300g	105	1.2	35	3.0	6.0	0.4	2.0
Chinese Style Chicken, GFY, Asda*	1 Pack/338g	362	5.8	107	6.0	17.0	1.7	1.5
Chinese Style Prawn, GFY, Asda*	1 Pack/400g	324	6.4	81	3.6	13.0	1.6	1.6
Chinese Style Turkey, Asda*	½ Pack/210g	321	6.0	153	23.8	8.1	2.9	0.8
Chinese Vegetables, Oriental Express*	½ Pack/200g	44	0.4	22	1.4	3.7	0.2	2.2
Chinese Vegetables, Tesco*	1 Serving/175g	93	0.7	53	1.6	10.8	0.4	1.3
Chunky Pepper & Butternut Squash, Finest, Tesco*	1 Pack/220g	68	0.9	31	1.6	4.2	0.4	2.0
Classic Medley, Veg Cuisine*	½ Pack/150g	45	0.6	30	2.5	4.1	0.4	2.1

	Measure INFO/WEIGHT	per Measure KCAL	FAT	Nutrition Values per 100g / 100ml KCAL	PROT	CARB	FAT	FIBRE
STIR FRY								
Edamame Bean, Morrisons*	½ Pack/175g	220	8.4	126	10.9	7.7	4.8	5.2
Edamame Bean & Ginger, Tesco*	1 Pack/290g	145	4.6	50	4.1	4.9	1.6	2.5
Green Vegetable, M & S*	1 Pack/220g	165	13.0	75	3.1	2.5	5.9	2.2
Hot & Spicy with Red Chillies, Cooked, Fresh Tastes, Asda*	½ Pack/125g	60	2.5	48	1.8	4.2	2.0	0.0
Mediterranean Style, Waitrose*	1 Pack/305g	82	1.2	27	1.6	4.6	0.4	2.2
Mexican Vegetables, Lidl*	1 Serving/100g	97	5.7	97	3.4	8.1	5.7	0.0
Mixed Pepper, Fresh Tastes, Asda*	½ Pack/160g	75	4.2	47	1.4	4.6	2.6	2.0
Mixed Pepper, HL, Tesco*	1 Pack/325g	62	0.3	19	1.9	2.6	0.1	1.5
Mixed Pepper, Just Stir Fry, Sainsbury's*	½ Pack/150g	117	8.4	67	1.5	4.6	4.8	1.2
Mixed Pepper, Sainsbury's*	1 Pack/300g	201	14.4	67	1.5	4.6	4.8	1.2
Mixed Pepper, Tesco*	1 Serving/34g	12	0.1	34	2.0	4.6	0.4	2.0
Mixed Pepper, Waitrose*	½ Pack/150g	52	0.6	35	1.9	4.8	0.4	1.9
Mixed Pepper & Vegetable, Asda*	½ Pack/150g	42	1.5	28	1.6	3.2	1.0	2.6
Mixed Vegetable, Asda*	1 Serving/200g	96	5.0	48	1.7	4.7	2.5	3.0
Mushroom, Tesco*	1 Portion/100g	34	0.5	34	2.6	3.9	0.5	2.0
Mushroom, Waitrose*	½ Pack/165g	43	0.7	26	2.3	3.3	0.4	1.6
Noodles & Bean Sprouts, Tesco*	½ Pack/125g	131	2.6	105	4.2	16.1	2.1	0.7
Orient Inspired, M & S*	1 Serving/250g	50	0.7	20	1.6	3.4	0.3	1.6
Oriental, Ready Prepared, M & S*	½ Pack/260g	65	1.6	25	2.3	2.1	0.6	1.9
Oriental Chinese, Waitrose*	1 Serving/150g	40	0.6	27	2.2	3.9	0.4	1.4
Oriental Leaf, M & S*	½ Pack/125g	25	0.6	20	1.9	2.5	0.5	2.2
Oriental Style Pak Choi, M & S*	1 Pack/220g	165	12.5	75	2.2	3.5	5.7	2.4
Oriental Vegetable, Frozen, Asda*	1 Serving/150g	115	6.7	77	2.1	7.0	4.5	1.7
Oriental Vegetable, Szechuan, Spicy, Sainsbury's*	1 Pack/350g	224	15.4	64	1.3	4.9	4.4	1.7
Spicy Thai Style Noodle, Tesco*	1 Pack/500g	335	13.0	67	2.6	8.4	2.6	1.3
Sweet & Sour, Tesco*	1 Pack/350g	161	1.0	46	1.8	9.1	0.3	1.3
Sweet & Sour Vegetable, Somerfield*	1 Pack/350g	248	3.5	71	2.0	14.0	1.0	0.0
Sweet Pepper, M & S*	1 Pack/400g	160	7.2	40	2.3	3.5	1.8	0.6
Thai Style, Tesco*	1 Pack/350g	301	17.8	86	3.9	6.2	5.1	1.9
Turkey, Fresh, Good Intentions, Somerfield*	½ Pack/150g	246	6.7	164	31.0	0.0	4.5	0.0
Vegetable, Asda*	1 Pack/300g	132	6.9	44	1.6	4.2	2.3	3.1
Vegetable, Cantonese, Sainsbury's*	1 Serving/150g	90	5.2	60	2.8	4.2	3.5	2.7
Vegetable, Chinese Style, Asda*	1 Pack/300g	81	2.1	27	1.6	3.6	0.7	2.8
Vegetable, Crunchy, Sainsbury's*	½ Pack/150g	85	5.8	57	1.4	4.1	3.9	2.1
Vegetable, Crunchy, Waitrose*	1 Pack/300g	81	0.3	27	1.6	4.8	0.1	2.4
Vegetable, Oriental, Frozen, Freshly, Asda*	1 Serving/100g	25	0.3	25	2.2	3.4	0.3	2.0
Vegetable, Premium, Sainsbury's*	½ Pack/150g	90	5.2	60	2.8	4.2	3.5	2.7
Vegetable, Ready Prepared, M & S*	½ Pack/150g	37	0.4	25	2.2	3.5	0.3	2.2
Vegetable, Sweet & Crunchy, Waitrose*	1 Pack/300g	69	0.3	23	1.8	3.6	0.1	1.4
Vegetable, Thai Style, Tesco*	½ Pack/135g	42	0.7	31	2.3	4.2	0.5	2.1
Vegetable & Beansprout, Tesco*	1 Pack/380g	129	1.9	34	2.0	5.4	0.5	2.2
Vegetable & Beansprout with Peanut Sauce, Tesco*	1 Serving/475g	408	23.7	86	3.9	6.2	5.0	1.9
Vegetable & Broccoli, Fresh Tastes, Asda*	½ Bag/175g	87	3.5	50	2.5	3.7	2.0	3.7
Vegetable & Noodle, Asda*	1 Pack/330g	465	14.8	141	4.0	21.0	4.5	3.0
Vegetable Noodles, BGTY, Sainsbury's*	1 Pack/455g	391	9.1	86	3.2	14.0	2.0	1.4
Water Chestnut & Bamboo Shoot, Fresh Tastes, Asda*	½ Pack/210g	82	2.9	39	1.4	4.3	1.4	1.7
STOCK								
Beef, As Sold, Stock Pot, Knorr*	1 Serving/5g	5	0.4	89	3.0	3.5	7.0	0.7
Beef, Cooks' Ingredients, Waitrose*	1 Jar/500g	74	0.5	15	3.0	0.3	0.1	0.8
Beef, Fresh, Tesco*	1 Serving/300ml	54	0.9	18	2.1	1.6	0.3	0.5
Beef, Made Up, Stock Pot, Knorr*	1 Serving/100ml	5	0.4	5	0.1	0.2	0.4	0.0
Beef, Pots, Unprepared, Sainsbury's*	1 Pot/28g	31	1.7	112	4.1	8.5	6.2	2.9
Beef, Signature, Sainsbury's*	1 Pack/500g	65	1.0	13	2.7	0.0	0.2	0.0

	Measure INFO/WEIGHT	per Measure		Nutrition Values per 100g / 100ml				
		KCAL	FAT	KCAL	PROT	CARB	FAT	FIBRE
STOCK								
Beef, Simply Stock, Knorr*	1 Serving/100ml	6	0.0	6	1.4	0.1	0.0	0.0
Beef, Slowly Prepared, Sainsbury's*	1 Serving/100g	7	0.3	7	0.7	0.3	0.3	0.5
Chicken, As Sold, Stock Pot, Knorr*	1 Serving/100ml	5	0.4	95	2.4	4.9	7.3	0.8
Chicken, Asda*	½ Pot/150g	25	1.3	17	1.8	0.7	0.9	0.2
Chicken, Concentrated, M & S*	1 Tsp/5g	16	0.9	315	25.6	12.2	18.1	0.8
Chicken, Cooks' Ingredients, Waitrose*	1 Pack/500ml	75	0.5	15	3.2	0.3	0.1	0.2
Chicken, Fresh, Sainsbury's*	½ Pot/142ml	23	0.1	16	3.7	0.1	0.1	0.3
Chicken, Fresh, Tesco*	1 Serving/300ml	27	0.3	9	1.6	0.5	0.1	0.5
Chicken, Granules, Knorr*	1 Tsp/5g	10	0.2	232	13.1	36.5	3.7	0.4
Chicken, Home Prepared, Average	*1 fl oz/30ml*	*7*	*0.3*	*24*	*3.8*	*0.7*	*0.9*	*0.3*
Chicken, Made Up, Stock Pot, Knorr*	1 fl oz/30ml	1	0.1	5	0.1	0.3	0.4	0.0
Chicken, Prepared, Tesco*	1 Serving/300ml	54	0.3	18	2.4	1.8	0.1	0.5
Chicken, Simply Stock, Knorr*	1 Pack/450ml	27	0.0	6	1.5	0.1	0.0	0.1
Chicken, Slowly Prepared, Sainsbury's*	1 Pot/300g	27	0.3	9	0.6	1.3	0.1	0.5
Fish, Fresh, Finest, Tesco*	1 Serving/100g	10	0.0	10	0.6	1.8	0.0	0.5
Fish, Home Prepared, Average	*1 Serving/250ml*	*42*	*2.0*	*17*	*2.3*	*0.0*	*0.8*	*0.0*
Vegetable, As Sold, Stock Pot, Knorr*	1 Serving/100ml	6	0.5	117	2.4	5.7	9.4	1.3
Vegetable, Campbell's*	1 Serving/250ml	37	1.7	15	0.3	2.0	0.7	0.0
Vegetable, Concentrated, M & S*	1 Tsp/5g	19	0.9	380	3.3	43.0	19.0	1.2
Vegetable, Cooks Ingredients, Waitrose*	1 Pouch/500ml	15	0.5	3	0.2	0.4	0.1	0.5
Vegetable, Granules, Knorr*	2 Tsp/9g	18	0.1	199	8.5	39.9	0.6	0.9
Vegetable, Made Up, Stock Pot, Knorr*	1 Serving/100ml	6	0.5	6	0.1	0.3	0.5	0.1
Vegetable, Tablets, Sainsbury's*	1 Tablet/11g	1	0.1	7	0.4	0.2	0.5	0.1
STOCK CUBES								
Basil, Herb Cubes, Knorr*	1 Cube/10g	47	3.4	472	6.1	35.9	33.8	0.6
Beef, Dry Weight, Bovril*	1 Cube/6g	12	0.2	197	10.8	29.3	4.1	0.0
Beef, Dry Weight, Oxo*	1 Cube/6g	15	0.3	265	17.3	38.4	4.7	1.5
Beef, Knorr*	1 Cube/10g	31	2.3	310	5.0	19.0	23.0	0.0
Beef, Organic, Kallo*	1 Cube/12g	25	1.0	208	16.7	16.7	8.3	0.0
Beef, Smart Price, Asda*	1 Cube/11g	31	2.5	279	10.0	8.0	23.0	0.0
Beef, Telma*	1 Serving/15g	20	1.0	133	0.0	0.0	6.7	0.0
Beef, Tesco*	1 Cube/7g	17	0.2	260	9.7	48.9	2.8	1.3
Chicken	1 Cube/6g	14	0.9	237	15.4	9.9	15.4	0.0
Chicken, Dry, Average	1 Cube/10g	29	1.8	293	7.3	25.5	18.0	0.4
Chicken, Dry, Oxo*	1 Cube/7g	17	0.2	249	10.9	44.0	3.3	0.9
Chicken, Just Bouillon, Kallo*	1 Cube/12g	30	1.3	247	11.8	26.1	10.6	1.0
Chicken, Knorr*	1 Cube/10g	31	2.0	310	4.0	29.0	20.0	0.0
Chicken, Made Up, Average	1 Pint/568ml	43	1.0	8	0.4	1.1	0.2	0.1
Chicken, Prepared, Oxo*	1 Cube/100ml	9	0.1	9	0.4	1.5	0.1	0.1
Chicken, Telma*	1 Cube/15g	25	0.1	167	0.0	0.0	1.0	0.0
Fish, Knorr*	1 Cube/10g	32	2.4	321	8.0	18.0	24.0	1.0
Fish, Sainsbury's*	1 Cube/11g	31	2.2	282	19.1	7.3	20.0	0.9
Garlic, Dry Weight, Oxo*	1 Cube/6g	18	0.3	298	13.4	48.5	5.5	3.6
Ham, Knorr*	1 Cube/10g	31	1.9	313	11.8	24.4	18.7	0.0
Indian, Dry Weight, Oxo*	1 Cube/6g	17	0.5	291	11.5	43.9	7.7	6.7
Italian, Dry Weight, Oxo*	1 Cube/6g	19	0.4	309	11.9	48.9	7.3	4.6
Lamb, Made Up, Knorr*	1 Cube/10g	32	2.5	320	11.0	14.0	25.0	0.0
Parsley & Garlic, Herb Cubes, Knorr*	1 Cube/10g	42	2.7	422	8.6	35.2	27.4	1.8
Vegetable, Average	1 Cube/7g	18	1.2	253	13.5	11.6	17.3	0.0
Vegetable, Dry, Oxo*	1 Cube/6g	17	0.3	251	10.4	41.4	4.9	1.4
Vegetable, Knorr*	1 Cube/10g	33	2.4	330	10.0	25.0	24.0	1.0
Vegetable, Low Salt, Organic, Made Up, Kallo*	1 Serving/500ml	50	3.5	10	0.3	0.7	0.7	0.2
Vegetable, Made Up, Organic, Kallo*	2 Cubes/100ml	7	0.4	7	0.1	0.5	0.4	0.1

	Measure INFO/WEIGHT	per Measure KCAL	FAT	Nutrition Values per 100g / 100ml KCAL	PROT	CARB	FAT	FIBRE
STOCK CUBES								
Vegetable, Made Up, Oxo*	1 Cube/100ml	9	0.2	9	0.4	1.4	0.2	0.1
Vegetable, Organic, Yeast Free, Dry, Kallo*	1 Cube/11g	37	3.1	334	11.4	8.2	27.8	2.3
Vegetable, Premium, Made Up, Kallo*	1 Serving/125ml	7	0.4	6	0.4	0.4	0.3	0.1
Vegetable, Yeast Free, Made Up, Kallo*	1 Cube/500ml	35	3.0	7	0.3	0.2	0.6	0.1
Vegetable Bouillon, Vegetarian, Amoy*	1 Cube/10g	30	2.0	300	0.0	20.0	20.0	0.0
Vegetable Bouillon, Yeast Free, Made Up, Marigold*	1 Serving/250ml	19	1.6	8	0.0	0.5	0.6	0.0
STOLLEN								
Slices, Average	1 Slice/42g	160	6.3	381	5.5	55.8	15.0	3.1
STRAWBERRIES								
& Creme Fraiche, Shapers, Boots*	1 Pack/100g	77	5.7	77	1.4	5.1	5.7	0.8
Fresh, Raw, Average	*1 Strawberry/12g*	*3*	*0.0*	*28*	*0.8*	*6.0*	*0.1*	*1.4*
Frozen, Average	*1 Serving/100g*	*29*	*0.2*	*29*	*0.8*	*6.3*	*0.2*	*1.0*
in Fruit Juice, Canned, Average	*1/3 Can/127g*	*58*	*0.0*	*45*	*0.4*	*11.0*	*0.0*	*1.0*
in Light Syrup, Canned, Drained, Tesco*	1 Can/149g	100	0.1	67	0.5	16.0	0.1	0.7
in Raspberry Sauce, WT5, Sainsbury's*	1 Serving/170g	110	0.2	65	0.7	15.3	0.1	2.3
in Syrup, Canned, Average	1 Serving/100g	63	0.0	63	0.4	15.2	0.0	0.6
STROGANOFF								
Beef, & Rice, TTD, Sainsbury's*	1 Pack/410g	595	20.9	145	9.6	15.2	5.1	1.7
Beef, 115, Oakhouse Foods Ltd*	1 Meal/400g	428	19.6	107	5.0	10.8	4.9	0.6
Beef, Asda*	1 Serving/120g	276	20.4	230	16.0	3.3	17.0	0.6
Beef, BGTY, Sainsbury's*	1 Pack/400g	416	10.4	104	5.6	14.6	2.6	0.6
Beef, Finest, Tesco*	½ Pack/200g	330	13.4	165	9.4	16.2	6.7	0.7
Beef, HL, Tesco*	1 Pack/400g	400	8.8	100	7.0	13.0	2.2	1.3
Beef, Low Fat with White & Wild Rice, Waitrose*	1 Pack/401g	429	6.4	107	7.9	15.3	1.6	1.0
Beef, Sainsbury's*	1 Can/200g	232	12.0	116	12.5	3.0	6.0	0.2
Beef, Weight Watchers*	1 Pack/330g	297	7.6	90	4.3	13.0	2.3	0.1
Beef, with Rice 'n' Peppers, Tesco*	1 Pack/450g	562	19.8	125	7.5	13.1	4.4	0.4
Beef, with White & Wild Rice, Classic, Tesco*	1 Pack/500g	770	29.6	154	9.5	15.5	5.9	2.3
Chicken, with Rice, BGTY, Sainsbury's*	1 Pack/415g	448	5.4	108	7.0	17.1	1.3	1.1
Chicken & Mushroom, COU, M & S*	1 Serving/400g	400	8.0	100	3.2	16.7	2.0	0.1
Mushroom, Diet Chef Ltd*	1 Pack/250g	202	14.7	81	2.6	4.5	5.9	1.7
Mushroom, Eat Smart, Morrisons*	1 Pack/400g	312	4.4	78	2.6	14.3	1.1	1.0
Mushroom, Solo Slim, Rosemary Conley*	1 Pack/251g	193	11.3	77	2.7	6.5	4.5	2.7
Mushroom, with Rice, BGTY, Sainsbury's*	1 Serving/450g	418	6.7	93	3.3	16.6	1.5	1.0
Mushroom, with Rice, Vegetarian, Light Choices, Tesco*	1 Pack/450g	420	7.5	95	2.6	16.4	1.7	1.1
STRUDEL								
Apple, Co-Op*	1 Slice/100g	225	12.0	225	3.0	28.0	12.0	3.0
Apple, Frozen, Sainsbury's*	1 Serving/100g	283	15.4	283	3.2	32.8	15.4	1.9
Apple, Tesco*	1 Serving/150g	432	21.6	288	3.3	36.4	14.4	2.8
Apple & Mincemeat, Tesco*	1 Serving/100g	322	16.7	322	3.3	39.6	16.7	2.0
Tesco*	1 Serving/150g	370	19.3	247	2.9	29.8	12.9	4.7
Woodland Fruit, Tesco*	1 Serving/100g	257	13.1	257	3.2	31.5	13.1	1.8
STUFFING								
Apricot & Walnut, Made Up, Celebrations, Paxo*	1 Serving/50g	80	1.7	161	4.3	28.0	3.5	2.8
Olde English Chestnut, Sainsbury's*	1 Serving/110g	216	12.8	196	9.4	13.5	11.6	2.1
Parsley, Thyme & Lemon Stuffing, Paxo*	1 Serving/45g	67	0.9	150	4.3	28.4	2.1	2.4
Parsley & Thyme, Co-Op*	1 Serving/28g	95	0.8	340	10.0	67.0	3.0	6.0
Sage & Onion, for Chicken, Paxo*	1 Serving/50g	61	0.9	123	3.6	23.0	1.8	1.7
Sage & Onion, Made Up, Paxo*	1 Serving/50g	71	0.6	143	3.2	29.9	1.2	1.9
Sage & Onion with Lemon, Paxo*	1 Serving/50g	61	0.6	122	3.4	24.2	1.2	1.9
Sausagemeat, Sainsbury's*	1 Serving/100g	175	4.2	175	7.0	27.0	4.2	2.3
Sausagemeat & Thyme, Made Up, Celebrations, Paxo*	1 Serving/50g	80	1.7	160	6.3	25.8	3.5	4.0

S

	Measure INFO/WEIGHT	per Measure KCAL	FAT	Nutrition Values per 100g / 100ml KCAL	PROT	CARB	FAT	FIBRE
STUFFING BALLS								
Pork, Sausagemeat, Aunt Bessie's*	1 Ball/26g	55	2.1	212	7.2	27.3	8.2	3.0
Sage & Onion, Aunt Bessie's*	1 Ball/26g	63	2.3	243	6.4	34.4	8.9	3.1
Sage & Onion, Meat-Free, Aunt Bessie's*	1 Ball/28g	54	1.9	193	5.4	28.0	6.7	1.7
Sage & Onion, Tesco*	1 Serving/20g	64	4.4	322	10.0	21.1	22.0	1.9
STUFFING MIX								
Apple, Mustard & Herb, Paxo*	1 Serving/50g	83	1.0	166	4.2	32.8	2.0	4.0
Apple & Herb, Special Recipe, Sainsbury's*	1 Serving/41g	68	0.9	165	3.8	32.4	2.2	2.2
Chestnut, Morrisons*	1 Serving/20g	33	0.7	165	4.6	29.1	3.4	3.7
Chestnut & Cranberry, Celebration, Paxo*	1 Serving/25g	35	0.5	141	4.0	26.7	2.0	2.4
Date, Walnut & Stilton, Special Recipe, Sainsbury's*	1 Serving/25g	49	2.1	196	5.2	25.0	8.4	2.0
Herb & Onion, Gluten Free, Allergycare*	1 Serving/12g	43	0.3	360	7.9	76.8	2.4	0.0
Parsley, Thyme & Lemon, Sainsbury's*	1 Pack/170g	240	2.2	141	4.2	28.2	1.3	1.3
Sage & Onion, Dry Weight, Tesco*	1 Std Pack/170g	578	4.1	340	10.3	69.3	2.4	6.3
Sage & Onion, Made Up, Paxo*	1 Serving/60g	74	1.1	123	3.6	23.0	1.8	1.7
Sage & Onion, Prepared, Tesco*	1 Serving/100g	50	0.4	50	1.5	10.1	0.4	0.9
Sausage Meat, Morrisons*	1 Serving/20g	35	0.5	174	6.8	30.8	2.6	2.9
SUET								
Beef, Shredded, Original, Atora*	1 Pack/200g	1592	163.0	796	1.1	14.6	81.5	0.5
Beef, Tesco*	1 Serving/100g	854	91.9	854	0.6	6.2	91.9	0.1
Vegetable, Average	*1oz/28g*	*234*	*24.6*	*836*	*1.2*	*10.1*	*87.9*	*0.0*
SUET PUDDING								
Average	*1oz/28g*	*94*	*5.1*	*335*	*4.4*	*40.5*	*18.3*	*0.9*
SUGAR								
Brown, Soft, Average	*1 Tsp/4g*	*15*	*0.0*	*382*	*0.0*	*96.5*	*0.0*	*0.0*
Brown, Soft, Light, Average	*1 Tsp/5g*	*20*	*0.0*	*393*	*0.2*	*97.8*	*0.1*	*0.0*
Caster, Average	*1 Tsp/5g*	*20*	*0.0*	*399*	*0.0*	*99.8*	*0.0*	*0.0*
Dark Brown, Muscovado, Average	*1 Tsp/7g*	*27*	*0.0*	*380*	*0.2*	*94.7*	*0.0*	*0.0*
Dark Brown, Soft, Average	*1 Tsp/5g*	*18*	*0.0*	*369*	*0.1*	*92.0*	*0.0*	*0.0*
Demerara, Average	*1 Tsp/5g*	*18*	*0.0*	*367*	*0.2*	*99.1*	*0.0*	*0.0*
Fructose, Fruit Sugar, Tate & Lyle*	1 Tsp/4g	16	0.0	400	0.0	100.0	0.0	0.0
Golden, Unrefined, Average	*1 Tsp/4g*	*16*	*0.0*	*399*	*0.0*	*99.8*	*0.0*	*0.0*
Granulated, Organic, Average	*1 Tsp/4g*	*16*	*0.0*	*398*	*0.2*	*99.7*	*0.0*	*0.0*
Icing, Average	*1 Tsp/4g*	*16*	*0.0*	*394*	*0.0*	*102.1*	*0.0*	*0.0*
Light Or Diet, Average	*1 Tsp/4g*	*16*	*0.0*	*394*	*0.0*	*98.5*	*0.0*	*0.0*
Muscovado, Light, Average	1 Tsp/5g	19	0.0	384	0.0	96.0	0.0	0.0
White, Granulated, Average	*1 Tsp/5g*	*20*	*0.0*	*398*	*0.0*	*100.0*	*0.0*	*0.0*
White Plus Stevia Blend, Light at Heart, Tate & Lyle*	1 Serving/2g	8	0.0	398	0.0	99.6	0.0	0.0
SULTANAS								
Average	*1oz/28g*	*82*	*0.1*	*291*	*2.8*	*69.2*	*0.4*	*2.0*
SUNDAE								
Banoffee, Perfectly Balanced, Waitrose*	1 Pot/115g	143	2.2	124	3.1	23.6	1.9	0.8
Blackcurrant, M & S*	1 Sundae/53g	212	10.2	400	3.0	54.2	19.2	1.9
Chocolate, Mini, Asda*	1 Pot/86g	199	12.9	231	3.1	21.0	15.0	1.7
Chocolate, Sainsbury's*	1 Pot/140g	393	29.8	281	2.5	19.3	21.3	0.6
Chocolate & Cookie, Weight Watchers*	1 Pot/82g	128	2.8	156	2.5	30.3	3.4	2.2
Chocolate & Sticky Toffee, Asda*	1 Sundae/215g	755	51.6	351	2.8	31.0	24.0	0.5
Chocolate & Vanilla, HL, Tesco*	1 Sundae/120g	193	3.1	161	2.8	31.5	2.6	0.6
Chocolate & Vanilla, Tesco*	1 Sundae/70g	140	6.0	199	2.8	27.5	8.6	0.5
Chocolate Brownie, Finest, Tesco*	1 Serving/215g	778	56.5	362	2.7	28.7	26.3	2.3
Chocolate Mint, COU, M & S*	1 Pot/90g	108	2.3	120	5.4	17.8	2.6	0.5
Chocolate Nut	1 Serving/70g	195	10.7	278	3.0	34.2	15.3	0.1
Galaxy Caramel, Eden Vale*	1 Serving/128g	300	15.9	234	4.8	26.5	12.4	0.7
Hot Fudge, Two Scoop, Baskin Robbins*	1 Serving/203g	530	29.0	261	3.9	30.5	14.3	0.0

	Measure INFO/WEIGHT	per Measure KCAL	FAT	Nutrition Values per 100g / 100ml KCAL	PROT	CARB	FAT	FIBRE
SUNDAE								
Ice Cream	1 Serving/170g	482	15.4	284	5.9	45.3	9.1	0.3
Raspberry, Perfectly Balanced, Waitrose*	1 Pot/175ml	150	1.0	86	1.7	18.9	0.6	0.0
Strawberry, M & S*	1 Sundae/45g	173	8.0	385	3.4	53.3	17.8	1.0
Strawberry, Tesco*	1 Sundae/48g	194	8.7	408	3.3	57.6	18.3	1.3
Strawberry & Vanilla, Tesco*	1 Serving/68g	120	3.9	177	2.0	29.5	5.7	0.1
Strawberry & Vanilla, Weight Watchers*	1 Pot/105g	148	2.2	141	1.2	29.1	2.1	0.3
Toffee, Asda*	1 Serving/120g	322	19.2	268	2.1	29.0	16.0	0.0
Toffee & Honeycomb, Weight Watchers*	1 Pot/98g	119	1.8	122	1.7	18.1	1.8	5.9
Toffee & Vanilla, Tesco*	1 Serving/70g	133	4.5	189	2.1	30.7	6.4	0.1
SUNNY DELIGHT*								
Californian Style, No Added Sugar, Sunny Delight*	1 Serving/200ml	20	0.4	10	0.1	1.4	0.2	0.1
Florida Style, Sunny Delight*	1 Serving/200ml	70	0.2	35	0.4	7.4	0.1	0.2
Original, Sunny Delight*	1 Glass/200ml	88	0.4	44	0.1	10.0	0.2	0.0
SUSHI								
& Edamame Beans, Boots*	1 Pack/89g	130	2.2	146	5.5	24.0	2.5	2.5
Aya Set, Waitrose*	1 Pack/110g	200	4.3	182	5.4	31.7	3.9	1.5
California Roll Box, M & S*	1 Pack/230g	391	12.0	170	7.0	22.0	5.2	1.1
California Roll Selection, Classics, M & S*	1 Pack/225g	326	6.1	145	7.0	23.2	2.7	1.1
California Rolls 8 Pack	1 Pack/206g	354	9.3	172	5.1	27.5	4.5	1.4
California Set, Waitrose*	1 Pack/120g	223	9.1	186	3.8	25.2	7.6	1.7
Californian, Yakatori, M & S*	1 Pack/200g	340	9.4	170	6.4	25.0	4.7	1.0
Californian Roll, Nigiri & Maki Selection, M & S*	1 Pack/210g	294	4.4	140	4.4	25.9	2.1	2.2
Californian Roll & Nigiri, Selection, M & S*	1 Pack/215g	355	5.8	165	7.1	28.0	2.7	1.1
Fish Nigiri, Adventurous, Tesco*	1 Pack/200g	270	4.4	135	7.1	21.7	2.2	0.5
Fish Roll, Nigiri & Maki Selection, M & S*	1 Pack/210g	315	4.8	150	6.5	25.8	2.3	1.0
Hagi Set, Waitrose*	1 Pack/370g	688	9.6	186	7.1	33.6	2.6	1.1
Hana Set, Waitrose*	1 Pack/175g	324	4.0	185	5.4	35.7	2.3	1.4
Irodori Set with Fish, Cucumber & Avocado, Waitrose*	1 Pack/281g	472	12.4	168	5.2	26.7	4.4	1.3
Komachi Set with Salmon, Whiting & Handroll, Waitrose*	1 Pack/257g	447	13.9	174	5.3	25.8	5.4	1.2
Large, Boots*	1 Pack/324g	480	5.8	148	5.0	28.0	1.8	0.7
Maki Rolls Box, Sainsbury's*	1 Pack/127g	197	2.2	155	4.5	30.5	1.7	0.8
Maki Selection, Shapers, Boots*	1 Pack/158g	225	2.1	142	3.5	29.0	1.3	1.1
Medium, Vegetarian, Taiko Foods*	1 Pack/267g	403	5.3	151	4.0	36.0	2.0	1.0
Medium Pack, Tesco*	1 Pack/139g	211	3.2	152	6.3	26.6	2.3	2.3
Mini, Boots*	1 Pack/99g	153	1.9	155	5.5	29.0	1.9	0.8
Mixed Box, Somerfield*	1 Pack/220g	339	2.4	154	4.6	31.4	1.1	0.0
Nigiri, M & S*	1 Pack/190g	303	5.9	159	7.3	25.3	3.1	0.6
Nigiri, Selection, Tesco*	1 Pack/152g	236	1.5	155	4.6	31.2	1.0	0.6
Nigiri Set, Taiko, Salmon & Tuna, Waitrose*	1 Pack/113g	174	2.3	154	6.3	26.0	2.0	0.6
Nigri, Californian Roll, Maki Roll, Sainsbury's*	1 Pack/195g	283	2.9	145	5.3	27.4	1.5	1.9
Oriental Fish Box, M & S*	1 Pack/205g	318	8.4	155	6.1	23.3	4.1	0.9
Prawn & Salmon Selection, M & S*	1 Pack/175g	255	2.9	146	5.5	27.4	1.7	0.6
Prawn Feast, M & S*	1 Pack/219g	350	8.1	160	5.7	25.8	3.7	1.1
Roll Selection, Sainsbury's*	1 Pack/217g	363	8.0	167	5.0	28.4	3.7	0.5
Roll Selection, Tesco*	1 Pack/214g	327	5.3	153	5.0	27.6	2.5	1.2
Rolls, Shapers, Boots*	1 Pack/168g	259	4.0	154	4.7	28.0	2.4	0.5
Salmon, Nigri Crayfish, Red Pepper, Sainsbury's*	1 Pack/150g	232	4.5	155	5.5	26.4	3.0	1.0
Salmon & Roll Set, Sainsbury's*	1 Serving/101g	167	2.6	165	4.9	30.4	2.6	0.8
Salmon Feast Box, M & S*	1 Pack/200g	330	5.8	165	5.6	27.0	2.9	1.0
Tokyo Set, M & S*	1 Pack/150g	240	4.6	160	7.3	25.3	3.1	0.6
Tuna, to Snack Selection, Food to Go, M & S*	1 Pack/150g	225	3.9	150	5.2	26.4	2.6	2.3
Veg Selection, Ichiban *	1 Pack/130g	198	1.7	152	2.7	32.3	1.3	1.2
Yasai Roll Set, Vegetarian, Wasabi Co Ltd*	1 Pack/498g	398	10.4	80	1.9	13.4	2.1	0.0

S

	Measure INFO/WEIGHT	per Measure KCAL	FAT	Nutrition Values per 100g / 100ml KCAL	PROT	CARB	FAT	FIBRE
SUSHI								
Yo!, Bento Box, Sainsbury's*	1 Pack/208g	530	6.2	255	8.4	48.7	3.0	0.9
Yo!, Salmon Lunch Set, Sainsbury's*	1 Pack/150g	241	4.2	161	5.9	28.1	2.8	0.8
SWEDE								
Boiled, Average	*1oz/28g*	*3*	*0.0*	*11*	*0.3*	*2.3*	*0.1*	*0.7*
Mash, COU, M & S*	1oz/28g	15	0.3	55	1.1	9.5	1.2	2.1
Raw, Flesh Only, Peeled	*1 Serving/100g*	*24*	*0.3*	*24*	*0.7*	*5.0*	*0.3*	*1.6*
Raw, Unprepared, Average	*1oz/28g*	*6*	*0.1*	*21*	*0.8*	*4.4*	*0.3*	*1.9*
SWEET & SOUR								
Beef, Feeling Great, New, Findus*	1 Pack/350g	420	8.7	120	4.5	20.0	2.5	1.3
Chicken, & Noodles, BGTY, Sainsbury's*	1 Pack/400g	356	2.4	89	7.5	13.3	0.6	0.7
Chicken, & Noodles, Chinese Takeaway, Tesco*	1 Pack/350g	350	0.7	100	5.7	18.8	0.2	0.2
Chicken, & Rice, Chilled, Tesco*	1 Pack/450g	540	5.8	120	4.9	21.9	1.3	0.9
Chicken, & Rice, Mega, Value, Tesco*	1 Pack/500g	675	9.5	135	4.4	25.0	1.9	1.9
Chicken, Breasts, Tesco*	1 Serving/185g	172	1.8	93	14.6	6.5	1.0	0.1
Chicken, Canned, Tesco*	1 Can/400g	408	6.4	102	9.6	12.4	1.6	1.1
Chicken, Chinese Takeaway, Sainsbury's*	1 Pack/264g	515	16.9	195	13.1	21.3	6.4	1.0
Chicken, Crispy, Fillets, Tesco*	1 Pack/350g	507	19.6	145	7.2	15.3	5.6	0.9
Chicken, Crispy, Iceland*	1 Serving/125g	221	6.5	177	18.3	14.2	5.2	1.2
Chicken, Healthy Options, Birds Eye*	1 Meal/348g	390	3.8	112	4.8	20.7	1.1	0.6
Chicken, in Batter, Cantonese, Chilled, Sainsbury's*	1 Pack/350g	560	21.0	160	8.9	22.4	6.0	0.9
Chicken, in Crispy Batter, Morrisons*	1 Pack/350g	511	13.6	146	10.1	17.6	3.9	1.2
Chicken, Take It Away, M & S*	1 Pack/200g	200	1.6	100	9.4	13.2	0.8	1.2
Chicken, Tinned, M & S*	1 Serving/481g	553	20.2	115	11.4	7.8	4.2	1.9
Chicken with Egg Fried Rice, M Kitchen, Morrisons*	1 Pack/450g	706	16.2	157	8.1	22.2	3.6	1.9
Chicken with Egg Fried Rice, Somerfield*	1 Pack/400g	428	2.8	107	8.5	16.7	0.7	2.0
Chicken with Egg Rice, Chilled, HL, Tesco*	1 Pack/450g	499	3.1	111	6.8	19.2	0.7	0.6
Chicken with Long Grain Rice, Weight Watchers*	1 Pack/330g	300	1.6	91	5.4	15.5	0.5	1.4
Chicken with Noodles, Feeling Great, Findus*	1 Pack/350g	385	8.7	110	5.0	17.0	2.5	1.5
Chicken with Rice, 233, Oakhouse Foods Ltd*	1 Meal/400g	488	10.4	122	6.1	18.5	2.6	0.7
Chicken with Rice, Chilled, BGTY, Sainsbury's*	1 Pack/400g	344	3.6	86	6.0	13.5	0.9	1.0
Chicken with Rice, Farmfoods*	1 Pack/300g	324	2.7	108	5.9	19.2	0.9	0.7
Chicken with Rice, Oriental Express*	1 Pack/340g	350	2.0	103	4.4	21.3	0.6	0.7
Chicken with Rice, Value, Tesco*	1 Pack/300g	348	0.9	116	5.9	22.3	0.3	0.7
Chicken with Vegetable Rice, COU, M & S*	1 Pack/400g	400	5.6	100	6.9	14.9	1.4	1.1
Chicken without Batter, Cantonese, Chilled, Sainsbury's*	1 Pack/350g	409	4.9	117	8.5	17.6	1.4	1.0
Pork	1oz/28g	48	2.5	172	12.7	11.3	8.8	0.6
Pork, Battered, Sainsbury's*	½ Pack/175g	306	8.7	175	7.3	25.1	5.0	0.6
Pork, Cantonese, & Egg Fried Rice, Farmfoods*	1 Pack/327g	520	19.0	159	4.8	22.0	5.8	0.1
Roasted Vegetables, Cantonese, Sainsbury's*	1 Pack/348g	327	4.2	94	1.1	19.6	1.2	0.9
Vegetables with Rice, Waitrose*	1 Pack/400g	384	4.4	96	1.9	19.5	1.1	1.1
SWEET POTATO								
Baked, Flesh Only, Average	*1 Med/130g*	*149*	*0.5*	*115*	*1.6*	*27.9*	*0.4*	*3.3*
Boiled in Salted Water, Average	*1 Med/200g*	*168*	*0.6*	*84*	*1.1*	*20.5*	*0.3*	*2.3*
Dried	1 Serving/100g	110	3.0	110	1.6	19.7	3.0	3.2
Raw, Peeled, Average	1 Sm Potato/130g	112	0.1	86	1.6	20.1	0.0	3.0
Raw, Unprepared, Average	*1 Potato/200g*	*174*	*0.6*	*87*	*1.2*	*21.3*	*0.3*	*2.4*
Steamed, Average	*1 Potato/200g*	*168*	*0.6*	*84*	*1.1*	*20.4*	*0.3*	*2.3*
SWEETBREAD								
Lamb, Fried	*1oz/28g*	*61*	*3.2*	*217*	*28.7*	*0.0*	*11.4*	*0.0*
SWEETCORN								
Baby, & Mangetout, Somerfield*	1 Pack/150g	42	0.4	28	3.2	3.0	0.3	1.9
Baby, Canned, Drained, Average	1 Serving/80g	18	0.3	23	2.0	2.0	0.4	1.5
Baby, Frozen, Average	*1oz/28g*	*7*	*0.1*	*24*	*2.5*	*2.7*	*0.4*	*1.7*

	Measure INFO/WEIGHT	per Measure KCAL	FAT	Nutrition Values per 100g / 100ml KCAL	PROT	CARB	FAT	FIBRE
SWEETCORN								
Boiled, Average	**1oz/28g**	*31*	*0.6*	*111*	*4.2*	*19.6*	*2.3*	*2.2*
Canned, No Sugar & Salt, Average	**½ Can/125g**	*99*	*1.3*	*79*	*2.7*	*14.9*	*1.1*	*1.6*
Canned with Sugar & Salt, Average	**1 Lge Can/340g**	*376*	*4.0*	*111*	*3.2*	*21.9*	*1.2*	*1.9*
Frozen, Average	**1 Sachet/115g**	*121*	*2.4*	*105*	*3.8*	*17.9*	*2.1*	*1.8*
Supersweet, Field Fresh, Birds Eye*	1 Portion/80g	67	0.6	84	2.6	16.9	0.7	2.4
Tinned, Weight Watchers*	1 Portion/143g	103	1.4	72	2.5	12.0	1.0	2.0
with Peppers, Canned, Average	**1 Serving/50g**	*39*	*0.1*	*79*	*2.6*	*16.4*	*0.3*	*0.6*
SWEETENER								
Aspartamo, Artificial Sugar, Zen*	1 Tbsp/2g	8	0.0	383	1.8	94.0	0.0	0.0
Calorie Free, Truvia*	1/3 Tsp/2g	0	0.0	0	0.0	99.0	0.0	0.0
Canderel, Spoonful, Canderel*	1 Tsp/0.5g	2	0.0	384	2.9	93.0	0.0	0.0
Canderel*	1 Tbsp/2g	8	0.0	379	24.7	7.0	0.0	5.3
Granulated, Asda*	1 Tsp/1g	4	0.0	400	0.0	100.0	0.0	0.0
Granulated, Low Calorie, Splenda*	1 Tsp/0.5g	2	0.0	391	0.0	97.7	0.0	0.0
Granulated, Silver Spoon*	1 Tsp/0.5g	2	0.0	387	1.0	96.8	0.0	0.0
Granulated, Tesco*	1 Tsp/1g	4	0.0	383	1.8	94.0	0.0	0.0
Low Calorie, Somerfield*	1 Tsp/1g	2	0.0	380	3.0	92.0	0.0	0.0
Lucuma Powder, Navitas*	1 Tbsp/15g	60	0.0	400	6.7	86.7	0.0	0.0
Silver Spoon*	1 Tablet/0.05g	0	0.0	325	10.0	71.0	0.0	0.0
Simply Sweet*	1 Tbsp/2g	7	0.0	375	1.4	92.3	0.0	0.0
Slendasweet, Sainsbury's*	1 Tsp/1g	4	0.0	395	1.8	97.0	0.0	0.1
Spoonfull, Low Calorie, SupaSweet*	1 Tsp/1g	4	0.0	392	3.0	95.0	0.0	0.0
Sweet' N Low*	1 Sachet/1g	3	0.0	368	0.0	92.0	0.0	0.0
Sweetex**	1oz/28g	0	0.0	0	0.0	0.0	0.0	0.0
Tablet, Average	1 Tablet/0.1g	0	0.0	355	8.7	73.0	0.0	0.8
Tablets, Low Calorie, Canderel*	1 Tablet/0.1g	0	0.0	342	13.0	72.4	0.0	0.0
Tablets, Splenda*	1 Tablet/0.1g	0	0.0	345	10.0	76.2	0.0	1.6
Tablets, Tesco*	1 Tablet/1g	0	0.0	20	2.0	2.0	0.5	0.0
Xylosweet, Xylitol*	1 Serving/4g	10	0.0	240	0.0	100.0	0.0	0.0
SWEETNER								
Natural, Pure Via*	1 Sachet/2g	3	0.0	149	0.0	95.7	0.0	0.0
Natural Syrup, Fruit, Sweet Freedom*	1 Tsp/5g	15	0.0	292	0.0	79.0	0.0	0.0
Slendersweet, Sainsbury's*	1 Tsp/1g	4	0.0	395	1.8	97.0	0.0	0.1
Tagatesse (Granulated), Damhert*	1 Serving/5g	14	2.0	275	0.0	79.8	39.9	20.1
Tagatesse (Tablet), Damhert*	1 Tablet/0.075g	0	0.0	266	2.7	76.3	0.0	0.0
SWEETS								
Almonds, Sugared, Dragee*	1 Sweet/4g	17	0.6	472	10.0	68.3	17.9	2.5
Alphabet Candies, Asda*	1 Pack/80g	306	0.0	382	0.5	95.0	0.0	0.0
Banana, Baby Foam, M & S*	1/3 Pack/34g	131	0.0	385	4.1	92.7	0.0	0.0
Big Purple One, Quality Street, Nestle*	1 Sweet/39g	191	9.9	490	4.7	60.5	25.5	0.7
Black Jacks & Fruit Salad, Bassett's*	1 Serving/190g	760	11.8	400	0.7	84.9	6.2	0.0
Blackcurrant & Liquorice, M & S*	1 Sweet/8g	32	0.3	400	0.6	89.0	4.3	0.0
Body Parts, Rowntree's*	1 Pack/42g	146	0.0	348	4.3	82.9	0.0	0.0
Butter Candies, Original, Werther's*	1 Sweet/5g	21	0.4	424	0.1	85.7	8.9	0.1
Butterscotch Candies, Weight Watchers*	1 Box/42g	95	0.0	226	0.0	81.9	0.0	14.5
Candy Floss, Asda*	1 Tub/75g	292	0.0	390	0.0	100.0	0.0	0.0
Cappuccino Cream, Sugar Free, Sula*	1 Sweet/3g	8	0.2	269	0.1	91.2	5.5	0.0
Cherry Lips, Chewits*	1 Serving/100g	319	0.2	319	5.6	72.1	0.2	0.0
Chewits, Blackcurrant	1 Pack/33g	125	0.9	378	0.3	86.9	2.7	0.0
Chewits, Blackcurrant, Leaf*	1 Chew/3g	12	0.1	385	0.2	87.5	3.0	0.0
Chewits, Cola, Leaf*	1 Chew/3g	12	0.1	385	0.2	87.5	3.0	0.0
Chewits, Fruit Salad, Leaf*	1 Chew/3g	12	0.1	385	0.2	87.5	3.0	0.0
Chewits, Strawberry, Leaf*	1 Chew/3g	12	0.1	385	0.2	87.5	3.0	0.0

SWEETS

INFO/WEIGHT	Measure KCAL	FAT	KCAL	PROT	CARB	FAT	FIBRE
Chews, Calcium, Ellactiva*	1 Sweet/7g	24	1.1	350	1.4	51.4	15.7	0.0
Chews, Just Fruit, Fruit-tella*	1 Serving/43g	170	2.8	400	0.9	79.5	6.5	0.0
Chews, Strawberry Mix, Starburst*	1 Sweet/4g	15	0.3	401	0.0	83.9	7.3	0.0
Choco Toffee, Sula*	1 Sweet/8g	21	1.2	267	3.3	31.7	15.8	0.0
Chocolate, Milk, Originals, Werther's*	1 Sweet/6g	35	2.5	593	5.8	47.6	42.2	1.8
Chocolate Eclairs, Cadbury*	1 Sweet/8g	36	1.4	455	4.5	68.9	17.9	0.0
Chocolate Limes, Pascall*	1 Sweet/8g	27	0.2	333	0.3	77.2	2.5	0.0
Cola Bottles, Fizzy, M & S*	1 Pack/200g	650	0.0	325	6.4	75.0	0.0	0.0
Cough, Herbs, Swiss, Orginal, Ricola*	1 Packet/37g	148	0.0	400	0.0	98.0	0.0	0.0
Crazy Crocs, Chewits*	1 Serving/100g	316	0.2	316	3.8	73.9	0.2	0.0
Cream Caramel, Sula*	1 Sweet/3g	10	0.0	297	0.4	86.1	0.0	0.0
Crunchies, Fruit, Fruit-tella*	1 Box/23g	90	1.1	390	0.7	86.0	5.0	0.0
Dolly Mix, Bassett's*	1 Bag/45g	171	1.4	380	3.0	85.1	3.1	0.4
Double Lolly, Swizzels Matlow*	1 Lolly/10g	41	0.3	409	0.0	93.2	3.4	0.0
Drops, Lemon & Orange, M & S*	1 Pack/42g	97	0.0	230	0.0	61.0	0.0	0.0
Drumstick, Matlow's*	1 Pack/40g	164	2.2	409	0.4	88.3	5.5	0.0
Edinburgh Rock, Gardiners of Scotland*	1 Piece/2g	8	0.0	380	0.1	94.4	0.3	0.8
Fizzy Lemon Fish, Asda*	1 Sweet/4g	14	0.0	325	5.0	76.0	0.1	0.0
Fizzy Mix, Tesco*	½ Bag/50g	166	0.0	332	5.2	75.2	0.0	0.0
Flumps, Bassett's*	1 Serving/5g	16	0.0	325	4.0	77.0	0.0	0.0
Flumps, Fluffy Mallow Twists, Fat Free, Bassett's*	1 Twist/13g	30	0.0	230	4.1	77.1	0.0	0.0
Foamy Mushrooms, Chewy, Asda*	1 Sweet/3g	9	0.0	347	4.2	82.0	0.2	0.0
Fruit, Mentos*	1 Sweet/3g	10	0.0	333	0.0	100.0	0.0	0.0
Fruit Gums & Jellies	1 Tube/33g	107	0.0	324	6.5	79.5	0.0	0.0
Fruit Tingles, Wonka*	1 Sweet/8g	8	0.0	104	0.0	26.0	0.0	0.0
Fruities, Lemon & Lime, Weight Watchers*	1 Sweet/2g	3	0.0	134	0.0	54.0	0.0	33.0
Fruity Babies, Bassett's*	1 Sweet/3g	10	0.0	310	4.6	72.7	0.2	0.0
Fruity Chews, Starburst*	1 Sweet/8g	34	0.6	404	0.0	83.4	7.4	0.0
Fruity Flutterbies, Chewits*	1 Serving/100g	316	0.2	316	3.8	73.9	0.2	0.0
Fruity Frogs, Rowntree's*	1 Serving/40g	128	0.1	321	4.7	74.5	0.2	0.0
Fruity Mallows, Fizzy, Asda*	1 Pack/400g	1252	0.0	313	4.3	74.0	0.0	0.0
Gobstoppers, Everlasting, Wonka*	1 Sweet/18g	60	0.0	333	0.0	93.3	0.0	0.0
Gummy Bears	10 Bears/22g	85	0.0	386	0.0	98.9	0.0	98.9
Gummy Mix, Tesco*	1 Pack/100g	327	0.1	327	5.9	75.7	0.1	0.0
Gummy Worms	10 Worms/74g	286	0.0	386	0.0	98.9	0.0	98.9
Gummy Zingy Fruits, Bassett's*	1 Sm Bag/40g	135	0.0	337	5.1	79.2	0.0	0.0
Hazardously Sour, Toxic Waste*	1 Sweet/3g	12	0.0	400	0.0	100.0	0.0	0.0
Jellies, Very Berry, Rowntrees*	1 Sweet/4g	12	0.0	326	5.0	74.8	0.2	0.1
Jelly Babies, Morrisons*	1 Serving/227g	781	0.0	344	5.3	80.7	0.0	0.0
Jelly Beans, Lucozade*	1 Packet/30g	111	0.0	370	0.0	92.0	0.0	0.0
Jelly Beans, Tesco*	¼ Bag/63g	243	0.2	385	0.1	94.5	0.3	0.3
Kisses, Hershey*	1 Sweet/5g	28	1.6	561	7.0	59.0	32.0	0.0
Lemon Mint Flavour, Herb Drops, Sugar Free, Ricola*	1 Sweet/3g	7	0.0	235	0.0	96.0	0.0	0.0
Liquorice & Fruit, Fruit-tella*	1 Sweet/4g	16	0.3	395	0.9	83.0	6.5	0.0
Liquorice Torpedoes, Sweets For Life*	1 Serving/100g	368	0.3	368	4.1	87.1	0.3	1.4
Lovehearts, Giant, Swizzels*	1 Pack/42g	165	0.0	393	0.0	100.0	0.0	0.0
Maynards Sours, Bassett's*	1 Pack/52g	169	0.0	325	6.1	75.0	0.0	0.0
Midget Gems, Maynards*	1 Sweet/1g	3	0.0	340	8.7	76.2	0.0	0.0
Milk Chocolate Eclairs, Sainsbury's*	1 Sweet/8g	33	1.1	442	2.1	75.7	14.5	0.5
Milk Duds, Hershey*	13 Pieces/33g	170	6.0	510	3.0	84.0	18.0	0.0
Mini Marti, Mushrooms, Asda*	1 Sweet/3g	10	0.0	340	3.8	81.1	0.1	0.0
Original, Chocolate Soft Caramel, Speciality, Werther's*	1 Piece/6g	30	1.5	480	5.1	61.5	23.5	1.0
Parma Violets, Swizzlers*	1 Small Tube/10g	41	0.0	406	0.9	99.1	0.0	0.0

	Measure INFO/WEIGHT	per Measure KCAL	FAT	Nutrition Values per 100g / 100ml KCAL	PROT	CARB	FAT	FIBRE
SWEETS								
Randoms, Rowntree's*	1 Pack/50g	164	0.1	328	4.9	75.7	0.3	0.6
Rhubarb & Custard, Sainsbury's*	1 Sweet/8g	28	0.0	351	0.1	87.7	0.0	0.0
Rotella, Haribo*	1 Sweet/13g	43	0.0	343	1.5	84.0	0.2	0.0
Scary Mix, Tesco*	1 Bag/100g	327	0.5	327	9.5	71.1	0.5	0.3
Scary Sours, Rowntree's*	1 Serving/100g	321	0.0	321	3.5	74.7	0.0	0.0
Sherbert Cocktails, Sainsbury's*	1 Sweet/9g	36	0.7	400	0.0	83.1	7.5	0.0
Sherbert Dib Dab, with Strawberry Lolly, Barratt*	1 Pack/23g	88	0.0	383	0.1	95.6	0.1	0.0
Sherbert Lemons, Weight Watchers*	1 Box/35g	84	0.2	239	0.0	94.7	0.5	0.0
Sherbet Lemons, Bassett's*	1 Sweet/7g	25	0.0	375	0.0	93.9	0.0	0.0
Shrimps & Bananas, Sainsbury's*	½ Pack/50g	188	0.0	376	2.5	91.3	0.1	0.5
Snakes, Bassett's*	1 Sweet/9g	30	0.0	320	3.5	76.8	0.1	0.0
Soft Fruits, Trebor*	1 Roll/45g	165	0.0	367	0.0	90.9	0.0	0.0
Sour Squirms, Bassett's*	1 Serving/7g	21	0.0	325	3.1	78.1	0.0	0.0
Strawberry & Cream, Sugar Free, Sula*	1 Sweet/3g	9	0.2	267	0.2	90.5	5.4	0.0
Sweetshop Favourites, Bassett's*	1 Sweet/5g	17	0.0	340	0.0	84.3	0.0	0.0
Tic Tac, Cool Cherry, Ferrero*	1 Pack/18g	69	0.1	382	0.2	92.2	0.7	0.0
Toffees, Value, Tesco*	3 Toffees/23g	101	3.3	450	2.1	77.3	14.8	0.3
Tooty Frooties, Rowntree's*	1 Bag/28g	111	1.0	397	0.1	91.5	3.5	0.0
Wazzly Wobble Drops, Wonka*	1 Bag/42g	186	6.8	443	3.0	71.6	16.1	0.2
Wiggly Worms, Sainsbury's*	1 Serving/10g	32	0.0	317	5.6	72.7	0.4	0.2
Wine Gummies, Matlow, Swizzels*	1 Pack/16g	52	0.0	324	0.0	58.7	0.0	0.0
Xtra Sour Spiders, Rowntree's*	1 Pack/35g	112	0.0	321	3.5	74.8	0.0	0.0
Yo Yo's, All Flavours, 100% Fruit, We Are Bear*	1 Roll/10g	27	0.0	275	1.9	63.4	0.2	12.0
Yo Yo's, Strawberry 100% Fruit, We Are Bear*	1 Roll/10g	27	0.0	275	1.9	63.4	0.2	12.0
SWORDFISH								
Grilled, Average	*1oz/28g*	*39*	*1.5*	*139*	*22.9*	*0.0*	*5.2*	*0.0*
Raw, Average	*1oz/28g*	*42*	*2.0*	*149*	*21.1*	*0.0*	*7.2*	*0.0*
SYRUP								
Amaretto, Fabbri*	1 Serving/20ml	70	0.0	349	0.0	86.0	0.0	0.0
Amaretto, Sugar Free, Monin*	1 Serving/30ml	0	0.0	0	0.0	13.3	0.0	0.0
Balsamic, Merchant Gourmet*	1 Tsp/5g	12	0.0	232	0.4	60.0	0.1	0.0
Butterscotch, Monin*	1 Serving/30ml	100	0.0	333	0.0	80.0	0.0	0.0
Caramel, for Coffee, Lyle's*	2 Tsp/10ml	33	0.0	329	0.0	83.0	0.0	0.0
Caramel, Sugar Free, Monin*	1 Serving/30ml	0	0.0	0	0.0	13.3	0.0	0.0
Chocolate Mint, Monin*	1 Serving/30ml	100	0.0	333	0.0	80.0	0.0	0.0
Cinnamon, Monin*	1 Serving/30ml	100	0.0	333	0.0	80.0	0.0	0.0
Corn, Dark, Average	*1 Tbsp/20g*	*56*	*0.0*	*282*	*0.0*	*76.6*	*0.0*	*0.0*
Gingerbread, Monin*	1 Serving/30ml	90	0.0	300	0.0	76.7	0.0	0.0
Golden, Average	*1 Tbsp/20g*	*61*	*0.0*	*304*	*0.4*	*78.2*	*0.0*	*0.0*
Hazelnut, Monin*	1 Serving/30ml	90	0.0	300	0.0	73.3	0.0	0.0
Maple, Average	*1 Tbsp/20g*	*52*	*0.0*	*262*	*0.0*	*67.2*	*0.2*	*0.0*
Organic Rice Malt, Clearspring*	2 Tbsp/42g	133	0.2	316	1.5	76.8	0.4	0.0
Peppermint, Monin*	1 Serving/30ml	96	0.0	320	0.0	80.0	0.0	0.0
Praline, Monin*	1 Serving/30ml	94	0.0	313	0.0	76.7	0.0	0.0
Sugar	1 Tbsp/20g	64	0.0	319	0.0	83.9	0.0	0.0

S

	Measure INFO/WEIGHT	per Measure KCAL	per Measure FAT	Nutrition Values per 100g / 100ml KCAL	PROT	CARB	FAT	FIBRE
TABOO*								
Average, Taboo*	1 Shot/35ml	80	0.0	230	0.0	33.0	0.0	0.0
TABOULEH								
Average	*1oz/28g*	*33*	*1.3*	*119*	*2.6*	*17.2*	*4.6*	*0.0*
TACO SHELLS								
Corn, Crunchy, Old El Paso*	1 Taco/10g	51	2.6	506	7.0	61.0	26.0	0.0
Old El Paso*	1 Taco/12g	57	2.7	478	7.4	60.8	22.8	0.0
Taco, Crunchy, Taco Bell *	1 Serving/78g	133	7.8	170	8.0	13.0	10.0	1.0
Traditional, Discovery*	1 Taco/11g	55	3.2	489	5.7	53.4	28.1	6.0
TAGINE								
Spicy Chermoula, Tasty Veg Pot, Innocent*	1 Pot/400g	356	9.6	89	3.4	13.8	2.4	5.0
Vegetable, Filo Topped, M & S*	1 Serving/282g	310	6.5	110	3.3	18.7	2.3	3.9
TAGLIATELLE								
Basil, M & S*	1 Serving/100g	365	2.8	365	15.1	69.0	2.8	4.0
Bicolore, Asda*	¼ Pack/125g	202	3.0	162	7.0	28.0	2.4	1.4
Carbonara, Average	1 Serving/400g	460	13.4	115	5.5	15.8	3.3	1.0
Carbonara, Low Fat, Bertorelli*	1 Pack/350g	301	7.7	86	5.3	12.0	2.2	0.9
Carbonara, Naturally Less 5% Fat, Asda*	1 Pack/400g	440	9.6	110	4.2	18.0	2.4	0.8
Chicken, Italia, M & S*	1 Pack/360g	342	6.5	95	8.1	12.1	1.8	1.2
Chicken, Italian, Sainsbury's*	1 Pack/450g	567	15.7	126	6.5	17.0	3.5	2.6
Chicken & Mushroom, GFY, Asda*	1 Pack/400g	359	7.0	90	7.2	11.2	1.7	0.7
Chicken & Tomato, Italiano, Tesco*	1 Pack/400g	416	8.4	104	6.6	14.8	2.1	0.8
Creamy Mushroom, Chosen By You, Asda*	1 Pak/400g	428	10.8	107	3.7	16.3	2.7	1.4
Dry, Average	*1 Serving/100g*	*356*	*1.8*	*356*	*12.6*	*72.4*	*1.8*	*1.0*
Egg, Dry, Average	*1 Serving/75g*	*271*	*2.5*	*362*	*14.2*	*68.8*	*3.3*	*2.3*
Egg, Fresh, Cooked, Tesco*	½ Pack/150g	415	3.1	277	9.6	52.8	2.1	3.2
Egg, Fresh, Dry, Average	*1 Serving/125g*	*345*	*3.5*	*276*	*10.6*	*53.0*	*2.8*	*2.1*
Egg & Spinach, M & S*	1 Serving/100g	365	2.7	365	15.5	69.6	2.7	3.0
Fresh, Dry, Average	*1 Serving/75g*	*211*	*2.0*	*281*	*11.4*	*53.3*	*2.6*	*2.6*
Fresh, Free Range, Morrisons*	¼ Pack/125g	331	2.5	265	11.5	50.2	2.0	3.4
Garlic & Herb, Fresh, Asda*	½ Pack/151g	202	6.0	134	3.5	21.0	4.0	2.1
Garlic & Herb, Fresh, Sainsbury's*	1 Serving/125g	184	2.2	147	6.5	26.2	1.8	1.9
Garlic & Herbs, Cooked, Pasta Reale*	1 Pack/250g	390	2.7	156	6.2	30.4	1.1	1.0
Garlic Mushroom, BGTY, Sainsbury's*	1 Pack/400g	416	9.2	104	4.7	16.2	2.3	2.0
Garlic Mushroom, Italiano, Tesco*	1 Pack/450g	738	40.9	164	5.2	15.2	9.1	0.6
Ham & Mushroom, Asda*	1 Pack/340g	469	12.9	138	6.0	20.0	3.8	0.2
Ham & Mushroom, BGTY, Sainsbury's*	1 Pack/450g	486	14.4	108	5.3	14.5	3.2	0.8
Ham & Mushroom, Light Choices, Tesco*	1 Pack/400g	400	8.8	100	6.0	13.8	2.2	1.8
Ham & Mushroom, M & S*	1 Pack/400g	400	18.8	100	4.0	15.1	4.7	0.7
Multigrain, BGTY, Uncooked, Sainsbury's*	1 Serving/190g	294	4.7	155	7.0	26.0	2.5	3.0
Mushroom & Bacon, BGTY, Sainsbury's*	1 Pack/400g	368	9.6	92	4.0	13.5	2.4	1.0
Nests, Dry Weight, Napolina*	1oz/28g	93	0.4	332	11.5	68.0	1.5	3.7
Prawn, Primavera, Sainsbury's*	1 Pack/400g	383	6.1	100	6.1	15.3	1.6	1.4
Red Pepper, Organic, Sainsbury's*	½ Bag/125g	182	1.9	146	5.4	27.8	1.5	1.4
Salmon, Hot Smoked, HL, Tesco*	1 Packet/400g	420	11.6	105	6.0	12.8	2.9	1.4
Salmon, Perfectly Balanced, Waitrose*	1 Pack/400g	376	10.8	94	5.4	11.7	2.7	0.8
Smoked Salmon, Ready Meals, M & S*	1 Pack/360g	612	40.3	170	6.2	10.6	11.2	0.9
Sundried Tomato, Fresh, Morrisons*	1 Pack/250g	747	8.2	299	11.1	56.4	3.3	3.5
Sweet Chilli & Prawn, Tesco*	1 Pack/400g	440	12.4	110	5.5	14.9	3.1	1.3
Tomato & Basil Chicken, Weight Watchers*	1 Pack/330g	322	4.0	98	7.5	14.1	1.2	0.3
Tricolore, Waitrose*	½ Pack/125g	351	3.6	281	12.0	51.6	2.9	1.6
Vegetables, Retail	1oz/28g	21	0.8	74	1.6	11.0	3.0	0.7
Verdi, Dry, Barilla*	1 Serving/150g	555	5.2	370	14.0	70.5	3.5	0.0
Verdi, Fresh, Average	*1 Serving/125g*	*171*	*1.8*	*137*	*5.5*	*25.5*	*1.5*	*1.8*

T

	Measure INFO/WEIGHT	per Measure KCAL	FAT	Nutrition Values per 100g / 100ml KCAL	PROT	CARB	FAT	FIBRE
TAHINI PASTE								
Average	*1 Tsp/6g*	*36*	*3.5*	*607*	*18.5*	*0.9*	*58.9*	*8.0*
TAMARIND								
Pulp	*1oz/28g*	*76*	*0.1*	*273*	*3.2*	*64.5*	*0.3*	*0.0*
Whole, Raw, Weighed with Pod, Average	*1oz/28g*	*67*	*0.2*	*239*	*2.8*	*62.5*	*0.6*	*5.1*
TANGERINES								
Fresh, Raw	*1oz/28g*	*10*	*0.0*	*35*	*0.9*	*8.0*	*0.1*	*1.3*
Fresh, Raw, Weighed with Peel, Average	*1 Med/70g*	*17*	*0.1*	*25*	*0.7*	*5.8*	*0.1*	*0.9*
TANGO*								
Cherry, Britvic*	1 Bottle/500ml	55	0.0	11	0.0	2.4	0.0	0.0
Orange, Britvic*	1 Can/330ml	63	0.0	19	0.1	4.4	0.0	0.0
TAPAS								
Basque Beef, (Estofado Vasco), Tapas at, Tesco*	½ Pack/80g	80	3.1	100	9.5	6.4	3.9	1.5
Champinones Al Ajillo, Tapas at, Tesco*	½ Pack/85g	123	11.6	145	2.3	2.5	13.6	1.5
Chorizo & Cheese Croquettes, Tapas at, Tesco*	½ Pack/117g	263	11.1	225	5.4	28.6	9.5	2.6
Paella De Verduras, Vegetable Paella, Tapas at, Tesco*	½ Pack/100g	105	4.2	105	2.3	14.6	4.2	2.1
Paella Valenciana, Tapas at, Tesco*	½ Pack/75g	105	4.1	140	9.0	12.6	5.5	1.3
Patatas Bravas, Tapas at, Tesco*	½ Pack/125g	169	6.4	135	2.5	18.7	5.1	3.0
Pollo Con Salsa, Tapas at, Tesco*	½ Pack/75g	94	6.5	125	9.4	2.1	8.7	0.7
TAPENADE								
Sundried Tomato & Jalapeno Pepper, Finest, Tesco*	1 Jar/90g	392	36.9	436	3.4	13.1	41.0	5.0
TAPIOCA								
Creamed, Ambrosia*	½ Can/213g	159	3.4	75	2.6	12.6	1.6	0.2
Raw	*1oz/28g*	*101*	*0.0*	*359*	*0.4*	*95.0*	*0.1*	*0.4*
TARAMASALATA								
Average	1 Tbsp/30g	143	14.4	478	4.2	7.9	47.9	1.1
BGTY, Sainsbury's*	1oz/28g	71	5.7	253	4.3	13.5	20.2	0.7
Reduced Fat, Tesco*	½ Pot/85g	256	23.0	301	3.8	10.5	27.1	1.5
Reduced Fat, Waitrose*	1 Pack/170g	522	48.3	307	4.0	8.9	28.4	1.5
Smoked Salmon, Tesco*	1 Serving/95g	474	48.2	499	3.0	7.7	50.7	0.3
TARRAGON								
Dried, Ground	*1 Tsp/2g*	*5*	*0.1*	*295*	*22.8*	*42.8*	*7.2*	*0.0*
Fresh, Average	*1 Tbsp/4g*	*2*	*0.0*	*49*	*3.4*	*6.3*	*1.1*	*0.0*
TART								
Apple & Custard, Asda*	1 Tart/84g	227	11.0	270	3.1	35.0	13.1	0.1
Apple & Fresh Cream, Asda*	½ Tart/50g	133	8.0	267	3.4	33.0	16.0	0.8
Apricot Lattice, Sainsbury's*	1 Slice/125g	321	14.2	257	3.4	35.3	11.4	2.6
Aubergine & Feta, Roast Marinated, Sainsbury's*	1 Serving/105g	227	15.2	216	4.8	16.6	14.5	1.7
Bakewell, Average	1 Tart/50g	228	14.8	456	6.3	43.5	29.7	1.9
Bakewell, Free From, Tesco*	1 Tart/50g	170	4.6	340	1.6	63.0	9.2	4.8
Bakewell, Lemon, Average	1 Tart/46g	206	9.7	447	3.7	60.9	21.1	0.9
Bakewell, Lemon, Holmefield Bakery*	1 Tart/46g	207	11.3	449	4.8	52.9	24.6	0.0
Bakewell, Lyons*	1/6 Tart/52g	205	8.9	397	3.8	56.7	17.2	0.9
Bakewell, Weight Watchers*	1 Tart/43g	156	5.0	363	3.6	65.2	11.7	3.2
Bannoffi, Finest, Tesco*	1/6 Tart/87g	291	16.8	334	3.0	37.2	19.3	0.5
Blackcurrant Sundae, Asda*	1 Tart/55g	227	10.4	413	3.5	57.0	19.0	2.3
Cherry Bakewell, Morrisons*	1 Tart/46g	198	9.8	430	4.6	54.9	21.4	1.3
Cherry Tomato & Mascarpone, Asda*	1 Tart/160g	290	18.0	181	4.4	15.6	11.2	1.1
Cherry Tomato & Mascarpone, Extra Special, Asda*	1 Tart/153g	290	18.3	190	4.6	16.0	12.0	1.1
Chocolate, Co-Op*	1 Tart/22g	102	6.8	465	4.0	42.0	31.0	0.7
Coconut, M & S*	1 Tart/53g	220	9.6	415	5.8	57.8	18.1	3.6
Coconut & Cherry, Asda*	1 Serving/50g	215	10.0	430	4.4	58.0	20.0	4.0
Coconut & Raspberry, Waitrose*	1 Tart/48g	204	11.5	426	5.0	45.0	24.0	3.9
Congress, Morrisons*	1 Tart/38g	149	5.5	393	6.0	59.7	14.4	2.4

T

	Measure INFO/WEIGHT	per Measure KCAL	FAT	Nutrition Values per 100g / 100ml KCAL	PROT	CARB	FAT	FIBRE
TART								
Custard, Individual, Average	1 Tart/94g	260	13.6	277	6.3	32.4	14.5	1.2
Date Pecan & Almond, Sticky, Sainsbury's*	1/8 Tart/75g	298	10.3	397	5.0	63.5	13.7	1.7
Feta Cheese & Spinach, Puff Pastry, Tesco*	1 Tart/108g	306	19.2	283	7.1	23.5	17.8	0.9
Filo Asparagus Tartlette, M & S*	1 Serving/15g	45	3.1	300	4.4	25.2	20.4	2.1
Frangipane, Lutowska Cherry Amaretto, Sainsbury's*	1 Serving/66g	264	12.9	400	6.0	50.0	19.5	1.3
Frangipane, Spiced Winter Fruit, Rustic Bake, Waitrose*	1 Slice/87g	315	13.6	363	7.2	48.3	15.7	2.1
Gruyere Pancetta & Balsamic Onion, Finest, Tesco*	1/4 Tart/106g	320	21.9	301	7.7	21.3	20.6	3.3
Italian Lemon & Almond, Sainsbury's*	1 Slice/49g	182	11.6	371	7.4	31.9	23.7	4.1
Jam, Assorted, VLH Kitchens	1 Serving/34g	44	42.4	130	3.4	56.0	14.4	1.3
Jam, Average	1 Slice/90g	342	13.4	380	3.3	62.0	14.9	1.6
Jam, Real Fruit, Mr Kipling*	1 Tart/35g	136	5.2	388	3.8	67.9	14.9	1.7
Leek & Stilton, Morrisons*	1 Serving/125g	392	26.9	314	6.9	23.1	21.5	0.3
Lemon, M & S*	1/6 Tart/50g	207	14.6	415	5.0	32.7	29.3	0.9
Lemon, Sainsbury's*	1/8 Tart/56g	258	15.8	459	4.4	47.0	28.1	0.6
Lemon & Raspberry, Finest, Tesco*	1 Tart/120g	360	16.8	300	5.2	38.4	14.0	2.9
Lemon Curd, Lyons*	1 Tart/30g	122	5.1	406	3.7	59.3	17.0	0.0
Mixed Fruit, Waitrose*	1 Tart/146g	318	16.4	218	2.3	27.3	11.2	1.0
Normandy Apple & Calvados, Finest, Tesco*	1/6 Tart/100g	256	7.6	256	3.2	41.4	7.6	1.9
Raspberry & Blueberry, Tesco*	1 Serving/85g	168	7.5	198	2.7	27.0	8.8	2.8
Raspberry Flavoured, Value, Tesco*	1 Tart/29g	113	4.8	389	3.8	56.6	16.4	1.6
Red Pepper, Serrano Ham & Goats Cheese, Waitrose*	1 Serving/100g	293	19.2	293	8.7	21.3	19.2	3.2
Roasted Vegetable, Finest, Tesco*	1/4 Tart/113g	226	13.2	200	3.1	20.6	11.7	2.3
Strawberries & Cream, Finest, Tesco*	1/6 Tart/74g	210	13.0	280	3.4	27.2	17.3	1.5
Strawberry, Fresh, M & S*	1 Tart/120g	305	18.4	255	3.1	26.4	15.4	2.4
Strawberry, Reduced Sugar, Asda*	1 Tart/37g	141	3.7	380	4.6	67.5	10.1	1.2
Strawberry, Sainsbury's*	1 Serving/206g	521	26.2	253	2.6	32.0	12.7	0.7
Strawberry & Fresh Cream, Finest, Tesco*	1 Tart/129g	350	19.1	271	3.3	31.1	14.8	1.2
Strawberry Custard, Asda*	1 Tart/100g	335	15.0	335	3.1	47.0	15.0	0.0
Strawberry Sundae, Asda*	1 Tart/46g	187	8.3	407	3.3	58.0	18.0	1.3
Toffee Apple, Co-Op*	1 Tart/20g	69	3.2	345	3.0	47.0	16.0	0.7
Toffee Bakewell, Sainsbury's*	1 Tart/45g	200	8.7	444	3.4	64.2	19.3	1.1
Toffee Pecan, M & S*	1 Tart/91g	414	24.1	455	6.0	48.5	26.5	2.0
Toffee Pecan, Waitrose*	1/4 Tart/133g	564	19.1	423	4.3	69.3	14.3	1.6
Tomato, Mozzarella & Basil Puff, Sainsbury's*	1/3 Tart/120g	318	25.0	265	9.2	10.2	20.8	0.9
Treacle, & Custard, Apetito*	1 Pack/142g	330	10.2	232	2.0	39.2	7.2	0.8
Treacle, Average	1 Portion/125g	460	17.6	368	3.7	60.4	14.1	1.1
Treacle, Lattice, Lyons*	1/6 Tart/70g	255	8.4	364	4.4	59.3	12.0	1.1
Treacle Lattice, Mr Kipling*	1/6 Tart/70g	255	8.5	365	4.4	59.8	12.1	1.1
Treacle with Custard	1 Serving/251g	586	23.5	233	3.1	36.1	9.4	0.8
Vegetable & Feta, Deli, M & S*	1/2 Tart/115g	315	18.4	274	5.0	20.0	16.0	6.0
Zesty Lemon, Tesco*	1/6 Tart/64g	260	15.5	405	5.3	41.0	24.2	0.7
TARTAR								
Cream of, Leavening Agent	*1 Tsp/3g*	*8*	*0.0*	*258*	*0.0*	*61.5*	*0.0*	*0.0*
TARTE								
Au Citron, Frozen, Tesco*	1/6 Tarte/81g	255	11.8	315	5.4	39.4	14.6	0.7
Au Citron, Frozen, TTD, Sainsbury's*	1/6 Tart/80g	232	13.4	290	4.7	40.7	16.8	7.7
Au Citron, Waitrose*	1 Tarte/100g	325	18.1	325	4.9	35.7	18.1	1.0
Aux Cerises, Finest, Tesco*	1 Serving/98g	219	7.0	225	4.9	35.4	7.2	0.6
Tatin, Sainsbury's*	1 Serving/120g	244	8.0	203	2.9	32.8	6.7	1.9
TARTLETS								
Caramelised Onion & Gruyere, Sainsbury's*	1 Tartlet/145g	381	27.5	263	5.8	17.3	19.0	1.3
TEA								
Assam, Blended, TTD, Sainsbury's*	1 Serving/2g	0	0.0	0	0.0	0.0	0.0	0.0

T

TEA

INFO/WEIGHT	Measure	per Measure		Nutrition Values per 100g / 100ml				
		KCAL	FAT	KCAL	PROT	CARB	FAT	FIBRE
Blackberry & Nettle, Twinings*	1 Cup/250ml	5	0.0	2	0.0	0.3	0.0	0.0
Blackcurrant, Fruit Creations, Typhoo*	1 Sm Cup/100ml	5	0.0	5	0.2	0.8	0.0	0.2
Camomile, Pure, Classic Herbal, Twinings*	1 Serving/200ml	4	0.0	2	0.0	0.3	0.0	0.0
Chai, Twinings*	1 Cup/200ml	2	0.0	1	0.1	0.0	0.0	0.0
Damask, Rose, Chinese, Choi Time*	1 Mug/500ml	0	0.3	0	0.0	0.0	0.1	0.0
Decaf, Tetley*	1 Cup/100ml	1	0.0	1	0.0	0.3	0.0	0.0
Earl Grey, Green, Twinings*	1 Cup/200ml	2	0.0	1	0.0	0.2	0.0	0.0
Earl Grey, Infusion with Water, Average	1 Mug/250ml	2	0.0	1	0.0	0.2	0.0	0.0
Fennel, Sweet, Twinings*	1 fl oz/30ml	1	0.0	2	0.0	0.3	0.0	0.0
Fennel Seeds & Peppermint, Refreshing Infusion, Twinings*	1 Cup/200ml	4	0.0	2	0.0	0.3	0.0	0.0
Fruit, Twinings*	1 Mug/227ml	4	0.0	2	0.0	0.4	0.0	0.0
Fruit Or Herbal, Made with Water, Twinings*	1 Mug/200ml	8	0.0	4	0.0	1.0	0.0	0.0
Fruits of the Forest, Westminster Tea*	1 Bag/250ml	5	0.0	2	0.0	0.6	0.0	0.0
Ginger, Herbal, Brit & Tang*	1 Tea Bag/2g	5	0.0	278	0.0	55.6	0.0	0.0
Green, Powder, Matcha*	1 Serving/10g	30	0.0	300	0.0	50.0	0.0	30.0
Green, Pure, Twinings*	1 Serving/100g	1	0.0	1	0.0	0.2	0.0	0.0
Green, with Citrus, Twinings*	1 Serving/200ml	0	0.0	0	1.0	0.2	0.0	0.0
Green, with Jasmine, Twinings*	1 Serving/100ml	1	0.0	1	0.0	0.2	0.0	0.0
Green, with Jasmine, Wellbeing Selection, Flavia*	1 Cup/200ml	0	0.0	0	0.0	0.0	0.0	0.0
Green, with Lemon, Jackson's*	1 Serving/200ml	2	0.0	1	0.0	0.2	0.0	0.0
Green, with Mango, Brewed with Water, Twinings*	1 Cup/200ml	2	0.0	1	0.0	0.2	0.0	0.0
Green, with Mint, Whittards of Chelsea*	1 Cup/100ml	1	0.0	1	0.2	0.1	0.0	0.0
Green, with Pomegranate, Twinings*	1 Serving/100ml	1	0.0	1	0.0	0.2	0.0	0.0
Herbal, Wellbeing Blends, Infusions, Twinings*	1 Serving/200ml	4	0.0	2	0.0	0.3	0.0	0.0
Ice with Lemon, Lipton*	1 Bottle/325ml	91	0.0	28	0.0	6.9	0.0	0.0
Ice with Mango, Lipton*	1 Bottle/500ml	165	0.0	33	0.0	8.1	0.0	0.0
Ice with Peach, Lipton*	1 Bottle/500ml	140	0.0	28	0.0	6.8	0.0	0.0
Iced, Green, Orange, Lipton*	1 Bottle/500ml	100	0.0	20	0.0	5.0	0.0	0.0
Iced, Lemon, San Benedetto*	1 Bottle/500ml	170	0.0	34	0.1	8.3	0.0	0.0
Iced, No Sugar Peach Flavour, Nestle*	1 Glass/100ml	1	0.0	1	0.0	0.1	0.0	0.0
Iced, Peach, Twinings*	1 Serving/200ml	60	0.2	30	0.1	7.3	0.1	0.0
Iced, Pickwick*	1 Serving/250ml	32	0.0	13	0.0	3.3	0.0	0.0
Iced, Powdered Mix, Crystal Light*	1/8 Tub/1g	5	0.0	500	0.0	0.0	0.0	0.0
Lemon, Instant, Original, Lift*	1 Serving/15g	53	0.0	352	0.0	87.0	0.0	0.0
Lemon, Instant, Tesco*	1 Serving/7g	23	0.0	326	1.0	80.5	0.0	0.0
Lemon & Ginger, Lipton*	1 Cup/200ml	8	0.0	4	0.5	0.5	0.0	0.0
Lemon & Limeflower, Infused, M & S*	1 Bottle/330ml	99	0.0	30	0.0	7.8	0.0	0.0
Light & Delicate, Green with Lemon, Twinings*	1 Cup/100ml	1	0.1	1	0.1	0.2	0.1	0.1
Made with Water	1 Mug/227ml	0	0.0	0	0.1	0.0	0.0	0.0
Made with Water with Semi-Skimmed Milk, Average	1 Cup/200ml	14	0.4	7	0.5	0.7	0.2	0.0
Made with Water with Skimmed Milk, Average	1 Mug/270ml	16	0.5	6	0.5	0.7	0.2	0.0
Made with Water with Whole Milk, Average	1 Cup/200ml	16	0.8	8	0.4	0.5	0.4	0.0
Morning Detox, Twinings*	1 Serving/200ml	5	0.0	2	0.0	0.3	0.0	0.0
Nettle & Peppermint, Twinings*	1 Cup/200ml	2	0.0	1	0.0	0.1	0.0	0.0
Nettle & Sweet Fennel, Twinings*	1 Cup/200ml	4	0.0	2	0.0	0.3	0.0	0.0
Peach Flavour, Lift*	1 Cup/15g	58	0.0	384	0.3	95.6	0.0	0.0
Raspberry & Cranberry, T of Life, Tetley*	1 Serving/100ml	36	0.0	36	0.0	9.0	0.0	0.0
Red Bush, Made with Water, Tetley*	1 Mug/250ml	2	0.0	1	0.0	0.1	0.0	0.0

TEACAKES

INFO/WEIGHT	Measure	per Measure		Nutrition Values per 100g / 100ml				
Average	1 Teacake/60g	178	4.5	296	8.0	52.5	7.5	0.0
Caramel, Highlights, Mallows, Cadbury*	1 Teacake/15g	61	1.9	408	6.2	69.1	12.4	3.6
Currant, Sainsbury's*	1 Teacake/72g	204	2.9	284	8.2	53.7	4.0	2.5
Fruit, Lidl*	1 Teacake/62g	166	2.7	267	10.6	46.3	4.4	2.2

	Measure INFO/WEIGHT	per Measure KCAL	FAT	Nutrition Values per 100g / 100ml KCAL	PROT	CARB	FAT	FIBRE
TEACAKES								
Fruited, Co-Op*	1 Teacake/62g	160	2.0	258	9.7	46.8	3.2	3.2
Fruited, M & S*	1 Teacake/60g	156	0.6	260	8.9	53.4	1.0	2.0
Fruity, Warburton's*	1 Teacake/63g	160	2.2	256	8.7	48.0	3.5	2.7
G H Sheldon*	1 Teacake/95g	274	2.6	288	8.5	57.4	2.7	0.0
Hovis*	1 Teacake/60g	155	1.5	258	9.0	49.9	2.5	3.0
Jam, Castello*	1 Teacake/13g	60	2.4	470	5.3	70.1	18.4	1.3
Jam with Biscuit & Mallow, Chocolate Covered, Burton's*	1 Teacake/13g	57	2.4	455	3.8	66.9	19.3	1.1
Lees*	1 Teacake/19g	81	2.9	426	4.2	67.7	15.4	0.0
Mallow, Tesco*	1 Teacake/14g	63	2.7	450	4.1	65.4	19.1	1.0
Mallow, Value, Tesco*	1 Teacake/14g	59	2.3	425	3.6	65.8	16.2	1.4
Marshmallow, Milk Chocolate, Tunnock's*	1 Teacake/24g	106	4.6	440	4.9	61.9	19.2	2.4
Richly Fruited, Waitrose*	1 Teacake/72g	205	2.7	285	7.8	55.0	3.7	2.2
Toasted, Average	1 Teacake/60g	197	5.0	329	8.9	58.3	8.3	0.0
Value, Tesco*	1 Teacake/68g	180	2.4	265	9.6	47.8	3.6	4.9
with Fruit, Morning Fresh, Aldi*	1 Teacake/65g	155	2.2	239	7.4	44.6	3.4	2.3
with Orange Filling, M & S*	1 Teacake/20g	80	2.8	410	4.5	66.6	14.2	0.9
TEMPEH								
Average	*1oz/28g*	*46*	*1.8*	*166*	*20.7*	*6.4*	*6.4*	*4.3*
Rashers, Cheatin, Redwood*	1 Pack/120g	232	7.8	193	16.0	12.0	6.5	0.0
TEQUILA								
Average	*1 Shot/35ml*	*78*	*0.0*	*224*	*0.0*	*0.0*	*0.0*	*0.0*
TERRINE								
Lobster & Prawn, Slices, M & S*	1 Serving/55g	107	7.4	195	18.2	0.7	13.4	0.7
Salmon, Poached, Tesco*	1 Pack/113g	349	30.6	309	15.5	0.8	27.1	0.0
Salmon, Three, M & S*	1 Serving/80g	168	12.2	210	17.6	0.8	15.3	0.9
Salmon & Crayfish, Slice, Finest, Tesco*	1 Serving/110g	148	5.7	135	21.9	0.1	5.2	0.1
Salmon & King Prawn, Waitrose*	1 Serving/75g	97	4.0	130	19.3	1.3	5.3	0.0
Salmon & Lemon, Luxury, Tesco*	1 Serving/50g	98	7.8	196	10.6	3.2	15.7	0.8
Salmon with Prawn & Lobster, M & S*	1 Serving/55g	107	7.4	195	18.2	0.7	13.4	0.7
THAI BITES								
Mild Thai Flavour, Jacob's*	1 Bag/25g	93	0.8	373	6.9	79.0	3.3	1.0
Roasted Chilli Flavour, Fusions, Jacob's*	1 Bag/30g	109	1.7	363	5.5	72.3	5.8	1.2
Seaweed Flavour, Jacob's*	1 Bag/25g	94	0.8	377	7.1	80.0	3.2	0.5
Sesame & Prawn, Fusions, Jacob's*	1 Bag/25g	91	1.5	366	6.3	71.2	5.9	1.3
Sweet Herb, Jacob's*	1 Bag/25g	93	0.8	372	7.1	78.8	3.2	0.2
THICKENING GRANULES								
McDougalls*	1 Tbsp/10g	46	1.9	463	0.0	73.7	18.7	0.0
THYME								
Dried, Ground, Average	*1 Tsp/1g*	*3*	*0.1*	*276*	*9.1*	*45.3*	*7.4*	*0.0*
Fresh, Average	*1 Tsp/1g*	*1*	*0.0*	*95*	*3.0*	*15.1*	*2.5*	*0.0*
TIA MARIA								
Original	*1 Shot/35ml*	*105*	*0.0*	*300*	*0.0*	*0.0*	*0.0*	*0.0*
TIC TAC								
Extra Strong Mint, Ferrero*	2 Tic Tacs/1g	4	0.0	381	0.0	95.2	0.0	0.0
Fresh Mint, Ferrero*	2 Tic Tacs/1g	4	0.0	390	0.0	97.5	0.0	0.0
Lime & Orange, Ferrero*	2 Tic Tacs/1g	4	0.0	386	0.0	95.5	0.0	0.0
Orange, Ferrero*	2 Tic Tacs/1g	4	0.0	385	0.0	95.5	0.0	0.0
Spearmint, Ferrero*	1 Box/16g	62	0.0	390	0.0	97.5	0.0	0.0
TIDGY PUDS								
Aunt Bessie's*	4 Puds/17g	55	2.5	326	9.6	38.4	14.8	2.1
TIDGY TOADS								
Aunt Bessie's*	1 Serving/45g	125	5.9	278	14.7	25.3	13.2	1.1

T

	Measure INFO/WEIGHT	per Measure KCAL	FAT	Nutrition Values per 100g / 100ml KCAL	PROT	CARB	FAT	FIBRE
TIKKA MASALA								
Chicken, & Pilau Basmati Rice, Frozen, Patak's*	1 Pack/400g	580	20.0	145	9.9	15.1	5.0	0.2
Chicken, & Pilau Rice, Asda*	1 Pack/400g	608	19.6	152	7.0	20.0	4.9	1.5
Chicken, & Pilau Rice, BGTY, Sainsbury's*	1 Pack/400g	380	4.8	95	8.1	13.0	1.2	1.1
Chicken, & Pilau Rice, GFY, Asda*	1 Pack/450g	495	9.0	110	6.0	17.0	2.0	0.8
Chicken, & Pilau Rice, Takeaway, Asda*	1 Pack/561g	852	27.5	152	7.0	20.0	4.9	1.5
Chicken, & Pilau Rice, Waitrose*	1 Pack/500g	797	34.5	159	8.2	16.1	6.9	0.8
Chicken, & Rice, Light Choices, Tesco*	1 Pack/450g	472	7.2	105	7.9	14.6	1.6	1.3
Chicken, & Rice, M & S*	1 Pack/400g	700	35.2	175	7.4	17.0	8.8	1.0
Chicken, & Vegetable, HL, Tesco*	1 Pack/450g	360	12.1	80	6.8	6.9	2.7	1.8
Chicken, Boiled Rice & Nan, Meal for One, GFY, Asda*	1 Pack/605g	823	18.8	136	6.0	21.0	3.1	0.0
Chicken, Breast, GFY, Asda*	1 Pack/380g	486	14.4	128	19.0	4.5	3.8	0.2
Chicken, COU, M & S*	1 Pack/400g	400	6.8	100	7.6	14.1	1.7	1.3
Chicken, Feeling Great, Findus*	1 Pack/350g	420	12.2	120	5.5	17.0	3.5	2.0
Chicken, Hot, Sainsbury's*	1 Pack/400g	604	37.2	151	13.2	3.6	9.3	1.5
Chicken, Hot, Tesco*	1 Pack/400g	588	34.4	147	8.7	8.6	8.6	1.0
Chicken, Indian, Medium, Sainsbury's*	1 Pack/400g	848	61.2	212	13.2	5.3	15.3	0.1
Chicken, Indian, Tesco*	1 Pack/350g	560	32.6	160	11.6	7.2	9.3	0.6
Chicken, Indian Takeaway, Iceland*	1 Pack/400g	484	28.4	121	8.9	6.0	7.1	1.9
Chicken, Low Fat, Iceland*	1 Pack/400g	360	4.0	90	7.8	12.5	1.0	0.5
Chicken, Microwave Meal, Good Choice, Iceland*	1 Pack/400g	488	6.0	122	6.6	20.4	1.5	0.6
Chicken, Mild, Diet Chef Ltd*	1 Pack/300g	291	6.6	97	10.4	9.0	2.2	0.6
Chicken, Morrisons*	1 Pack/340g	561	34.7	165	12.4	5.9	10.2	1.7
Chicken, Sharwood's*	1 Pack/375g	562	25.1	150	7.2	15.1	6.7	0.8
Chicken, Smart Price, Asda*	1 Pack/300g	414	18.0	138	13.0	8.0	6.0	1.6
Chicken, Somerfield*	1 Pack/350g	553	37.8	158	11.7	3.6	10.8	1.5
Chicken, Weight Watchers*	1 Pack/331g	344	4.6	104	7.0	15.8	1.4	0.2
King Prawn & Rice, Finest, Tesco*	1 Pack/475g	617	30.4	130	6.0	16.6	6.4	1.2
Prawn, COU, M & S*	1 Pack/400g	400	6.4	100	6.9	14.7	1.6	1.9
Vegetable, Asda*	1 Pack/340g	316	20.7	93	2.0	7.4	6.1	1.1
Vegetable, Canned, Waitrose*	1 Can/200g	152	4.4	76	3.6	10.5	2.2	0.0
Vegetable, Indian, Tesco*	1 Pack/225g	234	13.5	104	2.4	10.4	6.0	2.4
Vegetable, Waitrose*	1 Serving/196g	149	4.3	76	3.6	10.5	2.2	3.8
Vegetable with Rice, Tesco*	1 Pack/450g	499	19.3	111	2.6	15.5	4.3	0.9
Vegetarian with Pilau Rice, Tesco*	1 Serving/440g	519	17.2	118	5.0	15.6	3.9	1.5
TILAPIA								
Raw, Average	**1 Serving/100g**	**95**	**1.0**	**95**	**20.0**	**0.0**	**1.0**	**0.0**
TIME OUT								
Break Pack, Cadbury*	1 Serving/20g	108	6.3	530	6.2	58.3	30.7	0.0
Chocolate Fingers, Cadbury*	2 Fingers/35g	185	10.6	530	7.1	57.3	30.3	1.1
Orange, Snack Size, Cadbury*	1 Finger/11g	61	3.6	555	5.0	59.4	32.9	0.0
TIRAMISU								
BGTY, Sainsbury's*	1 Pot/90g	140	2.4	156	4.5	28.3	2.7	0.3
Choc & Mascarpone, Tiramigu, Gu*	1 Pud/90g	316	23.3	351	3.3	26.1	25.9	1.0
COU, M & S*	1 Tub/95g	138	2.6	145	3.7	26.9	2.7	0.6
Family Size, Tesco*	1 Serving/125g	356	18.1	285	4.3	34.5	14.5	4.3
Italian, Co-Op*	1 Pack/90g	229	9.0	255	5.0	37.0	10.0	0.4
Morrisons*	1 Pot/90g	248	9.9	276	4.0	38.0	11.0	0.0
Raspberry, M & S*	1 Serving/84g	197	12.1	235	3.8	22.9	14.4	0.2
Sainsbury's*	1 Serving/100g	263	10.0	263	4.4	40.2	10.0	0.1
Single Size, Tesco*	1 Pot/100g	290	12.9	290	3.8	35.1	12.9	4.5
Trifle, Sainsbury's*	1 Serving/100g	243	15.7	243	2.3	23.2	15.7	0.6
Waitrose*	1 Pot/90g	221	11.2	246	6.4	27.2	12.4	0.0

	Measure INFO/WEIGHT	per Measure		Nutrition Values per 100g / 100ml				
		KCAL	FAT	KCAL	PROT	CARB	FAT	FIBRE
TOAD IN THE HOLE								
& Potatoes, M & S*	1 Serving/100g	200	12.9	200	6.4	14.6	12.9	0.9
Average	1 Serving/231g	640	40.2	277	11.9	19.5	17.4	1.1
Vegetarian, Aunt Bessie's*	1 Pack/190g	502	19.4	264	15.6	27.5	10.2	2.7
Vegetarian, Linda McCartney*	1 Pack/190g	359	16.7	189	13.6	13.9	8.8	1.1
Vegetarian, Meat Free, Asda*	1 Serving/173g	407	19.0	235	9.0	25.0	11.0	3.1
Vegetarian, Tesco*	1 Pack/190g	471	19.0	248	13.1	26.5	10.0	2.8
TOFFEE APPLE								
Average	1 Sm Apple/141g	188	3.0	133	1.2	29.2	2.1	2.3
TOFFEE CRISP								
Biscuit, Nestle*	1 Original/44g	228	12.1	519	3.7	62.8	27.6	1.4
TOFFEES								
Assorted, Bassett's*	1 Toffee/8g	35	1.1	434	3.8	73.1	14.0	0.0
Brazil Nut, Diabetic, Thorntons*	1 Serving/20g	93	7.0	467	3.2	49.0	35.1	0.5
Butter, Smart Price, Asda*	1 Toffee/8g	37	1.3	440	1.3	75.0	15.0	0.0
Chewy, Werther's*	1 Toffee/5g	22	0.8	436	3.5	71.3	15.2	0.1
Dairy, Smart Price, Asda*	1 Sweet/9g	37	1.3	407	1.3	68.4	14.2	0.0
Dairy, Waitrose*	1 Toffee/14g	64	2.0	458	2.0	80.2	14.3	0.5
Devon Butter, Thorntons*	1 Sweet/9g	40	1.5	444	1.7	72.2	16.7	0.0
English Butter, Co-Op*	1 Toffee/8g	38	1.6	470	2.0	71.0	20.0	0.0
Liquorice, Thorntons*	1 Bag/100g	506	29.4	506	1.9	58.8	29.4	0.0
Milk Chocolate Covered, Thorntons*	1 Bag/215g	1120	66.0	521	4.1	57.2	30.7	0.9
Milk Chocolate Smothered, Thorntons*	1 Pack/125g	655	38.5	524	4.3	57.5	30.8	1.1
Mixed, Average	1oz/28g	119	5.2	426	2.2	66.7	18.6	0.0
No Added Sugar, Boots*	1 Serving/7g	23	1.0	324	1.3	52.0	14.0	0.0
Original, Hard Butter Candies, Sugar Free, Werther's*	1 Pack/80g	231	7.0	289	0.2	86.8	8.8	0.1
TOFU								
Average	*1 Pack/250g*	*297*	*16.5*	*119*	*13.4*	*1.4*	*6.6*	*0.1*
Beech Smoked, Organic, Cauldron Foods*	½ Pack/110g	124	7.8	113	10.9	1.0	7.1	0.5
Firm Silken Style, Blue Dragon*	1 Pack/216g	134	5.8	62	6.9	2.4	2.7	0.0
Fresh, Drained, Kong Nam*	1 Tub/575g	397	21.3	69	7.7	1.3	3.7	0.5
Fried, Average	*1oz/28g*	*75*	*4.0*	*268*	*28.6*	*9.3*	*14.1*	*0.0*
Original, Organic, Cauldron Foods*	¼ Pack/99g	84	4.2	85	10.0	1.9	4.2	0.9
Pieces, Marinated, Organic, Cauldron Foods*	1 Pack/160g	363	27.2	227	17.5	1.0	17.0	2.7
Smoked, Organic, Evernat*	1oz/28g	36	1.8	127	16.3	0.8	6.6	0.0
Traditional Luncheon, Bean Supreme*	1 Serving/100g	210	13.1	210	23.4	7.8	13.1	0.0
TOMATILLOS								
Raw	*1 Med/34g*	*11*	*0.3*	*32*	*1.0*	*5.8*	*1.0*	*1.9*
TOMATO PASTE								
Average	*1 Tbsp/20g*	*19*	*0.0*	*96*	*4.9*	*19.2*	*0.2*	*1.5*
Sun Dried, Average	*1 Heaped Tsp/10g*	*38*	*3.5*	*385*	*3.2*	*13.8*	*35.1*	*0.0*
TOMATO PUREE								
Average	*1 Tsp/5g*	*4*	*0.0*	*76*	*4.5*	*14.1*	*0.2*	*2.3*
Sun Dried, & Olive Oil & Herbs, GIA*	1 Serving/20g	41	4.3	204	2.6	0.5	21.6	0.0
TOMATOES								
Cherry, Average	*1 Tomato/15g*	*3*	*0.0*	*18*	*0.7*	*3.0*	*0.3*	*0.5*
Cherry, on the Vine, Average	*1 Serving/80g*	*15*	*0.3*	*18*	*0.7*	*3.1*	*0.3*	*1.2*
Cherry, Tinned, Napolina*	1 Can/400g	92	2.4	23	1.2	3.3	0.6	0.0
Chopped, Canned, Average	1 Serving/100g	19	0.2	19	1.1	3.3	0.2	0.9
Chopped, Canned, Branded Average	*1 Serving/130g*	*27*	*0.2*	*21*	*1.1*	*3.8*	*0.1*	*0.8*
Chopped, Canned, Parioli, Cucina*	½ Can/200g	50	0.4	25	1.4	4.0	0.2	0.9
Chopped, Italian, Average	*½ Can/200g*	*47*	*0.2*	*23*	*1.3*	*4.4*	*0.1*	*0.9*
Chopped, with Garlic, Average	*½ Can/200g*	*43*	*0.3*	*21*	*1.2*	*3.8*	*0.1*	*0.8*
Chopped, with Herbs, Average	*½ Can/200g*	*42*	*0.3*	*21*	*1.1*	*3.8*	*0.1*	*0.8*

T

	Measure INFO/WEIGHT	per Measure KCAL	FAT	Nutrition Values per 100g / 100ml KCAL	PROT	CARB	FAT	FIBRE
TOMATOES								
Chopped, with Onion & Herbs, Napolina*	1 Can/400g	84	0.4	21	1.0	4.0	0.1	0.4
Chopped, with Peppers & Onions, Sainsbury's*	½ Can/200g	40	0.2	20	1.2	3.5	0.1	0.9
Chopped, with Sliced Green & Black Olives, Sainsbury's*	1 Pack/390g	183	8.2	47	1.3	5.6	2.1	0.7
Creamed, Sainsbury's*	1oz/28g	6	0.0	22	1.5	5.0	0.1	1.6
Fresh, Raw, Average	*1 Med/123g*	*22*	*0.2*	*18*	*0.9*	*3.9*	*0.2*	*1.2*
Fried in Blended Oil	1 Med/85g	77	6.5	91	0.7	5.0	7.7	1.3
Green Tiger, Raw, M & S*	1 Serving/80g	16	0.2	20	0.7	3.1	0.3	1.0
Grilled, Average	1oz/28g	14	0.3	49	2.0	8.9	0.9	2.9
in Tomato Juice, Chopped, Heinz*	½ Can/200g	32	0.4	16	0.7	2.9	0.2	0.9
Peeled, Plum, Canned, Value, Tesco*	½ Can/200g	36	0.2	18	0.7	3.4	0.1	0.7
Plum, Baby, Average	*1 Serving/50g*	*9*	*0.2*	*18*	*1.5*	*2.3*	*0.3*	*1.0*
Plum, in Tomato Juice, Average	*1 Can/400g*	*71*	*0.4*	*18*	*0.9*	*3.3*	*0.1*	*0.7*
Plum, in Tomato Juice, Premium, Average	*1 Can/400g*	*93*	*1.2*	*23*	*1.3*	*3.8*	*0.3*	*0.7*
Ripened on the Vine, Average	*1 Med/123g*	*22*	*0.4*	*18*	*0.7*	*3.0*	*0.3*	*0.7*
Santini, M & S*	1 Serving/80g	16	0.2	20	0.7	3.1	0.3	1.0
Stuffed with Rice Based Filling, Average	1oz/28g	59	3.8	212	2.1	22.2	13.4	1.1
Sun Dried, Average	*3 Pieces/20g*	*43*	*3.2*	*213*	*4.7*	*12.9*	*15.9*	*3.3*
Sun Dried, in Oil, GIA*	1 Serving/10g	15	1.4	153	1.9	7.5	13.9	0.0
Sun Dried in Oil	1 Serving/100g	301	24.8	301	5.8	13.5	24.8	7.0
Sundried, Italian, Merchant Gourmet*	1 Serving/50g	55	0.3	111	5.7	20.4	0.7	1.3
TONGUE								
Lunch, Average	*1oz/28g*	*51*	*3.0*	*181*	*20.1*	*1.8*	*10.6*	*0.0*
Ox from Deli Counter, Sainsbury's*	1 Serving/100g	195	13.3	195	18.3	0.5	13.3	0.1
Slices, Average	*1oz/28g*	*56*	*3.9*	*201*	*18.7*	*0.0*	*14.0*	*0.0*
TONIC WATER								
Average	1 Glass/250ml	82	0.0	33	0.0	8.8	0.0	0.0
Diet, Asda*	1 Glass/200ml	2	0.0	1	0.0	0.0	0.0	0.0
Indian, Britvic*	1 Mini Can/150ml	39	0.1	26	0.1	6.2	0.1	0.1
Indian, Diet, Schweppes*	1 Glass/100ml	1	0.0	1	0.0	0.0	0.0	0.0
Indian, Fever Tree*	1 Bottle/200ml	76	0.0	38	0.0	9.0	0.0	0.0
Indian, Schweppes*	1 Serving/500ml	110	0.0	22	0.0	5.1	0.0	0.0
Indian, Slimline, Schweppes*	1 Serving/188ml	3	0.0	2	0.4	0.0	0.0	0.0
Indian, Sugar Free, Essential, Waitrose*	1 Serving/50ml	1	0.0	2	0.0	0.0	0.0	0.0
Indian, with a Hint of Lemon, Low Calorie, Asda*	1 Serving/300ml	3	0.3	1	0.0	0.0	0.1	0.0
Indian, with Lime, Low Calorie, Tesco*	1 Glass/250ml	5	0.0	2	0.0	0.0	0.0	0.0
Light, Royal Club*	1 Glass/250ml	2	0.0	1	0.0	0.0	0.0	0.0
Quinine, Schweppes*	1 Glass/125ml	46	0.0	37	0.0	9.0	0.0	0.0
Soda Stream*	1 Glass/100ml	15	0.0	15	0.0	3.2	0.0	0.0
TONIC WINE								
Original, Sanatogen*	1 Bottle/700ml	889	0.0	127	0.0	124.4	0.0	0.0
TOPIC								
Mars*	1 Bar/47g	234	12.3	498	6.2	59.6	26.2	1.7
TORTE								
Chocolate, Half Fat, Waitrose*	1/6 Torte/70g	135	4.1	193	5.4	29.7	5.8	2.2
Chocolate, Mint, Weight Watchers*	1 Pot/88g	174	4.1	198	4.7	34.3	4.7	5.2
Chocolate, Tesco*	1 Serving/50g	125	5.9	251	3.6	32.3	11.9	1.0
Chocolate & Pecan Brownie, Gu*	1/6 Torte/67g	292	17.7	436	5.3	45.1	26.4	3.1
Chocolate Fondant, Gu*	1/8 Tarte/63g	264	18.9	423	5.7	32.0	30.2	1.8
Chocolate Orange & Almond, Gu*	1 Serving/65g	273	19.8	420	5.0	28.2	30.5	2.7
Chocolate Truffle, Waitrose*	1 Serving/116g	359	20.1	309	4.6	30.1	17.3	1.4
Lemon, Somerfield*	1 Serving/45g	71	1.2	157	0.8	32.6	2.6	0.8
Lemon, Tesco*	1 Serving/62g	142	6.1	230	2.3	32.9	9.9	0.5
Lemon & Mango, Waitrose*	1 Serving/80g	142	2.4	177	3.9	33.6	3.0	0.6

T

INFO/WEIGHT	Measure	per Measure KCAL	FAT	Nutrition Values per 100g / 100ml KCAL	PROT	CARB	FAT	FIBRE

TORTE

	Measure INFO/WEIGHT	KCAL	FAT	KCAL	PROT	CARB	FAT	FIBRE
Raspberry, BGTY, Sainsbury's*	1 Serving/100g	154	3.9	154	2.6	27.0	3.9	1.2

TORTELLINI

	Measure INFO/WEIGHT	KCAL	FAT	KCAL	PROT	CARB	FAT	FIBRE
3 Cheese, Sainsbury's*	1 Serving/50g	195	4.3	391	14.4	63.8	8.7	3.0
Aubergine & Pecorino, Sainsbury's*	½ Pack/150g	354	6.4	236	8.9	40.3	4.3	3.2
Beef & Red Wine, Italian, Asda*	½ Pack/150g	242	4.2	161	9.0	25.0	2.8	0.0
Beef Bolognese, Rich, Italian, Giovanni Rana*	½ Pack/125g	222	9.0	178	7.6	20.6	7.2	4.1
Cheese, Fresh, Sainsbury's*	½ Pack/180g	329	9.0	183	7.6	26.8	5.0	1.7
Cheese, Tomato & Basil, Tesco*	1 Serving/150g	387	8.1	258	13.0	39.5	5.4	3.3
Cheese, Weight Watchers*	1 Can/395g	245	6.3	62	2.3	9.7	1.6	0.4
Cheese & Ham, Italiano, Tesco*	½ Pack/150g	396	12.3	264	12.8	34.8	8.2	3.0
Chicken, Spicy, Big Eat, Heinz*	1 Pot/350g	404	23.1	115	2.9	11.2	6.6	0.4
Four Cheese & Tomato, Italian, Asda*	1 Serving/150g	249	5.7	166	8.0	25.0	3.8	0.0
Four Cheese with Tomato & Basil Sauce, Tesco*	1 Pack/400g	500	14.8	125	6.1	16.9	3.7	0.6
Garlic, Basil & Ricotta, Asda*	½ Pack/175g	318	10.5	182	6.0	26.0	6.0	2.6
Garlic & Herb, Fresh, Sainsbury's*	½ Pack/150g	364	11.7	243	11.1	32.2	7.8	1.8
Ham & Cheese, Fresh, Asda*	½ Pack/150g	255	9.0	170	6.0	23.0	6.0	1.7
Italian, Diet Chef Ltd*	1 Pack/300g	234	1.5	78	2.3	16.0	0.5	0.2
Meat, Italian, Tesco*	1 Serving/125g	332	9.5	266	10.6	38.9	7.6	2.3
Mushroom, Asda*	1 Serving/125g	217	5.2	174	6.0	28.0	4.2	2.3
Mushroom, BGTY, Sainsbury's*	½ Can/200g	180	6.2	90	2.2	13.2	3.1	0.7
Pepperoni, Italian, Asda*	½ Pack/150g	250	6.0	167	6.7	26.0	4.0	0.0
Pesto & Goats Cheese, Fresh, Sainsbury's*	½ Pack/150g	310	12.1	207	8.9	24.6	8.1	2.6
Pork & Beef, BGTY, Sainsbury's*	½ Can/200g	148	3.0	74	3.7	11.2	1.5	0.6
Ricotta & Spinach, Giovanni Rana*	½ Pack/125g	340	13.6	272	10.1	34.6	10.9	10.0
Sausage & Ham, Italiano, Tesco*	1 Pack/300g	816	27.9	272	13.1	34.0	9.3	3.7
Smoked Bacon & Tomato, Asda*	1 Pack/300g	591	15.0	197	9.0	29.0	5.0	0.0
Spicy Pepperoni, Fresh, Asda*	½ Pack/150g	249	6.0	166	7.0	26.0	4.0	0.0
Spinach & Ricotta, Canned, Somerfield*	1 Can/250g	282	15.0	113	12.0	4.0	6.0	0.0
Spinach & Ricotta, Verdi, Asda*	1 Serving/125g	186	5.6	149	6.0	21.0	4.5	2.4
Tomato & Mozzarella, Fresh, Asda*	½ Pack/150g	235	4.2	157	8.0	25.0	2.8	0.0
Tomato & Mozzarella, Fresh, Sainsbury's*	½ Pack/150g	291	12.0	194	7.5	23.0	8.0	3.4

TORTELLONI

	Measure INFO/WEIGHT	KCAL	FAT	KCAL	PROT	CARB	FAT	FIBRE
Arrabbiata, Sainsbury's*	½ Pack/210g	407	11.8	194	7.1	28.8	5.6	2.6
Basil, Mozzarella & Tomato, Weight Watchers*	½ Pack/125g	278	3.4	222	9.0	40.5	2.7	4.8
Beef & Chianti, TTD, Sainsbury's*	½ Pack/125g	300	8.0	240	11.3	34.3	6.4	1.9
Beef & Pancetta, Aberdeen Angus, Grandi, Budgens*	½ Pack/125g	314	5.4	251	12.4	40.5	4.3	2.9
Bell Pepper & Sundried Tomato, Morrisons*	½ Pack/150g	375	6.5	250	12.1	40.7	4.3	2.9
Cheese, Garlic & Herb, Co-Op*	1 Serving/125g	331	7.5	265	10.0	43.0	6.0	0.0
Cheese, Tomato, & Basil, Sainsbury's*	½ Pack/150g	271	9.7	181	8.0	22.7	6.5	1.7
Cheese & Ham, Fresh, Budgens*	1 Serving/100g	268	6.5	268	12.6	42.0	6.5	2.2
Cheese & Smoked Ham, Tesco*	½ Pack/150g	315	10.6	210	8.9	26.5	7.1	1.7
Chicken & Bacon, Italiano, Tesco*	1 Pack/300g	660	21.9	220	7.8	29.8	7.3	2.1
Chorizo & Tomato, Morrisons*	1 Serving/150g	447	12.9	298	12.8	45.1	8.6	2.6
Five Cheese, Sainsbury's*	1 Serving/125g	285	11.6	228	10.8	25.2	9.3	2.9
Four Cheese, Asda*	½ Pack/150g	312	13.0	208	7.6	24.9	8.7	1.6
Four Cheese, Express, Dolmio*	1 Pack/220g	411	16.7	187	7.6	22.1	7.6	0.0
Four Cheese, Waitrose*	½ Pack/125g	297	8.4	238	10.3	34.2	6.7	1.6
Fresh, Ham & Cheese, Asda*	½ Pack/150g	315	11.4	210	8.8	26.7	7.6	1.4
Garlic & Herb, Cooked, Pasta Reale*	1 Pack/300g	546	11.7	182	6.7	30.1	3.9	0.9
Italian Style Sausage & Red Wine, Morrisons*	½ Pack/150g	420	10.8	280	11.1	45.5	7.2	2.7
Meat, Italian, Asda*	½ Pack/150g	265	6.7	177	7.0	27.0	4.5	2.4
Meat & Cheese, Fresh, Sainsbury's*	½ Pack/125g	304	10.5	243	13.5	28.3	8.4	2.6
Mediterranean Vegetable, Perfectly Balanced, Waitrose*	½ Pack/125g	286	4.5	229	9.1	40.1	3.6	2.5

	Measure INFO/WEIGHT	per Measure KCAL	per Measure FAT	Nutrition Values per 100g / 100ml KCAL	PROT	CARB	FAT	FIBRE
TORTELLONI								
Mozzarella, Tomato & Basil, Italian, Somerfield*	½ Pack/125g	314	5.1	251	10.5	43.1	4.1	1.9
Mushroom, Perfectly Balanced, Waitrose*	½ Pack/125g	300	4.0	240	10.9	41.8	3.2	2.2
Olive & Ricotta, Sainsbury's*	½ Pack/175g	403	18.4	230	8.8	25.1	10.5	2.3
Pasta, Fresh, Cream Cheese, Garlic & Herb, Morrisons*	1 Serving/150g	400	9.0	267	10.3	46.1	6.0	3.2
Pesto, Italian, Tesco*	1 Pack/300g	885	33.9	295	10.7	36.7	11.3	3.0
Pesto, Light Choices, Tesco*	½ Pack/150g	277	8.7	185	6.5	26.5	5.8	2.0
Ricotta & Basil, Asda*	½ Pack/150g	322	12.9	215	9.2	25.1	8.6	1.6
Sausage, Spicy, Italian, Asda*	½ Pack/150g	339	11.7	226	7.4	31.6	7.8	1.5
Sausage & Ham, Italiano, Tesco*	1 Serving/150g	285	10.5	190	8.5	22.5	7.0	1.8
Sicilian Style & Tuna, Morrisons*	½ Pack/150g	397	8.8	265	12.1	43.0	5.9	2.3
Smoked Ham, Bacon & Tomato, Tesco*	½ Packet/150g	450	17.5	300	12.0	35.7	11.7	2.5
Spicy Red Pepper & Tomato, Pasta Reale*	½ Pack/125g	310	5.5	248	10.0	42.0	4.4	3.3
Spinach & Ricotta, Chilled, Italiano, Tesco*	½ Pack/150g	412	12.7	275	10.4	38.1	8.5	3.3
Spinach & Ricotta, Sainsbury's*	½ Pack/150g	325	10.8	217	7.8	30.2	7.2	2.4
Spinach & Ricotta Cheese, Co-Op*	½ Pack/126g	315	6.3	250	10.0	41.0	5.0	4.0
Tomato & Mozzarella, Sainsbury's*	1 Serving/175g	339	14.0	194	7.5	23.0	8.0	3.4
Walnut & Gorgonzola, Fresh, Sainsbury's*	½ Pack/210g	414	12.2	197	8.4	27.8	5.8	2.4
Wild Mushroom, Italian, Sainsbury's*	½ Pack/150g	309	12.3	206	7.7	25.4	8.2	2.3
TORTIGLIONI								
Dry, Average	**1 Serving/75g**	**266**	**1.4**	**355**	**12.5**	**72.2**	**1.9**	**2.1**
TORTILLA CHIPS								
Black Pepper & Jalapeno, Love Life, Waitrose*	1 Bag/22g	92	1.9	420	6.7	76.0	8.8	3.2
Blazing BBQ, Sainsbury's*	1 Serving/50g	237	11.7	474	6.8	58.9	23.5	4.6
Blue, Organic, Sainsbury's*	1 Serving/50g	252	11.7	504	7.7	65.8	23.4	5.6
Chilli Flavour, Somerfield*	1 Serving/50g	242	12.0	484	6.8	60.1	24.1	5.3
Classic Mexican, Phileas Fogg*	1 Serving/35g	162	6.7	464	5.9	67.2	19.1	3.8
Cool, Salted, Sainsbury's*	1 Serving/50g	253	13.6	506	6.5	58.6	27.3	4.3
Cool, Tesco*	1 Serving/40g	190	9.9	474	6.3	56.7	24.7	7.8
Cool Flavour, Sainsbury's*	1 Serving/50g	231	9.3	463	5.7	68.1	18.7	3.7
Cool Sour Cream, Love Life, Waitrose*	1 Bag/22g	95	2.7	434	7.1	7.1	12.3	4.5
Easy Cheesy!, Sainsbury's*	1 Serving/50g	249	13.0	498	7.1	58.7	26.1	4.5
Honey BBQ, Love Life, Waitrose*	1 Bag/22g	93	2.2	425	6.6	76.0	9.8	3.3
Hot Chilli Flavour, Weight Watchers*	1 Bag/18g	83	3.3	461	4.6	67.7	18.2	4.2
Lightly Salted, M & S*	1 Serving/20g	98	4.8	490	7.2	61.5	24.1	4.5
Lightly Salted, Smart Price, Asda*	¼ Bag/50g	251	13.0	502	7.0	60.0	26.0	5.0
Lightly Salted, Tesco*	1 Serving/50g	247	13.8	495	4.8	56.8	27.6	7.5
Lightly Salted, Waitrose*	1 Serving/40g	187	8.6	468	7.1	61.2	21.6	6.5
Lighty Salted, Basics, Sainsbury's*	½ Pack/50g	241	11.9	483	6.5	60.7	23.8	5.3
Mexicana Cheddar, Kettle Chips*	1 Serving/50g	249	13.3	498	7.9	56.7	26.6	5.1
Nacho Cheese Flavour, M & S*	1 Serving/30g	144	6.7	480	7.5	62.0	22.4	4.2
Nacho Cheese Flavour, Weight Watchers*	1 Pack/18g	83	3.3	459	5.2	66.6	18.2	4.1
Plain	1 Serving/100g	486	21.1	486	6.8	62.0	21.1	4.2
Salsa, Asda*	1 Serving/25g	122	6.0	488	6.0	62.0	24.0	6.0
Salsa, M & S*	½ Bag/75g	364	18.8	485	5.7	59.1	25.1	6.1
TORTILLAS								
Corn, Gluten Free, Discovery*	1 Tortilla/22g	53	0.5	243	5.4	53.8	2.3	3.8
Corn, Soft, Old El Paso*	1 Tortilla/38g	129	2.6	343	10.0	60.0	7.0	0.0
Flour, 10 Pack, Asda*	1 Tortilla/30g	94	2.1	315	9.0	54.0	7.0	2.5
Flour, American Style, Sainsbury's*	1 Tortilla/35g	108	2.4	313	8.6	53.9	7.0	2.5
Flour, Bakery, Asda*	1 Tortilla/43g	129	3.0	303	9.1	50.9	7.1	2.6
Flour, From Dinner Kit, Old El Paso*	1 Tortilla/42g	144	4.9	344	8.7	51.1	11.7	0.0
Flour, Mexican Style, Morrisons*	1 Tortilla/33g	103	2.3	313	8.6	53.9	7.0	2.5
Flour, Salsa, Old El Paso*	1 Tortilla/41g	132	3.7	323	9.0	52.0	9.0	0.0

T

	Measure INFO/WEIGHT	per Measure KCAL	FAT	Nutrition Values per 100g / 100ml KCAL	PROT	CARB	FAT	FIBRE
TORTILLAS								
Flour, Soft, Chilli & Jalapeno, Discovery*	1 Tortilla/40g	131	5.2	328	7.8	44.8	13.1	2.2
Flour, Soft, Discovery*	1 Tortilla/40g	119	2.8	298	8.0	49.6	7.1	2.4
Flour, Soft, Garlic & Coriander, Discovery*	1 Tortilla/40g	116	2.4	289	8.1	50.6	6.0	1.7
Flour, Wheat, Waitrose*	1 Tortilla/62g	203	6.1	327	8.5	51.5	9.8	0.0
Made with Wheat Flour	1oz/28g	73	0.3	262	7.2	59.7	1.0	2.4
Plain, Morrisons*	1 Serving/35g	92	0.9	263	8.5	51.2	2.7	2.5
Plain, Wheat, Waitrose*	1 Tortilla/43g	134	3.5	311	8.1	51.5	8.1	3.0
Wholemeal, Discovery*	1 Wrap/40g	109	3.3	273	9.2	40.4	8.3	6.4
Wholewheat, Asda*	1 Tortilla/35g	88	2.7	252	9.8	35.7	7.8	7.1
Wholewheat, Magnifico*	1 Tortilla/34g	86	2.7	252	9.8	35.7	7.8	7.1
Wrap, 8 Pack, Asda*	1 Tortilla/50g	143	3.0	286	8.0	50.0	6.0	1.9
Wrap, 8 Pack, Light Choices, Tesco*	1 Tortilla/50g	135	1.0	270	7.1	53.2	2.1	3.5
Wrap, Bueno*	1 Tortilla/63g	171	3.6	272	6.9	48.2	5.7	2.0
Wrap, Flour, Soft, Old El Paso*	1 Tortilla/58g	200	7.2	343	9.3	48.6	12.4	1.7
Wrap, Garlic & Parsley, Sainsbury's*	1 Tortilla/60g	166	3.7	277	7.2	48.0	6.2	1.8
Wrap, Low Carb, Tesco*	1 Tortilla/17g	77	1.5	453	39.4	53.5	8.8	23.5
Wrap, Low Fat, M & S*	1 Serving/180g	225	4.0	125	6.3	20.6	2.2	1.9
Wrap, Morrisons*	1 Serving/60g	132	2.1	220	6.2	42.0	3.5	1.7
Wrap, Organic, Sainsbury's*	1 Tortilla/56g	167	4.3	298	8.6	48.7	7.7	2.1
Wrap, Organic, Tesco*	1 Tortilla/57g	173	4.4	306	8.1	51.0	7.7	2.0
Wrap, Plain, Mini, Morrisons*	1 Tortilla/34g	91	1.4	267	8.1	48.9	4.0	2.8
Wrap, Plain, Nannak*	1 Wrap/80g	134	3.5	167	8.9	62.2	4.4	0.0
Wrap, Spicy Tomato, Morrisons*	1 Tortilla/55g	158	3.1	288	8.6	50.5	5.7	0.7
Wrap, Spicy Tomato, Tesco*	1 Tortilla/63g	175	3.5	278	7.8	49.2	5.6	2.4
Wrap, Tomato & Herb, Tesco*	1 Serving/63g	165	3.5	262	7.9	45.1	5.5	2.1
Wrap, Tomato & Herbs, Sainsbury's*	1 Tortilla/52g	157	3.1	302	7.8	54.1	6.0	2.4
Wrap, Weight Watchers*	1 Wrap/42g	107	0.4	254	7.1	50.7	1.0	6.7
Wraps, Less Than 3% Fat, BGTY, Sainsbury's*	1 Tortilla/51g	127	1.1	250	7.8	50.1	2.2	2.9
Wraps, Mexican, Asda*	1 Tortilla/34g	100	2.8	295	7.9	47.2	8.3	3.9
Wraps, Multiseed, Discovery*	1 Tortilla/57g	160	2.8	280	8.7	50.1	5.0	3.6
Wraps, Plain, Sainsbury's*	1 Tortilla/56g	167	4.4	299	8.1	49.2	7.8	3.6
TREACLE								
Black, Average	**1 Tbsp/20g**	**51**	**0.0**	**257**	**1.2**	**67.2**	**0.0**	**0.0**
TRIFLE								
Average	1 Portion/170g	272	10.7	160	3.6	22.3	6.3	0.5
Banana & Mandarin, Co-Op*	¼ Trifle/125g	237	13.7	190	2.0	21.0	11.0	0.1
Black Forest, Asda*	1 Serving/100g	237	9.0	237	3.1	36.0	9.0	0.0
Blackforest, BGTY, Sainsbury's*	1 Pot/125g	171	5.6	137	2.1	21.9	4.5	1.6
Caramel, Galaxy, Mars*	1 Pot/100g	255	13.0	255	4.5	30.0	13.0	1.0
Cherry, Finest, Tesco*	¼ Trifle/163g	340	19.3	209	2.6	22.9	11.9	0.3
Cherry & Almond, Somerfield*	1 Trifle/125g	230	11.2	184	2.0	23.0	9.0	0.0
Chocolate, Cadbury*	1 Pot/100g	282	18.5	282	5.2	24.3	18.5	0.0
Chocolate, Light, Cadbury*	1 Pot/90g	166	6.7	185	5.5	23.4	7.5	0.0
Chocolate, Tesco*	1 Serving/125g	312	19.0	250	4.3	24.0	15.2	0.7
Fruit, Sainsbury's*	1 Serving/125g	232	12.5	186	2.3	21.7	10.0	0.3
Fruit Cocktail, COU, M & S*	1 Trifle/140g	175	3.2	125	2.8	23.1	2.3	0.5
Fruit Cocktail, Individual, Shape, Danone*	1 Trifle/115g	136	3.1	118	3.2	19.6	2.7	1.6
Fruit Cocktail, Individual, Tesco*	1 Pot/113g	175	8.8	155	1.7	19.6	7.8	0.6
Fruit Cocktail, Low Fat, Danone*	1 Pot/115g	140	2.1	122	2.2	24.0	1.8	0.4
Fruit Cocktail, M & S*	1 Serving/165g	272	13.7	165	2.4	19.6	8.3	0.9
Fruit Cocktail, Sainsbury's*	1 Trifle/150g	241	9.0	161	1.8	24.8	6.0	0.4
Peach & Zabaglione, COU, M & S*	1 Glass/130g	149	3.0	115	2.8	20.6	2.3	0.8
Raspberry, Asda*	1 Serving/100g	175	8.0	175	1.8	24.0	8.0	0.1

T

TRIFLE

	Measure INFO/WEIGHT	KCAL	FAT	KCAL	PROT	CARB	FAT	FIBRE
Raspberry, Sainsbury's*	1 Pot/125g	204	9.7	163	1.7	21.5	7.8	0.6
Raspberry, Tesco*	1 Pot/150g	210	9.7	140	1.7	18.5	6.5	1.0
Sherry, BGTY, Sainsbury's*	1 Pot/135g	146	2.3	108	3.0	20.2	1.7	0.5
Strawberry, BGTY, Sainsbury's*	1 Pot/125g	135	2.6	108	2.4	19.9	2.1	0.5
Strawberry, COU, M & S*	1 Pot/138g	145	2.9	105	2.7	19.2	2.1	1.2
Strawberry, Individual, Shape, Danone*	1 Pot/115g	137	3.1	119	3.3	19.8	2.7	1.6
Strawberry, Low Fat Goodies, Danone*	1 Pot/115g	148	2.1	129	2.2	26.0	1.8	0.3
Strawberry, Luxury Devonshire, St Ivel*	1 Trifle/125g	207	9.9	166	2.0	21.7	7.9	0.2
Strawberry, Sainsbury's*	¼ Tub/150g	261	15.4	174	2.2	18.1	10.3	1.0
Strawberry, St Ivel*	1 Trifle/113g	194	9.8	172	2.4	21.0	8.7	0.2
Summerfruit, BGTY, Sainsbury's*	1 Trifle/125g	151	5.5	121	1.2	19.2	4.4	0.5
Triple Chocolate, Farmfoods*	¼ Trifle/86g	223	15.7	259	2.1	21.6	18.2	1.2

TRIFLE MIX

Strawberry Flavour, Bird's*	1oz/28g	119	2.9	425	2.7	78.0	10.5	1.2

TRIFLE SPONGES

Sainsbury's*	1 Sponge/24g	77	0.4	323	5.3	71.9	1.6	1.1
Tesco*	1 Sponge/24g	75	0.6	311	5.3	66.6	2.6	1.1

TRIPE &

Onions, Stewed	1oz/28g	26	0.8	93	8.3	9.5	2.7	0.7

TROMPRETTI

Fresh, Waitrose*	1 Serving/125g	339	3.0	271	11.7	50.6	2.4	2.0
Tricolour, Fresh, Tesco*	1 Pack/250g	675	8.5	270	11.2	48.6	3.4	4.0

TROUT

Brown, Steamed, Average	*1 Serving/120g*	*162*	*5.4*	*135*	*23.5*	*0.0*	*4.5*	*0.0*
Grilled, Weighed with Bones & Skin	1 Serving/100g	98	3.9	98	15.7	0.0	3.9	0.0
Rainbow, Grilled, Average	*1 Serving/120g*	*162*	*6.5*	*135*	*21.5*	*0.0*	*5.4*	*0.0*
Rainbow, Raw, Average	*1oz/28g*	*36*	*1.4*	*127*	*20.5*	*0.0*	*5.1*	*0.0*
Rainbow, Smoked, Average	*1 Pack/135g*	*190*	*7.6*	*140*	*21.7*	*0.7*	*5.6*	*0.0*
Raw, Average	*1 Serving/120g*	*159*	*6.5*	*132*	*20.6*	*0.0*	*5.4*	*0.0*
Smoked, Average	*2 Fillets/135g*	*187*	*7.1*	*138*	*22.7*	*0.3*	*5.2*	*0.1*

TUMS

Extra 750, Sugar Free, Tums*	2 Tablets/2g	5	0.0	250	0.0	50.0	0.0	0.0
Extra 750, Tums*	2 Tablets/2g	10	0.0	500	0.0	100.0	0.0	0.0
Regular, Tums*	1 Tablet/2g	2	0.0	125	0.0	25.0	0.0	0.0
Smoothies, Extra Strength 750, Tums*	2 Tablets/2g	10	0.0	500	0.0	100.0	0.0	0.0

TUNA

Bluefin, Cooked, Dry Heat, Average	*1 Serving/100g*	*184*	*6.3*	*184*	*29.9*	*0.0*	*6.3*	*0.0*
Chunks, in Brine, Drained, Average	1 Can/130g	141	0.7	108	25.9	0.0	0.5	0.0
Chunks, in Spring Water, Average, Drained	*1 Can/130g*	*140*	*0.8*	*108*	*25.4*	*0.0*	*0.6*	*0.1*
Chunks, in Sunflower Oil, Average, Drained	*1 Can/138g*	*260*	*12.6*	*188*	*26.5*	*0.0*	*9.1*	*0.0*
Chunks, Skipjack, in Brine, Average	*1 Can/138g*	*141*	*0.8*	*102*	*24.3*	*0.0*	*0.6*	*0.0*
Chunks, with a Little Brine, No Drain, 120g, John West*	1 Can/120g	130	1.1	108	25.0	0.0	0.9	0.0
Chunks, with a Little Brine, No Drain, 60g, John West*	1 Can/60g	55	0.5	91	21.0	0.0	0.8	0.0
Chunks with a Little Sunflower Oil, No Drain, John West*	1 Can/120g	202	9.1	168	25.0	0.0	7.6	0.0
Coronation Style, Canned, Average	1 Can/80g	122	7.6	152	10.2	6.5	9.5	0.6
Fillets, in Tomato Sauce, Princes*	1 Can/120g	131	3.0	109	19.0	2.5	2.5	0.0
Flakes, in Brine, Average	*1oz/28g*	*29*	*0.2*	*104*	*24.7*	*0.0*	*0.5*	*0.0*
French Style, Light Lunch, John West*	1 Pack/240g	204	6.5	85	8.3	6.7	2.7	1.2
in a Light Lemon Mayonnaise, Slimming World, Princes*	1 Can/80g	99	3.8	124	16.8	3.5	4.8	0.0
in a Light Mayonnaise, Slimming World, Princes*	1 Can/80g	96	3.3	120	17.3	3.6	4.1	0.0
in a Red Chilli & Lime Dressing, Princes*	1 Sachet/85g	102	2.8	120	21.5	1.0	3.3	0.0
in a Tikka Dressing, Slimming World, Princes*	1 Can/80g	108	4.6	135	16.8	4.0	5.7	0.0
in Thousand Island Dressing, John West*	1 Can/185g	287	12.9	155	18.0	5.1	7.0	0.2

	Measure INFO/WEIGHT	per Measure KCAL	FAT	Nutrition Values per 100g / 100ml KCAL	PROT	CARB	FAT	FIBRE
TUNA								
in Thousand Island Dressing, Weight Watchers*	1 Can/79g	67	1.7	85	8.3	7.8	2.2	0.4
in Water, Average	*1 Serving/120g*	*126*	*1.0*	*105*	*24.0*	*0.1*	*0.8*	*0.0*
Lemon Pepper Flavour, Sensations, Sealord*	1 Can/95g	212	13.8	223	18.5	4.9	14.5	0.0
Light Lunch, Indian Style, John West*	1 Pack/240g	401	23.0	167	7.7	12.3	9.6	0.6
Light Lunch, Mediterranean Style, John West*	1 Pack/240g	218	6.0	91	7.9	9.3	2.5	1.7
Light Lunch, Nicoise Style, John West*	1 Pack/250g	245	5.7	98	10.3	9.0	2.3	2.7
Light Lunch, Tomato Salsa Style, John West*	1 Pack/250g	195	3.0	78	7.1	9.7	1.2	1.9
Lime & Black Pepper, John West*	1 Serving/85g	133	7.8	156	15.6	2.8	9.2	0.0
Puertorican Style, Tinned, Natura*	1 Can/185g	157	8.3	85	9.0	1.0	4.5	0.0
Steak, Control Chef, All About Weight*	1 Meal/270g	284	4.3	105	9.8	10.9	1.6	3.9
Steaks, in Brine, Average	*1 Sm Can/99g*	*106*	*0.5*	*107*	*25.6*	*0.0*	*0.5*	*0.0*
Steaks, in Olive Oil, Average	*1 Serving/111g*	*211*	*10.7*	*190*	*25.8*	*0.0*	*9.6*	*0.0*
Steaks, in Sunflower Oil, Average	*1 Can/150g*	*276*	*12.9*	*184*	*26.7*	*0.0*	*8.6*	*0.0*
Steaks, in Water, Average	*1 Serving/200g*	*215*	*0.8*	*107*	*25.6*	*0.0*	*0.4*	*0.0*
Steaks, John West*	1 Can/130g	140	0.4	108	26.2	0.0	0.3	0.0
Steaks, Raw, Average	*1 Serving/140g*	*185*	*2.8*	*132*	*28.5*	*0.1*	*2.0*	*0.2*
Steaks, Skipjack, in Brine, Average	*½ Can/75g*	*73*	*0.4*	*97*	*23.2*	*0.0*	*0.5*	*0.0*
Steaks, with a Little Brine, No Drain, John West*	1 Can/130g	140	0.4	108	26.2	0.0	0.3	0.0
Steaks, with a Little Olive Oil, No Drain, John West*	1 Can/130g	209	7.0	161	28.2	0.0	5.4	0.0
with a Twist, French Dressing, John West*	1 Pack/85g	135	8.2	159	15.2	2.8	9.7	0.1
with a Twist, Oven Dried Tomato & Herb, John West*	1 Pack/85g	129	6.8	152	16.1	3.9	8.0	0.1
with Lemon & Black Pepper, Tesco*	1 Can/85g	144	6.5	170	21.2	4.0	7.6	0.5
Yellowfin, Cooked, Dry Heat, Average	*1 Serving/100g*	*139*	*1.2*	*139*	*30.0*	*0.0*	*1.2*	*0.0*
Yellowfin, Steak, Chargrilled, in Thai Green Curry, Princes*	1 Pack/140g	151	1.7	108	20.5	3.9	1.2	0.0
TUNA IN								
Coronation Style Dressing, Weight Watchers*	1 Tin/80g	75	2.0	94	9.3	8.7	2.5	0.4
Tomato & Herb Dressing, Weight Watchers*	1 Can/80g	79	2.9	99	11.6	5.1	3.6	0.5
TUNA MAYONNAISE								
& Sweetcorn, Canned, BGTY, Sainsbury's*	1 Can/80g	78	1.8	97	15.2	4.0	2.3	0.7
Garlic & Herb, John West*	½ Can/92g	243	20.4	264	12.0	4.0	22.2	0.2
Light, Slimming World*	1 Serving/80g	96	3.3	120	17.3	3.6	4.1	0.0
with Sweetcorn, From Heinz, Weight Watchers*	1 Can/80g	114	6.3	142	11.5	6.2	7.9	0.1
with Sweetcorn, John West*	½ Can/92g	231	19.0	251	12.0	4.5	20.6	0.2
with Sweetcorn & Green Peppers, GFY, Asda*	1 Pack/100g	103	3.0	103	14.0	5.0	3.0	0.8
TURBOT								
Grilled	*1oz/28g*	*34*	*1.0*	*122*	*22.7*	*0.0*	*3.5*	*0.0*
Raw	*1oz/28g*	*27*	*0.8*	*95*	*17.7*	*0.0*	*2.7*	*0.0*
TURKEY								
Breast, 3% Fat, Bernard Matthews*	1 Slice/20g	21	0.5	103	19.2	0.9	2.5	0.5
Breast, Butter Basted, Average	*1 Serving/75g*	*110*	*3.6*	*146*	*23.7*	*1.9*	*4.9*	*0.4*
Breast, Canned, Average	*1 Can/200g*	*194*	*4.7*	*97*	*18.3*	*0.7*	*2.3*	*0.0*
Breast, Chunks, Bernard Matthews*	1 Serving/55g	64	0.5	116	26.1	0.9	0.9	1.6
Breast, Diced, Healthy Range, Average	*1oz/28g*	*30*	*0.4*	*107*	*23.8*	*0.0*	*1.3*	*0.0*
Breast, Honey Roast, Sliced, Average	*1 Serving/50g*	*57*	*0.7*	*114*	*24.0*	*1.6*	*1.3*	*0.2*
Breast, Joint, Raw, Average	*1 Serving/125g*	*134*	*2.6*	*107*	*21.3*	*0.7*	*2.1*	*0.6*
Breast, Joint, with Sage & Onion Stuffing, Waitrose*	1 Serving/325g	377	13.3	116	19.2	1.4	4.1	0.1
Breast, Raw, Average	*1oz/28g*	*33*	*0.6*	*117*	*24.1*	*0.5*	*2.0*	*0.1*
Breast, Roasted, Average	*1oz/28g*	*37*	*0.9*	*131*	*24.6*	*0.7*	*3.3*	*0.1*
Breast, Roll, Cooked, Average	*1 Slice/10g*	*9*	*0.1*	*92*	*17.6*	*3.5*	*0.8*	*0.0*
Breast, Slices, Cooked, Average	*1 Slice/20g*	*23*	*0.3*	*114*	*24.0*	*1.2*	*1.4*	*0.3*
Breast, Smoked, Sliced, Average	*1 Slice/20g*	*23*	*0.4*	*113*	*23.4*	*0.7*	*1.9*	*0.0*
Breast, Steaks, in Crumbs, Average	1 Steak/76g	217	14.1	286	13.7	16.4	18.5	0.2
Breast, Steaks, Raw, Average	*1oz/28g*	*30*	*0.3*	*107*	*24.3*	*0.0*	*1.1*	*0.0*

T

	Measure INFO/WEIGHT	per Measure		Nutrition Values per 100g / 100ml				
		KCAL	FAT	KCAL	PROT	CARB	FAT	FIBRE

TURKEY

	Measure INFO/WEIGHT	KCAL	FAT	KCAL	PROT	CARB	FAT	FIBRE
Breast, Steaks, Thai, Bernard Matthews*	1 Serving/175g	280	4.7	160	29.4	4.6	2.7	0.0
Breast, Strips, for Stir Fry, Average	*1 Serving/175g*	*205*	*2.7*	*117*	*25.6*	*0.1*	*1.6*	*0.0*
Breast, Wafer Thin, Chinese Style, Bernard Matthews*	1 Pack/100g	110	1.5	110	18.0	6.1	1.5	0.0
Breast Golden Norfolk, Bernard Matthews*	1 Slice/20g	22	0.2	109	23.8	0.9	1.1	0.8
Breast Slices, Bernard Matthews*	1 Slice/20g	21	0.5	103	19.2	0.9	2.5	0.5
Dark Meat, Raw, Average	*1oz/28g*	*29*	*0.7*	*104*	*20.4*	*0.0*	*2.5*	*0.0*
Drummers, Golden, Bernard Matthews*	1 Drummer/57g	147	10.3	258	13.1	11.0	18.0	1.1
Drummers, Golden, Grilled, Bernard Matthews*	1 Drummer/50g	147	10.6	294	15.6	10.0	21.2	1.0
Drumsticks, Tesco*	1 Serving/200g	272	12.6	136	19.9	0.0	6.3	0.0
Escalope, Average	*1 Escalope/138g*	*341*	*19.3*	*247*	*13.5*	*16.7*	*14.0*	*0.6*
Escalope, Lemon & Pepper, Average	1 Escalope/143g	371	22.6	259	12.6	16.7	15.8	0.4
Escalope, Spicy Mango, Bernard Matthews*	1 Escalope/136g	354	17.4	260	11.6	24.6	12.8	0.0
Escalope, Tomato & Herb, Bernard Matthews*	1 Escalope/143g	336	19.2	236	10.5	18.0	13.5	0.0
Fillets, Chinese Marinated, Bernard Matthews*	1 Pack/200g	304	6.6	152	23.4	7.2	3.3	0.0
Fillets, Tikka Marinated, 93% Fat Free, Bernard Matthews*	1 Pack/200g	310	10.4	155	21.8	5.2	5.2	1.5
Goujons, Cooked, Bernard Matthews*	4 Goujons/128g	355	23.3	277	11.8	16.6	18.2	1.1
Leg, Roast, Uncooked, Bernard Matthews*	1 Serving/283g	317	15.3	112	15.4	0.5	5.4	0.0
Light Meat, Raw, Average	*1oz/28g*	*29*	*0.2*	*105*	*24.4*	*0.0*	*0.8*	*0.0*
Light Meat, Roasted	*1 Cup/140g*	*220*	*4.5*	*157*	*29.9*	*0.0*	*3.2*	*0.0*
Mince, Average	*1oz/28g*	*45*	*2.0*	*161*	*23.9*	*0.0*	*7.2*	*0.0*
Mince, Lean, Healthy Range, Average	*1oz/28g*	*33*	*1.1*	*118*	*20.3*	*0.0*	*4.1*	*0.0*
Rashers, Average	*1 Rasher/26g*	*26*	*0.4*	*101*	*19.1*	*2.3*	*1.6*	*0.0*
Rashers, Smoked, Average	*1 Serving/75g*	*76*	*1.3*	*101*	*19.8*	*1.5*	*1.8*	*0.0*
Roast, Meat & Skin, Average	*1oz/28g*	*48*	*1.8*	*171*	*28.0*	*0.0*	*6.5*	*0.0*
Roast, Meat Only, Average	*1 Serving/100g*	*157*	*3.2*	*157*	*29.9*	*0.0*	*3.2*	*0.0*
Roll, Dinosaur, Cooked, Bernard Matthews*	1 Slice/10g	17	1.0	170	13.6	6.0	10.2	1.1
Schnitzel, Lidl*	1 Schnitzel/115g	210	8.0	183	19.0	11.0	7.0	0.0
Steaks, Breaded, Bernard Matthews*	1 Steak/110g	319	20.0	290	11.0	20.5	18.2	1.5
Strips, Stir-Fried, Average	1oz/28g	46	1.3	164	31.0	0.0	4.5	0.0
Thigh, Diced, Average	*1oz/28g*	*33*	*1.2*	*117*	*19.6*	*0.0*	*4.3*	*0.0*
Wafer Thin, Cooked, Average	1 Slice/10g	12	0.4	122	19.0	3.2	3.7	0.0
Wafer Thin, Honey Roast, Average	1 Slice/10g	11	0.2	109	19.2	4.2	1.7	0.2
Wafer Thin, Smoked, Average	1 Slice/10g	12	0.4	119	18.1	3.6	3.7	0.0
Whole, Raw, Average	*½ Joint/254g*	*389*	*16.8*	*153*	*22.5*	*0.8*	*6.6*	*0.0*

TURKEY DINNER

Roast, Asda*	1 Pack/400g	344	6.4	86	7.0	11.0	1.6	2.0
Roast, Iceland*	1 Meal/400g	374	7.2	93	8.4	10.9	1.8	1.3
Roast, Meal for One, M & S*	1 Pack/370g	462	16.3	125	9.1	12.4	4.4	2.7
Roast, Sainsbury's*	1 Pack/450g	354	9.0	79	6.8	8.4	2.0	1.9
Traditional, Birds Eye*	1 Pack/340g	292	7.8	86	6.1	10.3	2.3	1.7

TURKEY HAM

Average	*1 Serving/75g*	*81*	*2.9*	*108*	*15.6*	*2.8*	*3.9*	*0.0*

TURKEY IN

BBQ Marinade, Steaks, Asda*	1 Serving/225g	355	5.2	158	30.0	4.4	2.3	0.9
Pepper Sauce, Escalope, Bernard Matthews*	1 Escalope/143g	350	21.4	245	9.4	18.2	15.0	1.5

TURKISH DELIGHT

Assorted Flavours, Julian Graves*	1 Square/30g	110	0.0	366	0.5	91.1	0.1	0.0
Co-Op*	1 Bar/53g	207	4.2	390	2.0	78.0	8.0	0.1
Dark Chocolate Covered, Thorntons*	1 Chocolate/10g	39	1.1	390	2.7	69.0	11.0	2.0
Fry's*	1 Bar/51g	185	3.4	365	1.4	74.6	6.7	1.3
Milk Chocolate, M & S*	1 Pack/55g	220	4.7	400	1.6	79.0	8.5	0.0
Sultans*	1 Serving/16g	58	0.0	360	0.0	90.0	0.0	0.0
with Mixed Nuts, Hazer Baba*	1 Piece/12g	47	0.2	389	1.6	88.5	1.7	0.0

T

	Measure INFO/WEIGHT	per Measure KCAL	FAT	Nutrition Values per 100g / 100ml KCAL	PROT	CARB	FAT	FIBRE
TURKISH DELIGHT								
with Rose, Hazer Baba*	1 Square/18g	70	0.3	389	1.6	88.6	1.7	0.0
TURMERIC								
Powder	*1 Tsp/3g*	*11*	*0.3*	*354*	*7.8*	*58.2*	*9.9*	*0.0*
TURNIP								
Boiled, Average	*1oz/28g*	*3*	*0.1*	*12*	*0.6*	*2.0*	*0.2*	*1.9*
Mash, Direct Foods*	½ Pack/190g	49	3.4	26	0.6	2.0	1.8	1.9
Mashed, Mash Direct*	1 Pack/400g	148	2.3	37	0.7	6.0	0.6	2.5
Raw, Unprepared, Average	*1oz/28g*	*6*	*0.1*	*23*	*0.9*	*4.7*	*0.3*	*2.4*
TURNOVER								
Apple, Bramley, Tesco*	1 Turnover/88g	304	22.8	346	2.7	25.4	25.9	0.9
Apple, Co-Op*	1 Turnover/77g	308	20.8	400	4.0	35.0	27.0	1.0
Apple, Dutch, Sainsbury's*	1 Serving/33g	130	5.5	393	3.6	56.9	16.8	1.4
Apple, Fresh Cream, Sainsbury's*	1 Turnover/84g	292	20.9	347	4.1	26.9	24.8	2.5
Apple, Tesco*	1 Turnover/88g	294	19.7	334	3.2	29.8	22.4	0.9
Mincemeat, Fresh Cream, Tesco*	1 Turnover/83g	334	22.2	405	3.1	37.5	26.9	1.1
Raspberry, Fresh Cream, Asda*	1 Turnover/100g	411	23.0	411	6.0	45.0	23.0	2.1
Raspberry, Tesco*	1 Turnover/84g	290	20.2	345	4.0	27.2	24.1	2.1
TWIGLETS								
Curry, Jacob's*	1 Bag/30g	134	6.4	448	8.0	55.7	21.5	6.0
Original, Jacob's*	1 Bag/30g	115	3.5	383	12.7	57.0	11.6	11.8
Tangy, Jacob's*	1 Bag/30g	136	6.6	454	8.1	55.9	22.0	5.4
TWIRL								
Bites, Cadbury*	1 Bite/2g	11	0.6	530	7.7	56.5	30.3	0.8
Cadbury*	1 Finger/22g	118	6.8	535	7.6	56.0	30.9	0.8
Treat Size, Cadbury*	1 Bar/21g	115	6.6	535	7.6	56.0	30.9	0.8
TWISTS								
Black Olive & Basil, Finest, Tesco*	¼ Pack/31g	151	7.9	483	11.3	53.1	25.1	3.9
Gruyere & Poppy Seed, TTD, Sainsbury's*	1 Serving/8g	41	2.3	509	13.7	50.5	28.0	2.6
Parmesan, All Butter, TTD, Sainsbury's*	1 Serving/8g	38	2.0	487	13.8	51.0	25.3	2.8
Strawberry, Sainsbury's*	1 Serving/10g	37	0.3	375	1.7	82.7	3.0	0.1
Tomato & Herb, Shapers, Boots*	1 Pack/20g	94	4.2	468	3.7	66.0	21.0	3.9
TWIX								
Fun Size, Mars*	1 Bar/21g	103	5.0	492	4.7	65.5	23.7	1.5
Standard, Mars*	1 Pack/58g	284	13.7	490	4.7	65.5	23.7	1.5
Top, Mars*	1 Bar/28g	143	7.8	511	5.2	60.2	27.7	0.0
Twixels, Mars*	1 Finger/6g	31	1.6	513	5.0	64.0	26.1	0.0
Xtra, Mars*	1 Pack/85g	416	20.1	490	4.7	65.5	23.7	1.5
TZATZIKI								
Average	1 Tbsp/30g	20	1.5	66	3.7	2.0	4.9	0.2
Greek, Authentic, Total, Fage*	1 Serving/50g	49	3.5	99	4.9	4.1	7.0	1.0

T

	Measure INFO/WEIGHT	per Measure		Nutrition Values per 100g / 100ml				
		KCAL	FAT	KCAL	PROT	CARB	FAT	FIBRE
VANILLA								
Bean, Average	*1 Pod/2g*	*6*	*0.0*	*288*	*0.0*	*13.0*	*0.0*	*0.0*
Flavouring, Supercook*	1 Tsp/4g	2	0.0	50	6.2	0.0	0.0	0.0
VANILLA EXTRACT								
Average	*1 Tbsp/13g*	*37*	*0.0*	*288*	*0.1*	*12.6*	*0.1*	*0.0*
Pure, Nielsen Massey Vanillas*	1 Tsp/5ml	8	0.0	160	0.1	39.5	0.2	0.1
VEAL								
Chop, Loin, Raw, Weighed with Bone, Average	1 Chop/195g	495	27.8	254	29.5	0.0	14.3	0.0
Escalope, Fried, Average	1oz/28g	55	1.9	196	33.7	0.0	6.8	0.0
Escalopes, Breaded, M & S*	1 Escalope/130g	292	13.9	225	13.6	18.7	10.7	0.4
Mince, Raw, Average	*1oz/28g*	*40*	*2.0*	*144*	*20.3*	*0.0*	*7.0*	*0.0*
Shoulder, Lean & Fat, Roasted, Average	*1oz/28g*	*52*	*2.3*	*183*	*25.5*	*0.0*	*8.2*	*0.0*
Shoulder, Lean Only, Roasted, Average	*1oz/28g*	*46*	*1.6*	*164*	*26.1*	*0.0*	*5.8*	*0.0*
Sirloin, Lean & Fat, Roasted, Average	*1oz/28g*	*57*	*3.0*	*202*	*25.1*	*0.0*	*10.4*	*0.0*
Sirloin, Lean Only, Roasted, Average	*1oz/28g*	*48*	*1.8*	*168*	*26.3*	*0.0*	*6.2*	*0.0*
VEGEMITE								
Australian, Kraft*	1 Tsp/5g	9	0.0	173	23.5	19.7	0.0	0.0
VEGETABLE CHIPS								
Beetroot, Carrot & Parsnips, Hand Fried, Tyrrells*	½ Pack/25g	103	7.0	413	3.9	36.0	28.1	11.5
Cassava, Average	1oz/28g	99	0.1	353	1.8	91.4	0.4	4.0
Mixed Root, Tyrrells*	1oz/28g	133	8.3	476	5.7	35.4	29.8	12.8
Parsnip, Golden, Kettle Chips*	½ Pack/50g	257	18.8	515	4.6	39.5	37.6	8.4
Sweet Potato, Kettle Chips*	½ Pack/50g	241	16.4	483	2.4	44.4	32.8	9.3
VEGETABLE FAT								
Pure, Trex*	1 Tbsp/12g	108	12.0	900	0.0	0.0	100.0	0.0
VEGETABLE FINGERS								
Crispy, Birds Eye*	2 Fingers/60g	107	4.8	179	3.2	23.5	8.0	2.3
Crispy Crunchy, Dalepak*	1 Finger/28g	62	3.1	223	4.2	26.7	11.0	15.0
Sweetcorn, Tesco*	1 Finger/28g	66	3.5	236	7.7	23.0	12.6	3.0
VEGETABLE MEDLEY								
& New Potato, Asda*	½ Pack/175g	101	3.9	58	2.5	7.0	2.2	5.0
Asparagus Tips, Perfectly Balanced, Waitrose*	1 Serving/225g	121	7.6	54	1.3	4.6	3.4	1.4
Basil & Oregano Butter, Waitrose*	1 Serving/113g	59	3.8	52	1.7	3.7	3.4	1.9
Buttered, Sainsbury's*	½ Pack/175g	122	6.8	70	1.7	7.0	3.9	1.8
Carrot, Courgette, Fine Bean & Baby Corn, Tesco*	1 Serving/100g	36	2.4	36	1.1	2.4	2.4	3.0
Crunchy, M & S*	1 Pack/250g	75	2.0	30	3.1	2.8	0.8	2.5
Frozen, M & S*	1 Pack/500g	175	4.0	35	3.4	3.9	0.8	3.1
Green, HL, Tesco*	1 Serving/125g	59	2.2	47	3.7	4.1	1.8	4.1
Roast, Four Seasons*	1 Pack/375g	202	12.0	54	2.8	3.5	3.2	2.7
Roasted, Waitrose*	½ Pack/200g	282	15.6	141	1.2	16.4	7.8	3.7
VEGETABLES								
Asparagus & Tenderstem Broccoli, Finest, Tesco*	½ Pack/95g	28	0.4	29	3.7	2.7	0.4	2.7
Baby, Frozen, Asda*	1 Serving/100g	25	0.3	25	1.9	3.7	0.3	1.9
Baby Mix, Freshly Frozen, Iceland*	1 Serving/100g	26	0.3	26	1.8	3.9	0.3	1.9
Bean & Vegetable Layer, M & S*	1 Pack/285g	271	13.7	95	3.6	7.2	4.8	3.7
Broccoli, Leek & Cabbage, Fresh, Love Life, Waitrose*	1 Serving/100g	26	0.4	26	1.5	3.1	0.4	1.8
Broccoli & Cauliflower, Layered, M & S*	½ Pack/135g	94	4.6	70	1.5	7.6	3.4	1.2
Carrot & Sprouts, Microwaved, Fresh Tastes, Asda*	1 Pack/300g	150	0.9	50	1.9	8.7	0.3	2.3
Carrots, Peas & Sweetcorn, Steam, Tesco*	½ Pack/150g	150	4.2	100	3.4	15.0	2.8	3.2
Casserole, Cooks' Ingredients, Waitrose*	¼ Pack/125g	37	0.4	30	1.0	5.9	0.3	4.0
Casserole, Washed & Ready to Cook, Basics, Sainsbury's*	1 Bag/450g	121	0.4	27	0.7	4.2	0.1	3.1
Chinese Glazed, Tesco*	1 Pack/200g	110	4.4	55	1.3	7.7	2.2	1.2
Chinese Inspired, Crisp, M & S*	1 Pack/250g	62	0.7	25	1.7	4.6	0.3	1.9
Chunky, Somerfield*	1 Serving/100g	26	0.3	26	0.1	5.8	0.3	0.0

V

VEGETABLES

Measure INFO/WEIGHT	per Measure		Nutrition Values per 100g / 100ml				
	KCAL	FAT	KCAL	PROT	CARB	FAT	FIBRE
Classic Layered, M & S*							
1 Pack/320g	224	12.5	70	1.2	7.3	3.9	1.2
Crisp & Crunchy, Stir Fry, M & S*							
½ Pack/115g	29	0.2	25	1.9	3.9	0.2	1.7
Crispy, Ready to Cook, Sainsbury's*							
1 Serving/100g	24	0.3	24	1.8	3.6	0.3	2.2
Crush, Potato & Pea with Minted Butter, M & S*							
½ Pack/200g	180	6.8	90	3.9	9.6	3.4	3.9
Farmhouse, Mixed, Frozen, Boiled in Salted Water, Tesco*							
1 Portion/75g	31	0.5	42	3.2	5.8	0.7	3.3
Garden, Washed, Tesco*							
1 Bag/250g	65	1.7	26	3.0	1.9	0.7	2.0
Green, Medley, Fresh, Sainsbury's*							
1 Pack/160g	50	1.8	31	3.8	2.8	1.1	2.2
Green, Minted, Love Life, Waitrose*							
1 Pack/265g	154	6.9	58	3.0	4.1	2.6	3.2
Grilled, Frozen, Sainsbury's*							
1 Serving/80g	42	2.9	52	1.2	3.8	3.6	1.5
Grilled Mix, Frozen, Essential, Waitrose*							
1 Serving/80g	34	0.2	42	1.8	8.1	0.3	2.4
Italiano Marinated, Roasted, Tesco*							
½ Tub/100g	121	8.6	121	1.7	9.2	8.6	0.8
Julienne, Tesco*							
1 Serving/100g	30	0.3	30	1.1	5.7	0.3	1.9
Kale, Spinach, Pak Choi & Jagallo Nero, Asda*							
¼ Bag/45g	13	0.5	29	2.4	1.0	1.1	2.8
Layered, GFY, Asda*							
½ Pack/150g	81	4.2	54	1.2	6.0	2.8	2.0
Layered, Tesco*							
1 Serving/280g	202	14.6	72	1.6	4.8	5.2	1.6
Layered, with Butter, Waitrose*							
1 Pack/280g	207	16.2	74	1.7	3.6	5.8	2.4
Layered, with Seasoned Butter, Asda*							
½ Pack/163g	78	3.4	48	1.4	5.9	2.1	3.5
Mediterranean, in Tomato Sauce, COU, M & S*							
1 Pack/300g	105	2.1	35	2.5	4.3	0.7	2.2
Mediterranean, Ready to Roast, Waitrose*							
1 Serving/200g	128	8.0	64	1.3	5.6	4.0	1.6
Mediterranean, Sainsbury's*							
1 Pack/400g	180	9.6	45	1.2	4.5	2.4	3.1
Mediterranean Roasted, Sainsbury's*							
1 Serving/150g	118	5.4	79	2.2	9.5	3.6	3.4
Mediterranean Style, Asda*							
½ Pack/205g	113	3.7	55	1.7	7.9	1.8	1.3
Mediterranean Style, COOK!, M & S*							
½ Pack/200g	60	1.8	30	1.2	5.5	0.9	1.0
Mediterranean Style, Finest, Tesco*							
½ Pack/150g	155	12.2	103	1.5	5.5	8.1	3.0
Mediterranean Style, M & S*							
½ Pack/214g	75	1.9	35	1.2	5.5	0.9	1.0
Mediterranean Style, Ready to Roast, Sainsbury's*							
½ Pack/200g	138	4.4	69	2.3	9.9	2.2	2.2
Mediterranean Style, Roasting, Tesco*							
1 Serving/200g	72	2.0	36	1.1	5.7	1.0	1.3
Mixed, Carrot, Cauliflower, & Broccoli, Fresh, Tesco*							
1 Serving/80g	26	0.2	32	2.6	3.9	0.2	2.8
Mixed, Frozen, Chosen By You, Asda*							
1 Serving/80g	47	0.8	59	2.6	8.5	1.0	0.0
Mixed, Frozen, Sainsbury's*							
1 Serving/100g	50	0.7	50	2.9	7.9	0.7	3.5
Moroccan, COU, M & S*							
1 Pack/300g	165	4.5	55	2.4	8.2	1.5	1.7
Oriental, Waitrose*							
1 Pack/300g	108	0.6	36	0.8	7.8	0.2	1.4
Oriental Inspired, M & S*							
1 Pack/260g	78	1.3	30	1.9	4.6	0.5	2.7
Oriental Soup, TTD, Sainsbury's*							
1 Pack/200g	64	0.6	32	1.9	4.3	0.3	2.0
Oriental Stir Fry, Frozen, Sainsbury's*							
½ Pack/225g	142	8.8	63	1.5	5.4	3.9	1.5
Ready to Roast, Mediterranean Selection, Waitrose*							
½ Pack/200g	70	2.4	35	1.4	3.8	1.2	1.6
Ribbon, Pan Stir Fry, Love Life, Waitrose*							
½ Pack/134g	47	0.5	35	1.3	5.4	0.4	2.4
Roast, M & S*							
1 Pack/420g	273	17.6	65	1.4	4.9	4.2	0.4
Roasted, Italian, M & S*							
1 Serving/95g	218	19.9	230	1.8	7.1	21.0	1.7
Roasted, Selection, COU, M & S*							
1 Pack/250g	87	2.0	35	1.2	6.1	0.8	0.6
Roasted Mediterranean, The Best*							
1 Serving/125g	100	5.7	80	2.3	7.0	4.6	3.6
Roasted Root, Extra Special, Asda*							
½ Pack/205g	160	3.1	78	1.1	15.0	1.5	6.0
Roasted Winter, HL, Tesco*							
½ Pack/200g	160	5.0	80	1.9	12.7	2.5	3.6
Roasting, Tesco*							
1 Serving/350g	152	1.9	43	1.2	8.0	0.5	3.0
Root, Honey Roast, Sainsbury's*							
1 Pack/400g	748	34.8	187	0.0	25.8	8.7	5.2
Seasonal, Pack, Sainsbury's*							
1 Serving/261g	60	0.8	23	0.7	4.6	0.3	2.0
Selection, Baby Potatoes, Runner Beans & Broccoli, Tesco*							
1 Serving/100g	55	0.3	55	2.3	9.7	0.3	2.1
Sliced Carrots & Broccoli Florets, Fresh, Morrisons*							
1 Portion/100g	37	0.7	37	2.2	4.1	0.7	2.5
Soup Mix, Fresh, Classic, Prepared, Tesco*							
1/3 Pack/163g	60	1.0	37	1.1	5.3	0.6	2.8
Special Mix, Sainsbury's*							
1 Serving/80g	54	1.4	68	3.4	9.7	1.7	3.2
Steam & Serve, Morrisons*							
1 Serving/120g	66	1.3	55	2.4	8.8	1.1	2.6
Stew Pack, Budgens*							
1 Serving/80g	32	0.2	40	0.9	8.4	0.3	1.2
Summer, Rainbow, Roasting, Fresh Tastes, Asda*							
½ Pack/175g	84	4.7	48	1.4	3.5	2.7	0.0

	Measure INFO/WEIGHT	per Measure KCAL	FAT	Nutrition Values per 100g / 100ml KCAL	PROT	CARB	FAT	FIBRE
VEGETABLES								
Summer, Roasted, TTD, Sainsbury's*	½ Pack/200g	160	2.2	80	1.8	14.5	1.1	2.6
Sun Dried Tomato, Selection, Finest, Tesco*	1 Pack/340g	303	17.3	89	1.8	8.9	5.1	1.1
Sweet & Crunchy, Tesco*	1 Serving/50g	21	0.3	43	2.3	7.0	0.6	2.4
Szechuan Style, Ready Prepared, Waitrose*	1 Pack/300g	132	3.9	44	2.3	5.7	1.3	1.9
Tender, Green, Medley, Sainsbury's*	½ Pack/88g	35	0.5	40	3.6	5.1	0.6	3.3
Tender, Green, Selection, Waitrose*	½ Pack/140g	66	1.1	47	3.9	3.8	0.8	3.8
Tindora, Ivy Goud, Kovakkai, Dadoo's Market*	1 Serving/100g	27	0.1	27	0.0	5.2	0.1	0.0
Winter, Carrots, Brussels Sprouts & Broccoli Florets, Tesco*	1 Portion/100g	44	0.8	44	2.2	5.4	0.8	3.2
Winter, Fresh, Asda*	1 Bag/250g	75	2.5	30	3.0	2.2	1.0	2.3
Winter, Ready to Roast, Fresh, Sainsbury's*	1 Pack/272g	226	7.6	83	1.2	13.2	2.8	0.0
Winter, Sainsbury's*	1 Serving/125g	37	1.0	30	2.0	3.6	0.8	2.2
Winter Crunchy, M & S*	½ Pack/125g	31	1.0	25	2.0	3.1	0.8	2.7
Winter Soup Mix, Sainsbury's*	1 Portion/149g	61	0.3	41	1.1	7.9	0.2	1.7
with Sun Dried Tomato, Roasted, Finest, Tesco*	½ Pack/150g	153	10.8	102	1.9	7.3	7.2	1.2
Wok, Chinese, Stir Fry, Classic, Findus*	1 Pack/500g	150	2.5	30	1.0	5.0	0.5	3.5
Wok, Sambal Oelek, Findus*	1 Serving/200g	170	0.8	85	3.0	17.0	0.4	0.0
Wok, Thai, Findus*	½ Pack/250g	87	0.7	35	1.5	7.0	0.3	0.0
Wok Mix, Stir Fry, Frozen, Essential, Waitrose*	1 Serving/200g	60	0.4	30	1.2	4.0	0.2	3.4
VEGETARIAN								
Chicken Style Pieces, Sainsbury's*	1 Pack/375g	754	26.2	201	25.5	9.0	7.0	0.6
Fingers, Fish Style, Breaded, The Redwood Co*	1 Finger/36g	94	5.2	262	16.5	16.0	14.5	0.0
Nut & Date Roast with Gravy, Asda*	1 Serving/196g	300	12.7	153	4.7	16.1	6.5	5.5
Pepperoni Style, Cheatin', The Redwood Co*	1 Slice/10g	28	1.8	282	25.3	5.2	17.7	0.2
Roast, Chicken Style, Vegeroast, Realeat*	4 Slices/114g	211	10.2	186	23.0	3.2	9.0	1.5
Roast, Linda McCartney*	¼ Roast/114g	222	10.2	196	19.4	9.4	9.0	1.5
Slices, Sage & Onion, Vegi Deli, The Redwood Co*	1 Slice/10g	23	1.4	233	21.4	5.0	14.1	0.5
Slices, Vegetable, Tesco*	1 Slice/165g	452	30.5	274	5.6	21.4	18.5	3.3
VEGETARIAN MINCE								
Chicken Style Pieces, Realeat*	¼ Pack/88g	119	1.4	136	29.0	1.5	1.6	4.4
Easy Cook, Linda McCartney*	1oz/28g	35	0.1	126	21.4	9.3	0.4	1.7
Frozen, Meatfree, Improved Recipe, Sainsbury's*	1 Pack/454g	799	31.8	176	18.3	10.7	7.0	6.7
Meat Free, Boiled, Chosen By You, Asda*	1 Serving/75g	83	2.5	111	13.7	6.7	3.3	4.4
Meat Free, Tesco*	1 Serving/76g	113	3.8	150	19.0	7.0	5.0	6.0
Vegemince, Realeat*	1 Serving/125g	217	12.5	174	18.0	3.0	10.0	3.0
VENISON								
Grill Steak, Average	**1 Grillsteak/150g**	**178**	**3.7**	**119**	**19.0**	**5.0**	**2.5**	**0.9**
in Red Wine & Port, Average	1oz/28g	21	0.7	76	9.8	3.5	2.6	0.4
Minced, Cooked, Average	**1 Serving/100g**	**187**	**8.2**	**187**	**26.4**	**0.0**	**8.2**	**0.0**
Minced, Raw, Average	**1 Serving/100g**	**157**	**7.1**	**157**	**21.8**	**0.0**	**7.1**	**0.0**
Raw, Haunch, Meat Only, Average	1 Serving/100g	103	1.6	103	22.2	0.0	1.6	0.0
Roasted, Average	**1oz/28g**	**46**	**0.7**	**165**	**35.6**	**0.0**	**2.5**	**0.0**
Steak, Raw, Average	**1oz/28g**	**30**	**0.5**	**108**	**22.8**	**0.0**	**1.9**	**0.0**
VERMICELLI								
Dry	**1oz/28g**	**99**	**0.1**	**355**	**8.7**	**78.3**	**0.4**	**0.0**
Egg, Cooked, Average	**1 Serving/185g**	**239**	**2.6**	**129**	**5.0**	**24.0**	**1.4**	**1.0**
VERMOUTH								
Dry	**1 Shot/50ml**	**54**	**0.0**	**109**	**0.1**	**3.0**	**0.0**	**0.0**
Sweet	**1 Shot/50ml**	**75**	**0.0**	**151**	**0.0**	**15.9**	**0.0**	**0.0**
VIMTO*								
Cordial, No Added Sugar, Diluted, Vimto Soft Drinks*	1 Glass/250ml	6	0.2	2	0.1	0.4	0.1	0.0
Cordial, Original, Diluted, Vimto Soft Drinks*	1 Serving/200ml	60	0.0	30	0.0	7.4	0.0	0.0
VINAIGRETTE								
Balsamic, Hellmann's*	1 Tbsp/15ml	12	0.4	82	0.1	9.6	2.7	0.6

V

	Measure INFO/WEIGHT	per Measure KCAL	FAT	Nutrition Values per 100g / 100ml KCAL	PROT	CARB	FAT	FIBRE
VINAIGRETTE								
Balsamic Vinegar & Pistachio, Finest, Tesco*	1 Tbsp/15ml	55	5.9	370	0.2	2.8	39.2	0.0
Blush Wine, Briannas*	2 Tbsp/30ml	100	6.0	333	0.0	40.0	20.0	0.0
Fat Free, Hellmann's*	1 Serving/15ml	7	0.0	49	0.1	10.9	0.0	0.3
Frank Cooper*	1 Pot/28g	46	3.2	163	1.0	14.1	11.4	0.3
French, Real, Briannas*	2 Tbsp/30ml	150	17.0	500	0.0	0.0	56.7	0.0
French Style, Finest, Tesco*	1 Tbsp/15ml	93	9.8	620	0.6	6.3	65.3	0.2
Luxury French, Hellmann's*	1 Tsp/5ml	15	1.3	305	0.8	16.0	26.1	0.4
Olive Oil & Lemon, Amoy*	½ Sachet/15ml	37	3.6	250	0.3	3.0	24.0	0.0
Perfectly Balanced, Waitrose*	1 Tsp/5ml	4	0.0	89	0.4	20.9	0.4	0.5
Portuguese, Nando's*	1 Tbsp/15g	61	6.6	409	1.0	2.0	44.0	0.3
Waistline, 99% Fat Free, Crosse & Blackwell*	1 Tbsp/15ml	1	0.0	9	1.0	0.7	0.2	0.2
with Mustard, Delhaize*	1 Serving/20g	93	10.2	464	0.8	0.7	50.9	0.0
VINE LEAVES								
Preserved in Brine	**1oz/28g**	**4**	**0.0**	**15**	**3.6**	**0.2**	**0.0**	**0.0**
Stuffed, Mediterranean Deli, M & S*	1 Leaf/37g	39	1.5	105	2.6	14.2	4.1	1.2
Stuffed with Rice	1oz/28g	73	5.0	262	2.8	23.8	18.0	0.0
Stuffed with Rice, Palirria*	½ Pack/140g	186	9.0	133	2.2	16.6	6.4	0.0
VINEGAR								
Aged, Balsamic, Finest, Tesco*	1 Tbsp/15ml	34	0.0	230	0.5	51.4	0.0	0.0
Apple Balsamic, Aspall*	1 Serving/100g	123	0.1	123	0.5	26.1	0.1	0.0
Balsamic, Average	**1 Tsp/5ml**	**6**	**0.0**	**115**	**0.9**	**26.0**	**0.0**	**0.0**
Balsamic, of Modena, So Organic, Sainsbury's*	1 Tsp/5g	6	0.0	111	1.4	26.3	0.1	0.1
Balsamic Reduction, Secret Kitchen*	1 Tsp/5ml	15	0.0	309	0.4	50.0	0.1	0.0
Cider	**1 Tbsp/15ml**	**2**	**0.0**	**14**	**0.0**	**5.9**	**0.0**	**0.0**
Cyder, Aspall*	1 fl oz/30ml	5	0.0	18	0.0	0.1	0.0	0.0
Malt, Average	**1 Tbsp/15g**	**1**	**0.0**	**4**	**0.4**	**0.6**	**0.0**	**0.0**
Organic Red Wine, Aspall*	1 Serving/100g	20	0.0	20	0.3	0.0	0.0	0.0
Red Wine, Aspall*	1 Serving/100g	22	0.0	22	0.4	0.6	0.0	0.0
Red Wine, Average	1 Tbsp/15ml	3	0.0	19	0.0	0.3	0.0	0.0
Rice, Mizkan*	1 Tbsp/15ml	4	0.0	26	0.2	2.6	0.0	0.0
Rice, White, Amoy*	1 Tsp/5ml	0	0.0	4	0.0	1.0	0.0	0.0
Sushi Rice Seasoning, Organic, Clearspring*	1 Tsp/5ml	1	0.0	16	0.5	0.2	0.0	0.0
VODKA								
& Cranberry, Classic Combinations, Manchester Drinks Co*	1 Serving/200ml	146	0.0	73	0.0	11.3	0.0	0.0
37.5% Volume	**1 Shot/35ml**	**72**	**0.0**	**207**	**0.0**	**0.0**	**0.0**	**0.0**
40% Volume	**1 Shot/35ml**	**78**	**0.0**	**222**	**0.0**	**0.0**	**0.0**	**0.0**
Bullett & Cola, Premixed, Canned, Diageo*	1 Can/250ml	217	0.0	87	0.0	10.6	0.0	0.0
Cookies & Cream, Sidekick, Halewood International Ltd*	1 Serving/30ml	48	0.5	160	0.3	7.7	1.6	0.0
Smirnoff & Cola, Premixed, Canned, Diageo*	1 Can/250ml	177	0.0	71	0.0	8.9	0.0	0.0
Smirnoff & Cranberry, Premixed, Canned, Diageo*	1 Can/250ml	175	0.0	70	0.0	8.5	0.0	0.0
Smirnoff & Diet Cola, Premixed, Canned, Diageo*	1 Can/250ml	100	0.0	40	0.0	0.0	0.0	0.0
Smirnoff & Schweppes Tonic, Premixed, Canned, Diageo*	1 Can/250ml	157	0.0	63	0.0	6.4	0.0	0.0
VODKA &								
Tonic, Ready Mixed, M & S*	1 Can/250ml	202	0.0	81	0.0	6.3	0.0	0.0
VOL AU VENTS								
Garlic Mushroom, Mini, Asda*	1 Serving/17g	59	4.6	347	5.0	21.0	27.0	0.0
Ham & Cheese, M & S*	1oz/28g	106	7.5	380	8.8	25.7	26.7	1.8
Mushroom, Sainsbury's*	1 Serving/14g	49	3.1	350	6.9	30.8	22.1	1.4
Mushroom & Roast Garlic, M & S*	1 Serving/19g	65	4.6	345	6.2	25.2	24.3	1.9
Prawn, M & S*	1oz/28g	101	6.9	360	8.0	26.2	24.7	1.9
Seafood, Party, Youngs*	1 Serving/17g	60	4.2	354	8.3	26.0	24.8	1.0
Tomato, M & S*	1oz/28g	87	5.7	310	4.5	26.7	20.4	1.7

V

	Measure INFO/WEIGHT	per Measure KCAL	FAT	Nutrition Values per 100g / 100ml KCAL	PROT	CARB	FAT	FIBRE
WAFERS								
Apricot & Peach, Highlights, Cadbury*	1 Wafer/19g	80	2.7	430	5.2	70.6	14.3	1.4
Cafe Curls, Rolled, Askeys*	1 Wafer/5g	21	0.4	422	5.8	80.3	8.6	0.0
Caramel, Dark Chocolate, Tunnock's*	1 Wafer/26g	128	6.6	492	5.2	60.7	25.4	0.0
Caramel, Milk Chocolate, Farmfoods*	1 Wafer/22g	104	5.0	475	5.9	61.9	22.8	3.1
Caramel, Milk Chocolate Coated, Value, Tesco*	1 Wafer/23g	110	4.7	475	5.6	67.6	20.2	0.6
Caramel, Penguin, McVitie's*	1 Bar/21g	106	5.4	492	5.1	60.7	25.2	1.4
Caramel, Tunnock's*	1 Wafer/26g	116	4.5	448	3.6	69.2	17.4	2.5
Caramel Log, Tunnock's*	1 Wafer/32g	152	7.7	474	4.2	64.3	24.0	0.0
Caramel Mallow, Weight Watchers*	1 Mallow/17g	55	0.4	329	5.5	63.9	2.1	17.8
Cream, Tunnock's*	1 Wafer/20g	103	5.6	513	6.6	63.2	28.0	0.0
Desiree, Assortment of, Hans Freitag*	4 Biscuits/29g	161	9.6	555	3.6	59.5	33.2	2.1
Filled, Average	1oz/28g	150	8.4	535	4.7	66.0	29.9	0.0
Florida Orange, Tunnock's*	1 Wafer/20g	104	5.8	519	5.1	64.0	29.0	0.0
for Ice Cream, Askeys*	1 Wafer/2g	6	0.0	388	11.4	79.0	2.9	0.0
Hazelnut, Elledi*	1 Wafer/8g	38	1.9	493	6.3	62.4	24.3	0.0
Lemon, Sugar Free, Wawel*	3 Biscuits/35g	170	11.0	486	11.4	51.4	31.4	1.4
Milk Chocolate, Sainsbury's*	1 Wafer/10g	51	2.7	506	6.2	60.5	26.7	1.4
Orange, Highlights, Cadbury*	1 Wafer/19g	80	2.7	430	5.2	70.6	14.3	1.4
Stilton, Fudges*	¼ Pack/25g	133	9.8	533	15.8	34.7	39.2	1.6
WAFFLES								
Belgian, TTD, Sainsbury's*	1 Waffle/25g	122	7.3	490	6.0	50.6	29.3	1.2
Caramel, Asda*	1 Waffle/8g	37	1.8	459	3.3	62.0	22.0	1.1
Milk Chocolate, Tregroes*	1 Waffle/49g	220	20.5	450	4.5	57.0	42.0	0.5
Sweet, American Style, Sainsbury's*	1 Waffle/35g	160	8.9	457	7.2	50.6	25.3	1.1
Toasting, McVitie's*	1 Waffle/25g	118	6.3	474	6.0	52.6	25.5	0.6
Toffee, Tregroes, Aldi*	1 Waffle/35g	160	6.2	463	3.5	71.7	18.0	2.2
WAGON WHEEL								
Chocolate, Burton's*	1 Biscuit/39g	165	5.7	424	5.3	67.4	14.6	1.9
Jammie, Burton's*	1 Biscuit/40g	168	5.6	420	5.1	67.7	14.1	1.9
WALNUT WHIP								
Nestle*	1 Whip/35g	173	8.8	494	5.3	61.3	25.2	0.7
The, Classics, M & S*	1 Whip/26g	127	7.1	490	7.2	54.9	27.4	1.1
Vanilla, Nestle*	1 Whip/34g	165	8.4	486	5.7	60.5	24.6	0.0
WALNUTS								
Average	*1 Nut/7g*	*48*	*4.8*	*691*	*15.6*	*3.2*	*68.5*	*3.5*
Cocoa Cream, Dusted, Julian Graves*	1 Bag/200g	1124	70.6	562	8.2	52.9	35.3	2.0
Halves, Asda*	2 Halves/7g	48	4.8	689	14.7	3.3	68.5	3.5
Halves, Average	*1 Half/3g*	*23*	*2.3*	*669*	*17.4*	*6.3*	*65.0*	*4.7*
WATER								
Apple & Strawberry Flavoured, Morrisons*	1 Serving/200ml	3	0.0	2	0.2	0.1	0.0	0.0
Berry Blast, Revive, Volvic*	1 Bottle/500ml	9	0.0	2	0.3	0.4	0.0	0.0
Blackberry & Strawberry, Sparkling, Strathmore*	1 Glass/250ml	45	0.0	18	0.0	4.3	0.0	0.0
Blackcurrant Flavour, Still, Danone*	1 Serving/120ml	25	0.0	21	0.0	5.0	0.0	0.0
Blackcurrants, Juicy, Innocent*	1 Bottle/420ml	155	0.4	37	0.1	8.7	0.1	0.0
Cranberries & Raspberries, Spring Water, This Water*	1 Bottle/420ml	122	0.4	29	0.1	6.9	0.1	0.0
Cranberry & Blueberry, Lightly Sparkling, Waitrose*	1 Glass/250ml	10	0.0	4	0.0	0.7	0.0	0.0
Cranberry & Raspberry Flavoured, Morrisons*	1 Serving/200ml	3	0.0	2	0.2	0.1	0.0	0.0
Elderflower & Pear, Detox, V Water*	1 Bottle/500ml	40	0.0	8	0.0	1.9	0.0	0.0
Elderflower Presse, Bottle Green*	1 Serving/250ml	87	0.0	35	0.0	8.9	0.0	0.0
Ginger & Mango, Kick, V Water*	1 Bottle/500ml	40	0.0	8	0.0	1.9	0.0	0.0
Grapefruit, Slightly Sparkling, Tesco*	1 Serving/200ml	4	0.0	2	0.0	0.2	0.0	0.0
Green Tea, De-Stress, V Water*	1 Bottle/500ml	40	0.0	8	0.0	1.9	0.0	0.0
Juicy Spring, Blackcurrant & Apple, Drench*	1 Serving/250ml	97	0.0	39	0.0	9.2	0.0	0.0

W

	Measure INFO/WEIGHT	per Measure		Nutrition Values per 100g / 100ml				
		KCAL	FAT	KCAL	PROT	CARB	FAT	FIBRE
WATER								
Lemon, Vittel*	1 Bottle/500ml	5	0.0	1	0.0	0.0	0.0	0.0
Lemon & Lime, Shield, Sobe V Water*	1 Bottle/500ml	85	0.5	17	0.0	3.9	0.1	0.0
Lemon & Lime, Sugar Free, Touch of Fruit, Volvic*	1 Bottle/150ml	2	0.0	1	0.0	0.0	0.0	0.0
Lemon & Lime Flavour Sparkling Spring, Co-Op*	1 Serving/200ml	2	0.0	1	0.0	0.0	0.0	0.0
Lemon & Lime Flavoured, Strathmore*	1 Bottle/500g	85	0.0	17	0.0	4.0	0.0	0.0
Lemons & Limes, Spring Water, This Water*	1 Bottle/420ml	143	0.4	34	0.1	8.2	0.1	0.0
Mango Lime, Carbonated, Henniez, Nestle*	1 Bottle/50ml	7	0.0	14	0.0	3.2	0.0	0.0
Mangoes & Passion Fruits, Spring Water, This Water*	1 Bottle/420ml	147	0.4	35	0.1	8.3	0.1	0.0
Mineral, Apple & Elderflower, Hedgerow*	1 Serving/250ml	85	0.0	34	0.0	8.2	0.0	0.0
Mineral Or Tap	**1 Glass/200ml**	**0**	**0.0**	**0**	**0.0**	**0.0**	**0.0**	**0.0**
Orange & Passion Fruit, Vital V, V Water*	1 Bottle/500ml	45	0.0	9	0.0	2.1	0.0	0.0
Passion Fruit & Peaches, Spring Water, This Water*	1 Bottle/420g	155	0.4	37	0.2	8.2	0.1	0.0
Pomegranate & Blueberry, Glow, V Water*	1 Bottle/500ml	40	0.0	8	0.0	2.0	0.0	0.0
Pomegranates & Blackcurrants, Spring Water, This Water*	1 Bottle/420ml	147	0.2	35	0.0	8.7	0.0	0.0
Raspberry & Apple, Still, Shapers, Boots*	1 Serving/250ml	10	0.0	4	0.0	0.8	0.0	0.0
Skinny, Bo-Synergy*	1 Bottle/500ml	9	0.0	2	0.0	0.3	0.0	0.0
Sparkling, Blueberry & Pomegranate, M & S*	1 Glass/250ml	5	0.0	2	0.0	0.4	0.0	0.0
Sparkling, Fruit, Aqua Libra*	1 Glass/200ml	54	0.0	27	0.0	5.1	0.0	0.0
Sparkling, Perfectly Peachy, Sugar Free, Perfectly Clear*	1 Serving/250ml	2	0.0	1	0.0	0.0	0.0	0.0
Sparkling, San Pellegrino*	1 Glass/200ml	0	0.0	0	0.0	0.0	0.0	0.0
Sparkling, Strawberry & Kiwi, Sugar Free, Perfectly Clear*	1 Glass/250ml	1	0.0	1	0.0	0.0	0.0	0.0
Spring, Apple & Blackcurrant, Hadrian*	1 Bottle/365ml	3	0.0	1	0.1	0.1	0.0	0.0
Spring, Apple & Cherry Flavoured, Sparkling, Sainsbury's*	1 Glass/250ml	5	0.2	2	0.1	0.2	0.1	0.1
Spring, Apple & Mango, Sparkling, Asda*	1 Glass/200ml	2	0.0	1	0.0	0.2	0.0	0.0
Spring, Apple & Raspberry, Shapers, Boots*	1 Bottle/500ml	10	0.0	2	0.0	0.2	0.0	0.0
Spring, Blackberry & Blueberry Flavoured, Sainsbury's*	1 Serving/1000ml	20	1.0	2	0.1	0.2	0.1	0.1
Spring, Cranberry & Raspberry, Drench*	1 Bottle/440ml	146	0.4	33	0.1	7.7	0.1	0.0
Spring, Elderflower & Pear, Sainsbury's*	1 Glass/250g	5	0.2	2	0.1	0.2	0.1	0.1
Spring, Lemon & Lime, Slightly Sparkling, Tesco*	1 Serving/200ml	4	0.2	2	0.1	0.2	0.1	0.1
Spring, Lemon & Lime Flavoured, Sparkling, Sainsbury's*	1 Glass/250ml	4	0.2	2	0.1	0.1	0.1	0.1
Spring, Orange & Passionfruit, Drench*	1 Serving/250ml	95	0.5	38	0.1	9.0	0.2	0.0
Spring, Raspberry & Cranberry, Shapers, Boots*	1 Bottle/500ml	10	0.0	2	0.0	0.5	0.0	0.0
Spring, Strawberry, Sparkling, Tesco*	1 Bottle/1000g	20	0.0	2	0.0	0.2	0.0	0.0
Spring, Strawberry & Aloe Vera, Botanical, M & S*	1 Bottle/500ml	5	0.0	1	0.0	0.2	0.0	0.0
Spring, Strawberry & Kiwi, Still, Shapers, Boots*	1 Glass/250ml	2	0.0	1	0.0	0.1	0.0	0.9
Still, Raspberry & Mango, Shapers, Boots*	1 Bottle/500g	5	0.0	1	0.0	0.0	0.0	0.0
Still Raspberry & Apple Spring, WaterVit, Shapers, Boots*	1 Bottle/500ml	5	0.0	1	0.0	0.0	0.0	0.0
Strawberry, Original, Touch of Fruit, Volvic*	1 Bottle/500ml	99	0.0	20	0.0	4.8	0.0	0.0
Strawberry, Sugar Free, Touch of Fruit, Volvic*	1 Bottle/500ml	7	0.0	1	0.0	0.1	0.0	0.0
Strawberry & Guava, Still, M & S*	1 Glass/250ml	5	0.0	2	0.0	0.1	0.0	0.0
Touch of Fruit, Blackcurrant, Volvic*	1 250ml/250ml	42	0.0	17	0.0	4.0	0.0	0.0
Vitamin, Xxx, Triple Berry, Glaceau*	1 Bottle/500ml	95	0.0	19	0.0	4.6	0.0	0.0
WaterVit, Refresh & Revive, Shapers, Boots*	1 Bottle/500ml	10	0.0	2	0.0	0.2	0.0	0.0
WATER CHESTNUTS								
Raw, Average	**1oz/28g**	**10**	**0.0**	**34**	**1.0**	**7.8**	**0.0**	**0.1**
Whole, in Water, Drained, Sainsbury's*	1 Can/140g	25	0.1	18	0.8	3.4	0.1	0.4
with Bamboo Shoots, Sainsbury's*	1 Serving/50g	29	0.1	58	2.0	12.0	0.2	1.1
WATER ICE								
Cubes	1 Serving/100g	0	0.0	0	0.0	0.0	0.0	0.0
Orange, Iceland*	1 Ice/75ml	73	0.0	98	0.2	24.4	0.0	0.2
Raspberry, Iceland*	1 Ice/75ml	67	0.0	89	0.0	22.2	0.0	0.2
WATERCRESS								
Raw, Trimmed, Average	**1 Sprig/3g**	**1**	**0.0**	**22**	**3.0**	**0.4**	**1.0**	**1.5**

W

	Measure INFO/WEIGHT	per Measure KCAL	FAT	Nutrition Values per 100g / 100ml KCAL	PROT	CARB	FAT	FIBRE
WATERMELON								
Flesh Only, Average	**1 Serving/250g**	**75**	**0.7**	**30**	**0.4**	**7.0**	**0.3**	**0.4**
Raw	**1 Wedge/286g**	**92**	**1.2**	**32**	**0.6**	**7.2**	**0.4**	**0.5**
Raw, Weighed with Skin, Average	1 Serving/100g	30	0.3	30	0.4	7.0	0.3	0.4
WHEAT								
Whole Grain, Split, Average	**1 Serving/60g**	**205**	**1.0**	**342**	**11.3**	**75.9**	**1.7**	**12.2**
WHEAT BRAN								
Average	**1 Tbsp/7g**	**14**	**0.4**	**206**	**14.1**	**26.8**	**5.5**	**36.4**
Coarse, Holland & Barrett*	1 Tbsp/4g	8	0.2	206	14.1	26.8	5.5	36.4
Natural, Jordans*	1 Tbsp/7g	13	0.4	188	16.3	17.4	5.9	44.5
WHEAT CRUNCHIES								
Golden Wonder*	1 Pack/35g	172	8.7	491	11.1	55.9	24.8	0.0
Salt & Vinegar, Golden Wonder*	1 Bag/34g	165	8.5	484	10.5	54.5	24.9	2.8
Worcester Sauce, Golden Wonder*	1 Bag/35g	172	8.9	492	9.3	56.4	25.5	3.9
WHEAT GERM								
Average	**1oz/28g**	**100**	**2.6**	**357**	**26.7**	**44.7**	**9.2**	**15.6**
Natural, Jordans*	2 Tbsp/16g	54	1.5	340	28.0	36.0	9.3	13.1
Natural, Tree of Life*	1 Serving/100g	367	9.2	367	26.0	45.0	9.2	0.0
WHELKS								
Boiled, Weighed without Shell	**1oz/28g**	**25**	**0.3**	**89**	**19.5**	**0.0**	**1.2**	**0.0**
WHIPS								
Double Chocolate, M & S*	1 Whip/29g	140	7.3	485	6.6	57.8	25.3	1.0
WHISKEY								
Irish, Jameson*	1 Shot/25ml	58	0.0	233	0.0	0.0	0.0	0.0
Jack Daniel's*	1 Shot/35ml	78	0.0	222	0.0	0.0	0.0	0.0
WHISKY								
37.5% Volume	**1 Shot/35ml**	**72**	**0.0**	**207**	**0.0**	**0.0**	**0.0**	**0.0**
40% Volume	**1 Shot/35ml**	**78**	**0.0**	**222**	**0.0**	**0.0**	**0.0**	**0.0**
Bells & Ginger Ale, Premixed, Canned, Diageo*	1 Can/250ml	170	0.0	68	0.0	7.6	0.0	0.0
Scotch, 37.5% Volume	**1 Shot/35ml**	**72**	**0.0**	**207**	**0.0**	**0.0**	**0.0**	**0.0**
Scotch, 40% Volume	**1 Shot/35ml**	**78**	**0.0**	**222**	**0.0**	**0.0**	**0.0**	**0.0**
Teacher's*	1 Shot/35ml	78	0.0	222	0.0	0.0	0.0	0.0
WHITE PUDDING								
Average	**1oz/28g**	**126**	**8.9**	**450**	**7.0**	**36.3**	**31.8**	**0.0**
WHITEBAIT								
in Flour, Fried	**1oz/28g**	**147**	**13.3**	**525**	**19.5**	**5.3**	**47.5**	**0.2**
WHITECURRANTS								
Raw, Average	**1oz/28g**	**7**	**0.0**	**26**	**1.3**	**5.6**	**0.0**	**3.4**
WHITING								
in Crumbs, Fried in Blended Oil	1 Serving/180g	344	18.5	191	18.1	7.0	10.3	0.2
Raw	**1oz/28g**	**23**	**0.2**	**81**	**18.7**	**0.0**	**0.7**	**0.0**
Steamed	**1 Serving/85g**	**78**	**0.8**	**92**	**20.9**	**0.0**	**0.9**	**0.0**
WIENER SCHNITZEL								
Average	1oz/28g	62	2.8	223	20.9	13.1	10.0	0.4
WINE								
Cherry, Lambrini*	1 Glass/125ml	80	0.0	64	0.0	0.0	0.0	0.0
Diet, Lambrini*	1 Glass/125ml	43	0.0	35	0.0	0.0	0.0	0.0
Elderberry & Lemon, Ame*	1 Sml Glass/125ml	46	0.0	37	0.0	6.4	0.0	0.0
Fruit, Average	**1 Glass/125ml**	**115**	**0.0**	**92**	**0.0**	**5.5**	**0.0**	**0.0**
Grape & Apricot, Ame*	1 Glass/125ml	49	1.2	39	1.3	6.7	1.0	0.0
Madeira, Henriques & Henriques*	1 Glass/100ml	130	0.0	130	0.0	0.0	0.0	0.0
Mulled, Homemade, Average	**1 Glass/125ml**	**245**	**0.0**	**196**	**0.1**	**25.2**	**0.0**	**0.0**
Mulled, Sainsbury's*	1 Glass/125ml	112	0.0	90	0.0	8.6	0.0	0.0
Original, Lambrini*	1 Glass/125ml	88	0.0	70	0.0	0.0	0.0	0.0

W

	Measure INFO/WEIGHT	per Measure KCAL	FAT	Nutrition Values per 100g / 100ml KCAL	PROT	CARB	FAT	FIBRE
WINE								
Red, Amarone, Average*	1 Glass/125ml	120	0.0	96	0.1	3.0	0.0	0.0
Red, Average	*1 Glass/125ml*	*104*	*0.0*	*83*	*0.0*	*1.9*	*0.0*	*0.0*
Red, Burgundy, 12.9% Abv, Average	1 Glass/125ml	110	0.0	88	0.1	3.7	0.0	0.0
Red, Cabernet Sauvignon, 13.1% Abv, Average	1 Glass/125ml	105	0.0	84	0.1	2.6	0.0	0.0
Red, California, Blossom Hill*	1 Glass/175ml	132	0.0	75	0.0	0.9	0.0	0.0
Red, Claret, 12.8% Abv, Average	1 Glass/125ml	105	0.0	84	0.1	3.0	0.0	0.0
Red, Gamay, 12.3% Abv, Average	1 Glass/125ml	99	0.0	79	0.1	2.4	0.0	0.0
Red, Long Slim, Co-Op*	1 Glass/125ml	90	0.0	72	0.0	0.0	0.0	0.0
Red, Low Calorie, Asda*	1 Glass/125ml	49	0.0	39	0.0	0.1	0.0	0.0
Red, Merlot, 13.3% Abv, Average	1 Glass/125ml	105	0.0	84	0.1	2.5	0.0	0.0
Red, Non Alcoholic, Ame*	1 Glass/125ml	42	0.0	34	0.0	5.7	0.0	0.0
Red, Petit Sirah, 13.5% Abv, Average	1 Glass/125ml	107	0.0	86	0.1	2.7	0.0	0.0
Red, Pinot Noir, 13% Abv, Average	1 Glass/125ml	104	0.0	83	0.1	2.3	0.0	0.0
Red, Sangiovese, 13.6% Abv, Average	1 Glass/125ml	109	0.0	87	0.1	2.6	0.0	0.0
Red, Smooth, Weight Watchers*	1 Glass/125ml	75	0.1	60	0.1	1.4	0.1	0.1
Red, Syrah, 13.1% Abv, Average	1 Glass/125ml	105	0.0	84	0.1	2.6	0.0	0.0
Red, Zinfandel, 13.9% Abv, Average	1 Glass/125ml	111	0.0	89	0.1	2.9	0.0	0.0
Rose, Medium, Average	*1 Glass/125ml*	*98*	*0.0*	*79*	*0.0*	*2.1*	*0.0*	*0.0*
Rose, Refreshing, Weight Watchers*	1 Glass/125ml	80	0.0	64	0.0	1.6	0.0	0.0
Rose, Sparkling, Average	1 Glass/125ml	102	0.0	82	0.0	2.5	0.0	0.0
Rose, The Pink Chill, Co-Op*	1 Glass/125ml	85	0.0	68	0.0	0.0	0.0	0.0
Rose, Weight Watchers*	1 Bottle/187ml	112	0.2	60	0.1	1.8	0.1	0.1
Rose, White Grenache, Blossom Hill*	1 Glass/125ml	105	0.0	84	0.0	3.2	0.0	0.0
Rose, White Zinfandel, Ernest & Julio Gallo*	1 Glass/125ml	101	0.0	81	0.2	2.7	0.0	0.0
Sangria, Average	1 Glass/125ml	95	0.0	76	0.1	9.9	0.0	0.1
Strong Ale Barley	1 Can/440ml	290	0.0	66	0.7	6.1	0.0	0.0
White, Average	1 Glass/125ml	95	0.0	76	0.0	2.4	0.0	0.0
White, Californian, Chardonnay, Light Choices, Tesco*	1 Glass/125ml	96	0.0	53	0.0	1.8	0.0	0.0
White, Chardonnay, Low Alcohol, McGuigan*	1 Glass/125ml	75	0.1	60	0.1	2.2	0.1	0.0
White, Chardonnay, Southern Australia, Kissing Tree*	1 Bottle/185ml	85	0.0	46	0.0	0.0	0.0	0.0
White, Chenin Blanc, 12% Abv, Average	1 Glass/125ml	101	0.0	81	0.1	3.3	0.0	0.0
White, Dry, Average	*1 Glass/125ml*	*87*	*0.0*	*70*	*0.1*	*0.6*	*0.0*	*0.0*
White, Fume Blanc, 13.1% Abv, Average	1 Glass/125ml	104	0.0	83	0.1	2.3	0.0	0.0
White, Gewurztraminer, 12.6% Abv, Average	1 Glass/125ml	102	0.0	82	0.1	2.6	0.0	0.0
White, Late Harvest, 10.6% Abv, Average	1 Glass/125ml	141	0.0	113	0.1	13.4	0.0	0.0
White, Medium, Average	*1 Glass/125ml*	*92*	*0.0*	*74*	*0.1*	*3.0*	*0.0*	*0.0*
White, Muller-Thurgau, 11.3% Abv, Average	1 Glass/125ml	96	0.0	77	0.1	3.5	0.0	0.0
White, Muscat, 11% Abv, Average	1 Glass/125ml	104	0.0	83	0.1	5.2	0.0	0.0
White, Non Alcoholic, Ame*	1 Glass/125ml	47	0.0	38	0.0	9.5	0.0	0.0
White, Pinot Blanc, 13.3% Abv, Average	1 Glass/125ml	102	0.0	82	0.1	0.0	0.0	0.0
White, Pinot Grigio, 13.4% Abv, Average	1 Glass/125ml	105	0.0	84	0.1	2.1	0.0	0.0
White, Riesling, 11.9% Abv, Average	1 Glass/125ml	101	0.0	81	0.1	3.7	0.0	0.0
White, Sauvignon Blanc, 13.1% Abv, Average	1 Glass/125ml	102	0.0	82	0.1	2.0	0.0	0.0
White, Semillon, 12.5% Abv, Average	1 Glass/125ml	104	0.0	83	0.1	3.1	0.0	0.0
White, Sparkling, Average	*1 Glass/125ml*	*92*	*0.0*	*74*	*0.3*	*5.1*	*0.0*	*0.0*
White, Sweet, Average	*1 Glass/120ml*	*113*	*0.0*	*94*	*0.2*	*5.9*	*0.0*	*0.0*
WINE GUMS								
Average	1 Sweet/6g	19	0.0	315	5.0	73.4	0.2	0.1
Haribo*	1 Pack/175g	609	0.3	348	0.1	86.4	0.2	0.4
Light, Maynards*	1 Pack/42g	90	0.1	215	4.6	48.0	0.2	27.9
Mini, Co-Op*	1 Sweet/2g	7	0.0	330	6.0	76.0	0.1	0.0
Mini, Rowntree's*	1 Sm Bag/36g	125	0.0	348	6.7	80.5	0.0	0.0
Sour, Bassett's*	¼ Bag/50g	159	0.0	319	3.7	78.0	0.0	0.0

W

	Measure INFO/WEIGHT	per Measure KCAL	FAT	Nutrition Values per 100g / 100ml KCAL	PROT	CARB	FAT	FIBRE
WINKLES								
Boiled	*1oz/28g*	*20*	*0.3*	*72*	*15.4*	*0.0*	*1.2*	*0.0*
WISPA								
Bite, with Biscuit in Caramel, Cadbury*	1 Bar/47g	240	13.4	510	6.4	56.9	28.6	0.0
Cadbury*	1 Bar/40g	210	12.9	525	6.7	53.0	32.2	0.7
Gold, Cadbury*	1 Bar/52g	265	15.1	510	5.3	56.0	29.0	0.7
Mint, Cadbury*	1 Bar/50g	275	16.8	550	7.0	54.7	33.6	0.0
WONTON								
Prawn, Crispy from Selection, Modern Asian, M & S*	1 Wonton/25g	65	3.3	250	9.5	23.4	12.7	2.0
Prawn, Dim Sum Selection, Sainsbury's*	1 Wonton/10g	26	1.2	259	11.3	26.8	11.8	1.3
Prawn, Oriental Selection, Waitrose*	1 Wonton/18g	45	2.0	252	9.1	29.2	11.0	1.1
Prawn, Oriental Snack Selection, Sainsbury's*	1 Wonton/20g	53	2.7	265	10.6	25.6	13.4	2.0
WOTSITS								
Baked, Really Cheesy, Walkers*	1 Bag/23g	123	7.4	547	5.5	56.0	33.0	1.1
BBQ, Walkers*	1 Bag/21g	108	6.3	515	4.5	57.0	30.0	1.3
Flamin' Hot, Walkers*	1 Bag/19g	101	5.7	532	5.5	60.0	30.0	1.1
Prawn Cocktail, Walkers*	1 Bag/19g	99	5.7	522	4.5	58.0	30.0	1.1
Really Cheesy, Big Eat, Walkers*	1 Bag/36g	197	11.9	547	5.5	56.0	33.0	1.1
WRAP								
All Day Breakfast, M & S*	1 Pack/196g	529	31.4	270	10.8	21.2	16.0	1.4
American Deli, Shapers, Boots*	1 Pack/172g	249	4.5	145	9.5	21.0	2.6	2.0
BBQ Beef, Ginsters*	1 Pack/210g	404	12.2	192	6.7	28.4	5.8	1.8
Beef & Duck, Mouli with Salad, Eat Well, M & S*	1 Pack/88g	48	0.4	55	4.6	7.8	0.4	1.3
Beef Fajita, Boots*	1 Pack/200g	352	8.4	176	9.5	25.5	4.2	3.1
Beef in Black Bean, M & S*	1 Pack/150g	337	17.1	225	10.2	20.5	11.4	1.6
Bombay Potato, Whistlestop*	1 Wrap/180g	343	15.0	191	4.2	24.7	8.3	0.3
Brie & Cranberry, M & S*	1 Pack/225g	550	27.8	245	6.1	27.3	12.4	1.7
Butternut Squash, COU, M & S*	1 Pack/182g	245	4.7	135	4.3	22.2	2.6	2.9
Cajun, GFY, Asda*	1 Pack/176g	231	2.1	131	9.0	21.0	1.2	0.9
Cajun Chicken, Sandwich King*	1 Pack/138g	386	19.9	279	12.3	25.0	14.4	0.0
Cajun Chicken, Tesco*	1 Pack/184g	415	16.6	225	9.8	25.1	9.0	1.9
Chargrilled Chicken, Perfectly Balanced, Waitrose*	1 Pack/230g	361	6.7	157	10.3	22.7	2.9	2.9
Cheese & Bean, Tesco*	1 Pack/105g	235	9.4	224	7.0	28.6	9.0	1.0
Cheesy Gonzales, Cranks*	1 Pack/209g	501	22.3	240	8.0	27.3	10.7	1.1
Chicken, Barbecue, Shapers, Boots*	1 Pack/181g	283	4.9	156	10.0	23.0	2.7	3.3
Chicken, Cheddar & Peppers, Cajun, Sainsbury's*	1 Pack/242g	535	26.6	221	10.4	19.8	11.0	2.1
Chicken, Chilli, GFY, Asda*	1 Pack/194g	277	4.3	143	9.1	21.6	2.2	2.3
Chicken, M & S*	1 Pack/247g	530	24.9	215	8.2	23.4	10.1	1.6
Chicken, Mediterranean Style, Waitrose*	1 Pack/183g	296	11.0	162	8.3	18.6	6.0	2.3
Chicken, Southern Fried, Budgens*	1 Pack/195g	401	18.2	243	10.0	25.0	11.0	3.0
Chicken, Southern Fried, Fresh for You, Tesco*	1 Pack/206g	485	24.4	235	8.6	22.7	11.8	2.0
Chicken, Southern Style, Ginsters*	1 Wrap/210g	491	22.0	234	6.4	28.3	10.5	1.8
Chicken, Tasties*	1 Pack/149g	324	10.6	218	11.7	26.5	7.1	0.0
Chicken, Thai, Spiced, Salad, Eat Well, M & S*	1 Pack/122g	91	1.5	75	5.2	9.5	1.2	1.5
Chicken & Bacon, Simple Solutions, Tesco*	1 Pack/300g	474	23.4	158	20.7	1.2	7.8	0.5
Chicken & Bacon Caesar, COU, M & S*	1 Pack/170g	260	4.2	153	10.6	22.0	2.5	2.1
Chicken & Bacon Caesar Salad, Asda*	1 Pack/160g	565	35.2	353	18.0	20.8	22.0	0.9
Chicken Caesar, Tesco*	1 Pack/215g	516	24.3	240	11.6	23.0	11.3	1.2
Chicken Caesar, Weight Watchers*	1 Pack/173g	298	4.7	172	11.2	24.5	2.7	1.3
Chicken Fajita, Asda*	1 Pack/180g	369	16.9	205	9.4	20.6	9.4	0.4
Chicken Fajita, Daily Bread*	1 Pack/191g	392	10.5	205	9.4	29.4	5.5	0.0
Chicken Fajita, Finest, Tesco*	1 Pack/213g	422	15.6	198	9.0	24.0	7.3	1.9
Chicken Korma, Patak's*	1 Pack/150g	294	14.2	196	7.6	20.0	9.5	0.0
Chicken Louisiana, Benedicts*	1 Pack/250g	410	5.5	164	13.4	24.2	2.2	0.0

W

WRAP

	Measure INFO/WEIGHT	per Measure		Nutrition Values per 100g / 100ml				
		KCAL	FAT	KCAL	PROT	CARB	FAT	FIBRE
Chicken Nacho, HL, Tesco*	1 Pack/223g	390	10.0	175	12.3	21.2	4.5	2.6
Chicken Salad, Roast, Sainsbury's*	1 Pack/214g	443	19.9	207	10.0	20.9	9.3	2.5
Chicken Sweet & Sour, Ginsters*	1 Pack/150g	378	5.8	252	13.4	40.8	3.9	2.4
Chicken Thai Style, Boots*	1 Pack/156g	290	10.0	186	11.0	21.0	6.4	2.2
Chicken Tikka, Average	1 Wrap/183g	277	7.3	151	9.7	18.5	4.0	1.1
Chicken Tikka Masala, Patak's*	1 Pack/150g	252	9.9	168	7.8	19.3	6.6	0.0
Chilli Bean & Cheese, Meat Free, Asda*	1 Wrap/151g	263	7.1	174	7.9	25.1	4.7	4.9
Chilli Beef, Co-Op*	1 Pack/163g	310	9.8	190	10.0	26.0	6.0	2.0
Chilli Beef, COU, M & S*	1 Pack/179g	268	2.9	150	10.1	23.4	1.6	2.6
Chilli Chicken, BGTY, Sainsbury's*	1 Pack/180g	313	4.3	174	10.2	28.0	2.4	0.0
Crayfish, Lemon Dressing & Rocket, COU, M & S*	1 Pack/183g	274	4.9	150	9.5	22.5	2.7	1.2
Crayfish & Rocket, HL, Tesco*	1 Pack/164g	270	5.1	165	7.5	25.9	3.1	1.9
Crunchy Lunch, Cranks*	1 Pack/212g	463	21.2	218	5.7	25.0	10.0	2.8
Dhansak Prawn, M & S*	1 Pack/208g	385	15.0	185	7.1	23.3	7.2	2.4
Duck, Food to Go, M & S*	1 Pack/257g	475	13.9	185	8.5	25.5	5.4	1.0
Duck, Hoi Sin, Delicious, Boots*	1 Pack/160g	295	4.3	184	11.0	28.0	2.7	2.0
Duck, Hoisin, M & S*	1 Pack/225g	405	8.3	180	8.4	27.7	3.7	1.5
Duck, Hoisin, No Mayo, Tesco*	1 Pack/184g	340	8.5	185	9.4	26.1	4.6	1.8
Egg Mayonnaise, Tomato & Cress, Sainsbury's*	1 Pack/255g	592	38.2	232	7.3	17.7	15.0	0.0
Fajita, Steak, Delicatessen, Waitrose*	1 Pack/232g	489	21.1	211	10.5	22.7	9.1	2.7
Feta Cheese, GFY, Asda*	1 Pack/165g	256	7.1	155	7.0	22.0	4.3	2.1
Feta Cheese Flat Bread, COU, M & S*	1 Pack/180g	225	4.0	125	6.3	20.6	2.2	1.9
Fiery Cheese, Ginsters*	1 Pack/210g	424	17.6	202	6.8	24.8	8.4	1.8
Greek Salad, Sainsbury's*	1 Pack/167g	242	6.2	145	6.7	21.2	3.7	1.8
Green Thai Prawn, BGTY, Sainsbury's*	1 Pack/200g	237	3.0	118	7.0	19.2	1.5	1.5
Ham, Cheese & Pickle Tortilla, Weight Watchers*	1 Pack/170g	296	4.8	174	10.9	26.4	2.8	1.2
Houmous, Royal London Hospital*	1 Pack/200g	318	13.4	159	6.3	20.0	6.7	0.0
Houmous, Taste!*	1 Pack/170g	291	8.3	171	5.4	26.4	4.9	0.0
Mexican Three Bean, M & S*	1 Pack/188g	405	19.2	215	6.9	24.3	10.2	2.2
Mexican Tortilla, Ainsley Harriott*	1 Pack/230g	421	17.2	183	7.1	22.4	7.5	0.0
Mild Chicken Curry, Patak's*	1 Pack/150g	238	9.0	159	8.1	21.3	6.0	2.8
Monterey Jack & Ham, Tesco*	1 Pack/200g	522	28.2	261	7.9	25.9	14.1	0.2
Nacho Chicken, COU, M & S*	1 Pack/175g	280	4.2	160	10.2	24.4	2.4	2.0
Red Thai Chicken, Shapers, Boots*	1 Pack/172g	234	3.6	136	9.5	20.0	2.1	2.4
Selection, Chicken, BBQ Steak, Hoisin Duck, M & S*	1 Pack/334g	685	23.7	205	10.9	24.3	7.1	1.7
Sicilian Lemon & Roasted Vegetable, COU, M & S*	1 Pack/178g	240	3.7	135	4.9	23.8	2.1	1.9
Smoked Salmon, Finest, Tesco*	1 Pack/58g	113	8.4	194	15.5	0.6	14.4	0.3
Sunny Side Up, Cranks*	1 Pack/195g	423	18.9	217	7.8	23.3	9.7	1.7
Sushi Salmon & Cucumber, Waitrose*	1 Pack/180g	299	6.5	166	6.3	27.2	3.6	1.6
Sweet Chilli & King Prawn, COU, M & S*	1 Pack/155g	225	2.6	145	8.0	24.2	1.7	2.1
Sweet Chilli Chicken, Shapers, Boots*	1 Pack/195g	302	3.7	155	10.0	24.0	1.9	3.0
Sweet Chilli Chicken, Waitrose*	1 Pack/200g	390	14.7	195	10.2	22.0	7.3	2.4
Sweet Chilli King Prawn, M & S*	1 Pack/155g	225	3.1	145	8.0	24.2	2.0	2.1
Sweet Chilli Noodle, Sainsbury's*	1 Pack/210g	399	10.1	190	10.6	26.1	4.8	2.1
Tandoori Chicken, GFY, Asda*	1 Pack/167g	281	4.5	168	10.0	26.0	2.7	1.7
Thai Prawn, COU, M & S*	1 Pack/181g	235	2.9	130	8.3	20.4	1.6	1.9
Tuna Nicoise, BGTY, Sainsbury's*	1 Pack/181g	273	7.1	151	11.0	18.0	3.9	0.0
Tuna Salsa, Healthy Eating, Wild Bean Cafe*	1 Pack/159g	245	2.7	154	11.3	23.5	1.7	1.5
Turkey, Bacon & Cranberry, COU, M & S*	1 Pack/144g	230	2.2	160	9.6	27.1	1.5	2.3
Yellow Thai Prawn, COU, M & S*	1 Pack/171g	266	5.0	155	7.6	23.4	2.9	1.7

W

	Measure INFO/WEIGHT	per Measure		Nutrition Values per 100g / 100ml				
		KCAL	FAT	KCAL	PROT	CARB	FAT	FIBRE
YAM								
Baked	**1oz/28g**	**43**	**0.1**	**153**	**2.1**	**37.5**	**0.4**	**1.7**
Boiled, Average	**1oz/28g**	**37**	**0.1**	**133**	**1.7**	**33.0**	**0.3**	**1.4**
Raw	**1oz/28g**	**32**	**0.1**	**114**	**1.5**	**28.2**	**0.3**	**1.3**
YEAST								
Dried, Average	**1 Tbsp/6g**	**10**	**0.1**	**169**	**35.6**	**3.5**	**1.5**	**0.0**
Extract	**1 Tsp/9g**	**16**	**0.0**	**180**	**40.7**	**3.5**	**0.4**	**0.0**
YOGHURT								
0.1% Fat, Lidl*	1 Pot/150g	118	0.1	79	4.0	15.6	0.1	0.0
Activia, Danone*	1 Pot/132g	125	4.2	94	3.5	12.8	3.2	2.0
Apple, Light, Muller*	1 Pot/175g	94	0.2	54	4.4	9.0	0.1	0.0
Apple, Mango, Grape & Honey, Probiotic, Shapers, Boots*	1 Pack/140g	99	0.3	71	2.1	15.0	0.2	1.4
Apple, Raspberry & Banana, Smoothie, Sveltesse, Nestle*	1 Pot/125g	61	0.1	49	4.8	7.3	0.1	0.2
Apple, Spiced, 6% Fat, TTD, Sainsbury's*	1 Pot/15g	16	0.6	107	2.7	15.6	3.8	0.5
Apple, Strawberry & Peach, Smoothie, Sveltesse, Nestle*	1 Pot/125g	61	0.1	49	4.8	7.3	0.1	0.1
Apple & Blackberry, Bio, Sainsbury's*	1 Pot/125g	134	3.4	107	4.1	16.6	2.7	0.2
Apple & Blackberry, Custard Style, Co-Op*	1 Pot/150g	195	7.9	130	3.7	15.9	5.3	0.1
Apple & Blackberry, Organic, Yeo Valley*	1 Pot/125g	121	4.1	97	4.3	12.5	3.3	0.1
Apple & Blackcurrant, Low Fat, Stapleton*	1 Pot/150g	106	0.7	71	3.2	13.9	0.5	1.2
Apple & Cinnamon, Jubileum, Tine*	1 Pot/125g	166	6.5	133	3.2	18.5	5.2	0.0
Apple & Cinnamon Farmhouse, Twekkelo*	1 Bowl/125g	142	4.1	114	4.1	17.0	3.3	0.4
Apple & Cranberry, Smooth, Bio, Fat Free, Shape, Danone*	1 Pot/120g	86	0.1	72	4.2	13.5	0.1	0.0
Apple & Custard, Low Fat, Sainsbury's*	1 Pot/125g	116	1.9	93	4.3	15.5	1.5	0.2
Apple & Peach, Oatie Breakfast, Moma Foods*	1 Pot/234g	309	5.6	132	4.3	24.3	2.4	1.7
Apple & Pear, Low Fat, Sainsbury's*	1 Pot/125g	115	1.9	92	4.3	15.2	1.5	0.2
Apple & Prune, Fat Free, Yeo Valley*	1 Pot/125g	97	0.1	78	5.1	14.1	0.1	0.2
Apple & Spice Bio, Virtually Fat Free, Shape, Danone*	1 Pot/120g	67	0.1	56	5.6	7.3	0.1	0.2
Apricot, Bio, Low Fat, Benecol*	1 Pot/125g	98	0.8	78	3.9	14.3	0.6	0.0
Apricot, Bio Activia, Danone*	1 Pot/125g	121	4.0	97	3.7	13.3	3.2	1.7
Apricot, Fat Free, Activ8, Ski, Nestle*	1 Pot/120g	88	0.8	73	4.5	13.6	0.7	0.2
Apricot, Fat Free, Bio Live, Rachel's Organic*	1 Pot/142g	81	0.1	57	3.5	10.5	0.1	0.0
Apricot, Fat Free, Weight Watchers*	1 Pot/150g	62	0.2	42	4.1	4.9	0.1	0.2
Apricot, French Style Smooth, Tesco*	1 Pot/125g	122	3.7	98	3.6	14.1	3.0	0.0
Apricot, Fruity, Mullerlight, Muller*	1 Pot/175g	87	0.2	50	4.2	7.5	0.1	0.1
Apricot, HL, Tesco*	1 Pot/125g	67	0.4	54	5.1	7.9	0.3	1.1
Apricot, Layered Fruit, Thick & Creamy, Sainsbury's*	1 Pot/125g	141	3.4	113	4.1	18.0	2.7	0.2
Apricot, Light, Fat Free, Muller*	1 Pot/190g	93	0.2	49	4.1	7.3	0.1	0.1
Apricot, Light, HL, Tesco*	1 Pot/125g	54	0.2	43	4.1	6.3	0.2	0.9
Apricot, Low Fat, Organic, Average	1 Serving/100g	84	1.0	84	5.8	13.3	1.0	0.6
Apricot, Low Fat, Tesco*	1 Pot/125g	112	2.2	90	4.3	14.1	1.8	0.0
Apricot, Pro Activ, Flora*	1 Pot/125ml	70	0.6	56	4.0	7.9	0.5	1.8
Apricot, Smooth Set French, Sainsbury's*	1 Pot/125g	100	1.5	80	3.5	13.6	1.2	0.0
Apricot & Mango, 25% Extra Fruit, Low Fat, Asda*	1 Pot/125g	120	1.4	96	4.6	17.0	1.1	0.0
Apricot & Mango, Tropical Fruit, Activ8, Ski, Nestle*	1 Pot/120g	112	2.0	93	4.3	15.1	1.7	0.2
Apricot & Nectarine, Sunshine Selection, Sainsbury's*	1 Pot/125g	115	1.9	92	4.4	15.3	1.5	0.1
Apricot & Passion Fruit, Fat Free, Yeo Valley*	1 Pot/125g	94	0.1	75	5.3	13.2	0.1	0.1
Apricot Tart Style, Sveltesse, Nestle*	1 Pot/125g	97	0.2	78	4.8	14.2	0.2	0.1
Banana, Low Fat, Average	1 Serving/100g	98	1.4	98	4.6	16.7	1.4	0.1
Banana & Custard, Smooth, Mullerlight, Muller*	1 Pot/175g	94	0.2	54	4.1	8.6	0.1	0.6
Banana Choco Flakes, Crunch Corner, Muller*	1 Pot/150g	214	7.8	143	4.1	19.3	5.2	0.3
Banana Smooth, M & S*	1 Pot/150g	165	2.5	110	4.8	19.3	1.7	0.2
Banoffee, Low Fat, Asda*	1 Pot/125g	126	1.5	101	4.6	18.2	1.2	1.0
Banoffee, Snackpot, Activia, Danone*	1 Pot/155g	116	0.2	75	5.0	13.3	0.1	0.3
Bio, Low Fat, Spelga*	1 Pot/125g	125	2.1	100	3.9	17.0	1.7	0.0

YOGHURT

Measure INFO/WEIGHT	per Measure KCAL	FAT	Nutrition Values per 100g / 100ml KCAL	PROT	CARB	FAT	FIBRE
Black Cherry, Average	1 Serving/100g	96	2.2	96	3.4	16.5	2.2	0.1
Black Cherry, Fat Free, Benecol*	1 Pot/120g	78	0.6	65	3.0	11.0	0.5	2.1
Black Cherry, Greek Style, Corner, Muller*	1 Pot/150g	172	4.5	115	5.0	16.2	3.0	0.1
Black Cherry, Juicy, Shapers, Boots*	1 Pot/152g	91	1.7	60	4.0	8.4	1.1	0.5
Black Cherry, Low Fat, Average	1 Serving/100g	69	0.6	69	3.8	12.2	0.6	0.3
Black Cherry, Very Cherry, Activ8, Ski, Nestle*	1 Pot/120g	116	2.0	97	4.3	16.1	1.7	0.2
Black Cherry, Virtually Fat Free, Longley Farm Yoghurt*	1 Pot/150g	115	0.1	77	4.5	14.4	0.1	0.0
Black Cherry, Virtually Fat Free, Shapers, Boots*	1 Pot/125g	71	0.1	57	5.3	8.8	0.1	0.1
Black Cherry, VLH Kitchens	1 Serving/150g	188	2.5	125	3.7	19.6	3.7	1.0
Blackberry, Alpro Soya*	1 Pot/125g	99	2.6	79	3.7	9.2	2.1	1.2
Blackberry, Boysenberry & William Pear, M & S*	1 Pot/150g	187	9.7	125	4.0	13.6	6.5	2.4
Blackberry, Farmhouse, BGTY, Sainsbury's*	1 Pot/150g	106	0.6	71	3.4	13.5	0.4	1.6
Blackberry, Very Berry, Activ8, Ski, Nestle*	1 Pot/120g	114	2.0	95	4.4	15.5	1.7	0.7
Blackberry, Zer0% Fat, No Added Sugar, Shape, Danone*	1 Pot/120g	73	0.2	61	6.0	8.9	0.2	1.0
Blackberry & Apple, BGTY, Sainsbury's*	1 Pot/122g	61	0.2	50	4.7	7.2	0.2	0.3
Blackberry & Apple, HL, Tesco*	1 Pot/176g	86	0.2	49	2.1	10.0	0.1	1.5
Blackberry & Raspberry, Fruit Corner, Muller*	1 Pot/150g	157	5.8	105	3.8	13.1	3.9	0.9
Blackberry & Raspberry Flip, Morrisons*	1 Pot/175g	206	8.0	118	3.4	15.8	4.6	0.5
Blackcurrant, BGTY, Sainsbury's*	1 Pot/200g	100	0.4	50	4.8	7.3	0.2	0.1
Blackcurrant, Fruity, Mullerlight, Muller*	1 Pot/175g	89	0.2	51	4.1	7.9	0.1	0.8
Blackcurrant, Longley Farm*	1 Pot/150g	168	5.5	112	4.9	14.7	3.7	0.0
Blackcurrant, Low Fat, Chosen By You, Asda*	1 Pot/125g	104	1.6	83	3.6	14.2	1.3	0.0
Blackcurrant, Low Fat, Sainsbury's*	1 Pot/125g	116	1.7	93	4.2	15.9	1.4	0.6
Blackcurrant, Munch Bunch, Nestle*	1 Pot/100g	107	3.1	107	4.4	15.3	3.1	0.5
Blackcurrant, Probiotic, Organic, Yeo Valley*	1 Pot/150g	151	5.8	101	4.1	12.4	3.9	0.2
Blackcurrant, Thick & Creamy, Sainsbury's*	1 Pot/150g	171	5.4	114	4.3	15.9	3.6	0.4
Blackcurrant, Virtually Fat Free, Morrisons*	1 Pot/200g	114	0.4	57	5.4	8.4	0.2	0.2
Blackcurrant & Raspberry, Layers, Mullerlight, Muller*	1 Pot/175g	94	0.2	54	3.1	9.7	0.1	0.7
Blackcurrant with Liquorice, Tesco*	1 Pot/150g	138	1.6	92	4.6	15.8	1.1	0.4
Blueberries & Cream, Made Up, Easiyo*	1 Serving/100g	105	4.1	105	3.9	13.7	4.1	0.0
Blueberry, Extremely Fruity, Low Fat, Probiotic, M & S*	1 Pot/150g	142	2.1	95	4.7	14.7	1.4	1.5
Blueberry, Fat Free, Probiotic, Organic, Yeo Valley*	1 Serving/100g	73	0.1	73	5.1	12.9	0.1	0.4
Blueberry, Probiotic, Natural Balance, Asda*	1 Pot/125g	102	2.9	82	2.1	13.1	2.3	2.6
Blueberry, Wholemilk, Organic, Sainsbury's*	1 Pot/150g	123	5.2	82	3.5	9.2	3.5	0.1
Blueberry & Elderberry, Bio, with Wholegrains, Optifit*	1 Pot/250g	150	3.5	60	4.9	7.0	1.4	1.6
Blueberry & Loganberry, Bio, Layered, Sainsbury's*	1 Pot/125g	134	3.4	107	4.0	16.6	2.7	0.2
Blueberry Bio, Co-Op*	1 Pot/125g	141	3.5	113	4.5	16.5	2.8	0.4
Caramel, Smooth, Intensely Creamy, Activia, Danone*	1 Pot/165g	168	5.0	102	4.8	13.7	3.0	0.1
Caramel & Praline, Indulgent Greek Style, Somerfield*	1 Pot/125g	245	10.0	196	4.0	28.0	8.0	0.0
Cereals, Fibre, Bio Activia, Danone*	1 Pot/120g	119	4.1	99	3.7	13.5	3.4	3.0
Champagne Rhubarb & Vanilla, M & S*	1 Pot/150g	195	8.7	130	3.8	15.7	5.8	0.8
Cherry, Fat Free, M & S*	1 Pot/200g	170	0.2	85	4.3	16.7	0.1	0.5
Cherry, Fruity, Mullerlight, Muller*	1 Pot/175g	86	0.2	49	4.3	7.0	0.1	0.2
Cherry, Greek Style, Shape, Danone*	1 Pot/125g	143	3.4	114	6.0	16.4	2.7	0.0
Cherry, Light, Fat Free, Muller*	1 Pot/175g	87	0.2	50	3.9	7.9	0.1	0.2
Cherry, Low Fat, Asda*	1 Pot/125g	120	1.4	96	4.6	17.0	1.1	0.0
Cherry & Vanilla Flavour, Light, Brooklea*	1 Pot/200g	138	0.2	69	5.5	11.4	0.1	0.6
Cherry Bakewell Tart Flavour, M & S*	1 Pot/150g	315	13.2	210	3.0	17.0	8.8	1.0
Cherry Bakewell Tart Flavour, Muller*	1 Pot/175g	119	0.3	68	4.8	11.8	0.2	0.2
Cherry Bio, Co-Op*	1 Pot/125g	144	3.5	115	4.5	17.0	2.8	0.1
Cherry Flip, BFY, Morrisons*	1 Pot/175g	93	0.5	53	3.9	8.7	0.3	0.4
Choc Chip Granola, Naturally Creamy, Nom Dairy UK*	1 Pot/150g	196	8.5	131	4.2	15.8	5.7	0.4
Chocolate, Village Dairy*	1 Pot/125g	181	3.7	145	6.3	23.5	3.0	0.0

YOGHURT

INFO/WEIGHT	Measure per Measure KCAL	FAT	Nutrition Values per 100g / 100ml KCAL	PROT	CARB	FAT	FIBRE
Chocolate, Vitaline*	1 Pot/125g	102	0.6	82	3.5	15.8	0.5	0.0
Chocolate Cereal Flakes, Naturally Creamy, Nom Dairy UK*	1 Pot/150g	232	8.8	155	3.8	21.7	5.9	0.2
Chocolate Raisins, Naturally Creamy, Nom Dairy UK*	1 Pot/155g	245	9.5	158	3.4	22.4	6.1	0.2
Coconut, Biopot, Onken*	1 Pot/450g	562	23.4	125	3.9	15.6	5.2	0.9
Coconut, Malaysian, Thick & Creamy, Waitrose*	1 Pot/150g	241	15.9	161	3.9	12.6	10.6	0.3
Creamy Cranberry & Raspberry, Shapers, Boots*	1 Pot/150g	85	1.6	57	4.0	7.0	1.1	1.1
Dessert with Honey, Perfectly Balanced, Waitrose*	1 Pot/125ml	127	1.5	102	3.5	19.4	1.2	0.1
Devon Toffee, Low Fat, Sainsbury's*	1 Pot/126g	137	1.9	109	4.3	19.6	1.5	0.0
Devonshire Fudge, 0.06% Fat, TTD, Sainsbury's*	1 Pot/150g	219	9.0	146	3.5	19.5	6.0	0.0
Double Trouble, Chosen By You, Asda*	1 Pot/85g	93	2.2	109	5.0	16.4	2.6	0.0
Exotic, Alpro*	1 Pot/125g	97	2.4	78	3.6	11.1	1.9	0.9
Exotic Fruits, French Set, Wholemilk, Asda*	1 Pot/125g	125	4.0	100	3.6	14.1	3.2	0.0
Exotic Fruits, Soya, Savia, Danone*	1 Pot/125g	104	2.1	83	2.9	12.6	1.7	0.5
Fat Free, Vanilla, Onken*	½ Pot/225g	166	0.2	74	4.4	12.6	0.1	0.3
Fig, Bio, Activia, Danone*	1 Pot/125g	121	4.0	97	3.7	13.3	3.2	1.6
Fig, Date & Grape, Biopot, Lite, Wholegrain, Onken*	¼ Pot/120g	102	0.2	85	4.8	16.0	0.2	1.0
Forest Fruits, M & S*	1 Pot/150g	148	2.4	99	4.7	16.8	1.6	0.5
French Set, Low Fat, Iceland*	1 Pot/125g	100	1.5	80	3.6	13.6	1.2	0.0
French Set, Waitrose*	1 Pot/125g	120	3.9	96	3.5	13.4	3.1	0.0
French Style, Whole Milk, Smooth Set, Tesco*	1 Pot/125g	122	3.7	98	3.6	14.1	3.0	0.0
Fruit, Brooklea*	1 Pot/120g	97	0.1	81	2.7	15.0	0.1	0.0
Fruit, Low Fat	1 Pot/125g	112	0.9	90	4.1	17.9	0.7	0.0
Fruit Whole Milk	1 Pot/150g	157	4.2	105	5.1	15.7	2.8	0.0
Fruits of the Forest, Iced, Linessa, Lidl*	1 Pot/170g	168	3.9	99	2.5	17.0	2.3	0.0
Fruits of the Forest, Nestle*	1 Pot/125g	122	2.0	98	3.4	16.7	1.6	0.0
Fudge, Thick & Creamy, Waitrose*	1 Pot/150g	196	4.5	131	4.4	21.5	3.0	0.0
Garden Fruit, Strawberry & Rhubarb, Rachel's Organic*	1 Pot/120g	103	2.0	86	4.3	13.3	1.7	0.1
Garden Fruit, Wholemilk, Bio Live, Rachel's Organic*	1 Pot/125g	109	4.2	87	3.5	10.5	3.4	0.0
Goats Whole Milk	**1 Carton/150g**	**94**	**5.7**	**63**	**3.5**	**3.9**	**3.8**	**0.0**
Gooseberry, Custard Style, Somerfield*	1 Pot/125g	151	6.2	121	3.0	17.0	5.0	0.0
Gooseberry, Low Fat, Average	1 Serving/100g	90	1.4	90	4.5	14.5	1.4	0.2
Gooseberry, Low Fat, Chosen By You, Asda*	1 Pot/125g	102	1.7	82	3.6	13.7	1.4	0.0
Gooseberry, Virtually Fat Free, Longley Farm*	1 Pot/150g	121	0.1	81	4.2	15.7	0.1	0.0
Greek, with Honey, Strained, Authentic, Total, Fage*	1 Pot/150g	255	12.0	170	5.4	19.0	8.0	0.0
Greek, with Strawberry, 2% Fat, Total, Fage*	1 Pot/150g	139	2.4	93	6.7	12.9	1.6	0.0
Greek & Cranberry, Made Up, Easiyo*	1 Serving/100g	113	4.7	113	4.0	14.1	4.7	0.1
Greek 'n Coconut, Made Up, Easiyo*	1 Serving/100g	113	4.7	113	4.0	14.1	4.7	0.1
Greek Style, Fat Free, Natural, Chosen By You, Asda*	1 Tub/200g	114	0.4	57	7.9	5.8	0.2	0.1
Greek Style, Luxury, Loseley*	1 Pot/175g	226	17.8	129	4.8	4.5	10.2	0.0
Greek Style with Black Cherry Compote, M & S*	1 Pot/241g	205	3.4	85	3.4	15.0	1.4	0.5
Greek Style with Toffee & Hazelnuts, Asda*	1 Pot/125g	230	10.7	184	3.7	23.1	8.6	0.1
Greek Style with Tropical Fruits, Asda*	1 Pot/125g	164	8.2	131	3.3	14.5	6.6	0.3
Guava & Orange, Fat Free, Organic, Yeo Valley*	1 Pot/125g	92	0.1	74	5.3	13.0	0.1	0.2
Guava & Passion Fruit, Virtualy Fat Free, Tesco*	1 Pot/125g	56	0.2	45	4.2	6.7	0.2	1.2
Hazelnut, Longley Farm*	1 Pot/150g	201	8.5	134	5.5	16.0	5.7	0.0
Hazelnut, Low Fat, Average	1 Serving/100g	106	2.3	106	4.5	16.9	2.3	0.1
Honey, Greek Style, Co-Op*	1 Pot/150g	228	12.7	152	4.0	13.8	8.5	0.0
Honey & Ginger, Tesco*	1 Pot/150g	150	1.6	100	4.6	18.0	1.1	0.0
Honey & Ginger, Waitrose*	1 Pot/150g	240	12.9	160	3.8	16.8	8.6	0.1
Honey & Muesli, Breakfast Break, Tesco*	1 Pot/170g	207	4.6	122	3.9	20.5	2.7	0.6
Honey & Multigrain, Breakfast Selection, Sainsbury's*	1 Pot/125g	126	1.9	101	4.4	17.4	1.5	0.2
Honey Breakfast Pot, Activia, Danone*	1 Pot/160g	192	4.2	120	4.9	18.8	2.6	0.7
Juicy Raspberry, Intensely Creamy, Activia, Danone*	1 Pot/125g	121	3.7	97	4.8	12.7	3.0	0.6

Y

YOGHURT

	Measure INFO/WEIGHT	per Measure KCAL	per Measure FAT	Nutrition Values per 100g / 100ml KCAL	PROT	CARB	FAT	FIBRE
Kiwi, Activia, Danone*	1 Pot/125g	119	4.1	95	3.6	12.7	3.3	0.3
Lemon, Greek Style, GFY, Asda*	1 Pot/150g	124	4.3	83	4.1	10.0	2.9	0.1
Lemon, Greek Style, Shape, Danone*	1 Pot/125g	140	3.4	112	5.9	15.9	2.7	0.0
Lemon, Longley Farm*	1 Pot/150g	159	5.5	106	5.0	13.4	3.7	0.0
Lemon, Low Fat, Average	1 Serving/100g	95	0.9	95	4.6	17.3	0.9	0.1
Lemon, Smooth Set French, Low Fat, Sainsbury's*	1 Pot/125g	100	1.5	80	3.5	13.6	1.2	0.0
Lemon, Summer, Biopot, Onken*	1 Pot/150g	154	3.9	103	3.9	15.9	2.6	0.1
Lemon, Thick & Fruity, Citrus Fruits, Weight Watchers*	1 Pot/120g	47	0.1	39	4.1	4.9	0.1	0.9
Lemon Curd, Indulgent, Dessert, Waitrose*	1 Pot/150g	277	13.8	185	4.1	21.5	9.2	0.0
Lemon Curd, Very, Morrisons*	1 Pot/150g	262	13.6	175	4.1	19.2	9.1	0.0
Lemon Curd, West Country, TTD, Sainsbury's*	1 Pot/150g	243	10.0	162	3.7	21.6	6.7	0.5
Lemon Curd, Whole Milk, Yeo Valley*	1 Pot/120g	153	5.3	127	4.7	17.2	4.4	0.2
Lemon Curd with West Country Cream, Morrisons*	1 Pot/150g	244	12.7	163	3.4	17.9	8.5	0.5
Lemon Lime Mousse, Shapers, Boots*	1 Pot/90g	89	3.8	99	4.2	11.0	4.2	0.1
Loganberry, Sainsbury's*	1 Pot/150g	193	9.3	129	3.9	14.2	6.2	0.6
Low Calorie	1 Pot/120g	49	0.2	41	4.3	6.0	0.2	0.0
Luscious Cherry, Intensely Creamy, Activia, Danone*	1 Pot/120g	116	3.6	97	4.8	12.7	3.0	0.2
Mango, Bio Activia, Danone*	1 Pot/125g	121	4.0	97	3.7	13.4	3.2	1.6
Mango, Fat Free, Shape Danone*	1 Pot/120g	74	0.1	62	6.6	8.6	0.1	2.2
Mango, Light, Muller*	1 Pot/175g	96	0.2	55	4.3	9.2	0.1	0.0
Mango, Mouthwatering, Intensely Creamy, Activia, Danone*	1 Pot/125g	122	3.7	98	4.7	13.0	3.0	0.2
Mango, Zer0% Fat, No Added Sugar, Shape, Danone*	1 Pot/120g	72	0.1	60	6.0	8.8	0.1	0.9
Mango & Apple, Fat Free, Onken*	1 Serving/150g	132	0.1	88	4.4	16.0	0.1	0.2
Mango & Guava, Sunshine Selection, Sainsbury's*	1 Pot/125g	145	2.4	116	5.4	19.3	1.9	0.3
Mango & Passion Fruit, Creamy, Nom Dairy UK*	1 Pot/175g	189	6.6	108	3.1	15.4	3.8	0.3
Mango & Passion Fruit, Layered, Nom Dairy UK*	1 Pot/125g	114	3.0	91	3.2	14.2	2.4	0.3
Mango & Passion Fruit, Tropical Fruit, Activ8, Ski, Nestle*	1 Pot/120g	114	2.0	95	4.3	15.6	1.7	0.2
Mango & Pineapple, BGTY, Sainsbury's*	1 Pot/124g	63	0.2	51	4.6	7.6	0.2	0.2
Mixed Seeds, Probiotic, Yoplait*	1 Pot/125g	139	5.6	111	4.5	13.2	4.5	3.1
Morello Cherry, Amore Luxury, Muller*	1 Pot/150g	216	11.7	144	2.8	16.3	7.8	0.1
Morello Cherry, HL, Tesco*	1 Pot/125g	56	0.2	45	4.1	6.6	0.2	0.9
Muesli Nut, Low Fat	1 Pot/120g	134	2.6	112	5.0	19.2	2.2	0.0
Natural, 0.1% Fat, Stirred, Biopot, Onken*	1 Serving/100g	48	0.1	48	5.4	6.4	0.1	0.0
Natural, Bio Activia, Individual Pots, Danone*	1 Pot/125g	86	4.2	69	4.2	5.5	3.4	0.0
Natural, Bio Life, Easiyo*	1 Pot/150g	95	2.7	63	5.0	6.7	1.8	0.0
Natural, Bio Live, Low Fat, Organic, Waitrose*	¼ Pot/125g	81	1.2	65	5.8	8.3	1.0	0.0
Natural, Bio Live, Very Low Fat, Ann Forshaw's*	1 Pot/125g	52	0.1	42	5.0	5.5	0.1	0.0
Natural, Bio Set, Low Fat, Sainsbury's*	1 Pot/150g	78	2.2	52	3.9	5.7	1.5	0.0
Natural, Danone*	1 Pot/125g	71	3.6	57	3.2	3.8	2.9	0.0
Natural, Fat Free, Biopot, Dr Oetker*	¼ Pot/125g	60	0.1	48	5.4	6.4	0.1	0.0
Natural, Fat Free, Onken*	1 Serving/100g	48	0.1	48	5.4	6.3	0.1	0.0
Natural, Fat Free, Probiotic, Essential, Waitrose*	¼ Pot/125g	67	0.0	54	5.5	7.8	0.0	0.0
Natural, Fat Free, Rachel's Organic*	1 Pot/500g	180	0.5	36	3.9	4.8	0.1	0.0
Natural, Greek Style, Average	1 Serving/100g	138	10.6	138	4.7	6.1	10.6	0.0
Natural, Greek Style, Bio Live, Rachel's Organic*	1 Pot/450g	517	40.5	115	3.6	4.9	9.0	0.0
Natural, Greek Style, Less Than 3% Fat, BGTY, Sainsbury's*	¼ Pot/125g	99	3.4	79	5.6	8.1	2.7	0.0
Natural, Greek Style, Low Fat, Average	1 Serving/100g	77	2.7	77	6.1	7.3	2.7	0.2
Natural, Greek Style, with Honey Sauce, Sainsbury's*	1 Pot/140g	206	11.1	147	3.3	15.7	7.9	0.0
Natural, Longley Farm*	1 Pot/150g	118	5.2	79	4.8	7.0	3.5	0.0
Natural, Low Fat, Average	*1 Pot/125g*	*75*	*1.6*	*60*	*5.4*	*7.0*	*1.3*	*0.0*
Natural, Low Fat, Organic, Average	1 Serving/100g	87	1.2	87	5.7	7.7	1.2	0.0
Natural, Luxury, Bio Live, Jersey Dairy*	1 Pot/150g	225	12.0	150	4.6	8.2	8.0	0.0
Natural, Organic, Evernat*	1 Serving/100g	104	4.0	104	3.9	12.9	4.0	0.0

YOGHURT

	Measure INFO/WEIGHT	per Measure KCAL	FAT	Nutrition Values per 100g / 100ml KCAL	PROT	CARB	FAT	FIBRE
Natural, Organic, Yeo Valley*	1 Pot/150g	120	5.5	80	4.7	6.9	3.7	0.0
Natural, Pouring, Activia, Danone*	1 Carton/950g	484	16.1	51	4.1	4.9	1.7	0.0
Natural, Probiotic, Fat Free, Organic, Yeo Valley*	1 Pot/150g	87	0.1	58	5.9	8.4	0.1	0.0
Natural, Probiotic, Organic, Yeo Valley*	1 Pot/150g	123	6.3	82	4.5	6.6	4.2	0.0
Natural, Sojasun*	1 Serving/100g	51	2.7	51	4.6	2.0	2.7	0.0
Natural, Soya, Sojade*	1 Serving/100g	50	2.5	50	4.5	2.4	2.5	0.0
Natural, Whole Milk, Set, Biopot, Onken*	1 Pot/150g	108	5.5	72	3.9	5.7	3.7	0.0
Nectarine, Fat Free, Weight Watchers*	1 Pot/120g	48	0.1	40	4.1	4.7	0.1	0.4
Nectarine & Orange, Best There Is, Yoplait*	1 Pot/122g	131	2.0	107	4.7	18.0	1.6	0.0
Nectarine & Orange, Fat Free, Average	1 Serving/100g	46	0.1	46	4.4	6.7	0.1	0.0
Nectarine & Passion Fruit, 0.1% Fat, Shape, Danone*	1 Pot/120g	55	0.1	46	4.6	6.7	0.1	2.1
Nectarine & Passion Fruit, Low Fat, Stapleton Farm*	1 Pot/150g	120	0.7	80	3.2	16.3	0.5	0.6
Orange, Greek Style, Shape, Danone*	1 Pot/125g	140	3.4	112	6.0	16.0	2.7	0.1
Orange, Spanish, Amore Luxury, Muller*	1 Pot/150g	226	11.7	151	2.9	17.2	7.8	0.1
Orange, Sprinkled with Dark Chocolate, Light, Muller*	1 Pot/165g	84	0.8	51	4.0	7.1	0.5	0.1
Orange & Pineapple, Tropical Fruit, Activ8, Ski, Nestle*	1 Pot/120g	112	2.0	93	4.4	15.1	1.7	0.2
Peach, Bio, Fat Free, Snackpot, Activia, Danone*	1 Pot/165g	99	0.2	60	4.6	10.2	0.1	1.0
Peach, Biopot, Wholegrain, Onken*	1 Serving/100g	114	2.8	114	4.0	17.8	2.8	0.5
Peach, Forbidden Fruits, Rachel's Organic*	1 Pot/125g	156	7.6	125	3.4	14.0	6.1	0.0
Peach, Honeyed, Greek Style, Mullerlight, Muller*	1 Pot/120g	85	0.2	71	6.3	10.3	0.2	0.2
Peach, Low Fat, Average	1 Serving/100g	86	1.1	86	4.5	14.6	1.1	0.1
Peach, Luscious, Low Fat, Rachel's Organic*	1 Pot/125g	112	2.0	90	4.0	14.9	1.6	0.2
Peach, Smooth Style, Mullerlight, Muller*	1 Pot/125g	59	0.1	47	4.1	6.9	0.1	0.2
Peach & Apricot, 0.1% Fat, Shape, Danone*	1 Pot/120g	55	0.1	46	4.6	6.7	0.1	2.1
Peach & Apricot, Fruit Corner, Muller*	1 Pot/175g	189	6.8	108	3.8	13.6	3.9	0.5
Peach & Crunchy Clusters, Breakfast Pot, Activia, Danone*	1 Pot/160g	190	4.2	119	5.0	18.4	2.6	0.9
Peach & Lemon Balm, Biowild, Onken*	1 Pot/175g	157	2.6	90	4.3	14.9	1.5	0.1
Peach & Mango, 0.1% Actimel, Danone*	1 Serving/100g	29	0.1	29	2.7	3.6	0.1	0.1
Peach & Mango, Dairy Free, Organic, Yofu, Provamel*	1 Pot/125g	100	2.7	80	3.9	10.4	2.2	0.8
Peach & Maracuya, Mullerlight, Muller*	1 Pot/200g	102	0.2	51	4.5	8.1	0.1	0.0
Peach & Nectarine, Bio, Fat Free, Activia, Danone*	1 Pot/125g	70	0.1	56	4.5	9.3	0.1	1.0
Peach & Papaya, Fat Free, Yeo Valley*	1 Pot/125g	94	0.1	75	5.3	13.1	0.1	0.1
Peach & Passion Fruit, Average	1 Serving/100g	66	0.7	66	4.5	10.6	0.7	0.4
Peach & Passion Fruit, BGTY, Sainsbury's*	1 Pot/125g	69	0.1	55	4.9	8.6	0.1	0.1
Peach & Passion Fruit, Fat Free, Shape, Danone*	1 Pot/120g	74	0.1	62	6.6	8.6	0.1	2.3
Peach & Passion Fruit, Fruit Layered, Bio, GFY, Asda*	1 Pot/126g	77	0.1	61	4.0	11.0	0.1	0.5
Peach & Passion Fruit, Layers, Mullerlight, Muller*	1 Pot/175g	94	0.2	54	3.1	9.7	0.1	0.2
Peach & Passion Fruit, Lite Biopot, Onken*	1/5 Pot/100g	45	0.2	45	4.6	6.0	0.2	0.2
Peach & Passion Fruit, Low Fat, Somerfield*	1 Pot/150g	132	1.5	88	4.0	16.0	1.0	0.0
Peach & Pear, Low Fat, Somerfield*	1 Pot/125g	117	1.2	94	4.5	16.5	1.0	0.2
Peach & Pear, Seriously Fruity, Low Fat, Waitrose*	1 Pot/125g	110	1.2	88	4.5	15.3	1.0	0.3
Peach & Pineapple, Fat Free, Mullerlight, Muller*	1 Pot/175g	89	0.2	51	4.3	7.7	0.1	0.2
Peach & Vanilla, Average, Tesco*	1 Serving/100g	43	0.1	43	4.4	6.1	0.1	0.5
Peach & Vanilla, Thick & Creamy, Co-Op*	1 Pot/150g	180	6.9	120	3.6	16.0	4.6	0.1
Peach & Vanilla Flip, Morrisons*	1 Pot/175g	212	8.0	121	3.4	16.5	4.6	0.6
Peach Melba, Low Fat, Average	1 Serving/100g	75	0.7	75	2.6	14.5	0.7	0.0
Peach Melba, Sveltesse, Nestle*	1 Pot/126g	70	0.1	56	4.7	9.1	0.1	0.2
Peach Melba, Value, Tesco*	1 Pot/125g	100	0.9	80	2.3	16.0	0.7	0.1
Peaches, Farmhouse, BGTY, Sainsbury's*	1 Pot/150g	133	0.6	89	3.2	17.8	0.4	0.3
Peaches & Cream, Intensely Creamy, Activia, Danone*	1 Pot/120g	118	3.6	98	4.8	13.0	3.0	0.3
Peanut Toffee, Low Fat, Somerfield*	1 Pot/150g	130	1.5	87	4.0	15.0	1.0	0.0
Pear & Vanilla, Thick & Creamy, Weight Watchers*	1 Pot/120g	54	0.6	45	4.2	5.8	0.5	0.2
Pineapple, Average	1 Serving/100g	73	1.1	73	4.4	11.3	1.1	0.5

YOGHURT

Measure INFO/WEIGHT	per Measure KCAL	FAT	Nutrition Values per 100g / 100ml KCAL	PROT	CARB	FAT	FIBRE
Pineapple, Bio Activia, Fat Free, Danone*	1 Pot/125g	62	0.1	50	4.7	7.5	0.1	1.7
Pineapple, Channel Island, M & S*	1 Pot/150g	165	4.9	110	4.3	15.9	3.3	0.3
Pineapple, Extremely Fruity, M & S*	1 Pot/200g	200	2.8	100	4.3	17.6	1.4	0.2
Pineapple, Low Fat, Average	1 Serving/100g	89	1.2	89	4.6	14.7	1.2	0.0
Pineapple, Low Fat, Bio, Asda*	1 Pot/150g	144	1.6	96	4.6	17.0	1.1	0.1
Pineapple, Thick & Creamy, Waitrose*	1 Pot/125g	136	3.1	109	3.6	17.9	2.5	0.2
Pineapple, Tropical Fruit, Thick & Fruity, Weight Watchers*	1 Pot/120g	56	0.1	47	3.9	7.7	0.1	0.9
Pineapple, Virtually Fat Free, Tesco*	1 Pot/125g	55	0.2	44	4.1	6.5	0.2	0.9
Pineapple, Vitality, Low Fat, with Omega 3, Muller*	1 Pot/150g	138	2.8	92	4.2	13.8	1.9	0.7
Pineapple & Grapefruit, BGTY, Sainsbury's*	1 Pot/125g	67	0.1	54	4.4	8.8	0.1	0.1
Pineapple & Passion Fruit, Soya, Light, Alpro*	1 Pot/120g	62	1.3	52	2.1	7.3	1.1	0.8
Pineapple & Peach, Fruity, Mullerlight, Muller*	1 Pot/175g	89	0.2	51	4.2	7.7	0.1	0.2
Pink Grapefruit, Low Fat, Sainsbury's*	1 Pot/125g	116	1.7	93	4.2	15.9	1.4	0.1
Plain, Low Fat, Average	**1 Serving/100g**	**63**	**1.5**	**63**	**5.2**	**7.0**	**1.5**	**0.0**
Plain, Natural, Dairy Free, Organic, Yofu, Soya, Provamel*	1 Pot/125g	72	3.4	58	4.7	2.8	2.7	0.8
Plain, Soya, Average	**1oz/28g**	**20**	**1.2**	**72**	**5.0**	**3.9**	**4.2**	**0.0**
Plain, Whole Milk, Average	**1oz/28g**	**22**	**0.8**	**79**	**5.7**	**7.8**	**3.0**	**0.0**
Plum, BGTY, Sainsbury's*	1 Pot/125g	69	0.1	55	4.8	8.8	0.1	0.1
Plum, Low Fat, Sainsbury's*	1 Pot/125g	117	2.1	94	4.5	15.2	1.7	0.1
Plum, Probiotic, Summer Selection, Yeo Valley*	1 Pot/125g	126	4.9	101	4.1	12.4	3.9	0.1
Plum, Soya, Dairy Free, Organic, with Fibre, Provamel*	1 Serving/125g	90	2.5	72	3.7	7.5	2.0	4.0
Probiotic, Fat Free, Average	1 Tbsp/15g	8	0.0	56	5.4	7.7	0.3	0.6
Probiotic, Low Fat, Organic, Glenisk Organic Dairy Co*	1 Serving/150g	91	2.8	61	4.5	6.4	1.9	0.0
Prune, Bifidus, Activo, Mercadona*	1 Pot/125g	70	0.1	56	4.5	6.8	0.1	3.0
Prune, Bio Activia, Danone*	1 Pot/125g	110	3.5	88	3.5	12.2	2.8	0.2
Prune, Breakfast Selection, Sainsbury's*	1 Pot/125g	119	1.7	95	4.2	16.3	1.4	0.2
Prune, Fat Free, Natural Balance, Chosen By You, Asda*	1 Pot/125g	94	0.5	75	3.6	12.6	0.4	3.4
Prune, Probiotic, Natural Balance, Asda*	1 Pot/125g	105	2.9	84	2.1	13.8	2.3	0.8
Prune, Vitality, Low Fat, with Omega 3, Muller*	1 Pot/150g	144	2.8	96	4.7	15.0	1.9	1.1
Raspberry, Bio, Activia, Danone*	1 Pot/125g	112	3.5	90	3.5	12.8	2.8	2.0
Raspberry, Bio, Activia, Fat Free, Danone*	1 Pot/125g	67	0.1	54	4.7	7.2	0.1	2.6
Raspberry, Bio, Fat Free, Snackpot, Activia, Danone*	1 Pot/165g	81	0.2	48	4.6	6.9	0.1	2.5
Raspberry, Bio, Low Fat, Benecol*	1 Pot/125g	99	0.8	79	3.8	14.5	0.6	0.0
Raspberry, Bio, Low Fat, Sainsbury's*	1 Pot/150g	145	1.6	97	4.7	17.0	1.1	0.7
Raspberry, Bio, Pur Natur*	1 Pot/150g	150	4.6	100	1.4	14.5	3.1	0.0
Raspberry, Bio Live, Low Fat, Rachel's Organic*	1 Pot/125g	109	2.0	87	4.0	14.2	1.6	0.1
Raspberry, Economy, Sainsbury's*	1 Pot/125g	85	1.2	68	3.0	11.9	1.0	0.0
Raspberry, Extremely Fruity, M & S*	1 Pot/200g	190	3.0	95	5.0	15.6	1.5	0.5
Raspberry, Fat Free, Average	1 Serving/100g	64	0.1	64	4.9	11.0	0.1	1.7
Raspberry, Fat Free, Probiotic, Organic, Yeo Valley*	1 Pot/125g	97	0.1	78	5.2	14.0	0.1	0.4
Raspberry, Forbidden Fruit, Rachel's Organic*	1 Pot/125g	155	7.6	124	3.4	13.8	6.1	0.1
Raspberry, French Set, Waitrose*	1 Pot/125g	120	3.9	96	3.5	13.4	3.1	2.0
Raspberry, Incredibly Fruity, Fat Free, Tesco*	1 Pot/150g	112	0.1	75	4.8	13.1	0.1	1.0
Raspberry, Jubileum, Tine*	1 Pot/135g	163	6.5	121	3.2	16.1	4.8	0.0
Raspberry, Lactose Free, Lactofree, Arla*	1 Pot/125g	130	3.4	104	3.3	16.5	2.7	0.7
Raspberry, Light, HL, Tesco*	1 Pot/200g	88	0.2	44	3.9	7.0	0.1	1.7
Raspberry, Low Fat, Average	1 Serving/100g	83	1.1	83	4.1	14.1	1.1	0.8
Raspberry, Naturally Light, Nom Dairy UK*	1 Pot/180g	133	0.2	74	4.3	13.9	0.1	0.2
Raspberry, Organic, Yeo Valley*	1 Pot/150g	151	5.8	101	4.2	12.3	3.9	0.4
Raspberry, Probiotic, Live, Yeo Valley*	1 Pot/125g	106	1.2	85	5.1	14.0	1.0	0.4
Raspberry, Probiotic, Low Fat, Organic, M & S*	1 Pot/170g	127	2.4	75	4.4	11.5	1.4	0.4
Raspberry, Probiotic, Low Fat, Tesco*	1 Pot/170g	144	2.4	85	3.0	14.3	1.4	0.3
Raspberry, Scottish, The Best, Morrisons*	1 Pot/150g	208	10.3	139	3.6	15.6	6.9	1.3

YOGHURT

INFO/WEIGHT	Measure	per Measure		Nutrition Values per 100g / 100ml				
		KCAL	FAT	KCAL	PROT	CARB	FAT	FIBRE
Raspberry, Smooth, Activ8, Ski, Nestle*	1 Pot/120g	113	2.0	94	4.6	14.8	1.7	0.7
Raspberry, Smooth, Mullerlight, Muller*	1 Pot/125g	64	0.1	51	4.2	7.8	0.1	0.6
Raspberry, Soya, Alpro*	1 Pot/125g	99	2.4	79	3.7	10.4	1.9	1.2
Raspberry, Summer, Biopot, Onken*	1/5 Pot/90g	91	2.4	101	3.8	15.0	2.7	0.6
Raspberry, Thick & Creamy, Sainsbury's*	1 Pot/150g	178	5.5	119	4.4	17.2	3.7	0.2
Raspberry, Thick & Fruity, Probiotic, COU, M & S*	1 Pot/170g	76	0.2	45	4.2	6.9	0.1	0.6
Raspberry, Virtually Fat Free, Tesco*	1 Pot/125g	51	0.2	41	4.1	5.8	0.2	1.1
Raspberry, Vitality, Low Fat, with Omega 3, Muller*	1 Pot/125g	115	2.5	92	4.3	13.4	2.0	1.3
Raspberry, with Fruit Layer, Bio Activia, Danone*	1 Pot/125g	107	3.5	86	3.5	11.6	2.8	2.0
Raspberry, Zer0% Fat, No Added Sugar, Shape, Danone*	1 Pot/120g	68	0.1	57	6.0	8.1	0.1	0.3
Raspberry & Blackberry, Thick & Creamy, Co-Op*	1 Pot/150g	187	6.9	125	3.6	17.3	4.6	0.1
Raspberry & Cranberry, BGTY, Sainsbury's*	1 Pot/125g	65	0.1	52	4.4	8.4	0.1	0.5
Raspberry & Cranberry, Fat Free, Mullerlight, Muller*	1 Pot/175g	90	0.2	51	2.2	8.1	0.1	0.5
Raspberry & Cranberry, Light, HL, Tesco*	1 Pot/125g	55	0.2	44	4.2	6.3	0.2	1.1
Raspberry & Cranberry, Very Low Fat, Ann Forshaw's*	1 Pot/125g	91	0.1	73	4.6	14.2	0.1	0.2
Raspberry & Redcurrant, Low Fat, Morrisons*	1 Pot/125g	117	2.0	94	4.4	15.4	1.6	0.7
Raspberry & Redcurrant, Low Fat, Sainsbury's*	1 Pot/125g	109	1.7	87	4.2	14.5	1.4	0.5
Raspberry or Strawberry, Smooth (No Bits), Ski, Nestle*	1 Pot/120g	118	3.2	98	3.9	13.6	2.7	0.0
Raspberry Smooth, Favourites, Nom Dairy UK*	1 Pot/125g	111	3.0	89	3.2	13.7	2.4	0.3
Red Berry, Healthy Balance, Corner, Muller*	1 Pot/150g	178	4.0	119	5.0	18.0	2.7	0.5
Red Berry, Vitality, Low Fat, with Omega 3, Muller*	1 Pot/150g	138	2.8	92	4.3	13.8	1.9	0.7
Red Cherry, Dairy Free, Organic, Yofu, Soya, Provamel*	1 Pot/125g	101	2.7	81	3.9	10.5	2.2	0.8
Red Cherry, Fat Free, Ski, Nestle*	1 Pot/120g	97	0.1	81	4.5	15.6	0.1	0.1
Red Cherry, Fruit Corner, Muller*	1 Pot/150g	157	5.8	105	3.8	13.0	3.9	0.5
Red Cherry, Fruit Layered, GFY, Asda*	1 Pot/125g	75	0.1	60	3.7	11.0	0.1	0.1
Red Fruits, Crumble Style, Sveltesse, Nestle*	1 Pot/125g	100	0.2	80	4.9	14.6	0.2	0.4
Rhubarb, Bio Activia, Danone*	1 Pot/125g	112	4.0	90	3.5	11.8	3.2	2.2
Rhubarb, Bio Live, Low Fat, Luscious, Rachel's Organic*	1 Pot/125g	104	2.0	83	4.0	13.1	1.6	0.1
Rhubarb, Country, Naturally Light, Nom Dairy UK*	1 Pot/180g	131	0.2	73	4.3	13.8	0.1	0.4
Rhubarb, Custard Style, Co-Op*	1 Pot/150g	202	7.9	135	3.7	17.2	5.3	0.3
Rhubarb, Custard Style, Somerfield*	1 Pot/125g	149	6.2	119	3.0	16.0	5.0	0.0
Rhubarb, Eat Smart, Morrisons*	1 Pot/190g	79	0.2	42	4.1	6.1	0.1	1.4
Rhubarb, Extremely Fruity, Probiotic, Low Fat, M & S*	1 Pot/170g	153	1.7	90	4.4	15.5	1.0	0.7
Rhubarb, Fruity, Mullerlight, Muller*	1 Pot/175g	91	0.2	52	4.2	7.9	0.1	0.0
Rhubarb, Greek Style, Corner, Muller*	1 Pot/150g	169	4.5	113	5.0	15.8	3.0	0.1
Rhubarb, Live Bio, Low Fat, Perfectly Balanced, Waitrose*	1 Pot/150g	114	0.1	76	4.2	14.5	0.1	0.2
Rhubarb, Longley Farm*	1 Pot/150g	165	5.5	110	4.9	14.3	3.7	0.0
Rhubarb, Low Fat, Average	1 Serving/100g	83	1.2	83	4.6	13.3	1.2	0.2
Rhubarb, Spiced, Thick & Creamy, COU, M & S*	1 Pot/170g	68	0.2	40	4.3	5.8	0.1	0.5
Rhubarb, Very Low Fat, Somerfield*	1 Pot/125g	57	0.0	46	5.0	6.0	0.0	0.0
Rhubarb & Champagne, Truly Irresistible, Co-Op*	1 Pot/150g	195	8.2	130	3.5	16.6	5.5	0.2
Rhubarb & Orange, Tesco*	1 Pot/150g	145	1.6	97	4.6	17.1	1.1	0.5
Rhubarb & Vanilla, Summer, Biopot, Onken*	1/5 Pot/90g	94	2.4	104	3.7	16.0	2.7	0.3
Rhubarb Crumble, Crunch Corner, Muller*	1 Pot/150g	238	8.4	159	3.6	23.5	5.6	0.5
Sheep's Milk, Total, Fage*	1 Pot/200g	180	12.0	90	4.8	4.3	6.0	0.0
Smooth Toffee, Fat Free, Mullerlight, Muller*	1 Pot/175g	88	0.2	50	3.8	8.0	0.1	0.0
Smooth Toffee, Mullerlight, Muller*	1 Pot/190g	97	0.2	51	4.0	7.9	0.1	0.0
Smooth Toffee & Apple, Low Fat, Co-Op*	1 Pot/125g	150	1.2	120	6.0	22.0	1.0	0.1
Sticky Toffee Pudding, Dessert Style, Mullerlight, Muller*	1 Pot/175g	108	0.3	62	4.4	9.9	0.2	0.2
Strawberries & Cream, 0.06% Fat, TTD, Sainsbury's*	1 Pot/150g	183	8.2	122	3.5	14.7	5.5	0.4
Strawberries & Cream, Finest, Tesco*	1 Pot/150g	205	10.3	137	3.4	15.4	6.9	0.5
Strawberry, & Muesli, Breakfast, Tesco*	1 Pot/170g	192	4.8	113	4.1	17.9	2.8	0.5
Strawberry, & Whole Grain, Bio Break, Tesco*	1 Pot/175g	175	1.9	100	4.7	17.8	1.1	0.2

Y

YOGHURT

	Measure INFO/WEIGHT	per Measure KCAL	per Measure FAT	Nutrition Values per 100g / 100ml KCAL	PROT	CARB	FAT	FIBRE
Strawberry, Amore for Me, Muller*	1 Pot/150g	216	10.9	144	2.6	17.0	7.3	0.2
Strawberry, Balanced Lifestyle, Aldi*	1 Pot/150g	72	0.4	48	4.1	7.1	0.3	0.5
Strawberry, Bettabuy, Morrisons*	1 Pot/115g	91	1.5	79	4.4	12.8	1.3	0.3
Strawberry, BGTY, Sainsbury's*	1 Pot/125g	64	0.1	51	4.8	7.7	0.1	1.2
Strawberry, Bio, Co-Op*	1 Pot/125g	142	3.5	114	4.5	16.7	2.8	0.1
Strawberry, Bio, Fat Free, Snackpot, Activia, Danone*	1 Pot/165g	99	0.2	60	4.9	9.9	0.1	0.2
Strawberry, Bio, Granola, Corner, Muller*	1 Pot/135g	161	3.5	119	5.5	17.8	2.6	0.8
Strawberry, Bio, Low Fat, Dale Farm*	1 Pot/125g	125	2.1	100	3.9	17.0	1.7	0.2
Strawberry, Bio Activia, Danone*	1 Pot/125g	117	4.0	94	3.5	12.8	3.2	2.0
Strawberry, Biopot, Wholegrain, Onken*	1 Serving/100g	111	2.9	111	4.1	17.2	2.9	0.5
Strawberry, Cereals, Fibre, Bio Activia, Danone*	1 Pot/120g	113	3.8	94	3.7	12.7	3.2	3.0
Strawberry, Childrens, Co-Op*	1 Pot/125g	121	3.4	97	3.5	14.9	2.7	0.2
Strawberry, Custard Style, Shapers, Boots*	1 Pot/150g	117	1.0	78	3.9	14.0	0.7	0.5
Strawberry, Custard Style, Somerfield*	1 Pot/125g	152	6.2	122	3.0	17.0	5.0	0.0
Strawberry, Duo, Co-Op*	1 Pot/175g	219	8.7	125	3.0	17.0	5.0	0.7
Strawberry, Eat Smart, Morrisons*	1 Pot/200g	116	0.6	58	5.7	8.5	0.3	0.3
Strawberry, Everyday Low Fat, Co-Op*	1 Pot/125g	87	0.9	70	3.0	13.0	0.7	0.0
Strawberry, Farmhouse, BGTY, Sainsbury's*	1 Pot/150g	106	0.6	71	3.2	13.7	0.4	0.5
Strawberry, Fat Free, Average	1 Serving/100g	66	0.1	66	4.9	11.1	0.1	0.6
Strawberry, Fat Free, Probiotic, Organic, Yeo Valley*	1 Pot/125g	107	1.2	86	5.1	14.1	1.0	0.1
Strawberry, Fruit Corner, Snack Size, Muller*	1 Pot/95g	108	3.8	114	3.9	15.6	4.0	0.4
Strawberry, Fruit 'n' Creamy, Ubley*	1 Pot/151g	167	4.4	111	4.3	16.9	2.9	0.3
Strawberry, Fruity, Mullerlight, Muller*	1 Pot/175g	89	0.2	51	4.1	7.9	0.1	0.0
Strawberry, Granose*	1 Pot/120g	108	1.9	90	4.5	15.5	1.6	0.0
Strawberry, Great Stuff, Asda*	1 Pot/60g	58	1.5	97	4.7	14.0	2.5	0.5
Strawberry, Happy Shopper*	1 Pot/150g	130	0.4	87	3.0	18.5	0.3	0.0
Strawberry, Healthy Balance, Corner, Muller*	1 Pot/135g	161	3.5	119	5.4	17.9	2.6	0.8
Strawberry, Lactose Free, Lactofree, Arla*	1 Pot/125g	126	3.2	101	3.5	15.9	2.6	0.4
Strawberry, Light, Brooklea*	1 Pot/200g	154	0.2	77	6.1	12.9	0.1	0.4
Strawberry, Light, HL, Tesco*	1 Pot/200g	80	0.2	40	3.5	6.4	0.1	0.8
Strawberry, Light & Refreshing, Campina*	1 Pot/125g	110	1.4	88	2.5	16.9	1.1	0.0
Strawberry, Light Choices, Tesco*	1 Pot/200g	86	0.2	43	4.1	6.3	0.1	0.6
Strawberry, Little Town Dairy*	1 Pot/125g	82	2.0	66	2.9	9.9	1.6	0.0
Strawberry, Live, Turners Dairies*	1 Pot/125g	86	0.4	69	4.9	11.9	0.3	0.0
Strawberry, Low Fat, Average	1 Serving/100g	81	1.0	81	4.5	13.6	1.0	0.2
Strawberry, Low Fat, Probiotic, Organic, M & S*	1 Pot/170g	136	2.4	80	4.8	11.6	1.4	0.4
Strawberry, Luscious, Shapers, Boots*	1 Pot/150g	82	1.6	55	4.0	7.3	1.1	0.6
Strawberry, Luxury, Bio Live, Jersey Dairy*	1 Pot/150g	159	8.5	106	3.8	10.2	5.7	0.5
Strawberry, Naturally Creamy, Nom Dairy UK*	1 Pot/175g	185	6.6	106	3.1	15.0	3.8	0.3
Strawberry, Naturally Light, Nom Dairy UK*	1 Pot/180g	137	0.2	76	4.5	13.4	0.1	0.3
Strawberry, Organic, Yeo Valley*	1 Pot/150g	144	4.9	96	4.3	12.4	3.3	0.1
Strawberry, Perfectly Balanced, Waitrose*	1 Pot/150g	136	0.2	91	4.6	17.8	0.1	0.1
Strawberry, Pouring, Activia, Danone*	1 Serving/100g	59	1.6	59	3.9	7.3	1.6	0.1
Strawberry, Probiotic, Natural Balance, Asda*	1 Pot/125g	109	3.0	87	3.1	13.3	2.4	2.4
Strawberry, Probiotic, Organic, Yeo Valley*	1 Pot/125g	125	5.0	100	4.4	11.7	4.0	0.1
Strawberry, Redcurrant, Bio Layered, Sainsbury's*	1 Serving/125g	134	3.4	107	4.1	16.5	2.7	0.2
Strawberry, Smooth, Activ8, Ski, Nestle*	1 Pot/120g	113	2.0	94	4.6	14.8	1.7	0.7
Strawberry, Smooth Set French, Low Fat, Sainsbury's*	1 Pot/125g	112	4.0	90	3.7	11.8	3.2	0.0
Strawberry, Soya, Dairy Free, Organic, Yofu, Provamel*	1 Pot/125g	101	2.7	81	3.9	10.6	2.2	0.8
Strawberry, Soyage, GranoVita*	1 Pot/145g	112	0.6	77	1.8	16.5	0.4	0.0
Strawberry, Swiss, Emmi*	1 Pot/175g	177	4.4	101	3.5	16.0	2.5	0.3
Strawberry, Thick & Creamy, Co-Op*	1 Pot/150g	181	6.9	121	3.6	16.4	4.6	0.1
Strawberry, Thick & Creamy, Waitrose*	1 Pot/125g	135	3.1	108	3.7	17.6	2.5	0.4

YOGHURT

INFO/WEIGHT	Measure	per Measure KCAL	FAT	Nutrition Values per 100g / 100ml KCAL	PROT	CARB	FAT	FIBRE
Strawberry, Thick & Fruity, Probiotic, COU, M & S*	1 Pot/170g	76	0.2	45	4.1	7.3	0.1	0.4
Strawberry, Totally, Low Fat, Chosen By You, Asda*	1 Pot/125g	104	1.2	83	4.1	14.2	1.0	0.4
Strawberry, Very Berry, Activ8, Ski, Nestle*	1 Pot/120g	110	2.0	92	4.3	15.0	1.7	0.3
Strawberry, Very Low Fat, Bio, Somerfield*	1 Pot/200g	100	0.0	50	5.0	7.0	0.0	0.0
Strawberry, Virtually Fat Free, Average	1 Serving/100g	65	0.2	65	4.7	11.3	0.2	0.2
Strawberry, Vitality, Low Fat, with Omega 3, Muller*	1 Pot/150g	139	2.8	93	4.3	14.0	1.9	0.8
Strawberry, Wholemilk, Organic, Sainsbury's*	1 Pot/150g	123	5.2	82	3.5	9.2	3.5	0.1
Strawberry, Yoo Fruity Thing, Split Pot, Yoo, Nom Dairy UK*	1 Pot/175g	192	6.5	110	3.3	15.0	3.7	0.3
Strawberry, Yoplait*	1 Pot/125g	61	0.2	49	4.2	7.6	0.2	0.9
Strawberry, Zer0% Fat, No Added Sugar, Shape, Danone*	1 Pot/120g	71	0.1	59	6.0	8.5	0.1	0.9
Strawberry & Banana, Oatie Breakfast, Moma Foods*	1 Pot/235g	320	5.6	136	4.3	25.4	2.4	1.7
Strawberry & Clotted Cream, Luxury, Stapleton Farm*	1 Pot/150g	147	5.7	98	3.2	13.2	3.8	0.6
Strawberry & Cornish Clotted Cream, M & S*	1 Pot/150g	217	11.5	145	3.2	15.4	7.7	0.5
Strawberry & French Vanilla, Amore Luxury, Muller*	1 Pot/150g	225	11.7	150	2.9	17.0	7.8	0.1
Strawberry & Raspberry, HL, Tesco*	1 Pot/125g	57	0.1	46	4.2	7.0	0.1	0.0
Strawberry & Raspberry, Layered, Bio, GFY, Asda*	1 Pot/72g	43	0.1	60	3.8	11.0	0.1	0.4
Strawberry & Raspberry, Low Fat, Asda*	1 Pot/150g	142	1.5	95	4.6	17.4	1.0	0.2
Strawberry & Raspberry, Low Fat, Sainsbury's*	1 Pot/125g	109	1.7	87	4.2	14.3	1.4	0.2
Strawberry & Raspberry, Probiotic, Organic, Yeo Valley*	1 Pot/125g	125	4.9	100	4.2	12.0	3.9	0.1
Strawberry & Redcurrant, Farmhouse, Ann Forshaw's*	1 Pot/150g	193	7.3	129	3.8	17.4	4.9	0.2
Strawberry & Rhubarb, Channel Island, M & S*	1 Pot/150g	157	4.5	105	3.9	15.4	3.0	0.0
Strawberry & Rhubarb, Low Fat, Sainsbury's*	1 Pot/125g	107	1.7	86	4.2	14.1	1.4	0.2
Strawberry & Rhubarb, Low Fat, Somerfield*	1 Pot/125g	107	1.0	86	4.1	15.6	0.8	0.1
Strawberry & Rhubarb, Onken*	1 Serving/100g	85	0.1	85	4.6	16.2	0.1	0.4
Strawberry & Vanilla, Low Fat, Somerfield*	1 Pot/125g	109	1.0	87	4.0	15.9	0.8	0.1
Strawberry Crumble, Crunch Corner, Muller*	1 Pot/150g	234	8.4	156	3.6	22.9	5.6	0.5
Strawberry Mousse, Shapers, Boots*	1 Pot/91g	88	3.7	97	4.1	11.0	4.1	0.1
Strawberry Orange Balls, Crunch Corner, Muller*	1 Pot/150g	222	8.1	148	4.0	20.8	5.4	0.2
Strawberry Raspberry & Mint, Smoothie, Sveltesse, Nestle*	1 Pot/125g	62	0.1	50	4.8	7.4	0.1	0.2
Strawberry Rice, Low Fat, Muller*	1 Pot/190g	203	4.4	107	3.2	18.4	2.3	0.4
Strawberry Shortcake, Crunch Corner, Muller*	1 Pot/150g	232	8.7	155	3.9	21.0	5.8	0.1
Strawberry Smooth, Nom Dairy UK*	1 Pot/125g	112	3.0	90	3.2	13.8	2.4	0.3
Strawberry with Grains, Good Intentions, Somerfield*	1 Pot/125g	86	0.4	69	6.0	10.6	0.3	0.2
Strawbswirlmoo, Yoomoo*	1 Pot/150ml	134	1.2	89	1.7	17.7	0.8	2.3
Summer Berries, Biopot, Lite, Wholegrain, Onken*	¼ Pot/120g	100	0.2	83	4.6	15.8	0.2	1.4
Summer Berries, Fat Free, Mullerlight, Muller*	1 Pot/175g	87	0.2	50	4.1	7.6	0.1	0.4
Summer Berry Compote, Greek Style, & Granola, M & S*	1 Pot/205g	336	16.4	164	5.6	17.3	8.0	0.1
Summer Fruits, Greek Style, Corner, Muller*	1 Pot/150g	165	4.5	110	5.1	15.0	3.0	0.5
Summer Fruits, Light, Limited Edition, Muller*	1 Pot/175g	87	0.2	50	4.1	7.6	0.1	0.4
Summer Fruits, Light, Spelga*	1 Pot/175g	79	0.3	45	4.4	7.1	0.2	0.0
Summer Selection, Fat Free, Organic, Yeo Valley*	1 Pot/125g	89	0.1	71	5.2	12.3	0.1	0.2
Summer Selection, Thick & Fruity, COU, M & S*	1 Pot/145g	75	0.2	52	4.2	7.8	0.1	0.5
Summerfruits, Bio Live, Fat Free, Rachel's Organic*	1 Pot/125g	120	2.2	96	4.7	15.3	1.8	0.0
Summerfruits Bio, Boots*	1 Pot/150g	139	4.0	93	4.1	13.0	2.7	0.4
Sweet Treat, Low Fat, Tesco*	1 Pot/125g	131	2.9	105	3.1	18.0	2.3	0.3
Thick & Fruity Black Cherry, COU, M & S*	1 Pot/145g	72	0.1	50	4.2	7.8	0.1	0.5
Timperley Rhubarb, Seriously Fruity, Waitrose*	1 Pot/150g	127	1.5	85	4.6	14.4	1.0	0.0
Timperley Rhubarb, TTD, Sainsbury's*	1 Pot/150g	168	7.3	112	3.4	13.6	4.9	0.4
Toffee, Benecol*	1 Pot/125g	124	0.9	99	3.8	19.3	0.7	0.0
Toffee, COU, M & S*	1 Pot/145g	65	0.3	45	4.2	7.7	0.2	0.0
Toffee, Economy, Sainsbury's*	1 Pot/126g	91	1.3	72	3.0	12.8	1.0	0.0
Toffee, Light, HL, Tesco*	1 Pot/200g	80	0.2	40	3.9	5.9	0.1	1.0
Toffee, Live Bio, Perfectly Balanced, Waitrose*	1 Pot/150g	156	0.4	104	4.2	21.1	0.3	0.0

Y

YOGHURT

	Measure INFO/WEIGHT	per Measure KCAL	FAT	Nutrition Values per 100g / 100ml KCAL	PROT	CARB	FAT	FIBRE
Toffee, Low Fat, Budgens*	1 Pot/125g	145	1.5	116	4.7	21.6	1.2	0.0
Toffee, Low Fat, Co-Op*	1 Pot/150g	124	1.3	83	3.8	15.0	0.9	0.2
Toffee, Low Fat, M & S*	1 Pot/150g	180	2.5	120	4.9	21.6	1.7	0.0
Toffee, Low Fat, Somerfield*	1 Pot/150g	148	1.5	99	3.0	19.0	1.0	0.0
Toffee, Probiotic, You Count, Love Life, Waitrose*	1 Pot/131g	85	0.1	65	4.4	11.5	0.1	0.5
Toffee, Seriously Smooth, Low Fat, Waitrose*	1 Pot/150g	156	3.1	104	4.7	16.5	2.1	0.1
Toffee, Smooth & Creamy, Fat Free, Weight Watchers*	1 Pot/120g	48	0.1	40	3.9	5.9	0.1	0.8
Toffee, Virtually Fat Free, Boots*	1 Pot/125g	69	0.1	55	5.1	8.3	0.1	0.0
Toffee Fudge, Low Fat, Sainsbury's*	1 Pot/125g	146	2.5	117	4.3	20.4	2.0	0.0
Toffee with Chocolate Hoops, Crunch Corner, Muller*	1 Pot/150g	229	8.2	153	4.0	21.1	5.5	0.2
Treacle Toffee, Dessert, Low Fat, Sainsbury's*	1 Pot/125g	149	2.4	119	4.3	21.2	1.9	0.0
Tropical, Low Fat, Luscious, Rachel's Organic*	1 Pot/125g	115	2.0	92	4.0	15.3	1.6	0.0
Tropical Crunch, Healthy Balance, Fruit Corner, Muller*	1 Pot/150g	169	3.1	113	4.7	18.2	2.1	0.5
Tropical Fruit, Bio, Granola, Corner, Muller*	1 Pot/135g	161	3.2	119	5.4	18.2	2.4	0.6
Tropical Fruit, Greek Style, Asda*	1 Pot/125g	170	8.7	136	3.3	15.0	7.0	0.0
Tropical Fruit, Greek Style, Shapers, Boots*	1 Pot/150g	100	2.2	67	3.6	9.8	1.5	0.8
Vanilla, Average	1 Serving/120g	100	5.4	83	4.5	12.4	4.5	0.8
Vanilla, Benecol*	1 Serving/125g	99	0.8	79	3.7	14.6	0.6	0.0
Vanilla, BGTY, Sainsbury's*	1 Pot/200g	98	0.2	49	4.5	7.5	0.1	0.0
Vanilla, Bio, BFY, Morrisons*	1 Pot/150g	82	0.4	55	5.7	8.4	0.3	0.0
Vanilla, Bio, Fat Free, Snackpot, Activia, Danone*	1 Pot/165g	87	0.2	53	5.0	8.1	0.1	0.9
Vanilla, Bio, Very Low Fat, Somerfield*	1 Pot/200g	98	0.0	49	5.0	7.0	0.0	0.0
Vanilla, Bio Live, Wicked, Wholemilk, Rachel's Organic*	1 Pot/125g	125	4.4	100	5.2	12.1	3.5	0.0
Vanilla, Brooklea*	1 Pot/180g	135	0.4	75	4.8	13.4	0.2	0.0
Vanilla, Chocolate, & Black Cherry, Mullerlight, Muller*	1 Pot/175g	103	0.7	59	3.1	10.3	0.4	0.3
Vanilla, Creamy, Smarties, Nestle*	1 Pot/120g	200	7.4	167	4.1	23.7	6.2	0.0
Vanilla, Organic, Probiotic, Fat Free, Yeo Valley*	1 Pot/500g	400	0.5	80	5.4	14.2	0.1	0.0
Vanilla, Pouring, Activia, Danone*	1 Serving/100g	62	1.6	62	3.9	8.1	1.6	0.0
Vanilla, Smooth, Light, Fat Free, Muller*	1 Pot/175g	87	0.2	50	4.3	7.2	0.1	0.0
Vanilla, Smooth & Creamy, Fat Free, Weight Watchers*	1 Pot/120g	50	0.1	42	3.9	6.5	0.1	0.1
Vanilla, Soya, Dairy Free, Organic, Yofu, Provamel*	1 Pot/125g	114	2.7	91	3.8	13.3	2.2	0.7
Vanilla, Virtually Fat Free, Yeo Valley*	1 Pot/150g	121	0.1	81	5.1	15.0	0.1	0.0
Vanilla & Chocolate, Muller*	1 Pot/165g	86	0.8	52	4.0	7.2	0.5	0.1
Vanilla & Chocolate Sprinkles, Delights, Shape, Danone*	1 Pot/120g	88	0.6	74	5.4	11.8	0.5	0.5
Vanilla Choco Balls, Crunch Corner, Muller*	1 Pot/150g	223	8.2	149	4.1	20.2	5.5	0.2
Vanilla Flavour, Weight Watchers*	1 Pot/120g	47	0.1	39	4.2	5.2	0.1	0.2
Vanilla with Choc Flakes, Adore, Ehrmann*	1 Pot/150g	214	10.5	143	3.1	17.0	7.0	0.0
Vanilla with Dark Chocolate Flakes, Light, Brooklea*	1 Pot/180g	104	1.8	58	4.9	7.0	1.0	0.5
Velvety Vanilla, Intensely Creamy, Activia, Danone*	1 Pot/120g	116	3.6	97	4.8	12.7	3.0	0.1
Walnut & Greek Honey, Amore Luxury, Muller*	1 Pot/150g	241	13.0	161	3.0	17.6	8.7	0.1
White & Milk Chocolate Puffed Rice, Nom Dairy UK*	1 Pot/150g	226	8.8	151	3.8	20.7	5.9	0.1
Wholemilk, with Maple Syrup, Bio Live, Rachel's Organic*	1 Pot/142g	139	5.0	98	3.5	13.0	3.5	0.0
Wild Berry, Oatie Breakfast, Moma Foods*	1 Pot/235g	317	4.2	135	4.3	25.6	1.8	2.7
Wild Blueberry, Light, Fat Free, Muller*	1 Pot/175g	82	0.2	47	4.1	6.9	0.1	0.7
Winter Medley, COU, M & S*	1 Pot/150g	67	0.1	45	4.2	6.2	0.1	0.1
Yellow Fruit, Yoplait*	1 Pot/125g	139	3.6	111	3.3	18.0	2.9	0.0

YOGHURT DRINK

	Measure INFO/WEIGHT	per Measure KCAL	FAT	Nutrition Values per 100g / 100ml KCAL	PROT	CARB	FAT	FIBRE
Average	1 fl oz/30ml	19	0.0	62	3.1	13.1	0.0	0.0
Ayran, Gazi*	1 Can/330ml	34	1.9	10	0.5	0.8	0.6	0.0
Banana & Honey, Ski Up & Go, Nestle*	1 Bottle/250g	215	2.2	86	0.0	16.0	0.9	0.0
Blueberry, Low Fat, Prebiotic & Probiotic, Muller*	1 Pot/100g	66	1.4	66	2.6	10.3	1.4	2.2
Blueberry & Blackcurrant, Orchard Maid*	1 Carton/250ml	147	0.1	59	1.6	13.6	0.0	0.0
Fristi*	1 Carton/330g	191	0.3	58	2.6	13.6	0.1	0.0

YOGHURT DRINK

	Measure INFO/WEIGHT	KCAL	FAT	KCAL	PROT	CARB	FAT	FIBRE
Fruit, Mixed, Actimel, Danone*	1 Bottle/100ml	88	1.5	88	2.7	16.0	1.5	0.0
Light, Benecol*	1 Bottle/68g	40	1.4	60	2.8	7.3	2.1	0.1
Light, Yakult*	1 Bottle/65ml	27	0.0	42	1.4	10.2	0.0	1.8
Mango, Probiotic, Mundella Foods*	1 Glass/250g	191	2.5	76	2.4	12.3	1.0	1.4
Mixed Berry, Up & Go, Ski, Nestle*	1 Bottle/250g	217	2.2	87	3.1	16.0	0.9	0.2
Multi Fruit, Actimel, Danone*	1 Bottle/100g	85	1.5	85	2.7	14.4	1.5	0.1
Orange, Actimel, Danone*	1 Bottle/100g	74	1.5	74	2.9	11.5	1.5	0.0
Orange, Banana & Passion Fruit, One a Day, Muller*	1 Bottle/310ml	208	0.3	67	2.1	14.1	0.1	0.0
Orange, Pro Activ, Cholesterol, Flora*	1 Bottle/100g	45	1.5	45	3.2	5.6	1.5	1.1
Orange, Probiotic, Lidl*	1 Serving/125ml	105	2.0	84	2.5	14.7	1.6	0.0
Original, 0.1% Fat, Actimel, Danone*	1 Bottle/100g	28	0.1	28	2.8	3.3	0.1	1.9
Original, Actimel, Danone*	1 Bottle/100g	80	1.6	80	2.8	12.8	1.6	0.0
Original, Benecol*	1 Serving/70g	62	1.6	88	2.6	14.2	2.3	0.0
Original, Danacol, Danone*	1 Bottle/100ml	64	1.0	64	3.2	10.0	1.0	0.0
Original, Pro Activ, Cholesterol, Flora*	1 Bottle/100g	45	1.5	45	2.6	4.8	1.5	1.1
Peach & Apricot, Benecol*	1 Bottle/68g	38	1.5	56	2.8	6.2	2.2	0.0
Peach & Mango, Fristi*	1 Carton/330g	191	0.3	58	2.6	13.6	0.1	0.0
Pineapple, 0.1% Fat, Actimel, Danone*	1 Bottle/100g	33	0.0	33	2.7	5.5	0.0	1.8
Pomeganate & Raspberry Pro Active, Mini Drink, Flora*	1 Serving/100g	45	1.5	45	2.6	4.7	1.5	1.1
Raspberry, Apple, & Cranberry, Smooth, One a Day, Muller*	1 Bottle/330ml	155	0.3	47	2.0	9.0	0.1	0.5
Raspberry, Pro Biotic, Omega 3 Plus, Flora*	1 Bottle/100g	58	1.6	58	2.6	8.5	1.6	0.0
Raspberry & Passion Fruit, Everybody, Yoplait*	1 Bottle/90g	60	0.8	67	2.6	12.2	0.9	0.0
Strawberry, Actimel, Danone*	1 Bottle/100g	74	1.5	74	2.9	11.5	1.5	0.0
Strawberry, Benecol*	1 Bottle/68g	38	1.3	56	3.2	6.2	2.0	0.0
Strawberry, Danacol, Danone*	1 Bottle/100g	68	1.2	68	3.2	11.2	1.2	0.0
Strawberry, Fristi*	1 Carton/250g	165	0.2	66	2.6	13.6	0.1	0.0
Strawberry, Low Fat, Pre & Probiotic, Muller*	1 Pot/100g	67	1.4	67	2.5	10.7	1.4	2.4
Strawberry, Pro Activ, Cholesterol, Flora*	1 Bottle/100g	45	1.5	45	2.6	4.7	1.5	0.0
Strawberry, Probiotic, Mundella Foods*	1 Glass/250g	191	2.5	76	2.4	12.3	1.0	1.4
Strawberry, Yop, Yoplait*	1 Bottle/330g	261	4.3	79	2.8	14.0	1.3	0.0
Sveltesse, 0%, Nestle*	1 Pot/125g	61	0.1	49	4.8	7.3	0.1	0.1
Vanilla, Activate, Probiotic, Little Town Dairy*	1 Bottle/265g	167	3.7	63	2.7	10.0	1.4	0.2
Vanilla, Probiotic, Mundella Foods*	1 Glass/250g	191	2.5	76	2.4	12.3	1.0	1.4
Yakult*	1 Pot/65ml	43	0.1	66	1.3	14.7	0.1	0.0

YORK FRUITS

Terry's*	1 Sweet/9g	29	0.0	320	0.0	78.5	0.0	0.5

YORKIE

Honeycomb, Nestle*	1 Bar/65g	331	16.8	509	5.7	63.6	25.8	0.0
King Size, Nestle*	1 Bar/83g	445	26.1	537	6.1	57.3	31.5	0.0
Original, Nestle*	1 Bar/65g	365	21.4	537	6.1	57.3	31.5	0.7
Raisin & Biscuit, Nestle*	1 Bar/67g	331	17.4	497	5.5	59.7	26.2	0.9

YORKSHIRE PUDDING

& Beef Dripping, M & S*	4 Puddings/100g	410	30.4	410	9.4	25.2	30.4	3.2
3", Baked, Aunt Bessie's*	1 Pudding/36g	91	2.8	252	9.0	36.4	7.9	1.7
4 Minute, Aunt Bessie's*	1 Pudding/18g	52	2.0	291	10.5	36.6	11.3	2.2
7", Baked, Aunt Bessie's*	1 Pudding/110g	290	9.9	264	8.5	37.4	9.0	2.0
Average	1 Pudding/30g	62	3.0	208	6.6	24.7	9.9	0.9
Batters, in Foils, Ready to Bake, Frozen, Aunt Bessie's*	1 Pudding/17g	47	1.8	276	9.1	32.6	10.8	1.4
Chicken & Vegetable, COU, M & S*	1 Pudding/150g	195	3.3	130	12.2	14.3	2.2	1.3
Filled, Chicken Casserole, Farmfoods*	1 Pack/280g	347	6.4	124	6.5	19.3	2.3	1.3
Filled, with Beef, Morrisons*	1 Serving/350g	514	21.0	147	7.4	15.7	6.0	0.5
Filled, with Sausage, Sainsbury's*	1 Pack/300g	576	31.2	192	6.9	17.5	10.4	0.9
Filled with Beef, Tesco*	1 Pudding/300g	408	15.6	136	6.1	16.2	5.2	1.1

Y

	Measure INFO/WEIGHT	per Measure KCAL	FAT	Nutrition Values per 100g / 100ml KCAL	PROT	CARB	FAT	FIBRE
YORKSHIRE PUDDING								
Filled with Chicken, GFY, Asda*	1 Pack/381g	438	9.9	115	9.0	14.0	2.6	1.5
Filled with Chicken & Vegetable, GFY, Asda*	1 Pack/380g	376	9.9	99	6.0	13.0	2.6	1.1
Giant, Aunt Bessie's*	1 Pudding/110g	290	9.9	264	8.5	37.4	9.0	2.0
Giant VLH Kitchens	1 Serving/110g	284	9.1	259	8.5	33.6	10.0	2.3
Large, Aunt Bessie's*	1 Pudding/40g	111	4.6	277	8.5	35.3	11.4	1.5
Large, The Real Yorkshire Pudding Co*	1 Pudding/34g	103	4.1	304	11.5	37.3	12.1	2.5
Made From Batter Mix, Sainsbury's*	1 Pudding/100g	248	5.3	248	9.9	40.1	5.3	4.0
Minced Beef Filled, Waitrose*	1 Serving/350g	525	24.8	150	7.5	14.1	7.1	1.0
Ready Baked, Smart Price, Asda*	1 Pudding/12g	36	1.1	297	10.0	44.0	9.0	2.8
Ready to Bake, Aunt Bessie's*	1 Pudding/17g	42	1.4	246	8.5	35.1	8.0	1.7
Ready to Bake, Sainsbury's*	1 Pudding/18g	48	1.6	263	9.9	35.9	8.9	1.3
Roast Chicken Filled, COU, M & S*	1 Pudding/150g	210	4.0	140	12.6	15.7	2.7	0.9
Roberts Bakery*	1 Pudding/18g	48	1.6	263	9.9	35.9	8.9	1.3
Sage & Onion, Tesco*	1 Pudding/19g	53	2.3	280	8.0	35.0	12.0	2.6
Sausage Filled, Frozen, Tesco*	1 Pack/340g	510	19.7	150	6.6	17.8	5.8	1.8
Steak Filled, COU, M & S*	1 Serving/150g	187	3.7	125	11.0	14.7	2.5	0.8
with Beef, 214, Oakhouse Foods Ltd*	1 Meal/320g	381	13.4	119	5.4	15.5	4.2	1.0
with Beef in Gravy, Asda*	1 Serving/290g	406	10.1	140	7.0	20.0	3.5	0.7
with Sausage, 223, Oakhouse Foods Ltd*	1 Meal/320g	490	22.1	153	5.7	17.5	6.9	0.9
YULE LOG								
Chocolate, Sainsbury's*	1/8 Log/49g	186	9.5	382	5.1	46.5	19.6	0.7
Christmas Range, Tesco*	1 Serving/30g	131	6.4	442	4.9	56.8	21.7	2.8
Mini, M & S*	1 Cake/36g	165	8.4	460	5.7	56.9	23.3	1.1

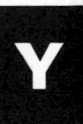

	Measure INFO/WEIGHT	per Measure KCAL	per Measure FAT	Nutrition Values per 100g / 100ml KCAL	PROT	CARB	FAT	FIBRE

ABOKADO
ABOWLAGO

	Measure INFO/WEIGHT	KCAL	FAT	KCAL	PROT	CARB	FAT	FIBRE
Chicken, Thai Red, Fragrant, Abokado*	1 Serving/448g	457	13.4	102	5.5	14.2	3.0	0.0
Chicken Teriyaki, & Brown Rice, Abokado*	1 Serving/430g	479	3.7	111	5.9	20.5	0.9	0.9
Chicken Teriyaki, & Noodles, Abokado*	1 Serving/369g	353	2.7	96	6.7	15.7	0.7	1.0
Shrimp, Red Thai, Fragrant, Abokado*	1 Serving/402g	368	8.6	92	4.5	14.5	2.1	0.0

BREAKFAST

Banana & Maple Syrup, Bowl, Abokado*	1 Bowl/220g	245	4.2	112	4.0	20.4	1.9	0.0
Muesli, Mango & Fig, Bircher, Abokado*	1 Serving/204g	240	4.1	117	4.0	20.0	2.0	2.3
Porridge, Organic, Abokado*	1 Serving/287g	250	6.3	87	3.7	12.2	2.2	1.9
Yoghurt, Greek Style, with Raspberry Compote, Abokado*	1 Serving/135g	78	1.3	58	4.5	8.3	1.0	0.0

SALAD

Chicken, Green Thai, & Brown Rice, Abokado*	1 Serving/310g	482	19.7	155	7.3	17.4	6.3	1.4
Chicken, Thai, Crystal Roll, Abokado*	1 Serving/313g	402	23.2	129	8.5	4.8	7.4	2.6
Crab, California, Crystal Roll, Abokado*	1 Serving/313g	438	31.1	140	6.2	4.3	9.9	2.5
Edamame & Avocado, Abokado*	1 Portion/140g	185	13.3	132	7.3	4.4	9.5	5.7
Edamame Beans, Abokado*	1 Serving/135g	181	8.2	134	11.5	0.0	6.1	4.2
Houmous & Falafel, & Brown Rice, Abokado*	1 Serving/234g	371	12.6	159	6.4	19.8	5.4	3.8
Peking Duck, Crystal Roll, Abokado*	1 Serving/293g	351	14.8	120	8.0	8.3	5.1	2.7
Seaweed, Sesame, Abokado*	1 Serving/60g	60	1.5	100	0.0	20.0	2.5	0.0
Superfood, Abokado*	1 Serving/181g	222	17.3	122	6.3	3.1	9.5	2.8

SOUP

Chicken, in Sizzling Coconut, Medium, Abokado*	1 Serving/302g	172	8.2	57	3.9	4.4	2.7	0.6
Salmon, Super, Detox, Medium, Abokado*	1 Pot/312g	149	4.8	48	3.8	5.1	1.5	0.0
Udon, Shrimp Dumpling, Large, Abokado*	1 Serving/635g	237	2.6	37	2.5	6.4	0.4	0.6
Udon, Vegetable Dumpling, Medium, Abokado*	1 Tub/312g	127	1.5	41	2.0	7.7	0.5	0.6

SUSHI

Avocado & Ginger, Shwrap, Abokado*	1 Wrap/106g	129	2.9	123	2.5	23.4	2.7	0.0
Chicken, Teriyaki, Shwrap, Abokado*	1 Serving/111g	145	0.7	130	6.6	26.0	0.6	0.4
Crab, California, Medium Set, Abokado*	1 Serving/234g	387	22.0	166	4.3	15.6	9.4	1.5
Deep Blue, Abokado*	1 Serving/331g	431	14.3	130	5.1	18.6	4.3	0.6
Goddess Goodness, Abokado*	1 Serving/209g	262	9.6	125	4.2	16.5	4.6	1.9
River Run, Abokado*	1 Serving/310g	412	14.2	133	7.4	15.8	4.6	0.6
Salad, California, Shwrap, Abokado*	1 Serving/137g	189	8.7	138	3.0	18.4	6.3	0.4
Salmon, Avocado & Chives, Medium Set, Abokado*	1 Serving/226g	313	12.6	138	6.0	15.4	5.6	1.5
Salmon, Sashimi, Medium Set, Abokado*	1 Serving/143g	175	9.0	122	11.7	2.3	6.3	1.4
Salmon, Scottish, Nigiri, Medium Set, Abokado*	1 Serving/222g	297	8.3	134	7.8	16.4	3.7	0.9
Salmon, Simply, Abokado*	1 Serving/297g	379	12.5	127	6.0	16.4	4.2	1.0
Salmon, Sweet Chilli, & Fresh Dill, Shwrap, Abokado*	1 Serving/123g	181	6.4	147	5.3	20.6	5.2	0.9
Scottish Salmon Tartare, Medium Set, Abokado*	1 Serving/133g	139	6.0	104	8.8	7.3	4.5	1.1
Super Omega 3, Abokado*	1 Serving/398g	531	16.5	133	6.9	17.7	4.1	0.4

WRAP

Chicken, Real Roast, Super Club, Abokado*	1 Wrap/122g	258	11.2	212	9.2	23.8	9.2	1.6
Falafel & Coriander, Abokado*	1 Wrap/169g	270	8.1	160	5.7	24.0	4.8	3.4
Peking Duck, Abokado*	1 Wrap/113g	194	2.6	171	6.9	32.1	2.3	1.9
Salmon, Super Food, Abokado*	1 Wrap/133g	181	2.9	136	6.9	23.4	2.2	1.9

BURGER KING
BURGERS

Angus, Double, Burger King*	1 Burger/323g	795	45.2	246	16.0	14.0	14.0	1.0
Angus, Mini, Burger King*	1 Burger/97g	272	10.7	280	14.0	31.0	11.0	1.0
Angus, Mini with Cheese, Burger King*	1 Burger/110g	321	15.4	292	15.0	27.0	14.0	1.0
Angus, Smoked Bacon & Cheddar, Burger King*	1 Burger/270g	678	37.8	251	14.0	17.0	14.0	1.0
Angus, Smoked Bacon & Cheddar, Dbl, Burger King*	1 Burger/354g	920	53.1	260	17.0	13.0	15.0	1.0
Angus, Steakhouse, Burger King*	1 Burger/239g	554	28.7	232	12.0	18.0	12.0	1.0

BURGER KING

	Measure INFO/WEIGHT	per Measure KCAL	FAT	Nutrition Values per 100g / 100ml KCAL	PROT	CARB	FAT	FIBRE
BURGERS								
BBQ Rodeo, Beef, Sandwich, Burger King*	1 Sandwich/270g	735	36.3	271	15.5	21.9	13.4	1.6
Bean, Veggie, Kids, Burger King*	1 Burger/116g	278	7.0	240	6.0	42.0	6.0	3.0
Big King, Burger King*	1 Burger/190g	503	26.6	265	15.0	17.0	14.0	1.0
Big King, XL, Burger King*	1 Burger/338g	902	54.1	267	16.0	14.0	16.0	1.0
Cheeseburger, Bacon Dbl, Extra Large, Burger King*	1 Burger/302g	927	54.4	307	21.0	15.0	18.0	1.0
Cheeseburger, Bacon Double, Burger King*	1 Burger/160g	478	25.6	299	19.0	19.0	16.0	1.0
Cheeseburger, Burger King*	1 Burger/123g	320	13.5	260	13.0	25.0	11.0	1.0
Cheeseburger, Double, Burger King*	1 Burger/173g	465	22.5	269	17.0	18.0	13.0	1.0
Cheeseburger, Kids, Burger King*	1 Burger/113g	318	13.6	281	14.0	27.0	12.0	1.0
Chicken, Chargrilled, Mini, Burger King*	1 Burger/109g	214	3.3	196	15.0	28.0	3.0	1.0
Chicken Royale, Burger King*	1 Burger/210g	607	31.5	289	11.0	25.0	15.0	1.0
Chicken Royale, Sweet Chilli, Burger King*	1 Burger/210g	542	23.1	258	11.0	28.0	11.0	1.0
Chicken Royale, with Cheese, Burger King*	1 Burger/263g	695	39.0	264	10.6	20.9	14.8	0.4
Hamburger, Burger King*	1 Burger/110g	275	8.8	250	13.0	28.0	8.0	1.0
Ocean Catch, Burger King*	1 Burger/188g	494	26.3	263	9.0	23.0	14.0	1.0
Whopper, Burger King*	1 Burger/274g	633	35.6	231	11.0	18.0	13.0	1.0
Whopper, Double, Burger King*	1 Burger/355g	877	53.2	247	14.0	14.0	15.0	1.0
Whopper, Double, with Cheese, Burger King*	1 Burger/380g	961	60.8	253	14.0	13.0	16.0	1.0
Whopper, Junior, Burger King*	1 Burger/148g	343	16.3	232	9.0	21.0	11.0	1.0
Whopper, with Cheese, Burger King*	1 Burger/299g	721	41.9	241	11.0	16.0	14.0	1.0
Whopper, with Cheese, Junior, Burger King*	1 Burger/161g	388	19.3	241	10.0	19.0	12.0	1.0
BUTTY								
Bacon, with Heinz Ketchup, Burger King*	1 Butty/77g	221	6.0	287	13.0	41.6	7.8	2.6
Bacon, with HP Sauce, Burger King*	1 Butty/77g	222	6.0	288	13.0	41.6	7.8	2.0
Bacon & Egg, with Heinz Ketchup, Burger King*	1 Butty/140g	362	17.0	259	12.9	25.0	12.1	11.4
Bacon & Egg, with HP Sauce, Burger King*	1 Butty/140g	363	17.0	259	12.9	25.0	12.1	1.4
Breakfast, Big, with Heinz Ketchup, Burger King*	1 Butty/297g	849	50.5	286	14.0	18.0	17.0	1.0
Egg & Cheese, with Heinz Ketchup, Burger King*	1 Butty/126g	300	17.6	238	10.3	27.0	14.0	1.6
Sausage, Cumberland, Egg, Ketchup, Burger King*	1 Butty/243g	668	38.9	275	11.0	21.0	16.0	1.0
Sausage, with Heinz Ketchup, Burger King*	1 Butty/119g	312	13.0	262	13.4	26.9	10.9	1.7
Sausage, with HP Sauce, Burger King*	1 Butty/119g	313	13.0	263	13.4	26.9	10.9	1.7
Sausage & Egg, with HP Sauce, Burger King*	1 Butty/182g	454	24.0	249	13.2	19.2	13.2	1.1
CHICKEN								
Bites, Burger King*	14 Bites/112g	317	15.0	283	16.1	25.0	13.4	0.9
Bites, Kids, Burger King*	1 Serving/56g	158	7.3	282	16.0	25.0	13.0	2.0
COFFEE								
Black, Large, Burger King*	1 Serving/284ml	6	0.0	2	0.0	0.0	0.0	0.0
Black, Regular, Burger King*	1 Serving/200ml	4	0.0	2	0.0	0.0	0.0	0.0
Cappuccino, Large, Burger King*	1 Serving/59g	81	2.9	137	10.0	15.0	5.0	0.0
Cappuccino, Regular, Burger King*	1 Serving/46g	64	1.8	139	9.0	15.0	4.0	0.0
Latte, Large, Burger King*	1 Serving/45g	60	1.8	133	11.0	13.0	4.0	0.0
Latte, Regular, Burger King*	1 Serving/62g	82	3.1	132	10.0	15.0	5.0	0.0
COLA								
Coca-Cola, Burger King*	1 Reg/400g	168	0.0	42	0.0	11.0	0.0	0.0
Coke, Diet, Burger King*	1 Reg/400g	4	0.0	1	0.0	0.0	0.0	0.0
DIP POT								
Barbeque Sauce, Heinz, Burger King*	1 Pot/40g	48	0.0	120	0.1	28.0	0.1	0.1
Sweet Chilli, Heinz, Burger King*	1 Pot/40g	96	0.0	240	0.0	60.0	0.0	0.0
DRESSING								
French, Burger King*	1 Sachet/40g	7	0.0	17	0.0	2.5	0.0	0.0
Honey & Mustard, Burger King*	1 Sachet/40g	32	1.0	80	2.5	15.0	2.5	0.0

BURGER KING

FANTA

	Measure INFO/WEIGHT	KCAL	FAT	KCAL	PROT	CARB	FAT	FIBRE
Orange, Burger King*	1 Reg/400g	156	0.4	39	0.1	10.0	0.1	0.0
Orange, Small, Burger King*	1 Sm/300g	117	0.3	39	0.1	10.0	0.1	0.0
FLATBREAD								
Lamb, Burger King*	1 Serving/330g	708	39.7	214	11.0	16.0	12.0	1.0
FRIES								
Large, Burger King*	1 Serving/141g	381	18.3	270	3.0	38.0	13.0	4.0
Regular, Burger King*	1 Serving/111g	300	15.5	270	3.0	39.0	14.0	4.0
Small, Burger King*	1 Serving/74g	200	10.4	270	3.0	38.0	14.0	4.0
Super, Burger King*	1 Serving/174g	470	22.6	270	3.0	39.0	13.0	4.0
HASH BROWNS								
Large, Burger King*	1 Serving/130g	403	27.3	310	3.0	27.0	21.0	4.0
Regular, Burger King*	1 Serving/102g	316	22.4	310	3.0	27.0	22.0	4.0
KETCHUP								
Heinz, Sachet, Burger King*	1 Sachet/10g	10	0.0	100	0.1	20.0	0.1	0.1
MAYONNAISE								
Heinz, Sachet, Burger King*	1 Sachet/12g	80	9.0	667	0.0	0.0	75.0	0.0
MILK								
Semi Skimmed, Kids, Burger King*	1 Carton/258g	117	3.9	47	3.5	4.6	1.5	0.0
MILK SHAKE								
Chocolate, Large, Burger King*	1 Serving/519g	612	10.4	118	3.0	22.0	2.0	0.0
Chocolate, Regular, Burger King*	1 Serving/401g	449	8.0	112	3.0	20.0	2.0	0.1
Chocolate, Small, Burger King*	1 Serving/276g	301	8.3	109	3.0	19.0	3.0	0.1
Strawberry, Large, Burger King*	1 Serving/519g	581	10.4	112	3.0	20.0	2.0	0.0
Strawberry, Regular, Burger King*	1 Serving/401g	433	8.0	108	3.0	19.0	2.0	0.0
Strawberry, Small, Burger King*	1 Serving/276g	293	8.3	106	3.0	18.0	3.0	0.0
Vanilla, Burger King*	1 Serving/124g	124	3.7	100	3.0	16.0	3.0	0.0
ONION RINGS								
Large, Burger King*	1 Serving/190g	697	36.0	367	6.3	43.2	18.9	4.7
Regular, Burger King*	1 Serving/126g	462	24.0	367	6.3	42.9	19.0	4.8
Super, Burger King*	1 Serving/253g	929	48.0	367	6.3	43.1	19.0	4.7
SALAD								
Chicken, Flame Grilled, Burger King*	1 Salad/240g	127	2.4	53	8.0	3.0	1.0	1.0
Garden, Burger King*	1 Serving/165g	33	1.6	20	1.0	4.0	1.0	1.0
SPRITE								
Burger King*	1 Reg/400g	148	0.0	37	0.0	9.0	0.0	0.0
TEA								
Regular, White, No Sugar, Burger King*	1 Reg/200ml	22	4.0	11	1.0	1.0	2.0	0.0
WRAP								
Sweet Chilli, Chicken, Burger King*	1 Wrap/160g	296	6.4	185	14.0	22.0	4.0	1.0

CAFFE NERO

BARS

	Measure INFO/WEIGHT	KCAL	FAT	KCAL	PROT	CARB	FAT	FIBRE
Fruit & Seed, Caffe Nero*	1 Serving/65g	197	5.8	303	7.5	48.2	8.9	8.7
Organic Granola, Caffe Nero*	1 Serving/64g	275	13.4	429	6.5	53.7	20.9	4.6
CHOCOLATE								
Coated Coffee Beans, Caffe Nero*	1 Serving/25g	117	6.5	469	8.5	50.0	26.2	11.9
Coin, Caffe Nero*	1 Serving/25g	129	6.9	516	6.3	59.7	27.8	2.1
Milk Bar, Caffe Nero*	1 Serving/40g	223	13.6	558	8.0	55.0	34.0	1.0
Milk Bar with Hazelnuts, Caffe Nero*	1 Serving/40g	229	15.2	572	8.0	49.5	38.0	1.8
COFFEE								
Cappuccino, Regular, Semi Skimmed Milk, Caffe Nero*	1 Serving/80g	37	1.4	46	3.5	4.7	1.7	0.0
Cappuccino, Regular, Skimmed Milk, Caffe Nero*	1 Serving/79g	27	0.1	34	3.5	4.8	0.1	0.0
Cappuccino, Regular, Soya Milk, Caffe Nero*	1 Serving/80g	36	1.8	45	3.7	2.5	2.2	0.6

	Measure INFO/WEIGHT	per Measure KCAL	FAT	Nutrition Values per 100g / 100ml KCAL	PROT	CARB	FAT	FIBRE

CAFFE NERO

COFFEE
Caramelatte, Semi Skimmed Milk, Caffe Nero*	1 Serving/422g	485	25.3	115	2.3	12.3	6.0	0.0
Latte, Regular, Semi Skimmed Milk, Caffe Nero*	1 Serving/150g	69	2.5	46	3.5	4.7	1.7	0.0
Latte, Regular, Skimmed Milk, Caffe Nero*	1 Serving/150g	36	0.3	24	2.5	3.4	0.2	0.0
Latte, Regular, Soya Milk, Caffe Nero*	1 Serving/151g	68	3.3	45	3.7	2.5	2.2	0.6
Mocha, No Cream, Regular, S/Skim Milk, Caffe Nero*	1 Serving/179g	174	3.4	97	3.8	16.6	1.9	0.8
Mocha, No Cream, Regular, Skimmed Milk, Caffe Nero*	1 Serving/179g	156	1.3	87	3.8	16.6	0.7	0.8
Mocha, White Chocolate, SS Milk, Caffe Nero*	1 Serving/402g	414	25.3	103	2.4	6.1	6.3	0.0

CROISSANT
Almond, Caffe Nero*	1 Serving/83g	350	19.8	422	10.0	41.7	23.9	2.6
Apricot, Caffe Nero*	1 Serving/100g	273	11.3	273	5.4	37.3	11.3	1.2
Butter, Caffe Nero*	1 Serving/52g	216	12.1	417	8.5	43.0	23.4	1.7
Cheese, Twist, Caffe Nero*	1 Serving/76g	316	18.4	416	13.4	36.1	24.2	2.6
Chocolate, Twist, Caffe Nero*	1 Serving/85g	314	13.3	369	6.8	42.2	15.6	2.9
Pain au Chocolat, Caffe Nero*	1 Serving/62g	269	15.0	435	8.3	46.0	24.2	1.8
Pain au Raisin, Caffe Nero*	1 Serving/90g	279	10.5	310	5.8	44.6	11.7	1.9

CUPCAKE
Chocolate, Caffe Nero*	1 Serving/68g	311	19.1	457	3.1	48.7	28.1	0.5
Lemon, Caffe Nero*	1 Serving/72g	340	19.6	472	2.9	54.0	27.2	0.3
Raspberry, Caffe Nero*	1 Serving/67g	295	15.1	440	3.4	55.7	22.5	0.5

DESSERTS
Tiramisu, Caffe Nero*	1 Serving/95g	311	20.6	327	3.9	28.4	21.7	1.0

FRAPPE
Double Chocolate, Caffe Nero*	1 Serving/455g	355	4.6	78	3.0	14.9	1.0	0.3
Frappe Latte, Mocha, Caffe Nero*	1 Serving/455g	355	4.6	78	3.0	14.9	1.0	0.3
Frappe Latte, Mocha, Skimmed Milk, Caffe Nero*	1 Serving/456g	328	1.4	72	3.0	15.0	0.3	0.3
Latte, Caffe Nero*	1 Serving/431g	267	3.9	62	2.8	11.1	0.9	0.0
Latte, Skimmed Milk, Caffe Nero*	1 Serving/429g	240	0.9	56	2.8	11.1	0.2	0.0
Latte, Soya Milk, Caffe Nero*	1 Serving/388g	101	5.0	26	2.2	1.5	1.3	0.4

HOT CHOCOLATE
Milano with Whipped Cream, Caffe Nero*	1 Serving/241g	424	22.6	176	3.5	19.3	9.4	2.0

JUICE
Apple & Mango, Caffe Nero*	1 Serving/250g	125	0.0	50	0.2	12.3	0.0	0.1
Orange, 100% Squeezed, Caffe Nero*	1 Serving/250g	95	0.0	38	0.5	8.8	0.0	0.1

LEMONADE
Sicilian, Still, Caffe Nero*	1 Serving/250g	115	0.0	46	0.0	11.2	0.0	0.0

MILKSHAKE
Banana, Frappe, Caffe Nero*	1 Serving/420g	315	4.6	75	3.0	13.5	1.1	0.0
Mint, Frappe, Semi Skimmed Milk, Caffe Nero*	1 Serving/419g	310	4.6	74	3.0	13.3	1.1	0.0
Strawberry, Frappe, Caffe Nero*	1 Serving/416g	316	4.6	76	3.0	13.6	1.1	0.0
Vanilla, Frappe, Caffe Nero*	1 Serving/420g	315	4.6	75	3.0	13.6	1.1	0.0

MINTS
Mints, Caffe Nero*	1 Serving/14g	35	0.1	249	0.6	97.0	0.8	0.0

MUFFINS
Apple, Spiced, & Pecan, Caffe Nero*	1 Serving/120g	474	26.5	395	4.7	43.5	22.1	1.5
Chocolate, Belgian, Triple, Caffe Nero*	1 Serving/120g	495	26.2	413	5.6	47.2	21.9	2.0
Raspberry, & White Chocolate, Caffe Nero*	1 Serving/120g	454	23.5	378	4.9	45.2	19.6	0.9

PANINI
Breakfast, All Day, Caffe Nero*	1 Panini/196g	389	15.9	198	9.0	21.3	8.1	1.6
Breakfast, Bacon & Tomato Sauce, Caffe Nero*	1 Panini/105g	263	9.7	251	11.1	30.6	9.3	1.4
Chicken, Bacon & Arrabbiata Sauce, Caffe Nero*	1 Panini/214g	346	8.5	162	11.2	20.2	4.0	1.3
Chicken Milanese, Caffe Nero*	1 Panini/249g	420	13.9	172	8.5	21.9	5.6	1.2
Ham, Mozzarella & Emmental, Tostati, Caffe Nero*	1 Panini/77g	172	7.1	223	15.6	19.4	9.2	0.8

	Measure INFO/WEIGHT		per Measure		Nutrition Values per 100g / 100ml				
			KCAL	FAT	KCAL	PROT	CARB	FAT	FIBRE
CAFFE NERO									
PANINI									
Ham & Mozzarella, Caffe Nero*	1 Panini/204g		421	16.1	206	13.0	20.7	7.9	1.1
Meatball & Mozzarella Napoletana, Caffe Nero*	1 Panini/218g		483	21.8	222	10.8	22.2	10.0	1.2
Mushroom, with Gorgonzola Cheese, Caffe Nero*	1 Panini/181g		377	17.4	208	7.0	23.4	9.6	1.5
Pesto Chicken, Caffe Nero*	1 Panini/210g		385	13.3	183	11.8	19.7	6.3	1.1
Salami, Napoli, & Mozzarella, Caffe Nero*	1 Panini/193g		404	17.8	209	10.1	21.5	9.2	1.2
Three Cheese & Roasted Tomato, Tostati, Caffe Nero*	1 Panini/71g		170	8.4	240	11.8	21.5	11.8	1.1
Tomato, Vine, Mozzarella & Basil, Caffe Nero*	1 Panini/212g		398	17.4	188	8.3	20.3	8.2	1.3
Tuna Melt, Caffe Nero*	1 Panini/201g		389	13.4	194	11.6	21.2	6.7	1.1
PASTA									
Penne, Red Pepper, Caffe Nero*	1 Serving/303g		197	3.0	65	2.8	11.4	1.0	1.3
SALADS									
Chicken, with Caesar Dressing, Caffe Nero*	1 Serving/170g		156	9.8	92	6.2	3.2	5.8	0.9
SANDWICH									
Cheddar, Mature, & Pickle, Caffe Nero*	1 Serving/186g		458	23.3	246	9.8	22.9	12.5	1.6
Egg Mayonnaise, Free Range, Caffe Nero*	1 Serving/159g		325	12.5	205	9.8	23.5	7.9	1.9
Ham & Cheddar, Caffe Nero*	1 Serving/179g		418	17.8	233	15.2	20.8	9.9	1.4
Salad, Chicken, Caffe Nero*	1 Serving/174g		368	16.9	211	10.1	20.9	9.7	1.7
Salad, Tuna, Caffe Nero*	1 Serving/147g		268	5.3	182	11.7	25.8	3.6	1.8
SCONES									
Fruit, Luxury, Caffe Nero*	1 Serving/100g		337	10.9	337	6.6	53.3	10.9	2.1
SOUP									
Tomato & Basil, Caffe Nero*	1 Serving/300g		144	6.9	48	2.2	4.7	2.3	0.5
TART									
Apple & Blackcurrant, Caffe Nero*	1 Serving/101g		279	12.9	276	2.9	37.4	12.8	2.2
Portuguese Custard, Caffe Nero*	1 Serving/69g		184	6.5	266	3.9	41.5	9.4	2.4
TEA									
Chai Latte, Semi Skimmed Milk, Caffe Nero*	1 Serving/406g		284	10.5	70	3.8	8.3	2.6	0.0
Chai Latte, Skimmed Milk, Caffe Nero*	1 Serving/405g		239	5.3	59	3.8	8.4	1.3	0.0
WRAP									
Caesar, Chicken, Caffe Nero*	1 Serving/165g		434	22.8	263	12.8	21.9	13.8	0.8
Falafel, Caffe Nero*	1 Serving/157g		424	21.8	270	8.7	29.4	13.9	1.8
CHOP'D									
DRESSING									
Balsamic, Chop'd*	1 Pot/55ml		253	27.0	460	0.0	4.1	49.2	0.0
Balsamic Vinegar, Chop'd*	1 Pot/35ml		49	0.0	140	0.3	32.6	0.0	0.0
Blue Cheese, Chop'd*	1 Pot/55ml		160	15.9	291	6.8	3.8	28.9	0.0
Caesar, Chop'd*	1 Pot/55ml		121	10.9	220	8.8	4.0	19.9	0.0
Creamy, Chop'd*	1 Pot/55ml		128	13.2	233	1.8	5.8	24.0	0.0
Mango, Chop'd*	1 Pot/55ml		151	15.8	275	0.1	3.3	28.8	0.0
SALAD									
Caesar, Chicken, Roast, Chop'd*	1 Serving/302g		232	10.0	77	8.3	3.6	3.3	0.0
Chicken, Avocado, Chop'd*	1 Serving/390g		311	17.0	80	5.9	5.1	4.4	0.0
Chicken, Bang Bang, No Dressing, Chop'd*	1 Serving/330g		269	9.8	82	6.9	7.4	3.0	0.0
Chicken, Jerk, Chop'd*	1 Serving/353g		215	3.0	61	4.8	9.2	0.8	0.0
Chorizo, Roasted, Feta & Couscous, Chop'd*	1 Serving/390g		595	19.5	153	4.1	5.2	5.0	0.0
Falafel & Hummus, Chop'd*	1 Serving/351g		521	28.0	148	5.0	11.2	8.0	0.0
Mackerel, Smoked, Kedgeree, Chop'd*	1 Serving/428g		579	25.5	135	6.0	14.9	5.9	0.0
New York Deli, Chop'd*	1 Serving/322g		522	29.0	162	9.9	9.0	9.0	0.0
Parma Ham & Mozzarella, Chop'd*	1 Serving/434g		563	23.0	130	5.3	17.0	5.3	0.0
Powerfoods, Chop'd*	1 Serving/316g		104	4.0	33	1.9	3.5	1.3	0.0
Tuna Nicoise, Chop'd*	1 Pack/393g		309	12.0	79	7.4	5.1	3.0	4.0

	Measure INFO/WEIGHT	per Measure KCAL	FAT	Nutrition Values per 100g / 100ml KCAL	PROT	CARB	FAT	FIBRE
CHOP'D								
STEW								
Butternut, Spinach & Lentil with Red Rice, Chop'd*	1 Serving/340g	373	17.0	110	2.6	14.1	5.0	0.0
Chicken & Chorizo, Chop'd*	1 Pack/340g	344	12.0	101	1.8	12.3	3.5	0.0
Chilli Con Carne with Red Rice, Chop'd*	1 Serving/340g	628	32.0	185	6.2	12.3	9.4	0.0
COSTA								
BISCUITS								
Gingerbread George, Costa*	1 Biscuit/55g	234	5.7	425	5.9	77.8	10.4	0.0
Stem Ginger, Costa*	1 Pack/60g	286	13.0	476	4.8	65.6	21.6	0.0
BROWNIES								
Bites, Costa*	1 Serving/72g	342	22.1	475	5.4	44.3	30.7	0.0
CAKE								
Carrot, Costa^	1 Slice/138g	514	23.4	374	5.1	48.6	17.0	0.0
Chocolate, Christmas, Costa*	1 Serving/162g	616	25.8	380	4.9	53.0	15.9	2.5
Chocolate, Costa*	1 Slice/150g	575	23.6	383	4.8	76.7	15.7	0.0
Lemon, Costa*	1 Slice/144g	576	25.4	399	3.6	56.0	17.6	0.0
Victoria Sandwich, Costa*	1 Slice/136g	546	25.6	401	3.5	54.0	18.8	0.0
CHOCOLATE								
Stirrer, Stick, Costa*	1 Stick/10g	53	3.6	531	4.8	46.7	36.1	6.6
COFFEE								
Americano, Massimo, No Added Milk, Costa*	1 Massimo/600ml	12	0.4	2	0.1	0.3	0.1	0.0
Americano, Medio, No Added Milk, Costa*	1 Medio/480ml	8	0.3	2	0.1	0.2	0.1	0.0
Americano, Primo, No Added Milk, Costa*	1 Primo/360ml	6	0.2	2	0.1	0.2	0.1	0.0
Babyccino, Full Fat, Solo, Costa*	1 Solo/30ml	101	4.3	337	14.0	38.3	14.3	0.0
Babyccino, Skimmed, Solo, Costa*	1 Solo/30ml	65	0.1	217	14.3	39.7	0.3	0.0
Babyccino, Soya, Solo, Costa*	1 Solo/30ml	70	2.2	233	13.0	28.7	7.3	0.0
Caffe Latte, Full Fat, Massimo, Costa*	1 Massimo/600ml	260	14.4	43	2.2	3.2	2.4	0.0
Caffe Latte, Full Fat, Medio, Costa*	1 Latte/480g	202	11.2	42	2.2	3.2	2.3	0.0
Caffe Latte, Full Fat, Primo, Costa*	1 Primo/360ml	151	8.5	42	2.2	3.1	2.4	0.0
Caffe Latte, Skimmed, Massimo, Costa*	1 Massimo/600ml	149	0.7	25	2.4	3.6	0.1	0.0
Caffe Latte, Skimmed, Medio, Costa*	1 Medio/480ml	114	0.5	24	2.3	3.5	0.1	0.0
Caffe Latte, Skimmed, Primo, Costa*	1 Primo/360ml	86	0.3	24	2.4	3.5	0.1	0.0
Caffe Latte, Soya, Massimo, Costa*	1 Massimo/600ml	165	7.7	27	2.1	1.8	1.3	0.0
Caffe Latte, Soya, Medio, Costa*	1 Medio/480ml	124	5.8	26	2.0	1.7	1.2	0.0
Caffe Latte, Soya, Primo, Costa*	1 Primo/360ml	93	4.4	26	2.0	1.6	1.2	0.0
Cappuccino, Full Fat, Massimo, Costa*	1 Massimo/568g	123	6.7	22	1.1	1.6	1.2	0.0
Cappuccino, Full Fat, Medio, Costa*	1 Medio/480g	160	8.8	33	1.7	2.5	1.8	0.0
Cappuccino, Full Fat, Primo, Costa*	1 Primo/360ml	94	5.1	26	1.4	2.0	1.4	0.0
Cappuccino, Skimmed, Massimo, Costa*	1 Massimo/600ml	113	0.7	19	1.8	2.7	0.1	0.0
Cappuccino, Skimmed, Medio, Costa*	1 Medio/480g	91	0.7	19	2.4	3.7	0.1	0.0
Cappuccino, Skimmed, Primo, Costa*	1 Primo/360ml	56	0.3	16	1.5	2.3	0.1	0.0
Cappuccino, Soya, Massimo, Costa*	1 Massimo/600ml	126	5.8	21	1.6	1.4	1.0	0.0
Cappuccino, Soya, Medio, Costa*	1 Medio/480ml	100	4.6	21	1.6	1.4	1.0	0.0
Cappuccino, Soya, Primo, Costa*	1 Primo/360ml	62	2.8	17	1.3	1.2	0.8	0.0
Espresso, Ristretto, Doppio, Costa*	1 Doppio/60ml	6	0.2	10	0.7	1.3	0.3	0.0
Espresso, Ristretto, Solo, Costa*	1 Solo/30ml	3	0.1	10	0.7	1.3	0.3	0.0
Light, Massimo, Costa*	1 Massimo/600ml	98	0.5	16	1.6	2.4	0.1	0.0
Light, Medio, Costa*	1 Medio/480ml	88	0.4	18	1.8	2.7	0.1	0.0
Light, Primo, Costa*	1 Primo/360ml	65	0.3	18	1.8	2.7	0.1	0.0
Mocha, Flake, Full Fat, Massimo, Costa*	1 Massimo/600ml	548	29.7	91	2.7	8.8	4.9	0.0
Mocha, Flake, Full Fat, Medio, Costa*	1 Medio/480ml	492	26.6	102	2.8	10.5	5.5	0.0
Mocha, Flake, Full Fat, Primo, Costa*	1 Primo/360ml	356	20.0	99	2.6	9.4	5.6	0.0
Mocha, Flake, Skimmed, Massimo, Costa*	1 Massimo/600ml	440	17.3	73	2.8	8.9	2.9	0.0
Mocha, Flake, Skimmed, Medio, Costa*	1 Medio/480ml	418	17.1	87	3.0	10.4	3.6	0.0

COSTA

	Measure INFO/WEIGHT	per Measure KCAL	per Measure FAT	Nutrition Values per 100g / 100ml KCAL	PROT	CARB	FAT	FIBRE
COFFEE								
Mocha, Flake, Skimmed, Primo, Costa*	1 Primo/360ml	303	13.5	84	2.7	9.6	3.7	0.0
Mocha, Flake, Soya, Massimo, Costa*	1 Massimo/600ml	461	23.6	77	2.6	7.4	3.9	0.0
Mocha, Flake, Soya, Medio, Costa*	1 Medio/480ml	433	22.3	90	2.8	8.8	4.6	0.0
Mocha, Flake, Soya, Primo, Costa*	1 Primo/360ml	314	17.0	87	2.6	8.2	4.7	0.0
Mocha, Full Fat, Massimo, Costa*	1 Massimo/600ml	373	15.7	62	2.5	7.0	2.6	0.0
Mocha, Full Fat, Medio, Costa*	1 Medio/480ml	316	12.6	66	2.5	7.8	2.6	0.0
Mocha, Full Fat, Primo, Costa*	1 Primo/360ml	206	6.3	57	1.7	5.0	1.7	0.0
Mocha, Skimmed, Massimo, Costa*	1 Massimo/600ml	264	3.3	44	2.5	7.1	0.5	0.0
Mocha, Skimmed, Medio, Costa*	1 Medio/480ml	242	3.1	50	2.7	8.2	0.6	0.0
Mocha, Skimmed, Primo, Costa*	1 Primo/360ml	153	1.9	42	2.4	6.9	0.5	0.0
Mocha, Soya, Massimo, Costa*	1 Massimo/600g	285	9.5	47	2.4	5.6	1.6	0.0
Mocha, Soya, Medio, Costa*	1 Medio/480ml	258	8.3	54	2.5	6.6	1.7	0.0
Mocha, Soya, Primo, Costa*	1 Primo/360ml	164	4.1	46	1.6	4.1	1.1	0.0
COFFEE COOLERS								
Mocha, with Full Fat Milk, Massimo, Costa*	1 Massimo/600ml	615	5.3	102	0.9	22.7	0.9	0.0
Mocha, with Full Fat Milk, Medio, Costa*	1 Medio/480ml	489	4.5	102	1.0	22.4	0.9	0.0
Mocha, with Full Fat Milk, Primo, Costa*	1 Primo/360ml	369	4.0	102	1.1	22.0	1.1	0.0
Mocha, with Skimmed Milk, Massimo, Costa*	1 Massimo/600ml	579	1.1	96	1.0	22.8	0.2	0.0
Mocha, with Skimmed Milk, Medio, Costa*	1 Medio/480ml	458	0.8	95	1.0	22.5	0.2	0.0
Mocha, with Skimmed Milk, Primo, Costa*	1 Primo/360ml	340	0.6	94	1.2	22.1	0.2	0.0
Mocha, with Soya Milk, Massimo, Costa*	1 Massimo/600ml	583	3.1	97	0.9	22.2	0.5	0.0
Mocha, with Soya Milk, Medio, Costa*	1 Medio/480ml	462	2.6	96	0.9	21.9	0.5	0.0
Mocha, with Soya Milk, Primo, Costa*	1 Primo/360ml	344	2.3	96	1.1	21.4	0.6	0.0
COOKIES								
Choc Chunk, Double, Costa*	1 Pack/60g	296	15.2	493	5.2	61.1	25.3	3.7
Fruit & Oat, Costa*	1 Pack/60g	283	12.7	472	5.1	65.2	21.2	2.0
CROISSANT								
Almond, Costa*	1 Croissant/88g	336	16.9	382	9.3	43.0	19.2	0.0
Butter, Costa*	1 Croissant/64g	276	16.7	431	8.3	40.6	26.1	0.0
Ham & Cheese, Costa*	1 Serving/100g	337	19.3	337	12.1	28.8	19.3	0.0
Tomato & Emmental, Costa*	1 Serving/98g	342	21.0	349	9.0	30.0	21.4	0.0
CUPCAKES								
Banoffee, Costa*	1 Cupcake/112g	431	17.7	385	3.7	56.7	15.8	0.0
Lemon, Costa*	1 Cupcake/97g	512	32.5	528	2.8	53.2	33.5	0.0
Rocky Road, Costa*	1 Cupcake/101g	427	17.7	421	5.1	58.9	17.5	0.0
FLAPJACK								
Fruity, Costa*	1 Serving/85g	353	12.1	415	4.9	67.0	14.2	12.5
Nutty, Costa*	1 Serving/85g	391	20.0	460	7.4	54.8	23.5	5.0
FLATBREAD								
Cheddar & Caramelised Onion Chutney, Costa*	1 Pack/118g	340	13.3	288	11.9	34.8	11.3	0.0
Chicken, Cajun, Costa*	1 Pack/168g	310	5.1	184	12.7	26.6	3.0	0.0
Chicken, Green Thai, Costa*	1 Pack/173g	325	6.4	188	12.2	26.6	3.7	0.0
Emmental & Mushroom, Costa*	1 Pack/158g	391	16.1	248	13.1	25.9	10.2	0.0
FRESCATO								
Coffee Caramel, Full Fat Milk, Medio, Costa*	1 Medio/454ml	488	7.9	107	1.5	21.5	1.7	0.0
Coffee Caramel, Skimmed Milk, Primo, Costa*	1 Primo/340ml	289	0.5	85	1.5	19.6	0.1	0.0
Coffee Caramel, Soya Milk, Primo, Costa*	1 Primo/340ml	300	2.8	88	1.4	18.6	0.8	0.0
Coffee Mocha, Full Fat Milk, Medio, Costa*	1 Medio/454ml	540	8.3	119	1.6	24.0	1.8	0.0
Coffee Mocha, Skimmed Milk, Medio, Costa*	1 Medio/454ml	477	1.2	105	1.7	24.1	0.3	0.0
Coffee Mocha, Skimmed Milk, Primo, Costa*	1 Primo/340ml	335	0.8	99	1.6	22.6	0.2	0.0
Coffee Vanilla, Full Fat Milk, Medio, Costa*	1 Medio/454ml	491	7.9	108	1.5	21.6	1.7	0.0
Coffee Vanilla, Full Fat Milk, Primo, Costa*	1 Primo/340ml	336	5.6	99	1.4	19.6	1.6	0.0

	Measure INFO/WEIGHT	per Measure KCAL	FAT	Nutrition Values per 100g / 100ml KCAL	PROT	CARB	FAT	FIBRE
COSTA								
FRESCATO								
Coffee Vanilla, Skimmed Milk, Medio, Costa*	1 Medio/454ml	427	0.7	94	1.6	21.7	0.1	0.0
Coffee Vanilla, Skimmed Milk, Primo, Costa*	1 Primo/340ml	290	0.5	85	1.5	19.7	0.1	0.0
FRUIT COOLERS								
Mango & Passionfruit, Massimo, Costa*	1 Massimo/600ml	290	0.6	48	0.1	11.6	0.1	0.0
Mango & Passionfruit, Medio, Costa*	1 Medio/480ml	232	0.5	48	0.1	11.6	0.1	0.0
Mango & Passionfruit, Primo, Costa*	1 Primo/360ml	173	0.3	48	0.1	11.6	0.1	0.0
Peach, Massimo, Costa*	1 Massimo/600ml	406	0.3	68	0.2	16.3	0.0	0.0
Peach, Medio, Costa*	1 Medio/480ml	325	0.2	68	0.2	16.3	0.0	0.0
Peach, Primo, Costa*	1 Primo/360ml	243	0.2	67	0.2	16.3	0.1	0.0
Red Berry, Massimo, Costa*	1 Massimo/600ml	409	0.6	68	0.2	16.3	0.1	0.0
Red Berry, Medio, Costa*	1 Medio/480ml	327	0.5	68	0.2	16.3	0.1	0.0
Red Berry, Primo, Costa*	1 Primo/360ml	245	0.3	68	0.2	16.3	0.1	0.0
Sicilian Lemonade, Medio, Costa*	1 Medio/454ml	264	0.2	59	0.0	14.0	0.0	0.0
Sicilian Lemonade, Primo, Costa*	1 Primo/340ml	197	0.2	58	0.1	14.0	0.1	0.0
HOT CHOCOLATE								
with Frothed Milk, Full Fat, Massimo, Costa*	1 Massimo/600ml	433	19.4	72	3.0	7.6	3.2	0.0
with Frothed Milk, Full Fat, Medio, Costa*	1 Medio/480ml	360	15.2	75	2.9	8.4	3.2	0.0
with Frothed Milk, Full Fat, Primo, Costa*	1 Primo/360ml	225	10.1	62	2.6	6.6	2.8	0.0
with Frothed Milk, Skimmed, Massimo, Costa*	1 Massimo/600ml	296	3.0	49	3.1	7.9	0.5	0.0
with Frothed Milk, Skimmed, Medio, Costa*	1 Medio/480ml	262	2.9	55	3.1	8.8	0.6	0.0
with Frothed Milk, Skimmed, Primo, Costa*	1 Primo/360ml	167	1.8	46	2.8	7.5	0.5	0.0
with Frothed Milk, Soya, Massimo, Costa*	1 Massimo/600ml	319	11.3	53	2.8	5.8	1.9	0.0
with Frothed Milk, Soya, Medio, Costa*	1 Medio/480ml	280	9.4	58	2.9	6.8	2.0	0.0
with Frothed Milk, Soya, Primo, Costa*	1 Primo/360ml	181	6.3	50	2.6	5.7	1.7	0.0
with Marshmallows & Cream, Soya, Massimo, Costa*	1 Massimo/600ml	468	21.0	78	3.0	8.2	3.5	0.0
with Marshmallows & Cream, Soya, Medio, Costa*	1 Medio/480ml	429	19.2	89	3.1	9.8	4.0	0.0
with Marshmallows & Cream, Soya, Primo, Costa*	1 Primo/360ml	305	13.6	85	2.8	9.5	3.8	0.0
ICE DESSERTS								
Double Choc Flake, Full Fat Milk, Medio, Costa*	1 Medio/454ml	786	29.9	173	2.1	26.4	6.6	0.0
Strawberry Shortcake, Full Fat Milk, Primo, Costa*	1 Primo/340ml	569	23.9	167	1.8	24.3	7.0	0.0
Strawberry Shortcake, Skimmed Milk, Medio, Costa*	1 Medio/454ml	694	19.0	153	1.9	27.2	4.2	0.0
Vanilla, Full Fat Milk, Medio, Costa*	1 Medio/454ml	421	7.8	93	1.4	17.9	1.7	0.0
Vanilla, Full Fat Milk, Primo, Costa*	1 Primo/340ml	301	5.6	89	1.4	17.1	1.6	0.0
Vanilla, Skimmed Milk, Primo, Costa*	1 Primo/340ml	255	0.5	75	1.5	17.1	0.1	0.0
Vanilla, Soya Milk, Medio, Costa*	1 Medio/454ml	373	3.8	82	1.4	17.0	0.8	0.0
Vanilla, Soya Milk, Primo, Costa*	1 Primo/340ml	267	2.7	79	1.4	16.2	0.8	0.0
LOAF								
Breakfast, Banana & Pecan, Costa*	1 Loaf/108g	422	22.3	391	5.1	44.0	20.7	0.0
MOCHA								
Iced, Full Fat Milk, Medio, Costa*	1 Medio/454ml	209	0.0	46	1.2	7.7	0.0	0.0
Iced, Full Fat Milk, Primo, Costa*	1 Primo/340ml	142	3.7	42	1.1	6.9	1.1	0.0
Iced, Skimmed Milk, Medio, Costa*	1 Medio/454ml	170	1.1	37	1.2	7.7	0.2	0.0
Iced, Skimmed Milk, Primo, Costa*	1 Primo/340ml	115	0.8	34	1.1	7.0	0.2	0.0
Iced, Soya Milk, Primo, Costa*	1 Primo/340ml	122	2.1	36	1.1	6.4	0.6	0.0
MUFFIN								
Banana & Pecan Breakfast Loaf, Costa*	1 Muffin/113g	442	23.4	391	5.1	44.0	20.7	0.0
Blueberry, Costa*	1 Muffin/132g	475	20.9	360	4.0	50.4	15.8	0.0
Chocolate, Mini, Costa*	1 Muffin/19g	73	3.9	383	4.3	44.5	20.5	0.0
Chocolate, Triple, Costa*	1 Muffin/130g	530	27.8	408	5.3	48.6	21.4	0.0
Lemon & Orange, Low Fat, Costa*	1 Muffin/135g	319	3.1	236	4.6	49.4	2.3	1.1
Lemon & Poppyseed, Costa*	1 Muffin/131g	532	28.0	406	4.3	49.0	21.4	0.0
Lemon & White Chocolate, Costa*	1 Muffin/129g	472	20.4	366	5.4	52.3	15.8	0.0

	Measure INFO/WEIGHT	per Measure KCAL	FAT	Nutrition Values per 100g / 100ml KCAL	PROT	CARB	FAT	FIBRE
COSTA								
MUFFIN								
Raspberry & White Chocolate, Costa*	1 Muffin/135g	511	26.0	376	4.8	46.4	19.1	0.0
Raspberry & White Chocolate, Mini, Costa*	1 Muffin/19g	72	3.7	379	4.1	45.9	19.4	0.0
PAIN AU RAISIN								
Costa*	1 Pastry/119g	356	13.7	299	5.1	43.7	11.5	0.0
PANETTINO								
Chocolate, Costa*	1 Cake/100g	423	19.8	423	9.7	50.8	19.8	0.0
Classic, Costa*	1 Serving/100g	365	12.7	365	7.6	54.3	12.7	0.0
PANINI								
Brie & Tomato Chutney, Costa*	1 Panini/177g	453	16.5	256	9.8	33.3	9.3	2.8
Chicken & Pesto, Costa*	1 Panini/209g	419	21.4	200	22.5	57.9	10.2	0.0
Chicken Roasted Pepper & Rocket, Costa*	1 Panini/185g	338	7.6	183	10.4	26.0	4.1	3.2
Goats Cheese & Caramelised Onion Chutney, Costa*	1 Panini/172g	431	5.3	251	4.9	19.5	3.1	0.0
Goats Cheese & Pepper, Costa*	1 Panini/197g	424	11.0	215	9.9	30.3	5.6	0.0
Ham & Cheese, Costa*	1 Panini/175g	461	21.2	263	12.5	26.2	12.1	0.0
Mozzarella, Tomato & Basil, Costa*	1 Panini/190g	400	11.0	211	8.3	29.8	5.8	0.0
Ragu Meatball, Costa*	1 Panini/190g	477	15.8	251	11.7	31.2	8.3	0.0
Steak & Cheese, Costa*	1 Panini/228g	492	16.4	216	11.3	25.7	7.2	0.0
Tuna Melt, Costa*	1 Panini/190g	462	14.3	243	14.4	29.5	7.5	0.0
SALAD								
Chicken & Pasta, Costa*	1 Serving/270g	427	11.1	158	8.4	21.9	4.1	0.0
Chicken & Pesto Pasta, Costa*	1 Pack/271g	420	11.4	155	7.8	21.3	4.2	1.7
Cous Cous, Moroccan Styles, Costa*	1 Pack/290g	392	7.3	135	3.6	24.6	2.5	2.2
Tomato, Sunblush, & Feta Pasta, Costa*	1 Pack/267g	360	13.6	135	4.4	17.1	5.1	2.2
Tuna, Costa*	1 Pack/181g	274	4.0	151	10.3	22.6	2.2	0.0
Vegetable, Chargrilled, & Cous Cous, Costa*	1 Serving/291g	352	7.6	121	3.0	21.5	2.6	0.0
SANDWICH								
Bacon & Tomato Sauce, Tostato, Costa*	1 Tostato/132g	316	6.6	239	8.5	40.2	5.0	0.0
BLT, Costa*	1 Pack/169g	397	15.7	235	11.0	26.8	9.3	0.0
Brie, Apple & Grape, Costa*	1 Serving/225g	535	24.5	238	8.3	28.7	10.9	0.0
Chicken, Coronation, Costa*	1 Pack/258g	600	26.1	232	12.5	23.0	10.1	2.5
Chicken, Roast, Costa*	1 Pack/177g	325	7.1	184	13.0	23.8	4.0	0.0
Club, Breakfast, All Day, Costa*	1 Pack/243g	592	20.9	244	11.0	30.6	8.6	0.0
Club, Chicken & Bacon, Costa*	1 Pack/213g	484	13.2	227	13.6	29.3	6.2	0.0
Egg, Free Range, Costa*	1 Pack/172g	377	14.6	219	9.7	25.9	8.5	0.0
Egg Mayonnaise & Tomato, Free Range, Costa*	1 Pack/174g	389	24.1	223	8.6	18.3	13.8	0.0
Houmous, Costa*	1 Pack/165g	263	4.7	160	6.4	25.9	2.8	0.0
Prawn, Tiger, with Lime & Chilli Dressing, Costa*	1 Pack/185g	367	19.0	198	8.2	21.2	10.2	0.0
Roll, Ham Hock & Mustard Pickle, Costa*	1 Pack/163g	286	5.2	176	10.6	26.1	3.2	0.0
Roll, Ploughman's, Cheese, Costa*	1 Pack/175g	431	21.3	247	9.4	25.0	12.2	0.0
Salmon, & Salad, Poached, Oatmeal, Costa*	1 Pack/151g	224	4.2	148	7.7	22.9	2.8	0.0
Sausage, Chorizo, & Vine Ripened Tomato, Costa*	1 Pack/181g	315	3.8	174	15.5	26.1	2.1	0.0
Tuna, & Salad, Costa*	1 Pack/177g	289	4.1	163	11.9	25.7	2.3	0.0
SCONE								
Fruit, Costa*	1 Serving/110g	370	11.8	336	5.6	55.1	10.7	0.0
SHORTBREAD								
Mini, Bag, Costa*	1 Bag/65g	316	15.7	486	4.1	63.0	24.1	0.0
SHORTCAKE								
Raspberry, Costa*	1 Shortcake/45g	215	10.7	477	2.4	63.5	23.7	0.0
SLICES								
Cheese, Twist, Pastry, Costa*	1 Pastry/103g	346	20.4	336	11.1	29.5	19.8	0.0
Cinnamon Swirl, Pastry, Costa*	1 Pastry/92g	341	22.8	369	4.0	31.9	24.7	0.0
Pecan, Pastry, Costa*	1 Pastry/105g	465	29.9	443	5.6	42.1	28.5	3.0

	Measure INFO/WEIGHT	per Measure KCAL	FAT	Nutrition Values per 100g / 100ml KCAL	PROT	CARB	FAT	FIBRE
COSTA								
SOUP								
Fish, Bouillabaisse, Costa*	1 Serving/400g	180	5.6	45	5.8	2.2	1.4	0.0
TART								
Chocolate & Orange, Costa*	1 Serving/78g	357	18.5	458	5.8	56.3	23.8	2.3
TEA								
Lemon, Iced, Costa*	1 Bottle/275ml	91	0.0	33	0.0	8.0	0.0	0.0
Original, Iced, Massimo, Costa*	1 Massimo/600ml	179	0.0	30	0.0	9.1	0.0	0.0
Original, Iced, Medio, Costa*	1 Medio/480ml	135	0.0	28	0.0	6.9	0.0	0.0
Original, Iced, Primo, Costa*	1 Primo/360ml	88	0.0	24	0.0	6.0	0.0	0.0
Peach, Iced, Massimo, Costa*	1 Massimo/600ml	121	0.0	20	0.0	4.8	0.0	0.0
Peach, Iced, Medio, Costa*	1 Medio/480ml	91	0.0	19	0.0	4.5	0.0	0.0
Peach, Iced, Primo, Costa*	1 Primo/360ml	60	0.0	17	0.0	4.0	0.0	0.0
Raspberry, Iced, Massimo, Costa*	1 Massimo/600ml	133	0.0	22	0.0	5.4	0.0	0.0
Raspberry, Iced, Medio, Costa*	1 Medio/480ml	100	0.0	21	0.0	5.1	0.0	0.0
Raspberry, Iced, Primo, Costa*	1 Primo/360ml	67	0.0	19	0.0	4.5	0.0	0.0
WRAP								
Caesar, Chicken, Costa*	1 Pack/194g	420	15.6	216	11.8	24.1	8.0	1.4
Chicken Fajita, Costa*	1 Wrap/186g	416	12.9	223	12.1	28.0	6.9	0.0
Three Bean, Spicy, Costa*	1 Pack/235g	456	14.3	194	7.1	27.7	6.1	0.0
YOGHURT								
Honey & Granola, Costa*	1 Pot/190g	303	6.1	159	5.3	27.3	3.2	0.0
Strawberry & Granola, Costa*	1 Pot/190g	253	7.4	133	5.4	19.0	3.9	0.0
CRUSSH JUICE BARS								
BREAKFAST CEREAL								
Muesli, Blueberry Bircher, Crussh Juice Bars*	1 Serving/190g	199	4.0	105	4.4	17.2	2.1	1.4
Muesli, Breakfast Berry, Pot, Crussh Juice Bars*	1 Serving/225g	294	13.7	131	5.1	13.9	6.1	1.3
Muesli, Strawberry, Bircher, Crussh Juice Bars*	1 Serving/190g	211	4.7	111	4.6	17.5	2.5	1.4
Porridge, Cinnamon, Large, Crussh Juice Bars*	1 Serving/400g	380	8.4	95	3.1	15.7	2.1	1.8
Porridge, Cinnamon, Medium, Crussh Juice Bars*	1 Serving/331g	314	6.9	95	3.1	15.7	2.1	1.8
Porridge, Summer, Large, Crussh Juice Bars*	1 Serving/460g	602	18.8	131	4.8	18.8	4.1	1.4
Porridge, Summer, Medium, Crussh Juice Bars*	1 Serving/330g	432	13.5	131	4.8	18.8	4.1	1.4
Porridge, Traditional, Organic, Lge, Crussh Juice Bars*	1 Serving/400g	380	8.4	95	3.1	15.7	2.1	1.8
Porridge, Traditional Organic, Med, Crussh Juice Bars*	1 Serving/331g	314	6.9	95	3.1	15.7	2.1	1.8
Strawberries & Blueberries, Crussh Juice Bars*	1 Serving/171g	60	0.2	35	0.8	8.0	0.1	1.8
FRUIT								
Seasonal, Crussh Juice Bars*	1 Serving/150g	61	0.3	41	0.5	10.0	0.2	1.1
JUICE								
Apple, Large, Crussh Juice Bars*	1 Serving/451g	185	0.5	41	0.1	9.8	0.1	0.0
Apple, Medium, Crussh Juice Bars*	1 Serving/339g	139	0.3	41	0.1	9.8	0.1	0.0
Carrot, Large, Crussh Juice Bars*	1 Serving/448g	112	0.4	25	0.5	5.4	0.1	0.8
Carrot, Medium, Crussh Juice Bars*	1 Serving/340g	85	0.3	25	0.5	5.4	0.1	0.8
Clean & Lean, Large, Crussh Juice Bars*	1 Serving/449g	211	0.4	47	0.4	11.1	0.1	2.4
Clean & Lean, Medium, Crussh Juice Bars*	1 Serving/338g	159	0.3	47	0.4	11.1	0.1	2.4
Energiser, Large, Crussh Juice Bars*	1 Serving/450g	180	0.9	40	0.5	9.0	0.2	2.9
Energiser, Medium, Crussh Juice Bars*	1 Serving/340g	136	0.7	40	0.5	9.0	0.2	2.9
Green Goddess, Large, Crussh Juice Bars*	1 Serving/449g	175	1.3	39	0.8	8.4	0.3	2.6
Green Goddess, Medium, Crussh Juice Bars*	1 Serving/338g	132	1.0	39	0.8	8.4	0.3	2.6
Love, Large, Crussh Juice Bars*	1 Serving/449g	193	0.4	43	0.6	9.9	0.1	0.5
Love, Medium, Crussh Juice Bars*	1 Serving/340g	146	0.3	43	0.6	9.9	0.1	0.5
Orange, Large, Crussh Juice Bars*	1 Serving/448g	148	0.0	33	0.6	7.7	0.0	0.1
Orange, Medium, Crussh Juice Bars*	1 Serving/339g	112	0.0	33	0.6	7.7	0.0	0.1
Purifier, Large, Crussh Juice Bars*	1 Serving/463g	162	0.9	35	0.6	7.6	0.2	2.8
Purifier, Medium, Crussh Juice Bars*	1 Serving/340g	119	0.7	35	0.6	7.6	0.2	2.8

CRUSSH JUICE BARS

	Measure INFO/WEIGHT	per Measure KCAL	FAT	Nutrition Values per 100g / 100ml KCAL	PROT	CARB	FAT	FIBRE
JUICE								
Super, Large, Crussh Juice Bars*	1 Serving/450g	144	1.3	32	0.8	6.5	0.3	2.7
Super, Medium, Crussh Juice Bars*	1 Serving/338g	108	1.0	32	0.8	6.5	0.3	2.7
Tropical Crussh, Large, Crussh Juice Bars*	1 Serving/451g	203	0.9	45	0.4	10.5	0.2	2.1
Tropical Crussh, Medium, Crussh Juice Bars*	1 Serving/340g	153	0.7	45	0.4	10.5	0.2	2.1
Zinger, Large, Crussh Juice Bars*	1 Serving/463g	162	0.9	35	0.6	7.6	0.2	1.9
Zinger, Medium, Crussh Juice Bars*	1 Serving/340g	119	0.7	35	0.6	7.6	0.2	1.9
SALADS								
NY:LON Cobb, Crussh Juice Bars*	1 Serving/215g	230	15.5	107	8.9	1.5	7.2	7.2
O-Me-Good Dressing, Crussh Juice Bars*	1 Serving/50g	55	3.8	111	3.2	7.3	7.6	0.7
Super Greens, Crussh Juice Bars*	1 Serving/230g	78	3.0	34	2.9	2.5	1.3	2.6
Tuna Nicoise, with New Potato, Crussh Juice Bars*	1 Serving/250g	135	5.2	54	6.7	4.5	2.1	1.2
Tuna Nicoise, with Zesty Dressing, Crussh Juice Bars*	1 Serving/40g	118	12.9	295	0.4	1.0	32.3	0.0
SANDWICH								
5 a Day Wheat Free, Crussh Juice Bars*	1 Pack/200g	326	14.6	163	4.2	22.2	7.3	1.2
Club, Chicken, Classic, Crussh Juice Bars*	1 Pack/235g	411	15.3	175	11.8	17.5	6.5	1.3
Ham, Swiss, Smokey, Crussh Juice Bars*	1 Pack/244g	490	19.3	201	12.1	20.2	7.9	3.0
Tu Cumber Mayo, Crussh Juice Bars*	1 Pack/180g	373	16.9	207	11.6	17.3	9.4	2.7
SMOOTHIES								
Bananarama, Large, Crussh Juice Bars*	1 Serving/450g	243	2.7	54	3.7	8.6	0.6	0.4
Bananarama, Medium, Crussh Juice Bars*	1 Serving/339g	183	2.0	54	3.7	8.6	0.6	0.4
Blueberry Hill, Large, Crussh Juice Bars*	1 Serving/449g	211	1.8	47	1.8	9.1	0.4	1.6
Blueberry Hill, Medium, Crussh Juice Bars*	1 Serving/338g	159	1.4	47	1.8	9.1	0.4	1.6
Brainstorm, Large, Super, Crussh Juice Bars*	1 Serving/449g	220	1.8	49	1.7	9.8	0.4	1.1
Brainstorm, Medium, Super, Crussh Juice Bars*	1 Serving/339g	166	1.4	49	1.7	9.8	0.4	1.1
Brazilian, Large, Super, Crussh Juice Bars*	1 Serving/450g	297	2.7	66	1.8	10.1	0.6	0.9
Brazilian, Medium, Super, Crussh Juice Bars*	1 Serving/339g	224	2.0	66	1.8	10.1	0.6	0.9
Breakfast Smoothie, Large, Super, Crussh Juice Bars*	1 Serving/450g	459	6.3	102	4.6	17.8	1.4	1.3
Breakfast Smoothie, Med, Super, Crussh Juice Bars*	1 Serving/339g	346	4.7	102	4.6	17.8	1.4	1.3
Crusshberry Blast, Large, Crussh Juice Bars*	1 Serving/449g	211	1.8	47	1.8	9.0	0.4	1.6
Crusshberry Blast, Medium, Crussh Juice Bars*	1 Serving/338g	159	1.4	47	1.8	9.0	0.4	1.6
Detox Cactus, Large, Super, Crussh Juice Bars*	1 Serving/400g	268	0.8	67	1.8	14.2	0.2	0.7
Detox Cactus, Medium, Super, Crussh Juice Bars*	1 Serving/330g	221	0.7	67	1.8	14.2	0.2	0.7
Energy Explosion, Large, Super, Crussh Juice Bars*	1 Serving/450g	243	1.8	54	1.7	10.8	0.4	0.9
Energy Explosion, Medium, Super, Crussh Juice Bars*	1 Serving/339g	183	1.4	54	1.7	10.8	0.4	0.9
Fat Burner, Large, Super, Crussh Juice Bars*	1 Serving/450g	207	1.8	46	1.7	9.0	0.4	1.4
Fat Burner, Medium, Super, Crussh Juice Bars*	1 Serving/339g	156	1.4	46	1.7	9.0	0.4	1.4
Good Morning, Large, Super, Crussh Juice Bars*	1 Serving/449g	220	0.9	49	1.9	9.5	0.2	1.2
Good Morning, Medium, Super, Crussh Juice Bars*	1 Serving/339g	166	0.7	49	1.9	9.5	0.2	1.2
Mango Madness, Large, Crussh Juice Bars*	1 Serving/449g	238	1.8	53	1.8	10.6	0.4	0.8
Mango Madness, Medium, Crussh Juice Bars*	1 Serving/340g	180	1.4	53	1.8	10.6	0.4	0.8
Peach Passion, Large, Crussh Juice Bars*	1 Serving/449g	211	1.3	47	2.0	9.0	0.3	0.6
Peach Passion, Medium, Crussh Juice Bars*	1 Serving/338g	159	1.0	47	2.0	9.0	0.3	0.6
Peach Performance, Large, Super, Crussh Juice Bars*	1 Serving/456g	310	6.4	68	12.0	13.8	1.4	0.7
Peach Performance, Med, Super, Crussh Juice Bars*	1 Serving/346g	235	4.8	68	12.0	13.8	1.4	0.7
Pineapple Pleasure, Large, Crussh Juice Bars*	1 Serving/450g	234	1.8	52	1.7	10.5	0.4	0.6
Pineapple Pleasure, Medium, Crussh Juice Bars*	1 Serving/338g	176	1.4	52	1.7	10.5	0.4	0.6
Protein Power, Large, Super, Crussh Juice Bars*	1 Serving/450g	306	5.4	68	9.9	14.0	1.2	0.8
Protein Power, Medium, Super, Crussh Juice Bars*	1 Serving/346g	235	4.1	68	9.9	14.0	1.2	0.8
Sporty Spicy, Large, Super, Crussh Juice Bars*	1 Serving/400g	280	1.2	70	1.8	14.8	0.3	0.6
Sporty Spicy, Medium, Super, Crussh Juice Bars*	1 Serving/329g	230	1.0	70	1.8	14.8	0.3	0.6
Strawberry Cool, Large, Crussh Juice Bars*	1 Serving/450g	207	1.3	46	1.9	8.9	0.3	0.9
Strawberry Cool, Medium, Crussh Juice Bars*	1 Serving/339g	156	1.0	46	1.9	8.9	0.3	0.9

	Measure INFO/WEIGHT	per Measure		Nutrition Values per 100g / 100ml				
		KCAL	FAT	KCAL	PROT	CARB	FAT	FIBRE

CRUSSH JUICE BARS

SNACKS & DESSERTS

	Measure INFO/WEIGHT	KCAL	FAT	KCAL	PROT	CARB	FAT	FIBRE
Cake, Carrot, Crussh Juice Bars*	1 Serving/167g	533	30.7	319	5.0	33.3	18.4	4.1
Cake, Chocolate, Crussh Juice Bars*	1 Serving/115g	469	22.3	408	4.2	54.7	19.4	0.0
Cookie, Oat & Raisin, Organic, Crussh Juice Bars*	1 Serving/50g	203	9.1	406	4.8	55.8	18.2	2.7
Crussh Brownie, Crussh Juice Bars*	1 Serving/75g	315	17.8	420	5.4	47.6	23.8	1.3
Organic Double Chocolate Cookie, Crussh Juice Bars*	1 Serving/50g	210	8.8	421	5.0	60.8	17.6	2.7
Peas, Wasabi, Natural, Crussh Juice Bars*	1 Serving/71g	294	6.3	412	15.7	66.6	8.8	10.8
Popcorn, Honey, Organic, Crussh Juice Bars*	1 Serving/30g	135	5.2	449	4.1	75.6	17.3	6.4
Popcorn, Sea Salt, Organic, Crussh Juice Bars*	1 Serving/30g	118	4.7	394	11.0	64.9	15.8	13.0

SOUP

	Measure INFO/WEIGHT	KCAL	FAT	KCAL	PROT	CARB	FAT	FIBRE
Bean & Vegetable Garden, Large, Crussh Juice Bars*	1 Serving/440g	295	2.2	67	3.2	10.6	0.5	3.9
Bean & Vegetable Garden, Med, Crussh Juice Bars*	1 Serving/330g	221	1.6	67	3.2	10.6	0.5	3.9
Beef & Vegetable Pot, Large, Crussh Juice Bars*	1 Serving/440g	198	2.2	45	2.9	7.1	0.5	1.2
Beef & Vegetable Pot, Medium, Crussh Juice Bars*	1 Serving/330g	148	1.6	45	2.9	7.1	0.5	1.2
Chicken, Farmhouse, Organic, Lge, Crussh Juice Bars*	1 Serving/400g	232	10.4	58	3.4	5.2	2.6	3.0
Chicken, Ginger, Miso, Crussh Juice Bars*	1 Serving/600g	204	6.6	34	2.8	3.3	1.1	0.7
Chicken, Gumbo, Louisiana, Large, Crussh Juice Bars*	1 Serving/411g	189	9.9	46	3.2	2.9	2.4	1.2
Chicken, Gumbo, Louisiana, Med, Crussh Juice Bars*	1 Serving/309g	142	7.4	46	3.2	2.9	2.4	1.2
Chickpea, Spinach & Dhal, Large, Crussh Juice Bars*	1 Serving/440g	246	7.5	56	3.5	6.6	1.7	1.4
Chickpea, Spinach & Dhal, Medium, Crussh Juice Bars*	1 Serving/330g	185	5.6	56	3.5	6.6	1.7	1.4
Chilli, Beef, Large, Crussh Juice Bars*	1 Serving/440g	321	14.1	73	5.4	5.6	3.2	1.6
Chilli, Beef, Medium, Crussh Juice Bars*	1 Serving/329g	240	10.5	73	5.4	5.6	3.2	1.6
Chilli, Chicken, Stew, Large, Crussh Juice Bars*	1 Serving/440g	238	1.8	54	6.7	5.1	0.4	1.4
Chilli, Chicken, Stew, Medium, Crussh Juice Bars*	1 Serving/330g	178	1.3	54	6.7	5.1	0.4	1.4
Chilli, Vegetable, Large, Crussh Juice Bars*	1 Serving/440g	211	7.0	48	2.3	6.3	1.6	2.2
Chilli, Vegetable, Medium, Crussh Juice Bars*	1 Serving/329g	158	5.3	48	2.3	6.3	1.6	2.2
Curry, Chicken, Green Thai, & Veg, Crussh Juice Bars*	1 Serving/499g	544	11.0	109	3.7	3.5	2.2	1.6
Dhal, Armenian, Organic, Large, Crussh Juice Bars*	1 Serving/440g	349	6.6	79	4.6	11.8	1.5	1.4
Dhal, Armenian, Organic, Medium, Crussh Juice Bars*	1 Serving/330g	262	5.0	79	4.6	11.8	1.5	1.4
Goulash, Hungarian, Large, Crussh Juice Bars*	1 Serving/439g	202	3.1	46	3.8	6.3	0.7	0.9
Goulash, Hungarian, Medium, Crussh Juice Bars*	1 Serving/330g	152	2.3	46	3.8	6.3	0.7	0.9
Leek & Potato, Large, Crussh Juice Bars*	1 Serving/440g	176	6.6	40	0.9	5.5	1.5	0.7
Leek & Potato, Medium, Crussh Juice Bars*	1 Serving/330g	132	4.9	40	0.9	5.5	1.5	0.7
Leek & Potato, Organic, Large, Crussh Juice Bars*	1 Serving/440g	242	12.3	55	1.2	6.5	2.8	1.0
Leek & Potato, Organic, Medium, Crussh Juice Bars*	1 Serving/329g	181	9.2	55	1.2	6.5	2.8	1.0
Lentil, Red, Thai, Large, Crussh Juice Bars*	1 Serving/440g	220	13.6	50	1.8	3.8	3.1	0.6
Lentil, Red, Thai, Medium, Crussh Juice Bars*	1 Serving/330g	165	10.2	50	1.8	3.8	3.1	0.6
Lentil & Herbs, Large, Crussh Juice Bars*	1 Serving/440g	229	1.8	52	3.8	8.3	0.4	1.4
Lentil & Herbs, Medium, Crussh Juice Bars*	1 Serving/330g	172	1.3	52	3.8	8.3	0.4	1.4
Meatballs, Sicilian Style, Fit, Crussh Juice Bars*	1 Serving/500g	635	18.5	127	45.6	17.5	3.7	1.3
Minestrone, Italian, Large, Crussh Juice Bars*	1 Serving/440g	172	1.3	39	2.1	6.8	0.3	2.0
Minestrone, Italian, Medium, Crussh Juice Bars*	1 Serving/330g	129	1.0	39	2.1	6.8	0.3	2.0
Mushroom, Wild, Organic, Large, Crussh Juice Bars*	1 Serving/439g	224	12.7	51	1.1	5.3	2.9	0.5
Mushroom, Wild, Organic, Medium, Crussh Juice Bars*	1 Serving/329g	168	9.6	51	1.1	5.3	2.9	0.5
Pea, & Homemade Pesto, Large, Crussh Juice Bars*	1 Serving/440g	238	13.6	54	2.4	4.0	3.1	1.7
Pea, & Homemade Pesto, Medium, Crussh Juice Bars*	1 Serving/330g	178	10.2	54	2.4	4.0	3.1	1.7
Pea, Mint & Lemon, Organic, Large, Crussh Juice Bars*	1 Serving/440g	164	2.6	37	1.9	4.6	0.6	2.7
Pea, Mint & Lemon, Organic, Med, Crussh Juice Bars*	1 Serving/330g	123	2.0	37	1.9	4.6	0.6	2.7
Tomato, Thai, Organic, Large, Crussh Juice Bars*	1 Serving/400g	324	24.8	81	0.9	5.4	6.2	1.6
Tomato, Thai, Organic, Medium, Crussh Juice Bars*	1 Serving/330g	267	20.5	81	0.9	5.4	6.2	1.6
Tomato & Lentil, Organic, Large, Crussh Juice Bars*	1 Serving/440g	231	4.0	52	2.9	8.3	0.9	11.4
Tomato & Lentil, Organic, Medium, Crussh Juice Bars*	1 Serving/330g	173	3.0	52	2.9	8.3	0.9	11.4
Vegetable, Spanish, Organic, Lge, Crussh Juice Bars*	1 Serving/440g	176	0.9	40	1.8	5.7	0.2	1.9

	Measure INFO/WEIGHT	per Measure KCAL	FAT	Nutrition Values per 100g / 100ml KCAL	PROT	CARB	FAT	FIBRE

CRUSSH JUICE BARS

SOUP

Vegetable, Spanish, Organic, Med, Crussh Juice Bars*	1 Serving/330g	132	0.7	40	1.8	5.7	0.2	1.9
Vegetable, Tuscan, Organic, Lge, Crussh Juice Bars*	1 Serving/441g	238	7.5	54	2.8	7.5	1.7	3.1

TOASTIES

Cheese, Cheddar, Tasty, Crussh Juice Bars*	1 Toastie/105g	310	10.0	295	14.5	37.9	9.5	0.0
Ham & Edam, Skinny, Crussh Juice Bars*	1 Toastie/130g	329	8.7	253	15.4	32.9	6.7	0.0
Jalapeno & Spinach, Melt, Crussh Juice Bars*	1 Toastie/150g	403	16.0	269	13.9	29.3	10.7	0.3
Pesto Chicken & Cheddar, Crussh Juice Bars*	1 Toastie/190g	541	26.8	285	17.8	21.7	14.1	0.0
Tuna, Swiss Melt, Crussh Juice Bars*	1 Toastie/170g	379	11.6	223	16.3	24.0	6.8	0.1

WRAP

Caesar, Simply, Crussh Juice Bars*	1 Wrap/190g	538	16.7	283	10.3	40.4	8.8	1.5
Chicken, Citrus, Herb & Yoghurt, Crussh Juice Bars*	1 Wrap/260g	426	15.9	164	20.3	18.0	6.1	0.8
Chicken, Tarragon, & Red Pepper, Crussh Juice Bars*	1 Wrap/247g	459	19.5	186	22.4	18.2	7.9	1.6
Salad, Beef, Vietnamese, Crussh Juice Bars*	1 Wrap/230g	375	10.8	163	9.1	18.7	4.7	1.4
Salad, Sweet Potato & Falafel, Crussh Juice Bars*	1 Wrap/245g	448	20.8	183	6.0	20.7	8.5	4.0
Salad, Tuna, Crussh Juice Bars*	1 Wrap/210g	365	10.3	174	12.0	20.4	4.9	0.4

DOMINO'S PIZZA

PIZZA

American Hot, Classic Crust, Large, Domino's Pizza*	1 Slice/87g	218	7.7	250	13.6	29.0	8.8	2.2
American Hot, Classic Crust, Medium, Domino's Pizza*	1 Slice/79g	194	7.0	245	13.3	28.0	8.9	2.2
American Hot, Classic Crust, Small, Domino's Pizza*	1 Slice/72g	182	6.6	253	14.0	28.5	9.2	2.2
American Hot, Dbl Decadence, Med, Domino's Pizza*	1 Slice/99g	298	15.1	301	13.0	27.8	15.3	1.7
American Hot, Dominator, Large, Domino's Pizza*	1 Slice/110g	307	12.1	279	13.2	31.7	11.0	1.9
American Hot, Personal, Domino's Pizza*	1 Slice/61g	161	5.1	264	14.7	32.6	8.3	2.2
American Hot, Thin Crust, Large, Domino's Pizza*	1 Slice/67g	203	9.7	303	14.7	28.4	14.5	2.2
American Hot, Thin Crust, Medium, Domino's Pizza*	1 Slice/62g	191	9.3	308	15.0	28.4	15.0	2.5
Americano, Classic Crust, Large, Domino's Pizza*	1 Slice/91g	268	8.4	295	15.7	37.2	9.3	1.9
Americano, Classic Crust, Medium, Domino's Pizza*	1 Slice/84g	248	7.8	295	15.7	37.2	9.3	1.9
Americano, Classic Crust, Small, Domino's Pizza*	1 Slice/76g	224	7.1	295	15.7	37.2	9.3	1.9
Americano, Dominator, Large, Domino's Pizza*	1 Slice/114g	334	11.4	293	14.1	37.0	10.0	1.8
Americano, Double Decadence, Med, Domino's Pizza*	1 Slice/103g	346	15.1	336	14.8	36.1	14.7	1.8
Americano, Personal, Domino's Pizza*	1 Slice/64g	184	4.9	287	19.4	35.0	7.7	2.5
Americano, Thin Crust, Large, Domino's Pizza*	1 Slice/71g	257	10.6	362	17.4	39.3	15.0	2.1
Americano, Thin Crust, Medium, Domino's Pizza*	1 Slice/67g	243	10.1	362	17.4	39.3	15.0	2.1
Bacon Double Cheese, Classic, Lge, Domino's Pizza*	1 Slice/89g	224	8.9	251	14.7	24.6	10.0	1.9
Bacon Double Cheese, Classic, Med, Domino's Pizza*	1 Slice/88g	221	8.8	251	14.7	24.6	10.0	1.9
Bacon Double Cheese, Classic, Small, Domino's Pizza*	1 Slice/80g	200	8.0	251	14.7	24.6	10.0	1.9
Bacon Double Cheese, Personal, Domino's Pizza*	1 Slice/68g	182	6.4	268	15.8	28.8	9.4	1.9
Bacon Double Cheese, Thin, Lge, Domino's Pizza*	1 Slice/78g	238	12.1	307	16.4	21.1	15.6	2.1
Bacon Double Cheese, Thin, Med, Domino's Pizza*	1 Slice/71g	218	11.1	307	16.4	21.1	15.6	2.1
Cheese & Tomato, Classic Crust, Lge, Domino's Pizza*	1 Slice/69g	183	5.4	265	14.0	34.7	7.8	2.4
Cheese & Tomato, Classic Crust, Med, Domino's Pizza*	1 Slice/63g	162	4.8	257	13.4	33.6	7.6	2.4
Cheese & Tomato, Classic Crust, Sm, Domino's Pizza*	1 Slice/56g	148	4.4	264	14.1	34.5	7.8	2.5
Cheese & Tomato, Dbl Dec, Lge, Domino's Pizza*	1 Slice/90g	284	13.9	316	12.6	31.7	15.5	2.5
Cheese & Tomato, Dominator, Large, Domino's Pizza*	1 Slice/92g	265	8.7	288	13.0	37.6	9.5	2.3
Cheese & Tomato, Personal, Domino's Pizza*	1 Slice/50g	140	3.6	278	15.1	38.3	7.2	2.4
Cheese & Tomato, Stuffed Crust, Lge, Domino's Pizza*	1 Slice/75g	216	7.3	288	14.4	34.6	9.8	2.3
Cheese & Tomato, Stuffed Crust, Med, Domino's Pizza*	1 Slice/69g	199	6.8	288	14.4	34.6	9.8	2.3
Cheese & Tomato, Thin, Classic, Lge, Domino's Pizza*	1 Slice/55g	131	3.9	239	11.3	31.5	7.1	2.2
Cheese & Tomato, Thin, Classic, Med, Domino's Pizza*	1 Slice/48g	114	3.4	239	11.3	31.5	7.1	2.2
Cheese & Tomato, Thin, Classic, Sm, Domino's Pizza*	1 Slice/41g	97	2.9	239	11.3	31.5	7.1	2.2
Cheese & Tomato, Thin Crust, Lge, Domino's Pizza*	1 Slice/49g	162	7.5	330	15.6	32.9	15.2	3.1
Cheese & Tomato, Thin Crust, Med, Domino's Pizza*	1 Slice/46g	160	7.1	347	15.7	36.2	15.5	2.9

DOMINO'S PIZZA

PIZZA

	Measure INFO/WEIGHT	per Measure KCAL	FAT	Nutrition Values per 100g / 100ml KCAL	PROT	CARB	FAT	FIBRE
Chicken Feast, Classic Crust, Large, Domino's Pizza*	1 Slice/89g	201	5.6	226	14.6	27.8	6.3	2.1
Chicken Feast, Classic Crust, Medium, Domino's Pizza*	1 Slice/81g	183	5.1	226	14.6	27.8	6.3	2.1
Chicken Feast, Classic Crust, Small, Domino's Pizza*	1 Slice/72g	163	4.5	226	14.6	27.8	6.3	2.1
Chicken Feast, Dbl Decadence, Med, Domino's Pizza*	1 Slice/100g	232	6.6	232	14.3	28.9	6.6	2.1
Chicken Feast, Dominator, Large, Domino's Pizza*	1 Slice/112g	289	9.2	258	13.9	32.3	8.2	2.0
Chicken Feast, Personal, Domino's Pizza*	1 Slice/62g	153	3.8	247	15.7	32.3	6.1	2.1
Chicken Feast, Thin Crust, Large, Domino's Pizza*	1 Slice/69g	195	8.0	283	16.5	28.1	11.6	2.4
Chicken Feast, Thin Crust, Medium, Domino's Pizza*	1 Slice/64g	181	7.4	283	16.5	28.1	11.6	2.4
Domino's Deluxe, Classic Crust, Large, Domino's Pizza*	1 Slice/84g	209	7.9	250	13.2	26.9	9.4	2.1
Domino's Deluxe, Classic Crust, Med, Domino's Pizza*	1 Slice/76g	191	7.2	250	13.2	26.9	9.4	2.1
Domino's Deluxe, Classic Crust, Small, Domino's Pizza*	1 Slice/70g	174	6.5	250	13.2	26.9	9.4	2.1
Domino's Deluxe, Personal, Domino's Pizza*	1 Slice/59g	159	5.4	270	14.4	31.4	9.1	2.1
Domino's Deluxe, Thin Crust, Large, Domino's Pizza*	1 Slice/65g	202	10.0	312	14.7	27.0	15.5	2.4
Domino's Deluxe, Thin Crust, Medium, Domino's Pizza*	1 Slice/60g	188	9.3	312	14.7	27.0	15.5	2.4
Domino's Meateor, Classic Crust, Lge, Domino's Pizza*	1 Slice/87g	278	11.1	319	14.5	36.7	12.7	1.8
Domino's Meateor, Classic Crust, Med, Domino's Pizza*	1 Slice/80g	255	10.2	319	14.5	36.7	12.7	1.8
Domino's Meateor, Classic Crust, Sm, Domino's Pizza*	1 Slice/73g	233	9.3	319	14.5	36.7	12.7	1.8
Domino's Meateor, Dbl Dec, Med, Domino's Pizza*	1 Slice/99g	352	17.3	356	13.9	35.7	17.5	1.8
Domino's Meateor, Dominator, Large, Domino's Pizza*	1 Slice/109g	341	13.8	313	13.3	36.6	12.7	1.8
Domino's Meateor, Personal, Domino's Pizza*	1 Slice/66g	204	7.8	310	18.4	32.5	11.8	2.3
Domino's Meateor, Thin Crust, Large, Domino's Pizza*	1 Slice/67g	236	11.9	352	15.3	32.8	17.7	1.7
Domino's Meateor, Thin Crust, Med, Domino's Pizza*	1 Slice/63g	247	12.2	392	16.0	38.6	19.3	2.0
Extravaganzza, Classic Crust, Large, Domino's Pizza*	1 Slice/104g	252	10.7	242	13.7	23.4	10.3	1.9
Extravaganzza, Classic Crust, Med, Domino's Pizza*	1 Slice/95g	230	9.8	242	13.7	23.4	10.3	1.9
Extravaganzza, Classic Crust, Small, Domino's Pizza*	1 Slice/86g	209	8.9	242	13.7	23.4	10.3	1.9
Extravaganzza, Dbl Decadence, Med, Domino's Pizza*	1 Slice/114g	328	17.7	287	13.1	23.7	15.5	2.1
Extravaganzza, Dominator, Large, Domino's Pizza*	1 Slice/127g	337	14.1	266	13.3	28.2	11.1	1.9
Extravaganzza, Personal, Domino's Pizza*	1 Slice/75g	195	7.8	262	15.2	26.7	10.4	1.9
Extravaganzza, Thin Crust, Large, Domino's Pizza*	1 Slice/84g	235	12.8	280	15.0	20.7	15.2	2.2
Extravaganzza, Thin Crust, Medium, Domino's Pizza*	1 Slice/78g	227	12.1	291	15.1	22.6	15.5	2.1
Farmhouse, Classic Crust, Large, Domino's Pizza*	1 Slice/88g	195	6.0	222	13.4	26.8	6.8	2.1
Farmhouse, Classic Crust, Medium, Domino's Pizza*	1 Slice/81g	180	5.5	222	13.4	26.8	6.8	2.1
Farmhouse, Classic Crust, Small, Domino's Pizza*	1 Slice/73g	162	5.0	222	13.4	26.8	6.8	2.1
Farmhouse, Dominator, Large, Domino's Pizza*	1 Slice/111g	283	9.4	255	13.0	31.7	8.5	2.0
Farmhouse, Double Decadence, Med, Domino's Pizza*	1 Slice/100g	277	13.4	277	12.7	26.5	13.4	2.3
Farmhouse, Personal, Domino's Pizza*	1 Slice/62g	151	4.0	244	14.8	31.5	6.5	2.1
Farmhouse, Thin Crust, Large, Domino's Pizza*	1 Slice/68g	180	8.1	265	14.8	24.6	11.9	2.5
Farmhouse, Thin Crust, Medium, Domino's Pizza*	1 Slice/63g	175	7.7	277	15.1	26.9	12.2	2.4
Firenze, Thin Crust, Fresh, Large, Domino's Pizza*	1 Slice/60g	193	8.6	323	15.3	32.0	14.4	1.7
Firenze, Thin Crust, Fresh, Medium, Domino's Pizza*	1 Slice/53g	172	7.7	323	15.3	32.0	14.4	1.7
Firenze, Thin Crust, Fresh, Small, Domino's Pizza*	1 Slice/46g	149	6.6	323	15.3	32.0	14.4	1.7
Florentine, Thin Crust, Fresh, Large, Domino's Pizza*	1 Slice/55g	152	5.5	277	12.6	33.3	10.0	1.7
Florentine, Thin Crust, Fresh, Medium, Domino's Pizza*	1 Slice/48g	133	4.8	277	12.6	33.3	10.0	1.7
Florentine, Thin Crust, Small, Fresh, Domino's Pizza*	1 Slice/41g	114	4.1	277	12.6	33.3	10.0	1.7
Four Seasons, Thin Crust, Fresh, Lge, Domino's Pizza*	1 Slice/71g	195	7.0	274	14.1	31.5	9.8	1.9
Four Seasons, Thin Crust, Fresh, Med, Domino's Pizza*	1 Slice/50g	137	4.9	274	14.1	31.5	9.8	1.9
Four Seasons, Thin Crust, Fresh, Sm, Domino's Pizza*	1 Slice/63g	173	6.2	274	14.1	31.5	9.8	1.9
Full House, Classic Crust, Large, Domino's Pizza*	1 Slice/111g	268	9.9	241	13.2	27.0	8.9	2.1
Full House, Classic Crust, Medium, Domino's Pizza*	1 Slice/102g	241	9.1	236	13.0	26.0	8.9	2.0
Full House, Classic Crust, Small, Domino's Pizza*	1 Slice/94g	227	8.6	242	13.5	26.3	9.2	2.1
Full House, Delight Mozzarella, Porc, Domino's Pizza*	1 Slice/70g	166	5.8	238	12.4	28.6	8.3	2.1
Full House, Dominator, Large, Domino's Pizza*	1 Slice/134g	351	13.0	262	12.6	31.0	9.7	2.0

DOMINO'S PIZZA

PIZZA

	Measure INFO/WEIGHT	per Measure KCAL	FAT	Nutrition Values per 100g / 100ml KCAL	PROT	CARB	FAT	FIBRE
Full House, Double Decadence, Med, Domino's Pizza*	1 Slice/121g	346	17.8	286	12.4	25.9	14.7	2.2
Full House, Personal, Domino's Pizza*	1 Slice/70g	180	6.4	257	14.6	29.2	9.1	2.0
Full House, Thin Crust, Large, Domino's Pizza*	1 Slice/91g	251	12.6	276	14.0	23.7	13.9	2.4
Full House, Thin Crust, Medium, Domino's Pizza*	1 Slice/85g	247	12.2	290	14.3	25.9	14.3	2.3
Ham & Pineapple, Classic Crust, Lge, Domino's Pizza*	1 Slice/84g	194	5.9	231	13.7	28.5	7.0	2.0
Ham & Pineapple, Classic Crust, Med, Domino's Pizza*	1 Slice/77g	178	5.4	231	13.7	28.5	7.0	2.0
Ham & Pineapple, Classic Crust, Sm, Domino's Pizza*	1 Slice/70g	162	4.9	231	13.7	28.5	7.0	2.0
Ham & Pineapple, Dbl Dec, Med, Domino's Pizza*	1 Slice/97g	278	13.4	287	12.9	27.8	13.8	2.2
Ham & Pineapple, Del Mozz, Pers, Domino's Pizza*	1 Slice/60g	137	3.4	229	12.4	32.3	5.6	2.2
Ham & Pineapple, Dominator, Large, Domino's Pizza*	1 Slice/107g	283	9.4	265	13.2	33.3	8.8	2.0
Ham & Pineapple, Personal, Domino's Pizza*	1 Slice/60g	150	4.0	251	14.9	33.0	6.6	2.1
Ham & Pineapple, Thin Crust, Large, Domino's Pizza*	1 Slice/64g	181	8.1	283	15.4	26.8	12.7	2.5
Ham & Pineapple, Thin Crust, Medium, Domino's Pizza*	1 Slice/60g	175	7.6	292	15.4	29.0	12.7	2.3
Hawaiian, Classic Crust, Large, Domino's Pizza*	1 Slice/90g	203	6.0	226	13.4	27.9	6.7	2.0
Hawaiian, Classic Crust, Medium, Domino's Pizza*	1 Slice/82g	180	5.4	219	13.1	26.8	6.6	2.0
Hawaiian, Classic Crust, Small, Domino's Pizza*	1 Slice/75g	168	5.0	224	13.7	27.2	6.7	2.1
Hawaiian, Del Mozzarella, Classic, Sm, Domino's Pizza*	1 Slice/79g	173	4.2	220	15.2	27.7	5.4	2.2
Hawaiian, Delight Mozzarella, Pers, Domino's Pizza*	1 Slice/66g	145	3.6	219	12.0	30.7	5.4	2.1
Hawaiian, Dominator, Large, Domino's Pizza*	1 Slice/113g	285	9.5	252	12.7	31.6	8.4	2.0
Hawaiian, Double Decadence, Med, Domino's Pizza*	1 Slice/101g	277	13.3	274	12.5	26.6	13.2	2.2
Hawaiian, Personal, Domino's Pizza*	1 Slice/63g	152	4.0	240	14.4	31.3	6.3	2.0
Hawaiian, Thin Crust, Large, Domino's Pizza*	1 Slice/70g	182	8.1	260	14.4	24.6	11.6	2.4
Hawaiian, Thin Crust, Medium, Domino's Pizza*	1 Slice/65g	177	7.7	273	14.6	26.9	11.9	2.3
Hot & Spicy, Classic Crust, Large, Domino's Pizza*	1 Slice/85g	202	6.5	238	12.7	29.5	7.7	2.3
Hot & Spicy, Classic Crust, Medium, Domino's Pizza*	1 Slice/77g	179	5.9	232	12.3	28.7	7.6	2.3
Hot & Spicy, Classic Crust, Small, Domino's Pizza*	1 Slice/69g	164	5.3	237	12.8	29.3	7.7	2.3
Hot & Spicy, Dominator, Large, Domino's Pizza*	1 Slice/107g	282	9.8	264	12.2	33.0	9.2	2.2
Hot & Spicy, Double Decadence, Med Domino's Pizza*	1 Slice/96g	276	13.7	288	11.8	28.0	14.3	2.4
Hot & Spicy, Personal, Domino's Pizza*	1 Slice/59g	150	4.3	254	13.9	33.3	7.2	2.3
Hot & Spicy, Thin Crust, Large, Domino's Pizza*	1 Slice/65g	182	8.6	280	9.3	26.5	13.3	2.7
Hot & Spicy, Thin Crust, Medium, Domino's Pizza*	1 Slice/60g	176	8.1	294	13.7	29.2	13.6	2.6
House Special, Classic Crust, Large, Domino's Pizza*	1 Slice/94g	232	8.8	247	15.8	23.8	9.4	1.9
House Special, Classic Crust, Medium, Domino's Pizza*	1 Slice/86g	212	8.1	247	15.8	23.8	9.4	1.9
House Special, Classic Crust, Small, Domino's Pizza*	1 Slice/77g	191	7.3	247	15.8	23.8	9.4	1.9
House Special, Personal, Domino's Pizza*	1 Slice/65g	170	5.6	262	16.6	28.4	8.6	1.9
House Special, Thin Crust, Large, Domino's Pizza*	1 Slice/75g	226	11.0	300	17.8	23.1	14.6	2.1
House Special, Thin Crust, Medium, Domino's Pizza*	1 Slice/70g	209	10.2	300	17.8	23.1	14.6	2.1
Meat Lovers, Classic Crust, Large, Domino's Pizza*	1 Slice/89g	235	9.3	264	16.1	26.5	10.4	1.9
Meat Lovers, Classic Crust, Medium, Domino's Pizza*	1 Slice/81g	214	8.4	264	16.1	26.5	10.4	1.9
Meat Lovers, Classic Crust, Small, Domino's Pizza*	1 Slice/74g	195	7.7	264	16.1	26.5	10.4	1.9
Meat Lovers, Dbl Decadence, Med, Domino's Pizza*	1 Slice/101g	314	16.5	311	14.9	26.3	16.3	2.1
Meat Lovers, Dominator, Large, Domino's Pizza*	1 Slice/111g	320	12.6	288	15.1	31.4	11.3	1.9
Meat Lovers, Personal, Domino's Pizza*	1 Slice/61g	171	5.7	280	16.8	31.8	9.4	2.0
Meat Lovers, Thin Crust, Large, Domino's Pizza*	1 Slice/69g	219	11.4	318	18.3	24.2	16.5	2.3
Meat Lovers, Thin Crust, Medium, Domino's Pizza*	1 Slice/64g	211	10.7	330	18.5	26.5	16.7	2.2
Meatilicious, Stuffed Crust, Large, Domino's Pizza*	1 Slice/82g	235	9.4	286	16.1	28.5	11.5	1.9
Meatilicious, Stuffed Crust, Medium, Domino's Pizza*	1 Slice/76g	217	8.7	286	16.1	28.5	11.5	1.9
Meatzza, Classic Crust, Large, Domino's Pizza*	1 Slice/87g	241	10.5	277	15.7	25.5	12.1	1.9
Meatzza, Classic Crust, Medium, Domino's Pizza*	1 Slice/81g	223	9.7	277	15.7	25.5	12.1	1.9
Meatzza, Classic Crust, Small, Domino's Pizza*	1 Slice/74g	205	9.0	277	15.7	25.5	12.1	1.9
Meatzza, Personal, Domino's Pizza*	1 Slice/59g	170	6.2	290	16.4	31.4	10.5	2.0
Meatzza, Thin Crust, Large, Domino's Pizza*	1 Slice/68g	234	12.6	343	17.7	25.2	18.5	2.1

DOMINO'S PIZZA

PIZZA

	Measure INFO/WEIGHT	per Measure KCAL	FAT	Nutrition Values per 100g / 100ml KCAL	PROT	CARB	FAT	FIBRE
Meatzza, Thin Crust, Medium, Domino's Pizza*	1 Slice/64g	221	11.9	343	17.7	25.2	18.5	2.1
Mexican Hot, Classic Crust, Large, Domino's Pizza*	1 Slice/86g	213	7.8	247	13.7	26.4	9.1	2.1
Mexican Hot, Classic Crust, Medium, Domino's Pizza*	1 Slice/79g	194	7.1	247	13.7	26.4	9.1	2.1
Mexican Hot, Classic Crust, Small, Domino's Pizza*	1 Slice/71g	175	6.4	247	13.7	26.4	9.1	2.1
Mexican Hot, Personal, Domino's Pizza*	1 Slice/59g	157	4.9	264	14.9	31.3	8.3	2.2
Mexican Hot, Thin Crust, Large, Domino's Pizza*	1 Slice/67g	206	10.0	306	15.3	26.4	14.9	2.4
Mexican Hot, Thin Crust, Medium, Domino's Pizza*	1 Slice/62g	191	9.3	306	15.3	26.4	14.9	2.4
Mighty Meaty, Classic Crust, Large, Domino's Pizza*	1 Slice/95g	243	9.7	256	15.0	26.1	10.2	2.0
Mighty Meaty, Classic Crust, Medium, Domino's Pizza*	1 Slice/87g	218	8.9	251	14.7	25.0	10.3	1.9
Mighty Meaty, Classic Crust, Small, Domino's Pizza*	1 Slice/80g	206	8.5	257	15.3	25.2	10.6	2.0
Mighty Meaty, Dbl Decadence, Lge, Domino's Pizza*	1 Slice/116g	350	18.2	302	13.7	25.3	15.7	2.1
Mighty Meaty, Dbl Decadence, Med, Domino's Pizza*	1 Slice/107g	319	16.9	298	13.8	25.1	15.8	2.1
Mighty Meaty, Del Mozz, Classic, Sm, Domino's Pizza*	1 Slice/80g	202	7.3	253	16.5	26.1	9.1	2.2
Mighty Meaty, Delight Mozzarella, Pers, Domino's Pizza*	1 Slice/66g	166	5.9	250	13.3	29.1	8.9	2.1
Mighty Meaty, Dominator, Large, Domino's Pizza*	1 Slice/118g	326	13.1	276	14.0	30.0	11.1	1.9
Mighty Meaty, Personal, Domino's Pizza*	1 Slice/66g	179	6.6	270	15.5	29.7	9.9	2.0
Mighty Meaty, Stuffed Crust, Large, Domino's Pizza*	1 Slice/100g	274	11.6	274	15.2	26.5	11.6	1.9
Mighty Meaty, Stuffed Crust, Medium, Domino's Pizza*	1 Slice/94g	258	10.9	274	15.2	26.5	11.6	1.9
Mighty Meaty, Thin Crust, Large, Domino's Pizza*	1 Slice/75g	222	11.8	296	16.2	22.6	15.7	2.3
Mighty Meaty, Thin Crust, Medium, Domino's Pizza*	1 Slice/70g	216	11.2	309	16.5	24.6	16.0	2.1
Mixed Grill, Classic Crust, Large, Domino's Pizza*	1 Slice/94g	244	10.6	259	13.5	25.0	11.2	2.0
Mixed Grill, Classic Crust, Medium, Domino's Pizza*	1 Slice/86g	224	9.7	259	13.5	25.0	11.2	2.0
Mixed Grill, Classic Crust, Small, Domino's Pizza*	1 Slice/79g	205	8.9	259	13.5	25.0	11.2	2.0
Mixed Grill, Personal, Domino's Pizza*	1 Slice/66g	182	6.9	275	14.8	29.6	10.4	2.0
Mixed Grill, Thin Crust, Large, Domino's Pizza*	1 Slice/74g	237	12.9	319	15.0	24.6	17.3	2.2
Mixed Grill, Thin Crust, Medium, Domino's Pizza*	1 Slice/70g	222	12.0	319	15.0	24.6	17.3	2.2
New Yorker, Classic Crust, Large, Domino's Pizza*	1 Slice/88g	225	8.2	257	15.5	26.7	9.4	2.0
New Yorker, Classic Crust, Medium, Domino's Pizza*	1 Slice/80g	206	7.5	257	15.5	26.7	9.4	2.0
New Yorker, Classic Crust, Small Domino's Pizza*	1 Slice/73g	188	6.9	257	15.5	26.7	9.4	2.0
New Yorker, Del Mozz, Classic, Lge, Domino's Pizza*	1 Slice/87g	225	7.1	258	17.5	27.9	8.1	2.2
New Yorker, Del Mozz, Classic, Med, Domino's Pizza*	1 Slice/80g	207	6.5	258	17.5	27.9	8.1	2.2
New Yorker, Del Mozz, Classic, Sm, Domino's Pizza*	1 Slice/73g	188	5.9	258	17.5	27.9	8.1	2.2
New Yorker, Del Mozzarella, Personal, Domino's Pizza*	1 Slice/60g	151	4.5	252	13.7	31.4	7.5	2.2
New Yorker, Personal, Domino's Pizza*	1 Slice/60g	165	5.1	275	16.3	32.1	8.5	2.0
New Yorker, Thin Crust, Large, Domino's Pizza*	1 Slice/67g	217	10.4	322	17.6	26.7	15.5	2.2
New Yorker, Thin Crust, Medium, Domino's Pizza*	1 Slice/63g	203	9.8	322	17.6	26.7	15.5	2.2
Pepperoni Passion, Classic, Med, Domino's Pizza*	1 Slice/72g	210	8.3	292	16.7	28.7	11.6	2.0
Pepperoni Passion, Classic Crust, Lge, Domino's Pizza*	1 Slice/78g	228	9.1	292	16.7	28.7	11.6	2.0
Pepperoni Passion, Classic Crust, Sm, Domino's Pizza*	1 Slice/65g	190	7.5	292	16.7	28.7	11.6	2.0
Pepperoni Passion, Dbl Dec, Med, Domino's Pizza*	1 Slice/91g	302	16.0	332	15.2	26.9	17.6	2.1
Pepperoni Passion, Dominator, Large, Domino's Pizza*	1 Slice/93g	310	16.4	332	15.2	26.9	17.6	2.1
Pepperoni Passion, Personal, Domino's Pizza*	1 Slice/59g	182	7.0	307	17.9	30.8	11.8	1.9
Pepperoni Passion, Stuff Crust, Med, Domino's Pizza*	1 Slice/96g	293	12.5	305	16.9	29.0	13.0	1.9
Pepperoni Passion, Stuffed Crust, Lge, Domino's Pizza*	1 Slice/100g	305	13.0	305	16.9	29.0	13.0	1.9
Pepperoni Passion, Thin Crust, Large, Domino's Pizza*	1 Slice/58g	210	10.9	362	19.0	27.5	18.8	2.2
Pepperoni Passion, Thin Crust, Med, Domino's Pizza*	1 Slice/55g	199	10.3	362	19.0	27.5	18.8	2.2
Rustica, Thin Crust, Fresh, Large, Domino's Pizza*	1 Slice/57g	164	5.0	287	15.4	35.7	8.8	2.1
Rustica, Thin Crust, Fresh, Medium, Domino's Pizza*	1 Slice/50g	144	4.4	287	15.4	35.7	8.8	2.1
Rustica, Thin Crust, Fresh, Small, Domino's Pizza*	1 Slice/43g	124	3.8	287	15.4	35.7	8.8	2.1
Scrummy, Classic Crust, Large, Domino's Pizza*	1 Slice/92g	253	11.4	275	17.0	22.8	12.4	1.7
Scrummy, Classic Crust, Medium, Domino's Pizza*	1 Slice/85g	233	10.5	275	17.0	22.8	12.4	1.7
Scrummy, Classic Crust, Small, Domino's Pizza*	1 Slice/77g	213	9.6	275	17.0	22.8	12.4	1.7

DOMINO'S PIZZA

PIZZA

	Measure INFO/WEIGHT	per Measure KCAL	FAT	Nutrition Values per 100g / 100ml KCAL	PROT	CARB	FAT	FIBRE
Scrummy, Personal, Domino's Pizza*	1 Slice/69g	198	7.6	288	17.7	28.1	11.1	1.8
Scrummy, Thin Crust, Large, Domino's Pizza*	1 Slice/72g	237	12.9	328	19.1	21.9	17.8	1.9
Scrummy, Thin Crust, Medium, Domino's Pizza*	1 Slice/68g	222	12.0	328	19.1	21.9	17.8	1.9
Tandoori Hot, Classic Crust, Large, Domino's Pizza*	1 Slice/89g	198	5.6	223	13.4	28.1	6.3	2.2
Tandoori Hot, Classic Crust, Medium, Domino's Pizza*	1 Slice/81g	176	5.0	217	13.0	27.2	6.2	2.2
Tandoori Hot, Classic Crust, Small, Domino's Pizza*	1 Slice/73g	162	4.6	222	13.5	27.9	6.3	2.3
Tandoori Hot, Dbl Decadence, Med, Domino's Pizza*	1 Slice/101g	276	13.0	273	12.4	26.9	12.9	2.3
Tandoori Hot, Del Mozz, Classic, Sm, Domino's Pizza*	1 Slice/73g	159	3.6	218	15.0	28.4	4.9	2.4
Tandoori Hot, Delight Mozzarella, Pers, Domino's Pizza*	1 Slice/62g	135	3.1	218	12.1	31.2	5.0	2.3
Tandoori Hot, Dominator, Large, Domino's Pizza*	1 Slice/112g	280	9.0	250	12.7	31.8	8.0	2.1
Tandoori Hot, Personal, Domino's Pizza*	1 Slice/62g	149	3.7	240	14.5	31.9	6.0	2.2
Tandoori Hot, Thin Crust, Large, Domino's Pizza*	1 Slice/69g	177	7.6	257	14.3	24.9	11.1	2.6
Tandoori Hot, Thin Crust, Medium, Domino's Pizza*	1 Slice/64g	173	7.3	270	14.5	27.4	11.4	2.5
Texas BBQ, Classic Crust, Large, Domino's Pizza*	1 Slice/87g	240	7.0	276	14.4	36.6	8.0	1.8
Texas BBQ, Classic Crust, Medium, Domino's Pizza*	1 Slice/79g	218	6.3	276	14.4	36.6	8.0	1.8
Texas BBQ, Classic Crust, Small, Domino's Pizza*	1 Slice/71g	196	5.7	276	14.4	36.6	8.0	1.8
Texas BBQ, Delight Mozzarella, Pers, Domino's Pizza*	1 Slice/61g	156	3.4	256	14.2	36.4	5.5	1.9
Texas BBQ, Dominator, Large, Domino's Pizza*	1 Slice/104g	293	9.5	283	12.9	37.3	9.2	1.8
Texas BBQ, Personal, Domino's Pizza*	1 Slice/61g	171	4.0	280	18.4	35.6	6.6	2.5
Texas BBQ, Stuffed Crust, Large, Domino's Pizza*	1 Slice/97g	252	8.8	261	15.3	28.6	9.1	2.0
Texas BBQ, Stuffed Crust, Medium, Domino's Pizza*	1 Slice/90g	234	8.2	261	15.3	28.6	9.1	2.0
Texas BBQ, Thin Crust, Large, Domino's Pizza*	1 Slice/63g	183	7.3	289	15.3	30.8	11.6	1.7
Texas BBQ, Thin Crust, Medium, Domino's Pizza*	1 Slice/59g	206	8.0	351	15.6	40.3	13.7	2.1
The Sizzler, Classic Crust, Large, Domino's Pizza*	1 Slice/95g	271	10.6	285	14.7	31.5	11.2	2.2
The Sizzler, Classic Crust, Medium, Domino's Pizza*	1 Slice/87g	248	9.7	285	14.7	31.5	11.2	2.2
The Sizzler, Classic Crust, Small, Domino's Pizza*	1 Slice/78g	222	8.7	285	14.7	31.5	11.2	2.2
The Sizzler, Dominator, Large, Domino's Pizza*	1 Slice/118g	346	13.5	293	13.7	34.1	11.4	2.1
The Sizzler, Double Decadence, Med, Domino's Pizza*	1 Slice/106g	334	17.0	315	13.5	29.3	16.0	2.3
The Sizzler, Personal, Domino's Pizza*	1 Slice/65g	177	5.7	271	15.6	32.6	8.7	2.4
The Sizzler, Thin Crust, Large, Domino's Pizza*	1 Slice/75g	227	10.9	303	14.7	28.4	14.5	2.2
The Sizzler, Thin Crust, Medium, Domino's Pizza*	1 Slice/70g	243	12.0	347	16.1	32.1	17.1	2.4
Tuna Delight, Classic Crust, Large, Domino's Pizza*	1 Slice/85g	203	5.9	238	13.1	29.6	6.9	2.2
Tuna Delight, Classic Crust, Medium, Domino's Pizza*	1 Slice/77g	184	5.3	238	13.1	29.6	6.9	2.2
Tuna Delight, Classic Crust, Small, Domino's Pizza*	1 Slice/69g	164	4.8	238	13.1	29.6	6.9	2.2
Tuna Delight, Personal, Domino's Pizza*	1 Slice/60g	155	3.9	259	14.5	34.1	6.6	2.2
Tuna Delight, Thin Crust, Large, Domino's Pizza*	1 Slice/65g	197	8.3	301	14.7	30.5	12.7	2.6
Tuna Delight, Thin Crust, Medium, Domino's Pizza*	1 Slice/60g	181	7.6	301	14.7	30.5	12.7	2.6
Veg-A-Roma, Classic Crust, Large, Domino's Pizza*	1 Slice/86g	240	8.9	279	12.3	34.3	10.4	2.4
Veg-A-Roma, Classic Crust, Medium, Domino's Pizza*	1 Slice/78g	218	8.1	279	12.3	34.3	10.4	2.4
Veg-A-Roma, Classic Crust, Small, Domino's Pizza*	1 Slice/70g	195	7.3	279	12.3	34.3	10.4	2.4
Veg-A-Roma, Del Mozz, Classic, Sm, Domino's Pizza*	1 Slice/70g	153	4.7	219	10.4	29.3	6.7	2.4
Veg-A-Roma, Delight Mozzarella, Pers, Domino's Pizza*	1 Slice/61g	143	4.1	237	11.2	33.2	6.7	2.0
Veg-A-Roma, Personal, Domino's Pizza*	1 Slice/60g	160	4.8	265	13.7	34.7	8.0	2.5
Veg-A-Roma, Thin Crust, Large, Domino's Pizza*	1 Slice/66g	180	7.8	273	12.5	29.2	11.8	2.8
Veg-A-Roma, Thin Crust, Medium, Domino's Pizza*	1 Slice/61g	167	7.2	273	12.5	29.2	11.8	2.8
Vegetarian Supreme, Classic, Lge, Domino's Pizza*	1 Slice/88g	192	5.5	218	11.5	29.1	6.3	2.3
Vegetarian Supreme, Classic, Med, Domino's Pizza*	1 Slice/80g	170	4.9	213	11.0	28.3	6.1	2.3
Vegetarian Supreme, Classic, Sm, Domino's Pizza*	1 Slice/72g	156	4.5	217	11.5	28.9	6.2	2.3
Vegetarian Supreme, Dbl Dec, Lge, Domino's Pizza*	1 Slice/96g	259	12.5	270	10.8	27.7	13.0	2.4
Vegetarian Supreme, Dbl Dec, Med, Domino's Pizza*	1 Slice/99g	267	12.9	270	10.8	27.7	13.0	2.4
Vegetarian Supreme, Del Mozz, Pers, Domino's Pizza*	1 Slice/61g	131	3.1	214	10.3	32.2	5.0	2.4
Vegetarian Supreme, Dominator, Lge, Domino's Pizza*	1 Slice/111g	274	8.9	247	11.2	32.6	8.0	2.2

	Measure INFO/WEIGHT	per Measure KCAL	FAT	Nutrition Values per 100g / 100ml KCAL	PROT	CARB	FAT	FIBRE

DOMINO'S PIZZA
PIZZA

	Measure INFO/WEIGHT	KCAL	FAT	KCAL	PROT	CARB	FAT	FIBRE
Vegetarian Supreme, Personal, Domino's Pizza*	1 Slice/61g	144	3.7	236	12.7	32.8	6.0	2.2
Vegetarian Supreme, Stuffed, Lge, Domino's Pizza*	1 Slice/93g	223	7.3	240	11.9	29.3	7.9	2.2
Vegetarian Supreme, Stuffed, Med, Domino's Pizza*	1 Slice/86g	206	6.8	240	11.9	29.3	7.9	2.2
Vegetarian Supreme, Thin Crust, Lge, Domino's Pizza*	1 Slice/68g	171	7.5	252	11.8	26.1	11.1	2.7
Vegetarian Supreme, Thin Crust, Med, Domino's Pizza*	1 Slice/63g	168	7.3	266	12.0	28.7	11.5	2.6
Vegi Lite, Classic Crust, Large, Domino's Pizza*	1 Slice/80g	177	5.1	220	11.4	28.2	6.3	2.3
Vegi Lite, Classic Crust, Medium, Domino's Pizza*	1 Slice/73g	160	4.6	220	11.4	28.2	6.3	2.3
Vegi Lite, Classic Crust, Small, Domino's Pizza*	1 Slice/65g	143	4.1	220	11.4	28.2	6.3	2.3
Vegi Lite, Personal, Domino's Pizza*	1 Slice/56g	137	3.4	243	13.0	32.8	6.1	2.3
Vegi Lite, Thin Crust, Large, Domino's Pizza*	1 Slice/62g	171	7.3	277	12.5	28.6	11.9	2.7
Vegi Lite, Thin Crust, Medium, Domino's Pizza*	1 Slice/57g	157	6.7	277	12.5	28.6	11.9	2.7
Vegi Volcano, Classic Crust, Large, Domino's Pizza*	1 Slice/91g	202	6.7	222	12.2	26.5	7.4	2.2
Vegi Volcano, Classic Crust, Medium, Domino's Pizza*	1 Slice/83g	184	6.1	222	12.2	26.5	7.4	2.2
Vegi Volcano, Classic Crust, Small, Domino's Pizza*	1 Slice/75g	167	5.6	222	12.2	26.5	7.4	2.2
Vegi Volcano, Dbl Decadence, Med, Domino's Pizza*	1 Slice/102g	282	14.0	276	11.7	26.3	13.7	2.3
Vegi Volcano, Del Mozz, Classic, Sm, Domino's Pizza*	1 Slice/75g	167	4.6	223	14.2	27.7	6.2	2.4
Vegi Volcano, Del Mozzarella, Pers, Domino's Pizza*	1 Slice/64g	141	3.9	222	11.3	30.4	6.1	2.3
Vegi Volcano, Dominator, Large, Domino's Pizza*	1 Slice/114g	288	10.2	253	12.1	31.1	9.0	2.1
Vegi Volcano, Personal, Domino's Pizza*	1 Slice/63g	154	4.5	243	13.7	31.0	7.1	2.2
Vegi Volcano, Thin Crust, Large, Domino's Pizza*	1 Slice/72g	189	9.0	262	13.3	23.9	12.5	2.6
Vegi Volcano, Thin Crust, Medium, Domino's Pizza*	1 Slice/66g	182	8.5	275	13.5	26.5	12.8	2.5

EAT
BAGEL

	Measure INFO/WEIGHT	KCAL	FAT	KCAL	PROT	CARB	FAT	FIBRE
Salmon & Cream Cheese, Large, EAT*	1 Serving/186g	399	12.7	214	13.3	26.0	6.8	1.2

BAGUETTE

	Measure INFO/WEIGHT	KCAL	FAT	KCAL	PROT	CARB	FAT	FIBRE
Egg & Bacon, Half, EAT*	1 Serving/112g	311	12.2	278	13.5	30.5	10.9	1.8
Egg & Tomato, EAT*	1 Serving/140g	304	12.2	217	9.0	24.8	8.7	1.7
Ham & Jarlsberg, Half, EAT*	1 Serving/123g	297	13.3	242	14.5	21.8	10.8	1.5

BREAKFAST CEREAL

	Measure INFO/WEIGHT	KCAL	FAT	KCAL	PROT	CARB	FAT	FIBRE
Grapenuts, Banana & Honey, EAT*	1 Serving/228g	349	6.4	153	6.3	25.4	2.8	1.5
Muesli, Apple, Almond & Cinnamon, Bircher, EAT*	1 Serving/210g	361	12.2	172	6.1	23.3	5.8	2.3
Muesli, Swiss, Bircher, EAT*	1 Serving/205g	246	3.1	120	4.7	21.7	1.5	2.0
Porridge, Plain, Big, EAT*	1 Serving/280g	227	3.4	81	4.4	13.3	1.2	1.2
Porridge, Plain, Small, EAT*	1 Serving/180g	146	2.2	81	4.4	13.3	1.2	1.2
Porridge, Plain, Super, Small, EAT*	1 Serving/219g	136	3.5	62	2.4	9.0	1.6	1.8
Porridge, with Apple & Blackberry, Compote, Big, EAT*	1 Serving/331g	291	3.6	88	3.9	16.0	1.1	1.5
Porridge, with Apple & Blackberry, Compote, Sm, EAT*	1 Serving/231g	210	2.3	91	3.6	17.2	1.0	1.7
Porridge, with Banana, Big, EAT*	1 Serving/301g	247	3.3	82	4.2	13.9	1.1	1.3
Porridge, with Banana, Small, EAT*	1 Serving/200g	166	2.2	83	4.1	14.2	1.1	1.3
Porridge, with Banana, Super, Big, EAT*	1 Serving/350g	224	5.2	64	2.3	9.8	1.5	1.8
Porridge, with Banana, Super, Small, EAT*	1 Serving/240g	156	3.6	65	2.3	10.1	1.5	1.9
Porridge, with Banana & Maple Syrup, Big, EAT*	1 Serving/315g	287	3.5	91	4.0	16.4	1.1	1.2
Porridge, with Banana & Maple Syrup, Small, EAT*	1 Serving/215g	206	2.4	96	3.8	17.8	1.1	1.2
Porridge, with Banana & Maple Syrup, Super, Big, EAT*	1 Serving/364g	266	5.5	73	2.2	12.0	1.5	1.8
Porridge, with Banana & Maple Syrup, Super, Sm, EAT*	1 Serving/254g	196	3.6	77	5.6	13.4	1.4	1.7
Porridge, with Berry Compote, Super, Big, EAT*	1 Serving/330g	284	3.3	86	3.8	15.5	1.0	1.2
Porridge, with Berry Compote, Super, Small, EAT*	1 Serving/30g	205	2.3	89	3.6	16.4	1.0	1.2
Porridge, with Maple Syrup, Big, EAT*	1 Serving/296g	266	3.5	90	4.2	16.0	1.2	1.1
Porridge, with Maple Syrup, Small, EAT*	1 Serving/195g	185	2.1	95	4.1	17.3	1.1	1.1
Porridge, with Maple Syrup, Super, EAT*	1 Serving/344g	244	5.5	71	2.3	11.4	1.6	1.7

EAT

	Measure INFO/WEIGHT	per Measure KCAL	FAT	Nutrition Values per 100g / 100ml KCAL	PROT	CARB	FAT	FIBRE
BRIOCHE								
Fruited without Butter, Toasted, EAT*	1 Serving/120g	414	13.4	345	7.3	50.2	11.2	2.2
CAKE								
Banana Toffee & Pecan, EAT*	1 Serving/79g	247	10.8	313	3.3	45.1	13.7	0.9
COFFEE								
Cappuccino, Skimmed Milk, EAT*	1 Tall/12oz	118	4.0	33	2.4	3.4	1.1	0.0
Cappuccino, Soya Milk, EAT*	1 Tall/12oz	131	4.9	37	3.2	3.5	1.4	0.9
Cappuccino, Whole Milk, EAT*	1 Tall/12oz	168	9.1	47	2.4	3.4	2.6	0.0
Espresso, Macchiato, Skimmed Milk, EAT*	1 Espresso/4oz	8	0.3	7	0.5	0.6	0.3	0.0
Espresso, Macchiato, Soya Milk, EAT*	1 Espresso/4oz	9	0.4	8	0.6	0.7	0.3	0.2
Espresso, Macchiato, Whole Milk, EAT*	1 Espresso/4oz	11	0.6	9	0.5	0.6	0.5	0.0
Latte, Chai, Skimmed Milk, EAT*	1 Tall/12oz	305	1.0	86	3.2	17.7	0.3	0.0
Latte, Chai, Soya Milk, EAT*	1 Tall/12oz	279	5.3	79	2.4	13.9	1.5	0.5
Latte, Chai, Whole Milk, EAT*	1 Tall/12oz	408	12.9	115	3.1	17.5	3.6	0.0
Latte, Chiller, Skimmed Milk, EAT*	1 Tall/12oz	241	3.3	68	3.1	11.9	0.9	0.0
Latte, Chiller, Whole Milk, EAT*	1 Tall/12oz	412	14.8	116	1.8	17.7	4.2	0.2
Latte, Iced, Skimmed Milk, EAT*	1 Tall/12oz	95	3.2	27	1.9	2.7	0.9	0.0
Latte, Iced, Soya Milk, EAT*	1 Tall/12oz	105	3.9	30	2.5	2.8	1.1	0.7
Latte, Matcha, Skimmed Milk, EAT*	1 Tall/12oz	204	1.0	57	3.0	10.6	0.3	0.3
Latte, Matcha, Soya Milk, EAT*	1 Tall/12oz	201	5.8	57	3.0	7.4	1.6	0.3
Latte, Matcha, Whole Milk, EAT*	1 Tall/12oz	297	11.8	84	3.0	10.4	3.3	0.3
Latte, Skimmed Milk, EAT*	1 Tall/12oz	142	4.8	42	3.0	4.2	1.4	0.0
Latte, Soya Milk, EAT*	1 Tall/12oz	157	5.9	46	4.0	4.3	1.7	1.1
Latte, Whole Milk, EAT*	1 Tall/12oz	202	10.9	59	3.0	4.2	3.2	0.0
Matcha, Chiller, Whole Milk, EAT*	1 Tall/12oz	418	14.9	118	1.9	18.2	4.2	0.3
Mocha, Chiller, Skimmed Milk, EAT*	1 Tall/12oz	243	3.4	68	2.5	12.6	0.9	0.0
Mocha, Chiller, Whole Milk, EAT*	1 Tall/12oz	283	7.5	80	2.5	12.6	2.1	0.0
Mocha, Skimmed Milk, EAT*	1 Tall/12oz	157	5.0	44	3.0	4.8	1.4	0.0
Mocha, Soya Milk, EAT*	1 Tall/12oz	173	6.1	49	4.0	5.0	1.7	1.2
Mocha, Whole Milk, EAT*	1 Tall/12oz	219	11.4	62	3.0	4.8	3.2	0.0
White, Flat, Skimmed Milk, EAT*	1 Tall/341ml	87	0.3	26	2.5	3.7	0.1	0.0
White, Flat, Soya Milk, EAT*	1 Tall/341ml	147	4.8	43	5.1	2.3	1.4	0.4
CROISSANT								
Almond, EAT*	1 Serving/83g	350	19.8	422	10.0	41.7	23.9	2.9
Chocolate, EAT*	1 Serving/81g	361	21.3	445	6.9	45.4	26.2	3.0
EAT*	1 Serving/71g	305	17.1	427	9.4	43.4	23.9	2.7
Ham & Jarlsberg, EAT*	1 Serving/128g	339	21.1	265	15.6	20.8	16.5	0.0
Tomato & Jarlsberg, EAT*	1 Serving/123g	291	19.1	236	9.0	22.6	15.5	0.4
DANISH PASTRY								
Maple Pecan, Plait, EAT*	1 Serving/83g	377	26.0	454	4.7	38.4	31.3	5.2
DESSERTS								
Cherries, Bag, EAT*	1 Serving/125g	55	0.1	44	0.8	9.0	0.1	1.8
JUICE DRINK								
Mango & Lime, Blast, EAT*	1 Tall/12oz	253	0.3	71	0.3	17.7	0.1	0.1
Peach & Mint, Blast, EAT*	1 Tall/12oz	216	0.2	61	0.2	15.1	0.1	0.0
Wild Berry, Blast, EAT*	1 Tall/12oz	330	0.2	93	0.2	23.5	0.1	0.5
MUFFIN								
Bacon Butty, Hot Toasted, EAT*	1 Serving/90g	291	10.9	324	17.1	36.1	12.1	0.8
Bacon Butty, Toasted, Hot, Large, EAT*	1 Serving/190g	589	18.4	310	15.4	39.7	9.7	0.9
Blueberry, Low Fat, EAT*	1 Serving/124g	324	3.8	261	5.5	51.6	3.1	2.2
Breakfast, Full English, EAT*	1 Serving/295g	687	24.5	233	10.7	28.4	8.3	0.7
Chocolate, Belgian, EAT*	1 Serving/124g	511	26.4	412	5.0	48.9	21.3	2.1
Egg, Mushroom & Cheddar, Hot Toasted, EAT*	1 Serving/125g	240	6.9	192	9.1	26.2	5.5	1.0

EAT

	Measure INFO/WEIGHT	per Measure KCAL	FAT	Nutrition Values per 100g / 100ml KCAL	PROT	CARB	FAT	FIBRE
MUFFIN								
Eggs Benedict, Hot Toasted, EAT*	1 Serving/120g	265	8.9	220	10.2	27.6	7.4	0.8
Salmon & Egg, Hot Toasted, EAT*	1 Serving/126g	325	10.0	258	11.8	37.1	7.9	1.5
Sunshine, EAT*	1 Serving/124g	498	25.1	402	5.7	47.2	20.3	3.8
PAIN AU CHOCOLATE								
EAT*	1 Serving/78g	329	18.4	422	9.8	42.6	23.6	3.6
PASTRY								
Cheese Twist, EAT*	1 Serving/74g	313	19.0	421	14.0	33.7	25.6	2.2
PIES								
Beef & Stilton, Pie Only, EAT*	1 Pie/270g	629	31.6	233	10.2	21.1	11.7	1.6
Beef & Stilton, with Mash & Gravy, EAT*	1 Pie/560g	885	40.3	158	5.9	15.9	7.2	1.9
Cheese & Onion, Pie Only, EAT*	1 Pie/270g	724	43.5	268	8.6	21.3	16.1	2.2
Cheese & Onion, with Mash & Gravy, EAT*	1 Pie/560g	980	52.6	175	5.1	16.0	9.4	2.2
Chicken & Mushroom, Pie Only, EAT*	1 Pie/270g	597	29.4	221	9.3	20.5	10.9	1.8
Chicken & Mushroom, with Mash & Gravy, EAT*	1 Pie/560g	851	38.6	152	5.4	15.6	6.9	2.0
Goats Cheese & Sweet Potato, Mash & Gravy, EAT*	1 Pie/560g	946	45.9	169	4.1	18.4	8.2	2.0
Goats Cheese & Sweet Potato, Pie Only, EAT*	1 Pie/270g	694	36.7	257	6.6	26.2	13.6	1.9
Steak & Ale, Pie Only, EAT*	1 Pie/270g	643	30.8	238	9.1	24.4	11.4	0.1
Steak & Ale, with Mash & Gravy, EAT*	1 Pie/560g	896	39.8	160	5.3	17.5	7.1	1.1
SALAD								
Beef, Thai, Spicy, with Dressing, EAT*	1 Serving/167g	174	6.0	104	10.0	8.0	3.6	1.4
Beef, Thai, Spicy, without Dressing, EAT*	1 Serving/142g	129	4.8	91	11.3	3.1	3.4	1.5
Chicken, Smoked, & Watercress, Dressing, Pot, EAT*	1 Salad/346g	516	37.7	149	6.0	6.2	10.9	1.1
Chicken, Smoked, & Watercress, No Dress, Pot, EAT*	1 Salad/316g	395	25.6	125	6.5	6.0	8.1	1.2
Chicken, Tandoori, Mango & Rice, no Dressing, EAT*	1 Serving/186g	227	3.9	122	8.7	16.5	2.1	1.7
Chicken, Tandoori, Mango & Rice, with Dressing, EAT*	1 Serving/206g	251	5.6	122	8.3	15.6	2.7	1.6
Ham, Summer, & Potato, with Dressing, EAT*	1 Serving/331g	480	36.7	145	6.0	4.9	11.1	0.8
Ham, Summer, & Potato, without Dressing, EAT*	1 Serving/303g	370	26.4	122	6.4	4.3	8.7	0.9
Houmous & Falafel Mezze, EAT*	1 Box/415g	577	28.6	139	4.6	15.0	6.9	3.9
Mexican Bean, Less Than 5% Fat, Veggie, Pot, EAT*	1 Salad/172g	192	4.0	111	5.2	17.1	2.3	4.1
Mezze, with Dressing, EAT*	1 Serving/306g	425	26.6	139	3.6	12.0	8.7	2.7
Mezze, without Dressing, EAT*	1 Serving/286g	349	20.3	122	3.8	11.0	7.1	2.9
Noodle, Chicken, Spicy, Less Than 5% Fat, EAT*	1 Serving/314g	406	8.8	129	8.9	16.2	2.8	1.6
Noodles, Crayfish, Spicy, Less Than 5% Fat, EAT*	1 Serving/285g	351	8.0	123	6.6	17.5	2.8	1.6
Pea & Mint, No Dressing, Pot, EAT*	1 Salad/106g	98	2.6	92	6.8	7.4	2.4	3.0
Pea & Mint, with Dressing, Pot, EAT*	1 Salad/125g	171	9.8	136	5.9	7.5	7.8	2.7
Prawn Cocktail, Pot, EAT*	1 Salad/129g	218	17.2	169	9.9	2.1	13.3	0.6
Prawn Cocktail, Side, EAT*	1 Serving/163g	346	29.5	212	9.6	2.4	18.1	0.7
Rainbow Superfood, with Dressing, EAT*	1 Serving/340g	520	24.8	153	5.4	15.2	7.3	2.6
Rainbow Superfood, without Dressing, EAT*	1 Serving/340g	439	16.0	129	5.9	14.2	4.7	2.8
SANDWICH								
Bacon, Lettuce & Tomato, EAT*	1 Pack/204g	479	25.1	235	11.1	19.9	12.3	1.7
Beef & Rocket, Baguette, EAT*	1 Baguette/228g	556	18.2	244	13.2	29.2	8.0	1.8
Chicken, Avocado & Basil, EAT*	1 Pack/233g	452	24.0	194	10.3	17.9	10.3	2.7
Chicken, Salad, Simple, Less Than 5% Fat, EAT*	1 Pack/203g	339	8.7	167	12.1	19.2	4.3	1.7
Chicken, Smoked, Tomato & Pesto EAT*	1 Pack/262g	517	21.3	197	11.2	19.0	8.1	1.4
Chicken & Bacon, EAT*	1 Pack/229g	483	23.1	211	12.2	17.7	10.1	1.6
Chicken Banh Mi, EAT*	1 Pack/299g	532	12.3	178	8.6	25.6	4.1	1.7
Club, EAT*	1 Pack/296g	624	28.7	211	12.9	17.7	9.7	1.3
Crayfish, Lemon & Rocket, EAT*	1 Pack/198g	348	13.6	176	9.4	19.9	6.9	1.4
Egg Mayo, Free Range, & Cress, EAT*	1 Pack/183g	410	20.9	224	8.7	21.6	11.4	1.8
Egg Mayo, Free Range, & Tomato, Bloomer, EAT*	1 Pack/262g	627	38.8	239	7.3	19.1	14.8	1.5
Ham, Tomato & Mustard, EAT*	1 Pack/203g	394	17.5	194	9.8	19.3	8.6	1.6

EAT

	Measure INFO/WEIGHT	per Measure KCAL	FAT	Nutrition Values per 100g / 100ml KCAL	PROT	CARB	FAT	FIBRE
SANDWICH								
Ham Brie & Cranberry, Baguette, EAT*	1 Baguette/295g	743	33.6	252	10.5	26.4	11.4	1.4
Houmous, Avocado & Harissa, EAT*	1 Pack/228g	397	20.5	174	5.0	21.5	9.0	3.9
Pastrami, New York EAT*	1 Pack/224g	358	11.4	160	9.9	18.6	5.1	1.3
Salmon, Scottish, Smoked, & Soft Cheese, EAT*	1 Pack/173g	362	12.8	209	13.8	22.2	7.4	1.6
Sticky BBQ, Banh Mi, Baguette, EAT*	1 Roll/269g	473	2.4	176	7.9	33.1	0.9	1.8
Tuna, Skipjack, & Cucumber, Less Than 5% Fat, EAT*	1 Pack/187g	305	7.1	163	10.8	21.3	3.8	1.7
SOUP								
Bacon, Smokey, & Lentil, Small, Simple, EAT*	1 Serving/300ml	249	3.9	83	5.9	11.4	1.3	1.2
Bacon & Sweetcorn, with Garnish, Sm, Bold, EAT*	1 Serving/314g	371	25.5	118	3.0	8.7	8.1	1.1
Beef & Potato, Massaman, Garnish, Sm, Bold, EAT*	1 Serving/312g	259	11.2	83	3.7	8.4	3.6	0.9
Beef & Potato, Massaman, No Garnish, Sm, Bold, EAT*	1 Serving/300g	255	11.1	85	3.8	8.7	3.7	0.9
Carrot, Parsnip & Ginger, Small, Simple, EAT*	1 Serving/300g	150	4.2	50	1.0	7.8	1.4	1.8
Cauliflower Cheese, Small, Simple, EAT*	1 Serving/300ml	216	13.8	72	2.5	5.1	4.6	1.0
Chicken, Creamy, Small, Simple, EAT*	1 Serving/300ml	237	14.4	79	4.2	4.5	4.8	0.6
Chicken, Leek & Bacon, Risotto with Garnish, EAT*	1 Serving/370ml	359	18.9	97	4.7	8.1	5.1	0.5
Chicken, Leek & Bacon, Risotto without Garnish, EAT*	1 Serving/400ml	344	23.2	86	5.2	3.0	5.8	0.4
Chicken & Garden Vegetable, Garnish, Sm, Bold, EAT*	1 Serving/320g	131	1.6	41	4.5	4.5	0.5	0.7
Chicken Laksa, with Garnish, Small, Bold, EAT*	1 Serving/310ml	276	15.2	89	4.9	5.0	4.9	0.2
Chicken Laksa, without Garnish, Big, EAT*	1 Serving/625ml	569	31.3	91	5.0	5.1	5.0	0.1
Chicken Laksa, without Garnish, Small, Bold, EAT*	1 Serving/300g	273	15.0	91	5.0	5.1	5.0	0.1
Chicken Pho, EAT*	1 Serving/786ml	291	4.7	37	3.7	3.6	0.6	0.3
Chicken Pot Pie, with Garnish, Small, Bold, EAT*	1 Serving/330ml	343	17.8	104	4.8	9.0	5.4	1.0
Chicken Pot Pie, without Garnish, Small, Bold, EAT*	1 Serving/300g	216	9.0	72	4.6	6.8	3.0	1.0
Chilli, Chicken, Mexican, with Garnish, EAT*	1 Serving/300ml	264	7.5	88	6.1	10.2	2.5	1.4
Chilli, Chicken, Mexican, without Garnish, EAT*	1 Serving/300ml	282	8.1	94	6.5	10.8	2.7	1.4
Chorizo & Chickpea, EAT*	1 Serving/402ml	358	16.5	89	5.0	8.1	4.1	1.6
Curry, Chicken, Thai Green, with Garnish, EAT*	1 Serving/340ml	306	15.0	90	4.3	6.9	4.4	0.6
Curry, Chicken, Thai Green, without Garnish, EAT*	1 Serving/300ml	246	14.1	82	4.5	3.8	4.7	0.5
Gazpacho, EAT*	1 Serving/279ml	78	1.4	28	1.0	4.5	0.5	1.0
Goan, Potato, Small, Simple, EAT*	1 Serving/300g	246	13.2	82	2.0	6.9	4.4	1.2
Goulash, Hungarian, with Garnish, EAT*	1 Serving/403ml	314	8.5	78	7.7	7.2	2.1	0.8
Goulash, Hungarian without Garnish, EAT*	1 Serving/400ml	312	8.4	78	7.7	7.2	2.1	0.8
Ham, Pea & Mint with Garnish, EAT*	1 Serving/321ml	202	4.5	63	4.8	7.5	1.4	1.1
Ham, Pea & Mint without Garnish, EAT*	1 Serving/626ml	388	8.8	62	4.7	7.4	1.4	0.6
Hoisin, Duck Gyoza Dumpling, EAT*	1 Serving/847ml	432	7.6	51	2.3	8.4	0.9	0.5
Minestrone, with Pesto, Chunky, with Garnish, EAT*	1 Serving/300ml	189	8.7	63	1.9	6.9	2.9	1.5
Minestrone, with Pesto, Chunky, without Garnish, EAT*	1 Serving/300ml	123	1.2	41	1.8	7.3	0.4	1.5
Mushroom, Wild, & Chestnut, Small, Simple, EAT*	1 Serving/300g	240	14.1	80	1.4	8.1	4.7	1.1
Mushroom, Wild Forest, EAT*	1 Serving/300ml	150	8.7	50	2.0	3.7	2.9	0.8
Onion, French, with Garnish, EAT*	1 Serving/316ml	136	3.8	43	1.6	6.2	1.2	0.5
Onion, French without Garnish, EAT*	1 Serving/400ml	112	1.2	28	0.7	5.4	0.3	0.5
Prawn Tom Yum, EAT*	1 Serving/814ml	285	9.0	35	1.8	4.1	1.1	0.5
Red Pepper, Roast, & Goats Cheese, Sm, Simple, EAT*	1 Serving300ml	147	8.1	49	1.9	4.0	2.7	0.9
Squash, Butternut, Thai, Small, Simple, EAT*	1 Serving/300ml	168	6.6	56	1.0	6.9	2.2	1.5
Sweet Potato & Chilli, Small, Simple, EAT*	1 Serving/300ml	261	13.2	87	1.3	9.6	4.4	1.7
Tomato, Slow Roasted, Small, Simple, EAT*	1 Serving/300ml	237	18.0	79	1.3	5.0	6.0	1.2
Tomato, Spicy, & Basil, Small, Simple, EAT*	1 Serving/300ml	78	0.9	26	0.9	4.6	0.3	0.9
Vegetable, Garden, EAT*	1 Serving/300ml	165	8.7	55	0.9	6.1	2.9	1.2
Vegetable, Moroccan, Spicy, Small, Simple, EAT*	1 Serving/300ml	138	2.1	46	1.7	7.8	0.7	1.9
Vegetarian, Gyoza Dumpling, EAT*	1 Serving/798ml	431	11.2	54	2.3	7.6	1.4	0.6
TEA								
Chai Latte, Soya, EAT*	1 Cup/355ml	208	6.4	59	4.2	7.1	1.8	0.0

	Measure INFO/WEIGHT	per Measure		Nutrition Values per 100g / 100ml				
		KCAL	FAT	KCAL	PROT	CARB	FAT	FIBRE

EAT
YOGHURT
Berries, Red, Mixed, EAT*	1 Serving/124g	131	3.6	106	5.6	14.1	2.9	0.3
Brownie Sundae, Frozen, EAT*	1 Serving/176g	308	6.0	175	3.6	34.1	3.4	2.0
Frozen, with Fresh Berries, EAT*	1 Serving/200g	190	0.4	95	2.7	22.0	0.2	2.5
Granola & Mixed Red Berries, EAT*	1 Serving/180g	306	8.8	170	5.8	26.1	4.9	2.4
Mango & Passionfruit, EAT*	1 Serving/124g	145	3.6	117	5.6	17.1	2.9	0.2
Plain, Frozen, EAT*	1 Serving/140g	169	0.3	121	3.5	29.0	0.2	2.0

GREGGS
BAGUETTE
Chicken, Sweet Chilli, Greggs*	1 Baguette/237g	520	3.0	219	10.3	39.7	1.3	0.0
Chicken & Sweetcorn, Greggs*	1 Baguette/235g	480	11.0	204	10.2	29.8	4.7	0.0
Chicken Fajita, Hot, Greggs*	1 Serving/185g	440	12.0	238	12.7	32.4	6.5	0.0
Chicken Pesto, Greggs*	1 Baguette/214g	520	16.0	243	11.7	32.5	7.5	0.0
Chicken Tikka, Greggs*	1 Baguette/250g	490	10.5	196	10.2	29.0	4.2	0.0
Club, Chicken, Chargrill, Hot, Greggs*	1 Serving/167g	450	16.0	269	14.1	31.7	9.6	0.0
Club, Chicken, Greggs*	1 Baguette/265g	600	18.5	226	10.6	29.0	7.0	0.0
Ham, Honey Roast, & Mature Cheddar, Greggs*	1 Baguette/216g	580	19.0	269	14.3	32.2	8.8	0.0
Ham & Cheese, Greggs*	1 Baguette/219g	560	17.0	256	13.7	32.4	7.8	0.0
Ham & Cheese, Hot, Greggs*	1 Serving/156g	566	15.5	363	14.1	28.2	9.9	0.0
Meatball Melt, Hot, Greggs*	1 Serving/200g	440	16.0	220	12.0	24.0	8.0	0.0
Mozzarella & Tomato, Hot, Greggs*	1 Serving/154g	420	14.5	273	12.3	34.7	9.4	0.0
Prawn, Mayonnaise, Greggs*	1 Baguette/235g	500	15.0	213	8.7	4.5	6.4	0.0
Tuna, Crunch, Greggs*	1 Baguette/235g	530	12.5	226	10.6	32.5	5.3	0.0
Tuna, Crunch Melt, Hot, Greggs*	1 Serving/187g	440	13.0	235	13.4	29.9	6.9	0.0

BAKE
Chicken, Curry, Greggs*	1 Bake/131g	400	25.5	305	7.6	21.4	19.5	0.0
Chicken, Fajita Flavour, The Spicy One, Greggs*	1 Bake/138g	450	31.0	326	9.1	20.6	22.5	0.0
Chicken, Freshly Baked, Greggs*	1 Bake/138g	450	29.0	326	8.3	25.4	21.0	0.0
Sausage, & Bean Melt, Greggs*	1 Bake/140g	450	28.5	321	7.1	25.4	20.4	0.0
Steak, Freshly Baked, Greggs*	1 Bake/136g	430	27.5	316	12.1	20.6	20.2	0.0

BLOOMERS
Chicken, Bacon & Sweetcorn on Malt Brown, Greggs*	1 Bloomer/235g	520	18.0	221	11.3	26.8	7.7	0.0
Chicken, Bacon & Sweetcorn on White, Greggs*	1 Bloomer/235g	520	18.5	221	11.1	27.0	7.9	0.0
Chicken, Mango, on Malted Brown, Greggs*	1 Bloomer/217g	510	18.5	235	11.3	28.3	8.5	0.0
Chicken, Mango, on White, Greggs*	1 Bloomer/217g	510	19.5	235	11.3	26.7	9.0	0.0
Chicken, Sweet Chilli, on White, No Mayo, Greggs*	1 Bloomer/255g	460	3.0	180	10.8	31.0	1.2	0.0
Ham, Cheese & Pickle, on Malted Brown, Greggs*	1 Bloomer/228g	540	19.0	237	11.2	28.9	8.3	0.0
Ham, Cheese & Pickle, on White, Greggs*	1 Bloomer/228g	510	18.0	224	11.2	27.4	7.9	0.0
Tuna, Crunch, on Malted Brown, Greggs*	1 Bloomer/235g	520	15.0	221	11.1	28.9	6.4	0.0
Tuna, Crunch, on White, Greggs*	1 Bloomer/217g	430	13.5	198	10.8	24.6	6.2	0.0

CAKE
Belgian Bun, Greggs*	1 Bun/135g	420	5.0	311	4.8	64.1	3.7	0.0
Brownies, Chocolate, Mini, Greggs*	1 Brownie/18g	90	5.0	500	8.3	58.3	27.8	0.0
Christmas Slice, Greggs*	1 Slice/86g	360	11.5	419	5.8	67.4	13.4	0.0
Cupcake, Lemon, Sweet, Greggs*	1 Cake/81g	380	16.0	469	0.0	71.6	19.7	0.0
Doughnut, Blueberry Burst, Greggs*	1 Doughnut/96g	340	10.5	355	6.3	56.9	11.0	0.0
Doughnut, Jam Filled, Greggs*	1 Doughnut/74g	250	7.5	338	7.4	53.4	10.1	0.0
Doughnut, Lemon Drizzle, Lemon Curd Filled, Greggs*	1 Doughnut/97g	360	12.5	371	6.2	56.2	12.9	0.0
Doughnut, Strawberry Milkshake, Filled, Greggs*	1 Doughnut/91g	360	15.0	397	6.3	54.0	16.5	0.0
Doughnut, Triple Chocolate Vanilla Filled, Greggs*	1 Doughnut/91g	340	12.0	374	6.6	57.1	13.2	0.0
Finger Bun, Iced, Greggs*	1 Bun/35g	111	3.0	316	7.0	52.4	8.7	1.6
Flapjacks, Fruity, Mini, Greggs*	1 Flapjack/22g	110	5.0	500	6.8	59.1	22.7	0.0
Mince Pie, Sweet, Greggs*	1 Pie/70g	290	11.0	414	4.3	61.4	15.7	0.0

GREGGS

	Measure INFO/WEIGHT	per Measure KCAL	FAT	Nutrition Values per 100g / 100ml KCAL	PROT	CARB	FAT	FIBRE
CAKE								
Mince Pie, Sweet, Iced, Greggs*	1 Pie/63g	230	6.5	365	2.4	62.7	10.3	0.0
Muffin, Sicilian Lemon, Greggs*	1 Muffin/116g	460	23.0	397	5.2	49.1	19.8	0.0
Muffin, Triple Chocolate, Greggs*	1 Muffin/129g	530	28.5	411	5.0	46.1	22.1	0.0
Tart, Strawberry, Greggs*	1 Tart/65g	180	7.5	277	2.3	41.5	11.5	0.0
Tart, Strawberry, with Fresh Cream, Greggs*	1 Tart/94g	300	16.5	319	3.2	35.1	17.5	0.0
Yum Yum, Glazed, Greggs*	1 Yum Yum/73g	290	15.5	397	4.8	45.2	21.2	0.0
Yum Yum, Toffee Topping, Greggs*	1 Yum Yum/73g	290	16.5	397	5.5	43.1	22.6	0.0
COLD DRINKS								
Capri-Sun, Greggs*	1 Serving/330ml	143	0.0	43	0.0	10.5	0.0	0.0
Cola, Coca-Cola, Diet, Greggs*	1 Serving/330ml	2	0.0	1	0.0	0.0	0.0	0.0
Cola, Coca-Cola, Greggs*	1 Serving/330ml	139	0.0	42	0.0	10.6	0.0	0.0
Cola, Coca-Cola, Greggs*	1 Serving/500ml	210	0.0	42	0.0	10.6	0.0	0.0
Cola, Coke Zero, Greggs*	1 Serving/500ml	3	0.0	1	0.0	0.0	0.0	0.0
Dr Pepper, Greggs*	1 Serving/500ml	210	0.0	42	0.0	2.1	0.0	0.0
Fanta, Orange, Greggs*	1 Serving/500ml	150	0.0	30	0.0	7.1	0.0	0.0
Irn-Bru, Diet, Greggs*	1 Serving/330ml	2	0.0	1	0.0	0.0	0.0	0.0
Irn-Bru, Greggs*	1 Serving/330ml	145	0.0	44	0.0	10.5	0.0	0.0
Juice, Apple, Fairtrade, Greggs*	1 Serving/500ml	220	0.0	44	0.0	11.0	0.0	0.0
Juice, Orange, Fairtrade, Greggs*	1 Serving/500ml	220	0.0	44	0.1	10.2	0.0	0.0
Lucozade, Orange, Energy, Greggs*	1 Serving/500ml	350	0.0	70	0.0	17.2	0.0	0.0
Lucozade, Sport, Greggs*	1 Serving/500ml	140	0.0	28	0.0	6.4	0.0	0.0
Oasis, Citrus Punch, Greggs*	1 Serving/500ml	90	0.0	18	0.0	4.1	0.0	0.0
Oasis, Summer Fruits, Greggs*	1 Serving/500ml	90	0.0	18	0.0	4.2	0.0	0.0
Ribena, Greggs*	1 Serving/288ml	124	0.0	43	0.0	10.5	0.0	0.0
Smoothie, Mango & Orange, Greggs*	1 Serving/250ml	145	0.0	58	0.6	13.2	0.0	0.0
Smoothie, Raspberry & Banana, Greggs*	1 Serving/250ml	135	0.0	54	0.6	12.2	0.0	0.0
Sprite, Greggs*	1 Serving/500ml	220	0.0	44	0.0	10.6	0.0	0.0
Water, Cranberry or Raspberry, Greggs*	1 Serving/500ml	5	0.0	1	0.0	0.0	0.0	0.0
HOT DRINKS								
Coffee, Black, Regular, Greggs*	1 Serving/455ml	18	0.0	4	0.0	0.8	0.0	0.0
Coffee, Black, Small, Greggs*	1 Serving/340ml	17	0.0	5	0.0	0.8	0.0	0.0
Coffee, Cappuccino, No Chocolate Top, Reg, Greggs*	1 Serving/455ml	180	5.0	40	1.7	5.6	1.1	0.0
Coffee, Cappuccino, No Chocolate Top, Sm, Greggs*	1 Serving/340ml	130	3.6	38	1.3	5.9	1.1	0.0
Coffee, Espresso, Double Shot, Greggs*	1 Serving/60ml	10	0.1	17	0.0	3.3	0.2	0.0
Coffee, Latte, Regular, Greggs*	1 Serving/455ml	190	5.2	42	0.9	6.1	1.1	0.0
Coffee, Latte, Small, Greggs*	1 Serving/340ml	130	3.7	38	0.5	6.6	1.1	0.0
Coffee, White, Regular, Greggs*	1 Serving/455ml	87	2.3	19	0.4	3.3	0.5	0.0
Coffee, White, Small, Greggs*	1 Serving/340ml	68	2.0	20	0.3	3.5	0.6	0.0
Hot Chocolate, Regular, Greggs*	1 Serving/455ml	390	10.0	86	2.3	11.3	2.2	0.0
Hot Chocolate, Small, Greggs*	1 Serving/340ml	280	7.7	82	2.4	11.3	2.3	0.0
Tea, White, Large, Greggs*	1 Serving/455ml	32	1.4	7	0.4	0.5	0.3	0.0
Tea, White, Regular, Greggs*	1 Serving/340ml	20	0.0	6	0.3	0.7	0.0	0.0
PAIN AU CHOCOLAT								
with Belgian Chocolate, Greggs*	1 Pain/81g	340	18.5	420	8.6	45.1	22.8	0.0
PASTY								
Cheese & Onion, Freshly Baked, Greggs*	1 Pasty/126g	390	26.0	310	5.9	23.4	20.6	0.0
Cornish, Freshly Baked, Greggs*	1 Pasty/180g	500	31.5	278	7.2	21.9	17.5	0.0
PIZZA								
Cheese & Tomato, Freshly Baked, Greggs*	1 Pizza/106g	290	8.5	274	11.3	36.8	8.0	0.0
Chicken, Chargrill, Greggs*	1 Pizza/124g	310	9.0	250	13.7	31.8	7.3	0.0
Pepperoni, Freshly Baked, Greggs*	1 Pizza/116g	350	14.5	302	12.5	34.0	12.5	0.0

	Measure INFO/WEIGHT	per Measure KCAL	FAT	Nutrition Values per 100g / 100ml KCAL	PROT	CARB	FAT	FIBRE
GREGGS								
ROLLS								
Bacon, Breakfast, Greggs*	1 Roll/124g	320	14.5	258	10.9	26.0	11.7	0.0
Bacon & Sausage, Breakfast, Greggs*	1 Serving/174g	510	26.0	293	12.9	27.0	14.9	0.0
Sausage, Breakfast, Greggs*	1 Roll/164g	420	19.0	256	11.9	24.4	11.6	0.0
SANDWICH								
BLT, with Sweetcure Bacon on Brown, Malt, Greggs*	1 Pack/213g	550	28.0	258	8.9	24.2	13.1	0.0
Cheese & Tomato, on Brown, Malted, Greggs*	1 Pack/187g	490	23.0	262	9.9	26.7	12.3	0.0
Cheese Savoury, on White, Seeded, Greggs*	1 Pack/174g	510	24.0	293	11.2	27.0	13.8	0.0
Chicken & Sweetcorn, with Red Fat Mayo, Greggs*	1 Pack/166g	310	5.5	187	11.4	25.9	3.3	0.0
Christmas Dinner, Greggs*	1 Pack/205g	365	18.5	178	12.2	35.4	9.0	0.0
Egg Mayo, Free Range, with Black Pepper, Greggs*	1 Pack/166g	410	16.0	247	9.6	29.5	9.6	0.0
Egg Mayonnaise, Greggs*	1 Pack/166g	410	16.0	247	9.6	29.5	9.6	0.0
Egg Mayonnaise, on White, Seeded, Greggs*	1 Pack/174g	420	17.5	241	11.2	26.7	10.1	0.0
Festive Oval Bite, Greggs*	1 Sandwich/160g	410	18.0	256	13.4	23.7	11.2	0.0
Salad, Chicken, on Brown, Malted, Greggs*	1 Pack/248g	520	23.0	210	9.9	20.6	9.3	0.0
Salad, Ham, Oval Bite, Greggs*	1 Sandwich/175g	320	10.5	183	9.1	21.7	6.0	0.0
Tuna Mayo, on Brown, Malted, Greggs*	1 Pack/203g	440	13.5	217	12.3	26.6	6.6	0.0
Tuna Mayo, with Cucumber, on Oatmeal, Greggs*	1 Pack/194g	400	11.0	206	12.1	25.5	5.7	0.0
SAUSAGE ROLL								
Freshly Baked, Greggs*	1 Serving/103g	358	22.4	348	8.7	29.9	21.7	0.0
SOUP								
Tomato, Heinz, Greggs*	1 Serving/296ml	200	7.4	68	0.9	10.5	2.5	0.0
SUB ROLL								
Chicken Mayonnaise, on White, Plain, Greggs*	1 Roll/186g	400	15.0	215	11.5	22.3	8.1	0.0
Egg Mayonnaise, & Bacon, on White, Plain, Greggs*	1 Roll/181g	430	16.5	238	12.1	26.2	9.1	0.0
Ham Salad, on White, Plain, Greggs*	1 Roll/220g	440	16.5	200	10.2	22.9	7.5	0.0
Tuna Mayonnaise, on White, Mixed Seeded, Greggs*	1 Roll/222g	410	12.0	185	11.7	20.9	5.4	0.0
TART								
Egg Custard, Greggs*	1 Tart/90g	257	13.0	286	5.5	33.2	14.5	0.0
WRAP								
Caesar, Chicken, Greggs*	1 Pack/189g	410	20.0	217	11.9	18.8	10.6	0.0
Cheese & Bacon, Greggs*	1 Wrap/91g	390	29.5	429	14.3	19.8	32.4	0.0
Salad, Chicken, Chargrill, Greggs*	1 Pack/192g	360	14.5	187	9.9	19.8	7.5	0.0
ITSU								
HOT DISHES								
Detox 7 Vegetables, Itsu*	1 Serving/100g	184	0.7	184	1.2	3.5	0.7	0.8
Potsu, Chicken, Itsu*	1 Serving/100g	497	10.4	497	27.7	73.0	10.4	3.5
Potsu, Vegetable Dumpling, Itsu*	1 Serving/406g	326	2.9	80	2.1	2.1	0.7	0.0
Rice Bowl, Chicken, Medium, Itsu*	1 Bowl/100g	499	3.0	499	2.0	12.5	3.0	0.2
Rice Bowl, Prawn, Medium, Itsu*	1 Bowl/100g	414	3.2	414	4.3	12.6	3.2	0.2
Rice Bowl, Prawn, Original, Itsu*	1 Bowl/100g	517	3.8	517	3.6	12.2	3.8	0.3
Rice Bowl, Vegetable, Medium, Itsu*	1 Bowl/100g	385	3.7	385	2.5	15.2	3.7	0.3
Rice Bowl, Vegetable, Original, Itsu*	1 Bowl/100g	481	4.0	481	2.4	14.4	4.0	0.3
PUDDING								
Lemon Zinger, Itsu*	1 Pudding/70g	234	16.3	334	1.3	29.8	23.3	0.3
RICE CAKES								
Chocolate, Dark, Itsu*	1 Pack/50g	255	25.2	510	16.8	196.8	50.4	23.4
Chocolate, Milk, Itsu*	1 Pack/50g	249	11.4	498	6.0	65.4	22.8	3.0
Yoghurt, Itsu*	1 Pack/50g	240	9.6	480	9.0	66.0	19.2	3.0
RICE CRACKERS								
Peanut, Itsu*	1 Pack/70g	239	16.1	342	17.0	55.0	23.0	0.0
SALAD BOXES								
Low Carb Salmon & Tuna Tartar, Itsu*	1 Box/137g	173	5.3	126	8.2	3.6	3.9	0.8

	Measure INFO/WEIGHT	per Measure KCAL	FAT	Nutrition Values per 100g / 100ml KCAL	PROT	CARB	FAT	FIBRE

ITSU

SUSHI

	Measure INFO/WEIGHT	KCAL	FAT	KCAL	PROT	CARB	FAT	FIBRE
Health & Happiness, Itsu*	1 Serving/100g	500	26.8	500	32.4	33.3	26.8	5.6
Salmon, Omega 3, Supreme, Itsu*	1 Pack/100g	459	25.7	459	25.5	32.3	25.7	2.9
Salmon, Slim, Itsu*	1 Serving/100g	405	21.7	405	24.3	31.4	21.7	5.1
Salmon, Sushi, Itsu*	1 Serving/100g	203	8.4	203	14.2	17.8	8.4	0.4
Salmon 3 Ways, Super, Itsu*	1 Serving/100g	474	21.0	474	29.1	44.3	21.0	4.2
Tuna & Salmon, Junior, Itsu*	1 Serving/100g	174	4.7	174	15.3	18.0	4.7	0.4
Tuna & Salmon, Sushi, Itsu*	1 Serving/100g	245	6.4	245	12.6	14.9	6.4	1.3

J D WETHERSPOON

BAGUETTE

BLT, Malted Grain, J D Wetherspoon*	1 Baguette/399g	823	45.5	206	8.3	17.8	11.4	1.3
Chicken, Southern Fried, Creole, J D Wetherspoon*	1 Meal/250g	817	35.7	327	12.6	37.7	14.3	2.0
Club, Malted Grain, J D Wetherspoon*	1 Baguette/388g	768	36.8	198	9.8	18.5	9.5	1.4
Crayfish, Malted Grain, J D Wetherspoon*	1 Baguette/314g	594	25.5	189	6.1	23.2	8.1	1.7
Ham, Wiltshire, J D Wetherspoon*	1 Baguette/346g	536	13.1	155	9.9	20.4	3.8	1.5
Hot Sausage & Tomato Chutney, J D Wetherspoon*	1 Meal/250g	839	33.4	336	14.1	40.7	13.4	3.8
Ploughman's, Lloyds, J D Wetherspoon*	1 Baguette/346g	778	34.3	225	8.6	25.5	9.9	2.2
Tuna Mayonnaise, Malted Grain, J D Wetherspoon*	1 Baguette/401g	710	31.3	177	8.9	18.1	7.8	1.3

BHAJI

Onion, J D Wetherspoon*	1 Bhaji/30g	43	2.2	143	5.3	18.7	7.3	5.7

BIRYANI

Chicken, without Naan, J D Wetherspoon*	1 Meal/614g	700	24.6	114	4.7	14.8	4.0	1.3

BREAD

Garlic, Ciabatta, J D Wetherspoon*	1 Serving/142g	406	17.9	286	8.0	1.0	12.6	1.5
Naan, J D Wetherspoon*	1 Naan/90g	197	2.5	219	7.6	41.0	2.8	1.4

BREAKFAST

Baguette, Quorn Sausage, J D Wetherspoon*	1 Baguette/285g	622	18.3	218	10.5	29.4	6.4	3.4
Blueberry Muffin, J D Wetherspoon*	1 Muffin/124g	467	25.8	374	4.7	43.2	20.7	0.4
Bran, Fruit & Nut Muffin, J D Wetherspoon*	1 Serving/145g	571	31.7	394	7.2	43.0	21.9	1.1
Children's, J D Wetherspoon*	1 Serving/341g	613	37.1	180	10.4	10.8	10.9	2.3
Chocolate Muffin, J D Wetherspoon*	1 Muffin/125g	490	28.4	392	5.0	43.6	22.7	4.8
Farmhouse, with Toast, J D Wetherspoon*	1 Serving/796g	1647	101.8	207	9.4	14.0	12.8	1.9
Morning Roll, with Bacon, J D Wetherspoon*	1 Roll/183g	546	34.6	298	11.1	21.7	18.9	1.1
Morning Roll, with Fried Egg, J D Wetherspoon*	1 Roll/143g	400	21.3	280	9.7	27.8	14.9	1.4
Morning Roll, with Quorn Sausage, J D Wetherspoon*	1 Roll/143g	367	16.1	257	10.1	29.5	11.3	2.6
Morning Roll, with Sausage, J D Wetherspoon*	1 Roll/158g	517	28.0	327	13.8	30.1	17.7	2.3
Scrambled Egg, on Toast, J D Wetherspoon*	1 Serving/265g	503	24.9	190	8.4	17.4	9.4	1.1
Toast & Preserves, J D Wetherspoon*	1 Serving/148g	420	15.2	284	5.7	41.8	10.3	3.2
Traditional, J D Wetherspoon*	1 Breakfast/523g	904	60.1	173	8.4	9.4	11.5	1.8
Vegetarian, J D Wetherspoon*	1 Breakfast/562g	804	47.2	143	6.7	10.2	8.4	2.1

BURGERS

Beef, Double, & Chips, J D Wetherspoon*	1 Serving/598g	1382	81.6	231	16.8	11.4	13.6	0.5
Beef, Double, Cheese, & Chips, J D Wetherspoon*	1 Serving/654g	1565	91.4	239	17.2	10.7	14.0	0.5
Beef, with Bacon, Cheese & Chips, J D Wetherspoon*	1 Serving/531g	1295	78.9	244	15.2	12.6	14.8	0.5
Beef, with Cheese, & Chips, J D Wetherspoon*	1 Serving/456g	966	53.8	212	13.7	13.8	11.8	0.5
Beef, with Chips, J D Wetherspoon*	1 Serving/428g	881	46.4	206	12.8	15.7	10.8	0.6
Chicken, Fillet, with Chips, J D Wetherspoon*	1 Serving/465g	727	17.1	156	10.9	16.7	3.7	0.8
Lamb, Double, Minted, with Chips, J D Wetherspoon*	1 Serving/598g	1077	47.2	180	14.6	14.1	7.9	0.9
Lamb, Minted, with Chips, J D Wetherspoon*	1 Serving/428g	712	27.8	166	11.3	17.2	6.5	0.9
Vegetable, with Chips, J D Wetherspoon*	1 Meal/488g	839	25.9	172	4.7	27.2	5.3	2.0

BUTTY

Bacon, Brown Bloomer, J D Wetherspoon*	1 Serving/309g	869	39.6	281	23.3	18.3	12.8	1.2
Bacon & Egg, Brown Bloomer, J D Wetherspoon*	1 Serving/269g	702	31.1	261	18.2	21.0	11.6	1.4

J D WETHERSPOON

	Measure INFO/WEIGHT	per Measure KCAL	FAT	Nutrition Values per 100g / 100ml KCAL	PROT	CARB	FAT	FIBRE
BUTTY								
Bacon & Egg, White Bloomer, J D Wetherspoon*	1 Serving/269g	689	32.7	256	16.7	20.9	12.2	1.2
Chip, Brown Bloomer, J D Wetherspoon*	1 Serving/204g	478	14.7	234	7.6	35.7	7.2	1.9
Chip, White Bloomer, J D Wetherspoon*	1 Serving/204g	465	16.3	228	5.6	35.6	8.0	1.6
Chip & Cheese, Brown Bloomer, J D Wetherspoon*	1 Serving/232g	593	24.4	256	9.7	31.4	10.5	1.6
Chip & Cheese, White Bloomer, J D Wetherspoon*	1 Serving/232g	580	26.0	250	7.9	31.3	11.2	1.4
Sausage & Egg, Brown Bloomer, J D Wetherspoon*	1 Serving/331g	885	49.0	267	16.8	20.8	14.8	1.3
Sausage & Egg, White Bloomer, J D Wetherspoon*	1 Serving/331g	872	50.6	263	11.4	20.7	15.3	1.1
CAKE								
Chocolate Fudge, & Ice Cream, J D Wetherspoon*	1 Serving/239g	822	47.3	344	4.0	37.6	19.8	0.4
CAULIFLOWER CHEESE								
J D Wetherspoon*	1 Portion/220g	275	15.2	125	4.1	3.6	6.9	0.8
CHEESECAKE								
Chocolate Chip, J D Wetherspoon*	1 Serving/100g	270	11.5	270	4.9	36.8	11.5	0.5
White Chocolate & Raspberry, J D Wetherspoon*	1 Serving/175g	656	36.9	375	5.6	40.8	21.1	0.9
CHICKEN								
Wings, Buffalo, J D Wetherspoon*	1 Portion/328g	636	42.9	194	15.2	4.0	13.1	0.5
CHICKEN ALFREDO								
Pasta, with Dressed Side Salad, J D Wetherspoon*	1 Meal/576g	950	52.4	165	8.7	12.0	9.1	0.3
Pasta, with Garlic Bread, J D Wetherspoon*	1 Meal/501g	1007	47.6	201	10.8	13.0	9.5	0.3
Pasta, without Garlic Bread, J D Wetherspoon*	1 Meal/430g	804	38.7	187	11.3	15.0	9.0	0.1
CHICKEN FORESTIERRE								
J D Wetherspoon*	1 Serving/684g	626	26.0	91	7.7	8.7	3.8	1.0
CHICKEN ROAST								
& Chips, Peas, Toms, Mushrooms, J D Wetherspoon*	1 Meal/742g	904	38.6	122	13.0	5.6	5.2	1.2
with BBQ Sauce, J D Wetherspoon*	1 Meal/742g	948	37.5	128	11.3	9.2	5.0	0.6
with Chips & BBQ Sauce, J D Wetherspoon*	1 Meal/768g	1183	53.0	154	11.5	12.2	6.9	0.9
with Chips & Salad, J D Wetherspoon*	1 Meal/695g	983	52.1	141	13.1	5.9	7.5	0.6
with Dressed Salad & BBQ Sauce, J D Wetherspoon*	1 Meal/666g	913	46.0	137	12.2	6.0	6.9	0.9
with Jacket Potato, Salad, & Salsa, J D Wetherspoon*	1 Meal/785g	1193	57.3	152	12.2	10.2	7.3	1.3
with Piri Piri Sauce, J D Wetherspoon*	1 Serving/994g	994	47.1	100	8.4	5.8	4.7	0.8
CHICKEN VINDALOO								
J D Wetherspoon*	1 Meal/500g	704	18.9	141	6.4	21.0	3.8	1.3
CHILLI								
Con Carne, Rice, & Tortilla Chips, J D Wetherspoon*	1 Serving/585g	744	20.0	127	6.5	17.8	3.4	1.6
CHIPS								
Bowl, J D Wetherspoon*	1 Serving/300g	750	30.4	250	3.5	36.5	10.1	2.9
with Cheese, J D Wetherspoon*	1 Serving/501g	1002	51.6	200	5.2	21.9	10.3	1.8
with Roast Gravy, J D Wetherspoon*	1 Serving/400g	392	12.4	98	2.5	17.6	3.1	0.0
CHUTNEY								
Mango, J D Wetherspoon*	1 Serving/25g	47	0.2	188	0.4	44.8	0.8	0.4
CIABATTA								
BBQ Chicken & Bacon Melt, J D Wetherspoon*	1 Ciabatta/333g	716	33.6	215	11.3	20.4	10.1	1.8
BLT, J D Wetherspoon*	1 Ciabatta/390g	789	47.3	202	8.2	15.4	12.1	1.5
Club, J D Wetherspoon*	1 Ciabatta/378g	734	38.6	194	9.7	16.1	10.2	1.6
Crayfish, J D Wetherspoon*	1 Ciabatta/305g	561	27.4	184	5.8	20.3	9.0	1.9
Mature Cheddar Cheese & Pickle, J D Wetherspoon*	1 Ciabatta/350g	662	31.5	189	7.8	19.4	9.0	1.7
Tuna Mayonnaise, J D Wetherspoon*	1 Ciabatta/391g	676	32.8	173	8.8	15.8	8.4	1.5
Wiltshire Ham, J D Wetherspoon*	1 Ciabatta/335g	503	14.8	150	9.8	17.7	4.4	1.7
CURRY								
Beef, Malaysian, Rendang, Naan, J D Wetherspoon*	1 Meal/706g	1144	41.0	162	6.8	20.1	5.8	1.1
Goan, Vegetable, without Naan, J D Wetherspoon*	1 Meal/748g	1017	41.9	136	3.1	18.3	5.6	1.3
Kashmiri, Lamb, with Naan, J D Wetherspoon*	1 Meal/704g	1021	33.1	145	7.2	19.5	4.7	1.2

J D WETHERSPOON

	Measure INFO/WEIGHT	per Measure KCAL	FAT	Nutrition Values per 100g / 100ml KCAL	PROT	CARB	FAT	FIBRE
CURRY								
Kashmiri, Lamb, without Naan, J D Wetherspoon*	1 Meal/615g	824	30.7	134	7.1	16.3	5.0	1.1
Kerala, Fish, with Naan, J D Wetherspoon*	1 Meal/706g	1066	36.0	151	7.0	20.0	5.1	1.0
Kerala, Fish, without Naan, J D Wetherspoon*	1 Meal/616g	869	33.3	141	6.9	16.9	5.4	0.9
Mushroom Dopiaza, with Naan, J D Wetherspoon*	1 Serving/719g	899	24.5	125	3.5	21.5	3.4	1.5
Royal Thali, with Naan, J D Wetherspoon*	1 Meal/948g	1336	48.3	141	7.1	16.8	5.1	1.3
Thai, Green Chicken, without Naan, J D Wetherspoon*	1 Meal/617g	1037	46.9	168	7.5	17.6	7.6	0.5
Vegetable, Goan, with Naan Bread, J D Wetherspoon*	1 Meal/707g	1032	36.8	146	3.6	21.2	5.2	1.3
Vegetarian, Thali, with Naan, J D Wetherspoon*	1 Meal/950g	1320	42.7	139	5.3	20.3	4.5	2.4
DHANSAK								
Lamb, Meal, J D Wetherspoon*	1 Serving/720g	983	26.1	137	7.2	19.6	3.6	0.8
FISH & CHIPS								
Haddock, J D Wetherspoon*	1 Meal/496g	806	40.7	162	7.2	14.4	8.2	2.4
Plaice, Breaded, & Peas, J D Wetherspoon*	1 Serving/460g	550	15.6	120	6.8	15.0	3.4	1.7
Traditional, J D Wetherspoon*	1 Serving/495g	804	40.6	162	7.2	14.4	8.2	2.4
FISH CAKES								
Salmon & Lime, with Tartare Sauce, J D Wetherspoon*	1 Serving/355g	569	31.3	160	5.8	14.5	8.8	1.0
GAMMON								
Steak, 8oz, Eggs, Chips & Pineapple, J D Wetherspoon*	1 Meal/609g	1036	51.8	170	13.4	10.2	8.5	0.8
Steak, Egg, Chips & Side Salad, J D Wetherspoon*	1 Meal/593g	801	41.5	135	10.2	9.0	7.0	0.3
Steak, Pineapple, Chips & Salad, J D Wetherspoon*	1 Meal/654g	830	41.8	127	9.3	9.3	6.4	0.3
GAMMON &								
Chips, Peas, Tomato, & Egg, J D Wetherspoon*	1 Meal/564g	844	41.2	150	15.0	6.7	7.3	1.3
Chips, Peas, Tomato, & Pineapple, J D Wetherspoon*	1 Meal/575g	799	36.2	139	13.6	7.8	6.3	1.4
HAGGIS								
with Neeps & Tatties, J D Wetherspoon*	1 Meal/682g	982	52.5	144	4.6	15.0	7.7	1.9
HAM								
& Eggs, J D Wetherspoon*	1 Serving/396g	253	12.7	64	4.9	3.5	3.2	0.0
ICE CREAM								
Bombe, Mint Chocolate, J D Wetherspoon*	1 Portion/135g	300	13.4	222	2.6	30.6	9.9	0.8
Chocolate, Bomb, J D Wetherspoon*	1 Portion/100g	259	13.4	259	5.9	34.3	13.4	5.4
Neopolitan, Movenpick, J D Wetherspoon*	1 Bowl/100g	181	9.6	181	3.0	20.0	9.6	0.0
JALFREZI								
Chicken, Meal, with Naan Bread, J D Wetherspoon*	1 Meal/705g	916	19.7	130	6.8	19.9	2.8	1.3
Chicken, without Naan Bread, J D Wetherspoon*	1 Meal/615g	719	17.2	117	6.7	16.9	2.8	1.3
KORMA								
Chicken, Meal, without Naan, J D Wetherspoon*	1 Meal/617g	944	38.2	153	6.4	17.0	6.2	0.8
Chicken, with Naan, J D Wetherspoon*	1 Meal/704g	1141	40.8	162	6.6	20.1	5.8	0.9
LASAGNE								
Al Forno with Dressed Side Salad, J D Wetherspoon*	1 Meal/658g	823	40.8	125	5.5	11.4	6.2	0.8
MASALA								
Chicken, Hot, with Naan, J D Wetherspoon*	1 Meal/707g	1033	31.1	146	6.9	20.1	4.4	1.2
Chicken, Hot, without Naan, J D Wetherspoon*	1 Meal/614g	835	28.2	136	6.8	17.1	4.6	1.1
Vegetable, Tandoori, Meal, J D Wetherspoon*	1 Serving/720g	1020	36.0	142	3.4	20.7	5.0	2.3
MEATBALLS								
with Linguine Pasta, J D Wetherspoon*	1 Serving/512g	614	24.0	120	6.3	13.1	4.7	1.9
MELT								
BBQ Chicken, & Chips, & Salad, J D Wetherspoon*	1 Serving/643g	849	42.4	132	10.4	8.2	6.6	0.4
MIXED GRILL								
with Chips, & Dressed Side Salad, J D Wetherspoon*	1 Serving/784g	1324	87.0	169	12.0	5.6	11.1	0.3
MOUSSAKA								
Vegetarian, J D Wetherspoon*	1 Serving/555g	582	38.8	105	2.7	7.6	7.0	2.7

	Measure	per Measure		Nutrition Values per 100g / 100ml				
	INFO/WEIGHT	KCAL	FAT	KCAL	PROT	CARB	FAT	FIBRE

J D WETHERSPOON

NACHOS

J D Wetherspoon*	1 Serving/366g	1139	67.3	311	7.0	29.2	18.4	3.2
with Chilli Con Carne, J D Wetherspoon*	1 Meal/570g	1505	88.9	264	8.6	22.2	15.6	1.8
with Fajita Chicken, J D Wetherspoon*	1 Serving/486g	1225	70.5	252	5.7	24.7	14.5	2.9
with Five Bean Chilli, J D Wetherspoon*	1 Serving/571g	1399	81.1	245	7.3	21.8	14.2	2.7

NOODLES

Thai, with Chicken, J D Wetherspoon*	1 Serving/100g	516	20.8	516	20.8	39.0	20.8	4.4

PANINI

BBQ Chicken & Bacon, Melt, J D Wetherspoon*	1 Panini/337g	650	27.6	193	9.9	19.9	8.2	1.7
Cheese, Tomato, & Bacon, J D Wetherspoon*	1 Panini/261g	630	29.0	241	14.3	21.6	11.1	0.8
Cheese & Tuna, J D Wetherspoon*	1 Panini/221g	551	22.3	249	15.5	24.9	10.1	0.7
Club, J D Wetherspoon*	1 Panini/378g	734	38.6	194	9.7	16.1	10.2	1.6
Fajita Chicken, J D Wetherspoon*	1 Panini/235g	359	6.1	153	4.4	28.8	2.6	1.7
Mature, Cheddar Cheese & Tomato, J D Wetherspoon*	1 Panini/330g	750	27.1	227	10.4	18.0	8.2	1.7
Pepperoni & Mozzarella, J D Wetherspoon*	1 Panini/205g	617	33.4	301	11.6	27.5	16.3	1.0
Tomato, Mozzarella & Green Pesto, J D Wetherspoon*	1 Panini/245g	502	22.9	205	7.3	23.0	9.3	1.4

PASTA BAKE

Mediterranean, J D Wetherspoon*	1 Serving/450g	577	22.1	128	4.3	16.4	4.9	0.9

PEAS

& Ham, with Poppy Seed Bloomer, J D Wetherspoon*	1 Portion/456g	474	17.8	104	4.4	12.5	3.9	2.0

PIE

Aberdeen Angus, Chips, & Veg, J D Wetherspoon*	1 Serving/780g	1356	86.6	174	5.5	15.7	11.1	0.9
Cottage, with Chips & Peas, J D Wetherspoon*	1 Meal/682g	846	33.4	124	3.7	15.6	4.9	1.9
Fish, Carrot & Broccoli, in Butter, J D Wetherspoon*	1 Serving/550g	612	37.9	111	4.6	9.7	6.9	2.4
Scotch, J D Wetherspoon*	1 Serving/145g	302	15.4	208	13.1	7.8	10.6	0.9
Scotch, with Chips & Beans, J D Wetherspoon*	1 Serving/435g	603	22.2	139	6.8	14.9	5.1	1.5

PLATTER

Italian Style, J D Wetherspoon*	1 Platter/1020g	1985	75.5	195	10.4	22.9	7.4	0.6
Mexican, Chilli, Sour Cream, J D Wetherspoon*	1 Platter/1062g	2560	141.2	241	7.5	22.6	13.3	2.8
Mexican, with Five Bean Chilli, J D Wetherspoon*	1 Platter/1002g	2358	123.2	235	6.2	25.6	12.3	3.6
Western, J D Wetherspoon*	1 Platter/1454g	2973	168.7	204	16.9	9.1	11.6	0.4

POPPADOMS

& Dips, J D Wetherspoon*	1 Serving/134g	425	10.9	317	4.6	28.4	8.1	2.5
J D Wetherspoon*	1 Poppadom/12g	35	0.2	281	6.7	45.0	1.9	10.0

POTATO BOMBAY

J D Wetherspoon*	1 Serving/300g	285	14.7	95	1.8	10.8	4.9	2.5

POTATO SKINS

Cheese & Bacon, Loaded, J D Wetherspoon*	1 Serving/439g	949	58.4	216	8.9	15.2	13.3	1.5
Cheese & Red Onion, Loaded, J D Wetherspoon*	1 Serving/414g	835	51.3	202	6.0	16.5	12.4	1.6
Chilli Con Carne, Loaded, J D Wetherspoon*	1 Serving/503g	735	35.7	146	5.0	15.7	7.1	1.9

POTATO WEDGES

Spicy, J D Wetherspoon*	1 Serving/270g	434	15.7	161	2.2	27.7	5.8	1.8
Spicy, with Sour Cream, J D Wetherspoon*	1 Serving/330g	558	27.4	169	2.3	23.4	8.3	1.5

POTATOES

Baked, Jacket, Coleslaw, J D Wetherspoon*	1 Meal/596g	918	48.9	154	2.3	17.1	8.2	1.8
Mashed, Creamy, J D Wetherspoon*	1 Portion/279g	349	21.2	125	1.5	15.0	7.6	1.1
Roast, J D Wetherspoon*	1 Portion/200g	290	9.4	145	2.5	23.0	4.7	2.3

RIBS

Double, J D Wetherspoon*	1 Serving/350g	767	40.9	219	16.7	11.9	11.7	0.4
Double, with Chips, J D Wetherspoon*	1 Serving/500g	949	46.5	190	12.5	14.9	9.3	0.3
Double, with Jacket Potato, J D Wetherspoon*	1 Serving/590g	1159	50.7	196	11.4	19.2	8.6	1.3

RICE

Basmati, Yellow, J D Wetherspoon*	1 Portion/200g	286	1.2	143	3.4	31.1	0.6	0.2

J D WETHERSPOON

	Measure INFO/WEIGHT	per Measure KCAL	FAT	Nutrition Values per 100g / 100ml KCAL	PROT	CARB	FAT	FIBRE
RICE								
J D Wetherspoon*	1 Serving/200g	274	0.4	137	2.9	30.9	0.2	0.2
ROGAN JOSH								
Lamb, Meal, without Naan, J D Wetherspoon*	1 Meal/617g	820	27.7	133	7.1	17.0	4.5	1.0
Lamb, with Naan, J D Wetherspoon*	1 Meal/706g	1017	30.4	144	7.2	20.1	4.3	1.1
SALAD								
Caesar, Chicken, J D Wetherspoon*	1 Meal/230g	507	36.4	220	14.3	5.1	15.8	0.8
Caesar, J D Wetherspoon*	1 Meal/211g	448	38.0	212	6.8	5.8	18.0	1.1
Chicken, BBQ, Croutons & Dressing, J D Wetherspoon*	1 Portion/350g	315	8.4	90	9.4	7.5	2.4	0.8
Chicken & Bacon, Warm, J D Wetherspoon*	1 Meal/426g	600	41.3	141	9.8	3.8	9.7	0.6
Crayfish, J D Wetherspoon*	1 Meal/317g	247	18.0	78	4.4	2.7	5.7	0.6
Side, No Dressing, J D Wetherspoon*	1 Salad/195g	125	4.5	64	2.0	8.9	2.3	1.1
Side, with Dressing, J D Wetherspoon*	1 Salad/215g	263	19.6	122	2.2	8.1	9.1	1.0
Side, with Dressing & Croutons, J D Wetherspoon*	1 Portion/140g	221	18.3	158	2.1	8.6	13.1	1.1
Side, with Dressing & No Croutons, J D Wetherspoon*	1 Portion/129g	145	14.0	112	1.0	3.2	10.8	0.9
Side, without Croutons, J D Wetherspoon*	1 Portion/111g	157	10.8	141	9.8	3.8	9.7	0.6
Thai Noodle, J D Wetherspoon*	1 Portion/394g	433	21.3	110	2.7	12.7	5.4	1.4
Thai Noodle, with Chicken, J D Wetherspoon*	1 Meal/554g	637	27.7	115	9.2	9.6	5.0	1.4
Tiger Prawn, Dressing, & Chilli Jam, J D Wetherspoon*	1 Portion/340g	500	33.0	147	4.7	10.1	9.7	0.9
Tuna, Eggs, Olives, & Croutons, J D Wetherspoon*	1 Portion/395g	679	51.7	172	10.3	3.2	13.1	0.7
SAMOSAS								
Lamb, J D Wetherspoon*	1 Samosa/90g	160	3.8	178	7.9	29.9	4.2	3.9
Vegetable, J D Wetherspoon*	1 Samosa/50g	92	3.1	184	5.4	28.4	6.2	2.2
SANDWICH								
Beef, Hot, Brown Bloomer, J D Wetherspoon*	1 Sandwich/299g	618	27.2	207	11.4	19.9	9.1	1.3
Beef, Hot, Poppy Seed Bloomer, J D Wetherspoon*	1 Sandwich/299g	605	28.7	202	10.0	19.8	9.6	1.1
BLT, Brown Bloomer, J D Wetherspoon*	1 Sandwich/404g	885	39.6	219	18.0	14.6	9.8	1.2
BLT, White Bloomer, J D Wetherspoon*	1 Sandwich/404g	872	32.7	216	17.0	14.6	8.1	1.0
Cheddar, & Pickle, Brown Bloomer, J D Wetherspoon*	1 Sandwich/260g	665	31.9	256	11.0	25.4	12.3	1.9
Cheddar, & Pickle, White Bloomer, J D Wetherspoon*	1 Sandwich/260g	638	32.8	245	9.2	0.0	12.6	1.5
Chicken, Cheese, Bacon, Mayo, J D Wetherspoon*	1 Sandwich/312g	710	39.6	228	13.5	18.8	12.7	1.2
Chicken, Half Fat Mayo, Brown, Hot, J D Wetherspoon*	1 Sandwich/289g	628	28.3	217	11.8	20.7	9.8	1.7
Chicken, Half Fat Mayo, White, Hot, J D Wetherspoon*	1 Sandwich/289g	615	29.8	213	11.3	20.6	10.3	1.5
Egg Mayonnaise, Brown Bloomer, J D Wetherspoon*	1 Sandwich/295g	704	39.5	239	10.1	19.7	13.4	1.3
Egg Mayonnaise, White Bloomer, J D Wetherspoon*	1 Sandwich/295g	692	41.0	235	8.7	19.6	13.9	1.1
Ham, & Tomato, Brown Bloomer, J D Wetherspoon*	1 Sandwich/239g	514	17.2	215	11.4	24.4	7.2	1.8
Ham, & Tomato, White Bloomer, J D Wetherspoon*	1 Sandwich/239g	501	18.6	210	9.7	24.4	7.8	1.5
Prawn Mayonnaise, Brown, J D Wetherspoon*	1 Sandwich/244g	579	26.6	237	11.0	23.8	10.9	1.6
Prawn Mayonnaise, White Bloomer, J D Wetherspoon*	1 Sandwich/244g	567	28.3	232	9.3	23.7	11.6	1.4
Salmon, Lemon Mayo, Brown, J D Wetherspoon*	1 Sandwich/229g	637	33.7	278	11.4	25.4	14.7	1.7
Tuna Mayo, Half Fat Mayo, White, J D Wetherspoon*	1 Sandwich/389g	828	47.1	213	11.2	15.6	12.1	1.0
SAUSAGE & MASH								
with Red Wine Gravy, J D Wetherspoon*	1 Portion/677g	887	50.8	131	6.0	10.2	7.5	1.8
SAUSAGES WITH								
Bacon & Egg, J D Wetherspoon*	1 Serving/582g	1040	57.6	179	11.7	11.3	9.9	1.0
Chips & Beans, J D Wetherspoon*	1 Meal/554g	897	42.6	162	7.3	16.4	7.7	2.3
SCAMPI								
Breaded, Chips, Peas, Tartare, J D Wetherspoon*	1 Serving/561g	987	43.7	176	5.2	19.9	7.8	2.3
SORBET								
Mango & Passionfruit, J D Wetherspoon*	1 Serving/135g	115	0.1	85	0.2	20.0	0.1	0.2
SOUP								
Leek & Potato, no Bread & Butter, J D Wetherspoon*	1 Bowl/420g	105	0.8	25	0.9	5.1	0.2	1.0
Mushroom, No Bread, J D Wetherspoon*	1 Serving/305g	252	16.5	83	2.8	5.5	5.4	0.4

J D WETHERSPOON

	Measure INFO/WEIGHT	per Measure KCAL	FAT	Nutrition Values per 100g / 100ml KCAL	PROT	CARB	FAT	FIBRE
SOUP								
Mushroom, with Brown Bloomer, J D Wetherspoon*	1 Serving/429g	561	23.7	131	3.4	16.0	5.5	1.2
Mushroom, with White Bloomer, J D Wetherspoon*	1 Serving/429g	549	25.2	128	3.4	15.9	5.9	1.1
Tomato, No Bread, J D Wetherspoon*	1 Serving/305g	198	14.0	65	0.9	3.9	4.6	0.6
Tomato, with Brown Bloomer, J D Wetherspoon*	1 Serving/429g	576	25.8	134	3.7	15.7	6.0	1.3
Tomato, with White Bloomer, J D Wetherspoon*	1 Serving/429g	563	27.3	131	2.8	15.6	6.4	1.2
Tomato & Basil, Organic, J D Wetherspoon*	1 Serving/491g	584	23.1	119	2.9	15.8	4.7	1.2
Tomato & Basil, Organic, no Bread, J D Wetherspoon*	1 Bowl/350g	199	15.0	57	0.7	3.0	4.3	0.6
SPONGE PUDDING								
Treacle, with Hot Custard, J D Wetherspoon*	1 Serving/515g	1267	71.1	246	2.3	41.8	13.8	0.2
SQUASH								
Butternut, Roast Dinner, J D Wetherspoon*	1 Meal/847g	1211	55.9	143	4.9	17.5	6.6	2.9
STEAK								
Ribeye, 8oz, Chips & Side Salad, J D Wetherspoon*	1 Meal/562g	1006	71.9	179	8.0	8.9	12.8	0.3
STEAK &								
Breaded Scampi, Chips, & Peas, J D Wetherspoon*	1 Serving/816g	1369	72.6	168	10.1	11.3	8.9	1.2
STEAK WITH								
Chips, & Dressed Side Salad, Rump, J D Wetherspoon*	1 Meal/634g	922	60.2	145	9.5	6.3	9.5	0.3
Chips, & Dressed Side Salad, Sirloin, J D Wetherspoon*	1 Meal/577g	979	73.3	170	7.6	6.9	12.7	0.3
Jacket, Salad, & Salsa, Rump, J D Wetherspoon*	1 Meal/724g	1132	64.4	156	9.0	10.9	8.9	1.1
Jacket Pot, Salad, & Salsa, Sirloin, J D Wetherspoon*	1 Meal/667g	1189	77.4	178	7.3	11.8	11.6	1.2
STEW								
Irish, J D Wetherspoon*	1 Serving/600g	516	23.4	86	7.3	5.6	3.9	0.9
STUFFING BALLS								
Sage & Onion, J D Wetherspoon*	1 Portion/70g	137	1.1	196	6.6	32.3	1.6	3.6
TART								
Apple, with Ice Cream, J D Wetherspoon*	1 Serving/235g	464	20.0	197	1.6	29.8	8.5	0.4
TIKKA								
Mixed Grill, Starter, J D Wetherspoon*	1 Portion/374g	460	23.9	123	13.4	3.2	6.4	0.9
TIKKA MASALA								
Chicken with Rice & No Naan Bread, J D Wetherspoon*	1 Meal/614g	872	33.2	142	6.9	16.9	5.4	1.2
WAFFLES								
Belgian, Ice Cream & Maple Syrup, J D Wetherspoon*	1 Serving/395g	934	33.6	236	13.8	28.4	8.5	0.8
WRAP								
Caesar, & Potato Wedges, J D Wetherspoon*	1 Serving/289g	687	40.2	238	5.0	25.2	13.9	1.6
Caesar, Tortillas & Salsa, J D Wetherspoon*	1 Serving/244g	624	38.8	256	5.7	23.4	15.9	1.6
Caesar Wetherwrap, J D Wetherspoon*	1 Wrap/159g	478	32.6	301	7.0	23.1	20.5	1.5
Chicken, Cheese, & Potato Wedges, J D Wetherspoon*	1 Serving/401g	762	34.1	190	8.0	22.2	8.5	1.5
Chicken, Cheese, Tortillas, Salsa, J D Wetherspoon*	1 Serving/356g	699	32.4	196	8.8	20.6	9.1	1.5
Chicken, Guacamole, Tortilla, Salsa, J D Wetherspoon*	1 Serving/273g	474	16.9	174	8.2	21.9	6.2	2.0
Chicken, Guacamole, Wedges, J D Wetherspoon*	1 Serving/318g	537	18.4	169	7.2	23.7	5.8	2.0
Chicken, with Chicken Breast, J D Wetherspoon*	1 Wrap/292g	450	21.6	154	9.4	14.5	7.4	1.5
Chicken, with Potato Wedges, J D Wetherspoon*	1 Serving/373g	647	24.2	173	6.7	23.9	6.5	1.7
Chicken, with Tortilla Chips & Salsa, J D Wetherspoon*	1 Serving/328g	584	23.0	178	7.5	22.3	7.0	1.6
Chicken & Cheese, J D Wetherspoon*	1 Wrap/271g	553	26.3	204	10.7	19.6	9.7	1.4
Club, with Potato Wedges, J D Wetherspoon*	1 Serving/381g	822	43.1	216	10.9	19.2	11.3	1.2
Fajita Chicken, J D Wetherspoon*	1 Wrap/228g	345	14.1	151	3.8	21.2	6.2	1.9
Fajita Chicken, Tortilla Chips, Salsa, J D Wetherspoon*	1 Serving/313g	491	20.3	157	3.5	21.9	6.5	1.9
Fajita Chicken, with Potato Wedges, J D Wetherspoon*	1 Serving/358g	554	21.8	155	3.2	23.5	6.1	1.9
Poached Salmon, Tortillas, Salsa, J D Wetherspoon*	1 Serving/203g	573	32.9	282	9.9	25.8	16.2	1.6
Poached Salmon, with Wedges, J D Wetherspoon*	1 Serving/298g	656	34.3	220	7.1	24.2	11.5	1.5
Poached Salmon & Prawn Salad, J D Wetherspoon*	1 Wrap/355g	512	34.1	144	9.8	4.5	9.6	0.5
Reggae Reggae Chicken, Slices, J D Wetherspoon*	1 Meal/100g	364	9.6	364	24.4	42.0	9.6	2.7

	Measure INFO/WEIGHT	per Measure KCAL	FAT	Nutrition Values per 100g / 100ml KCAL	PROT	CARB	FAT	FIBRE

J D WETHERSPOON

YORKSHIRE PUDDING

	Measure INFO/WEIGHT	KCAL	FAT	KCAL	PROT	CARB	FAT	FIBRE
J D Wetherspoon*	2 Puddings/56g	132	4.6	236	8.2	32.9	8.2	1.1

KFC

BEANS

BBQ, Large, KFC*	1 Serving/188g	158	1.4	84	5.3	15.1	0.7	0.0
BBQ, Regular, KFC*	1 Serving/130g	200	1.5	154	6.1	30.0	1.1	6.9

BURGERS

Fillet, KFC*	1 Burger/245g	479	19.8	196	11.1	19.5	8.1	0.0
Fillet, Mini, KFC*	1 Burger/114g	275	11.2	241	14.8	23.9	9.8	0.0
Fillet Tower Burger, KFC*	1 Burger/163g	617	21.0	378	24.3	41.4	12.9	0.0
Mini Fillet, Kids, KFC*	1 Burger/114g	253	6.4	222	15.8	27.0	5.6	0.0
Tower, KFC*	1 Burger/210g	628	20.8	299	15.9	30.0	9.9	0.0
Tower, Zinger, KFC*	1 Burger/264g	655	32.7	248	11.2	24.3	12.4	0.0
Zinger, Fillet, KFC*	1 Burger/185g	445	19.6	241	13.9	22.4	10.6	1.4
Zinger, KFC*	1 Burger/219g	481	20.8	220	12.2	22.0	9.5	0.0

CHEESECAKE

Boysenberry, Chateau, KFC*	1 Serving/85g	196	9.3	230	4.0	30.0	11.0	0.0
Cookies & Cream, KFC*	1 Serving/80g	261	17.1	326	4.3	29.1	21.4	0.0

CHICKEN

Breast, Original Recipe, KFC*	1 Breast/137g	285	13.3	207	24.9	5.6	9.7	0.0
Drumsticks, Original Recipe, KFC*	1 Drumstick/95g	161	9.5	170	11.9	9.1	10.0	0.0
Fillet, Mini, Not In a Bun, KFC*	1 Fillet/50g	116	4.0	232	26.6	14.0	8.0	0.0
Popcorn, Kids, KFC*	1 Portion/66g	144	8.4	219	14.1	13.2	12.7	0.0
Popcorn, Large, KFC*	1 Serving/189g	494	29.8	262	17.5	13.5	15.8	0.0
Ribs, Original Recipe, KFC*	1 Rib/126g	238	13.4	188	19.8	4.1	10.6	0.0
Strips, Crispy, KFC*	1 Strip/46g	112	5.4	243	15.4	20.4	11.7	0.0
Thighs, Original Recipe, KFC*	1 Thigh/134g	218	14.2	162	12.6	4.4	10.6	0.0
Wings, Hot, KFC*	1 Wing/58g	102	7.0	175	9.4	7.5	12.1	0.0
Wings, Original Recipe, KFC*	1 Wing/48g	126	3.8	262	25.0	8.3	8.0	0.0

COLESLAW

Large, KFC*	1 Serving/200g	268	22.4	134	0.8	9.5	11.2	0.0
Regular, KFC*	1 Serving/100g	134	11.2	134	0.8	9.5	11.2	0.0

CORN

Cobs, Cobette, KFC*	1 Serving/70g	141	8.5	201	4.3	20.1	12.1	0.0

DRESSING

Caesar, KFC*	1 Sachet/35g	103	10.9	295	19.2	2.7	31.1	0.0
French, KFC*	1 Sachet/45g	30	1.3	66	0.2	2.9	2.9	0.0
Vinaigrette, Low Fat, KFC*	1 Sachet/35g	21	0.8	59	0.5	8.9	2.2	0.0
Yoghurt, Coriander & Chilli, KFC*	1 Sachet/45g	166	16.2	369	2.2	9.3	36.0	0.0

FRIES

Large, KFC*	1 Serving/162g	375	19.3	231	3.1	32.4	11.9	0.0
Regular, KFC*	1 Serving/111g	257	13.2	232	3.1	32.4	11.9	0.0

GRAVY

Large, KFC*	1 Serving/204g	144	8.0	71	2.3	7.3	3.9	0.0
Regular, KFC*	1 Serving/102g	72	4.0	71	2.3	7.3	3.9	0.0

ICE CREAM

Avalanche, KFC*	1 Pot/28g	114	5.1	407	10.4	51.4	18.2	0.0
Soft, KFC*	1 Serving/110g	171	7.0	155	3.7	20.6	6.4	0.0

PIE

Apple Slice, Colonel's Pies, KFC*	1 Slice/113g	310	13.9	274	1.7	38.9	12.3	0.0
Strawberry Creme, Slice, KFC*	1 Slice/78g	279	15.0	358	5.4	41.0	19.2	2.5

SALAD

Chicken, Original Recipe, No Dressing, KFC*	1 Salad/292g	270	9.5	92	9.0	7.0	3.3	0.0

	Measure INFO/WEIGHT	per Measure KCAL	FAT	Nutrition Values per 100g / 100ml KCAL	PROT	CARB	FAT	FIBRE
KFC								
SALAD								
Chicken, Zinger, No Dressing, KFC*	1 Salad/285g	307	14.8	108	7.8	8.0	5.2	0.0
Potato, KFC*	1 Portion/160g	229	13.9	143	2.5	14.3	8.7	1.8
WRAP								
Twister, Salsa, Toasted, KFC*	1 Wrap/222g	516	24.9	232	8.7	24.6	11.2	0.0
Twister, Toasted, KFC*	1 Wrap/217g	509	24.8	235	8.9	24.6	11.5	0.0
Wrapstar, KFC*	1 Wrapstar/239g	642	36.6	269	11.4	25.9	15.3	0.0
KRISPY KREME								
DOUGHNUTS								
Blueberry, Powdered, Filled, Krispy Kreme*	1 Doughnut/86g	307	17.2	357	7.0	36.0	20.0	5.0
Butterscotch Fudge, Krispy Kreme*	1 Doughnut/93g	372	16.7	400	6.0	53.0	18.0	0.0
Chocolate, Glazed, Krispy Kreme*	1 Doughnut/80g	309	13.6	387	4.0	55.0	17.0	3.0
Chocolate Dreamcake, Krispy Kreme*	1 Doughnut/92g	358	19.3	389	6.0	43.0	21.0	0.0
Chocolate Iced, Creme Filled, Krispy Kreme*	1 Doughnut/87g	339	17.4	390	6.0	47.0	20.0	4.0
Chocolate Iced, Custard Filled, Krispy Kreme*	1 Doughnut/87g	307	14.8	353	6.0	43.0	17.0	2.0
Chocolate Iced, Glazed, Krispy Kreme*	1 Doughnut/66g	270	13.2	410	5.0	51.0	20.0	3.0
Chocolate Iced, with Creme Filling, Krispy Kreme*	1 Doughnut/87g	350	20.9	402	3.0	42.0	24.0	1.0
Chocolate Iced, with Sprinkles, Krispy Kreme*	1 Doughnut/71g	293	13.5	413	5.0	56.0	19.0	3.0
Cinnamon Apple, Filled, Krispy Kreme*	1 Doughnut/81g	269	14.6	332	7.0	37.0	18.0	5.0
Cookies & Kreme, Krispy Kreme*	1 Doughnut/93g	379	16.7	408	4.0	57.0	18.0	0.0
Cruller, Glazed, Krispy Kreme*	1 Doughnut/54g	254	15.6	471	4.0	49.0	29.0	3.0
Glazed, with a Creme Filling, Krispy Kreme*	1 Doughnut/86g	309	15.5	359	5.0	44.0	18.0	4.0
Lemon Filled, Glazed, Krispy Kreme*	1 Doughnut/66g	218	10.5	331	5.0	41.0	16.0	4.0
Lemon Meringue Pie, Krispy Kreme*	1 Doughnut/83g	290	14.9	350	6.0	40.0	18.0	0.0
Maple Iced, Krispy Kreme*	1 Doughnut/66g	279	15.2	422	5.0	49.0	23.0	3.0
Original, Glazed, Krispy Kreme*	1 Doughnut/52g	217	13.0	417	6.0	43.0	25.0	4.0
Raspberry, Glazed, Krispy Kreme*	1 Doughnut/86g	307	13.8	357	6.0	47.0	16.0	4.0
Sour Cream, Krispy Kreme*	1 Doughnut/80g	340	18.4	425	4.0	53.0	23.0	1.0
Strawberries & Kreme, Krispy Kreme*	1 Doughnut/90g	323	15.3	359	5.0	45.0	17.0	0.0
Strawberry Filled, Powdered, Krispy Kreme*	1 Doughnut/74g	248	13.3	335	7.0	36.0	18.0	5.0
Vanilla, Krispy Kreme*	1 Doughnut/80g	315	13.7	391	4.0	57.0	17.0	2.0
MCDONALD'S								
BAGEL								
Toasted, with Strawberry Jam, McDonald's*	1 Bagel/105g	260	1.0	248	8.0	52.0	1.0	3.0
with Bacon, Egg & Cheese, McDonald's*	1 Bagel/173g	455	22.5	263	13.0	26.0	13.0	2.0
with Butter & Jam, McDonald's*	1 Bagel/122g	399	10.2	326	5.9	58.8	8.3	2.2
with Flora & Jam, McDonald's*	1 Bagel/120g	369	6.9	305	6.0	59.4	5.7	2.2
with Philadelphia, McDonald's*	1 Bagel/125g	317	5.9	254	7.7	47.5	4.7	2.1
with Sausage, Egg & Cheese, McDonald's*	1 Bagel/203g	540	28.4	266	14.0	22.0	14.0	2.0
with Sausage & Egg, McDonald's*	1 Bagel/207g	551	26.5	266	13.3	23.3	12.8	1.6
BREAD								
Bagel, Plain, Toasted, McDonald's*	1 Bagel/85g	210	0.8	248	9.0	50.0	1.0	3.0
BREAKFAST								
Big Breakfast, McDonald's*	1 Breakfast/264g	595	37.0	225	11.0	15.0	14.0	1.0
Big Breakfast Bun, McDonald's*	1 Bun/242g	571	32.2	236	13.0	15.1	13.3	0.9
BREAKFAST CEREAL								
Porridge, Oatso Simple, & Jam, McDonald's*	1 Serving/232g	246	5.3	106	4.0	17.0	2.3	0.9
Porridge, Oatso Simple, & Sugar, McDonald's*	1 Serving/215g	205	5.4	95	4.3	13.7	2.5	0.9
Porridge, Oatso Simple, Plain, McDonald's*	1 Serving/212g	195	4.2	92	5.0	13.0	2.0	1.0
BROWNIE								
Belgian Bliss, McDonald's*	1 Serving/85g	390	22.1	459	6.0	51.0	26.0	2.0
BURGERS								
1955 Burger, McDonald's*	1 Burger/281g	655	33.7	233	14.0	18.0	12.0	2.0

MCDONALD'S

	Measure INFO/WEIGHT	per Measure KCAL	FAT	Nutrition Values per 100g / 100ml KCAL	PROT	CARB	FAT	FIBRE
BURGERS								
Bacon, Chicken & Onion, McDonald's*	1 Burger/255g	660	33.1	259	14.0	22.0	13.0	2.0
Big Mac, McDonald's*	1 Burger/214g	491	25.7	229	13.0	19.0	12.0	2.0
Big Mac, No Sauce, No Cheese, McDonald's*	1 Burger/181g	400	16.0	221	12.1	23.8	8.8	1.1
Big Tasty, McDonald's*	1 Burger/346g	835	52.0	241	13.0	14.0	15.0	1.0
Big Tasty, with Bacon, McDonald's*	1 Burger/359g	890	57.4	248	14.0	14.0	16.0	1.0
Bigger Big Mac, McDonald's*	1 Burger/325g	714	34.0	220	12.9	18.5	10.5	1.6
Cheeseburger, Bacon, McDonald's*	1 Burger/127g	336	15.3	264	16.0	24.0	12.0	2.0
Cheeseburger, Double, McDonald's*	1 Burger/169g	440	23.7	260	17.0	19.0	14.0	1.0
Cheeseburger, McDonald's*	1 Burger/119g	300	12.0	253	14.3	26.2	10.1	2.5
Chicken Fiesta, McDonald's*	1 Burger/240g	610	26.4	254	14.0	24.0	11.0	2.0
Chicken Legend, Bacon, & Tom Salsa, McDonald's*	1 Serving/233g	555	16.3	238	15.0	29.0	7.0	2.0
Chicken Legend, with Bacon, Cool Mayo, McDonald's*	1 Burger/227g	590	22.7	260	15.0	27.0	10.0	2.0
Festive, Deluxe, McDonald's*	1 Burger/284g	770	45.5	271	16.0	17.0	16.0	1.0
Filet-O-Fish, McDonald's*	1 Burger/150g	350	18.1	232	10.0	24.0	12.0	1.0
Filet-O-Fish, No Tartar Sauce, McDonald's*	1 Burger/124g	290	9.0	234	12.1	30.6	7.3	0.8
Hamburger, McDonald's*	1 Burger/104g	250	8.3	240	13.0	29.0	8.0	2.0
Mayo Chicken, McDonald's*	1 Burger/122g	310	13.4	254	10.0	30.0	11.0	2.0
McChicken Sandwich, McDonald's*	1 Sandwich/171g	385	17.2	224	9.0	26.0	10.0	2.0
Quarter Pounder, Bacon with Cheese, McDonald's*	1 Burger/230g	592	33.2	259	16.5	15.4	14.5	1.3
Quarter Pounder, Deluxe, McDonald's*	1 Burger/253g	521	26.8	206	11.4	16.1	10.6	1.7
Quarter Pounder, Double, with Cheese, McDonald's*	1 Burger/275g	710	40.3	259	19.5	12.2	14.7	1.1
Quarter Pounder, McDonald's*	1 Burger/178g	424	19.0	238	14.5	20.9	10.7	2.1
Quarter Pounder, with Cheese, McDonald's*	1 Burger/194g	490	25.3	252	16.0	19.0	13.0	2.0
Summer Chorizo, McDonald's*	1 Burger/238g	650	35.7	273	17.0	17.0	15.0	1.0
The M, McDonald's*	1 Serving/240g	580	28.8	242	16.0	18.0	12.0	1.0
The M with Bacon, McDonald's*	1 Serving/249g	620	32.4	249	17.0	18.0	13.0	1.0
BURGERS VEGETARIAN								
Vegetable, Deluxe, McDonald's*	1 Burger/181g	411	16.3	227	6.0	30.0	9.0	6.0
BUTTER								
Country Life, McDonald's*	1 Pack/11g	85	9.0	752	0.0	0.0	80.0	0.0
CAKE								
Birthday, McDonald's*	1 Portion/158g	640	22.6	405	2.7	65.4	14.3	1.0
CARROTS								
Sticks, McDonald's*	1 Bag/80g	30	0.0	38	0.0	8.0	0.0	2.0
CHEESE								
Soft, Philadelphia, Light, McDonald's*	1 Serving/35g	55	3.9	157	9.0	3.0	11.0	0.0
CHICKEN								
McNuggets, 4 Pieces, McDonald's*	4 Pieces/70g	170	9.1	243	13.0	19.0	13.0	1.0
McNuggets, 6 Pieces, McDonald's*	6 Pieces/105g	250	13.7	238	13.0	19.0	13.0	1.0
McNuggets, 9 Pieces, McDonald's*	9 Pieces/157g	375	20.4	239	13.0	19.0	13.0	1.0
Selects, 3 Pieces, McDonald's*	3 Pieces/130g	365	19.6	280	16.0	20.0	15.0	1.0
Selects, 5 Pieces, McDonald's*	5 Pieces/219g	612	32.8	280	16.0	20.0	15.0	1.0
COFFEE								
Black, Large, McDonald's*	1 Serving/428ml	0	0.0	0	0.0	0.0	0.0	0.0
Black, Regular, McDonald's*	1 Serving/312ml	0	0.0	0	0.0	0.0	0.0	0.0
Cappuccino, Large, McDonald's*	1 Serving/307ml	120	3.1	39	3.0	4.0	1.0	0.0
Cappuccino, Regular, McDonald's*	1 Serving/231ml	90	2.3	39	3.0	4.0	1.0	0.0
Espresso, Single Shot, McDonald's*	1 Serving/30ml	0	0.0	0	0.0	0.0	0.0	0.0
Latte, Large, McDonald's*	1 Serving/451ml	185	4.5	41	3.0	4.0	1.0	0.0
Latte, Regular, McDonald's*	1 Serving/337ml	135	3.4	40	3.0	4.0	1.0	0.0
White, Large, McDonald's*	1 Serving/428ml	30	0.0	7	0.0	1.0	0.0	0.0
White, Regular, McDonald's*	1 Serving/313ml	25	0.0	8	1.0	1.0	0.0	0.0

MCDONALD'S

	Measure INFO/WEIGHT	per Measure KCAL	FAT	Nutrition Values per 100g / 100ml KCAL	PROT	CARB	FAT	FIBRE
COLA								
Coca-Cola, Diet, McDonald's*	1 Med/405ml	4	0.0	1	0.0	0.0	0.0	0.0
Coca-Cola, McDonald's*	1 Med/405ml	170	0.0	42	0.0	10.0	0.0	0.0
Coke, Zero, McDonald's*	1 Serving/200ml	2	0.0	1	0.0	0.0	0.0	0.0
CREAMER								
Uht, McDonald's*	1 Cup/14ml	17	1.4	123	4.2	4.2	10.0	0.0
CROUTONS								
McDonald's*	1 Sachet/14g	60	2.0	426	11.8	63.4	14.0	2.7
DIP								
BBQ, McDonald's*	1 Pot/50g	83	0.0	166	0.0	37.0	0.0	0.0
Caramelised Onion, McDonald's*	1 Dip/31g	45	1.9	144	3.0	19.0	6.0	3.0
Sour Cream & Chive, McDonald's*	1 Pot/50g	150	16.0	300	2.0	2.0	32.0	4.0
Sweet Chilli, McDonald's*	1 Pot/31g	80	0.9	256	0.0	58.0	3.0	0.0
DOUGHNUTS								
Chocolate Donut, McDonald's*	1 Donut/79g	345	16.2	437	5.7	43.8	20.5	1.0
Chocolate Donut, McMini, McDonald's*	1 Donut/17g	64	3.0	375	6.8	46.9	17.8	1.6
Cinnamon Donut, McDonald's*	1 Donut/72g	302	18.1	419	5.1	43.1	25.1	3.8
Sugared Donut, McDonald's*	1 Donut/49g	205	14.7	418	6.0	35.0	30.0	4.0
DRESSING								
Balsamic, Low Fat, McDonald's*	1 Sachet/33g	20	1.0	60	0.0	9.0	3.0	0.0
Caesar, Low Fat, McDonald's*	1 Sachet/80g	55	1.6	68	2.0	10.0	2.0	0.0
French, Low Fat, McDonald's*	1 Serving/22g	13	0.6	58	0.5	7.1	2.6	1.0
FANTA								
Orange, McDonald's*	1 Super/750ml	315	0.0	42	0.0	10.0	0.0	0.0
FISH FINGERS								
McDonald's*	3 Fingers/84g	195	9.2	232	15.0	19.0	11.0	1.0
FRIES								
French, Large, McDonald's*	1 Serving/160g	460	22.4	288	3.0	38.0	14.0	4.0
French, Medium, McDonald's*	1 Serving/114g	330	16.0	289	3.0	37.0	14.0	4.0
French, Small, McDonald's*	1 Serving/80g	230	11.2	288	2.0	38.0	14.0	4.0
FRUIT								
Bag, McDonald's*	1 Pack/80g	40	0.8	50	0.0	12.0	1.0	2.0
FRUIT DRINK								
Fruitizz, Sparkling, McDonald's*	1 Drink/250ml	160	0.0	64	0.4	15.6	0.0	0.0
FRUIT SHOOT								
Robinsons, McDonald's*	1 Bottle200ml	10	0.0	5	0.0	1.0	0.0	0.0
HASH BROWNS								
McDonald's*	1 Hash Brown/53g	140	9.0	264	2.0	26.0	17.0	2.0
HOT CHOCOLATE								
McDonald's*	1 Serving/330ml	164	3.6	50	0.7	8.8	1.1	0.0
HOT DOG								
& Ketchup, McDonald's*	1 Serving/116g	296	14.6	255	9.6	25.8	12.6	1.3
ICE CREAM								
Smartie, McDonald's*	1 Pot/120g	260	9.5	216	3.4	33.3	7.9	1.0
ICE CREAM CONE								
McDonald's*	1 Cone/90g	141	4.5	156	4.5	24.4	5.0	0.0
with Flake, McDonald's*	1 Cone/107g	204	7.7	191	4.8	27.0	7.2	0.0
JAM								
Strawberry, McDonald's*	1 Pack/20g	50	0.0	250	0.0	60.0	0.0	0.0
JUICE								
Tropicana, McDonald's*	1 Bottle/250ml	107	0.0	43	1.0	9.0	0.0	0.4
KETCHUP								
Tomato, McDonald's*	1 Portion/23g	25	0.0	109	0.0	26.0	0.0	0.0

MCDONALD'S	Measure INFO/WEIGHT	per Measure KCAL	FAT	Nutrition Values per 100g / 100ml KCAL	PROT	CARB	FAT	FIBRE
LEMONADE								
Sprite, Z, McDonald's*	1 Lge/500ml	5	0.0	1	0.0	0.0	0.0	0.0
MARGARINE								
Flora, Original, McDonald's*	1 Portion/10g	55	6.0	550	0.0	0.0	60.0	0.0
MCFLURRY								
After Eight, McDonald's*	1 Serving/206g	400	16.5	194	3.0	27.0	8.0	1.0
Cadbury, Shortcake, Limited Edition, McDonald's*	1 Serving/206g	385	14.4	187	3.0	28.0	7.0	1.0
Chocolate, Cornetto, McDonald's*	1 Serving/207g	400	16.6	193	3.0	29.0	8.0	1.0
Cornetto, Mint Choc, McDonald's*	1 Serving/207g	400	16.6	193	3.0	29.0	8.0	1.0
Creme Egg, Cadbury's, McDonald's*	1 Serving/203g	381	12.9	188	2.9	29.8	6.3	0.5
Crunchie, McDonald's*	1 Serving/185g	330	11.1	178	3.0	28.0	6.0	1.0
Dairy Milk, McDonald's*	1 Serving/184g	340	12.9	184	3.0	28.0	7.0	1.0
Dairy Milk, with Caramel, McDonald's*	1 Serving/206g	385	13.0	187	2.9	29.1	6.3	0.0
Flake, Chocolate, McDonald's*	1 Serving/206ml	400	14.4	194	3.0	29.0	7.0	0.0
Flake, Raspberry, McDonald's*	1 Serving/205ml	370	12.3	180	3.0	27.0	6.0	0.0
Jammie Dodger, McDonald's*	1 Serving/128g	256	8.2	200	3.9	33.6	6.4	0.3
Raspberry, McDonald's*	1 Serving/206ml	370	12.3	180	3.0	27.0	6.0	0.0
Rolo, McDonald's*	1 Serving/205g	390	13.3	190	4.0	29.2	6.5	0.1
Smarties, McDonald's*	1 Serving/185g	330	11.1	178	3.0	28.0	6.0	1.0
Strawberry, Cornetto, McDonald's*	1 Serving/207g	375	12.4	181	3.0	29.0	6.0	0.0
Terry's Chocolate Orange, McDonald's*	1 Serving/204g	405	16.3	199	3.0	28.0	8.0	0.0
Toffee Swirl, Oreo Cookie, McDonald's*	1 Serving/206ml	400	12.4	194	3.0	31.0	6.0	1.0
Wispa Gold, McDonald's*	1 Serving/206g	395	14.0	192	2.9	29.1	6.8	0.5
Yorkie, McDonald's*	1 Serving/204g	379	14.9	186	3.4	27.0	7.3	0.8
MCMUFFIN								
Bacon & Egg, Double, McDonald's*	1 McMuffin/161g	395	21.0	244	15.0	16.0	13.0	1.0
Bacon & Egg, McDonald's*	1 McMuffin/146g	345	17.5	237	14.0	18.0	12.0	1.0
Egg, Scrambled, McDonald's*	1 McMuffin/147g	294	14.1	200	10.9	17.5	9.6	1.3
Sausage & Egg, Double, McDonald's*	1 McMuffin/222g	560	35.6	252	16.0	12.0	16.0	1.0
Sausage & Egg, McDonald's*	1 McMuffin/174g	420	24.3	242	14.0	16.0	14.0	1.0
MELT								
Toasted Ham & Cheese, McDonald's*	1 Serving/100g	239	8.0	239	11.2	30.6	8.0	1.8
MILK								
Fresh, Portion, McDonald's*	1 Portion/14ml	10	0.0	69	0.0	7.0	0.0	0.0
Organic, McDonald's*	1 Bottle/250ml	117	5.0	47	4.0	5.0	2.0	0.0
MILKSHAKE								
Banana, Large, McDonald's*	1 Serving/432ml	545	13.0	126	3.0	21.0	3.0	0.0
Banana, Medium, McDonald's*	1 Serving/338ml	425	10.1	126	3.0	21.0	3.0	0.0
Banana, Small, McDonald's*	1 Serving/178ml	226	5.3	127	3.0	21.0	3.0	0.0
Cadburys Dairy Milk, Caramel, Large, McDonald's*	1 Serving/417ml	505	16.7	121	3.0	19.0	4.0	1.0
Cadburys Dairy Milk, Caramel, Medium, McDonald's*	1 Serving/394ml	480	15.8	122	3.0	19.0	4.0	1.0
Cadburys Dairy Milk, Caramel, Small, McDonald's*	1 Serving/177ml	220	5.3	124	3.0	20.0	3.0	1.0
Chocolate, Large, McDonald's*	1 Serving/431ml	530	12.9	123	3.0	20.0	3.0	0.0
Chocolate, Medium, McDonald's*	1 Serving/337ml	425	10.1	126	3.0	21.0	3.0	0.0
Chocolate, Small, McDonald's*	1 Serving/177ml	225	5.3	127	3.0	21.0	3.0	0.0
Starburst Mixed Berry Flavour, McDonald's*	1 Small/177ml	200	4.0	113	2.8	20.3	2.3	0.0
Strawberry, Large, McDonald's*	1 Serving/432ml	540	13.0	125	3.0	21.0	3.0	0.0
Strawberry, Medium, McDonald's*	1 Serving/336ml	420	10.1	125	3.0	21.0	3.0	0.0
Strawberry, Small, McDonald's*	1 Serving/177ml	220	5.3	124	3.0	21.0	3.0	0.0
Vanilla, Large, McDonald's*	1 Serving/431ml	535	12.9	124	3.0	21.0	3.0	0.0
Vanilla, Medium, McDonald's*	1 Serving/336ml	420	10.1	125	3.0	21.0	3.0	0.0
Vanilla, Small, McDonald's*	1 Serving/177ml	220	5.3	124	3.0	21.0	3.0	0.0

MCDONALD'S

	Measure INFO/WEIGHT	per Measure KCAL	per Measure FAT	Nutrition Values per 100g / 100ml KCAL	PROT	CARB	FAT	FIBRE
MOZZARELLA								
Dippers, McDonald's*	3 Dippers/85g	265	13.6	312	13.0	27.0	16.0	1.0
MUFFIN								
Blueberry, Low Fat, McDonald's*	1 Muffin/126g	300	3.8	238	5.0	50.0	3.0	2.0
Double Chocolate, McDonald's*	1 Muffin/123g	515	28.3	419	6.0	46.0	23.0	2.0
ONION RINGS								
McDonald's*	1 Serving/99g	245	11.9	247	4.0	31.0	12.0	3.0
PANCAKE								
& Sausage, with Syrup, McDonald's*	1 Portion/223g	615	20.1	275	8.0	42.0	9.0	2.0
& Syrup, McDonald's*	1 Pack/175g	515	14.0	294	4.0	52.0	8.0	2.0
PIE								
Apple, McDonald's*	1 Pie/80g	231	12.8	289	2.0	35.0	16.0	0.0
POTATO WEDGES								
McDonald's*	1 Portion/177g	349	17.7	197	3.3	23.3	10.0	2.8
QUORN*								
Burger, Premiere, McDonald's*	1 Burger/210g	311	6.1	148	9.1	24.2	2.9	2.7
ROLL								
Bacon, McBacon, McDonald's*	1 Roll/122g	349	14.0	286	13.5	30.5	11.5	1.7
Bacon, with Brown Sauce, McDonald's*	1 Roll/126g	350	8.8	278	15.0	37.0	7.0	2.0
Bacon, with Tomato Ketchup, McDonald's*	1 Roll/126g	345	8.8	273	15.0	36.0	7.0	2.0
SALAD								
Chicken, Crispy, No Bacon, McDonald's*	1 Salad/281g	270	11.2	96	8.0	6.0	4.0	1.0
Chicken, Crispy, with Bacon, McDonald's*	1 Serving/292g	326	14.6	111	10.0	7.0	5.0	1.0
Chicken, No Bacon, Grilled, McDonald's*	1 Salad/255g	115	2.6	45	7.0	2.0	1.0	1.0
Chicken, with Bacon, Grilled, McDonald's*	1 Salad/266g	164	5.3	62	9.0	2.0	2.0	1.0
Garden, Side, No Dressing, McDonald's*	1 Salad/91g	10	0.0	11	1.0	2.0	0.0	1.0
Garden, Side, with Balsamic Dressing, McDonald's*	1 Salad/128g	91	3.8	71	1.0	11.0	3.0	1.0
Garden, Side, with Low Fat Caesar, McDonald's*	1 Salad/63g	40	1.3	63	2.0	8.0	2.0	2.0
SANDWICH								
Deli, Chicken, Salad, McDonald's*	1 Sandwich/216g	350	8.6	162	7.0	24.0	4.0	2.0
Deli, Chicken, Sweet Chilli, McDonald's*	1 Sandwich/250g	570	22.5	228	12.0	28.0	9.0	2.0
Deli, Chicken & Bacon, McDonald's*	1 Sandwich/192g	405	13.4	211	10.0	27.0	7.0	2.0
Deli, Spicy Veggie, McDonald's*	1 Sandwich/216g	555	21.6	257	6.0	36.0	10.0	4.0
SAUCE								
Barbeque, McDonald's*	1 Portion/50g	85	1.0	170	0.0	38.0	2.0	0.0
Curry, Sweet, McDonald's*	1 Portion/29g	50	0.9	171	0.0	38.0	3.0	3.0
Mustard, Mild, McDonald's*	1 Portion/30g	64	3.6	212	1.0	24.8	12.1	0.0
Sweet & Sour, McDonald's*	1 Portion/29g	50	0.0	172	0.0	38.0	0.0	0.0
SUNDAE								
Hot Caramel, McDonald's*	1 Sundae/189g	357	8.3	189	3.8	33.9	4.4	0.0
Hot Fudge, McDonald's*	1 Sundae/187g	352	10.7	188	4.5	30.0	5.7	0.0
No Topping, McDonald's*	1 Sundae/149g	219	7.6	147	4.2	21.6	5.1	0.0
Strawberry, McDonald's*	1 Sundae/214g	360	8.6	168	2.0	33.0	4.0	0.0
Toffee, McDonald's*	1 Sundae/182g	350	9.1	192	3.0	34.0	5.0	1.0
SYRUP								
Pancake, McDonald's*	1 Pot/55g	190	0.0	345	0.0	84.0	0.0	0.0
TEA								
with Milk, McDonald's*	1 Serving/333ml	10	3.3	3	0.0	1.0	1.0	0.0
WRAP								
Breakfast with Brown Sauce, McDonald's*	1 Wrap/235g	595	30.6	253	11.0	23.0	13.0	2.0
Breakfast with Tomato Ketchup, McDonald's*	1 Wrap/235g	595	30.6	253	11.0	23.0	13.0	2.0
Chicken, BBQ, Snack, McDonald's*	1 Wrap/115g	300	12.0	261	10.4	30.4	10.4	1.7
Chicken, Cajun, McDonald's*	1 Wrap/222g	585	33.4	263	9.0	22.0	15.0	2.0

MCDONALD'S

	Measure INFO/WEIGHT	per Measure KCAL	FAT	Nutrition Values per 100g / 100ml KCAL	PROT	CARB	FAT	FIBRE
WRAP								
Chicken, Cheese & Bacon Snack, McDonald's*	1 Wrap/100g	360	18.0	360	14.0	33.0	18.0	2.0
Chicken, Grilled, Salad, McDonald's*	1 Wrap/221g	335	11.0	152	7.2	19.9	5.0	1.8
Chicken, Snack, McDonald's*	1 Wrap/112g	266	11.2	237	10.0	29.0	10.0	2.0
Chicken Fajita, McDonald's*	1 Wrap/259g	647	31.1	250	8.9	26.7	12.0	1.2
Garlic & Herb, Snack, McDonald's*	1 Wrap/121g	335	18.2	276	12.0	25.0	15.0	2.0
Oriental, Snack, McDonald's*	1 Wrap/127g	265	10.1	209	10.0	25.0	8.0	2.0
Spicy Vegetable, McDonald's*	1 Wrap/203g	445	16.3	219	5.0	29.0	8.0	5.0

NANDO'S

	Measure INFO/WEIGHT	per Measure KCAL	FAT	Nutrition Values per 100g / 100ml KCAL	PROT	CARB	FAT	FIBRE
BREAD								
Garlic, Nando's*	1 Portion/101g	330	15.5	327	8.5	38.8	15.3	1.7
BURGERS								
Bean, Nando's*	1 Burger/235g	468	13.4	199	9.5	26.5	5.7	2.4
Chicken, Breast, Double, Nando's*	1 Burger/275g	446	6.9	162	20.2	15.0	2.5	0.7
Chicken, Breast, Fillet, Nando's*	1 Burger/195g	333	5.3	171	15.9	21.0	2.7	1.9
Veggie, Nando's*	1 Burger/246g	387	6.5	157	8.2	23.2	2.6	3.1
CHICKEN								
¼, Breast, Peri Peri, Nando's*	¼ Breast/90g	135	2.4	150	28.1	3.4	2.7	0.0
¼, Leg, Peri Peri, Nando's*	1 Portion/95g	218	13.2	229	25.9	0.1	13.9	0.0
½, Peri Peri, Nando's*	½ Chicken/185g	353	15.6	191	27.0	1.7	8.4	0.0
Breast, Fillet Strips, Nando's*	1 Serving/108g	152	2.2	141	30.6	0.2	2.0	0.0
Peri Peri, Butterfly, Flame Grilled, Nando's*	1 Portion/193g	315	9.1	163	30.1	0.1	4.7	0.5
Whole, Nando's*	1 Chicken/370g	705	31.3	191	27.0	1.7	8.5	0.0
Wings, 10, Nando's*	10 Wings/246g	593	34.7	241	28.4	0.1	14.1	0.2
Wings, 3, Nando's*	3 Wings/71g	189	11.3	267	30.8	0.1	16.0	0.6
Wings, 5, Nando's*	5 Wings/123g	296	17.3	241	28.4	0.1	14.1	0.0
CHIPS								
Large, Nando's*	1 Serving/480g	1071	43.7	223	2.9	33.6	9.1	2.5
Peri Peri, Large, Nando's*	1 Serving/482g	1074	43.7	223	2.9	33.6	9.1	2.5
Peri Peri, Regular, Nando's*	1 Portion/161g	359	14.6	223	2.9	33.5	9.1	2.5
Regular, Nando's*	1 Serving/160g	357	14.6	223	2.9	33.6	9.1	2.5
COLESLAW								
Large, Nando's*	1 Serving/100g	531	45.9	177	0.8	6.3	15.3	1.1
Regular, Nando's*	1 Serving/150g	265	23.0	177	0.8	6.3	15.3	1.1
CORN								
On The Cob, Large, Nando's*	1 Serving/69g	99	1.9	144	5.6	26.7	2.7	4.6
DESSERT								
Cake, Carrot, Nando's*	1 Serving/191g	726	30.6	380	4.0	32.0	16.0	1.0
Cake, Choc-a-Lot, Nando's*	1 Serving/157g	534	31.4	340	5.0	40.0	20.0	2.0
Cheesecake, Chocolate, Nando's*	1 Serving/134g	496	34.8	370	6.0	29.0	26.0	1.0
Cheesecake, Mango & Passion Fruit, Nando's*	1 Serving/131g	419	26.2	320	50.4	29.0	20.0	0.0
Cheesecake, White Choc Raspberry Swirl, Nando's*	1 Serving/137g	493	34.3	360	5.0	28.0	25.0	1.0
Tart, Bolo De Coco, Nando's*	1 Serving/70g	277	16.0	396	11.9	35.6	22.9	6.6
Tart, Custard, Nata, Nando's*	1 Serving/75g	210	8.1	280	5.5	40.3	10.8	2.0
HOUMOUS								
with Peri Peri Drizzle & Pitta, Nando's*	1 Serving/295g	876	32.1	297	9.5	40.9	10.9	6.2
ICE CREAM								
Chocolate, Nando's*	1 Serving/90g	194	8.8	216	4.4	27.6	9.8	0.6
Rum & Raisin Flavour, Nando's*	1 Serving/95g	210	8.4	221	2.9	32.6	8.8	0.5
Strawberry, Nando's*	1 Serving/105g	223	11.5	212	3.1	25.3	10.9	0.5
Vanilla Chilli & Toffee Flavour Sauce, Nando's*	1 Serving/100g	219	10.4	219	3.2	28.1	10.4	0.5
LOLLY								
Chilly Billy, Apple & Blackcurrant, Nando's*	1 Lolly/115g	49	0.1	43	0.2	10.1	0.1	0.0

	Measure INFO/WEIGHT	per Measure KCAL	FAT	Nutrition Values per 100g / 100ml KCAL	PROT	CARB	FAT	FIBRE

NANDO'S
MASH
Creamy, Large, Nando's*	1 Serving/100g	544	31.6	136	1.7	13.0	7.9	2.5
Creamy, Regular, Nando's*	1 Serving/200g	272	15.8	136	1.7	13.0	7.9	2.5
Sweet Potato, Fino Side, Nando's*	1 Serving/200g	236	4.2	118	2.2	22.7	2.1	2.7

OLIVES
Spicy, Mixed, Nando's*	1 Bowl/100g	106	10.4	106	0.9	0.6	10.4	3.0

PEAS
Macho, Large, Nando's*	1 Serving/280g	316	20.7	113	4.7	7.0	7.4	4.2
Macho, Regular, Nando's*	1 Serving/140g	158	10.4	113	4.7	7.0	7.4	4.2

PITTA
Bean, Nando's*	1 Pitta/235g	477	12.9	203	8.5	28.8	5.5	2.4
Chicken Breast, Nando's*	1 Pitta/223g	386	5.1	173	17.7	20.4	2.3	0.9
Veggie, Nando's*	1 Pitta/235g	384	5.9	163	7.6	26.3	2.5	3.2

RATATOUILLE
Fino Side, Nando's*	1 Serving/180g	185	13.0	103	1.2	6.3	7.2	4.1

RICE
Spicy, Large, Nando's*	1 Serving/100g	398	10.7	153	3.1	25.9	4.1	3.0
Spicy, Regular, Nando's*	1 Regular/130g	199	5.3	153	3.1	25.9	4.1	3.0

ROLL
Portuguese with Chicken Livers, Nando's*	1 Serving/251g	641	29.8	255	21.2	16.0	11.9	0.9
Prego Steak, Nando's*	1 Roll/230g	435	11.4	189	18.3	17.7	5.0	0.9

SALAD
Caesar, no Chicken, Nando's*	1 Serving/220g	265	21.3	120	3.4	4.9	9.7	1.2
Couscous, with Chicken, Nando's*	1 Salad/270g	371	24.8	137	2.9	10.2	9.2	1.9
Mediterranean, Nando's*	1 Salad/240g	230	17.4	96	3.8	3.0	7.2	1.8
Mixed Leaf, Fino Side, Nando's*	1 Portion/115g	17	0.4	15	0.7	0.3	0.3	1.1
Mixed Leaf, Nando's*	1 Portion/115g	17	0.4	15	0.7	0.3	0.3	1.1

SORBET
Mango, Nando's*	1 Serving/135g	186	0.3	138	0.3	33.4	0.2	0.7

WRAP
Beanie, Nando's*	1 Wrap/320g	698	29.2	218	7.2	25.3	9.1	2.1
Chicken, Breast, Double, Fillet, Nando's*	1 Wrap/426g	774	23.7	182	18.4	13.8	5.6	0.7
Chicken, Breast, Fillet, Nando's*	1 Wrap/308g	608	21.4	197	13.7	19.1	6.9	1.0
Mushroom, Portobello, & Halloumi Cheese, Nando's*	1 Wrap/303g	618	33.1	204	5.5	19.7	10.9	1.3
Veggie, Nando's*	1 Wrap/320g	605	22.2	189	6.5	23.4	6.9	2.7

YOGHURT
Banana, Frozen, Nando's*	1 Serving/100g	87	0.1	87	3.3	18.2	0.1	0.1
Chocolate, Frozen, Nando's*	1 Serving/100g	107	0.3	107	4.0	22.3	0.3	0.8
Strawberry, Frozen, Nando's*	1 Serving/100g	87	0.1	87	3.3	18.2	0.1	0.1
Vanilla, Frozen, Nando's*	1 Serving/100ml	87	0.1	87	3.3	18.2	0.1	0.1

PIZZA HUT
BACON BITS
Pizza Hut*	1 Serving/12g	60	3.6	496	8.3	48.7	29.8	0.0

BEANS
Chocolate Coated, Ice Cream Factory, Pizza Hut*	1 Serving/30g	142	5.4	475	5.5	72.2	18.1	0.0

BEETROOT
Pizza Hut*	1 Portion/25g	14	0.0	55	0.9	12.0	0.1	0.0

BREAD
Garlic, Ciabatta, Pizza Hut*	2 Pieces/253g	820	32.1	324	9.1	43.4	12.7	0.0
Garlic, Dipsters, Pizza Hut*	1 Piece/90g	308	14.2	342	6.8	43.1	15.8	0.0
Garlic, Pizza Hut*	1 Slice/30g	95	4.6	318	6.8	38.1	15.4	0.0
Garlic, with Cheese, Pizza Hut*	4 Pieces/187g	568	34.0	304	15.9	19.0	18.2	0.0

PIZZA HUT

	Measure INFO/WEIGHT	per Measure KCAL	FAT	Nutrition Values per 100g / 100ml KCAL	PROT	CARB	FAT	FIBRE
BREADSTICKS								
Garlic, Pizza Hut*	1 Stick/50g	173	6.7	347	9.8	46.9	13.4	1.0
BRUSCHETTA								
Light Lunch, Pizza Hut*	3 Pieces/211g	369	16.0	175	4.1	22.4	7.6	0.0
CAKE								
Chocolate Fudge, Dessert, Pizza Hut*	1 Piece/178g	684	31.9	384	4.2	51.4	17.9	0.0
CARBONARA								
Ham, Buffet, Pizza Hut*	1 Portion/200g	180	4.6	90	3.4	14.4	2.3	0.0
CHEESE								
4 & Vegetable, Buffet, Pizza Hut*	1 Portion/200g	210	8.6	105	4.0	12.6	4.3	0.0
Hard, Grated, Pizza Hut*	1 Serving/30g	121	9.0	404	33.0	0.1	30.0	0.0
Parmesan Reggiano, Grated at table, Pizza Hut*	1 Serving/5g	20	1.4	400	34.0	0.0	28.0	0.0
Three Cheese Melt, Starter, Pizza Hut*	3 Pieces/209g	546	38.1	261	11.1	12.3	18.2	0.0
CHEESECAKE								
Chocolate, Pizza Hut*	1 Serving/63g	228	11.1	360	5.6	44.9	17.5	0.0
Clotted Cream, Pizza Hut*	1 Serving/64g	205	10.4	323	4.6	39.3	16.4	0.0
Lemon & Ginger, Pizza Hut*	1 Serving/64g	205	9.7	323	4.2	42.4	15.2	0.0
New York Style, Baked, Pizza Hut*	1 Slice/113g	442	16.2	391	6.6	62.3	14.3	0.0
Vanilla, Madagascan, Dessert, Pizza Hut*	1 Serving/133g	397	18.1	298	4.8	39.2	13.6	0.0
CHICKEN								
Cheesy Jalapeno Poppers, Pizza Hut*	6 Pieces/150g	408	19.9	272	5.2	32.8	13.3	0.0
Dippin, Pizza Hut*	1 Serving/155g	332	14.4	214	15.7	17.1	9.3	0.0
Goujons, Pizza Hut*	5 Pieces/169g	311	13.5	184	17.0	11.0	8.0	1.5
Strips, Breaded, (Five Strips), Pizza Hut*	5 Pieces/175g	283	13.2	162	15.9	8.9	7.5	0.0
Strips, Breaded, with Wedges, 2, Kids, Pizza Hut*	1 Serving/231g	386	11.6	167	6.7	23.9	5.0	0.0
Strips, Breaded, with Wedges, 3, Kids, Pizza Hut*	1 Serving/265g	451	14.3	170	8.1	22.2	5.4	0.0
Strips, Breaded, Wrap Factory, 2, Kids, Pizza Hut*	1 Serving/247g	434	12.1	176	8.3	24.8	4.9	0.0
Strips, Breaded, Wrap Factory, 3, Kids, Pizza Hut*	1 Serving/325g	617	17.9	190	9.2	25.9	5.5	0.0
Strips, Hot n Kicking, Pizza Hut*	7 Pieces/140g	276	12.6	197	17.0	12.0	9.0	0.0
Wings, BBQ, (Delivery Only), Pizza Hut*	6 Pieces/156g	303	14.4	194	23.2	4.6	9.2	0.0
Wings, BBQ, Pizza Hut*	6 Pieces/171g	306	14.5	179	21.3	4.4	8.5	0.0
Wings, BBQ, Saucy, Pizza Hut*	6 Wings/159g	355	21.8	223	21.4	3.6	13.7	0.0
Wings, Buffalo, Saucy, Pizza Hut*	6 Wings/181g	380	22.2	209	21.0	3.7	12.2	0.0
Wings, Spicy, Crunch, (Delivery Only), Pizza Hut*	1 Portion/218g	510	30.5	234	17.0	10.0	14.0	0.0
Wings, Texan BBQ Chicken, Pizza Hut*	6 Pieces/159g	355	21.8	223	21.4	3.6	13.7	0.0
Wings, with Sour Cream & Chive Dip, Pizza Hut*	1 Pack/178g	680	56.1	382	22.8	1.9	31.5	1.3
COLESLAW								
Pizza Hut*	1 Pot/38g	54	4.6	143	0.9	7.1	12.3	0.0
CREAM								
Single, Dessert, Pizza Hut*	1 Serving/40g	75	7.2	188	2.6	3.9	18.0	0.0
UHT, Portion, Pizza Hut*	1 Portion/12g	23	2.2	188	2.7	3.9	18.0	0.0
CROUTONS								
Pizza Flavoured, Pizza Hut*	1 Serving/12g	23	3.1	196	10.1	55.2	26.1	0.0
Salad, Large, Pizza Hut*	1 Portion/20g	94	4.2	470	11.0	59.1	21.1	0.0
DESSERT								
Cherries in Sauce, Pizza Hut*	1 Serving/20g	28	0.0	142	0.5	34.9	0.1	0.0
Chocolate Obsession, Pizza Hut*	1 Serving/100g	157	6.8	157	2.0	22.1	6.8	0.0
Toffee Apple Meltdown, Pizza Hut*	1 Serving/120g	325	11.0	271	3.3	43.7	9.2	0.0
DIP								
BBQ Sauce Portion In Restaurant, Pizza Hut*	1 Pot/28g	34	0.0	121	1.4	29.3	0.1	0.0
BBQ Tabasco, Pizza Hut*	1 Serving/25g	36	0.1	142	1.2	33.6	0.2	0.0
Garlic & Herb, Pizza Hut*	1 Serving/28g	93	9.2	331	1.4	7.6	32.6	0.0
Mayonnaise, Light, Restaurant Only, Pizza Hut*	1 Dippot/50g	163	16.5	326	0.6	6.0	33.0	0.0

PIZZA HUT

	Measure INFO/WEIGHT	per Measure KCAL	FAT	Nutrition Values per 100g / 100ml KCAL	PROT	CARB	FAT	FIBRE
DIP								
Sour Cream & Chive, Restaurant Only, Pizza Hut*	1 Serving/28g	83	8.7	296	0.7	3.6	31.1	0.0
Sweet Chilli Sauce, Restaurant Only, Pizza Hut*	1 Pot/28g	48	0.2	171	0.4	32.9	0.7	0.0
Tomato Ketchup, Restaurant Only, Pizza Hut*	1 Pot/28g	39	0.0	139	1.4	34.3	0.0	0.0
DOUGH BALLS								
Cheese & Jalapeno, (Delivery Only), Pizza Hut*	1 Portion/198g	495	16.2	250	9.7	33.8	8.2	0.0
DRESSING								
1000 Island, Pizza Hut*	1 Serving/38g	107	9.7	280	0.7	11.5	25.5	0.0
Blue Cheese, Pizza Hut*	1 Serving/35g	91	8.0	258	1.7	11.5	22.7	0.0
Caesar, Pizza Hut*	1 Serving/40g	27	1.1	68	1.5	8.9	2.8	0.0
Ranch, Pizza Hut*	1 Serving/32g	163	18.0	510	1.2	1.5	56.4	0.0
Vinaigrette, Low Fat, Pizza Hut*	1 Serving/30ml	23	0.1	77	0.3	17.2	0.5	0.0
FISH								
Goujons (5 Strips), Pizza Hut*	5 Strips/210g	416	20.9	198	9.9	17.1	9.9	0.0
FRIES								
Savoury Seasoned, Pizza Hut*	1 Serving/144g	238	11.5	165	2.4	20.8	8.0	0.0
Seasoned, Savoury, (Express Only), Pizza Hut*	1 Portion/145g	247	11.1	171	2.3	23.0	7.7	0.0
FUDGE BROWNIE								
Pizza Hut*	1 Serving/105g	418	16.4	398	4.3	60.1	15.6	0.0
ICE CREAM								
Coco Mango, Pizza Hut*	1 Serving/100g	88	1.8	88	0.6	17.3	1.8	0.0
Cookie Craving, Pizza Hut*	1 Serving/100g	149	6.9	149	1.6	20.1	6.9	0.0
Dairy, Dessert, Pizza Hut*	1 Portion/142g	272	12.6	192	4.6	23.3	8.9	0.2
Mix, Pizza Hut*	1 Serving/100g	147	6.2	147	4.0	18.8	6.2	0.0
Traditional, Kids, Pizza Hut*	1 Serving/89g	171	9.2	193	2.6	22.4	10.4	0.0
Traditional, Pizza Hut*	1 Serving/132g	254	13.7	193	2.6	22.4	10.4	0.0
KETCHUP								
Heinz, Pizza Hut*	1 Serving/12g	14	0.0	119	0.5	28.4	0.1	0.0
MACARONI CHEESE								
Pizza Hut*	1 Serving/41g	57	2.4	140	4.9	16.6	6.0	0.0
MARSHMALLOWS								
Mini, Ice Cream Factory, Pizza Hut*	1 Serving/30g	96	0.0	320	5.4	74.3	0.0	0.0
MAYONNAISE								
Sachet, Pizza Hut*	1 Sachet/12g	88	9.8	731	1.3	1.8	81.2	0.0
MEATBALLS								
in Pomodoro Sauce, Light Lunch, Pizza Hut*	1 Portion/253g	342	18.2	135	6.6	11.0	7.2	0.0
MILK								
Half Fat, Portions, Pizza Hut*	1 Portion/14g	6	0.2	45	6.0	5.1	1.6	0.0
MILKSHAKE								
Strawberry Cheesecake, Pizza Hut*	1 Serving/236g	371	14.1	157	3.4	22.3	5.9	0.0
The Chocoholic, Pizza Hut*	1 Serving/248g	442	20.4	178	3.6	22.8	8.2	0.0
Toffee Banoffee Shake, Pizza Hut*	1 Serving/404g	763	22.6	189	2.4	32.3	5.6	0.0
MUFFIN								
Cheesecake, Sicilian Lemon, Pizza Hut*	1 Portion/130g	508	24.2	391	5.1	50.9	18.6	0.0
Fruity, Pizza Hut*	1 Serving/115g	366	13.7	318	4.1	48.4	11.9	0.0
Mixed Berry, Pizza Hut*	1 Muffin/108g	402	22.6	372	4.4	41.6	20.9	0.0
Sicilian Lemon Cheesecake, Pizza Hut*	1 Serving/130g	508	24.2	391	5.1	50.9	18.6	0.0
Strawberry & White Chocolate, Pizza Hut*	1 Muffin/108g	402	22.6	372	4.4	41.6	20.9	0.0
MUSHROOMS								
Blue Cheese, Pizza Hut*	1 Serving/256g	514	40.7	201	7.2	7.5	15.9	0.0
Breaded, Pizza Hut*	6 Mushrooms/180g	410	14.4	228	4.5	26.1	8.0	0.0
Garlic, 2, Pizza Hut*	1 Serving/230g	570	43.4	248	7.9	7.0	18.9	0.0
Garlic, Crispy Coated, Pizza Hut*	1 Portion/135g	240	10.1	178	4.1	23.4	7.5	0.0

PIZZA HUT

	Measure INFO/WEIGHT	per Measure KCAL	FAT	Nutrition Values per 100g / 100ml KCAL	PROT	CARB	FAT	FIBRE
MUSHROOMS								
Garlic, with BBQ Dip, Pizza Hut*	1 Portion/112g	263	11.2	234	6.2	30.5	10.0	3.4
Garlic, with Sour Cream & Chive Dip, Pizza Hut*	1 Portion/112g	426	34.6	380	6.4	20.0	30.8	3.4
NACHOS								
Chilli, Pizza Hut*	1 Serving/190g	550	33.1	289	8.8	27.2	17.4	0.0
Sharing Starters, Pizza Hut*	1 Serving/356g	1087	76.3	305	7.9	24.6	21.4	0.0
Side, Delivery Only, Pizza Hut*	1 Serving/222g	669	40.3	301	7.7	30.2	18.1	0.0
OLIVES								
Mixed, Pizza Hut*	1 Serving/70g	140	9.0	200	1.5	19.6	12.8	0.0
ONION RINGS								
Chilli, (Delivery Only), Pizza Hut*	1 Ring/13g	26	1.2	212	3.2	28.2	9.6	0.0
Chilli, Pizza Hut*	8 Rings/100g	212	9.6	212	3.2	28.2	9.6	0.0
ONIONS								
White, Pizza Hut*	1 Serving/24g	10	0.0	42	1.0	10.0	0.0	0.0
PANCAKE								
Fruity, Kids, Pizza Hut*	1 Serving/156g	227	3.3	146	1.9	30.6	2.1	0.0
PASTA								
3 Cheese & Vegetable, Pizza Hut*	1 Serving/300g	315	12.9	105	4.0	12.6	4.3	0.0
4 Cheese, Sharing, Pizza Hut*	1 Serving/1200g	1860	102.0	155	6.1	13.5	8.5	0.0
Alfredo, Chicken, Sharing, (Delivery Only), Pizza Hut*	1 Pack/1200g	1680	40.8	140	8.1	19.1	3.4	0.0
Alfredo, Light Lunch, Pizza Hut*	1 Portion/226g	294	5.0	130	4.1	23.3	2.2	0.0
Alfredo, Pizza Hut*	1 Portion/400g	520	8.8	130	4.1	23.3	2.2	0.0
Arrabiata, Pizza Hut*	1 Portion/450g	441	13.0	98	2.9	15.0	2.9	0.0
Bolognese, Sharing, (Delivery Only), Pizza Hut*	1 Pack/1200g	1500	64.8	125	7.2	11.9	5.4	0.0
Bolognese, Sharing, Pizza Hut*	1 Serving/1200g	1500	64.8	125	7.2	11.9	5.4	0.0
Cannelloni, Spinach & Ricotta, Pizza Hut*	1 Portion/404g	566	27.5	140	6.2	13.1	6.8	0.0
Chicken Alfredo, Sharing, Pizza Hut*	1 Serving/1200g	1680	40.8	140	8.1	19.1	3.4	0.0
Ham & Mushroom, Pizza Hut*	1 Serving/450g	473	10.4	105	4.2	17.0	2.3	0.0
Lasagne, Traditional, Pizza Hut*	1 Portion/460g	589	26.7	128	5.9	13.0	5.8	0.0
Macaroni Cheese, Kids, Pizza Hut*	1 Portion/250g	332	16.2	133	4.0	14.8	6.5	0.0
Mezzaluna, Tomato & Mozzarella, Pizza Hut*	1 Portion/350g	339	10.1	97	3.1	14.7	2.9	0.0
Penne, Mediterranean Vegetable, Pizza Hut*	1 Portion/448g	592	19.7	132	3.7	18.3	4.4	0.0
Salmone Penne Al Forno, Pizza Hut*	1 Serving/496g	832	49.1	168	7.5	10.6	9.9	0.0
Spaghetti Bolognese, Kids, New, Pizza Hut*	1 Serving/234g	211	3.5	90	7.6	14.6	1.5	0.0
Spaghetti Bolognese, Pizza Hut*	1 Portion/475g	745	31.3	157	6.2	17.8	6.6	0.0
Tagliatelle, Alla Carbonara, Pizza Hut*	1 Serving/400g	548	32.4	137	5.6	10.4	8.1	0.0
Tagliatelle, Meatball, Italian Recipe, Pizza Hut*	1 Portion/240g	324	10.6	135	6.9	16.6	4.4	0.0
Tomato & Pepperoni, Pizza Hut*	1 Serving/300g	312	8.1	104	3.6	16.3	2.7	0.0
PASTA BAKE								
Salmon, Pizza Hut*	1 Portion/400g	692	42.8	173	7.9	11.3	10.7	0.0
PASTA SALAD								
Sweetcorn & Pepper, Pizza Hut*	1 Serving/47g	75	2.5	159	4.6	23.1	5.3	0.0
Tomato, Dressed, Med, Pizza Hut*	1 Serving/100g	112	1.5	112	3.5	21.2	1.5	0.0
Tomato & Basil, Pizza Hut*	1 Serving/50g	50	0.7	100	3.7	17.8	1.5	0.0
PEPPERS								
Red & Green Wedges, Pizza Hut*	1 Serving/40g	6	0.1	15	0.8	2.6	0.3	0.0
Romano, Stuffed, Pizza Hut*	1 Serving/208g	250	13.3	120	2.7	13.3	6.4	0.0
PIE								
Banoffee, Dessert, Pizza Hut*	1 Serving/125g	428	25.3	340	2.5	37.3	20.1	0.0
Banoffee, Pizza Hut*	1 Serving/100g	350	21.5	350	4.2	34.9	21.5	0.0
PIZZA								
BBQ Deluxe, Cheesy Bites, Pizza Hut*	1 Slice/143g	358	11.6	251	11.7	34.4	8.1	0.0
BBQ Deluxe, Italian, Individual, Pizza Hut*	1 Slice/78g	185	6.1	238	10.9	34.3	7.9	0.0

PIZZA HUT

PIZZA

	Measure INFO/WEIGHT	per Measure KCAL	FAT	Nutrition Values per 100g / 100ml KCAL	PROT	CARB	FAT	FIBRE
BBQ Deluxe, Italian, Large, Pizza Hut*	1 Slice/95g	239	8.0	252	14.3	29.7	8.4	0.0
BBQ Deluxe, Italian, Medium, Pizza Hut*	1 Slice/105g	253	8.0	241	12.0	31.1	7.6	0.0
BBQ Deluxe, Pan, Individual, Pizza Hut*	1 Slice/79g	200	7.9	253	12.7	28.0	10.0	0.0
BBQ Deluxe, Pan, Large, Pizza Hut*	1 Slice/122g	306	12.1	251	11.8	28.6	9.9	0.0
BBQ Deluxe, Pan, Medium, Pizza Hut*	1 Slice/107g	276	11.3	257	11.7	28.8	10.5	0.0
BBQ Deluxe, Stuffed Crust, Pizza Hut*	1 Serving/155g	337	10.4	217	11.6	31.9	6.7	0.0
Cajun Chicken, Hot One, Italian, Medium, Pizza Hut*	1 Slice/100g	250	9.3	250	12.5	29.1	9.3	0.0
Cajun Chicken, Hot One, Pan, Large, Pizza Hut*	1 Slice/125g	321	14.7	257	12.9	24.7	11.8	0.0
Cajun Chicken, Hot One, Pan, Medium, Pizza Hut*	1 Slice/105g	273	12.3	259	12.7	25.6	11.7	0.0
Cajun Chicken, Hot One, Stuffed Crust, Pizza Hut*	1 Slice/135g	331	10.8	245	13.3	30.0	8.0	0.0
Cheese Feast, Italian, Medium, Pizza Hut*	1 Slice/96g	260	11.3	272	12.3	29.1	11.8	0.0
Cheese Feast, Pan, Medium, Pizza Hut*	1 Slice/106g	299	15.0	283	14.6	24.2	14.2	0.0
Cheese Feast, Stuffed Crust, Pizza Hut*	1 Slice/132g	361	13.8	273	14.3	30.5	10.4	0.0
Chicken, Hi Light, Medium, Pizza Hut*	1 Slice/83g	189	5.5	230	13.2	29.2	6.7	0.0
Chicken Feast, Italian, Medium, Pizza Hut*	1 Slice/100g	249	8.6	248	14.1	28.6	8.6	0.0
Chicken Feast, Pan, Medium, Pizza Hut*	1 Slice/109g	283	12.0	259	15.5	24.6	11.0	0.0
Chicken Feast, Stuffed Crust, Pizza Hut*	1 Slice/133g	337	12.6	254	14.8	27.3	9.5	0.0
Chicken Supreme, Cheesy Bites, Pizza Hut*	1 Slice/148g	322	10.0	218	11.8	29.5	6.8	0.0
Chicken Supreme, Express, Pizza Hut*	1 Serving/65g	143	5.8	221	10.1	28.1	9.0	0.0
Chicken Supreme, Italian, Individual, Pizza Hut*	1 Slice/74g	169	4.4	229	10.7	35.4	5.9	0.0
Chicken Supreme, Italian, Large, Pizza Hut*	1 Slice/111g	217	6.4	196	9.8	29.3	5.8	0.0
Chicken Supreme, Italian, Medium, Pizza Hut*	1 Slice/102g	220	6.3	215	10.3	31.9	6.2	0.0
Chicken Supreme, Pan, Individual, Pizza Hut*	1 Slice/81g	186	8.0	231	11.6	26.9	9.9	0.0
Chicken Supreme, Pan, Large, Pizza Hut*	1 Slice/124g	271	11.6	219	10.9	26.1	9.4	0.0
Chicken Supreme, Pan, Medium, Pizza Hut*	1 Slice/115g	251	9.9	219	11.2	26.6	8.6	0.0
Chicken Supreme, Stuffed Crust, Pizza Hut*	1 Slice/153g	367	11.0	240	11.6	34.8	7.2	0.0
Country Feast, Italian, Medium, Pizza Hut*	1 Slice/109g	252	9.6	232	9.7	28.6	8.8	0.0
Country Feast, Pan, Medium, Pizza Hut*	1 Slice/115g	279	12.1	243	11.4	25.8	10.5	0.0
Country Feast, Stuffed Crust, Pizza Hut*	1 Slice/144g	326	10.8	227	11.5	28.4	7.5	0.0
Express, Supreme, Pizza Hut*	1 Serving/68g	165	7.6	242	10.7	27.8	11.2	0.0
Farmhouse, Cheesy Bites, Pizza Hut*	1 Slice/133g	332	12.6	250	13.2	30.7	9.5	0.0
Farmhouse, Italian, Individual, Pizza Hut*	1 Slice/74g	188	6.0	253	11.8	33.1	8.1	0.0
Farmhouse, Italian, Large, Pizza Hut*	1 Slice/92g	206	6.7	224	10.2	34.0	7.3	0.0
Farmhouse, Italian, Medium, Pizza Hut*	1 Slice/84g	192	5.4	229	10.2	35.7	6.4	0.0
Farmhouse, Pan, Individual, Pizza Hut*	1 Slice/70g	179	7.4	256	11.3	31.6	10.6	0.0
Farmhouse, Pan, Large, Pizza Hut*	1 Slice/106g	257	11.0	242	11.4	29.7	10.4	0.0
Farmhouse, Pan, Medium, Pizza Hut*	1 Slice/100g	242	10.4	242	11.3	28.6	10.4	0.0
Farmhouse, Stuffed Crust, Pizza Hut*	1 Slice/132g	387	10.0	293	11.8	30.0	7.6	0.0
Ham, Hi Light, Medium, Pizza Hut*	1 Slice/82g	184	5.5	225	12.1	29.1	6.7	0.0
Happy Hour, Chicken & Mushroom, Pizza Hut*	1 Serving/80g	165	5.4	207	9.6	27.6	6.8	0.0
Happy Hour, Ham & Sweetcorn, Pizza Hut*	1 Serving/86g	174	5.6	202	9.4	27.0	6.5	0.0
Happy Hour, Pepper & Tomato, Pizza Hut*	1 Serving/86g	163	5.4	189	8.0	26.1	6.3	0.0
Happy Hour, Pepperoni & Onion, Pizza Hut*	1 Serving/80g	179	6.9	224	9.4	28.2	8.6	0.0
Hawaiian, Cheesy Bites, Pizza Hut*	1 Slice/136g	316	10.6	232	11.6	31.2	7.8	0.0
Hawaiian, Express, Pizza Hut*	1 Serving/60g	147	6.4	245	10.5	29.9	10.6	0.0
Hawaiian, Italian, Individual, Pizza Hut*	1 Serving/71g	164	4.2	229	9.8	37.9	5.8	0.0
Hawaiian, Italian, Large, Pizza Hut*	1 Slice/99g	221	7.0	223	10.0	33.2	7.1	0.0
Hawaiian, Italian, Medium, Pizza Hut*	1 Slice/92g	201	5.6	219	9.8	33.3	6.1	0.0
Hawaiian, Pan, Individual, Pizza Hut*	1 Serving/73g	175	6.5	240	10.9	32.2	8.9	0.0
Hawaiian, Pan, Large, Pizza Hut*	1 Slice/112g	293	12.7	262	10.6	32.6	11.4	0.0
Hawaiian, Pan, Medium, Pizza Hut*	1 Slice/109g	245	9.7	224	10.1	28.5	8.9	0.0
Hawaiian, Stuffed Crust, Pizza Hut*	1 Slice/141g	306	10.3	217	11.0	30.7	7.3	0.0

PIZZA HUT

PIZZA

	Measure INFO/WEIGHT	per Measure KCAL	per Measure FAT	Nutrition Values per 100g / 100ml KCAL	PROT	CARB	FAT	FIBRE
Hot 'n' Spicy, Cheesy Bites, Pizza Hut*	1 Slice/127g	331	12.6	261	12.6	33.7	9.9	0.0
Hot 'n' Spicy, Italian, Individual, Pizza Hut*	1 Slice/66g	180	6.9	272	11.0	36.5	10.4	0.0
Hot 'n' Spicy, Italian, Large, Pizza Hut*	1 Slice/93g	236	9.4	254	11.2	32.7	10.1	0.0
Hot 'n' Spicy, Italian, Medium, Pizza Hut*	1 Slice/86g	222	8.4	259	11.0	34.5	9.8	0.0
Hot 'n' Spicy, Pan, Individual, Pizza Hut*	1 Slice/71g	183	7.9	259	10.9	30.4	11.2	0.0
Hot 'n' Spicy, Pan, Large, Pizza Hut*	1 Slice/105g	266	11.4	254	12.0	30.2	10.9	0.0
Hot 'n' Spicy, Pan, Medium, Pizza Hut*	1 Slice/93g	237	10.6	254	11.5	29.2	11.4	0.0
Hot 'n' Spicy, Stuffed Crust, Pizza Hut*	1 Slice/139g	329	11.0	236	11.8	33.1	7.9	0.0
Margherita, Cheesy Bites, Pizza Hut*	1 Serving/128g	337	12.9	263	12.8	33.1	10.1	0.0
Margherita, Fingers, Kids, Pizza Hut*	1 Serving/95g	258	12.1	273	11.0	28.4	12.8	0.0
Margherita, Italian, Individual, Pizza Hut*	1 Slice/67g	177	5.4	264	11.9	39.2	8.0	0.0
Margherita, Italian, Large, Pizza Hut*	1 Slice/91g	229	8.6	252	10.4	34.2	9.5	0.0
Margherita, Italian, Medium, Pizza Hut*	1 Slice/80g	205	7.0	256	11.0	35.7	8.8	0.0
Margherita, Pan, Individual, Pizza Hut*	1 Slice/71g	189	8.1	268	11.6	32.4	11.5	0.0
Margherita, Pan, Large, Pizza Hut*	1 Slice/105g	273	12.4	261	11.6	29.8	11.9	0.0
Margherita, Pan, Medium, Pizza Hut*	1 Serving/97g	256	11.4	265	11.6	30.6	11.8	0.0
Margherita, Stuffed Crust, Pizza Hut*	1 Slice/140g	349	12.4	248	14.0	31.6	8.8	0.0
Margherita, Thick, Kids, Pizza Hut*	1 Serving/202g	506	17.9	251	9.0	33.0	8.9	0.0
Meat Feast, Cheesy Bites, Pizza Hut*	1 Slice/142g	387	16.2	272	13.9	30.3	11.4	0.0
Meat Feast, Italian, Individual, Pizza Hut*	1 Slice/81g	220	8.8	270	13.9	32.3	10.8	0.0
Meat Feast, Italian, Large, Pizza Hut*	1 Slice/111g	279	12.7	251	12.9	27.3	11.4	0.0
Meat Feast, Italian, Medium, Pizza Hut*	1 Slice/100g	257	11.0	258	13.0	30.0	11.0	0.0
Meat Feast, Pan, Individual, Pizza Hut*	1 Slice/84g	220	9.9	262	13.3	27.6	11.8	0.0
Meat Feast, Pan, Large, Pizza Hut*	1 Slice/124g	344	16.4	277	12.6	29.1	13.2	0.0
Meat Feast, Pan, Medium, Pizza Hut*	1 Slice/112g	294	13.9	262	12.2	28.0	12.4	0.0
Meat Feast, Stuffed Crust, Pizza Hut*	1 Slice/152g	376	15.8	247	13.5	28.0	10.4	0.0
Meaty, The Edge, Medium, Pizza Hut*	1 Slice/36g	110	5.7	308	17.0	20.4	16.1	0.0
Meaty BBQ, Cheesy Bites, Delivery, Pizza Hut*	1 Serving/115g	282	10.8	245	11.3	31.1	9.4	0.0
Meaty BBQ, Italian, Medium, Delivery, Pizza Hut*	1 Serving/70g	154	5.0	220	10.9	30.0	7.2	0.0
Meaty BBQ, Pan, Medium, Delivery, Pizza Hut*	1 Serving/92g	215	8.7	234	11.1	25.9	9.5	0.0
Mediterranean Meat Deluxe, Italian, Medium, Pizza Hut*	1 Slice/91g	245	9.4	270	12.8	33.5	10.4	0.0
Mediterranean Meat Deluxe, Italian, Pizza Hut*	1 Slice/72g	206	8.8	288	12.6	34.7	12.3	0.0
Mediterranean Meat Deluxe, Pan, Individual, Pizza Hut*	1 Slice/75g	212	10.4	284	13.5	29.5	13.9	0.0
Mediterranean Meat Deluxe, Pan, Medium, Pizza Hut*	1 Slice/98g	245	11.2	249	11.7	28.1	11.4	0.0
Mountain Fantastico, Italian, Individual, Pizza Hut*	1 Slice/75g	183	6.3	245	9.3	36.4	8.5	0.0
Pepperoni Feast, Cheesy Bites, Pizza Hut*	1 Slice/135g	382	16.7	284	15.8	29.6	12.4	0.0
Pepperoni Feast, Italian, Individual, Pizza Hut*	1 Slice/73g	205	8.4	282	11.4	36.3	11.6	0.0
Pepperoni Feast, Italian, Large, Pizza Hut*	1 Slice/103g	286	13.3	278	12.2	30.9	12.9	0.0
Pepperoni Feast, Italian, Medium, Pizza Hut*	1 Slice/93g	254	9.8	273	12.3	35.0	10.5	0.0
Pepperoni Feast, Pan, Individual, Pizza Hut*	1 Slice/79g	227	10.8	286	12.3	30.3	13.6	0.0
Pepperoni Feast, Pan, Large, Pizza Hut*	1 Slice/115g	347	20.2	302	12.0	26.4	17.6	0.0
Pepperoni Feast, Pan, Medium, Pizza Hut*	1 Slice/106g	297	15.9	279	12.6	26.2	14.9	0.0
Pepperoni Feast, Stuffed Crust, Pizza Hut*	1 Slice/143g	375	16.2	261	13.1	30.4	11.3	0.0
Seafood Fantastico, Italian, Individual, Pizza Hut*	1 Slice/81g	173	4.6	213	15.3	25.1	5.7	0.0
Seafood Fantastico, Italian, Large, Pizza Hut*	1 Slice/106g	228	6.6	215	15.1	24.6	6.2	0.0
Seafood Lovers, Italian, Individual, Pizza Hut*	1 Slice/66g	170	5.4	258	9.8	38.4	8.2	0.0
Seafood Lovers, Italian, Large, Pizza Hut*	1 Slice/90g	215	6.8	239	10.2	35.3	7.6	0.0
Seafood Lovers, Italian, Medium, Pizza Hut*	1 Slice/82g	202	6.6	245	10.1	35.3	8.0	0.0
Seafood Lovers, Pan, Individual, Pizza Hut*	1 Slice/69g	160	6.0	232	10.7	31.3	8.7	0.0
Seafood Lovers, Pan, Medium, Pizza Hut*	1 Slice/98g	233	10.4	237	9.7	28.3	10.6	0.0
Seafood Lovers, Stuffed Crust, Pizza Hut*	1 Slice/131g	314	10.9	239	12.3	31.8	8.3	0.0
Spicy, Hot One, Pan, Medium, Pizza Hut*	1 Slice/115g	274	13.0	239	11.2	23.1	11.3	0.0

PIZZA HUT

	Measure INFO/WEIGHT	per Measure KCAL	FAT	Nutrition Values per 100g / 100ml KCAL	PROT	CARB	FAT	FIBRE

PIZZA

	Measure INFO/WEIGHT	per Measure KCAL	FAT	KCAL	PROT	CARB	FAT	FIBRE
Stuffed Crust, Italian, Large, Delivery, Pizza Hut*	1 Serving/85g	198	8.6	234	11.7	26.9	10.2	0.0
Stuffed Crust, Italian, Medium, Delivery, Pizza Hut*	1 Serving/76g	170	7.8	225	11.0	25.3	10.3	0.0
Stuffed Crust, Pan, Large, Delivery, Pizza Hut*	1 Serving/120g	289	14.5	241	10.9	25.0	12.1	0.0
Stuffed Crust, Pan, Medium, Delivery, Pizza Hut*	1 Serving/100g	234	12.0	234	11.6	22.9	12.0	0.0
Super Supreme, Cheesy Bites, Pizza Hut*	1 Slice/162g	393	16.2	242	12.4	26.9	10.0	0.0
Super Supreme, Italian, Individual, Pizza Hut*	1 Slice/97g	260	11.0	267	13.9	27.3	11.3	0.0
Super Supreme, Italian, Large, Pizza Hut*	1 Slice/128g	281	13.2	219	10.6	24.4	10.3	0.0
Super Supreme, Italian, Medium, Pizza Hut*	1 Slice/119g	267	11.5	225	11.1	26.3	9.7	0.0
Super Supreme, Pan, Individual, Pizza Hut*	1 Slice/96g	228	10.9	237	11.9	24.8	11.3	0.0
Super Supreme, Pan, Large, Pizza Hut*	1 Slice/148g	346	17.7	234	11.4	22.5	12.0	0.0
Super Supreme, Pan, Medium, Pizza Hut*	1 Slicc/127g	323	18.5	255	11.4	22.8	14.6	0.0
Super Supreme, Stuffed Crust, Pizza Hut*	1 Slice/165g	397	14.3	241	11.7	29.0	8.7	0.0
Supreme, Italian, Individual, Pizza Hut*	1 Slice/81g	204	7.5	251	10.9	33.5	9.2	0.0
Supreme, Italian, Large, Pizza Hut*	1 Slice/113g	264	11.0	233	9.7	29.6	9.7	0.0
Supreme, Pan, Individual, Pizza Hut*	1 Slice/84g	209	9.6	248	11.0	28.0	11.4	0.0
Supreme, Stuffed Crust, Pizza Hut*	1 Slice/160g	371	13.8	232	11.9	29.7	8.6	0.0
The Sizzler, Cajun Chicken, Italian, Large, Pizza Hut*	1 Serving/83g	177	6.1	213	11.2	28.1	7.4	0.0
The Sizzler, Cajun Chicken, Italian, Medium, Pizza Hut*	1 Serving/67g	147	4.8	220	11.8	30.2	7.2	0.0
The Sizzler, Cajun Chicken, Pan, Large, Pizza Hut*	1 Serving/90g	215	7.9	238	10.8	27.2	8.8	0.0
The Sizzler, Cajun Chicken, Pan, Medium, Pizza Hut*	1 Serving/75g	166	7.0	221	10.3	27.3	9.3	0.0
The Sizzler, Cajun Chicken, Stuffed Crust, Pizza Hut*	1 Serving/114g	270	9.8	236	11.7	31.7	8.6	0.0
The Sizzler, Spicy Beef, Italian, Large, Pizza Hut*	1 Serving/80g	179	5.9	223	9.6	33.1	7.4	0.0
The Sizzler, Spicy Beef, Italian, Medium, Pizza Hut*	1 Serving/68g	163	6.1	240	10.9	31.6	9.0	0.0
The Sizzler, Spicy Beef, Pan, Large, Pizza Hut*	1 Serving/96g	240	11.0	250	10.5	29.1	11.5	0.0
The Sizzler, Spicy Beef, Pan, Medium, Pizza Hut*	1 Serving/76g	173	7.7	228	10.3	32.0	10.1	0.0
The Sizzler, Spicy Mushroom, Italian, Large, Pizza Hut*	1 Serving/79g	165	5.5	209	9.3	31.2	7.0	0.0
The Sizzler, Spicy Mushroom, Italian, Med, Pizza Hut*	1 Serving/66g	146	5.4	223	10.5	30.1	8.2	0.0
The Sizzler, Spicy Mushroom, Stuffed Crust, Pizza Hut*	1 Serving/116g	244	7.9	210	9.7	31.7	6.8	0.0
The Works, The Edge, Medium, Pizza Hut*	1 Slice/64g	150	6.7	235	12.7	19.5	10.4	0.0
Tortilla, Thin, Kids, Pizza Hut*	1 Serving/108g	264	14.4	245	9.1	20.9	13.4	0.0
Tuscani, Chicken & Mushroom, Pizza Hut*	1 Serving/491g	1032	55.0	210	10.5	16.9	11.2	0.0
Tuscani, Mediterranean Meat, Pizza Hut*	1 Serving/379g	1065	56.8	281	13.6	21.8	15.0	0.0
Tuscani, Rocket & Prosciutto, Pizza Hut*	1 Serving/434g	829	36.9	191	9.2	19.2	8.5	0.0
Tuscani, Verde, Pizza Hut*	1 Serving/460g	878	42.3	191	8.0	18.6	9.2	0.0
Tuscani Caprina, Pizza Hut*	1 Serving/474g	990	45.5	209	9.0	20.6	9.6	0.0
Vegetable Supreme, Cheesy Bites, Pizza Hut*	1 Slice/145g	312	10.0	215	10.0	30.7	6.9	0.0
Vegetable Supreme, Italian, Individual, Pizza Hut*	1 Slice/77g	160	4.7	207	8.7	32.4	6.1	0.0
Vegetable Supreme, Italian, Large, Pizza Hut*	1 Slice/111g	222	6.3	200	7.4	32.5	5.7	0.0
Vegetable Supreme, Italian, Medium, Pizza Hut*	1 Slice/99g	196	6.0	198	8.3	30.7	6.1	0.0
Vegetable Supreme, Pan, Individual, Pizza Hut*	1 Slice/84g	180	7.6	214	8.6	27.7	9.0	0.0
Vegetable Supreme, Pan, Large, Pizza Hut*	1 Slice/126g	258	11.6	204	8.1	25.7	9.2	0.0
Vegetable Supreme, Pan, Medium, Pizza Hut*	1 Slice/109g	263	11.2	241	9.9	30.0	10.3	0.0
Vegetable Supreme, Stuffed Crust, Pizza Hut*	1 Slice/156g	307	10.8	197	9.3	27.8	6.9	0.0
Vegetarian, Hi Light, Medium, Pizza Hut*	1 Slice/77g	170	5.1	221	10.3	30.0	6.6	0.0
Vegetarian Hot One, Cheesy Bites, Pizza Hut*	1 Slice/142g	302	10.1	212	9.8	30.3	7.1	0.0
Vegetarian Hot One, Italian, Individual, Pizza Hut*	1 Slice/78g	164	4.5	211	8.1	34.6	5.8	0.0
Vegetarian Hot One, Italian, Large, Pizza Hut*	1 Slice/114g	165	6.7	145	7.5	19.1	5.9	0.0
Vegetarian Hot One, Italian, Medium, Pizza Hut*	1 Slice/98g	188	5.4	192	9.3	29.5	5.5	0.0
Vegetarian Hot One, Pan, Individual, Pizza Hut*	1 Slice/82g	174	6.0	211	8.8	29.6	7.3	0.0
Vegetarian Hot One, Pan, Large, Pizza Hut*	1 Slice/126g	290	12.1	231	9.4	29.7	9.6	0.0
Vegetarian Hot One, Pan, Medium, Pizza Hut*	1 Slice/115g	234	9.9	204	8.4	26.6	8.6	0.0
Vegetarian Hot One, Stuffed Crust, Pizza Hut*	1 Slice/161g	334	11.1	208	10.1	30.2	6.9	0.0

PIZZA HUT

	Measure INFO/WEIGHT	per Measure KCAL	per Measure FAT	Nutrition Values per 100g / 100ml KCAL	PROT	CARB	FAT	FIBRE
PIZZA								
Veggie, The Edge, Medium, Pizza Hut*	1 Slice/60g	136	5.4	227	11.2	22.2	9.0	0.0
PLATTER								
Favourites, Pizza Hut*	1 Platter/732g	1385	82.4	189	8.7	13.5	11.3	0.0
POTATO SKINS								
Cheese & Bacon (6 Skins), Pizza Hut*	6 Skins/246g	408	17.8	166	6.4	20.1	7.2	0.0
Jacket, Loaded, with Cheese, Pizza Hut*	1 Portion/267g	571	34.2	214	13.6	11.2	12.8	0.0
Jacket, Pizza Hut*	1 Portion/224g	571	37.2	255	3.4	23.0	16.6	2.1
Jacket, with Sour Cream & Chive Dip, Pizza Hut*	1 Portion/224g	311	24.1	139	1.4	9.3	10.8	0.8
POTATO WEDGES								
without Dip, Pizza Hut*	1 Serving/390g	569	23.8	146	2.5	20.3	6.1	0.0
PROFITEROLES								
Dessert, Pizza Hut*	1 Serving/100g	381	31.3	381	4.6	20.1	31.3	0.0
Pizza Hut*	1 Serving/100g	381	31.3	381	4.6	20.1	31.3	0.0
PUDDING								
Sticky Toffee, Pizza Hut*	1 Serving/105g	400	18.2	380	5.5	50.6	17.3	0.0
RAISINS								
Chocolate, Ice Cream Factory, Pizza Hut*	1 Serving/30g	121	4.3	405	5.4	63.3	14.2	0.0
SALAD								
4 Leaf Mix, Pizza Hut*	1 Serving/100g	14	0.5	14	0.8	1.7	0.5	0.0
Apple & Grape, Fresh, Mix, Pizza Hut*	1 Portion/80g	39	0.8	49	0.4	12.0	1.0	0.0
Caesar, Chicken, Pizza Hut*	1 Portion/175g	297	14.9	170	11.5	11.7	8.5	0.0
Caesar, Classic, Pizza Hut*	1 Serving/194g	366	23.1	189	7.2	13.0	11.9	0.0
Caesar, Classic, Small, Light Lunch, Pizza Hut*	1 Portion/97g	183	11.5	189	7.2	13.0	11.9	0.0
Caesar, Pizza Hut*	1 Salad/195g	344	20.2	177	6.0	14.8	10.4	0.0
Caesar, Prawn, Pizza Hut*	1 Portion/345g	459	24.1	133	9.6	7.6	7.0	0.0
Caesar, with Chicken & Bacon, Pizza Hut*	1 Serving/375g	588	29.6	157	14.4	6.8	7.9	0.0
Carrot, Grated, Fresh, Pizza Hut*	1 Serving/17g	5	0.1	30	0.7	6.0	0.5	0.0
Cheese, Goats, Pizza Hut*	1 Serving/341g	525	40.2	154	7.5	4.4	11.8	0.0
Cheese, Hard, Grated, Pizza Hut*	1 Serving/50g	202	15.0	404	33.0	0.0	30.0	0.0
Chicken, Warm, Pizza Hut*	1 Salad/342g	403	17.4	118	11.0	6.8	5.1	0.0
Chicken & Bacon, Pizza Hut*	1 Serving/323g	514	32.0	159	10.3	6.9	9.9	0.0
Cucumber, Slices, Fresh, Pizza Hut*	1 Serving/80g	8	0.1	10	0.7	1.5	0.1	0.0
Dressed, Tabbouleh, Pizza Hut*	1 Serving/100g	189	8.1	189	4.2	24.9	8.1	0.0
Leaf Mix, Pizza Hut*	1 Serving/41g	7	0.5	17	2.9	6.3	1.1	0.0
Mozzarella & Tomato, Light Lunch, Pizza Hut*	1 Serving/188g	387	30.6	206	12.3	2.4	16.3	0.0
Mozzarella & Tomato, Pizza Hut*	1 Salad/160g	234	19.0	146	7.7	2.1	11.9	0.0
Olive & Feta, Pizza Hut*	1 Portion/406g	345	26.0	85	3.8	3.6	6.4	0.0
Onion, Red, Slices, Fresh, Pizza Hut*	1 Portion/80g	29	0.2	36	1.2	7.9	0.2	0.0
Potato, Whole, Pizza Hut*	1 Serving/100g	154	10.1	154	1.6	13.5	10.1	0.0
Seasonal, Fresh, Pizza Hut*	1 Serving/80g	12	0.5	15	0.7	1.8	0.6	0.0
Tomatoes, Cherry, Fresh, Pizza Hut*	1 Serving/80g	15	0.3	19	0.8	3.0	0.4	0.0
Tuna, Pizza Hut*	1 Portion/461g	378	8.8	82	10.4	5.9	1.9	2.0
SALAD BAR								
Adults Pasta, Pizza Hut*	1 Serving/100g	250	10.9	250	5.7	16.8	10.9	0.0
Baby Potatoes, Pizza Hut*	1 Serving/80g	63	1.4	79	1.2	14.6	1.8	0.0
Beetroot & Carrot, with Balsamic, Pizza Hut*	1 Serving/80g	24	0.2	30	1.1	5.7	0.3	0.0
Carrot Batons, Fresh, Pizza Hut*	1 Serving/80g	28	0.2	35	0.6	7.9	0.3	0.0
Coleslaw, Pizza Hut*	1 Serving/80g	149	14.6	186	1.1	4.5	18.2	0.0
Cous Cous, Pizza Hut*	1 Serving/100g	219	9.0	219	5.0	30.0	9.0	0.0
Lettuce, Cos, Fresh, Pizza Hut*	1 Serving/80g	10	0.2	13	0.7	1.9	0.3	0.0
Melon, Pieces, Fresh, Pizza Hut*	1 Serving/80g	27	0.0	34	0.8	8.2	0.0	0.0
Pasta, Gemelli, Pizza Hut*	1 Serving/100g	155	4.4	155	4.3	26.0	4.4	0.0

	Measure INFO/WEIGHT		per Measure		Nutrition Values per 100g / 100ml				
			KCAL	FAT	KCAL	PROT	CARB	FAT	FIBRE
PIZZA HUT									
SALAD BAR									
Pasta, Kids, Pizza Hut*	1 Serving/100g		180	9.4	180	6.9	16.5	9.4	0.0
Pasta, Tomato, Pizza Hut*	1 Serving/80g		149	7.4	186	3.7	21.8	9.3	0.0
Peppers, Mixed, Fresh, Pizza Hut*	1 Serving/80g		12	0.2	15	0.8	2.6	0.3	0.0
Potato Salad, Pizza Hut*	1 Serving/80g		123	9.5	154	1.7	10.0	11.9	0.0
Sweetcorn, Fresh, Pizza Hut*	1 Serving/80g		63	0.6	79	1.8	16.8	0.8	0.0
Tomato, Slices, Fresh, Pizza Hut*	1 Serving/80g		14	0.2	17	0.7	3.1	0.3	0.0
SAUCE									
Caramel, Ice Cream Factory, Pizza Hut*	1 Serving/25g		77	1.0	307	0.7	67.2	3.9	0.0
Chocolate, Ice Cream Factory, Pizza Hut*	1 Serving/25g		74	0.6	298	2.0	66.8	2.5	0.0
Strawberry, Ice Cream Factory, Pizza Hut*	1 Serving/25g		70	0.0	280	0.0	69.5	0.0	0.0
SMOOTHIE									
BananaBerry Split, Pizza Hut*	1 Serving/171g		258	0.4	151	1.5	33.6	0.2	0.0
Truly Tropical, Pizza Hut*	1 Serving/239g		234	0.3	98	0.6	24.0	0.1	0.0
Very Berry, Pizza Hut*	1 Serving/220g		189	0.3	86	0.6	20.4	0.1	0.0
SUNDAE									
Chocolate, Double, Pizza Hut*	1 Sundae/145g		307	16.2	212	3.1	27.0	11.2	0.0
SWEETCORN									
Pizza Hut*	1 Serving/30g		24	0.2	79	1.8	16.8	0.8	0.0
TIRAMISU									
Delivery, Pizza Hut*	1 Serving/75g		223	10.3	297	3.9	39.5	13.7	0.0
Pizza Hut*	1 Serving/84g		248	11.4	297	3.9	39.5	13.7	0.0
TOPPINGS									
Chocolate Raisins, Pizza Hut*	1 Serving/100g		405	14.2	405	5.4	63.3	14.2	0.0
Coated Chocolate Beans, Pizza Hut*	1 Serving/100g		475	18.1	475	5.5	72.2	18.1	0.0
Marshmallows, Mini, Pizza Hut*	1 Serving/100g		320	0.0	320	5.4	74.3	0.0	0.0
Sauce, Caramel, Pizza Hut*	1 Serving/100g		307	3.9	307	0.7	67.2	3.9	0.0
Sauce, Chocolate, Pizza Hut*	1 Serving/100g		298	2.5	298	2.0	66.8	2.5	0.0
Sauce, Lemon, Pizza Hut*	1 Serving/100g		280	0.0	280	0.1	69.0	0.0	0.0
Sauce, Strawberry, Pizza Hut*	1 Serving/100g		280	0.0	280	0.0	69.5	0.0	0.0
PRET A MANGER									
BAGUETTE									
Bang Bang Chicken, Pret a Manger*	1 Baguette/229g		451	14.8	197	11.0	23.4	6.5	1.8
Brie, Tomato & Basil, Pret a Manger*	1 Pack/225g		396	14.1	176	8.0	21.9	6.3	1.6
Caesar, Chicken & Bacon, on Artisan, Pret a Manger*	1 Pack/230g		619	29.4	269	14.2	24.0	12.8	1.8
Cheddar & Pickle, Posh, Artisan, Pret a Manger*	1 Slim Pret/249g		611	28.1	245	8.4	26.8	11.3	1.8
Chicken, Chilli & Coriander, Baguette, Pret a Manger*	1 Pack/210g		390	11.4	186	10.2	23.8	5.4	1.5
Italian Prosciutto, Artisan, Baguette, Pret a Manger*	1 Pack/268g		567	25.1	212	9.1	22.0	9.4	1.9
Salmon & Watercress, Artisan, Pret a Manger*	1 Baguette/238g		459	15.5	193	9.0	24.1	6.5	2.1
BARS									
Choc Bar, Pret a Manger*	1 Slice/76g		380	21.7	500	4.7	54.3	28.5	3.5
Chocolate Brownie, Pret a Manger*	1 Slice/64g		369	27.5	577	5.3	40.5	43.0	3.9
Love Bar, Pret a Manger*	1 Bar/72g		324	18.3	450	6.0	49.2	25.4	3.5
Pret Bar, Pret a Manger*	1 Bar/65g		265	15.6	408	6.8	41.4	24.0	6.1
BISCUITS									
Fruit & Oat, Pret a Manger*	1 Pack/40g		187	9.8	467	8.2	50.0	24.5	6.2
BREAD									
Artisan Soup, Pret a Manger*	1 Serving/80g		175	0.6	219	7.2	45.6	0.7	2.0
BREAKFAST CEREAL									
Honey & Granola, Pret Pot, Pret a Manger*	1 Pot/133g		263	7.8	198	7.3	28.8	5.9	1.3
Hot & Cold Granola, Pret a Manger*	1 Serving/226g		579	19.9	256	6.4	38.4	8.8	3.5
Muesli, Bircher, Bowl, Pret a Manger*	1 Bowl/206g		304	9.7	148	6.3	20.2	4.7	1.4
Porridge, Pret a Manger*	1 Serving/300g		242	8.4	81	3.0	9.6	2.8	1.7

PRET A MANGER

	Measure INFO/WEIGHT	per Measure KCAL	FAT	Nutrition Values per 100g / 100ml KCAL	PROT	CARB	FAT	FIBRE
BREAKFAST CEREAL								
Porridge, with Compote, Pret a Manger*	1 Serving/324g	267	8.4	82	2.8	10.8	2.6	1.7
Porridge, with Honey, Pret a Manger*	1 Serving/321g	307	8.4	96	2.8	14.0	2.6	1.6
CAKE								
Apple, Slice, Pret a Manger*	1 Slice/100g	303	14.7	303	3.8	38.8	14.7	1.9
Banana, Slice, Pret a Manger*	1 Slice/103g	345	18.3	335	4.6	39.0	17.8	1.9
Carrot, Slice, Pret a Manger*	1 Slice/112g	402	22.3	359	4.0	41.0	19.9	2.3
Chocolate, Slice, Pret a Manger*	1 Slice/88g	354	20.9	402	5.3	41.7	23.7	1.4
Lemon, Slice, Pret a Manger*	1 Slice/100g	330	15.1	330	4.2	44.0	15.1	0.9
CHEESECAKE								
Lemon, Pot, Pret a Manger*	1 Pot/120g	390	25.9	325	2.7	29.3	21.6	1.4
CHOCOLATE								
Dark, with Sea Salt, Pret a Manger*	1 Bar/25g	136	9.0	544	4.0	44.0	36.0	8.0
COFFEE								
Americano, Pret a Manger*	1 Serving/360ml	35	1.3	10	0.7	0.9	0.4	0.0
Cappuccino, Pret a Manger*	1 Serving/280ml	280	9.7	100	7.0	10.1	3.5	0.0
Espresso, Pret a Manger*	1 Serving/137ml	0	0.0	0	0.0	0.0	0.0	0.0
Filter, made with Semi Skimmed Milk, Pret a Manger*	1 Serving/350ml	14	0.5	4	0.3	0.4	0.1	0.0
Flat White, Pret a Manger*	1 Serving/250ml	75	2.7	30	2.2	2.9	1.1	0.0
Latte, Pret a Manger*	1 Serving/330ml	112	4.1	34	2.4	3.3	1.2	0.0
Mocha, Pret a Manger*	1 Serving/330ml	177	4.4	54	2.5	7.9	1.3	0.0
COOKIES								
Chocolate, Chunk, Pret a Manger*	1 Cookie/90g	319	12.2	354	4.8	52.6	13.6	3.7
Chocolate, White, & Orange, Pret a Manger*	1 Cookie/90g	369	13.3	410	4.9	62.3	14.8	2.6
CRISPS								
Chilli, Spicy Piri, Pret a Manger*	1 Pack/40g	190	10.1	475	5.2	56.7	25.2	5.2
Parsnip, Beetroot & Carrot, Pret a Manger*	1 Pack/25g	120	8.6	480	4.4	38.4	34.4	15.2
Sea Salt, & Organic Cider Vinegar, Pret a Manger*	1 Pack/40g	178	9.7	445	5.2	52.0	24.2	7.0
Sea Salt, Maldon, Pret a Manger*	1 Pack/40g	184	10.4	460	5.5	51.2	26.0	7.5
Sweet Potato & Chipotle Chilli, Pret a Manger*	1 Pack/25g	123	8.2	492	5.2	44.8	32.8	9.6
CROISSANT								
Almond, Pret a Manger*	1 Croissant/100g	365	21.1	365	8.8	34.9	21.1	1.1
Chocolate, Pret a Manger*	1 Croissant/95g	406	24.3	427	7.9	45.2	25.6	3.6
Egg & Bacon, Pret a Manger*	1 Croissant/167g	483	20.1	289	11.3	20.6	12.0	1.8
French Butter, Pret a Manger*	1 Croissant/80g	304	15.9	380	8.5	41.7	19.9	2.6
Ham, Bacon & Cheese, Pret a Manger*	1 Croissant/110g	352	22.5	320	13.2	20.6	20.4	1.5
Mozzarella & Tomato, Pret a Manger*	1 Croissant/110g	373	24.6	339	13.4	20.2	22.4	1.3
Pain au Raisin, Pret a Manger*	1 Croissant/110g	311	13.5	283	5.1	37.4	12.3	1.6
DRIED FRUIT								
Mango, Pret a Manger*	1 Serving/60g	200	0.2	333	1.5	84.5	0.3	3.7
FRUIT								
Five Berry, Bowl, Pret a Manger*	1 Bowl/219g	368	15.1	168	5.2	20.3	6.9	1.4
Five Berry, Pot, Pret a Manger*	1 Pot/148g	147	4.7	99	6.0	11.6	3.2	0.2
Grapes, Seedless, Pret a Manger*	1 Serving/150g	96	0.2	64	0.4	15.4	0.1	1.0
Kid's, Pot, Pret a Manger*	1 Pot/140g	43	0.1	31	0.5	7.4	0.1	1.0
Mango & Lime, Pret a Manger*	1 Serving/135g	70	0.3	52	0.7	12.0	0.2	2.3
Salad, Pret a Manger*	1 Serving/250g	115	0.3	46	0.7	11.0	0.1	1.6
Superfruit, Bowl, Pret a Manger*	1 Serving/155g	71	0.2	46	0.8	11.0	0.1	2.0
Tropical, Sticks, Pret a Manger*	1 Serving/200g	78	0.4	39	0.6	8.9	0.2	1.4
GINGER BEER								
Pret a Manger*	1 Serving/330ml	152	0.0	46	0.0	11.4	0.0	0.0
GINGERBREAD								
Godfrey, Gingerbread Man, Pret a Manger*	1 Serving/54g	198	7.5	367	4.8	55.7	13.9	1.8

PRET A MANGER

	Measure INFO/WEIGHT	per Measure KCAL	FAT	Nutrition Values per 100g / 100ml KCAL	PROT	CARB	FAT	FIBRE
HOT CHOCOLATE								
Pret a Manger*	1 Serving/305ml	268	5.9	88	3.5	14.1	1.9	0.0
JELLY								
Jelly, Elderflower & Raspberry, Pret a Manger*	1 Serving/135g	96	0.0	71	0.3	17.5	0.0	0.4
JUICE								
Carrot, Pret a Manger*	1 Serving/250ml	60	0.3	24	0.5	5.7	0.1	0.0
Orange, Large, Pret a Manger*	1 Serving/520ml	229	0.0	44	0.6	11.0	0.0	0.1
Orange, Pret a Manger*	1 Serving/260ml	114	0.0	44	0.6	11.0	0.0	0.1
JUICE DRINK								
Apple, Pure Pret, Pret a Manger*	1 Serving/330ml	159	0.0	48	0.0	11.6	0.0	0.0
Grape & Elderflower, Pure Pret, Pret a Manger*	1 Serving/330ml	146	0.0	44	0.0	10.6	0.0	0.0
Orange, Pure Pret, Pret a Manger*	1 Serving/330ml	200	0.0	61	0.1	3.1	0.0	0.0
MOUSSE								
Chocolate, Pret a Manger*	1 Serving/100g	375	29.2	375	3.4	24.6	29.2	1.2
MUFFIN								
Double Berry, Pret a Manger*	1 Muffin/140g	537	26.8	384	5.5	46.0	19.1	2.1
High Fibre, Pret a Manger*	1 Muffin/130g	455	23.4	350	7.2	36.0	18.0	7.4
POPCORN								
Rock Salt, Skinny, Topcorn, Pret a Manger*	1 Pack/23g	115	6.1	500	8.3	53.5	26.5	10.4
Savoury, Skinny, Topcorn, Pret a Manger*	1 Pack/23g	96	3.0	417	9.6	65.3	12.9	12.0
Sweet 'n' Salt, Skinny, Topcorn, Pret a Manger*	1 Pack/25g	123	6.1	492	7.1	60.0	24.6	9.5
PRETZELS								
Pret a Manger*	1 Serving/120g	371	7.8	309	10.9	51.6	6.5	2.5
SALAD								
Chicken, Chef's Italian, Pret a Manger*	1 Serving/303g	323	23.5	107	6.7	2.6	7.8	1.9
Chicken & Pasta, Pret a Manger*	1 Serving/267g	507	21.9	190	7.4	21.0	8.2	1.3
Crayfish & Avocado, No Bread, Pret a Manger*	1 Serving/206g	182	15.0	88	4.7	1.5	7.3	2.2
Crayfish & Thai Noodle, Pret a Manger*	1 Serving/239g	174	5.2	73	4.7	8.4	2.2	1.5
Edamame, Bowl, Pret a Manger*	1 Serving/125g	125	5.6	100	8.4	6.5	4.5	0.0
Ham, Wiltshire, & Potato Salad, Pret a Manger*	1 Serving/294g	272	14.2	93	6.4	6.0	4.8	1.1
Hoisin Duck, no Bread, Pret a Manger*	1 Pack/183g	117	10.9	64	7.4	5.9	6.0	1.7
Moroccan Chickpea, no Bread, Pret a Manger*	1 Serving/322g	610	28.0	189	9.1	18.8	8.7	7.5
Salmon, Smoke Roast, Pret a Manger*	1 Serving/323g	455	30.5	141	5.8	8.4	9.4	1.5
Superfood, Pret a Manger*	1 Serving/327g	345	15.9	105	4.5	11.1	4.9	1.9
Tuna Nicoise, Pole & Line Caught, Pret a Manger*	1 Serving/281g	138	3.8	49	6.7	2.7	1.3	1.0
SANDWICH								
All Day Breakfast, Pret a Manger*	1 Pack/329g	654	37.7	199	9.9	14.1	11.5	1.4
BLT, Beech Smoked, Pret a Manger*	1 Pack/248g	493	28.8	199	8.5	15.4	11.6	1.6
Cheddar, Mature, & Pret Pickle, Pret a Manger*	1 Pack/266g	486	25.2	183	7.1	17.5	9.5	1.6
Cheese, Kid's, Pret a Manger*	1 Pack/127g	399	20.2	314	13.9	28.9	15.9	2.2
Cheese Salad, Emmental, Pret a Manger*	1 Pack/239g	494	28.2	207	8.3	16.9	11.8	1.8
Chicken & Pesto, Bloomer, Pret a Manger*	1 Pack/273g	477	17.1	175	10.2	18.0	6.3	1.9
Chicken Avocado, Pret a Manger*	1 Pack/244g	463	24.8	190	8.6	16.0	10.2	2.8
Chilli, Crayfish & Mango, Bloomer, Pret a Manger*	1 Pack/215g	401	12.2	187	9.3	24.6	5.7	2.3
Club, Chicken, Ham & Swiss Cheese, Pret a Manger*	1 Pack/318g	492	20.0	155	11.5	12.9	6.3	1.3
Club, Classic, Super, Pret a Manger*	1 Pack/274g	551	30.3	201	10.8	14.6	11.1	1.5
Coronation Chicken & Fruit Chutney, Pret a Manger*	1 Pack/290g	529	27.3	182	7.9	16.5	9.4	1.7
Egg Mayo, Free-Range, Pret a Manger*	1 Pack/185g	426	23.4	231	9.1	19.9	12.7	1.6
Egg Salad, Cracking, Pret a Manger*	1 Pack/262g	439	23.6	168	6.6	15.1	9.0	1.5
Falafel & Houmous, Moroccan, Pret a Manger*	1 Pack/285g	525	17.6	184	5.8	22.9	6.2	3.3
Ham, Kid's, Pret a Manger*	1 Pack/127g	289	8.2	228	13.4	28.9	6.5	2.2
Ham & Eggs, Classic, Bloomer, Pret a Manger*	1 Pack/225g	598	25.7	266	14.1	21.3	11.4	2.0
Houmous, Crunchy, Bloomer, Pret a Manger*	1 Pack/224g	511	17.5	228	10.1	30.1	7.8	7.0

PRET A MANGER

	Measure INFO/WEIGHT	per Measure		Nutrition Values per 100g / 100ml				
		KCAL	FAT	KCAL	PROT	CARB	FAT	FIBRE
SANDWICH								
Prawn Cocktail, King, Pret a Manger*	1 Pack/199g	362	14.4	182	9.0	19.3	7.2	1.8
Red Pepper Tapenade & Soft Cheese, Pret a Manger*	1 Pack/225g	394	18.3	175	6.0	19.5	8.1	2.7
Salmon, Scottish, Smoked, Pret a Manger*	1 Pack/158g	348	11.5	220	16.5	21.8	7.3	1.7
Spring Houmous & Feta, Granary, Pret a Manger*	1 Pack/216g	404	17.4	187	7.4	21.5	8.1	3.2
The New York, Bloomer, Pret a Manger*	1 Pack/223g	525	23.9	235	11.9	25.2	10.7	2.5
Tuna & Rocket, Bloomer, Pret a Manger*	1 Pack/237g	534	26.5	226	11.0	20.0	11.2	2.0
Tuna Mayo, Kid's, Pret a Manger*	1 Pack/150g	372	17.3	248	10.9	24.9	11.5	1.9
Wensleydale, & Chutney, Bloomer, Pret a Manger*	1 Pack/276g	564	26.1	204	8.9	20.9	9.5	2.2
Wild Crayfish & Rocket, Pret a Manger*	1 Pack/195g	370	17.1	190	8.3	19.4	8.8	1.6
SMOOTHIE								
Mango, Pret a Manger*	1 Serving/250ml	143	0.5	57	0.6	13.7	0.2	3.0
Strawberry, Pret a Manger*	1 Serving/250ml	128	0.8	51	0.9	11.2	0.3	0.0
Vitamin Volcano, Pret a Manger*	1 Serving/250ml	135	0.8	54	4.6	12.4	0.3	2.3
SOUP								
Beef, Ale & Barley, Pret a Manger*	1 Serving/370g	230	6.7	62	3.3	6.3	1.8	1.4
Beef, Chilli, & Rice, Pret a Manger*	1 Serving/370g	270	9.2	73	5.4	7.3	2.5	2.8
Carrot & Coriander, Pret a Manger*	1 Serving/370g	181	10.7	49	0.9	4.5	2.9	0.7
Cauliflower Cheese, Pret a Manger*	1 Serving/370g	293	13.5	79	3.3	5.2	3.6	0.9
Celeriac & Smoked Pancetta, Pret a Manger*	1 Pot/370g	215	15.6	58	2.5	2.1	4.2	0.9
Chicken, Moroccan, Pret a Manger*	1 Serving/370g	304	9.9	82	4.5	8.8	2.7	2.4
Chicken, Spicy, & Bean, Pret a Manger*	1 Pot/370g	281	5.9	76	5.2	8.3	1.6	3.8
Chicken & Mushroom, Pret a Manger*	1 Serving/370g	269	14.4	73	6.6	2.7	3.9	0.5
Chorizo, Spanish, & Butterbean, Pret a Manger*	1 Serving/370g	233	8.9	63	3.8	6.1	2.4	1.1
Leek & Potato, Pret a Manger*	1 Serving/370g	189	9.3	51	1.2	5.5	2.5	0.9
Lentil & Coconut Curry, Pret a Manger*	1 Pack/370g	403	15.9	109	5.4	11.5	4.3	1.5
Lentil & Smoked Bacon, Pret a Manger*	1 Serving/370g	274	11.5	74	5.9	6.3	3.1	1.2
Malaysian Chicken Curry, Pret a Manger*	1 Serving/370g	270	14.8	73	2.7	5.5	4.0	2.0
Meatball, Italian, Pret a Manger*	1 Serving/370g	263	15.5	71	2.4	5.8	4.2	1.0
Miso, Pret a Manger*	1 Serving/20g	32	1.0	160	10.0	0.0	5.0	0.0
Mushroom, Cream of, Pret a Manger*	1 Pack/370g	148	8.8	40	1.3	2.8	2.4	0.6
Mushroom Risotto, Pret a Manger*	1 Serving/347g	215	9.9	62	1.6	7.5	2.8	1.3
Pea, Garden, & Mint, Pret a Manger*	1 Serving/370g	215	8.9	58	2.4	5.9	2.4	1.8
Sag Aloo, Pret a Manger*	1 Serving/375g	245	11.5	65	1.6	7.9	3.1	0.2
Sausage Hot Pot, Pret a Manger*	1 Serving/370g	230	13.0	62	4.0	2.6	3.5	2.0
Tomato, Pret's Classic, Pret a Manger*	1 Serving/370g	259	17.8	70	1.6	4.7	4.8	0.7
Veg, Root, & Bean, Pret a Manger*	1 Serving/370g	178	3.0	48	2.3	6.5	0.8	2.3
SUSHI								
California Rolls, Pret a Manger*	1 Pack/206g	354	9.3	172	5.1	27.5	4.5	1.4
Deluxe Bento Box, Pret a Manger*	1 Serving/267g	369	10.9	138	5.9	19.3	4.1	1.1
Maki & Nigiri, Pret a Manger*	1 Serving/200g	314	8.4	157	5.4	23.4	4.2	1.0
Salmon & Prawn, Pret a Manger*	1 Serving/232g	382	9.3	165	6.2	25.8	4.0	1.3
TART								
Bakewell, Pret a Manger*	1 Serving/68g	315	17.7	463	7.2	50.0	26.0	2.2
TEA								
Iced, Peach, Still, Pret a Manger*	1 Serving/500ml	78	0.0	16	0.0	3.8	0.0	0.0
Red Berries, Pret a Manger*	1 Serving/60ml	0	0.0	0	0.0	0.0	0.0	0.0
Tropical Green, Pret a Manger*	1 Serving/60ml	0	0.0	0	0.0	0.0	0.0	0.0
TOASTIE								
Ham, Cheese & Mustard, Pret a Manger*	1 Serving/215g	601	29.0	280	17.8	21.8	13.5	2.1
Italian Mozzarella & Pesto, Pret a Manger*	1 Serving/233g	498	23.2	214	10.3	20.6	10.0	2.1
New York Deli, Pret a Manger*	1 Serving/233g	586	28.0	251	15.2	21.3	12.0	2.4
Tuna Melt, Pret a Manger*	1 Serving/218g	561	25.3	257	16.8	21.3	11.6	2.4

	Measure INFO/WEIGHT	per Measure KCAL	FAT	Nutrition Values per 100g / 100ml KCAL	PROT	CARB	FAT	FIBRE
PRET A MANGER								
WRAP								
Avocado & Herb Salad, Pret a Manger*	1 Wrap/252g	458	29.3	182	4.7	14.2	11.6	2.6
Chunky Houmous Salad, Pret a Manger*	1 Wrap/207g	335	17.4	162	5.1	16.1	8.4	1.2
Falafel & Halloumi, Hot, Pret a Manger*	1 Wrap/275g	567	22.6	206	6.5	21.6	8.2	1.2
Hoisin Duck, Pret a Manger*	1 Wrap/211g	448	21.5	212	8.6	20.3	10.2	1.5
Indian Summer, Pret a Manger*	1 Wrap/225g	358	12.0	159	5.5	22.5	5.3	1.6
Italian Pizza Hot, Pret a Manger*	1 Wrap/200g	391	17.2	195	8.7	20.8	8.6	2.4
Jalapeno Chicken, Hot, Pret a Manger*	1 Wrap/243g	431	16.4	177	11.8	17.2	6.7	1.5
Salad, Sweet Chilli Crayfish, Pret a Manger*	1 Wrap/223g	282	10.1	126	5.9	15.5	4.5	1.3
Salad, Sweet Chilli Prawn, Pret a Manger*	1 Wrap/219g	298	10.3	136	7.7	15.5	4.7	1.5
Swedish Meatball, Hot, Pret a Manger*	1 Wrap/219g	566	26.0	259	13.3	24.9	11.9	2.2
YOGHURT								
Yoga Bunny, Bowl, Pret a Manger*	1 Serving/233g	210	5.0	90	5.2	10.9	2.1	1.0
Yoga Bunny, Pure Pret, Pret a Manger*	1 Serving/330g	132	0.0	40	0.0	9.7	0.0	0.0
Yoghurt Nuts, Pret a Manger*	1 Pack/75g	430	33.2	573	6.9	29.7	44.3	6.9
YOGHURT DRINK								
Blueberry Probiotic, Pret a Manger*	1 Serving/250ml	185	4.3	74	2.3	12.4	1.7	0.0
Vanilla Probiotic, Pret a Manger*	1 Serving/250ml	200	4.5	80	2.5	13.2	1.8	0.0
STARBUCKS								
BAGEL								
Salmon, Smoked, with Cream Cheese, Starbucks*	1 Bagel/165g	370	11.1	224	12.7	27.2	6.7	1.7
BARS								
Chocolate, Dark, Fairtrade, Starbucks*	1 Bar/45g	259	20.8	575	6.7	27.6	46.3	10.7
Chocolate, Milk, Fairtrade, Starbucks*	1 Bar/45g	242	17.4	537	6.4	49.0	38.6	2.2
Fruit & Nut, Cranberry, Seed & Blueberry, Starbucks*	1 Bar/50g	235	12.4	470	12.3	49.5	24.8	1.0
Granola, Starbucks*	1 Bar/85g	398	22.0	468	7.2	48.9	25.9	5.1
BISCUITS								
Ginger Snaps, Starbucks*	1 Biscuit/30g	133	4.6	445	4.8	71.9	15.4	1.5
BREAKFAST CEREAL								
Porridge, Dairy, Starbucks*	1 Serving/230g	244	6.2	106	4.1	17.4	2.7	1.8
Porridge, Soy, Starbucks*	1 Serving/230g	205	4.8	89	4.6	13.9	2.1	2.2
Topping, Compote, Very Berry, Starbucks*	1 Serving/50g	59	0.1	119	0.6	29.7	0.2	2.1
Topping, Granola, Maple & Honey, Starbucks*	1 Serving/25g	112	4.0	448	9.0	64.5	15.9	5.6
Topping, Sauce, Maple & Honey, Starbucks*	1 Serving/40g	120	0.0	300	0.1	74.8	0.1	0.2
BROWNIES								
Belgian Chocolate, Gluten Free, Fairtrade, Starbucks*	1 Cake/72g	370	22.8	514	4.1	51.9	31.7	2.6
BUTTIE								
Bacon, Starbucks*	1 Buttie/118g	414	18.2	351	19.1	33.3	15.4	1.4
CAKE								
Chocolate Chilli, Starbucks*	1 Cake/38g	170	8.7	448	5.3	57.6	22.8	4.4
Loaf, Banana Nut, Starbucks*	1 Cake/103g	431	25.7	418	6.5	40.5	25.0	2.8
Loaf, Chocolate Hazelnut, Starbucks*	1 Cake/85g	331	20.8	389	4.0	38.4	24.5	3.2
Loaf, Lemon, Starbucks*	1 Cake/86g	365	20.2	424	5.0	47.3	23.5	1.6
Loaf, Raspberry & Coconut, Starbucks*	1 Cake/89g	402	22.8	452	4.5	49.9	25.6	2.1
Marshmallow Twizzle, Chocolate, Starbucks*	1 Cake/40g	193	8.6	483	4.4	66.9	21.6	1.8
Marshmallow Twizzle, Red White & Blue, Starbucks*	1 Cake/35g	147	4.9	421	4.4	68.8	13.9	1.6
Rocky Road, Starbucks*	1 Cake/78g	423	27.1	542	4.3	51.5	34.8	2.7
Strawberry Shortcake, Petites, Starbucks*	1 Cake/41g	207	11.3	501	4.7	60.2	27.4	2.5
CHEWING GUM								
Sugar Free, Starbucks*	1 Chew/3g	5	0.0	166	0.0	80.0	0.0	0.0
COFFEE								
Caffe Americano, Grande, Starbucks*	1 Grande/473ml	17	0.0	4	0.2	0.6	0.0	0.0
Caffe Americano, Short, Starbucks*	1 Short/236ml	6	0.0	2	0.2	0.4	0.0	0.0

STARBUCKS

INFO/WEIGHT	Measure	per Measure		Nutrition Values per 100g / 100ml				
		KCAL	FAT	KCAL	PROT	CARB	FAT	FIBRE

COFFEE

	Measure INFO/WEIGHT	KCAL	FAT	KCAL	PROT	CARB	FAT	FIBRE
Caffe Americano, Tall, Starbucks*	1 Tall/355ml	11	0.0	3	0.2	0.6	0.0	0.0
Caffe Americano, Venti, Starbucks*	1 Venti/591ml	23	0.0	4	0.2	0.7	0.0	0.0
Caffe Latte, Grande, Semi Skimmed Milk, Starbucks*	1 Grande/473ml	188	7.0	40	2.6	3.9	1.5	0.0
Caffe Latte, Grande, Skimmed Milk, Starbucks*	1 Grande/473ml	131	0.3	28	2.7	4.1	0.1	0.0
Caffe Latte, Grande, Soy, Starbucks*	1 Grande/473ml	148	5.3	31	2.2	2.7	1.1	0.3
Caffe Latte, Grande, Whole Milk, Starbucks*	1 Grande/473ml	223	11.5	47	2.6	3.8	2.4	0.0
Caffe Latte, Short, Skimmed Milk, Starbucks*	1 Short/236ml	67	0.1	28	2.7	4.2	0.0	0.0
Caffe Latte, Short, Soy, Starbucks*	1 Short/236ml	75	2.7	32	2.2	2.8	1.1	0.3
Caffe Latte, Short, Whole Milk, Starbucks*	1 Short/236ml	113	5.8	48	2.6	3.9	2.5	0.0
Caffe Latte, Short, Semi Skimmed Milk, Starbucks*	1 Short/236ml	95	3.5	40	2.7	4.0	1.5	0.0
Caffe Latte, Tall, Semi Skimmed Milk, Starbucks*	1 Tall/355ml	143	5.1	40	2.7	4.2	1.4	0.0
Caffe Latte, Tall, Skimmed Milk, Starbucks*	1 Tall/355ml	102	0.2	29	2.7	4.3	0.1	0.0
Caffe Latte, Tall, Soy, Starbucks*	1 Tall/355ml	110	4.0	31	2.2	2.8	1.1	0.3
Caffe Latte, Tall, Whole Milk, Starbucks*	1 Tall/355ml	172	8.4	48	2.6	4.2	2.4	0.0
Caffe Latte, Venti, Semi Skimmed Milk, Starbucks*	1 Venti/591ml	248	9.2	42	2.8	4.2	1.6	0.0
Caffe Latte, Venti, Skimmed Milk, Starbucks*	1 Venti/591ml	174	0.4	29	2.8	4.4	0.1	0.0
Caffe Latte, Venti, Soy, Starbucks*	1 Venti/591ml	184	6.7	31	2.2	2.8	1.1	0.3
Caffe Latte, Venti, Whole Milk, Starbucks*	1 Venti/591ml	299	15.0	51	2.6	4.2	2.5	0.0
Caffe Misto, Grande, Semi Skimmed Milk, Starbucks*	1 Grande/473ml	106	4.1	22	1.5	2.1	0.9	0.0
Caffe Misto, Grande, Skimmed Milk, Starbucks*	1 Grande/473ml	73	0.2	15	1.5	2.2	0.0	0.0
Caffe Misto, Grande, Soy, Starbucks*	1 Grande/473ml	82	3.2	17	1.2	1.4	0.7	0.2
Caffe Misto, Grande, Whole Milk, Starbucks*	1 Grande/473ml	126	6.8	27	1.5	2.0	1.4	0.0
Caffe Misto, Short, Semi Skimmed Milk, Starbucks*	1 Short/236ml	54	2.1	23	1.5	2.1	0.9	0.0
Caffe Misto, Short, Skimmed Milk, Starbucks*	1 Short/236ml	37	0.1	16	1.6	2.2	0.0	0.0
Caffe Misto, Short, Soy, Starbucks*	1 Short/236ml	42	1.6	18	1.3	1.4	0.7	0.2
Caffe Misto, Short, Whole Milk, Starbucks*	1 Short/236ml	65	3.5	27	1.5	2.0	1.5	0.0
Caffe Misto, Tall, Semi Skimmed Milk, Starbucks*	1 Tall/355ml	81	3.2	23	1.5	2.1	0.9	0.0
Caffe Misto, Tall, Skimmed Milk, Starbucks*	1 Tall/355ml	56	0.2	16	1.6	2.2	0.1	0.0
Caffe Misto, Tall, Soy, Starbucks*	1 Tall/355ml	63	2.4	18	1.3	1.4	0.7	0.2
Caffe Misto, Tall, Whole Milk, Starbucks*	1 Tall/355ml	97	5.2	27	1.5	2.0	1.5	0.0
Caffe Misto, Venti, Semi Skimmed Milk, Starbucks*	1 Venti/591ml	134	5.2	23	1.5	2.1	0.9	0.0
Caffe Misto, Venti, Skimmed Milk, Starbucks*	1 Venti/591ml	92	0.3	16	1.6	2.2	0.1	0.0
Caffe Misto, Venti, Soy, Starbucks*	1 Venti/591ml	104	4.0	18	1.3	1.4	0.7	0.2
Caffe Misto, Venti, Whole Milk, Starbucks*	1 Venti/591ml	160	8.6	27	1.5	2.0	1.5	0.0
Caffe Mocha, Cream, Grande, Skim Milk, Starbucks*	1 Grande/473ml	288	9.5	61	2.8	9.3	2.0	0.4
Caffe Mocha, Cream, Grande, Soy, Starbucks*	1 Grande/473ml	302	13.7	64	2.5	8.1	2.9	0.6
Caffe Mocha, Cream, Grande, SS Milk, Starbucks*	1 Grande/473ml	335	15.0	71	2.8	9.1	3.2	0.4
Caffe Mocha, Cream, Grande, Whole Milk, Starbucks*	1 Grande/473ml	364	18.7	77	2.7	9.0	4.0	0.4
Caffe Mocha, Cream, Short, Skim Milk, Starbucks*	1 Short/236ml	160	6.4	68	2.9	9.5	2.7	0.4
Caffe Mocha, Cream, Short, Soy, Starbucks*	1 Short/236ml	167	8.5	71	2.5	8.3	3.6	0.6
Caffe Mocha, Cream, Short, SS Milk, Starbucks*	1 Short/236ml	184	9.1	78	2.8	9.3	3.9	0.4
Caffe Mocha, Cream, Short, Whole Milk, Starbucks*	1 Short/236ml	198	11.0	84	2.8	9.2	4.7	0.4
Caffe Mocha, Cream, Tall, Skimmed Milk, Starbucks*	1 Tall/355ml	239	8.5	67	2.8	9.5	2.4	0.4
Caffe Mocha, Cream, Tall, Soy, Starbucks*	1 Tall/355ml	247	11.8	70	2.5	8.4	3.3	0.7
Caffe Mocha, Cream, Tall, SS Milk, Starbucks*	1 Tall/355ml	273	12.7	77	2.8	9.4	3.6	0.4
Caffe Mocha, Cream, Tall, Whole Milk, Starbucks*	1 Tall/355ml	297	15.5	84	2.7	9.4	4.4	0.4
Caffe Mocha, Cream, Venti, Skimmed Milk, Starbucks*	1 Venti/591ml	359	10.9	61	2.8	9.3	1.8	0.4
Caffe Mocha, Cream, Venti, Soy, Starbucks*	1 Venti/591ml	372	15.8	63	2.5	8.4	2.7	0.7
Caffe Mocha, Cream, Venti, SS Milk, Starbucks*	1 Venti/591ml	417	17.7	70	2.7	9.2	3.0	0.4
Caffe Mocha, Cream, Venti, Whole Milk, Starbucks*	1 Venti/591ml	456	22.3	77	2.7	9.2	3.8	0.4
Cappuccino, Grande, Semi Skimmed Milk, Starbucks*	1 Grande/473ml	115	4.1	24	1.6	2.5	0.9	0.0
Cappuccino, Grande, Skimmed Milk, Starbucks*	1 Grande/473ml	82	0.2	17	1.6	2.6	0.0	0.0

STARBUCKS
COFFEE

INFO/WEIGHT	Measure	per Measure		Nutrition Values per 100g / 100ml				
		KCAL	FAT	KCAL	PROT	CARB	FAT	FIBRE
Cappuccino, Grande, Soy, Starbucks*	1 Grande/473ml	92	3.2	19	1.4	1.8	0.7	0.2
Cappuccino, Grande, Whole Milk, Starbucks*	1 Grande/473ml	136	6.8	29	1.6	2.4	1.4	0.0
Cappuccino, Short, Semi Skimmed Milk, Starbucks*	1 Short/236ml	78	2.8	33	2.2	3.3	1.2	0.0
Cappuccino, Short, Skimmed Milk, Starbucks*	1 Short/236ml	55	0.1	23	2.2	3.4	0.0	0.0
Cappuccino, Short, Soy, Starbucks*	1 Short/236ml	62	2.2	26	1.8	2.3	0.9	0.3
Cappuccino, Short, Whole Milk, Starbucks*	1 Short/236ml	92	4.7	39	2.1	3.2	2.0	0.0
Cappuccino, Tall, Semi Skimmed Milk, Starbucks*	1 Tall/355ml	97	3.4	27	1.8	2.9	1.0	0.0
Cappuccino, Tall, Skimmed Milk, Starbucks*	1 Tall/355ml	69	0.1	20	1.8	3.0	0.0	0.0
Cappuccino, Tall, Soy, Starbucks*	1 Tall/355ml	74	2.5	21	1.4	2.0	0.7	0.2
Cappuccino, Tall, Whole Milk, Starbucks*	1 Tall/355ml	116	5.6	33	1.7	2.9	1.6	0.0
Cappuccino, Venti, Semi Skimmed Milk, Starbucks*	1 Venti/591ml	161	5.7	27	1.8	2.8	1.0	0.0
Cappuccino, Venti, Skimmed Milk, Starbucks*	1 Venti/591ml	115	0.2	19	1.8	2.9	0.0	0.0
Cappuccino, Venti, Soy, Starbucks*	1 Venti/591ml	123	4.2	21	1.4	1.9	0.7	0.2
Cappuccino, Venti, Whole Milk, Starbucks*	1 Venti/591ml	192	9.3	33	1.7	2.8	1.6	0.0
Espresso, Con Panna, Doppio, Starbucks*	1 Doppio/60ml	36	2.5	61	1.5	4.5	4.2	0.0
Espresso, Con Panna, Solo, Starbucks*	1 Solo/30ml	31	2.5	103	1.7	5.7	8.3	0.0
Espresso, Doppio, Starbucks*	1 Doppio/60ml	11	0.0	19	1.2	3.3	0.0	0.0
Espresso, Solo, Starbucks*	1 Solo/30ml	6	0.0	19	1.3	3.3	0.0	0.0
Espresso Macchiato, Doppio, Skimmed Milk, Starbucks*	1 Doppio/60ml	13	0.0	22	1.7	4.0	0.0	0.0
Espresso Macchiato, Doppio, Soy, Starbucks*	1 Doppio/60ml	13	0.1	22	1.5	3.3	0.2	0.0
Espresso Macchiato, Doppio, SS Milk, Starbucks*	1 Doppio/60ml	14	0.1	23	1.5	3.8	0.2	0.0
Espresso Macchiato, Doppio, Whole Milk, Starbucks*	1 Doppio/60ml	15	0.2	24	1.5	3.8	0.3	0.0
Espresso Macchiato, Solo, Skimmed Milk, Starbucks*	1 Solo/30ml	7	0.0	24	1.7	4.0	0.0	0.0
Espresso Macchiato, Solo, Soy, Starbucks*	1 Solo/30ml	7	0.1	25	1.7	3.7	0.3	0.0
Espresso Macchiato, Solo, SS Milk, Starbucks*	1 Solo/30ml	8	0.1	27	1.7	4.0	0.3	0.0
Espresso Macchiato, Solo, Whole Milk, Starbucks*	1 Solo/30ml	8	0.2	28	1.7	4.0	0.7	0.0
Filter, Grande, Starbucks*	1 Grande/473ml	5	0.1	1	0.1	0.0	0.0	0.0
Filter, Short, Starbucks*	1 Short/236ml	3	0.1	1	0.1	0.0	0.0	0.0
Filter, Tall, Starbucks*	1 Tall/355ml	4	0.1	1	0.1	0.0	0.0	0.0
Filter, Venti, Starbucks*	1 Venti/591ml	6	0.1	1	0.1	0.0	0.0	0.0
Flat White, Short, Whole Milk, Starbucks*	1 Short/236ml	119	5.8	50	2.8	4.3	2.5	0.0
Iced, Caffe Americano, Grande, Starbucks*	1 Grande/473ml	17	0.0	4	0.2	0.6	0.0	0.0
Iced, Caffe Americano, Tall, Starbucks*	1 Tall/335ml	11	0.0	3	0.2	0.6	0.0	0.0
Iced, Caffe Americano, Venti, Starbucks*	1 Venti/591ml	23	0.0	4	0.2	0.7	0.0	0.0
Iced, Caffe Latte, Grande, Skimmed Milk, Starbucks*	1 Grande/473ml	90	0.2	19	1.8	2.8	0.0	0.0
Iced, Caffe Latte, Grande, Soy, Starbucks*	1 Grande/473ml	104	3.6	22	1.5	2.0	0.8	0.2
Iced, Caffe Latte, Grande, SS Milk, Starbucks*	1 Grande/473ml	126	4.5	27	1.8	2.7	1.0	0.0
Iced, Caffe Latte, Grande, Whole Milk, Starbucks*	1 Grande/473ml	149	7.5	32	1.7	2.6	1.6	0.0
Iced, Caffe Latte, Tall, Semi Skimmed Milk, Starbucks*	1 Tall/335ml	87	3.0	26	1.7	2.8	0.9	0.0
Iced, Caffe Latte, Tall, Skimmed Milk, Starbucks*	1 Tall/335ml	63	0.1	19	1.7	2.8	0.0	0.0
Iced, Caffe Latte, Tall, Soy, Starbucks*	1 Tall/335ml	71	2.4	21	1.5	2.0	0.7	0.2
Iced, Caffe Latte, Tall, Whole Milk, Starbucks*	1 Tall/335ml	104	4.9	31	1.6	2.8	1.5	0.0
Iced, Caffe Latte, Venti, Semi Skimmed Milk, Starbucks*	1 Venti/591ml	132	4.6	22	1.5	2.4	0.8	0.0
Iced, Caffe Latte, Venti, Skimmed Milk, Starbucks*	1 Venti/591ml	95	0.2	16	1.5	2.4	0.0	0.0
Iced, Caffe Latte, Venti, Soy, Starbucks*	1 Venti/591ml	109	3.7	18	1.3	1.7	0.6	0.2
Iced, Caffe Latte, Venti, Whole Milk, Starbucks*	1 Venti/591ml	158	7.5	27	1.4	2.4	1.3	0.0
Iced, Caffe Mocha, Whip, Grande, Skim, Starbucks*	1 Grande/473ml	289	13.6	61	2.0	8.2	2.9	0.4
Iced, Caffe Mocha, Whip, Grande, Soy, Starbucks*	1 Grande/473ml	300	16.1	63	1.8	7.6	3.4	0.5
Iced, Caffe Mocha, Whip, Grande, SS Milk, Starbucks*	1 Grande/473ml	316	16.8	67	2.0	8.1	3.6	0.4
Iced, Caffe Mocha, Whip, Grande, Whole, Starbucks*	1 Grande/473ml	332	18.9	70	1.9	8.1	4.0	0.4
Iced, Caffe Mocha, Whip, Tall, Skim Milk, Starbucks*	1 Tall/335ml	208	9.8	62	2.0	8.5	2.9	0.4
Iced, Caffe Mocha, Whip, Tall, SS Milk, Starbucks*	1 Tall/335ml	225	11.8	67	1.9	8.4	3.5	0.4

	Measure INFO/WEIGHT	per Measure		Nutrition Values per 100g / 100ml				
		KCAL	FAT	KCAL	PROT	CARB	FAT	FIBRE

STARBUCKS

COFFEE

Iced, Caffe Mocha, Whip, Tall, Whole Milk, Starbucks*	1 Tall/335ml	236	13.1	71	1.9	8.4	3.9	0.4
Iced, Caffe Mocha, Whip, Venti, Skim Milk, Starbucks*	1 Venti/591ml	315	14.1	53	1.7	7.7	2.4	0.4
Iced, Caffe Mocha, Whip, Venti, SS Milk, Starbucks*	1 Venti/591ml	340	17.0	58	1.7	7.6	2.9	0.4
Iced, Caffe Mocha, Whip, Venti, Whole Milk, Starbucks*	1 Venti/591ml	357	19.0	60	1.6	7.6	3.2	0.4
Iced, Caffe Mocha, with Whip, Tall, Soy, Starbucks*	1 Tall/335ml	214	11.3	64	1.8	7.9	3.4	0.5
Iced, Caffe Mocha, with Whip, Venti, Soy, Starbucks*	1 Venti/591ml	325	16.4	55	1.5	7.2	2.8	0.5
Iced, Cappuccino, Grande, Skimmed Milk, Starbucks*	1 Grande/473ml	96	0.2	20	1.9	3.0	0.0	0.0
Iced, Cappuccino, Grande, Soy, Starbucks*	1 Grande/473ml	111	4.0	23	1.6	2.1	0.8	0.2
Iced, Cappuccino, Grande, SS Milk, Starbucks*	1 Grande/473ml	135	4.9	29	1.9	2.9	1.0	0.0
Iced, Cappuccino, Grande, Whole Milk, Starbucks*	1 Grande/473ml	163	8.1	34	1.8	2.9	1.7	0.0
Iced, Cappuccino, Tall, Semi Skimmed Milk, Starbucks*	1 Tall/335ml	94	3.3	28	1.9	3.0	1.0	0.0
Iced, Cappuccino, Tall, Skimmed Milk, Starbucks*	1 Tall/335ml	68	0.1	20	1.9	3.0	0.0	0.0
Iced, Cappuccino, Tall, Soy, Starbucks*	1 Tall/335ml	78	2.7	23	1.6	2.2	0.8	0.2
Iced, Cappuccino, Tall, Whole Milk, Starbucks*	1 Tall/335ml	113	5.4	34	1.8	3.0	1.6	0.0
Iced, Cappuccino, Venti, Semi Skim Milk, Starbucks*	1 Venti/591ml	141	4.9	24	1.6	2.5	0.8	0.0
Iced, Cappuccino, Venti, Skimmed Milk, Starbucks*	1 Venti/591ml	101	0.2	17	1.6	2.6	0.0	0.0
Iced, Cappuccino, Venti, Soy, Starbucks*	1 Venti/591ml	116	3.9	20	1.4	1.8	0.7	0.2
Iced, Cappuccino, Venti, Whole Milk, Starbucks*	1 Venti/591ml	168	8.1	28	1.5	2.5	1.4	0.0
Iced, Caramel Macchiato, Grande, Skim, Starbucks*	1 Grande/473ml	188	1.3	40	2.1	7.2	0.3	0.0
Iced, Caramel Macchiato, Grande, Soy, Starbucks*	1 Grande/473ml	206	5.3	43	1.8	6.3	1.1	0.2
Iced, Caramel Macchiato, Grande, SS Milk, Starbucks*	1 Grande/473ml	231	6.3	49	2.0	7.1	1.3	0.0
Iced, Caramel Macchiato, Grande, Whole, Starbucks*	1 Grande/473ml	257	9.8	54	2.0	7.0	2.1	0.0
Iced, Caramel Macchiato, Tall, SkimMilk, Starbucks*	1 Tall/335ml	124	1.1	37	1.6	6.8	0.3	0.0
Iced, Caramel Macchiato, Tall, Soy, Starbucks*	1 Tall/335ml	134	3.3	40	1.4	6.1	1.0	0.2
Iced, Caramel Macchiato, Tall, SS Milk, Starbucks*	1 Tall/335ml	146	3.7	43	1.6	6.8	1.1	0.0
Iced, Caramel Macchiato, Tall, Whole Milk, Starbucks*	1 Tall/335ml	161	5.5	48	1.5	6.8	1.6	0.0
Iced, Caramel Macchiato, Venti, Skim Milk, Starbucks*	1 Venti/591ml	189	1.2	32	1.3	6.2	0.2	0.0
Iced, Caramel Macchiato, Venti, Soy, Starbucks*	1 Venti/591ml	201	4.2	34	1.1	5.6	0.7	0.1
Iced, Caramel Macchiato, Venti, SS Milk, Starbucks*	1 Venti/591ml	221	5.0	37	1.3	6.1	0.8	0.0
Iced, Caramel Macchiato, Venti, Whole Milk, Starbucks*	1 Venti/591ml	243	7.5	41	1.3	6.1	1.3	0.0
Iced, Grande, Starbucks*	1 Grande/473ml	4	0.1	1	0.1	0.0	0.0	0.0
Iced, Tall, Starbucks*	1 Tall/335ml	3	0.1	1	0.1	0.0	0.0	0.0
Iced, Venti, Starbucks*	1 Venti/591ml	5	0.1	1	0.1	0.0	0.0	0.0
Macchiato, Caramel, Grande, Skim Milk, Starbucks*	1 Grande/473ml	193	1.1	41	2.3	7.4	0.2	0.0
Macchiato, Caramel, Grande, Soy, Starbucks*	1 Grande/473ml	207	5.3	44	1.9	6.2	1.1	0.2
Macchiato, Caramel, Grande, SS Milk, Starbucks*	1 Grande/473ml	240	6.7	51	2.2	7.2	1.4	0.0
Macchiato, Caramel, Grande, Whole Milk, Starbucks*	1 Grande/473ml	269	10.5	57	2.2	7.1	2.2	0.0
Macchiato, Caramel, Short, Skimmed Milk, Starbucks*	1 Short/236ml	97	0.9	41	2.4	7.1	0.4	0.0
Macchiato, Caramel, Short, Soy, Starbucks*	1 Short/236ml	104	3.0	44	1.9	5.9	1.3	0.3
Macchiato, Caramel, Short, SS Milk, Starbucks*	1 Short/236ml	122	3.8	52	2.3	6.9	1.6	0.0
Macchiato, Caramel, Short, Whole Milk, Starbucks*	1 Short/236ml	137	5.7	58	2.2	6.8	2.4	0.0
Macchiato, Caramel, Tall, Skimmed Milk, Starbucks*	1 Tall/355ml	165	1.0	46	2.9	8.1	0.3	0.0
Macchiato, Caramel, Tall, Soy, Starbucks*	1 Tall/355ml	167	4.6	47	2.1	6.5	1.3	0.3
Macchiato, Caramel, Tall, SS Milk, Starbucks*	1 Tall/355ml	209	6.3	59	2.8	7.9	1.8	0.0
Macchiato, Caramel, Tall, Whole Milk, Starbucks*	1 Tall/355ml	240	9.8	68	2.7	7.9	2.8	0.0
Macchiato, Caramel, Venti, Skimmed Milk, Starbucks*	1 Venti/591ml	261	1.2	44	2.6	8.0	0.2	0.0
Macchiato, Caramel, Venti, Soy, Starbucks*	1 Venti/591ml	280	7.4	47	2.1	6.6	1.3	0.3
Macchiato, Caramel, Venti, SS Milk, Starbucks*	1 Venti/591ml	329	9.3	56	2.6	7.8	1.6	0.0
Macchiato, Caramel, Venti, Whole Milk, Starbucks*	1 Venti/591ml	376	14.6	64	2.5	7.8	2.5	0.0
Mocha, White Choc, Cream, Grande, Milk, Starbucks*	1 Grande/473ml	500	22.1	106	3.1	13.2	4.7	0.0
Mocha, White Choc, Cream, Grande, Skim, Starbucks*	1 Grande/473ml	425	12.9	90	3.2	13.4	2.7	0.0
Mocha, White Choc, Cream, Grande, Soy, Starbucks*	1 Grande/473ml	439	17.0	93	2.8	12.3	3.6	0.2

	Measure INFO/WEIGHT	per Measure		Nutrition Values per 100g / 100ml				
		KCAL	FAT	KCAL	PROT	CARB	FAT	FIBRE

STARBUCKS

COFFEE

	Measure INFO/WEIGHT	KCAL	FAT	KCAL	PROT	CARB	FAT	FIBRE
Mocha, White Choc, Cream, Grande, SS, Starbucks*	1 Grande/473ml	471	18.4	100	3.2	13.3	3.9	0.0
Mocha, White Choc, Cream, Short, Skim, Starbucks*	1 Short/236ml	229	8.0	97	3.3	13.7	3.4	0.0
Mocha, White Choc, Cream, Short, Soy, Starbucks*	1 Short/355ml	236	10.1	66	1.9	8.3	2.8	0.2
Mocha, White Choc, Cream, Short, SS Milk, Starbucks*	1 Short/236ml	252	10.8	107	3.2	13.5	4.6	0.0
Mocha, White Choc, Cream, Short, Whole, Starbucks*	1 Short/236ml	267	12.7	113	3.2	13.4	5.4	0.0
Mocha, White Choc, Cream, Tall, Skim Milk, Starbucks*	1 Tall/355ml	327	10.4	92	3.2	13.5	2.9	0.0
Mocha, White Choc, Cream, Tall, Soy, Starbucks*	1 Tall/355ml	465	20.4	131	4.7	15.3	5.7	0.2
Mocha, White Choc, Cream, Tall, SS Milk, Starbucks*	1 Tall/355ml	323	14.5	91	3.2	13.4	4.1	0.0
Mocha, White Choc, Cream, Tall, Whole, Starbucks*	1 Tall/355ml	385	17.1	108	3.1	13.4	4.8	0.0
Mocha, White Choc, Cream, Venti, Skim, Starbucks*	1 Venti/591ml	515	14.3	87	3.2	13.4	2.4	0.0
Mocha, White Choc, Cream, Venti, Soy, Starbucks*	1 Venti/591ml	530	19.5	90	2.8	12.3	3.3	0.2
Mocha, White Choc, Cream, Venti, SS Milk, Starbucks*	1 Venti/591ml	573	21.2	97	3.2	13.3	3.6	0.0
Mocha, White Choc, Cream, Venti, Whole, Starbucks*	1 Venti/591ml	613	25.8	104	3.1	13.3	4.4	0.0

COOKIES

	Measure INFO/WEIGHT	KCAL	FAT	KCAL	PROT	CARB	FAT	FIBRE
Chocolate Chunk, Starbucks*	1 Cookie/107g	499	20.5	466	7.4	65.0	19.2	1.7
Fruit & Oat, Starbucks*	1 Cookie/50g	216	8.8	433	4.4	64.3	17.6	3.1

CRISPS

	Measure INFO/WEIGHT	KCAL	FAT	KCAL	PROT	CARB	FAT	FIBRE
Pepperoni, Potato Chips, Starbucks*	1 Pack/50g	239	14.1	478	6.0	53.6	28.2	4.9
Sea Salt, Potato Chips, Starbucks*	1 Pack/50g	244	15.0	488	5.6	53.3	30.0	4.5
Sea Salt & Cider Vinegar, Potato Chips, Starbucks*	1 Pack/50g	248	14.1	496	6.2	54.2	28.3	4.3

CROISSANT

	Measure INFO/WEIGHT	KCAL	FAT	KCAL	PROT	CARB	FAT	FIBRE
Almond, Starbucks*	1 Croissant/104g	433	21.8	416	6.4	50.1	21.0	2.0
Butter, Starbucks*	1 Croissant/70g	267	15.7	381	5.8	38.2	22.5	1.3
Cinnamon Swirl, Starbucks*	1 Croissant/115g	371	11.7	323	7.4	49.1	10.2	2.6
Ham & Emmental, Starbucks*	1 Croissant/120g	378	21.0	315	13.8	25.2	17.5	0.9

DOUGHNUT

	Measure INFO/WEIGHT	KCAL	FAT	KCAL	PROT	CARB	FAT	FIBRE
Apple Fritter, Starbucks*	1 Doughnut/115g	473	24.3	411	6.0	47.5	21.1	3.1

DRIED FRUIT

	Measure INFO/WEIGHT	KCAL	FAT	KCAL	PROT	CARB	FAT	FIBRE
Starbucks*	1 Serving/30g	90	0.1	299	1.9	73.0	0.4	2.0

FRAPPUCCINO

	Measure INFO/WEIGHT	KCAL	FAT	KCAL	PROT	CARB	FAT	FIBRE
Caramel, with Whip, Grande, Skimmed Milk, Starbucks*	1 Grande/473ml	375	11.9	79	0.9	13.4	2.5	0.0
Caramel, with Whip, Grande, Soy, Starbucks*	1 Grande/473ml	325	13.9	69	0.9	9.7	2.9	0.1
Caramel, with Whip, Grande, SS Milk, Starbucks*	1 Grande/473ml	338	14.4	72	1.1	10.1	3.0	0.0
Caramel, with Whip, Grande, Whole Milk, Starbucks*	1 Grande/473ml	400	15.0	85	0.8	13.3	3.2	0.0
Caramel, with Whip, Tall, Skimmed Milk, Starbucks*	1 Tall/335ml	238	8.7	71	1.2	10.8	2.6	0.0
Caramel, with Whip, Tall, Soy, Starbucks*	1 Tall/335ml	278	9.9	83	0.9	13.3	3.0	0.1
Caramel, with Whip, Tall, SS Milk, Starbucks*	1 Tall/335ml	286	10.2	85	1.0	13.6	3.0	0.0
Caramel, with Whip, Tall, Whole Milk, Starbucks*	1 Tall/335ml	294	11.2	88	1.0	13.6	3.3	0.0
Caramel, with Whip, Venti, Skimmed Milk, Starbucks*	1 Venti/591ml	427	10.9	72	0.8	13.2	1.8	0.0
Caramel, with Whip, Venti, Soy, Starbucks*	1 Venti/591ml	377	13.4	64	0.9	10.0	2.3	0.1
Caramel, with Whip, Venti, SS Milk, Starbucks*	1 Venti/591ml	393	14.0	67	1.0	10.4	2.4	0.0
Caramel, with Whip, Venti, Whole Milk, Starbucks*	1 Venti/591ml	409	16.0	69	1.0	10.4	2.7	0.0
Coffee, No Whip, Grande, Skimmed Milk, Starbucks*	1 Grande/473ml	216	0.1	46	0.7	10.6	0.0	0.0
Coffee, No Whip, Grande, Soy, Starbucks*	1 Grande/473ml	222	1.6	47	0.6	10.3	0.3	0.1
Coffee, No Whip, Grande, SS Milk, Starbucks*	1 Grande/473ml	232	1.9	49	0.7	10.6	0.4	0.0
Coffee, No Whip, Grande, Whole Milk, Starbucks*	1 Grande/473ml	241	3.2	51	0.7	10.5	0.7	0.0
Coffee, No Whip, Tall, Semi Skimmed Milk, Starbucks*	1 Tall/335ml	169	1.6	51	0.8	10.7	0.5	0.0
Coffee, No Whip, Tall, Skimmed Milk, Starbucks*	1 Tall/335ml	157	0.1	47	0.9	10.8	0.0	0.0
Coffee, No Whip, Tall, Soy, Starbucks*	1 Tall/335ml	162	1.3	48	0.7	10.4	0.4	0.1
Coffee, No Whip, Tall, Whole Milk, Starbucks*	1 Tall/335ml	177	2.6	53	0.8	10.7	0.8	0.0
Coffee, No Whip, Venti, Semi Skimmed Milk, Starbucks*	1 Venti/591ml	286	2.1	48	0.6	10.6	0.4	0.0
Coffee, No Whip, Venti, Skimmed Milk, Starbucks*	1 Venti/591ml	268	0.1	45	0.7	10.7	0.0	0.0

STARBUCKS

FRAPPUCCINO

	Measure INFO/WEIGHT	per Measure KCAL	FAT	Nutrition Values per 100g / 100ml KCAL	PROT	CARB	FAT	FIBRE
Coffee, No Whip, Venti, Soy, Starbucks*	1 Venti/591ml	275	1.7	46	0.6	10.3	0.3	0.1
Coffee, No Whip, Venti, Whole Milk, Starbucks*	1 Venti/591ml	296	3.5	50	0.6	10.6	0.6	0.0
Cream, Choc with Whip, Grande, Skim Milk, Starbucks*	1 Grande/473ml	314	12.2	66	1.3	10.3	2.6	0.2
Cream, Choc with Whip, Grande, SS Milk, Starbucks*	1 Grande/473ml	335	14.7	71	1.2	10.2	3.1	0.2
Cream, Choc with Whip, Grande, Whole, Starbucks*	1 Grande/473ml	349	16.3	74	1.2	10.2	3.4	0.2
Cream, Choc with Whip, Tall, Skim Milk, Starbucks*	1 Tall/335ml	226	8.7	67	1.4	10.4	2.6	0.2
Cream, Choc with Whip, Tall, SS Milk, Starbucks*	1 Tall/335ml	243	10.7	72	1.3	10.3	3.2	0.2
Cream, Choc with Whip, Tall, Whole Milk, Starbucks*	1 Tall/335ml	253	12.0	75	1.3	10.3	3.6	0.2
Cream, Choc with Whip, Venti, Skim Milk, Starbucks*	1 Venti/591ml	361	11.5	61	1.2	10.4	1.9	0.2
Cream, Choc with Whip, Venti, SS Milk, Starbucks*	1 Venti/591ml	386	14.4	65	1.2	10.3	2.4	0.2
Cream, Choc with Whip, Venti, Whole Milk, Starbucks*	1 Venti/591ml	401	16.4	68	1.2	10.3	2.8	0.2
Cream, Chocolate with Whip, Grande, Soy, Starbucks*	1 Grande/473ml	322	14.2	68	1.1	9.8	3.0	0.3
Cream, Chocolate with Whip, Tall, Soy, Starbucks*	1 Tall/335ml	232	10.3	69	1.2	9.9	3.1	0.3
Cream, Chocolate with Whip, Venti, Soy, Starbucks*	1 Venti/591ml	370	13.8	63	1.0	9.9	2.3	0.3
Espresso, No Whip, Grande, Skimmed Milk, Starbucks*	1 Grande/473ml	200	0.1	42	0.6	9.9	0.0	0.0
Espresso, No Whip, Grande, Soy, Starbucks*	1 Grande/473ml	204	1.1	43	0.5	9.7	0.2	0.1
Espresso, No Whip, Grande, SS Milk, Starbucks*	1 Grande/473ml	210	1.3	44	0.6	9.9	0.3	0.0
Espresso, No Whip, Grande, Whole Milk, Starbucks*	1 Grande/473ml	217	2.1	46	0.6	9.9	0.4	0.0
Espresso, No Whip, Tall, Skimmed Milk, Starbucks*	1 Tall/335ml	136	0.0	41	0.6	9.5	0.0	0.0
Espresso, No Whip, Tall, Soy, Starbucks*	1 Tall/335ml	139	0.7	41	0.5	9.3	0.2	0.1
Espresso, No Whip, Tall, SS Milk, Starbucks*	1 Tall/335ml	143	0.9	43	0.6	9.5	0.3	0.0
Espresso, No Whip, Tall, Whole Milk, Starbucks*	1 Tall/335ml	148	1.5	44	0.6	9.4	0.4	0.0
Espresso, No Whip, Venti, Skimmed Milk, Starbucks*	1 Venti/591ml	250	0.1	42	0.5	10.0	0.0	0.0
Espresso, No Whip, Venti, Soy, Starbucks*	1 Venti/591ml	254	1.2	43	0.5	9.8	0.2	0.1
Espresso, No Whip, Venti, SS Milk, Starbucks*	1 Venti/591ml	262	1.5	44	0.5	9.9	0.3	0.0
Espresso, No Whip, Venti, Whole Milk, Starbucks*	1 Venti/591ml	270	2.5	46	0.5	9.9	0.4	0.0
Light, No Whip, Grande, Skimmed Milk, Starbucks*	1 Grande/473ml	118	0.1	25	0.7	5.4	0.0	0.1
Light, No Whip, Tall, Skimmed Milk, Starbucks*	1 Tall/335ml	83	0.1	25	0.8	5.3	0.0	0.1
Light, No Whip, Venti, Skimmed Milk, Starbucks*	1 Venti/591ml	139	0.1	24	0.7	5.0	0.0	0.1
Mango Passion, Grande, Starbucks*	1 Grande/473ml	191	0.3	40	0.2	9.8	0.1	0.3
Mango Passion, Tall, Starbucks*	1 Tall/335ml	157	0.2	47	0.2	11.4	0.1	0.3
Mango Passion, Venti, Starbucks*	1 Venti/591ml	228	0.3	39	0.2	9.4	0.1	0.3
Mocha, No Whip, Grande, Skimmed Milk, Starbucks*	1 Grande/473ml	143	0.8	30	0.8	6.7	0.2	0.2
Mocha, No Whip, Tall, Skimmed Milk, Starbucks*	1 Tall/335ml	96	0.5	29	0.9	6.3	0.1	0.1
Mocha, No Whip, Venti, Skimmed Milk, Starbucks*	1 Venti/591ml	179	0.9	30	0.9	6.7	0.2	0.2
Mocha, with Whip, Grande, Skimmed Milk, Starbucks*	1 Grande/473ml	346	12.0	73	1.0	12.2	2.5	0.1
Mocha, with Whip, Grande, Soy, Starbucks*	1 Grande/473ml	352	13.3	74	0.9	11.9	2.8	0.2
Mocha, with Whip, Grande, SS Milk, Starbucks*	1 Grande/473ml	361	13.7	76	1.0	12.2	2.9	0.1
Mocha, with Whip, Grande, Whole Milk, Starbucks*	1 Grande/473ml	370	14.8	78	1.0	12.1	3.1	0.1
Mocha, with Whip, Tall, Semi Skimmed Milk, Starbucks*	1 Tall/335ml	266	10.0	79	1.1	12.6	3.0	0.1
Mocha, with Whip, Tall, Skimmed Milk, Starbucks*	1 Tall/335ml	254	8.6	76	1.1	12.7	2.6	0.1
Mocha, with Whip, Tall, Soy, Starbucks*	1 Tall/335ml	258	9.7	77	1.0	12.3	2.9	0.2
Mocha, with Whip, Tall, Whole Milk, Starbucks*	1 Tall/335ml	274	11.0	82	1.1	12.6	3.3	0.1
Mocha, with Whip, Venti, Skimmed Milk, Starbucks*	1 Venti/591ml	410	11.3	69	0.9	12.7	1.9	0.2
Mocha, with Whip, Venti, Soy, Starbucks*	1 Venti/591ml	416	12.8	70	0.8	12.4	2.2	0.2
Mocha, with Whip, Venti, SS Milk, Starbucks*	1 Venti/591ml	427	13.2	72	0.9	12.7	2.2	0.2
Mocha, with Whip, Venti, Whole Milk, Starbucks*	1 Venti/591ml	437	14.6	74	0.9	12.7	2.5	0.2
Raspberry, Grande, Starbucks*	1 Grande/473ml	192	0.1	41	0.1	10.0	0.0	0.1
Raspberry, Tall, Starbucks*	1 Tall/335ml	158	0.1	47	0.1	11.6	0.0	0.2
Raspberry, Venti, Starbucks*	1 Venti/591ml	229	0.1	39	0.1	9.5	0.0	0.1
Strawberries & Cream, Whip, Grande, Soy, Starbucks*	1 Grande/473ml	391	13.1	83	0.9	13.7	2.8	0.2
Strawberries & Cream, Whip, Grande, SS, Starbucks*	1 Grande/473ml	403	13.6	85	1.0	14.1	2.9	0.1

STARBUCKS

	Measure INFO/WEIGHT	per Measure		Nutrition Values per 100g / 100ml				
		KCAL	FAT	KCAL	PROT	CARB	FAT	FIBRE
FRAPPUCCINO								
Strawberries & Cream, Whip, Tall, Skim, Starbucks*	1 Tall/335ml	300	8.1	90	1.2	16.1	2.4	0.1
Strawberries & Cream, Whip, Tall, Soy, Starbucks*	1 Tall/335ml	306	9.6	91	1.0	15.6	2.9	0.2
Strawberries & Cream, Whip, Tall, SS Milk, Starbucks*	1 Tall/335ml	316	9.9	94	1.2	16.0	3.0	0.1
Strawberries & Cream, Whip, Tall, Whole, Starbucks*	1 Tall/335ml	326	11.2	97	1.1	16.0	3.3	0.1
Strawberries & Cream, Whip, Venti, Skim, Starbucks*	1 Venti/591ml	422	10.3	71	0.9	13.2	1.7	0.1
Strawberries & Cream, Whip, Venti, Soy, Starbucks*	1 Venti/591ml	431	12.5	73	0.8	12.8	2.1	0.2
Strawberries & Cream, Whip, Venti, SS, Starbucks*	1 Venti/591ml	445	13.0	75	0.9	13.1	2.2	0.1
Strawberries & Cream, Whip, Venti, Whole, Starbucks*	1 Venti/591ml	459	14.9	78	0.9	13.1	2.5	0.1
Vanilla, with Whip, Grande, Skimmed Milk, Starbucks*	1 Grande/473ml	305	11.3	65	1.1	9.8	2.4	0.0
Vanilla, with Whip, Grande, Soy, Starbucks*	1 Grande/473ml	313	13.4	66	0.9	9.3	2.8	0.1
Vanilla, with Whip, Grande, SS Milk, Starbucks*	1 Grande/473ml	327	13.9	69	1.1	9.7	2.9	0.0
Vanilla, with Whip, Grande, Whole Milk, Starbucks*	1 Grande/473ml	341	15.6	72	1.1	9.7	3.3	0.0
Vanilla, with Whip, Tall, Semi Skimmed Milk, Starbucks*	1 Tall/335ml	233	10.0	69	1.2	9.6	3.0	0.0
Vanilla, with Whip, Tall, Skimmed Milk, Starbucks*	1 Tall/335ml	216	8.1	64	1.2	9.6	2.4	0.0
Vanilla, with Whip, Tall, Soy, Starbucks*	1 Tall/335ml	222	9.7	66	1.0	9.1	2.9	0.1
Vanilla, with Whip, Tall, Whole Milk, Starbucks*	1 Tall/335ml	243	11.4	73	1.1	9.5	3.4	0.0
Vanilla, with Whip, Venti, Skimmed Milk, Starbucks*	1 Venti/591ml	347	10.4	59	1.0	9.8	1.8	0.0
Vanilla, with Whip, Venti, Soy, Starbucks*	1 Venti/591ml	346	12.4	59	0.7	9.2	2.1	0.1
Vanilla, with Whip, Venti, SS Milk, Starbucks*	1 Venti/591ml	372	13.4	63	1.0	9.7	2.3	0.0
Vanilla, with Whip, Venti, Whole Milk, Starbucks*	1 Venti/591ml	388	15.4	66	1.0	9.7	2.6	0.0
FRUIT								
Banana, Fairtrade, Starbucks*	1 Banana/120g	108	0.5	90	0.8	22.6	0.4	2.7
HOT CHOCOLATE								
Classic, with Whip, Grande, Skimmed Milk, Starbucks*	1 Grande/473ml	277	9.5	58	2.7	8.8	2.0	0.4
Classic, with Whip, Grande, Soy, Starbucks*	1 Grande/473ml	291	13.7	62	2.3	7.7	2.9	0.6
Classic, with Whip, Grande, SS Milk, Starbucks*	1 Grande/473ml	323	15.0	68	2.6	8.7	3.2	0.4
Classic, with Whip, Grande, Whole Milk, Starbucks*	1 Grande/473ml	352	18.7	74	2.6	8.6	4.0	0.4
Classic, with Whip, Short, Skimmed Milk, Starbucks*	1 Short/236ml	155	6.4	66	2.8	9.1	2.7	0.4
Classic, with Whip, Short, Soy, Starbucks*	1 Short/236ml	162	8.5	69	2.3	7.9	3.6	0.6
Classic, with Whip, Short, SS Milk, Starbucks*	1 Short/236ml	178	9.1	75	2.7	8.9	3.9	0.4
Classic, with Whip, Short, Whole Milk, Starbucks*	1 Short/236ml	193	11.0	82	2.6	8.8	4.7	0.4
Classic, with Whip, Tall, Semi Skimmed Milk, Starbucks*	1 Tall/335ml	260	12.5	78	3.0	9.5	3.7	0.4
Classic, with Whip, Tall, Skimmed Milk, Starbucks*	1 Tall/335ml	222	8.0	66	3.0	9.7	2.4	0.4
Classic, with Whip, Tall, Soy, Starbucks*	1 Tall/335ml	234	11.4	70	2.6	8.4	3.4	0.7
Classic, with Whip, Tall, Whole Milk, Starbucks*	1 Tall/335ml	284	15.5	85	3.0	9.4	4.6	0.4
Classic, with Whip, Venti, Skimmed Milk, Starbucks*	1 Venti/591ml	336	10.2	57	2.8	8.9	1.7	0.4
Classic, with Whip, Venti, Soy, Starbucks*	1 Venti/591ml	355	15.7	60	2.4	7.7	2.7	0.6
Classic, with Whip, Venti, SS Milk, Starbucks*	1 Venti/591ml	398	17.5	67	2.8	8.7	3.0	0.4
Classic, with Whip, Venti, Whole Milk, Starbucks*	1 Venti/591ml	437	22.5	74	2.7	8.6	3.8	0.4
Signature, with Whip, Grande, Skim Milk, Starbucks*	1 Grande/473ml	505	27.0	107	3.3	12.6	5.7	1.4
Signature, with Whip, Grande, Soy, Starbucks*	1 Grande/473ml	515	29.8	109	3.0	11.8	6.3	1.6
Signature, with Whip, Grande, SS Milk, Starbucks*	1 Grande/473ml	537	30.7	113	3.2	12.5	6.5	1.4
Signature, with Whip, Grande, Whole Milk, Starbucks*	1 Grande/473ml	556	33.5	118	3.2	12.5	7.1	1.4
Signature, with Whip, Short, Skimmed Milk, Starbucks*	1 Short/236ml	267	15.0	113	3.3	12.7	6.4	1.4
Signature, with Whip, Short, Soy, Starbucks*	1 Short/236ml	272	16.4	115	3.1	11.9	6.9	1.6
Signature, with Whip, Short, SS Milk, Starbucks*	1 Short/236ml	283	16.9	120	3.3	12.6	7.2	1.4
Signature, with Whip, Short, Whole Milk, Starbucks*	1 Short/236ml	293	18.1	124	3.2	12.5	7.7	1.4
Signature, with Whip, Tall, Skimmed Milk, Starbucks*	1 Tall/335ml	393	21.3	117	3.6	13.6	6.4	1.5
Signature, with Whip, Tall, Soy, Starbucks*	1 Tall/335ml	401	23.5	120	3.3	12.8	7.0	1.7
Signature, with Whip, Tall, SS Milk, Starbucks*	1 Tall/335ml	418	24.2	125	3.5	13.5	7.2	1.5
Signature, with Whip, Tall, Whole Milk, Starbucks*	1 Tall/335ml	433	26.1	129	3.5	13.4	7.8	1.5
Signature, with Whip, Venti, Skimmed Milk, Starbucks*	1 Venti/591ml	624	32.4	106	3.3	12.7	5.5	1.4

STARBUCKS

	Measure INFO/WEIGHT	per Measure KCAL	FAT	Nutrition Values per 100g / 100ml KCAL	PROT	CARB	FAT	FIBRE
HOT CHOCOLATE								
Signature, with Whip, Venti, Soy, Starbucks*	1 Venti/591ml	637	36.0	108	3.0	12.0	6.1	1.6
Signature, with Whip, Venti, SS Milk, Starbucks*	1 Venti/591ml	665	37.2	113	3.3	12.7	6.3	1.4
Signature, with Whip, Venti, Whole Milk, Starbucks*	1 Venti/591ml	690	40.4	117	3.2	12.5	6.8	1.4
LOLLIPOPS								
Starbucks*	1 Lolly/13g	50	0.0	388	0.0	97.0	0.0	0.0
MILK								
Steamed, Grande, Semi Skimmed Milk, Starbucks*	1 Grande/473ml	203	8.0	43	2.8	4.0	1.7	0.0
Steamed, Grande, Skimmed Milk, Starbucks*	1 Grande/473ml	138	0.3	29	2.9	4.2	0.1	0.0
Steamed, Grande, Soy, Starbucks*	1 Grande/473ml	157	6.1	33	2.3	2.7	1.3	0.3
Steamed, Grande, Whole Milk, Starbucks*	1 Grande/473ml	244	13.2	52	2.8	3.9	2.8	0.0
Steamed, Short, Semi Skimmed Milk, Starbucks*	1 Short/236ml	102	4.0	43	2.9	4.1	1.7	0.0
Steamed, Short, Skimmed Milk, Starbucks*	1 Short/236ml	70	0.2	30	2.9	4.3	0.1	0.0
Steamed, Short, Soy, Starbucks*	1 Short/236ml	79	3.1	34	2.4	2.7	1.3	0.3
Steamed, Short, Whole Milk, Starbucks*	1 Short/236ml	123	6.7	52	2.8	3.9	2.8	0.0
Steamed, Tall, Semi Skimmed Milk, Starbucks*	1 Tall/335ml	155	6.1	46	3.1	4.4	1.8	0.0
Steamed, Tall, Skimmed Milk, Starbucks*	1 Tall/335ml	106	0.3	32	3.1	4.6	0.1	0.0
Steamed, Tall, Soy, Starbucks*	1 Tall/335ml	120	4.7	36	2.5	2.9	1.4	0.4
Steamed, Tall, Whole Milk, Starbucks*	1 Tall/335ml	187	10.1	56	3.0	4.2	3.0	0.0
Steamed, Venti, Semi Skimmed Milk, Starbucks*	1 Venti/591ml	258	10.2	44	2.9	4.1	1.7	0.0
Steamed, Venti, Skimmed Milk, Starbucks*	1 Venti/591ml	175	0.4	30	2.9	4.3	0.1	0.0
Steamed, Venti, Soy, Starbucks*	1 Venti/591ml	199	7.8	34	2.4	2.7	1.3	0.3
Steamed, Venti, Whole Milk, Starbucks*	1 Venti/591ml	309	16.7	52	2.8	3.9	2.8	0.0
MINTS								
After Coffee, Starbucks*	1 Mint/2g	5	0.0	250	0.0	100.0	0.0	0.0
MUFFIN								
Blueberry, Skinny, Starbucks*	1 Muffin/141g	372	5.5	264	4.1	51.9	3.9	2.3
Chocolate & Belgian Choc Sauce, Starbucks*	1 Muffin/119g	430	17.8	361	6.6	48.7	15.0	2.6
Classic Blueberry, Starbucks*	1 Muffin/110g	481	18.6	437	5.6	47.4	16.9	1.6
Lemon & Poppyseed, Skinny, Iced, Starbucks*	1 Muffin/139g	399	6.1	287	3.9	56.6	4.4	2.6
Peach & Raspberry, Skinny, Starbucks*	1 Muffin/136g	369	3.9	271	6.2	53.9	2.9	2.3
Rise & Shine, Starbucks*	1 Muffin/124g	448	18.8	361	7.1	47.8	15.2	2.3
NUTS								
Almonds, Roasted, Starbucks*	1 Pack/75g	484	41.4	646	21.2	17.7	55.2	10.5
Mixed, Starbucks*	1 Pack/75g	401	25.2	535	17.7	41.1	33.6	6.7
PAIN AU CHOCOLAT								
Starbucks*	1 Pastry/65g	269	15.9	414	5.7	42.2	24.4	2.6
PAIN AU RAISIN								
Starbucks*	1 Pastry/110g	373	19.2	339	4.7	40.3	17.5	1.4
PANINI								
All Day Breakfast, Starbucks*	1 Panini/158g	338	15.2	214	11.5	19.7	9.6	1.4
Cheese & Marmite, Starbucks*	1 Panini/130g	373	17.8	287	14.3	26.0	13.7	1.1
Chicken, Roast, & Tomato, Starbucks*	1 Panini/223g	375	8.0	168	10.2	23.1	3.6	1.4
Croque Monisieur, Starbucks*	1 Panini/190g	456	17.7	240	12.8	25.9	9.3	0.9
Meatball, Starbucks*	1 Panini/216g	521	22.5	241	11.2	25.0	10.4	1.4
Mozzarella, Italian, & Slow Roast Tomato, Starbucks*	1 Panini/178g	470	20.5	264	11.2	28.0	11.5	1.5
Steak, Cheese & Caramelised Onion, Starbucks*	1 Panini/210g	525	20.4	250	14.9	25.3	9.7	1.0
Tuna Melt, & Mature Cheddar, Starbucks*	1 Panini/200g	492	21.0	246	13.3	24.2	10.5	0.9
SALAD								
Chicken, & Red Pesto, Bistro Box, Starbucks*	1 Salad/296g	275	13.9	93	5.1	7.1	4.7	1.1
Falafel Mezze, Bistro Box, Starbucks*	1 Salad/329g	493	14.5	150	5.0	20.9	4.4	3.6
Ham, Hock, Cured, Bistro Box, Starbucks*	1 Salad/302g	387	20.5	128	7.9	8.2	6.8	1.3
Tuna, Potato & Pea, Bistro Box, Starbucks*	1 Salad/286g	320	14.6	112	6.3	9.5	5.1	1.7

STARBUCKS

INFO/WEIGHT	Measure	per Measure KCAL	per Measure FAT	Nutrition Values per 100g / 100ml KCAL	PROT	CARB	FAT	FIBRE
SANDWICH								
Cheese & Pickle, Gluten Free, Starbucks*	1 Sandwich/197g	552	32.5	280	7.5	23.9	16.5	2.9
Chicken, Roasted, with Herb Mayonnaise, Starbucks*	1 Sandwich/201g	314	7.2	156	10.6	19.2	3.6	2.1
Egg Mayonnaise, Free Range, Starbucks*	1 Sandwich/191g	365	15.3	191	10.3	18.6	8.0	1.9
SHORTBREAD								
Chocolate Chunk, Fairtrade, Starbucks*	1 Shortbread/96g	497	29.0	518	6.2	53.5	30.2	3.1
SYRUP								
1 Pump, Starbucks*	1 Pump/10g	20	0.0	202	0.0	50.0	0.0	0.0
Bar Mocha, 1 Pump, Starbucks*	1 Pump/17g	26	0.6	156	3.5	37.6	3.5	5.9
TEA								
Brewed, Grande, Starbucks*	1 Grande/473ml	0	0.0	0	0.0	0.0	0.0	0.0
Brewed, Short, Starbucks*	1 Short/236ml	0	0.0	0	0.0	0.0	0.0	0.0
Brewed, Tall, Starbucks*	1 Tall/335ml	0	0.0	0	0.0	0.0	0.0	0.0
Brewed, Venti, Starbucks*	1 Venti/591ml	0	0.0	0	0.0	0.0	0.0	0.0
Chai, Latte, Grande, Semi Skimmed Milk, Starbucks*	1 Grande/473ml	236	4.0	50	1.6	9.3	0.8	0.0
Chai, Latte, Grande, Skimmed Milk, Starbucks*	1 Grande/473ml	204	0.2	43	1.6	9.4	0.0	0.0
Chai, Latte, Grande, Soy, Starbucks*	1 Grande/473ml	213	3.2	45	1.3	8.6	0.7	0.2
Chai, Latte, Grande, Whole Milk, Starbucks*	1 Grande/473ml	255	6.5	54	1.5	9.2	1.4	0.0
Chai, Latte, Short, Semi Skimmed Milk, Starbucks*	1 Short/236ml	119	2.0	50	1.6	9.3	0.8	0.0
Chai, Latte, Short, Skimmed Milk, Starbucks*	1 Short/236ml	103	0.1	44	1.7	9.4	0.0	0.0
Chai, Latte, Short, Soy, Starbucks*	1 Short/236ml	108	1.6	46	1.4	8.6	0.7	0.2
Chai, Latte, Short, Whole Milk, Starbucks*	1 Short/236ml	129	3.3	55	1.6	9.3	1.4	0.0
Chai, Latte, Tall, Semi Skimmed Milk, Starbucks*	1 Tall/335ml	179	3.0	53	1.7	9.9	0.9	0.0
Chai, Latte, Tall, Skimmed Milk, Starbucks*	1 Tall/335ml	154	0.2	46	1.7	10.0	0.1	0.0
Chai, Latte, Tall, Soy, Starbucks*	1 Tall/335ml	162	2.4	48	1.4	9.1	0.7	0.2
Chai, Latte, Tall, Whole Milk, Starbucks*	1 Tall/335ml	194	5.0	58	1.6	9.8	1.5	0.0
Chai, Latte, Venti, Semi Skimmed Milk, Starbucks*	1 Venti/591ml	296	5.0	50	1.6	9.3	0.8	0.0
Chai, Latte, Venti, Skimmed Milk, Starbucks*	1 Venti/591ml	256	0.3	43	1.6	9.4	0.1	0.0
Chai, Latte, Venti, Soy, Starbucks*	1 Venti/591ml	268	4.0	45	1.3	8.6	0.7	0.2
Chai, Latte, Venti, Whole Milk, Starbucks*	1 Venti/591ml	322	8.3	54	1.5	9.2	1.4	0.0
Iced, Chai, Latte, Grande, Skimmed Milk, Starbucks*	1 Grande/473ml	205	0.2	43	1.6	9.4	0.0	0.0
Iced, Chai, Latte, Grande, Soy, Starbucks*	1 Grande/473ml	219	3.4	46	1.4	8.6	0.7	0.2
Iced, Chai, Latte, Grande, SS Milk, Starbucks*	1 Grande/473ml	238	4.2	50	1.6	9.3	0.9	0.0
Iced, Chai, Latte, Grande, Whole Milk, Starbucks*	1 Grande/473ml	259	6.9	55	1.5	9.2	1.5	0.0
Iced, Chai, Latte, Tall, Semi Skimmed Milk, Starbucks*	1 Tall/335ml	176	3.0	52	1.6	9.7	0.9	0.0
Iced, Chai, Latte, Tall, Skimmed Milk, Starbucks*	1 Tall/335ml	152	0.2	45	1.6	9.9	0.1	0.0
Iced, Chai, Latte, Tall, Soy, Starbucks*	1 Tall/335ml	162	2.4	48	1.4	9.1	0.7	0.2
Iced, Chai, Latte, Tall, Whole Milk, Starbucks*	1 Tall/335ml	191	5.0	57	1.6	9.7	1.5	0.0
Iced, Chai, Latte, Venti, Semi Skimmed Milk, Starbucks*	1 Venti/591ml	277	4.4	47	1.3	9.0	0.7	0.0
Iced, Chai, Latte, Venti, Skimmed Milk, Starbucks*	1 Venti/591ml	242	0.3	41	1.4	9.0	0.1	0.0
Iced, Chai, Latte, Venti, Soy, Starbucks*	1 Venti/591ml	256	3.5	43	1.2	8.5	0.6	0.2
Iced, Chai, Latte, Venti, Whole Milk, Starbucks*	1 Venti/591ml	299	7.2	51	1.3	9.0	1.2	0.0
TOPPING								
Caramel, Starbucks*	1 Serving/4ml	15	0.6	372	0.0	62.5	15.0	0.0
Chocolate, Starbucks*	1 Serving/4ml	6	0.1	152	2.5	37.5	2.5	2.5
Sprinkles, Starbucks*	1 Serving/1ml	4	0.0	380	0.0	100.0	0.0	0.0
Whipped Cream, Cold, Grande, Starbucks*	1 Grande/32g	114	11.2	356	1.9	9.4	35.0	0.0
Whipped Cream, Cold, Tall, Starbucks*	1 Tall/25g	81	8.0	324	1.6	8.0	32.0	0.0
Whipped Cream, Cold, Venti, Starbucks*	1 Venti/35g	104	10.2	297	1.7	8.6	29.1	0.0
Whipped Cream, Hot, Grande, Starbucks*	1 Serving/21g	72	7.0	343	1.9	9.5	33.3	0.0
Whipped Cream, Hot, Short, Starbucks*	1 Short/16g	52	5.1	325	1.9	6.2	31.9	0.0
Whipped Cream, Hot, Tall, Starbucks*	1 Tall/19g	62	6.1	326	1.6	10.5	32.1	0.0

	Measure INFO/WEIGHT	per Measure		Nutrition Values per 100g / 100ml				
		KCAL	FAT	KCAL	PROT	CARB	FAT	FIBRE
STARBUCKS								
WAFFLES								
Caramel, Large, Starbucks*	1 Waffle/80g	354	16.2	443	3.2	62.2	20.3	1.1
YOGHURT								
Apple, Oats & Berries, Breakfast Pot, Starbucks*	1 Pot/180g	319	11.9	177	4.1	24.3	6.6	2.1
Natural, Creamy, Starbucks*	1 Serving/140g	132	6.4	94	5.5	7.5	4.6	0.0
SUBWAY								
BACON								
2 Strips, Subway*	2 Strips/9g	40	2.9	444	33.3	0.0	32.2	0.0
BREAD								
6 inch, 9 Grain Honey Oat, Subway*	1 Bread/89g	237	1.9	266	11.2	47.2	2.1	6.5
6 inch, 9 Grain Wheat, Subway*	1 Bread/78g	198	1.5	254	11.5	44.9	1.9	6.7
6 inch, Hearty Italian, Subway*	1 Bread/75g	201	1.5	268	10.7	50.7	2.0	2.8
6 inch, Italian Herbs & Cheese, Subway*	1 Bread/82g	234	4.3	285	12.2	46.3	5.2	2.3
6 inch, Italian White, Subway*	1 Bread/71g	190	1.3	268	9.9	50.7	1.8	2.3
Wrap, Subway*	1 Wrap/101g	328	6.6	325	7.8	58.4	6.5	2.0
CHEESE								
American, Subway*	1 Serving/11g	40	3.4	364	18.2	9.1	30.9	0.0
Cheddar, Monterey, Subway*	1 Serving/14g	57	4.4	407	25.0	0.0	31.4	0.0
Peppered, Subway*	1 Serving/11g	39	3.1	355	18.2	0.0	28.2	0.0
COOKIES								
Chocolate Chip, Subway*	1 Cookie/45g	218	10.3	484	4.4	64.4	22.9	2.4
Chocolate Chunk, Subway*	1 Cookie/45g	224	11.7	498	4.4	62.2	26.0	2.0
Double Choc Chip, Subway*	1 Cookie/45g	221	11.7	491	4.4	60.0	26.0	2.7
Oatmeal Raisin,, Subway*	1 Cookie/45g	190	8.8	422	4.4	55.6	19.6	4.2
Rainbow, Subway*	1 Cookie/45g	215	10.4	478	4.4	62.2	23.1	2.0
White Chip Mac Nut, Subway*	1 Cookie/45g	222	11.7	493	4.4	60.0	26.0	1.6
DOUGHNUTS								
Chocolate Donut, Subway*	1 Doughnut/55g	243	15.5	442	7.3	38.2	28.2	2.2
Sugared Donut, Subway*	1 Doughnut/49g	207	11.6	422	6.1	42.9	23.7	1.0
MEATBALLS								
Bowl, Subway*	1 Serving/206g	311	18.4	151	9.2	9.2	8.9	2.0
MUFFIN								
Blueberry, Subway*	1 Muffin/111g	352	20.6	317	4.5	36.0	18.6	2.7
Chocolate Chunk, Subway*	1 Muffin/111g	394	22.9	355	5.4	39.6	20.6	2.6
NACHOS								
Cheese, Melted, Snacking, Subway*	1 Serving/126g	415	24.3	329	8.7	28.6	19.3	2.1
SALADS								
Beef, Subway*	1 Salad/328g	118	2.4	36	4.9	1.8	0.7	1.1
Chicken, Breast, Subway*	1 Salad/342g	139	2.4	41	5.8	2.0	0.7	1.1
Chicken Teriyaki, Sweet Onion, Subway*	1 Salad/385g	189	2.6	49	5.5	4.9	0.7	1.0
Club, Subway*	1 Salad/361g	145	2.8	40	6.1	1.9	0.8	1.0
Garden, Side, Subway*	1 Toastie/135g	21	0.2	16	0.7	2.2	0.1	1.3
Ham, Subway*	1 Salad/328g	104	2.9	32	3.7	2.1	0.9	1.1
Turkey Breast, & Ham, Subway*	1 Salad/338g	113	2.3	33	4.7	1.8	0.7	1.1
Turkey Breast, Subway*	1 Salad/328g	104	1.6	32	4.6	1.8	0.5	1.1
Veggie Delite, Subway*	1 Salad/271g	49	1.0	18	1.1	1.8	0.4	1.3
SAUCE								
BBQ, Low Fat, Subway*	1 Serving/21g	37	0.1	176	0.0	42.9	0.5	0.9
Chipotle Southwest Sauce, Subway*	1 Serving/21g	90	9.2	429	0.0	9.5	43.8	0.5
Honey Mustard, Low Fat, Subway*	1 Serving/21g	32	0.2	152	0.0	33.3	0.9	0.5
Mayonnaise, Light, Subway*	1 Serving/15g	56	6.0	373	0.0	6.7	40.0	0.0
Onion, Sweet, Low Fat, Subway*	1 Serving/21g	34	0.1	162	0.0	38.1	0.5	0.5
Ranch Dressing, Subway*	1 Serving/21g	44	4.5	210	0.0	4.8	21.4	0.0

SUBWAY

	Measure INFO/WEIGHT	per Measure KCAL	FAT	Nutrition Values per 100g / 100ml KCAL	PROT	CARB	FAT	FIBRE
SOUP								
Beef Goulash, Subway*	1 Serving/250g	199	11.8	80	3.3	6.0	4.7	0.9
Carrot & Coriander, Subway*	1 Serving/250g	81	1.8	32	0.9	5.6	0.7	1.1
Chicken, Cream of, Subway*	1 Serving/250g	160	11.3	64	2.7	3.1	4.5	0.0
Country Chicken & Vegetable, Subway*	1 Serving/250g	168	11.0	67	2.7	4.2	4.4	0.2
Leek & Potato, Subway*	1 Serving/250g	124	3.0	50	1.7	8.0	1.2	1.1
Lentil & Bacon, Subway*	1 Serving/250g	182	5.0	73	4.4	9.3	2.0	1.1
Minestrone, Subway*	1 Serving/250g	81	3.3	32	0.7	4.4	1.3	0.7
Mushroom, Cream of, Subway*	1 Serving/250g	150	10.8	60	1.0	4.4	4.3	0.3
Mushroom, Wild, Subway*	1 Serving/250g	101	5.5	40	1.0	4.1	2.2	0.3
Red Pepper & Tomato, Subway*	1 Serving/250g	96	3.5	38	1.4	5.0	1.4	0.9
Tomato, Subway*	1 Serving/250g	103	3.8	41	0.8	6.1	1.5	0.3
Vegetable, Highland, Subway*	1 Serving/250g	73	0.3	29	1.5	5.5	0.1	0.9
Vegetable, Thai Style, Subway*	1 Serving/250g	87	1.0	35	1.1	6.7	0.4	0.8
SUBS								
Beef, Kids, Subway*	1 Sub/156g	210	2.2	135	10.3	18.6	1.4	3.1
Beef, Low Fat, Subway*	1 Sub/219g	282	3.0	129	10.5	17.3	1.4	2.9
Breakfast, Bacon, Egg & Cheese, Subway*	1 Sub/133g	334	12.0	251	12.8	27.1	9.0	4.1
Breakfast, Bacon, Subway*	1 Sub/96g	279	7.4	291	15.6	36.5	7.7	5.4
Breakfast, Egg & Cheese, Subway*	1 Sub/124g	294	9.0	237	11.3	29.0	7.3	4.3
Breakfast, Mega Melt, Subway*	1 Sub/209g	510	23.1	244	13.9	21.0	11.0	3.0
Breakfast, Sausage, Egg & Cheese, Subway*	1 Sub/200g	470	20.1	235	12.5	22.0	10.0	3.1
Breakfast, Sausage, Subway*	1 Sub/154g	374	12.6	243	13.0	27.3	8.2	4.0
Chicken, & Bacon Ranch Melt, Subway*	1 Sub/292g	503	19.2	172	13.0	13.7	6.6	2.2
Chicken, Breast, Low Fat, Subway*	1 Sub/233g	304	3.0	130	11.6	16.7	1.3	2.7
Chicken, Temptation, Subway*	1 Sub/262g	406	8.7	155	10.3	19.8	3.3	2.4
Chicken Tikka, Low Fat, Subway*	1 Sub/233g	302	3.0	130	11.6	16.3	1.3	2.7
Club, Low Fat, Subway*	1 Sub/252g	310	3.4	123	11.5	15.1	1.3	2.5
Ham, Kids, Subway*	1 Sub/147g	192	2.2	131	8.2	19.7	1.5	3.3
Italian, B.M.T., Subway*	1 Sub/226g	396	16.8	175	9.3	16.8	7.4	2.8
Meatball Marinara, Subway*	1 Sub/300g	431	15.1	144	8.0	16.3	5.0	3.1
Melt, Includes Cheese, Subway*	1 Sub/249g	359	9.3	144	11.2	15.7	3.7	2.5
Spicy Italian, Subway*	1 Sub/222g	471	25.3	212	9.5	17.1	11.4	2.8
Steak & Cheese, with Peppers & Onions, Subway*	1 Sub/245g	343	8.5	140	10.6	16.3	3.5	2.7
Sweet Onion Chicken Teriyaki, Low Fat, Subway*	1 Sub/276g	354	3.3	128	10.1	18.1	1.2	2.4
Tuna, Subway*	1 Sub/233g	359	12.6	154	9.0	16.7	5.4	2.7
Turkey, Breast, & Ham, Low Fat, Subway*	1 Sub/228g	278	3.0	122	9.6	16.7	1.3	2.8
Turkey, Breast, Kids, Subway*	1 Sub/156g	201	1.6	129	9.6	18.6	1.0	3.1
Turkey, Breast, Low Fat, Subway*	1 Sub/219g	269	2.2	123	10.0	17.3	1.0	2.9
Veggie Delite, Kids, Subway*	1 Sub/118g	164	1.2	139	5.9	24.6	1.0	4.1
Veggie Delite, Low Fat, Subway*	1 Sub/162g	213	1.6	131	5.6	22.8	1.0	3.9
Veggie Patty, Subway*	1 Sub/247g	380	8.7	154	8.9	18.6	3.5	2.6
Ham, Low Fat, Subway*	1 Sub/219g	269	3.5	123	8.7	17.3	1.6	2.9
TOASTIE								
Cheese, Subway*	1 Toastie/64g	210	9.5	328	17.2	29.7	14.8	1.2
Pepperoni Pizza, Subway*	1 Toastie/93g	247	12.4	266	11.8	23.7	13.3	1.4
WRAPS								
Beef, Subway*	1 Wrap/242g	412	8.1	170	9.1	25.6	3.3	1.3
Chicken, Breast, Subway*	1 Wrap/256g	434	8.1	170	10.2	24.6	3.2	1.2
Chicken, Temptation, Subway*	1 Wrap/285g	536	13.8	188	9.1	27.0	4.8	1.1
Chicken & Bacon, Ranch Melt, Subway*	1 Wrap/315g	633	24.3	201	11.7	20.6	7.7	1.0
Chicken Tikka, Subway*	1 Wrap/256g	432	8.1	169	10.2	24.6	3.2	1.2
Club, Subway*	1 Wrap/275g	440	8.5	160	10.2	22.9	3.1	1.1

SUBWAY

	Measure INFO/WEIGHT	per Measure KCAL	FAT	KCAL	PROT	CARB	FAT	FIBRE
WRAPS								
Ham, Subway*	1 Wrap/242g	399	8.6	165	7.9	26.0	3.6	1.3
Italian B.M.T., Subway*	1 Wrap/249g	526	21.8	211	8.4	25.3	8.8	1.2
Meatball Marinara, Subway*	1 Wrap/323g	561	20.2	174	7.1	22.9	6.3	1.9
Melt with Cheese, Subway*	1 Wrap/272g	489	14.3	180	9.9	23.2	5.3	1.1
Spicy Italian, Subway*	1 Wrap/245g	602	30.4	246	8.2	25.3	12.4	1.3
Steak & Cheese, with Peppers & Onions, Subway*	1 Wrap/268g	473	13.6	176	9.3	24.3	5.1	1.3
Sweet Onion Chicken Teriyaki, Subway*	1 Wrap/299g	484	8.3	162	9.0	25.1	2.8	1.2
Tuna, Subway*	1 Wrap/256g	489	17.7	191	7.8	25.0	6.9	1.2
Turkey, Breast, Subway*	1 Wrap/242g	399	7.3	165	8.7	25.6	3.0	1.3
Turkey, Breast & Ham, Subway*	1 Wrap/251g	408	8.1	163	8.8	25.1	3.2	1.2
Veggie Delite, Subway*	1 Wrap/185g	343	6.7	185	4.9	33.5	3.6	1.7
Veggie Patty, Subway*	1 Wrap/270g	510	13.8	189	7.8	26.3	5.1	1.1

THE REAL GREEK FOOD COMPANY LTD

	Measure INFO/WEIGHT	per Measure KCAL	FAT	KCAL	PROT	CARB	FAT	FIBRE
COLD MEZE								
Crudites, The Real Greek Food Company Ltd*	1 Serving/231g	37	0.4	16	0.6	3.1	0.2	1.6
Dolmades, The Real Greek Food Company Ltd*	1 Serving/131g	254	15.7	194	2.9	18.8	12.0	0.8
Flatbread, Greek, The Real Greek Food Company Ltd*	1 Serving/200g	615	15.7	307	6.6	52.6	7.8	7.4
Gigandes Plaki, The Real Greek Food Company Ltd*	1 Serving/210g	183	11.7	87	2.3	7.4	5.6	2.5
Htipiti, The Real Greek Food Company Ltd*	1 Serving/140g	305	24.8	218	8.0	7.8	17.7	3.5
Hummus, The Real Greek Food Company Ltd*	1 Serving/140g	298	19.1	213	7.6	15.6	13.6	5.2
Koliosalata, The Real Greek Food Company Ltd*	1 Serving/140g	506	47.8	361	12.1	1.6	34.1	0.3
Melitzanasalata, The Real Greek Food Company Ltd*	1 Serving/140g	236	21.8	168	1.2	7.1	15.5	3.2
Revithia, The Real Greek Food Company Ltd*	1 Serving/160g	286	20.1	179	4.8	11.9	12.6	4.0
Salad, Tabouleh, The Real Greek Food Company Ltd*	1 Serving/165g	117	8.2	71	1.3	6.3	5.0	1.9
Taramasalata, The Real Greek Food Company Ltd*	1 Serving/140g	913	99.0	652	2.5	2.1	70.7	0.0
Tzatziki, The Real Greek Food Company Ltd*	1 Serving/141g	163	14.1	116	3.5	3.1	10.0	0.4
DESSERTS								
Loukoumia, The Real Greek Food Company Ltd*	1 Serving/66g	211	1.7	320	0.8	74.2	2.6	0.4
DIPS								
Aioli, Parsley, The Real Greek Food Company Ltd*	1 Serving/35g	176	18.8	504	2.3	2.3	53.8	0.6
Dip, Selection, The Real Greek Food Company Ltd*	1 Serving/140g	589	56.5	421	1.8	9.9	40.4	0.8
Relish, Chilli, The Real Greek Food Company Ltd*	1 Serving/35g	42	0.1	119	1.1	30.0	0.3	0.6
HOT MEZE								
Asparagus, The Real Greek Food Company Ltd*	1 Serving/110g	140	9.8	127	3.3	9.3	8.9	2.3
Bifteki & Yoghurt, The Real Greek Food Company Ltd*	1 Serving/250g	252	60.3	101	21.6	3.7	24.2	0.0
Chicken, Skewer, The Real Greek Food Company Ltd*	1 Serving/144g	177	7.6	123	3.1	1.3	5.3	0.7
Fish, Cod, Salt, The Real Greek Food Company Ltd*	1 Serving/152g	346	1.5	227	21.1	34.2	1.0	0.6
Halloumi, Grilled, The Real Greek Food Company Ltd*	1 Serving/86g	151	11.8	175	10.3	74.5	13.7	0.9
Halloumi, Skewer, The Real Greek Food Company Ltd*	1 Serving/128g	118	8.5	92	6.8	49.7	6.6	0.5
Lamb, Cutlets, The Real Greek Food Company Ltd*	1 Serving/260g	881	79.1	339	16.3	0.0	30.4	0.0
Lamb, Kefte, The Real Greek Food Company Ltd*	1 Serving/216g	344	24.8	159	12.0	2.2	11.5	0.3
Lamb, Skewer, The Real Greek Food Company Ltd*	1 Serving/166g	255	18.8	154	11.8	1.1	11.3	0.6
Octopus, Grilled, The Real Greek Food Company Ltd*	1 Serving/128g	447	25.4	349	39.3	3.2	19.8	0.3
Pork, Skewer, The Real Greek Food Company Ltd*	1 Serving/165g	281	21.7	170	11.8	1.1	13.1	0.6
Potatoes, New, The Real Greek Food Company Ltd*	1 Serving/386g	293	5.2	76	1.7	15.2	1.3	1.4
Rice, Saffron, The Real Greek Food Company Ltd*	1 Serving/259g	406	2.8	157	3.2	32.2	1.1	0.3
Sardines, Grilled, The Real Greek Food Company Ltd*	1 Serving/360g	619	32.8	172	22.2	0.3	9.1	0.1
Tiropitakia, The Real Greek Food Company Ltd*	1 Serving/120g	416	21.2	344	10.0	37.3	17.5	1.3
KIDS MENU								
Chicken, Skewer, The Real Greek Food Company Ltd*	1 Serving/72g	88	3.8	123	3.2	1.4	5.3	0.7
Lamb, Skewer, The Real Greek Food Company Ltd*	1 Serving/82g	127	9.4	154	11.9	1.2	11.4	0.6
Pork Skewer, The Real Greek Food Company Ltd*	1 Skewer/82g	140	10.9	170	11.9	1.2	13.2	0.6

	Measure INFO/WEIGHT	per Measure KCAL	FAT	Nutrition Values per 100g / 100ml KCAL	PROT	CARB	FAT	FIBRE

THE REAL GREEK FOOD COMPANY LTD

NIBBLES

	Measure INFO/WEIGHT	KCAL	FAT	KCAL	PROT	CARB	FAT	FIBRE
Nuts, Athenian, The Real Greek Food Company Ltd*	1 Serving/75g	479	45.4	638	17.7	6.1	60.5	9.2
Olives, The Real Greek Food Company Ltd*	1 Serving/110g	317	33.2	288	1.7	2.4	30.2	4.3

TOBY CARVERY

BEEF

Tewkesbury, Toby Carvery*	1 Serving/100g	176	5.6	176	31.4	0.1	5.6	0.0

DRESSING

Sauce, Mint, Toby Carvery*	1 Serving/100g	67	0.1	67	1.1	15.6	0.1	0.0
Sauce, Parsley, Toby Carvery*	1 Serving/100g	42	1.3	42	1.6	5.9	1.3	0.0

GRAVY

Beef, Toby Carvery*	1 Serving/100g	22	0.2	22	0.6	4.5	0.2	0.0
Caramelised Onion, Toby Carvery*	1 Serving/100g	80	0.8	80	1.7	16.4	0.8	0.0
Poultry, Toby Carvery*	1 Serving/100g	29	0.1	29	1.1	6.1	0.1	0.0
Vegetarian, Toby Carvery*	1 Serving/100g	18	0.1	18	1.2	3.2	0.1	0.0

PORK

Horseshoe of, Toby Carvery*	1 Serving/100g	203	8.4	203	31.7	0.1	8.4	0.0

POTATOES

Mashed, Toby Carvery*	1 Serving/100g	70	2.4	70	1.3	10.8	2.4	0.0
New, Toby Carvery*	1 Spoonful/100g	73	0.5	73	1.8	15.4	0.5	0.0
Roasted, Toby Carvery*	1 Serving/80g	137	3.7	171	2.7	28.9	4.6	0.0

TURKEY

with Orange Glaze, Toby Carvery*	1 Serving/100g	145	1.8	145	32.0	0.1	1.8	0.0

VEGETABLES

Broccoli, Toby Carvery*	1 Spoon/100g	60	2.1	60	2.7	7.6	2.1	0.0
Cabbage, Toby Carvery*	1 Serving/80g	34	1.1	43	1.7	6.0	1.4	0.0
Carrots, Toby Carvery*	1 Serving/100g	46	1.1	46	1.1	3.0	1.1	0.0
Carrots, Toby Carvery*	1 Serving/100g	46	1.1	46	1.1	3.0	1.1	0.0
Leeks, Toby Carvery*	1 Serving/100g	32	0.1	32	0.8	7.1	0.1	0.0
Parsnips, Honey Glazed, Toby Carvery*	1 Serving/100g	148	3.2	148	1.7	28.1	3.2	0.0
Peas, Toby Carvery*	1 Spoonful/100g	107	1.8	107	6.2	16.6	1.8	0.0

YORKSHIRE PUDDING

New Muffin Style, Toby Carvery*	1 Serving/100g	331	11.7	331	15.3	41.0	11.7	0.0

URBAN EAT

CROISSANT

Gammon Ham, Cheese & Tomato, Urban Eat*	1 Croissant/154g	369	19.8	240	12.1	18.8	12.9	0.9
Tomato, Mozzarella Cheese & Spinach, Urban Eat*	1 Croissant/150g	368	21.5	245	9.1	19.9	14.3	1.0

FRUIT

Citrus, Pot, Urban Eat*	1 Pot/200g	94	0.2	47	0.8	10.7	0.1	1.9
Grape, Pot, Urban Eat*	1 Pot/150g	96	0.1	64	0.4	15.4	0.1	1.0
Melon & Grape, Pot, Urban Eat*	1 Pot/178g	80	0.4	45	0.6	10.2	0.2	0.8
Pineapple, Chunks, Pot, Urban Eat*	1 Pot/160g	69	0.3	43	0.4	9.8	0.2	1.2
Salad, Classic, Pot, Urban Eat*	1 Pot/170g	68	0.2	40	0.6	9.2	0.1	1.5
Tropical Fingers, Urban Eat*	1 Pot/161g	71	0.2	44	0.6	10.2	0.1	1.5

PANINI

Ciabatta, All Day Breakfast, Urban Eat*	1 Pack/202g	521	26.0	258	10.6	24.8	12.9	1.5
Ciabatta, Chicken Fajita, Urban Eat*	1 Pack/215g	498	20.6	232	10.4	26.0	9.6	1.3
Ciabatta, Three Cheese & Roasted Tomato, Urban Eat*	1 Pack/206g	431	16.7	209	9.7	24.3	8.1	1.4
Ciabatta, Tuna Melt, Urban Eat*	1 Pack/180g	397	12.6	221	13.0	26.4	7.0	1.3

SALAD

Caesar, Chicken, Urban Eat*	1 Pack/210g	332	20.4	158	11.4	4.6	9.7	0.8
Noodle, Prawn, Oriental, & Mango, Ultimate, Urban Eat*	1 Pack/297g	217	6.8	73	3.6	8.9	2.3	1.3
Pasta, Cheese & Tomato, Urban Eat*	1 Pack/238g	612	41.4	257	7.4	17.3	17.4	1.1
Pasta, Chicken & Bacon, Urban Eat*	1 Pack/240g	503	27.3	210	9.5	16.7	11.4	1.2

URBAN EAT

	Measure INFO/WEIGHT	per Measure KCAL	FAT	Nutrition Values per 100g / 100ml KCAL	PROT	CARB	FAT	FIBRE
SALAD								
Tabbouleh, & Roast Vegetable, Ultimate, Urban Eat*	1 Pack/280g	414	21.3	148	2.8	15.0	7.6	4.1
SANDWICH								
All Day Breakfast, on White, Urban Eat*	1 Pack/192g	368	15.1	192	9.2	21.1	7.9	1.7
Bap, Cheddar, Mature, & Onion Salad, Urban Eat*	1 Bap/225g	668	40.5	297	7.5	26.1	18.0	1.3
Bap, Chicken Mayo & Salad, Urban Eat*	1 Bap/232g	556	26.1	239	9.0	25.4	11.2	1.2
Beef, Rare, Scottish, & Horseradish, Urban Eat*	1 Pack/149g	373	17.5	250	10.3	25.8	11.7	1.3
BLT on Malted Wheat, Urban Eat*	1 Pack/177g	485	30.6	274	9.0	20.5	17.3	1.6
Cheddar, Mature, & Pickle, Wholemeal, Urban Eat*	1 Pack/125g	333	14.9	266	12.6	27.1	11.9	4.0
Cheddar, Mature, Ploughman's, Wheatgrain, Urban Eat*	1 Pack/197g	476	25.8	242	9.3	21.7	13.1	1.6
Cheddar, Onion, & Chutney, Wheatgrain, Urban Eat*	1 Pack/177g	581	36.8	328	10.6	24.5	20.8	1.8
Cheese, Two, & Onion, Urban Eat*	1 Sandwich/130g	456	29.0	351	9.8	27.7	22.3	2.0
Chicken, Bacon & Avocado, on Wheatgrain, Urban Eat*	1 Pack/199g	485	26.5	243	10.7	19.8	13.3	1.5
Chicken, Tuna, on Wheatgrain, Triple Pack, Urban Eat*	1 Pack/267g	623	34.2	233	8.7	20.6	12.8	1.6
Chicken & Bacon, on Malted Wheatgrain, Urban Eat*	1 Pack/170g	530	30.9	312	13.4	23.7	18.2	1.7
Chicken & Stuffing, on White, Urban Eat*	1 Pack/175g	497	28.0	284	11.9	23.1	16.0	1.1
Chicken & Sweetcorn, on Wheatgrain, Urban Eat*	1 Pack/160g	422	20.5	264	12.1	25.1	12.8	1.7
Chicken Mayo, on Malted Wheatgrain, Urban Eat*	1 Pack/155g	466	27.0	300	12.0	24.1	17.4	1.6
Coronation Chicken, on Malted Wheatgrain, Urban Eat*	1 Pack/160g	475	25.9	297	10.4	27.2	16.2	2.0
Egg & Cress, Free Range, on Wheatgrain, Urban Eat*	1 Pack/151g	327	14.5	216	8.9	23.6	9.6	2.3
Egg & Salad Cream, on Wholemeal, Urban Eat*	1 Pack/187g	252	7.3	135	7.7	17.4	3.9	3.4
Egg & Spinach, Double, on Wheatgrain, Urban Eat*	1 Pack/184g	374	16.7	193	9.7	19.2	8.6	1.9
Egg & Tomato, Free Range, on Wheatgrain, Urban Eat*	1 Pack/155g	262	7.8	169	7.5	23.5	5.0	2.1
Egg Mayo, & Bacon, Free Range, on White, Urban Eat*	1 Pack/155g	369	18.4	238	9.8	22.8	11.9	1.5
Egg Mayo, & Cress, Halal, on Oatmeal, Urban Eat*	1 Pack/145g	312	13.4	215	8.8	23.0	9.2	2.6
Egg Mayonnaise, & Bacon on Wheatgrain, Urban Eat*	1 Pack/192g	276	26.5	144	10.7	19.2	13.8	2.0
French Brie & Cranberry on Softgrain, Urban Eat*	1 Pack/164g	399	18.9	243	8.5	26.6	11.5	1.6
Gammon, Cheddar, & Pickle, Softgrain, Urban Eat*	1 Pack/154g	384	15.9	249	13.1	25.9	10.3	1.4
Gammon, Irish Cheddar, & Pickle, White, Urban Eat*	1 Pack/180g	393	15.7	218	12.2	22.8	8.7	1.2
Gammon & English Mustard Mayo, White, Urban Eat*	1 Pack/150g	319	11.5	213	12.1	23.6	7.7	1.3
Gammon & Tomato Salad, on Wheatgrain, Urban Eat*	1 Pack/173g	247	3.3	143	9.6	21.8	1.9	2.2
Houmous & Roast Veg, on Wheatgrain, Urban Eat*	1 Pack/194g	289	4.8	149	5.6	25.9	2.5	3.0
Mixed Triple Pack on Malted Wheatgrain, Urban Eat*	1 Pack/233g	578	27.3	248	11.0	24.9	11.7	1.9
Ploughman's, Cheddar, on Wheatgrain, Urban Eat*	1 Pack/17g	445	23.4	251	8.3	24.9	13.2	1.9
Prawn Mayonnaise, on Oatmeal, Urban Eat*	1 Pack/160g	439	27.6	274	8.9	21.1	17.2	1.8
Prawns with Mayonnaise, on Oatmeal, Urban Eat*	1 Pack/170g	388	20.8	228	10.2	19.4	12.2	1.7
Roll, Cheese, Cheddar, Urban Eat*	1 Roll/119g	351	13.4	295	12.4	36.1	11.3	1.7
Roll, Chicken Mayo, Urban Eat*	1 Roll/134g	383	16.3	286	11.3	32.7	12.2	1.5
Roll, Egg Mayo, Free Range, Urban Eat*	1 Roll/134g	325	11.9	243	9.9	30.8	8.9	4.9
Roll, Ham, Smoked, Urban Eat*	1 Roll/121g	278	6.2	230	10.2	35.7	5.1	1.7
Roll, Tuna Mayonnaise, Urban Eat*	1 Roll/130g	386	17.9	295	9.9	33.1	13.7	1.5
Salad, Chicken, Roast, on Wheatgrain, Urban Eat*	1 Pack/189g	380	16.3	201	11.4	19.4	8.6	1.6
Salad, Chicken & Tomato, on Wheatgrain, Urban Eat*	1 Pack/177g	245	2.0	138	10.5	21.3	1.1	2.1
Salad, Tuna, on Malted Wheatgrain, Urban Eat*	1 Pack/178g	302	7.8	170	9.4	23.1	4.4	2.4
Salmon, Smoked, & Soft Cheese, Oatmeal, Urban Eat*	1 Pack/140g	304	11.6	217	11.1	24.5	8.3	2.1
Sausage & Red Onion Chutney, Softgrain, Urban Eat*	1 Pack/155g	416	18.5	268	9.1	31.1	11.9	2.6
Sub, Chicken, Bacon & Mayonnaise, Urban Eat*	1 Sub/233g	667	31.7	286	11.7	29.1	13.6	1.3
Sub, Gammon Ham & Salad, Urban Eat*	1 Sub/256g	438	8.5	171	8.9	26.6	3.3	1.4
Sub, Mature Cheddar, Spring Onion & Tom, Urban Eat*	1 Sub/257g	710	36.0	276	8.6	28.8	14.0	2.2
Sub, Tuna Mayo & Cucumber, Urban Eat*	1 Sub/260g	636	30.0	244	8.8	26.2	11.5	1.3
Tomato, Mozzarella & Pesto, Wheatgrain, Urban Eat*	1 Pack/1179g	404	20.9	226	8.8	21.3	11.7	2.2
Tuna Mayo & Cucumber, on Softgrain, Urban Eat*	1 Pack/170g	423	23.8	249	9.2	21.4	14.0	1.4
Tuna Mayo & Sweetcorn, Halal, on White, Urban Eat*	1 Pack/149g	390	18.8	262	11.2	25.4	12.6	1.2

	Measure INFO/WEIGHT	per Measure KCAL	FAT	Nutrition Values per 100g / 100ml KCAL	PROT	CARB	FAT	FIBRE

URBAN EAT

SANDWICH
Tuna Mayo & Sweetcorn, on White, Urban Eat*	1 Pack/149g	266	4.3	178	11.4	26.5	2.9	1.7
Vegetarian, Triple Pack, Urban Eat*	1 Pack/209g	538	28.3	257	9.8	24.1	13.5	2.2

TOASTIES
Gammon & Irish Mature Cheddar, on White, Urban Eat*	1 Toastie/140g	364	16.0	260	14.4	24.9	11.4	1.1
Irish Mature Cheddar & Tomato, on White, Urban Eat*	1 Toastie/142g	333	14.9	235	9.8	25.3	10.5	1.3

WRAP
Chicken, with Caesar Mayonnaise, Urban Eat*	1 Pack/208g	647	39.3	311	11.6	23.6	18.9	0.9
Chicken Fajita, with Tomato Salsa, Urban Eat*	1 Pack/229g	423	10.7	185	9.2	26.3	4.7	1.4
Egg, Bombay, Salsa, Tortilla, Ultimate, Urban Eat*	1 Pack/218g	534	30.6	244	8.5	19.1	14.0	3.5
Shredded Duck, with Hoisin Sauce, Urban Eat*	1 Pack/220g	446	14.5	203	8.1	27.6	6.6	1.0

YOGHURT
Granola, & Blueberry Compote, Urban Eat*	1 Pot/165g	218	13.5	132	5.3	9.5	8.2	1.0
Granola, & Strawberry Compote, Urban Eat*	1 Pot/165g	218	13.5	132	5.2	9.3	8.2	0.8

WAGAMAMA

BEANS
Edamame with Salt, Wagamama*	1 Serving/202g	179	6.3	89	6.6	3.7	3.1	9.9

CAKE
Chocolate Fudge, with Vanilla Ice Cream, Wagamama*	1 Serving/203g	671	36.9	331	4.0	37.6	18.2	0.4

CHA HAN
Chicken, & Prawn, Rice, Wagamama*	1 Dinner/778g	972	24.9	125	5.1	18.6	3.2	0.8
Chicken, with Fried Rice & Veg, Mini, Wagamama*	1 Serving/245g	429	11.5	175	8.2	24.9	4.7	0.4

CHICKEN
Firecracker, Stir Fried with Vegetables, Wagamama*	1 Portion/720g	1056	27.4	147	7.7	20.1	3.8	0.6
Grilled, Katsu Curry, Wagamama*	1 Serving/569g	871	30.2	153	6.0	20.1	5.3	0.5
Raisukaree, in Coconut Curry Sauce, Wagamama*	1 Serving/774g	1276	58.0	165	5.7	18.4	7.5	0.5
Tama Rice, Wagamama*	1 Meal/810g	917	25.9	113	4.5	16.4	3.2	0.5
Tebasaki, Wagamama*	1 Serving/105g	274	15.5	261	21.7	9.8	14.8	1.3
with Sauce & Rice, Mini, Wagamama*	1 Serving/295g	484	13.9	164	8.0	22.2	4.7	0.5

CHICKEN
Itame, Chicken & Noodle, in Coconut, Wagamama*	1 Portion/829g	850	51.4	103	4.5	6.6	6.2	1.1

COD
Cubes, Deep Fried, with Rice & Veg, Wagamama*	1 Serving/344g	582	19.3	169	6.4	22.9	5.6	0.7

CURRY
Chicken, Chu Chee, Wagamama*	1 Serving/824g	1350	61.7	164	4.9	18.8	7.5	0.7
Chicken, Katsu, Wagamama*	1 Serving/619g	1103	45.2	178	7.5	20.5	7.3	0.5

EBI KATSU
Prawns, Deep Fried, in Breadcrumbs, Wagamama*	1 Serving/129g	289	18.2	224	9.4	14.5	14.1	0.9

FROZEN YOGHURT
Chocolate, Chilli & Ginger, Wagamama*	1 Serving/195g	300	3.7	154	5.0	28.7	1.9	1.4
Citrus Yuzu, Wagamama*	1 Serving/133g	196	2.8	147	4.7	27.3	2.1	0.2

GYOZA
Chicken & Vegetable, Dumplings, Wagamama*	1 Serving/149g	236	10.6	158	7.6	15.0	7.1	2.0
Duck Dumplings, with Hoi Sin Sauce, Wagamama*	1 Serving/115g	299	12.3	260	10.4	29.2	10.7	2.8
Ebi, Prawn & Vegetable Dumplings, Wagamama*	1 Serving/112g	219	8.4	195	8.3	22.0	7.5	3.2

ICE CREAM
Coconut Reika, Wagamama*	1 Serving/195g	417	21.4	214	3.5	25.0	11.0	0.7

JUICE
Apple, Mint, Celery & Lime, Wagamama*	1 Serving/273g	153	0.3	56	0.2	13.8	0.1	0.3
Apple & Orange, Wagamama*	1 Serving/271g	129	0.3	48	0.4	11.2	0.1	0.6
Blueberry, Apple & Ginger, Wagamama*	1 Serving/359g	183	0.4	51	0.4	11.2	0.1	2.0
Carrot with a Hint of Ginger, Wagamama*	1 Serving/312g	72	0.0	23	0.2	5.0	0.0	1.1
Fruit, Refreshing Cleansing Blend, Wagamama*	1 Serving/311g	128	0.0	41	0.4	9.9	0.0	0.3

	Measure INFO/WEIGHT	per Measure KCAL	FAT	Nutrition Values per 100g / 100ml KCAL	PROT	CARB	FAT	FIBRE
WAGAMAMA								
KUSHIYAKI								
Lollipop Prawn, Wagamama*	1 Serving/122g	228	16.6	187	10.4	5.6	13.6	0.4
NOODLES								
Amai Udon, Teppan Fried, Wagamama*	1 Serving/676g	865	35.1	128	5.5	13.9	5.2	1.7
Chicken, Breast, Grilled, with Vegetables, Wagamama*	1 Serving/273g	373	7.4	137	12.1	15.9	2.7	0.4
Chicken, Stir Fried, Chilli Men, Wagamama*	1 Serving/703g	944	40.8	134	6.0	14.2	5.8	0.8
Chicken Ramen, with Vegetables in Soup, Wagamama*	1 Serving/816g	519	13.1	64	5.1	7.0	1.6	0.4
Fish, Grilled, Mini, & Vegetables, Wagamama*	1 Serving/248g	309	6.7	125	7.5	17.4	2.7	0.5
Pad Thai, Chicken & Prawn, Wagamama*	1 Serving/648g	794	31.0	123	5.4	13.8	4.8	1.4
Udon, Ginger Chicken, Wagamama*	1 Serving/605g	752	28.4	124	7.0	12.6	4.7	1.6
PRAWNS								
Firecracker, Stir Fried with Vegetables, Wagamama*	1 Serving/659g	906	24.4	138	3.8	21.9	3.7	0.7
RAMEN								
Chilli Beef, Wagamama*	1 Serving/989g	680	22.7	69	5.1	6.7	2.3	0.6
Chilli Chicken, Wagamama*	1 Serving/949g	597	16.1	63	4.6	6.9	1.7	0.6
Grilled Fish, Seafood & Noodles, Wagamama*	1 Bowl/685g	463	4.8	68	5.6	9.5	0.7	0.4
SALAD								
Chicken Mandarin & Sesame, Wagamama*	1 Serving/393g	790	54.2	201	11.0	7.7	13.8	1.1
Ginger Beef & Coriander, Wagamama*	1 Serving/433g	686	54.6	158	8.4	2.5	12.6	1.0
SQUID								
Deep Fried with Shichimi & Chilli Sauce, Wagamama*	1 Serving/208g	493	33.3	237	8.7	14.3	16.0	0.4
SUSHI								
California Roll, Inside Out, with Surimi, Wagamama*	1 Serving/93g	132	3.3	142	2.0	25.1	3.5	0.8
Hosomaki, Avocado, Wagamama*	1 Serving/113g	176	4.5	157	1.7	28.0	4.0	1.0
Hosomaki, Cucumber, Wagamama*	1 Serving/108g	138	0.6	129	1.5	29.2	0.6	0.5
Uramaki, Asparagus & Shiitake, Wagamama*	1 Serving/87g	112	0.8	129	2.1	27.4	0.9	1.2
Uramaki, Mango, Avocado & Cucumber, Wagamama*	1 Serving/84g	114	2.4	136	1.7	25.2	2.9	0.9
Uramaki, Salmon Skin with Avocado, Wagamama*	1 Serving/95g	169	6.3	178	6.0	23.3	6.7	0.7
WASABI CO LTD								
BEEF								
Sukiyaki Don, Wasabi Co Ltd*	1 Portion/592g	758	16.0	128	7.4	18.4	2.7	0.0
CHICKEN								
Gyoza, Steamed, Side Dish, Wasabi Co Ltd*	1 Portion/20g	43	2.6	215	8.3	16.3	13.0	0.0
Karaage, Wasabi Co Ltd*	1 Portion/210g	468	18.5	223	24.5	11.4	8.8	0.0
Katsu, Wasabi Co Ltd*	1 Portion/160g	421	9.0	263	26.9	26.3	5.6	0.0
Spicy, Don, Wasabi Co Ltd*	1 Portion/671g	825	18.8	123	7.8	16.5	2.8	0.0
Sweet Chilli, Wasabi Co Ltd*	1 Portion/350g	843	18.5	241	24.7	23.7	5.3	0.0
Sweet Chilli Don, Wasabi Co Ltd*	1 Portion/652g	991	28.0	152	7.6	20.7	4.3	0.0
Teriyaki, Wasabi Co Ltd*	1 Portion/350g	388	7.7	111	14.7	8.2	2.2	0.0
Teriyaki Don, Wasabi Co Ltd*	1 Portion/684g	732	9.6	107	6.9	16.6	1.4	0.0
with Spicy Sauce, Wasabi Co Ltd*	1 Portion/350g	402	8.4	115	14.0	9.3	2.4	0.0
CHICKEN								
Karaage, Side Dish, Wasabi Co Ltd*	1 Portion/70g	156	6.2	223	24.5	11.4	8.8	0.0
Yakitori, Side Dish, Wasabi Co Ltd*	1 Portion/40g	65	5.2	163	0.0	11.8	12.9	0.0
CURRY								
Chicken, Katsu Don, Wasabi Co Ltd*	1 Portion/668g	1136	34.7	170	8.3	22.5	5.2	0.0
Chicken, Wasabi Co Ltd*	1 Portion/350g	535	30.4	153	11.0	7.7	8.7	0.0
Chicken Katsu, Wasabi Co Ltd*	1 Portion/360g	774	33.5	215	13.4	19.5	9.3	0.0
Tofu, Wasabi Co Ltd*	1 Portion/350g	535	37.4	153	3.6	10.5	10.7	0.0
Tofu Don, Wasabi Co Ltd*	1 Portion/552g	707	25.4	128	2.9	18.9	4.6	0.0
NOODLES								
Roasted Veg Yakisoba, Wasabi Co Ltd*	1 Portion/630g	554	19.5	88	3.6	11.5	3.1	0.0
Stir Fry, Chicken Katsu Yakisoba, Wasabi Co Ltd*	1 Portion/568g	710	8.0	125	13.7	14.2	1.4	0.0

WASABI CO LTD

	Measure INFO/WEIGHT	per Measure KCAL	FAT	Nutrition Values per 100g / 100ml KCAL	PROT	CARB	FAT	FIBRE
NOODLES								
Stir Fry, Chicken Yakisoba, Wasabi Co Ltd*	1 Portion/450g	459	3.6	102	12.4	11.3	0.8	0.0
Stir Fry, Tofu Yakisoba, Wasabi Co Ltd*	1 Portion/450g	553	24.3	123	7.1	11.4	5.4	0.0
PRAWNS								
Fried Don, Wasabi Co Ltd*	1 Portion/555g	666	15.0	120	2.2	21.8	2.7	0.0
RICE								
Steamed, Wasabi Co Ltd*	1 Portion/250g	297	0.7	119	2.3	26.6	0.3	0.0
SALMON								
Teriyaki, Wasabi Co Ltd*	1 Portion/150g	339	19.2	226	20.5	7.0	12.8	0.0
SOUP								
Miso, Side Dish, Wasabi Co Ltd*	1 Portion/170ml	17	0.5	10	0.6	1.3	0.3	0.0
SUSHI								
Avocado Hosomaki, Wasabi Co Ltd*	1 Portion/40g	2	0.0	6	0.1	1.5	0.1	0.0
California Hand Roll, Wasabi Co Ltd*	1 Portion/119g	23	0.2	19	0.3	2.8	0.2	0.0
California Roll, Wasabi Co Ltd*	1 Portion/59g	4	0.1	7	0.1	2.9	0.2	0.0
California Roll Set, Mixed, Wasabi Co Ltd*	1 Portion/470g	248	15.5	53	7.5	20.5	3.3	0.0
Chicken Bento, Sweet & Spicy, Wasabi Co Ltd*	1 Portion/917g	923	22.9	101	15.1	21.4	2.5	0.0
Chicken Karaage Set, Wasabi Co Ltd*	1 Portion/818g	520	28.6	64	17.7	36.4	3.5	0.0
Chicken Katsu Salad, Wasabi Co Ltd*	1 Portion/858g	770	29.2	90	15.3	29.1	3.4	0.0
Chicken Teriyaki Hand Roll, Wasabi Co Ltd*	1 Portion/107g	21	0.2	20	2.1	2.3	0.2	0.0
Chicken Teriyaki Onigiri, Wasabi Co Ltd*	1 Portion/147g	47	0.6	32	6.8	1.1	0.4	0.0
Chicken Teriyaki Roll, Wasabi Co Ltd*	1 Portion/54g	4	0.1	7	1.0	2.5	0.2	0.0
Chirashi, with Japanese Dressing, Wasabi Co Ltd*	1 Portion/660g	484	8.6	73	12.2	26.4	1.3	0.0
Chirashi Set, Mini, Wasabi Co Ltd*	1 Portion/487g	248	9.3	51	13.6	22.0	1.9	0.0
Chirashi Set, Spicy, Mini, Wasabi Co Ltd*	1 Portion/487g	291	9.7	60	14.2	17.3	2.0	0.0
Chirashi Sushi, Spicy, Wasabi Co Ltd*	1 Portion/660g	519	9.2	79	12.6	23.5	1.4	0.0
Crabmeat & Chive, Hosomaki, Wasabi Co Ltd*	1 Portion/39g	2	0.0	6	0.1	1.0	0.1	0.0
Crabmeat & Cucumber Roll, Wasabi Co Ltd*	1 Portion/60g	5	0.2	8	0.2	2.5	0.4	0.0
Cucumber Hosomaki, Wasabi Co Ltd*	1 Portion/29g	2	0.0	6	0.1	0.2	0.1	0.0
Edamame, Wasabi Co Ltd*	1 Portion/208g	25	6.0	12	1.1	9.2	2.9	0.0
Hana Set, Wasabi Co Ltd*	1 Portion/538g	411	6.5	76	1.9	16.1	1.2	0.0
Harmony Set, Wasabi Co Ltd*	1 Portion/534g	403	7.5	75	3.1	17.1	1.4	0.0
Hosomaki Set, Mini, Wasabi Co Ltd*	1 Portion/310g	146	2.5	47	2.6	8.2	0.8	0.0
Maki Set, Mixed, Wasabi Co Ltd*	1 Portion/393g	205	4.3	52	2.9	14.4	1.1	0.0
Omelette, Japanese, Nigiri, Wasabi Co Ltd*	1 Portion/38g	3	0.1	7	0.8	0.7	0.2	0.0
Prawn, Fried, Hand Roll, Wasabi Co Ltd*	1 Portion/115g	26	0.6	22	0.3	1.9	0.5	0.0
Prawn, Fried, Roll, Wasabi Co Ltd*	1 Portion/46g	3	0.1	7	0.4	1.6	0.3	0.0
Prawn Mayo Gunkan, Wasabi Co Ltd*	1 Portion/48g	3	0.2	5	0.1	1.7	0.5	0.0
Pumpkin Korokke Set, Wasabi Co Ltd*	1 Portion/517g	299	15.0	58	22.6	26.6	2.9	0.0
Rainbow Set, Wasabi Co Ltd*	1 Portion/618g	436	7.4	70	1.8	24.7	1.2	0.0
Salmon & Masago Roll, Wasabi Co Ltd*	1 Portion/59g	4	0.2	7	0.1	2.8	0.3	0.0
Salmon Gunkan, Spicy, Wasabi Co Ltd*	1 Portion/54g	4	0.2	7	1.7	1.7	0.4	0.0
Salmon Hosomaki, Wasabi Co Ltd*	1 Portion/35g	2	0.0	6	0.1	0.6	0.1	0.0
Salmon Nigiri, Wasabi Co Ltd*	1 Portion/42g	2	0.0	6	0.1	1.1	0.1	0.0
Salmon Nigiri Set, Wasabi Co Ltd*	1 Portion/255g	96	1.8	38	2.4	6.7	0.7	0.0
Salmon Onigiri, Wasabi Co Ltd*	1 Portion/168g	44	0.7	26	0.5	3.7	0.4	0.0
Salmon Roll, Spicy, Wasabi Co Ltd*	1 Portion/60g	4	0.1	6	0.4	2.7	0.1	0.0
Salmon Sashimi Set, Wasabi Co Ltd*	1 Portion/282g	50	8.5	18	6.3	11.2	3.0	0.0
Salmon Sesame Gunkan, Wasabi Co Ltd*	1 Portion/58g	3	0.1	5	0.1	3.5	0.1	0.0
Sashimi Set, Wasabi Co Ltd*	1 Portion/251g	2	0.0	1	0.8	15.4	0.0	0.0
Seaweed Onigiri, Wasabi Co Ltd*	1 Portion/172g	46	1.2	27	1.1	3.6	0.7	0.0
Seaweed Salad Gunkan, Wasabi Co Ltd*	1 Portion/39g	3	0.2	8	2.7	0.5	0.5	0.0
Shrimp Nigiri, Wasabi Co Ltd*	1 Portion/28g	2	0.1	6	0.1	0.1	0.2	0.0

	Measure INFO/WEIGHT	per Measure		Nutrition Values per 100g / 100ml				
		KCAL	FAT	KCAL	PROT	CARB	FAT	FIBRE

WASABI CO LTD
SUSHI
Snomono Salad, Wasabi Co Ltd*	1 Portion/279g	83	14.2	30	14.6	9.6	5.1	0.0
Tobiko Cucumber Gunkan, Wasabi Co Ltd*	1 Portion/26g	2	0.1	6	0.7	0.1	0.2	0.0
Tofu Nigiri, Wasabi Co Ltd*	1 Portion/49g	3	0.0	6	0.2	1.7	0.1	0.0
Tofu Roll, Wasabi Co Ltd*	1 Portion/46g	3	0.0	6	0.5	1.6	0.1	0.0
Tuna & Mustard Onigiri, Wasabi Co Ltd*	1 Portion/171g	48	0.7	28	2.2	2.5	0.4	0.0
Tuna & Sweetcorn Roll, Wasabi Co Ltd*	1 Portion/51g	3	0.2	7	0.5	0.7	0.3	0.0
Tuna Hosomaki, Wasabi Co Ltd*	1 Portion/33g	2	0.0	6	0.1	0.3	0.1	0.0
Tuna Nigiri, Wasabi Co Ltd*	1 Portion/38g	2	0.0	6	0.1	0.5	0.1	0.0
Veg Set, Mixed, Wasabi Co Ltd*	1 Portion/312g	149	3.1	48	10.1	9.8	1.0	0.0
Wakame Seaweed Salad, Wasabi Co Ltd*	1 Portion/339g	143	34.2	42	22.9	8.7	10.1	0.0
Wasabi Special Bento, Wasabi Co Ltd*	1 Portion/614g	423	18.4	69	7.4	22.9	3.0	0.0

TANMEN
Chicken, Spicy, Wasabi Co Ltd*	1 Portion/864g	475	13.0	55	3.4	7.0	1.5	0.0
Chicken, Wasabi Co Ltd*	1 Portion/833g	425	11.7	51	3.4	6.1	1.4	0.0
Chicken Dumpling, Wasabi Co Ltd*	1 Portion/833g	458	14.2	55	1.9	7.9	1.7	0.0
Prawn Tempura, Wasabi Co Ltd*	1 Portion/813g	382	9.8	47	1.1	8.0	1.2	0.0
Veg, Wasabi Co Ltd*	1 Portion/819g	385	9.8	47	1.9	7.1	1.2	0.0

WIMPY
BREAKFAST
Breakfast Roll, Bacon, Wimpy*	1 Roll/144g	278	5.1	193	13.3	24.7	3.5	0.0
Breakfast Roll, Bacon & Egg, Wimpy*	1 Roll/194g	368	12.1	190	13.4	18.3	6.2	0.0
Breakfast Roll, Sausage, Wimpy*	1 Roll/161g	437	21.5	271	11.3	26.6	13.4	0.0
Breakfast Roll, Sausage & Egg, Wimpy*	1 Roll/211g	527	28.4	250	11.8	20.3	13.5	0.0
Hash brown, Wimpy*	1 Serving/424g	545	41.1	129	4.1	8.7	9.7	1.9
The Country Breakfast, Wimpy*	1 Serving/271g	392	23.1	145	9.4	6.9	8.5	1.7
The Great Wimpy Breakfast, Wimpy*	1 Serving/459g	910	53.6	198	10.7	12.7	11.7	1.2
Toast, with Jam, Extra, Wimpy*	1 Serving/89g	276	8.3	310	7.3	52.6	9.3	1.7
Wimpy Club, Wimpy*	1 Serving/330g	767	38.6	232	14.7	18.2	11.7	0.8

BURGERS
BBQ, Wimpy*	1 Burger/236g	644	30.5	273	14.1	24.6	12.9	1.6
Cheeseburger, Bacon, Classic, Wimpy*	1 Burger/192g	405	19.0	211	13.6	16.8	9.9	0.0
Chicken, in a Bun, Wimpy*	1 Burger/191g	449	21.4	235	10.4	22.7	11.2	1.3
Chicken & Bacon Melt, Wimpy*	1 Burger/172g	443	20.2	258	12.6	25.4	11.7	0.0
Chicken Fillet, in a Bun, Hot & Spicy, Wimpy*	1 Burger/193g	398	18.5	206	10.6	19.1	9.6	1.8
Chicken Fillet, in a Bun, Savoury, Wimpy*	1 Burger/218g	356	13.8	163	10.4	16.1	6.3	1.1
Chicken Fillet, Wimpy*	1 Burger/327g	380	16.8	116	6.7	11.1	5.1	0.0
Classic, Wimpy*	1 Burger/159g	337	15.1	212	12.4	19.9	9.5	0.0
Halfpounder, with Bacon & Cheese, Wimpy*	1 Burger/312g	892	50.5	286	19.2	15.5	16.2	0.8
Kingsize, Classic, Wimpy*	1 Burger/227g	551	31.1	243	16.2	14.2	13.7	0.0
Mega Burger, Wimpy*	1 Burger/206g	594	36.0	288	15.3	18.0	17.5	0.0
Quarterpounder, Wimpy*	1 Burger/200g	538	31.3	269	15.0	18.0	15.6	0.0
Quarterpounder, with Bacon & Cheese, Wimpy*	1 Burger/237g	658	33.4	278	16.8	20.5	14.1	1.1
Quarterpounder, with Cheese, Wimpy*	1 Burger/213g	578	34.6	271	15.1	17.2	16.2	0.0
Spicy Bean, Wimpy*	1 Burger/233g	611	29.4	262	5.9	30.5	12.6	2.7
Spicy Bean, with Cheese, Wimpy*	1 Burger/245g	1459	98.3	596	24.2	35.5	40.1	2.7
with Cheese, Classic, Wimpy*	1 Burger/175g	379	18.5	217	12.7	17.3	10.6	1.1

CHICKEN
Chunks, with Chips, Wimpy*	1 Serving/333g	779	46.8	234	8.3	19.0	14.0	1.5

DESSERT
Apple Tart, Deep Filled, Wimpy*	1 Serving/164g	339	10.2	207	1.7	36.2	6.2	0.0
Brown Derby, with Dairy Ice Cream, Wimpy*	1 Serving/180g	431	20.6	239	4.5	31.3	11.4	1.4
Brownie Sundae, Wimpy*	1 Sundae/252g	574	21.8	228	3.8	34.7	8.6	0.6

WIMPY

	Measure INFO/WEIGHT	per Measure KCAL	FAT	Nutrition Values per 100g / 100ml KCAL	PROT	CARB	FAT	FIBRE
DESSERT								
Cheese Cake, Wimpy*	1 Serving/144g	412	18.3	286	4.5	38.5	12.7	0.0
Chocolate Fudge Cake, Wimpy*	1 Serving/100g	371	12.4	371	4.7	60.2	12.4	0.0
Chocolate Waffle, with Dairy Ice Cream, Wimpy*	1 Serving/178g	691	37.0	388	5.1	45.3	20.8	0.0
Chocolate Waffle, with Squirty Cream, Wimpy*	1 Serving/158g	667	36.9	422	5.1	47.7	23.4	0.0
Dairy Ice Cream, with Chocolate Sauce, Wimpy*	1 Serving/88g	200	8.1	227	3.4	32.5	9.2	0.0
Dairy Ice Cream, with Strawberry Sauce, Wimpy*	1 Serving/88g	199	7.9	226	3.0	34.3	9.0	0.0
Eskimo Waffle, Wimpy*	1 Serving/228g	694	30.2	304	4.6	42.7	13.2	1.3
Half Chocolate Waffle, with Dairy Ice Cream, Wimpy*	1 Serving/116g	395	18.8	341	4.0	44.7	16.2	0.0
Ice Cream Sundae, Plain, Wimpy*	1 Sundae/170g	190	8.8	112	3.1	15.0	5.2	0.0
Knickerbocker Glory, Mini, with Ice Cream, Wimpy*	1 Serving/194g	190	8.5	98	1.6	13.2	4.4	0.0
Spotted Dick Pudding, Wimpy*	1 Serving/130g	400	16.5	308	4.1	44.2	12.7	0.0
Toffee Sundae, Wimpy*	1 Sundae/239g	537	23.6	225	3.8	30.8	9.9	0.8
Treacle Sponge Pudding, Wimpy*	1 Serving/130g	504	21.3	388	3.9	56.1	16.4	0.0
EXTRAS								
Bacon, Wimpy*	1 Serving/91g	267	22.0	294	24.2	0.0	24.2	0.0
Baked Beans, Heinz, Wimpy*	1 Portion/110g	85	0.2	77	4.4	12.5	0.2	3.5
Cheese, Slice, Wimpy*	1 Slice/12g	40	3.3	333	18.3	5.0	27.5	0.0
Chips, Large Portion, Wimpy*	1 Portion/143g	333	17.1	233	3.0	30.4	12.0	3.0
Chips, Standard Portion, Wimpy*	1 Portion/114g	267	13.7	234	3.0	30.5	12.0	3.0
Coleslaw, Wimpy*	1 Serving/50g	49	3.8	98	1.4	6.2	7.6	0.8
Egg, Wimpy*	1 Egg/50g	90	7.0	180	13.6	0.0	14.0	0.0
Hash Browns, Wimpy*	1 Serving/55g	93	7.8	169	2.2	19.6	14.2	1.8
Mozzarella Meltz 3, Wimpy*	3 Meltz/79g	253	15.4	320	15.4	25.7	19.5	2.5
Mozzarella Meltz 6, Wimpy*	6 Meltz/157g	506	30.8	322	15.6	25.9	19.6	2.5
Onion Rings, Large (12), Wimpy*	1 Portion/180g	401	23.2	223	3.2	23.6	12.9	0.0
Onion Rings, Standard (6), Wimpy*	1 Portion/90g	201	11.6	223	3.2	23.6	12.9	3.0
Side Salad, Wimpy*	1 Portion/145g	44	0.3	30	1.4	6.1	0.2	0.8
FISH								
Haddock, & Chips, with Peas, Wimpy*	1 Serving/314g	674	37.9	215	6.6	21.2	12.1	2.4
Scampi, & Chips with Peas, Wimpy*	1 Serving/303g	577	29.8	190	5.2	22.7	9.8	2.3
GRILL								
Bacon, classic, Wimpy*	1 Serving/321g	722	45.3	225	11.5	14.0	14.1	0.0
BBQ Rib Rack Platter, Wimpy*	1 Serving/439g	713	35.2	162	5.6	17.5	8.0	1.4
Chicken, Platter, Gourmet, Wimpy*	1 Serving/392g	525	21.4	134	11.4	10.0	5.5	1.4
Sausage, Egg & Chips, Wimpy*	1 Serving/244g	597	38.8	245	9.0	17.4	15.9	1.7
Steak Platter, Wimpy*	1 Serving/424g	719	38.0	170	9.9	12.9	9.0	0.0
The International Grill, Wimpy*	1 Serving/416g	1010	71.3	243	13.9	9.9	17.1	0.9
Wimpy All-Day Breakfast, Wimpy*	1 Serving/410g	731	39.7	178	8.3	14.5	9.7	0.0
ICE CREAMS								
Banana Longboat, with Soft Ice Cream, Wimpy*	1 Serving/209g	260	6.0	124	2.3	23.9	2.9	0.0
Brown Derby, with Dairy Ice Cream, Wimpy*	1 Serving/125g	397	19.7	318	5.6	38.9	15.8	0.0
Choc Nut Sundae, Wimpy*	1 Serving/83g	196	6.2	236	4.6	38.4	7.5	0.0
Fruit & Nut Sundae, Wimpy*	1 Serving/83g	138	5.8	166	4.2	23.3	7.0	0.0
Ice Cream, Portion, Soft with Chocolate Sauce, Wimpy*	1 Serving/71g	137	3.2	193	2.8	36.1	4.5	0.0
Ice Cream, Soft with Strawberry Sauce, Wimpy*	1 Serving/71g	137	3.0	193	2.4	38.3	4.2	0.0
Knickerbockerglory, with Ice Cream, Wimpy*	1 Serving/138g	196	6.0	142	2.7	24.7	4.3	0.0
Triple Strawberry Sundae, with Ice Cream, Wimpy*	1 Serving/170g	123	3.3	72	1.4	13.1	1.9	0.0
KIDS								
Cheese Toastie, with Salad, Wimpy*	1 Serving/250g	367	8.8	147	5.9	24.2	3.5	1.2
Cheeseburger Meal, with Chips, Wimpy*	1 Serving/191g	497	23.5	260	10.0	27.7	12.3	2.1
Chicken Chunks Meal, with Chips, Wimpy*	1 Serving/172g	440	26.1	256	8.4	22.1	15.2	1.8
Chicken Chunks Meal, with Salad, Wimpy*	1 Serving/187g	265	16.8	142	6.8	8.4	9.0	0.7

	Measure INFO/WEIGHT	per Measure		Nutrition Values per 100g / 100ml				
		KCAL	FAT	KCAL	PROT	CARB	FAT	FIBRE

WIMPY
KIDS
Fish Bites Meal, with Chips, Wimpy*	1 Serving/160g	380	20.9	237	6.7	24.7	13.1	2.1
Fish Bites Meal, with Salad, Wimpy*	1 Serving/175g	205	11.6	117	5.2	9.8	6.6	0.9
Hamburger Meal, with Chips, Wimpy*	1 Serving/184g	457	20.0	248	9.0	29.9	10.9	0.0
Hamburger Meal, with Salad, Wimpy*	1 Serving/199g	283	10.7	142	7.5	16.4	5.4	0.0
Hot Dog, with Salad, Wimpy*	1 Serving/241g	425	21.1	176	7.0	17.3	8.8	0.0
Sausage Meal, with Chips, Wimpy*	1 Serving/160g	428	27.7	267	8.9	19.9	17.3	1.9

MUFFIN
Giant Blueberry, Wimpy*	1 Muffin/108g	470	25.6	435	5.9	48.9	23.7	0.0

NUTS
Nibbed (for desserts), Wimpy*	1 Serving/5g	32	2.8	640	26.0	6.0	56.0	12.0

PANINI
Cheese, with Red Onion, Wimpy*	1 Panini/205g	673	22.8	329	14.6	42.7	11.1	1.9
Cheese & Tomato, Wimpy*	1 Panini/225g	694	25.1	309	14.6	37.4	11.1	2.2
Ham, Tomato & Cheese, Wimpy*	1 Panini/275g	1145	39.0	417	33.0	38.4	14.2	2.2
Ham & Cheese, Wimpy*	1 Panini/235g	944	33.3	402	32.0	35.7	14.2	1.4
Steak, Cheese & Onion, Wimpy*	1 Panini/305g	688	28.6	226	13.8	21.4	9.4	0.9

POTATO JACKET
with Baked Beans, Wimpy*	1 Serving/452g	549	7.9	121	3.4	23.5	1.7	2.7
with Beans & Cheese, Wimpy*	1 Serving/577g	1069	51.5	185	8.4	18.4	8.9	2.1
with Butter, Wimpy*	1 Serving/327g	453	7.6	139	3.5	27.7	2.3	2.4
with Coleslaw, Wimpy*	1 Serving/452g	576	17.1	127	2.9	21.7	3.8	2.0
with Grated Cheese, Wimpy*	1 Serving/452g	973	51.2	215	9.6	20.0	11.3	1.7
with Tuna Mayo, Wimpy*	1 Serving/452g	764	34.2	169	5.9	20.6	7.6	1.7

RIBS
Pork Rib, Wimpy*	1 Rib/189g	463	22.4	245	13.0	21.6	11.9	0.0

ROLL
Bacon, in a Bun, Wimpy*	1 Roll/125g	341	16.1	273	16.0	22.6	12.9	1.4
Bacon & Egg, in a Bun, Wimpy*	1 Roll/155g	702	41.7	453	29.6	22.6	26.9	1.4

SALAD
Chicken, Gourmet, Wimpy*	1 Serving/358g	251	4.3	70	11.9	2.7	1.2	0.4
Chicken, Hot & Spicy, Wimpy*	1 Serving/290g	283	15.2	98	6.1	6.7	5.2	0.9
Fish, Wimpy*	1 Serving/356g	389	21.3	109	4.6	9.9	6.0	0.0
Scampi, Wimpy*	1 Serving/356g	376	19.1	106	4.2	10.7	5.4	0.0
Steak, Wimpy*	1 Serving/355g	329	16.9	93	10.0	2.7	4.8	0.4

SAUCE
Chocolate, (for sundae), Wimpy*	1 Serving/28g	80	0.4	286	1.4	66.1	1.4	1.1
Strawberry, (for dessert), Wimpy*	1 Serving/28g	78	0.0	279	0.0	69.6	0.0	0.4
Syrup, Maple Flavoured (for dessert), Wimpy*	1 Serving/28g	74	0.1	264	0.0	67.9	0.4	0.0

SWEETS
Mini Marshmallows, (for desserts), Wimpy*	1 Serving/10g	33	0.0	330	4.0	83.0	0.0	0.0

TEACAKE
Toasted, with Butter, Wimpy*	1 Teacake/66g	227	2.3	344	1.7	10.4	3.4	0.4

VEGETARIAN
Quorn, Lemon Pepper, Wimpy*	1 Serving/239g	586	26.5	245	8.0	29.2	11.1	0.0
Spicy Beanburger, Wimpy*	1 Serving/233g	593	29.2	255	5.4	30.8	12.5	0.0

WRAPID
WRAP
All Day Breakfast (W22), Wrapid*	1 Wrap/223g	569	27.9	255	14.0	23.1	12.5	1.5
Chicken, Stir Fry, with Noodles, (W23), Wrapid*	1 Wrap/251g	411	8.6	164	8.0	24.8	3.4	1.5
Chicken Fajita (W18), Wrapid*	1 Wrap/226g	485	19.2	215	13.3	22.0	8.5	1.3
Chicken Tikka Balti (W15), Wrapid*	1 Wrap/266g	476	13.7	179	8.5	24.4	5.2	1.5
Chicken Tikka Massala Pot (WPOT004), Wrapid*	1 Pot/310g	487	14.7	157	5.4	20.8	4.7	1.2

WRAPID

WRAP

	Measure INFO/WEIGHT	per Measure KCAL	FAT	Nutrition Values per 100g / 100ml KCAL	PROT	CARB	FAT	FIBRE
Chilli Cheese Bean (T8 & W46), Wrapid*	1 Wrap/189g	411	13.9	217	7.8	29.9	7.3	2.8
Chilli Con Carne & Rice (W19), Wrapid*	1 Wrap/286g	505	13.9	176	3.9	28.8	4.8	1.2
Chilli Con Carne Pot (WPOT001), Wrapid*	1 Wrap/310g	412	12.9	133	2.2	20.9	4.1	0.4
Croques Monsier, Ham & Cheese (W30), Wrapid*	1 Wrap/231g	648	30.5	281	15.4	27.1	13.2	0.7
Ham & Pineapple Pizza (W28), Wrapid*	1 Wrap/270g	510	17.5	189	12.5	21.3	6.5	2.1
Meat Balls Pasta Pot (WPOT002), Wrapid*	1 Pot/291g	349	9.1	120	4.8	19.0	3.1	1.4
Mushroom, Cheese & Egg (W20), Wrapid*	1 Wrap/210g	531	29.6	253	9.6	22.0	14.1	1.4
Panini, Breakfast, (W35), Wrapid*	1 Wrap/181g	466	20.2	257	12.9	27.6	11.2	1.8
Panini, Fajita Chicken (W39), Wrapid*	1 Wrap/181g	336	8.4	186	10.0	25.5	4.6	1.6
Panini, Ham & Cheddar (W34), Wrapid*	1 Wrap/176g	501	21.4	284	13.1	30.9	12.2	1.5
Panini, Margerita (W36), Wrapid*	1 Wrap/173g	441	18.7	255	11.6	28.6	10.8	2.2
Panini, Pepperoni Pizza (W37), Wrapid*	1 Wrap/194g	570	30.7	294	13.9	25.0	15.8	1.8
Panini, Tuna Melt, (W33), Wrapid*	1 Wrap/178g	430	15.1	241	14.2	27.7	8.5	1.3
Panini, Vegetable, Breakfast, (W43), Wrapid*	1 Wrap/204g	366	11.0	180	7.0	25.8	5.4	1.8
Panini, Vegetable, Red Thai (W45), Wrapid*	1 Wrap/185g	360	12.8	194	6.8	30.1	6.9	2.1
Pepperoni Pizza (W26), Wrapid*	1 Wrap/249g	688	36.8	276	16.5	21.2	14.8	2.3
Pizza, Roasted Peppers (W27), Wrapid*	1 Wrap/261g	502	18.7	192	11.9	21.3	7.2	2.5
Roast Vegetable Pasta Pot (WPOT003), Wrapid*	1 Pot/311g	294	3.5	94	3.4	18.1	1.1	1.7
Steak & Mash, Wrapid*	1 Wrap/246g	424	9.7	172	6.6	26.2	4.0	1.0
Tuna Melt (W29), Wrapid*	1 Wrap/237g	538	21.3	227	16.3	21.2	9.0	1.3

Useful Resources

Weight Loss
Weight Loss Resources is home to the UK's largest calorie and nutrition database along with diaries, tools and expert advice for weight loss and health.
Tel: 01733 345592   Email: helpteam@weightlossresources.co.uk
Website: www.weightlossresources.co.uk

Exercise Equipment for Home
Diet and Fitness Resources has a range of equipment for exercise at home, from pedometers to treadmills and fitballs to weights. As well as diet tools such as food diaries, a weight loss kit and diet plates.
Tel: 01733 345592   Email: helpteam@dietandfitnessresources.co.uk
Website: www.dietandfitnessresources.co.uk

Dietary Advice
The British Dietetic Association has helpful food fact leaflets and information on how to contact a registered dietitian.
Tel: 0121 200 8080 Email: webmaster@bda.uk.com
Website: www.bda.uk.com

Healthy Eating
The British Nutrition Foundation has lots of in depth scientifically based nutritional information, knowledge and advice on healthy eating for all ages.
Tel: 0207 404 6504 Email: postbox@nutrition.org.uk
Website: www.nutrition.org.uk

Healthy Heart
The British Heart Foundation provides advice and information for all on all heart aspects from being healthy, to living with heart conditions, research and fundraising.
Tel: 0207 554 000   Email: via their website
Website: www.bhf.org.uk

Cancer Research
Cancer Research UK is the leading UK charity dedicated to research, education and fundraising for all forms of cancer.
Tel: 0207 242 0200 Email: via their website
Website: www.cancerresearchuk.org

Diabetes Advice

Diabetes UK is the leading charity working for people with diabetes. Their mission is to improve the lives of people with diabetes and to work towards a future without diabetes
Tel : 0845 120 2960 Email: info@diabetes.org.uk
Website: www.diabetes.org.uk

Beating Bowel Cancer

Beating Bowel Cancer is a leading UK charity for bowel cancer patients, working to raise awareness of symptoms, promote early diagnosis and encourage open access to treatment choice for those affected by bowel cancer.Tel: 08450 719301 Email: nurse@beatingbowelcancer.org
Website: http://www.beatingbowelcancer.org

Safety and Standards

The Food Standards Agency is an independent watchdog, set up to protect the public's health and consumer interests in relation to food.
Tel: 0207 276 8829 Email: helpline@foodstandards.gsi.gov.uk
Website: www.food.gov.uk

Feedback

If you have any comments or suggestions about The Calorie, Carb & Fat Bible, or would like further information on Weight Loss Resources, please call, email, or write to us:

Tel: 01733 345592
Email: helpteam@weightlossresources.co.uk
Address: Pat Wilson,
             Weight Loss Resources Ltd,
             29 Metro Centre,
             Woodston,
             Peterborough,
             PE2 7UH.

Reviews for The Calorie Carb & Fat Bible

'What a brilliant book. I know I'll be sinking my teeth into it.'
GMTV Nutritionist Amanda Ursell, BSc RD

'To help you make low-cal choices everyday, invest in a copy.'
ZEST magazine

'There is no doubt that the food listings are extremely helpful
for anyone wishing to control their calorie intake in order to lose
pounds or maintain a healthy weight.'
Women's Fitness magazine

'Useful if you don't want to exclude any overall food groups.'
Easy Living magazine

'Quite simply an astonishing achievement by the authors.'
Evening Post, Nottingham

'The book gives you all the basic information so you can work out
your daily calorie needs.'
Woman magazine

'This is a welcome resource in view of the 'national epidemic of obesity.'

Bryony Philip, Bowel Cancer UK

'The authors seem to understand the problems of slimming.'

Dr John Campion

'Jam-packed with info on dieting, and full to bursting point with the calorie, carbohydrate and fat values of thousands of different foods, it's the perfect weight loss tool.'

Evening Express, Aberdeen

'Excellent resource tool - used by myself in my role as a Practice Nurse.'

Pam Boal, Sunderland

'I recently bought your book called the Calorie, Carb & Fat Bible and would love to tell you what a brilliant book it is. I have recently started a weight management programme and I honestly don't know where I'd be without your book. It has helped me a lot and given me some really good advice.'

Rachel Mitchell

About Weight Loss Resources

weightlossresources.co.uk

"What this does is put you in control with no guilt, no awful groups and no negativity! Fill in your food diary, get support on the boards and watch it fall off!"

LINDAB, Weight Loss Resources Member

How Does It Work?

Weight Loss Resources is home to the UK's biggest online calorie and nutrition database. You simply tap in your height, weight, age and basic activity level - set a weight loss goal, and the programme does all the necessary calculations.

What Does It Do?

The site enables you to keep a food diary which keeps running totals of calories, fat, fibre, carbs, proteins and portions of fruit and veg. You can also keep an exercise diary which adds the calories you use during exercise. At the end of a week, you update your weight and get reports and graphs on your progress.

How Will It Help?

You'll learn a great deal about how your eating and drinking habits affect your weight and how healthy they are. Using the diaries and other tools you'll be able to make changes that suit your tastes and your lifestyle. The result is weight loss totally tailored to your needs and preferences. A method you can stick with that will help you learn how to eat well for life!

Try It Free!

Go to **www.weightlossresources.co.uk** and take a completely free, no obligation, 24 hour trial. If you like what you see you can sign up for membership from £6.95 per month.